Vol 43, No 1 January 2006

Seminars in HEMATOLOGY

Neal S. Young · Photis Beris
Editors

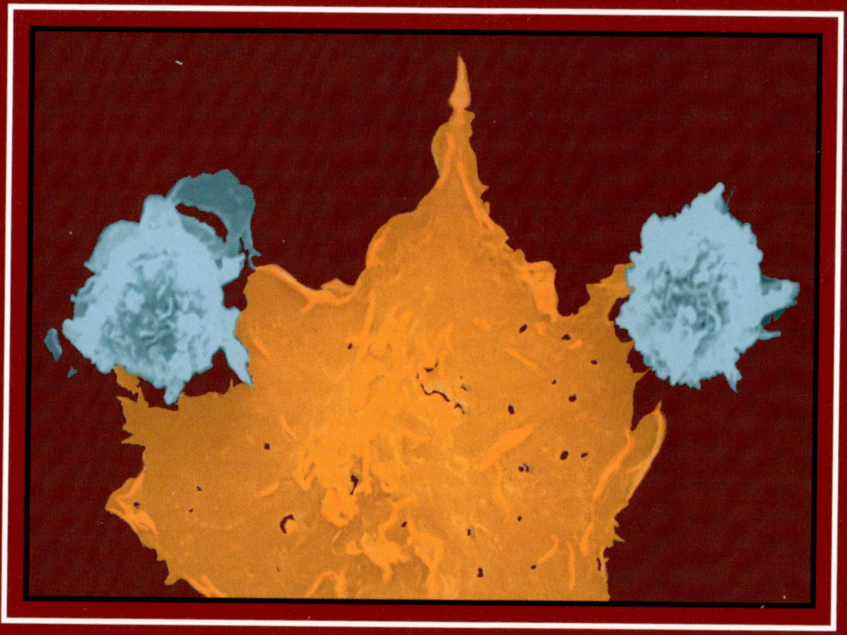

Graft-Versus-Host Disease

James L.M. Ferrara and John E. Levine
Guest Editors

W.B. Saunders

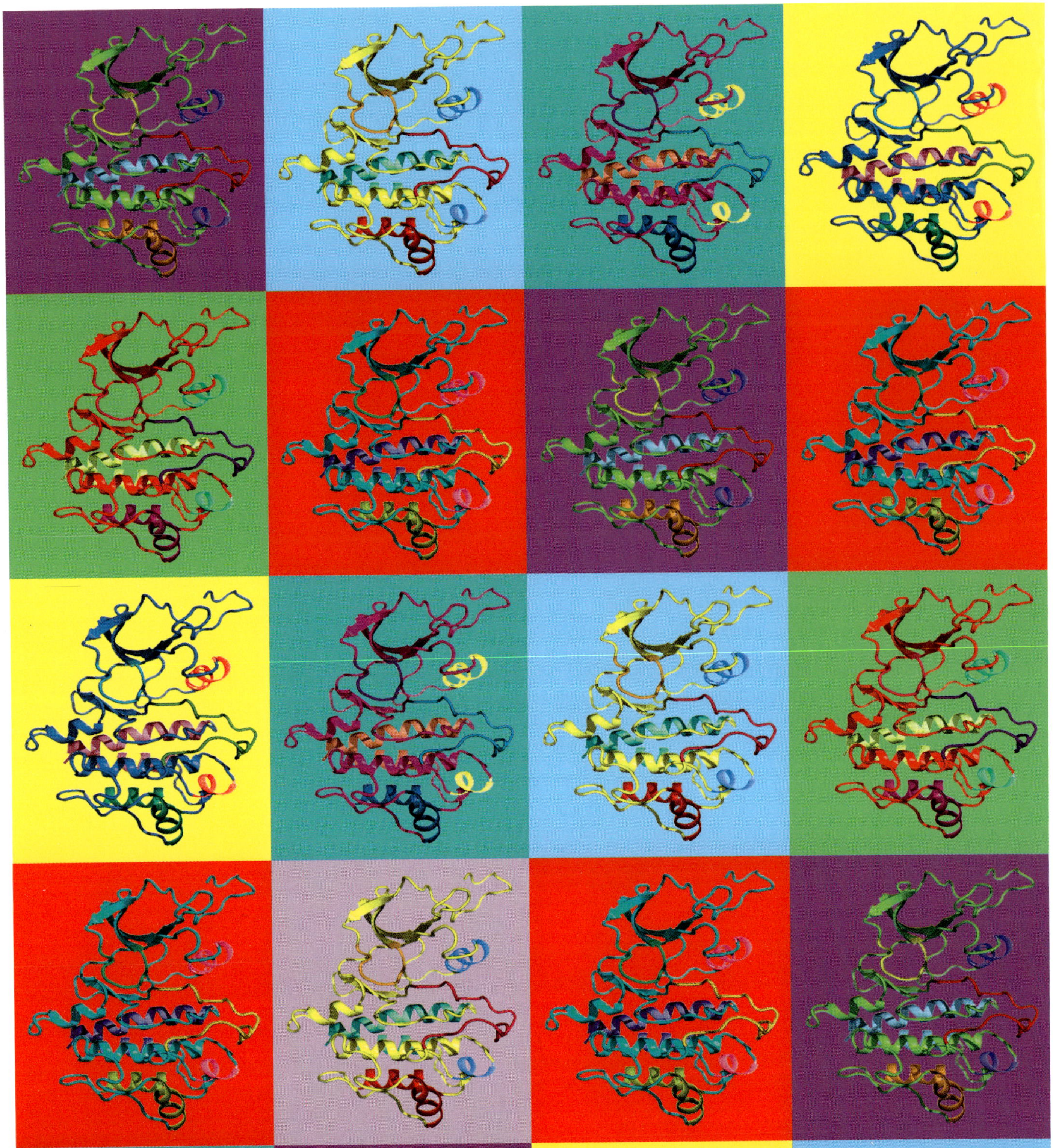

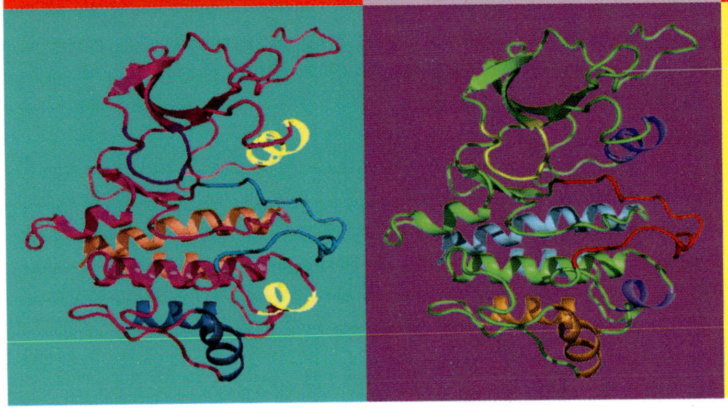

References: 1. Melo JV, Deininger MWN. *Hematol Oncol Clin North Am.* 2004;18:545-568. 2. Deininger MWN, Buchunger E, Druker BJ. *Blood.* 2005;105:2640-2653. 3. Branford S, Rudzki Z, Walsh S, et al. *Blood.* 2003;102:276-283. 4. Hochhaus A, La Rosée P. *Leukemia.* 2004;188:1321-1331. 5. Roche-Lestienne C, Soenen-Cornu V, Grardel-Duflos N, et al. *Blood.* 2002;100:1014-1018. 6. Gorre ME, Skaggs BJ, Sawyers CL. Presented at: Annual Meeting of the American Society of Hematology; December 2-6, 2004; San Diego, Calif. Abstract 556. 7. Donato NJ, Wu JY, Stapley J, et al. *Blood.* 2003;101:690-698. 8. Martinelli G, Soverini S, Rosti G, Cillani D, Baccarani M. *Haematologica.* 2005;90:534-541. 9. Pasquet J-M, Pocaly M, Lagarde V, et al. Presented at: Annual Meeting of the American Society of Hematology; December 2-6, 2004; San Diego, Calif. Abstract 1981. 10. Gorre ME, Ellwood-Yen K, Chiosis G, Rosen N, Sawyers CL. *Blood.* 2002;100:3041-3044. 11. Deininger MWN, Goldman JM, Melo JV. *Blood.* 2000:96:3343-3356.

CML: A Disease of Increasing Molecular Complexity

At present, there is a considerable amount of knowledge on the molecular biology of chronic myeloid leukemia (CML), providing an unparalleled platform for molecularly targeted therapy. While the *BCR-ABL* gene remains the driving force in CML, ongoing research into the inhibition of additional molecular targets, including mutations of the *BCR-ABL* kinase, may lead to new therapies.[1,2]

CML Is a Disease With More Than One Target

BCR-ABL Kinase Mutations within the *ABL* kinase domain are emerging as the most frequent mechanism for the reactivation of *BCR-ABL* activity and, thus, represent important potential targets in CML.[2-5] The development of *BCR-ABL* mutations can occur through either genetic instability or secondary mutational events over the course of the disease and is not limited to late-stage disease.[5]

Recent evidence has also shown that certain mutations may bind and phosphorylate substrates distinct from wild-type *BCR-ABL* and have the potential to activate alternative signaling pathways, providing additional insight into why certain mutations are associated with poor prognosis.[6]

SRC-Family Kinases are independent oncogenic pathways that are believed to be involved in late-stage disease progression. Two members of the *SRC* family in particular, *LYN* and *HCK*, are highly overexpressed and activated in patients with blast crisis and have been implicated in leukemic tumor cell growth, apoptotic protection, and kinase inhibitory activity.[7,8]

Heat-Shock Family Proteins (Hsp) are molecular chaperones capable of maintaining the stability and function of *BCR-ABL*.[9,10]

Downstream BCR-ABL Signal Transduction Pathways are responsible for the development and proliferation of malignant cells through a signaling cascade of multiple oncogenic kinase events.[11] These pathways represent potential new targets for molecular therapy.[1]

BCR-ABL Mitogenic Signaling Pathways*[11]

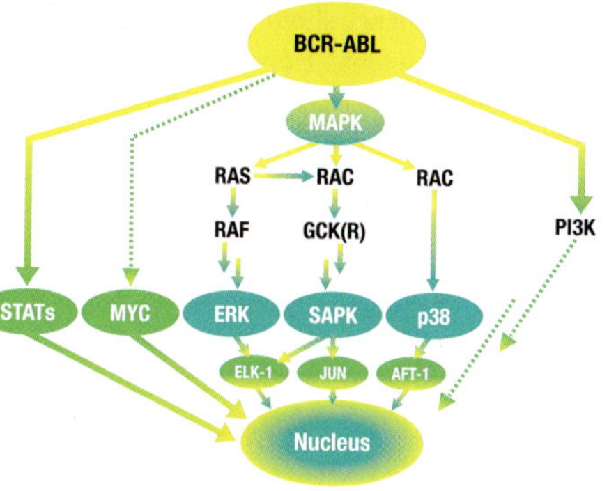

Reprinted with permission from Deininger MWN, et al.

* Note: This is a simplified diagram of the *BCR-ABL* signaling pathways. Numerous additional downstream targets have been reported.

Potential Multi-Targeted Approaches to CML Therapy

Significant progress has been made in the development of therapeutic agents directed against molecular targets specifically expressed or abnormally activated in patients with CML.[1] While *BCR-ABL* remains the primary target for CML therapy, there is hope that new research investigating synergistic approaches, simultaneously addressing multiple targets, may lead to new therapies for patients with CML.

Bristol-Myers Squibb is committed to investigating the molecular causes of cancer and developing potential new treatment alternatives to help address the needs of people living with cancer.

Bristol-Myers Squibb

Seminars in HEMATOLOGY

Neal S. Young · Photis Beris
Editors

Peter A. Miescher, *Founding Editor* Ernst R. Jaffé, *Co-Editor Emeritus*

Seminars in Hematology (ISSN 0037-1963) is published quarterly by Elsevier, 1600 John F. Kennedy Blvd, Ste 1800, Philadelphia, PA 19103-2899. (For Post Office use only: Volume 43 issue 1 of 4.) Months of issue are January, April, July, and October. Corporate and Editorial Offices: 6277 Sea Harbor Dr, Orlando, FL 32887-4800. Periodicals postage paid at Orlando, FL 32887-4800, and at additional mailing officies.

POSTMASTER: Send change of address to *Seminars in Hematology*, Elsevier, Periodicals Department, 6277 Sea Harbor Dr, Orlando, FL 32887-4800.

Editorial correspondence should be addressed to Photis Beris, MD, Division d'Hématologie, Hôpital Cantonal Universitaire, 25 rue Micheli-du-Crest, 1211 Geneve 14, Switzerland, or Neal S. Young, MD, 4400 17th Street, NW, Washington, DC 20011.

Business correspondence (subscriptions, change of address) should be addressed to the Publisher, Elsevier, 6277 Sea Harbor Dr, Orlando, FL 32887-4800; Email elspcs@elsevier.com.

Change of address notices, including both the old and new addresses of the subscriber, should be sent at least one month in advance.

Customer Service: 1-800-654-2452; outside the United States and Canada, (407) 345-4000.

Yearly subscription rates: United States and possessions: individual, $169.00; institution, $267.00; single issues, $81.00. All other countries: individual, $239.00; institution, $339.00; single issues, $81.00. Student and resident: United States and possessions, and Canada: $85.00; all other countries: $122.00. To receive student/resident rate, orders must be accompanied by name of affiliated institution, date of term, and the *signature* of program/residency coordinator on institution letterhead. Orders will be billed at individual rate until proof of status is received. Current prices are in effect for back volumes and back issues. Single issues, both current and back, exist in limited quantities and are offered for sale subject to availability. Back issues sold in conjunction with a subscription are on a prorated basis. Prices are subject to change without notice. *Checks* should be made payable to Elsevier and sent to *Seminars in Hematology*, Elsevier, Periodicals Department, PO Box 628239, Orlando, FL 32862-8239.

Other correspondence (copyediting, production) should be addressed to Elsevier, 1600 John F. Kennedy Blvd, Ste 1800, Philadelphia, PA 19103-2899.

Reprints: For 100 or more copies of an article in this publication, please contact the Commercial Reprints Department, Elsevier, 360 Park Ave South, New York, NY 10010-1710. Telephone (212) 633-3813, fax (212) 633-3820; e-mail, reprints@elsevier.com.

Advertising Representative: Cunningham Associates, PO Box 308, Park Ridge, NJ 07656. Telephone (201) 767-4170.

The contents of *Seminars in Hematology* are indexed in *Index Medicus* and *MEDLINE, Current Contents/Clinical Medicine, Current Contents/Life Sciences,* Science Citation Index, and *EMBASE/* Excerpta Medica.

The *Seminars in Hematology* home page is located at *www.seminhematol.org*.

W.B. Saunders **Philadelphia, PA**

Seminars in
HEMATOLOGY

Vol 43, No 1, January 2006

Graft-Versus-Host Disease

James L.M. Ferrara and John E. Levine
Guest Editors

Graft-Versus-Host Disease in the 21st Century: New Perspectives on an Old Problem 1
John E. Levine and James L.M. Ferrara

Pathophysiology of Graft-Versus-Host Disease 3
James L.M. Ferrara and Pavan Reddy

Genetics of Risk Factors for Graft-Versus-Host Disease 11
Effie W. Petersdorf and Mari Malkki

The Clinical Spectrum of Acute Graft-Versus-Host Disease 24
H. Joachim Deeg and Joseph H. Antin

Prophylaxis and Treatment of Acute Graft-Versus-Host Disease 32
Nelson J. Chao and Benny J. Chen

The Lung as a Target Organ of Graft-Versus-Host Disease 42
Gregory Yanik and Kenneth R. Cooke

Graft-Versus-Host Disease and Graft-Versus-Leukemia After Donor Leukocyte Infusion 53
David Porter and John E. Levine

Continued on following page

Cover Illustration: Dendritic cell interacting with two T cells.

$CD4^+CD25^+$ Regulatory T Cells and Graft-Versus-Host Disease 62
Petra Hoffmann and Matthias Edinger

Diagnosis and Treatment of Chronic Graft-Versus-Host Disease 70
Andrew L. Gilman and Jonathan Serody

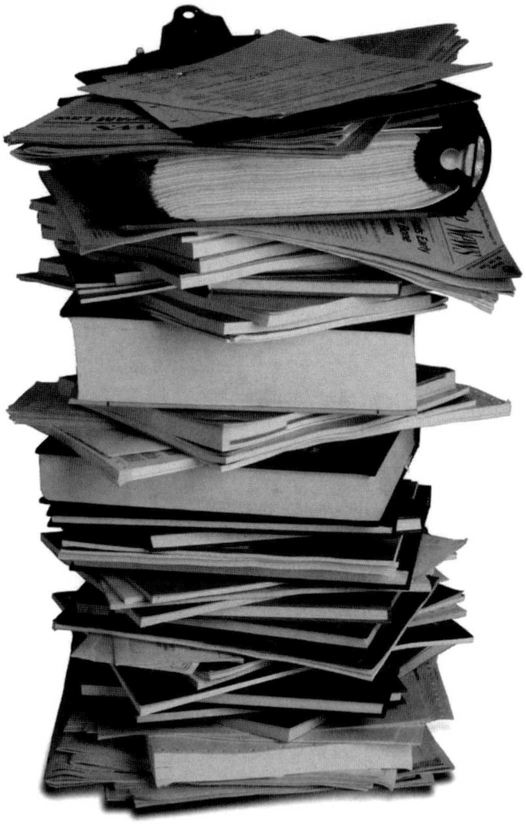

Seminars in HEMATOLOGY

Previous Issues

2005

Vol 42, No 1, January	**von Willebrand Factor in Hemostasis and Thrombosis** *Pier M. Mannucci, Guest Editor*
Vol 42, No 2, April	**Immune Hemolytic Anemia** *George Garratty, Guest Editor*
Vol 42, No 3, July	**Transplant Immunobiology** *Effie W. Petersdorf, Guest Editor*
Vol 42, No 4, October	**Chronic Myeloproliferative Disorders** *Radek Skoda and Josef T. Prchal, Guest Editors*

2004

Vol 41, No 1, January	**Thrombotic Thrombocytopenic Purpura: Advances in Pathophysiology, Diagnosis, and Treatment** *Bernhard Lämmle and James N. George, Guest Editors*
Vol 41, No 2, April	**Erythrocyte Membrane Proteins and Their Diseases** *Narla Mohandas, Guest Editor*
Vol 41, No 3, July	**Chronic Lymphocytic Leukemia** *Kanti R. Rai and Jacques Louis Binet, Guest Editors*
Vol 41, No 4, October	**Gene Therapy in Hematology** *Cynthia E. Dunbar, Guest Editor*

2003

Vol 40, No 1, January	**Management of Chronic Myeloid Leukemia** *John M. Goldman, Guest Editor*
Vol 40, No 2, April	**Herpesvirus in Hematology** *Giovanna Tosato, Guest Editor*
Vol 40, No 3, July	**Hematologic Malignancies of Cytotoxic Cells** *Thomas P. Loughran Jr, Guest Editor*
Vol 40, No 4, October	**Genomics in Hematology** *Louis M. Staudt, Guest Editor*

Seminars in HEMATOLOGY

Future Topics

Vol 43, No 2, April	**Acute Leukemia in the Elderly** *Eli Estey, Guest Editor*
Vol 43, No 3, July	**Constitutional Marrow Failure** *Grover Bagby, Guest Editor*
Vol 43, No 4, October	**Aggressive Treatment of Aggressive Lymphomas** *Richard Fisher*
Vol 44, No 1, January	**Transfusion Medicine in the Early 21st Century** *Harvey Klein, Guest Editor*

Seminars in
HEMATOLOGY

Forthcoming Issue
April 2006

Acute Leukemia in the Elderly
Elihu H. Estey, ***Guest Editor***

General Therapeutic Approach to the Older Patient With AML — *Elihu H. Estey*

Biologic Features of AML in the Elderly: Emphasis on Gene Expression Studies — *Cheryl L. Willman*

Management of Acute Lymphoblastic Leukemia in Older Patients — *Richard A. Larson*

Increasing Role of Transplantation for Older Patients With Acute Leukemia — *Sergio Giralt*

Approach to the Complications of Treatment for Acute Leukemia in the Elderly — *Joel Gingerich and Eric Bow*

Treatment of Older Patients—New Agents — *Alan K. Burnett*

Etiology of AML in the Elderly — *David T. Bowen*

Immunologic Approaches to Acute Leukemia in the Elderly — *Sherif Farag and Michael Caligiuri*

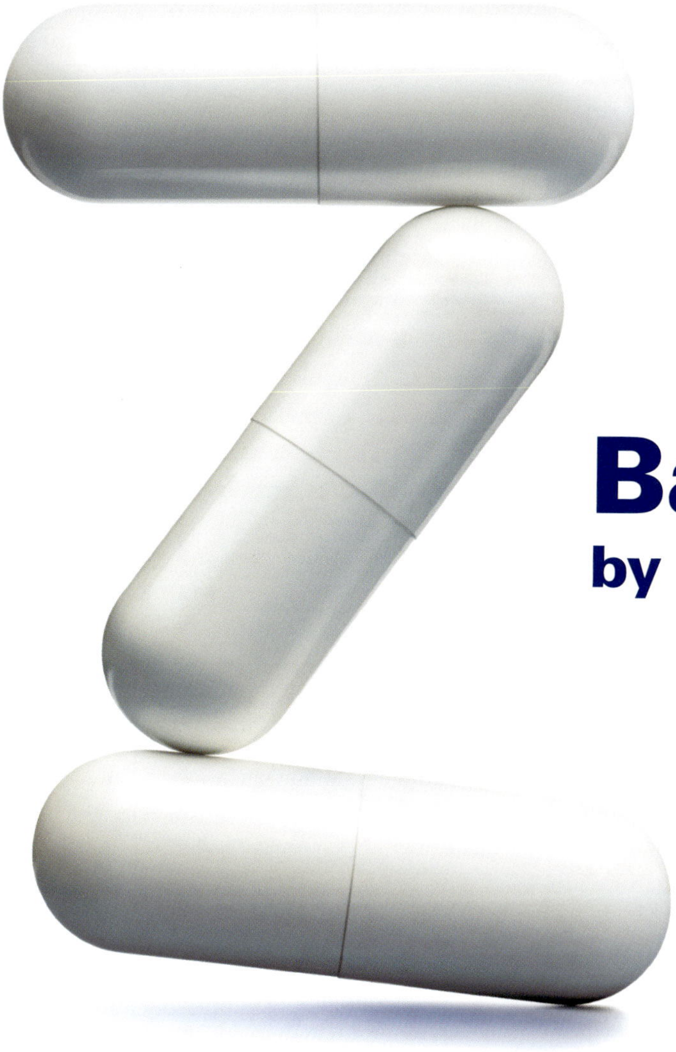

For adults with mild-to-moderate ***type 1 Gaucher disease*** *for whom enzyme replacement therapy is not an option*

Balance
by Substrate Reduction

Substrate Reduction Therapy (SRT) With Zavesca Provides Important Benefits

- Liver and spleen volume reductions seen as early as month 6—continued reductions over 24 months
- Hemoglobin concentration and platelet count improvements seen as early as month 6—significant improvements seen at 24 months

Zavesca Maintained Benefits of Long-Term Enzyme Replacement Therapy (ERT)

- In patients on ERT for a mean of 5.6 years, liver and spleen volume, as well as hemoglobin concentration and platelet count, were maintained after 6 months of Zavesca monotherapy

Important Safety Information

- Peripheral neuropathy has been reported in patients receiving Zavesca
- Zavesca may cause fetal harm if administered to a pregnant woman
- There is a risk of impaired fertility in men

Convenient Oral Dosing

- Recommended at 100 mg tid
- May be taken with or without food

Zavesca may be prescribed only by physicians knowledgeable in the management of Gaucher disease

- **Visit www.ZAVESCA.com or call 1.866.228.3546**

ZAVESCA® 100mg
(miglustat) capsules

Please see brief summary of full prescribing information on following page.

ACTELION

ELSEVIER

Seminars in HEMATOLOGY

Volume 43, Number 1 **January 2006**

Graft-Versus-Host Disease in the 21st Century: New Perspectives on an Old Problem

This volume of *Seminars* focuses on graft-versus-host disease (GVHD), a highly morbid toxicity of allogeneic hematopoietic stem cell transplant (HSCT). The toxicity of GVHD limits the accessibility of HSCT to patients whose underlying disease is either incurable with standard chemotherapy or who have already failed standard approaches. An improved understanding of the pathophysiology of GVHD should lead to better preventive, diagnostic, and therapeutic strategies, thus making allogeneic HSCT more widely available. Hence the timeliness of this volume.

Acute GVHD occurs in up to 40% of patients undergoing related donor HSCT[1,2] and in up to 70% of patients undergoing unrelated donor HSCT.[3] The clinical manifestations of GVHD, reviewed by Deeg and Antin, usually become manifest within the first month following stem cell infusion. Less than 40% of patients with acute GVHD experience complete responses to high-dose corticosteroids,[4,5] leading to significant morbidity and mortality from chronic corticosteroid therapy. The severity of acute GVHD continues to be measured by changes in three primary target organs (skin, liver and intestines),[4,6] but a strong case can be made to also consider the lung a target of GVHD, as reviewed in the chapter by Yanik and Cooke.

The initial models for GVHD pathophysiology were based, logically enough, on a paradigm of solid organ rejection mediated by cytotoxic T lymphocytes. This useful model has led to effective strategies for GVHD prevention, as well as establishing a role for donor leukocytes to treat relapse after transplant, as reviewed in the chapter by Porter and Levine. Recent scholarship considers acute GVHD to be the result of more complex interactions between donor T cells, host antigen-presenting cells, and target tissues, influenced by networks of regulatory cells and shifting balances of pro- and anti-inflammatory signals. As reviewed by Ferrara and Reddy, new insights into mechanisms underlying GVHD suggest additional therapeutic strategies, such as neutralization of inflammatory cytokines or infusions of regulatory cells. Chao and Chen provide an overview of the current clinical state of the art regarding GVHD prevention and treatment, and Hoffmann and Edinger summarize cutting edge studies of regulatory T cells to control GVHD. The genetic typing of both donor and host that predicts the development of GVHD is elegantly reviewed by Petersdorf and Malkki, who also examine the implications of improvements in human leukocyte antigen (HLA) typing.

Finally, Gilman and Serody deftly summarize chronic GVHD, a poorly understood toxicity of allogeneic bone marrow transplantation whose natural history continues to defy easy characterization. With increased numbers of patients suffering from chronic GVHD, it continues as an important arena for clinical and laboratory research, as illustrated by a recent National Institutes of Health consensus conference.

By the next time *Seminars* focuses a volume on GVHD, we fully expect that the insights provided in these pages will have produced new standards of care for our patients, and that we will have made significant progress in making allogeneic HSCT a safer and more effective therapy for all patients who could benefit from it.

James L.M. Ferrara
John E. Levine
University of Michigan Medical School
Ann Arbor, MI
Guest Editors

References

1. Brown RA, Adkins D, Khoury H, Vij R, Goodnough LT, Shenoy S, DiPersio JF. Long-term follow-up of high-risk allogeneic peripheral-blood stem-cell transplant recipients: graft-versus-host disease and transplant-related mortality. J Clin Oncol 17:806-812, 1999
2. Storb R, Deeg HJ, Farewell V, Doney K, Appelbaum F, Beatty P, et al. Marrow transplantation for severe aplastic anemia: methotrexate alone compared with a combination of methotrexate and cyclosporine for prevention of acute graft-versus-host disease. Blood 68:119-125, 1986
3. Nash RA, Antin JH, Karanes C, Fay JW, Avalos BR, Yeager AM, et al. Phase 3 study comparing methotrexate and tacrolimus with methotrexate and cyclosporine for prophylaxis of acute graft-versus-host

doi:10.1053/j.seminhematol.2005.11.028

disease after marrow transplantation from unrelated donors. Blood 96:2062-2068, 2000
4. Glucksberg H, Storb R, Fefer A, Buckner CD, Neiman PE, Clift RA, et al. Clinical manifestations of graft-versus-host disease in human recipients of marrow from HL-A-matched sibling donors. Transplantation 18:295-304, 1974
5. Ferrara JL. Cytokine dysregulation as a mechanism of graft versus host disease. Curr Opin Immunol 5:794-799, 1993
6. Przepiorka D, Weisdorf D, Martin P, Klingemann HG, Beatty P, Hows J, et al. 1994 Consensus Conference on Acute GVHD Grading. Bone Marrow Transplant 15:825-828, 1995

Seminars in
HEMATOLOGY

Pathophysiology of Graft-Versus-Host Disease

James L.M. Ferrara and Pavan Reddy

Complications of allogeneic hematopoietic stem cell transplantation (HSCT) remain barriers to its wider application for a variety of diseases. Graft-versus-host disease (GVHD) is the major cause of morbidity and mortality following allogeneic HSCT. GVHD can be considered an exaggerated, undesirable manifestation of a normal inflammatory mechanism, in which donor lymphocytes encounter foreign antigens in a milieu that fosters inflammation. Recent advances in the study of cytokine networks, chemokine gradients, and the direct mediators of cellular cytotoxicity have led to improved understanding of this complex syndrome. The pathophysiology of acute GVHD can be considered as a three-step process in which the innate and adaptive immune systems interact: (1) tissue damage to the recipient by the radiation/chemotherapy pretransplant conditioning regimen; (2) donor T-cell activation and clonal expansion; and (3) cellular and inflammatory factors. Here we review the immunologic interactions that cause clinical GVHD and discuss the risk factors and prophylactic strategies for acute GVHD according to this model.
Semin Hematol 43:3-10

Graft-versus-host disease (GVHD) is the major cause of morbidity and mortality after allogeneic hematopoietic stem cell transplantation (HSCT). GVHD has traditionally been classified by the time of its clinical manifestations: acute GVHD occurs within the first 100 days after HSCT; chronic GVHD occurs after day 100. This simple classification is increasingly unsatisfactory, particularly as reduced intensity conditioning regimens gain wider acceptance. The clinical manifestations of acute GVHD after such conditioning often occur much later, blurring the sharp day 100 demarcation between acute and chronic. Nevertheless, extensive clinical data has been codified according to this classification and it will be used throughout this article.

In 1966, Billingham formulated the three requirements necessary for GVHD. First, the transplanted graft must contain immunologically competent cells; second, the recipient must be incapable of rejecting the transplanted cells; and third, the recipient must express tissue antigens that are not present in the transplant donor that could thus be recognized as foreign.[1]

University of Michigan Medical School, Ann Arbor, MI.
Supported by National Institutes of Health Grants No. K08 AI052863-01 (P.R.) and PO1 CA 49542 (J.L.M.F.). P.R. is the recipient of the Alaina J. Enlow Scholar Award from Amy Strelzer Manasevit-National Marrow Donor Program and the New Investigator Award from American Society of Blood and Marrow Transplantation. J.L.M.F. is the recipient of the Doris Duke Distinguished Clinical Scientist Award.
Address correspondence to James L.M. Ferrara, MD, Professor of Pediatrics and Medicine, University of Michigan Medical School, 1500 E Medical Center Dr, 6308 CCGC, Ann Arbor, MI 48109-0942. E-mail: ferrara@umich.edu

Mature T lymphocytes are the immunocompetent cells in the graft that fulfill the first precondition for GVHD.[2] After allogeneic HSCT, the severity of GVHD correlates with the number of donor T cells transfused.[3] Because experimental models have shown that the ability of marrow T cells to induce GVHD is much less potent than for mature circulating T cells,[4] contamination of bone marrow with peripheral blood at the time of marrow harvest may significantly contribute to the development of GVHD.

The second precondition for GVHD stipulates that the recipient must be immuno-compromised; a normal immune system will usually reject T cells from a foreign donor. Immuno-compromise commonly follows allogeneic HSCT, as patients historically have received immuno-ablative doses of chemotherapy and/or radiation before stem cell infusion. During solid organ allografts and with blood transfusion, recipients are often immuno-suppressed. There are, however, exceptions for this requirement. GVHD can occur in an immuno-competent recipient of tissues from a donor who is homozygous for one haplotype of the recipient (as with transfusion of blood from a human leukocyte antigen [HLA] homozygous parent to a heterozygous child). This genetic situation prevents the recipient from rejecting the donor cells despite immune competence.[5]

The third precondition for GVHD, the expression of recipient tissue antigens not present in the donor, became the focus of intensive research with the discovery of the major histocompatibility complex (MHC). HLAs are the gene products of the MHC. HLAs are expressed on the cell surfaces of all nucleated cells in the human body and are essential to the

0037-1963/06/$-see front matter
doi:10.1053/j.seminhematol.2005.09.001

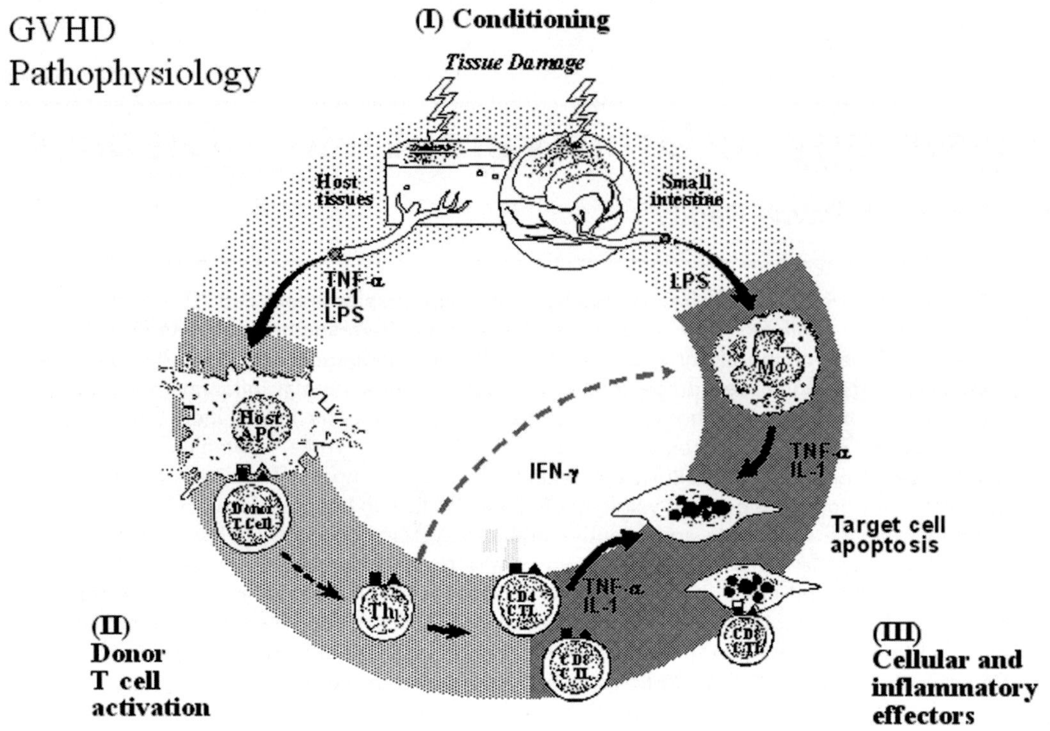

Figure 1 The pathophysiology of acute GVHD. GVHD pathophysiology can be summarized in a three-step process. In step I, the conditioning regimen (irradiation, chemotherapy, or both) leads to the damage and activation of host tissues, especially the intestinal mucosa. This allows the translocation of LPS from the intestinal lumen to the circulation, stimulating the secretion of the inflammatory cytokines TNF-α and IL-1 from host tissues, particularly macrophages. These cytokines increase the expression of MHC antigens and adhesion molecules on host tissues, enhancing the recognition of MHC and mHags by mature donor T cells. Donor T-cell activation in step II is characterized by the predominance of Th1 cells and the secretion of IFN-γ, which activates mononuclear phagocytes. In step III, effector functions of activated mononuclear phagocytes are triggered by the secondary signal provided by LPS and other stimulatory molecules that leak through the intestinal mucosa damaged during steps I and II. Activated macrophages, along with CTL, secrete inflammatory cytokines that cause target cell apoptosis. $CD8^+$ CTL also lyse target cells directly. Damage to the GI tract in this phase, principally by inflammatory cytokines, amplifies LPS release and leads to the "cytokine storm" characteristic of severe acute GVHD. This damage results in the amplification of local tissue injury, and it further promotes an inflammatory response.

activation of allogeneic T cells.[6] During lymphocyte development, T cells are selected in the thymus to recognize self-MHC molecules, but when confronted with allogeneic (non-self) MHC molecules, the activated T cells mount a formidable attack that culminates in the destruction of the allogeneic tissues. MHC differences between donor and recipient are the most important risk factor for the induction of GVHD. In addition, there are minor histocompatibility antigens (mHag) derived from the expression of polymorphic genes.

The pathophysiology of acute GVHD after HSCT can be considered as a three-step process in which the innate and adaptive immune systems interact (Fig 1): (I) tissue damage to the recipient by the radiation/chemotherapy pretransplant conditioning regimen; (II) donor T-cell activation and clonal expansion; and (III) cellular and inflammatory factors. In step I, the conditioning regimen leads to damage and activation of host antigen-presenting cells (APCs) by inflammatory cytokines. In step II, host APCs present alloantigen to the resting T cells and activate them. Donor T-cell activation is characterized by cellular proliferation and the secretion of cytokines, including interleukin (IL)-2 and interferon (IFN)-γ. In step III, mononuclear phagocytes and neutrophils cause inflammation, triggered by mediators such as lipopolysaccharides (LPS) that leak through the intestinal mucosa damaged during step I. Inflammation recruits effector cells into target organs, amplifying local tissue injury with further secretion of inflammatory cytokines which, together with cytotoxic T lymphocytes (CTL), lead to target tissue destruction.[7,8]

Step I: Effects of HSCT Conditioning

The first step of acute GVHD begins before donor cells are infused. Prior to HSCT, a patient's tissues have been damaged by a number of factors, including the underlying disease and its treatment, infection, and drugs and radiation used in the conditioning regimen. High-intensity chemoradiotherapy, characteristic of many HSCT conditioning regimens, activates host APCs that are critical to the stimulation of donor T cells infused in the stem cell inoculum. Total body irradiation (TBI) is particularly important because it activates host tissues to secrete inflammatory cytokines, such as tumor necrosis factor (TNF)-α and IL-1, and induces endothelial apoptosis that leads to epithelial cell damage in the gastrointestinal (GI) tract.[9,10] GVHD damage to the GI tract amplifies GVHD by allowing the translocation of microbial products such as LPS into the systemic circulation. This model helps to explain the increased risk of GVHD associated with intensive conditioning regimens.[11,12]

Step II: Donor T-Cell Activation and Cytokine Secretion

Murine studies have demonstrated that host APCs alone are both necessary and sufficient to stimulate donor T cells to proliferate as early as day 3, 12 hours after HSCT, preceding the engraftment of donor stem cells.[13–15] Inflammatory cytokines and microbial products such as LPS may all be considered "danger signals"[16] that help to activate T cells, and they may make the difference between an immune response and tolerance.[17] When T cells are exposed to antigens in the presence of an adjuvant such as LPS, the migration and survival of T cells are dramatically enhanced in vivo.[18] The effect of advanced age in enhancing allo-stimulatory activity of host APCs may also contribute to the increased incidence of acute GVHD in older recipients.[19] The elimination of host APCs by activated natural killer (NK) cells can prevent GVHD in experimental models.[20] This suppressive effect of NK cells on GVHD has been confirmed in humans: HLA class I differences driving donor NK-mediated alloreactions in the GVHD direction mediate potent graft-versus-leukemia (GVL) effects and produce higher engraftment rates without causing severe, acute GVHD.[20,21]

CD4 and CD8 proteins are co-receptors for constant portions of MHC class II and MHC class I molecules, respectively. MHC class I (HLA-A, -B, -C) differences stimulate $CD8^+$ T cells and MHC class II (HLA-DR, -DP, -DQ) differences stimulate $CD4^+$ T cells.[22] After HLA-identical HSCT, GVHD is induced by mHAg, peptides derived from polymorphic cellular proteins presented on the cell surface by MHC molecules.[23] Because the genes for these proteins are located outside of the MHC, two siblings often will have many different peptides in the same MHC that can be recognized by donor T cells and lead to GVHD. How many of these peptides behave as mHAg remains unclear, although more than 50 different minor histocompatability genetic loci have been defined among inbred strains of mice.[24] In humans, of five previously characterized mHAg (HA-1, -2, -3, -4, -5) recognized by T cells in association with HLA-A1 and -A2, only mismatching of HA-1 significantly correlated with acute grade II to IV GVHD.[23] Several mHags are encoded on the male-specific Y chromosome and there is an increased risk of GVHD when male recipients are transplanted from female donors.[25]

Cytokines secreted by activated T cells are generally classified as Th1 (secreting IL-2 and IFN-α) or Th2 (secreting IL-4, IL-5, IL-10, and IL-13).[26] Dendritic cells (DC) can modulate the function of T cells which, in turn, have multiple effects, including: (1) amplification of cytokine secretion, (2) lysis of target cells by Fas/FasL interactions, (3) activation of macrophages, (4) activation of endothelium to induce macrophage binding and extravasation, and (5) recruitment of macrophages by secreting monocyte chemo-attractant protein-1 (MCP-1).[18,20]

Monoclonal antibodies (mAb) against IL-2 or its receptor prevent GVHD when administered shortly after the infusion of T cells,[27,28] but this strategy was only moderately successful in reducing established GVHD.[29] Cyclosporine (CSP) and FK506 dramatically reduce IL-2 production and effectively prevent GVHD. IL-15 is another critical cytokine in initiating allogeneic T-cell division in vivo, and elevated serum levels of IL-15 are associated with acute GVHD in humans.[30] IFN-γ increases the expression of numerous molecules involved in GVHD, including adhesion molecules, chemokines, MHC antigens, and Fas, resulting in enhanced antigen presentation and the recruitment of effector cells into target organs.[31,32] IFN-γ also alters target cells in the GI tract and skin so that they are more vulnerable to damage during GVHD; the administration of anti–IFN-α mAbs prevents GI GVHD[33] and high levels of both IFN-γ and TNF-α correlate with the most intense cellular damage in skin.[34] IFN-γ mediates GVHD-associated immuno-suppression in several experimental HSCT systems, in part by the induction of nitric oxide (NO),[35,36] and primes macrophages to produce pro-inflammatory cytokines and NO in response to LPS.[37] Paradoxically, at early time points after HSCT, IFN-γ can reduce GVHD by enhancing Fas-mediated apoptosis of activated donor T cells.[13,38]

Subpopulations of regulatory donor T cells can prevent GVHD. Repeated in vitro stimulation of donor $CD4^+$ T cells with alloantigens results in the emergence of a population of regulatory T-cell (Treg) clones that secretes high amounts of IL-10 and tissue growth factor-β (TGF-β). The immunosuppressive properties of these cytokines are explained by their ability to inhibit APC function and to suppress proliferation of responding T cells directly. Natural suppressor (NS) cells and NK1.1+ T cells (NKT) also prevent GVHD in experimental models.[4,39]

Step III: Cellular and Inflammatory Effectors

The pathophysiology of acute GVHD culminates in the generation of multiple cytotoxic effectors of target tissue injury, including several inflammatory cytokines, specific anti-host CTLs, NK cells, and NO. Experimental and clinical data suggest that soluble inflammatory mediators act in conjunction with direct cell-mediated cytolysis by CTL and NK cells to cause the full spectrum of deleterious effects observed in acute GVHD. As such, the effector phase of GVHD involves aspects of both the innate and adaptive immune responses and the synergistic interactions of components generated during step I and step II.

The Fas/Fas ligand (FasL) and the perforin/granzyme (or granule exocytosis) pathways are the principal effector mechanisms used by CTLs and NK cells to lyse their target cells.[40,41] Perforin is stored together with granzymes and other proteins in cytotoxic granules of CTLs and NK cells; perforin inserts itself into the target cell membrane forming "perforin pores" that allow granzymes to enter the cell and induce apoptosis through various downstream effector pathways. FasL binds Fas, which results in the formation of the death-inducing signaling complex (DISC) and the subsequent activation of caspases.[42] A number of T-cell surface proteins also possess the capability to trimerize TNF receptor-like death receptors (DR) that also induce apoptosis in their targets.[43] $CD4^+$ CTLs preferentially use the Fas/FasL pathway during acute GVHD, while $CD8^+$ CTLs primarily use the perforin/granzyme pathway, consistent with other conditions involving cell-mediated cytolysis. FasL-defective donor T cells markedly reduce experimental GVHD in liver, skin, and lymphoid organs. The Fas/FasL pathway is particularly important in hepatic GVHD, consistent with the marked sensitivity of hepatocytes to Fas-mediated cytotoxicity in models of murine hepatitis.[44]

In the effector phase of acute GVHD, inflammatory cytokines synergize with CTLs, resulting in amplification of local tissue injury and development of target organ dysfunction in the transplant recipient. A central role for inflammatory cytokines in acute GVHD was confirmed by recent murine experiments using bone marrow chimeras; GVHD-target organ injury was induced, even in the absence of epithelial alloantigens, and mortality and organ injury were prevented by the neutralization of TNF-α and IL-1.[45] TNF-α plays a central role in intestinal GVHD in murine and human studies.[46–48] Experimentally, neutralization of TNF-α alone or in combination with IL-1 resulted in a significant reduction of GVHD.[45,49] However, while neutralization of IL-1 with an IL-1 receptor antagonist was able to prevent GVHD in mice, its use in a randomized clinical trial did not prevent GVHD.[50]

Macrophages secrete cytokines after ligation of Toll-like receptors (TLRs) by LPS and other microbial products that have leaked though a damaged intestinal mucosa. Since the GI tract is particularly sensitive to the injurious effects of cytokines,[46,51] organ damage incurred during the effector phase can lead to a positive feedback loop, wherein increased translocation of LPS results in further cytokine production and progressive intestinal injury. Thus, the GI tract may be critical to propagating the "cytokine storm" characteristic of acute GVHD.[52] Elevated serum levels of LPS correlate directly with the degree of intestinal histopathology occurring after allogeneic HSCT,[51,53] and gram-negative gut decontamination during HSCT reduces GVHD.[54,55]

LPS can stimulate inflammatory chemokine expression in inflamed tissues; these tendencies are specialized to recruit effector cells, such as T cells, neutrophils, and monocytes.[56] Chemokine receptors that are differentially expressed on activated T cells can rapidly switch chemokine receptor expression to acquire new migratory capacity.[18,57] $CCR5^+$ $CD8^+$ T cells migrate into the liver, lung, and spleen during GVHD,[58] and levels of several chemokines are elevated in GVHD-associated lung injury.[59] The expression of chemokines and their receptors may help to explain the unusual cluster of GVHD target organs (skin, gut, and liver).

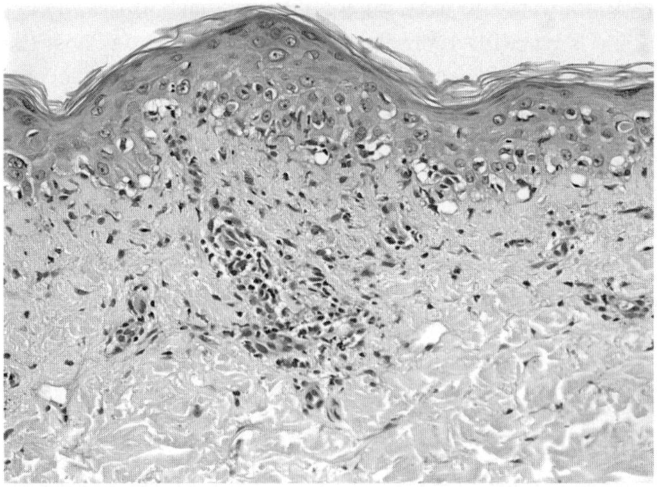

Figure 2 Skin, grade 2 acute GVHD (histopathology): interface vacuolar change, lymphocytic infiltrate, and dyskeratotic cells in the epidermis. Damaged epithelial cells occasionally surrounded by two or more lymphocytes in a process known as "satellite cell necrosis."

Risk Factors and Prevention

GVHD can thus be considered an exaggerated and dysregulated response of a normal immune system (that of the donor) to tissue damage that is intrinsic to transplantation. The donor's immune system reacts as if there is a massive and uncontrolled infection, and its efforts to deal with this injury result in the clinical manifestations of GVHD. Tissue injury intrinsic to the administration of high-dose chemo-radiotherapy initiates the breakdown of mucosal barriers, allowing endotoxin into tissues. TLRs on DCs bind to endotoxin and activate signal transduction pathways that lead to DC maturation and induce inflammation.[60] The upregulation of costimulatory molecules, MHC molecules, adhesion molecules, cytokines, chemokines, prostanoids, and other inflammatory mediators prime and trigger attack on target tissues, fueling the fire. Likely danger signals[16] contribute to the "cytokine storm," making GVHD a disorder of dysregulated innate and adaptive immune responses. Risk factors and prophylactic strategies for acute GVHD can be considered according to this three-step model.

Reduced Intensity Conditioning Regimens

The three cardinal organs affected by GVHD are skin, intestinal tract, and liver (Fig 2). One common link among them is exposure to the environment. Skin and gut have very obvious barrier functions and a well-developed reticulo-endothelial system; the liver is the first line of defense downstream of the gut. The lung would be a similar target by this criterion, and elsewhere in this volume an argument is forwarded for its involvement in GVHD; less intense exposure to organisms, particularly gram-negative rods, may reduce pulmonary manifestations of acute GVHD. All of these organs are rich in DC, a probable prerequisite for antigen presentation and the generation of injurious cytokines. They are all subject to injury from conditioning, and breaches of the barrier would allow organisms or endotoxin into the circulation.

One prediction of the model is that less intense conditioning regimens would be associated with less GVHD. When donor lymphocyte infusions were administered without pharmacologic GVHD prophylaxis, the resultant GVHD has been less frequent and severe than would be expected in the absence of immunosuppressive drugs. Similarly, the GVHD after reduced intensity conditioning regimens should be less severe, as a result of diminished cellular injury from reduced endotoxin exposure due to less mucosal injury. Although clinical data on reducing colonization with bacteria after less intense regimens are suggestive and support the basic concepts described above, the effect is insufficient to control GVHD adequately in human transplantation.

Modulation of Donor T Cells

Histocompatibility differences between donor and recipient are major determinants of donor T cell activation, and increased HLA disparity is one of the most important risk factors for acute GVHD. Female donors, particularly those with multiple pregnancies, cause greater GVHD in male recipients because proteins encoded on the Y chromosome serve as mHags.

The number of T cells in donor marrow is directly associated with the severity of acute GVHD, and T-cell depletion is one of the most effective forms of GVHD prophylaxis. A T-cell dose $\leq 10^5$ per kg was associated with complete control of GVHD if an HLA-identical sibling served as the donor.[3] The combination of very high stem cell numbers and CD3 T-cell numbers less than 3×10^4 per kg allowed haploidentical transplantation without GVHD.[61] Unfortunately, the nonspecific removal or clearance of T cells results in increased fatal opportunistic infections, and equivalent overall survival.[62,63]

The first generally prescribed GVHD preventive regimen was the administration of intermittent low-dose methotrexate (MTX) immediately after HSCT, when T cells start to divide on exposure to allogeneic antigens.[64] The introduction of cyclosporine (CSP) in the late 1970s was a significant advance in GVHD prevention. As a single agent, CSP is about as effective as MTX alone, but in combination with MTX, CSP significantly reduces GVHD and improves survival.[65] A similar agent, tacrolimus, shows comparable control of GVHD.

More recently, mycophenolate mofetil (MMF), an inhibitor of the de novo pathway of guanosine nucleotide synthesis, has been studied. MMF does not inhibit the activation of T cells but blocks the coupling of activation to DNA synthesis and proliferation.[66]

Blockade of Inflammatory Stimuli and Effectors

Elimination of intestinal colonization with bacteria reduces GVHD by minimizing the triggering signal for monocytes and macrophages, thus reducing activation of APCs. The first indication that elimination of exposure to microorganisms could prevent GVHD was in germ-free experiments in mice; GVHD was not observed until the animals were colonized with gram-negative organisms.[67] Later, gut decontamination and use of a laminar air flow environment was associated with less GVHD and better survival in patients with severe aplastic anemia.[54]

An important role for TNF-α in clinical acute GVHD was suggested by the elevated levels of TNF-α in serum during acute GVHD and other endothelial complications such as veno-occlusive disease.[68,69] Time of first appearance of increased levels predicted the severity of complications and overall survival; patients with higher serum TNF-α levels during the conditioning regimen had a 90% incidence of grade II or greater acute GVHD and an overall mortality of 70%, compared with a mortality of 20% in patients without TNF-α elevations.[68] Murine monoclonal antibodies or $F(ab)_2$ fragments directed at TNF-α have been studied either as therapy for steroid-resistant GVHD (47) or as prophylaxis,[70] and some partial responses were observed. Therapy of GVHD with humanized anti–TNF-α (infliximab)[71] or a dimeric fusion protein consisting of the extracellular ligand-binding portion of the human TNF-α receptor (TNFR) linked to the constant (Fc) portion of human IgG1 (etanercept) have shown promise.

The second major pro-inflammatory cytokine with an important role in the effector phase of acute GVHD is IL-1. This cytokine is produced mainly by activated mononuclear phagocytes, and it shares with TNF-α a wide variety of biologic activities.[72] In a murine model, secretion of IL-1 occurred predominantly during the effector phase of GVHD in the spleen and skin, two major GVHD target organs.[73] IL-1 receptor antagonist (IL-1RA) is a naturally occurring pure competitive inhibitor of IL-1 that is produced by monocytes/macrophages and keratinocytes. The IL-1RA gene is polymorphic, and the presence in the donor of the allele that is linked to higher secretion of IL-1RA was associated with less acute GVHD.[74] In a murine model of GVHD to multiple mHags, intraperitoneal administration of recombinant IL-1RA for 10 days after HSCT prevented the development of GVHD in the majority of animals.[75] Although clinical trials of IL-1RA were promising, a subsequent randomized trial of the addition of IL-1RA or placebo to cyclosporine and methotrexate beginning at the time of conditioning and continuing through day 14 after stem cell infusion failed to demonstrate any protective effect of the drug.[64] Thus, at least as administered in that study, IL-1 inhibition by IL-1RA was insufficient to prevent GVHD in humans. IL-11 was also able to protect the GI tract in animal models and prevent GVHD,[76,77] but it did not prevent clinical GVHD in humans. Not all preclinical results successfully translate to effective therapies.

IL-6 might be expected to play a role in the pathophysiology of GVHD, particularly since it has inflammatory properties and is induced in monocytes after stimulation by IFN-γ and TNF-α. Little experimental work has been done in animal models, but serum IL-6 levels are elevated in patients with acute GVHD and hepatorenal syndrome[78] and with transplant-related toxicities after autologous HSCT.[79] However, IL-6 levels may respond to many stimuli, and lack of specificity may limit the utility of blood measurements. IL-8, also called neutrophil-activating peptide (NAP-1), may also figure in GVHD. IL-8 is produced in response to inflammatory mediators such as endotoxin, IL-1, and TNF-α, and its systemic administration inhibits the adhesion of leukocytes to endothelial surfaces. In a recent study of patients receiving HSCT for β-thalassemia, those with GVHD showed significantly elevated IL-8 blood levels compared to cases without GVHD.[80] One interesting implication is that granulocytes and macrophages may contribute to GVHD pathology, and most GVHD does occur after leukocyte recovery. These kinetics are typically interpreted as a reflection of the time necessary for lymphocytes to expand to a critical mass; they might equally suggest that the inflammatory cytokine network also activates and recruits neutrophils, and that these newly produced myeloid cells follow chemotactic signals to injured epithelium where they contribute to tissue injury by releasing activated oxygen metabolites as well as cytotoxic and proteolytic enzymes.

Conclusion

Complications of HSCT, particularly GVHD, remain major barriers to the wider application of allogeneic HSCT for a variety of diseases. Recent advances in the study of cytokine networks as well as the direct mediators of cellular cytotoxicity have led to improved understanding of this complex disease process. GVHD can be considered an exaggerated, undesirable manifestation of a normal inflammatory mechanism, in which donor lymphocytes encounter foreign antigens in an environment that fosters inflammation. Tissue injury related to the conditioning regimen or infection is then amplified by direct cytotoxicity via perforin-granzyme and Fas-FasL pathways, through direct cytokine-induced damage, and by recruitment of secondary effectors such as granulocytes and monocytes. Cytokine dysregulation may further result in the production of secondary mediators such as NO. The net effects of this complex system are the severe inflammatory manifestations that we recognize as clinical GVHD.

References

1. Billingham RE: The biology of graft-versus-host reactions. Harvey Lecture 62:21-78, 1966
2. Korngold R, Sprent J: T cell subsets in graft-vs.-host disease, in Burakoff SJ, Deeg HJ, Ferrara J (eds): Graft-vs.-Host Disease: Immunology, Pathophysiology, and Treatment. New York, NY, Dekker, 1990, pp 31-50
3. Kernan NA, Collins NH, Juliano L, Cartagena T, Dupont B, O'Reilly RJ: Clonable T lymphocytes in T cell-depleted bone marrow transplants correlate with development of graft-v-host disease. Blood 68:770-773, 1986
4. Zeng D, Lewis D, Dejbakhsh-Jones S, Lan F, Garcia-Ojeda M, Sibley R, et al: Bone marrow NK1.1(-) and NK1.1(+) T cells reciprocally regulate acute graft versus host disease. J Exp Med 189:1073-1081, 1999
5. Anderson KC.: Transfusion-associated graft-versus-host disease, in Ferrara JLM, Deeg HJ, Burakoff SJ (eds): Graft-vs.-Host Disease. New York, NY, Dekker, 1997, pp 587-605
6. Krensky AM, Weiss A, Crabtree G, Davis MM, Parham P: T-lymphocyte-antigen interactions in transplant rejection. N Engl J Med 322:510-517, 1990
7. Antin JH, Ferrara JLM: Cytokine dysregulation and acute graft-versus-host disease. Blood 80:2964-2968, 1992
8. Wang H, Clouthier S, Galchev V, Misek DE, Duffner U, Min CK, et al: Intact-protein based high-resolution three-dimensional quantitative analysis system for proteome profiling of biological fluids. Mol Cell Proteomics 4:618-625, 2005
9. Shlomchik WD, Couzens MS, Tang CB, McNiff J, Robert ME, Liu J, et al: Prevention of graft versus host disease by inactivation of host antigen-presenting cells. Science 285:412-415, 1999
10. Korngold R, Sprent J: Negative selection of T cells causing lethal graft-versus-host disease across minor histocompatibility barriers. Role of the H-2 complex. J Exp Med 151:1114-1124, 1980
11. Clift RA, Buckner CD, Appelbaum FR, Bearman SI, Petersen FB, Fisher LD, et al: Allogeneic marrow transplantation in patients with acute myeloid leukemia in first remission: A randomized trial of two irradiation regimens. Blood 76:1867-1871, 1990
12. Hill GR, Crawford JM, Cooke KR, Brinson YS, Pan L, Ferrara JL: Total body irradiation and acute graft-versus-host disease: The role of gastrointestinal damage and inflammatory cytokines. Blood 90:3204-3213, 1997
13. Dey BR, Yang YG, Szot GL, Pearson DA, Sykes M: Interleukin-12 inhibits graft-versus-host disease through an Fas-mediated mechanism associated with alterations in donor T-cell activation and expansion. Blood 91:3315-3322, 1998
14. Reddy P, Teshima T, Kukuruga M, Ordemann R, Liu C, Lowler K, et al: Interleukin-18 regulates acute graft-versus-host disease by enhancing Fas-mediated donor T cell apoptosis. J Exp Med 194:1433-1440, 2001
15. Teshima T, Reddy P, Lowler KP, KuKuruga MA, Liu C, Cooke KR, et al: Flt3 ligand therapy for recipients of allogeneic bone marrow transplants expands host CD8 alpha(+) dendritic cells and reduces experimental acute graft-versus-host disease. Blood 99:1825-1832, 2002
16. Matzinger P: The danger model: A renewed sense of self. Science 296: 301-305, 2002
17. Roncarolo MG, Levings MK, Traversari C: Differentiation of T regulatory cells by immature dendritic cells. J Exp Med 193:F5-F9, 2001
18. Reinhardt RL, Khoruts A, Merica R, Zell T, Jenkins MK: Visualizing the generation of memory CD4 T cells in the whole body. Nature 410:101-105, 2001
19. Ordemann R, Hutchinson R, Friedman J, Burakoff SJ, Reddy P, Duffner U: Enhanced allostimulatory activity of host antigen-presenting cells in old mice intensifies acute graft-versus-host disease. J Clin Invest 109: 1249-1256, 2002
20. Ruggeri L, Capanni M, Urbani E, Perruccio K, Shlomchik WD, Tosti A, et al: Effectiveness of donor natural killer cell alloreactivity in mismatched hematopoietic transplants. Science 295:2097-2100, 2002
21. Ruggeri L, Capanni M, Martelli MF, Velardi A: Cellular therapy: Exploiting NK cell alloreactivity in transplantation. Curr Opin Hematol 8:355-359, 2001
22. Sprent J, Schaefer M, Gao EK, Korngold R: Role of T cell subsets in lethal graft-versus-host disease (GVHD) directed to class I versus class II H-2 differences. I. L3T4+ cells can either augment or retard GVHD elicited by Lyt-2+ cells in class I different hosts. J Exp Med 167:556-569, 1988
23. Goulmy E, Schipper R, Pool J, Blokland E, Falkenburg JH, Vossen J, et al: Mismatches of minor histocompatibility antigens between HLA-identical donors and recipients and the development of graft-versus-host disease after bone marrow transplantation. N Engl J Med 334:281-285, 1996
24. Doolittle DP, Davisson MT, Guidi JN, Green MC: Catalog of mutant genes and polymorphic loci, in Lyon MF, Rastan S, Brown SDM (eds): Genetic Variants and Strains of the Laboratory Mouse (ed 3). Oxford, UK, Oxford University Press, 1996, pp 12-403
25. Hansen JA, Gooley TA, Martin PJ, Appelbaum F, Chauncey TR, Clift RA, et al: Bone marrow transplants from unrelated donors for patients with chronic myeloid leukemia. N Engl J Med 338:962-968, 1998
26. Mosmann TR, Cherwinski H, Bond MW, Giedlin MA, Coffman RL: Two types of murine helper T cell clone. I. Definition according to

profiles of lymphokine activities and secreted proteins. J Immunol 136:2348-2357, 1986

27. Ferrara JLM, Cooke KR, Pan L, Krenger W: The immunopathophysiology of acute graft-versus-host disease. Stem Cells 14:473-489, 1996
28. Herve P, Wijdenes J, Bergerat JP, Bordigoni P, Milpied N, Cahn JY, et al: Treatment of corticosteroid-resistant acute graft-versus-host disease by in vivo administration of anti-interleukin-2 receptor monoclonal antibody (B-B10). Blood 75:1017-1023, 1990
29. Belanger C, Esperou-Bourdeau H, Bordigoni P, Jouet JP, Souillet G, Milpied N, et al: Use of an anti-interleukin-2 receptor monoclonal antibody for GVHD prophylaxis in unrelated donor BMT. Bone Marrow Transplant 11:293-297, 1993
30. Kumaki S, Minegishi M, Fujie H, Sasahara Y, Ohashi Y, Tsuchiya S, et al: Prolonged secretion of IL-15 in patients with severe forms of acute graft-versus-host disease after allogeneic bone marrow transplantation in children. Int J Hematol 67:307-312, 1998
31. Dufour JH, Dziejman M, Liu MT, Leung JH, Lane TE, Luster AD: IFN-gamma-inducible protein 10 (IP-10; CXCL10)-deficient mice reveal a role for IP-10 in effector T cell generation and trafficking. J Immunol 168:3195-3204, 2002
32. Mohan K, Ding Z, Hanly J, Issekutz TB: IFN-gamma-inducible T cell alpha chemoattractant is a potent stimulator of normal human blood T lymphocyte transendothelial migration: Differential regulation by IFN-gamma and TNF-alpha. J Immunol 168:6420-6428, 2002
33. Mowat A: Antibodies to IFN-gamma prevent immunological mediated intestinal damage in murine graft-versus-host reactions. Immunology 68:18-24, 1989
34. Dickinson AM, Sviland L, Dunn J, Carey P, Proctor SJ: Demonstration of direct involvement of cytokines in graft-versus-host reactions using an in vitro skin explant model. Bone Marrow Transplant 7:209-216, 1991
35. Klimpel GR, Annable CR, Cleveland MG, Jerrells TR, Patterson JC: Immunosuppression and lymphoid hypoplasia associated with chronic graft-versus-host disease is dependent upon IFN-g production. J Immunol 144:84-93, 1990
36. Krenger W, Falzarano G, Delmonte J Jr, Snyder KM, Byon JC, Ferrara JL: Interferon-g suppresses T-cell proliferation to mitogen via the nitric oxide pathway during experimental acute graft-versus-host disease. Blood 88:1113-1121, 1996
37. Nestel FP, Price KS, Seemayer TA, Lapp WS: Macrophage priming and lipopolysaccharide-triggered release of tumor necrosis factor alpha during graft-versus-host disease. J Exp Med 175:405-413, 1992
38. Haskill S, Martin G, Van Le L, Morris J, Peace A, Bigler CF: cDNA cloning of an intracellular form of the human interleukin-1 receptor antagonist associated with epithelium. Proc Natl Acad Sci USA 88: 3681-3685, 1991
39. Eberl G, MacDonald HR: Rapid death and regeneration of NKT cells in anti-CD3epsilon- or IL-12-treated mice: A major role for bone marrow in NKT cell homeostasis. Immunity 9:345-353, 1998
40. Kagi D, Vignaux F, Ledermann B, Burki K, Depraetere V, Nagata S, et al: Fas and perforin pathways as major mechanisms of T cell-mediated cytotoxicity. Science 265:528-530, 1994
41. Lowin B, Hahne M, Mattmann C, Tschopp J: Cytolytic T-cell cytotoxicity is mediated through perforin and Fas lytic pathways. Nature 370: 650-652, 1994
42. Krammer PH: CD95's deadly mission in the immune system. Nature 407:789-795, 2000
43. Aggarwal BB: Signalling pathways of the TNF superfamily: A double-edged sword. Nat Rev Immunol 3:745-756, 2003
44. Kondo T, Suda T, Fukuyama H, Adachi M, Nagata S: Essential roles of the Fas ligand in the development of hepatitis. Nat Med 4:409-413, 1997
45. Teshima T, Ordemann R, Reddy P, Gagin S, Liu C, Cooke KR, et al: Acute graft-versus-host disease does not require alloantigen expression on host epithelium. Nat Med 8:575-581, 2002
46. Piguet PF, Grau GE, Allet B, Vassalli P: Tumor necrosis factor/cachectin is an effector of skin and gut lesions of the acute phase of graft-versus-host disease. J Exp Med 166:1280-1289, 1987
47. Herve P, Flesch M, Tiberghien P, Wijdenes J, Racadot E, Bordigoni P, et al: Phase I-II trial of a monoclonal anti-tumor necrosis factor alpha antibody for the treatment of refractory severe acute graft-versus-host disease. Blood 79:3362-3368, 1992
48. Hattori K, Hirano T, Miyajima H, Yamakawa N, Tateno M, Oshimi K, et al: Differential effects of anti-Fas ligand and anti-tumor necrosis factor-alpha antibodies on acute graft-versus-host disease pathologies. Blood 91:4051-4055, 1998
49. Cooke KR, Hill GR, Gerbitz A, Kobzik L, Martin TR, Crawford JM, et al: Tumor necrosis factor-alpha neutralization reduces lung injury after experimental allogeneic bone marrow transplantation. Transplantation 70:272-279, 2000
50. Pan G, O'Rourke K, Chinnaiyan AM, Gentz R, Ebner R, Ni J, et al: The receptor for the cytotoxic ligand TRAIL. Science 276:111-113, 1997
51. Cooke KR, Hill G, Crawford JM, Bungard D, Brinson YS, Delmonte J Jr, et al: Tumor necrosis factor-a production to lipopolysaccharide stimulation by donor cells predicts the severity of experimental acute graft versus host disease. J Clin Invest 102:1882-1891, 1998
52. Hill G, Ferrara J: The primacy of the gastrointestinal tract as a target organ of acute graft-versus-host disease: Rationale for the use of cytokine shields in allogeneic bone marrow transplantation. Blood 95: 2754-2759, 2000
53. Fegan C, Poynton CH, Whittaker JA: The gut mucosal barrier in bone marrow transplantation. Bone Marrow Transplant 5:373-377, 1990
54. Storb R, Prentice RL, Buckner CD, Clift RA, Appelbaum F, Deeg J, et al: Graft-versus-host disease and survival in patients with aplastic anemia treated by marrow grafts from HLA-identical siblings. Beneficial effect of a protective environment. N Engl J Med 308:302-307, 1983
55. Beelen DW, Elmaagacli A, Muller KD, Hirche H, Schaefer UW: Influence of intestinal bacterial decontamination using metronidazole and ciprofloxacin or ciprofloxacin alone on the development of acute graft-versus-host disease after marrow transplantation in patients with hematologic malignancies: Final results and long term follow-up of an open-label prospective randomized trial. Blood 93:3267-3275, 1999
56. Moser B, Loetscher P: Lymphocyte traffic control by chemokines. Nat Immunol 2:123-128, 2001
57. Sallusto F, Lenig D, Forster R, Lipp M, Lanzaveccia A: Two subsets of memory T lymphocytes with distinct homing potentials and effector functions. Nature 401:708-712, 1999
58. Murai M, Yoneyama H, Harada A, Yi Z, Vestergaard C, Guo B, et al: Active participation of CCR5(+)CD8(+) T lymphocytes in the pathogenesis of liver injury in graft-versus-host disease. J Clin Invest 104:49-57, 1999
59. Panoskaltsis-Mortari A, Strieter RM, Hermanson JR, Fegeding KV, Murphy WJ, Farrell CL, et al: Induction of monocyte- and T-cell-attracting chemokines in the lung during the generation of idiopathic pneumonia syndrome following allogeneic murine bone marrow transplantation. Blood 96:834-839, 2000
60. Schnare M, Barton GM, Holt AC, Takeda K, Akira S, Medzhitov R: Toll-like receptors control activation of adaptive immune responses. Nat Immunol 2:947-950, 2001
61. Aversa F, Tabilio A, Velardi A, Cunningham I, Terenzi A, Falzette F, et al: Treatment of high-risk acute leukemia with T-cell-depleted stem cells from related donors with one fully mismatched HLA haplotype. N Engl J Med 339:1186-1193, 1998
62. Martin P, Schoch G, Fisher L, Byers V, Anasetti C, Appelbaum FR, et al: A retrospective analysis of therapy for acute graft-versus-host diesase: Initial Treatment. Blood 76:1464-1472, 1990
63. Cragg L, Blazar BR, Defor T, Kolatker N, Miller W, Kersey J, et al: A randomized trial comparing prednisone with antithymocyte globulin/prednisone as an initial systemic therapy for moderately severe acute graft-versus-host disease. Biol Blood Marrow Transplant 6:441-447, 2000
64. Antin J.H, Weisdorf D, Neuberg D, Nixklow R, Clouthier S, Lee SJ, et al: Interleukin-1 blockade does not prevent acute graft-versus-host disease: results of a randomized, double-blind, placebo-controlled trial of interleukin-1 receptor antagonist in allogeneic bone marrow transplantation. Blood 100:3479-3482, 2002
65. Storb R, Deeg HJ, Pepe M, Appelbaum F, Anasetti C, Beatty P, et al: Methotrexate and cyclosporine versus cyclosporine alone for prophy-

laxis of graft-versus-host disease in patients given HLA-identical marrow grafts for leukemia: Long-term follow-up of a controlled trial. Blood 73:1729-1734, 1989
66. Allison AC, Eugui EM: Mycophenolate mofetil and its mechanisms of action. Immunopharmacology 47:85-118, 2000
67. van Bekkum DW, Roodenburg J, Heidt PJ, van der Waaij D: Mitigation of secondary disease of allogeneic mouse radiation chimeras by modification of the intestinal microflora. J Natl Cancer Inst 52:401-404, 1974
68. Holler E, Kolb HJ, Moller A, Kempeni J, Liesenfeld S, Pechumer H, et al: Increased serum levels of tumor necrosis factor alpha precede major complications of bone marrow transplantation. Blood 75:1011-1016, 1990
69. Huang XJ, Wan J, Lu DP: Serum TNF alpha levels in patients with acute graft-versus-host disease after bone marrow transplantation. Leukemia 15:1089-1091, 2001
70. Holler E, Kolb HJ, Mittermueller J, Kaul M, Ledderose G, Duell T, et al: Modulation of acute graft-versus-host disease after allogeneic bone marrow transplantation by tumor necrosis factor alpha (TNFalpha) release in the course of pretransplant conditioning: Role of conditioning regimens and prophylactic application of a monoclonal antibody neutralizing human TNFalpha (MAK 195F). Blood 86:890-899, 1995
71. Kobbe G, Schneider P, Rohr U, Fenk R, Neumann F, Aivado M, et al: Treatment of severe steroid refractory acute graft-versus-host disease with infliximab, a chimeric human/mouse antiTNFalpha antibody. Bone Marrow Transplant 28:47-49, 2001
72. Dinarello CA: Interleukin-1 and interleukin-1 antagonism. Blood 77: 1627-1652, 1991
73. Abhyankar S, Gilliland DG, Ferrara JLM: Interleukin 1 is a critical effector molecule during cytokine dysregulation in graft-versus-host disease to minor histocompatibility antigens. Transplantation 56:1518-1523, 1993
74. Cullup H, Dickinson AM, Jackson GH, Taylor PR, Cavet J, Middleton PG: Donor interleukin 1 receptor antagonist genotype associated with acute graft-versus-host disease in human leucocyte antigen-matched sibling allogeneic transplants. Br J Haematol 113:807-813, 2001
75. McCarthy PL Jr, Abhyankar S, Neben S, Newman G, Sieff C, Thompson RC, et al: Inhibition of interleukin-1 by an interleukin-1 receptor antagonist prevents graft-versus-host disease. Blood 78:1915-1918, 1991
76. Hill GR, Cooke KR, Teshima T, Crawford JM, Keith JC Jr, Brinson YS, et al: Interleukin-11 promotes T cell polarization and prevents acute graft-versus-host disease after allogeneic bone marrow transplantation. J Clin Invest 102:115-123, 1998
77. Antin JH, Lee SJ, Neuberg D, Alyea E, Soiffer RJ, Sonis S, et al: A phase I/II double-blind, placebo-controlled study of recombinant human interleukin-11 for mucositis and acute GVHD prevention in allogeneic stem cell transplantation. Bone Marrow Transplant 29:373-377, 2002
78. Symington FW, Symington BE, Liu PY, Viguet H, Santhanam U, Sehgal PB: The relationship of serum IL-6 levels to acute graft-versus-host disease and hepatorenal disease after human bone marrow transplantation. Transplantation 54:457-462, 1992
79. Rabinowitz J, Petros WP, Stuart AR, Peters WP: Characterization of endogenous cytokine concentrations after high-dose chemotherapy with autologous bone marrow support. Blood 81:2452-2459, 1993
80. Uguccioni M, Meliconi R, Nesci S, Lucarelli G, Ceska M, Gasbarrini G, et al: Elevated interleukin-8 serum concentrations in beta-thalassemia and graft-versus-host disease. Blood 81:2252-2256, 1993

ELSEVIER

Seminars in HEMATOLOGY

Genetics of Risk Factors for Graft-Versus-Host Disease

Effie W. Petersdorf[a,b] and Mari Malkki[b]

Modern understanding of the genetic basis of graft-versus-host disease (GVHD) in allogeneic hematopoietic stem cell transplantation (HSCT) involves knowledge of human leukocyte antigen (HLA), killer immunoglobulin-like receptors (KIR), cytokine genes, and their interactions. Insights into the immunogenetic basis of GVHD come from long-standing clinical experience in the use of myeloablative conditioning regimens and donor bone marrow as the grafting source. Under these circumstances, donor T-cell recognition of host HLA can cause GVHD. The recent elucidation of HLA class I as ligands for natural killer (NK) cell inhibitory KIR demonstrates that GVHD is the result of a complex interplay between the innate and adaptive immune responses. The extent to which T cells and NK cells contribute to clinical GVHD is a function of the host post-conditioning environment, immunosuppressive treatments, and the content of the graft source. The contribution of donor and host genetic differences in cytokine genes in modulating risks of GVHD has recently been recognized.
Semin Hematol 43:11-23

At the core of the immunogenetic basis for graft-versus-host disease (GVHD) is the diversity of human leukocyte antigen (HLA), killer immunoglobulin-like receptors (KIR), and cytokine genes. In the DNA era, the elucidation of the polymorphism of the HLA system has had implications to the study of the "HLA barrier" in transplantation. The mapping to chromosome 19 of the KIR family of natural killer (NK) receptors has now reformed the concepts underlying host-versus-graft and graft-versus-host allorecognition. The relevance of sequence polymorphism in donor and recipient cytokine genes in inducing and augmenting clinical GVHD has direct relevance to clinical results of related and unrelated transplantation. This review will describe the role of HLA, KIR and cytokine gene polymorphisms in the risk of GVHD after allogeneic hematopoietic stem cell transplantation (HSCT). Since a summary of the vast literature in this field is beyond the scope of this review, the selected clinical studies from recent publications presented must necessarily describe patients and donors from ethnically diverse populations, and a spectrum of transplant conditioning and immunosuppressive regimens.

The HLA Barrier

The major histocompatibility complex (MHC) is the most comprehensively studied multi-megabase region of the human genome. Interest in the MHC has been motivated by its biomedical importance in transplantation, autoimmunity, and infectious diseases. More than 421 loci are now identified within the 7.6 Mb extended MHC region, an estimated 40% of which are involved in immune function, including inflammation, leukocyte maturation, complement cascade, nonclassical class I, immunoregulation, stress response, and the immunoglobulin superfamily. Of the 252 expressed genes, more than 20% reside within the class III region, making this the densest region in the entire human genome. As transplantation determinants, HLA-A, -B, -C, -DR, -DQ, and -DP control T-cell recognition and determine histocompatibility. A hallmark of HLA genes is their extensive polymorphism[1] and the high degree of nonrandom association of alleles at two or more HLA loci, a phenomenon termed "linkage disequilibrium."[2]

Unrelated donor transplantation is an acceptable treatment for patients who do not have a matched donor in the

[a]Department of Medicine, University of Washington, Seattle, WA.
[b]Division of Clinical Research, Fred Hutchinson Cancer Research Center, Seattle, WA.
E.W.P. is supported by Grants No. CA18029, CA100019, CA15704, AI33484, and AI49213 from the National Institutes of Health (NIH). M.M. is supported by CA18029, AI33484, and AI49213 from the NIH and by the Amy Strelzer Manasevit Scholars Program from the National Marrow Donor Program (NMDP).
Address correspondence to Effie W. Petersdorf, MD, Professor of Medicine, University of Washington, Member, Fred Hutchinson Cancer Research Center, Division of Clinical Research, 1100 Fairview Ave North, D4-100, Seattle, WA 98109. E-mail: epetersd@fhcrc.org

0037-1963/06/$-see front matter
doi:10.1053/j.seminhematol.2005.09.002

Table 1 Paradigm for Donor HLA Matching and GVHD Risk in Unrelated Donor HSCT

Effect	Observations	References
Tally	Multiple class I mismatches increase GVHD risk	4-6,15
	Multiple class II mismatches increase GVHD risk	5,7,9,10
	Combined class I and II mismatches increased GVHD risk	4-6
Class	Class I mismatching is a risk factor for GVHD	4,6,8,15
	Class II mismatching is a risk factor for GVHD	5,7,11,13,17,23
Allele and antigen	Antigen mismatches confer higher risks than allele mismatches	15
Epitope	Sequence of coding region defines GVHD risk	8,24

family.[3-18] In unrelated donors, use of an HLA allele-matched donor can offer comparable disease-free survival (DFS) compared to a haploidentical mismatched related donor for certain good-risk patients.[14,19,20] Methodologic advances in tissue typing have revolutionized HLA in its applications to transplantation. Polymerase chain reaction (PCR)-based technology has provided the tools needed to elucidate the clinical importance of HLA-A, -B, -C, -DRB1, -DQB1, and -DPB1 genes in unrelated HSCT. In general, (1) high-resolution (allele) DNA typing methods can uncover functionally relevant transplant determinants, and therefore these methods are required for donor evaluation[6,15,17]; (2) the risks of graft rejection, GVHD, and mortality are increased with increasing numbers of HLA mismatches, and therefore selection of the donor with the fewest mismatches may reduce complications[4-6,15]; (3) the risks of graft rejection, GVHD, and mortality may be greater with mismatches detectable by low-level (antigen) resolution techniques than for mismatches only detectable by high-resolution methods, and therefore allele-mismatched donors should be prioritized over antigen-mismatched donors[15] (Table 1). These concepts provide an approach for the selection of an optimal unrelated donor. When we cannot identify well-matched donors, identification of permissive locus- and allele-specific mismatches should enable more patients to benefit from unrelated HSCT.

Large-Scale Analyses of High-Resolution Donor Matching in Unrelated HSCT

The largest comprehensive analysis of donor-recipient low-resolution (antigen) and high-resolution (allele) HLA matching to date was performed by the NMDP in 1,874 transplants.[15] Three major findings emerged from the National Marrow Donor Program (NMDP) study. First, mismatches at HLA-A, -B, -C, and -DRB1 each had a statistically significantly increased risk of mortality when compared to patients matched at the appropriate locus, after adjusting for a variety of demographic factors (including disease stage). Compared to patients matched for DQB1, patients mismatched at DQB1 had a similar hazard of mortality; no increase in adverse events was associated with DPB mismatching. Second, allele mismatches at each of HLA-A, -B, -C, and -DRB1 were less detrimental when compared to patients matched at the appropriate antigen for mortality, suggesting that antigen mismatches confer a higher risk of mortality than do allele mismatches. However, definitive conclusions are difficult due to the relatively small numbers in the various groups. Third, when compared to HLA-A, HLA-B antigen-matched, and HLA-DRB1–matched patients, those with an allele mismatch at HLA-A or -B or any mismatch at HLA-C had poorer survival and a higher incidence of acute GVHD.

A recent single center study approached the analysis of HLA and the impact of mismatching on outcome differently than did the NMDP.[17] The impact of a mismatch on outcome depended on severity of disease, and the impact of a mismatch at a specific locus depended on the total number of mismatches. Due to the latter observation, initial analyses were focused on single mismatches. Among patients considered to have low-risk disease (chronic-phase chronic myelogenous leukemia [CML] transplanted within 2 years of diagnosis), patients with a single mismatch had a higher hazard compared to patients matched at HLA-A, -B, -C, -DRB1, and -DQB1, while the impact of a single mismatch among patients with higher risk disease (all other stages of CML; acute leukemia, myelodysplastic syndrome [MDS]) was minimal.

A second observation from the Seattle study was that single antigen mismatches did not appear to confer a higher risk of mortality compared to single allele mismatches. Although the number of locus-specific mismatches was small in the two disease risk groups, single mismatches among the low-risk group were associated with an increased hazard of mortality for each locus, as compared to matching for 10 alleles at HLA-A, -B, -C, -DRB1,and -DQB1 (10/10 matches). In particular, there was a statistically significant increased risk associated with single allele mismatches at HLA-C. The impact of a single mismatch among the patients with higher risk disease was minimal for each locus, with the possible exception of HLA-C. The number of mismatches at HLA-C was sufficiently small that this question warrants further study. Lastly, among patients with multiple mismatches (both low-risk and higher risk), those involving a particular locus had similar hazards of death compared to those not involving that locus, this observation holding for HLA-A, -B, -C, and -DRB1. Multiple mismatches involving DQB1, however, had a hazard 1.50 times that of patients with multiple mismatches that did not involve DQB1.

Conclusions drawn from the NMDP and Seattle studies are seemingly contradictory in some respects. However, because each study made different assumptions, it is not possible to directly compare their results and conclusions. The NMDP analysis was conducted among all patients, regardless of disease risk and level of HLA matching; each of these factors was included in the multivariable regression models, with other factors; implicit is the assumption that the impact of a mismatch at a particular locus is the same across all levels of disease risk and HLA mismatching. Because the Seattle analysis suggested that this assumption is not necessarily true, antigen versus allele mismatches were compared among single mismatches and separately according to disease. Taken together, the question of the impact of locus-specific mismatches is still unresolved. Furthermore, whether single mismatches lead to similar outcome compared to 10/10 allele matches among patients with higher risk disease requires further exploration.

The studies described above demonstrate that HLA matching can diminish the early risks of acute GVHD. Complete and precise donor matching has also been shown to lower risks of late GVHD events,[21,22] including a higher rate of discontinuation of immunosuppressive therapy in HLA-matched transplants and less prolonged treatment compared to HLA mismatching. Therefore, prospective efforts to match donors should translate to improved outcome from both lowered early and late complications.

The risk of acute GVHD is increased with donor-recipient mismatching for HLA-A, -B, -C, and -DRB1. The relevance of HLA-DQ and HLA-DP mismatching to GVHD is less clear.[5,6,10-13,15,23,34] In the case of HLA-DQ, the strong linkage disequilibrium between HLA-DR and HLA-DQ yields few HLA-DRB1–matched donor-recipient pairs with a single HLA-DQ mismatch. The converse is observed at HLA-DP, where the relatively weak degree of linkage disequilibrium yields match:mismatch ratios that are 20:80 in most populations tested.[6,10,15] Given the low probability of successful matching at the HLA-DP locus, the practical approach would be to define the rules that govern acceptable HLA-DP mismatches.

As described above for HLA-A, -B, and -DRB1, various studies have asked different questions and employed different study design to measure independent effects contributed by HLA-DQ and HLA-DP. In the NMDP study, risks associated with HLA-DQ mismatching were measured among all pairs with an HLA-DQ mismatch.[15] This population was then divided into those pairs that were class I–matched and a second group that was class I–mismatched. There were no significant differences in risk of GVHD between the two groups. Another question was addressed in the Seattle study[17]: whether patients with HLA-DQ mismatching, in addition to mismatching at other HLA loci, had increased GVHD and mortality as compared to patients with multi-locus mismatches not involving HLA-DQ. A population of multi-locus mismatched pairs was divided into pairs that had an HLA-DQ mismatch and pairs that did not. Compared to pairs that did not have an HLA-DQ mismatch, the HLA-DQ–mismatched pairs had an increased hazard ratio of mortality. These data suggest a trend for an additive HLA-DQ effect when there is additional HLA mismatching at other loci; one inference is that selection of an HLA-DQB1–matched donor over a mismatched donor may lower post-transplant complications for patients who only have multi-locus donors from which to chose. Similar approaches have been used to study GVHD risk associated with HLA-DP mismatching. Comparing patients with an HLA-DP mismatch to those without a mismatch, and controlling for other HLA mismatches,[4,6,15] there was no increased GVHD risk associated with HLA-DP mismatching. Other studies have examined HLA-DP among pairs matched for all other HLA genes[10,13,16,23] and have measured independent effects conferred by HLA-DP on GVHD and survival.

Additive Effects of Multiple Mismatches

The total number of HLA mismatches on transplant outcome is an important predictor of risk[4-6,15] (Table 1). Mismatching for HLA-A, -B, and/or -C within class I, HLA-DR, -DQ, and/or -DP within class II, as well as the combination of class I and class II mismatches, have additive and synergistic effects that can be appreciated at a single locus. Mismatching for both determinants at a locus can amplify the risk of GVHD.[10]

HLA Factors That Govern Permissibility of Mismatches

Nucleotide substitutions that define unique HLA class I and II alleles are concentrated at residues that result in a change in the protein sequence, and which contact either bound peptide or the T-cell receptor (TCR)[2] (Table 1). Increased risk of acute GVHD and mortality is associated with donor mismatching for residue 116 of class I (predicted to participate in peptide binding at P9).[8] Recently, functional epitopes of the HLA-DP molecule have been described.[24] Although these observations suggest that mismatching for residues that contact the bound peptide or the TCR are associated with increased transplant complications, more data are needed to determine the rules that govern acceptable mismatches.

One strategy to understand the clinical ramifications of HLA diversity on function has been to examine a wide array of HLA allele and antigen mismatches in racially diverse transplant populations (www.ihwg.org). An analysis by the International Histocompatibility Working Group (IHWG) in HSCT of 2,399 unrelated transplants from North America, Europe, Asia, and Australia has enabled testing of the hypothesis that permissibility of HLA mismatches is in part governed by the locus and the combination of mismatched alleles or antigens.[25] An increased hazard of death was associated with the number of mismatched alleles compared to 10/10 allele matches, regardless of the race or ethnicity of the recipient or donor. Locus-specific effects on mortality were examined for transplant pairs with a single HLA mismatch. Among Caucasian recipients, the presence of a single HLA-C mismatch conferred an increased hazards ratio of mortality compared to matching, whereas an HLA-A mismatch was not associated with a statistically significant increase in risk. In contrast, Japanese recipients had an increased risk of mortality associated with an HLA-A mismatch but not with HLA-C mismatching. Examination of the specific HLA-A and HLA-C mismatch combinations represented in the Japanese and Caucasian recipients and donors revealed major differences between the allele combinations mismatched for a given antigen. Similar findings at each HLA locus were uncovered, indicating that the study of permissible mismatches will require large numbers of ethnically and racially diverse transplant populations who have been characterized at high genetic resolution.

Locus-specific and antigen-specific differences may affect whether certain combinations of mismatches are permissible. Consideration for the specific residues of the HLA molecule that are known to influence the peptide binding repertoire or that contact the TCR represents a different level of discrimination of mismatches. For this purpose, a very large number of HLA allele-typed donor-recipient pairs is needed due to the extreme diversity of HLA alleles and the sharing of common epitopes.[8] Permissible epitopes have been sought in functional assays.[26] Most recently, alloreactive cytotoxic T lymphocytes against epitopes of the HLA-DP molecule have been used to test the hypothesis that mismatching at certain residues confers a greater risk of GVHD and mortality.[24] The evaluation of permissible HLA mismatches must take a multipronged approach to understand how the sequence motifs relate to functional differences among HLA allotypes at a given locus, and HLA loci.

HLA Mismatching in Nonmyeloablative HSCT

The extensive experience in myeloablative unrelated HSCT donor HLA matching has also provided donor selection criteria for nonmyeloablative transplant regimens. However, the impact of donor-recipient HLA mismatching in nonmyeloablative HSCT is largely unknown. In a series of 52 patients receiving a fludarabine/low-dose total body irradiation (TBI) conditioning regimen, an association between class I mismatching and risk of severe acute GVHD was present.[27]

Nongenetic Factors That Impact Permissibility of HLA Mismatching

Many nongenetic factors influence transplant outcome.[3,28] Understanding the risks associated with them is important in the interpretation of HLA effects. One of the most significant predictors of transplant outcome is the stage of the underlying malignancy at the time of transplantation.[3,4] Transplantation during active or advanced stages of malignancy has a higher likelihood of post-transplant disease recurrence compared to disease that is well controlled prior to transplantation. For advanced or active malignancy, a prolonged donor search may increase the time during which the disease may advance—a situation faced by patients who do not have common HLA phenotypes or haplotypes.[29] For this group, whether the potential gain of extending a search for a fully compatible donor offsets the harm of lengthening the time from diagnosis to transplantation remains to be determined. If the donor search is extended, the four possible outcomes are: 1) a better matched donor is identified and the disease remains stable; (2) a better matched donor is identified, but the disease advances; (3) a better matched donor is not identified, but the disease remains stable; and (4) a better matched donor is not identified and the disease progresses. The clinical outcomes of patients receiving an unrelated donor transplant for CML in the Seattle program were compared.[17] In brief, the overall survival of a patient receiving a transplant in early chronic phase from a mismatched donor was similar to the survival of patients transplanted in late chronic phase from an HLA-identical donor, suggesting that the potential benefit of HLA matching was indeed reduced by the negative impact of proression. If a donor search for a patient in late chronic phase was extended in the hope of identifying a matched donor, survival using an HLA-matched donor in late chronic phase was similar to that using an HLA-mismatched donor in late chronic phase. If a matched donor was identified, but the disease progressed beyond CP, survival was lower; if a matched donor could not be identified, and transplantation was conducted using a mismatched donor in late CP, survival was similarly compromised. These results suggest that when a donor search is highly unlikely to yield matched donors for newly diagnosed CML, the increased mortality associated with a longer time interval from diagnosis to transplantation must be carefully weighed against the increased mortality with earlier transplantation with a mismatched donor, and also against the probability of disease progression to advanced-phase CML during the time required to perform a donor search. Similar information on the impact of disease stage and permissibility of donor mismatching is needed for other diagnoses.

Role of HLA in Cord Blood Transplantation

To date, the studies described above indicate the importance of HLA genes in the standard myeloablative conditioning and donor bone marrow or peripheral blood stem cells (PBSC) transplantation. Under these conditions, the presence of donor-recipient mismatching is associated with increased risk of acute and chronic GVHD and mortality. These risks are increased with multiple HLA mismatches. For the majority of patients who lack HLA-matched unrelated donors, options include extending the search in the hope of identifying a better matched donor. However, as described above, prolongation of the search may delay transplantation and allow the disease to advance. The use of human cord blood as a source of hematopoietic stem cells provides patients who lack unrelated donors an alternative for transplantation with low risk of severe GVHD despite a higher degree of HLA disparity. In addition to the advantages of higher tolerability of HLA mismatching, cord blood units are associated with lower risks of transmission of cytomegalovirus and other viruses. Cord blood units are readily available. For these reasons, cord blood as a source of stem cells is particularly attractive for patients with higher risk or advanced disease in whom earlier transplantation is advisable.[30] The first successful cord blood transplant was performed in 1988 for a child with Fanconi anemia[31] and demonstrated that a single cord blood unit could successfully engraft. Wider application of cord blood transplant in children and adults for malignant and nonmalignant blood disorders followed.[32-36]

Because few patients have cord blood from an HLA-identical sibling, cord blood transplantation is mainly performed from unrelated donors. There is a lower incidence and rate of severity of acute and chronic GVHD from an unrelated cord blood donor donor compared to use of an HLA-matched unrelated donor bone marrow or haploidentical related family member.[32-34] In pediatrics, the incidence of grades II to IV acute GVHD ranges from 33% to 44%, grades III to IV from 11% to 22%, and chronic GVHD from 0% to 25%; GVHD in adult unrelated cord blood transplants is more consistent, with a 40% to 60%, 20% to 22%, and 26% to 90% incidence, respectively.

Cell dose correlates with the probability and speed of neutrophil and platelet recovery, and is the single most important factor associated with optimal cord blood transplant outcome.[33,34,37] The role of donor HLA mismatching in cord blood transplant is more difficult to analyze than in unrelated bone marrow transplantation, because allele level typing of cord blood units for HLA-A, -B, -C, -DRB1, and -DQB1 is not routine. The standard for HLA typing of cord blood units considers serologic-level discrimination of HLA-A and -B gene products, and HLA-DRB1 molecular typing. With this level of HLA resolution, comparison of unrelated cord blood and unrelated bone marrow/PBSC demonstrates that higher degrees of HLA disparity are tolerable with cord blood transplantation. Unlike the unrelated donor bone marrow/PBSC transplant, in the majority of cord blood studies there is a less dramatic association between HLA mismatching and risk of GVHD[32,34,35]; however, HLA disparity is an independent predictor of transplant-related mortality and survival.[33,34]

The total number of HLA disparities between recipient and the cord blood unit correlates with risk of acute GVHD.[33,37,38] Transplant-related events are associated with underlying disease, patient age, cell dose of the graft, and degree of HLA mismatching in the cord blood unit.[33] The frequency of severe acute GVHD was lower in patients transplanted from 6/6 antigen-matched units. Multivariate analysis for GVHD demonstrated trends for significant risks conferred by HLA mismatching (0 *v* 1 or more antigen mismatches). In a more recent update, the incidence of grades III to IV acute GVHD was found to increase with increasing numbers of mismatched HLA antigens: 8%, 19%, and 28% with 0, 1, and 2 or more antigen mismatches, respectively ($P = .006$).[38]

Pronounced effects of multi-locus HLA mismatching have been described in the Eurocord experience of 550 unrelated cord blood transplants for children and adults younger than 21 years for acute myeloid leukemia (AML), acute lymphoid leukemia (ALL), chronic leukemia, lymphoma, and meylodysplastic syndrome.[37] In this study, HLA matching was defined by serology for HLA-A and -B and for HLA-DRB1 by DNA, and ranged from 1, 2, 3, or 4 mismatches. Both the number and type of HLA mismatches correlated with engraftment, GVHD, and relapse, but not with transplant-related mortality or survival. Although neither the number of HLA mismatches nor the number of $CD34^+$ cells infused correlated with risk of grades II to IV acute GVHD, the presence of both a class I and a class II mismatch, with a high $CD34^+$ cell dose in the graft, was associated with severe grades III to IV acute GVHD. A higher number of HLA mismatches was associated with lower hazard of relapse, indicating a potential graft-versus-leukemia effect in patients receiving HLA-mismatched cord blood transplants. Although acute GVHD was not associated with HLA match status or class of disparity, in another study multivariate analysis demonstrated that the presence of HLA mismatching with low $CD34^+$ cell dose and grades III to IV acute GVHD correlated with lowered survival.[34]

At the Interface Between HLA and KIR Genetics: The Role of NK Inhibitory Receptors and Their Ligands in Clinical Transplantation

The recognition of the relationship between HLA class I alloantigens and the NK cell KIR receptors was an important advance in immunology. Since the first demonstration that NK cells can be activated by the downregulation of self HLA antigens on target cells in a model known as "missing self," the KIR family of receptors has been most comprehensively studied.[39-41] Encoded on chromosome 19q13.4, a total of 16 KIR genes have been mapped, and they show extensive allelic and haplotypic diversity.[39,40] The most functionally relevant difference between KIR haplotypes is the number of activating and inhibitory genes[39,41] and lower GVHD risk has been attributed to donor inhibitory KIR alloreactivity. Nine inhibitory receptors have thus far been described; of these, KIR2DL1, 2DL2, 2DL3, and 3DL1 are the best studied with respect to their known HLA ligand. HLA class I gene products serve as the ligands for the KIR2DL1, 2DL2, and 2DL3 receptors.[42] Receptor-ligand specificity is governed by residues 77 and 80 of HLA-C and by the HLA-Bw4 epitope present on some HLA-B and -A molecules.[39,41] Most individuals have the full complement of inhibitory KIRs that recognize HLA-C group 1, group 2, and Bw4 ligands.[39,41]

Two models have been proposed for HLA-KIR allorecognition by donor NK cells following HSCT: the "mismatched ligand" model and the "missing ligand" model (Table 2). Both models are supported by clinical observations, albeit in patients receiving very different transplant and immunosuppressive regimens. Analysis of outcome after haploidentical transplantation with ex vivo T-cell depletion and infusion of very large doses of donor stem cells has been the basis of the mismatched ligand model. Donor-recipient ligand disparity leads to release of donor NK inhibition and subsequent killing of host cells, including residual leukemic cells (resulting in a lowered rate of relapse) and antigen-presenting cells (lower GVHD).[43,44] Furthermore, donor alloreactive NK clones were identified only from patients who were HLA class

Table 2 HLA-KIR Models in Transplantation

Model	Mechanism of NK Cell Alloreactivity	Examples of Release of NK Cell Inhibition and Target Cell Cytotoxicity		References
		Recipient	Donor	
Mismatched ligand	Donor NK cells recognize recipient target cells that lack the class I allotype present in the donor	C1,Bw4 C2,C2,Bw4,Bw6	C1,C2,Bw4,Bw6* C1,C2,Bw6†	43-51
Missing ligand	Donor NK cell inhibition is released when host cells lack the correct HLA ligand to provide the inhibitory signal	C1,Bw4 C2,Bw6	KIR2DL1; C1,Bw4‡ KIR2DL2/3DL1;C1,Bw6§	52,53,54

Abbreviations: C1, HLA-C group 1 allotypes: KIR2DL2 and 2DL3 receptors recognize Ser77 and Asn80; C2, HLA-C group 2 allotypes: KIR2DL1 receptor recognize HLA-C allotypes encoding Asn77 and Lys80; Bw4: the inhibitory receptor KIR3DL1 recognizes the HLA-Bw4 epitope expressed on certain HLA-B and HLA-A molecules.
*Patient is missing the HLA-C group 2 ligand for donor KIR.
†Donor is missing the HLA-Bw4 ligand present in the recipient.
‡Patient is missing the HLA-C group 2 ligand for KIR2DL1 receptor in the donor.
§Patient is missing both the HLA-C group 1 and the Bw4 ligands for the KIR2DL2 and KIR3DL1 receptors in the donor.

I–mismatched for the ligand present in their donor, and not in patients who were matched; NK lysis of Epstein-Barr virus–transformed B-cell lines and phytohemagglutinin-stimulated recipient target cells could be blocked by target cells expressing the missing ligand.[45] These clinical observations were supported by independent studies of related and unrelated donor transplants, in which donor-recipient ligand disparity was associated with lower relapse[46] and improved disease-free survival and overall survival,[47] but they have not been confirmed by other investigators.[48-51] In the NMDP, ligand mismatching between the donor and recipient was associated with increased risk of severe GVHD and lower survival.[51] Differences in results and conclusions may reflect the varying conditioning and immunosuppressive regimens, as well as patient characteristics for the nongenetic variables that also affect transplant outcome.

The mismatched ligand model is operational when the donor and the recipient are mismatched for HLA class I. The alternative "missing ligand" model of NK alloreactivity in transplantation is based on two findings: (1) since HLA and KIR genes families are encoded on different chromosomes and are inherited in classical Mendelian fashion, individuals may lack KIR receptors for their HLA ligands, and in turn they may lack HLA ligands for their KIR receptors; and (2) the KIR genotype, rather than the HLA genotype, governs the expression of KIR.[39,41,52] The missing ligand model assumes that the transplant donor encodes a complete repertoire of inhibitory KIR receptors; indeed, the frequencies of KIR2DL2, 2DL3, 2DL1, and 3DL1 are very close to 90% in most populations tested.[53] The frequencies of the HLA-C group 1 and group 2 epitopes and the HLA-Bw4 epitope vary significantly from population to population. These frequencies imply that even between HLA-matched individuals (including siblings), the patient may be missing one or more HLA ligands for donor inhibitory KIR, leading to loss of donor NK inhibition and killing of host target cells, and ultimately lower relapse and GVHD and improved survival.

In the clinic, information on donor genotype for inhibitory KIR receptors along with recipient genotype for HLA class I ligand predicted improved transplant outcome when recipients were missing the ligand for the donor KIR.[52] In a single-center analysis of 178 T-cell–depleted HLA identical sibling transplants, patients transplanted for acute myelogenous leukemia (AML), MDS, and high-risk CML, but not patients with acute lymphoblastic leukemia (ALL), had a significantly lower risk of relapse and higher disease-free and overall survival compared to recipients who had all ligands present.[53] A dose-effect of improved disease-free survival and overall survival occurred with increasing number of missing ligands (HLA-B and HLA-C ligands both missing). In a side-by-side comparison of the mismatched ligand and the missing ligand models in a large transplant population from the IHWG in HSCT (www.ihwg.org), among 1,765 T-replete transplants for CML, AML, MDS, and ALL, there was a significant reduction in relapse and improved survival among AML patients lacking ligand but not among the ALL patients.[54] The effect was contributed strongly by patients missing the group 2 HLA-C ligand. Among 633 HLA-B and/or HLA-C mismatched pairs, there was no effect of KIR ligand incompatibility on relapse or survival; however, AML recipients who were missing ligand had a lower risk of relapse.

The Cytokine Genes: Genetic Diversity and GVHD Risk

The interactions between HLA genes and between HLA and KIR genes have profound effects on donor-versus-host and host-versus-donor allorecognition. GVHD is a consequence of donor recognition of host HLA alleles or antigens not present in the donor. Donor NK cells may lower risks of GVHD by loss of inhibition, resulting in killing of recipient antigen presenting cells. A third mechanism in the pathogenesis of GVHD is the modulation of the intensity of tissue injury and inflammation through effects of cytokine genes.[55] Allelic diversity within coding and promoter regions of cytokine genes is basic to the hypothesis that cytokine genetic polymorphism in either patient or donor or both, may explain individual risks of GVHD[56-73] (Table 3).

As with HLA and KIR,[1,40] the cataloguing of cytokine genetic polymorphism requires a common nomenclature to facilitate communication and reference to complex variation. Furthermore, comparison of clinical results necessitates complete information on the transplant conditioning regimen, immunosuppressive agents, and graft source. Accordingly, each cytokine that has thus far been examined in clinical transplantation is provided in Table 3 with reference to the single nucleotide polymorphism (SNP), microsatellite (Msat), allele, and haplotype tested, officially recognized names and aliases, and the transplant demographics.

Sequence Polymorphism of Cytokine Genes

Cytokine gene variation in SNPs, variable number of tandem repeat (VNTR) sequences, microsatellite (Msat) markers, and allele and haplotype frequencies have been described among racially diverse transplant populations.[74,75] A recent analysis of African-, Cuban-, and caucasian Americans found similar frequencies of the tumor necrosis factor-α (TNF-α) proinflammatory cytokine in all three. However, pronounced differences in allele and haplotype frequencies of interleukin (IL)-10, IL-6 and interferon-γ (IFN-γ) were present between African-Americans and both caucasian and Cuban-Americans.[74] The majority of African-Americans encoded the high-expression G/G allele of proinflammatory IL-6, whereas the frequency of the low-expression C/C genotype was significantly lower compared to Cuban- and caucasian Americans. In Japanese individuals, the TNF-α–308 polymorphism was at a lower frequency compared to that in caucasians.[73] These studies demonstrate the need for comprehensive analysis of racially and ethnically diverse populations to fully appreciate the extent of genetic diversity of cytokine genes and the impact of structure on function.

The Proinflammatory Cytokine: TNF-α

TNF-α is among the best-characterized cytokines. TNF-α is produced by macrophages, monocytes, NK and T cells, and it has multiple roles in the pathogenesis of GVHD. TNF-α induces apoptosis in target tissues, increases expression of HLA alloantigens, and promotes further production of the IL-1, IL-6, IL-10, and interleukin receptor antagonist cytokines.[55]

The TNF locus is comprised of the TNF-α gene and the lymphotoxin-α (also known as LTα, TNF-β) gene within the class III region of the MHC. Because of their physical location, TNF-α and LTα display strong linkage disequilibrium with HLA-B and HLA-DRB1 genes.[76] Msat-defined alleles of TNF-α are referred to as "TNF a, b, c, d, e, and f."[77] In addition to Msat polymorphisms, SNPs located in the promoter have been characterized, with the best known involving a single base change at TNF-308G/A and TNF-863C/A.[58,61,63,64,69,70,77] An intron 1 LTα polymorphism located at +252 defines a 5.5-kb ("TNFB*1") and a 10.5-kb ("TNFB*2") allele. The TNF-308A allele ("TNFA*02") and the 5.5-kb LTA allele are associated with high production of cytokine observed on HLA-A1–, HLA-B8–, HLA-DR3–, and HLA-DR4–positive haplotypes.[76]

The clinical importance of TNF-α in the development of GVHD has been demonstrated in several studies. However, direct comparison of results is difficult different polymorphisms of the TNF-α locus have been evaluated in different clinical populations (HLA-identical sibling transplants, T-cell depleted unrelated donor transplants, and cord blood transplants) (Table 3). Association of TNF-α polymorphism and acute GVHD has been described with recipient or donor A allele, or with recipient homozygosity for the d3 Msat allele.[56,67,69,70] Correlation to serum levels sometimes links increased risk of grades III to IV acute GVHD with higher levels of TNF-α.[78] Among TCD transplants and cord blood recipients, however, no association between the d4 allele[68] or the d3 allele[71] and GVHD was observed.

The TNFRII receptor has an arginine (R) or methionine (M) substitution at residue 196. There is allelic diversity of the TNF locus and striking differences in TNF SNP frequencies between Japanese and caucasian populations.[73] Polymorphism of residue 196 of the TNFRII receptor was examined in matched sibling[65] and unrelated[73] transplants. Patients positive for the MR or RR genotype had an increased risk of acute GVHD, and recipients whose donors were homozygous for RR were at increased risk for chronic extensive GVHD.

IL-10: T_H2 Cytokine

A member of the interferon receptor superfamily, IL-10 is produced by monocytes and functions as an anti-inflammatory cytokine. IL-10 maps to chromosome 1q31-32. There are SNPs at positions −3575, −2763, −1082, −819, and −592 and an Msat repeat at −1064 of the promoter. Genotypes of one or more of these promoter SNPs have been assessed in donors and recipients.[61,63-65,67-71] Another approach has been to evaluate the −1082, −819, and −592 SNPs collectively as a haplotype and measure GVHD risks associated with the haplotype.[58,61,63,65,68] Table 3 summarizes the findings for each SNP and haplotype. Studies that have taken the haplotype approach for −1082, −819, and −592 have reported increased risk of acute GVHD for recipients positive for the GCC/GCC haplotype and for donors positive for haplotypes other than the GCC/GCC haplotype. When −592A SNP was used to mark the haplotype, recipients homozygous for C/C at this position were at increased risk for acute GVHD compared to patients with A/A (protective).[61]

In addition to promoter polymorphisms, Msats can define the clinical role of IL-10 polymorphism.[56,67-71] IL-10 −1064 is a $(CA)_n$-repeat; longer Msat alleles (alleles 12, 13, 14, and 15) in the recipient have been associated with increased risk of acute GVHD.[56,67,70] Information in the setting of cord blood transplantation is limited. In a multicenter study of cord blood transplants, neither donor nor recipient IL-10 −1064[11-16] genotype was associated with development of grade II to IV acute GVHD or severity of GVHD.[71]

IL-10 high- and low-producing genotypes have been described in African-, caucasian, and Hispanic-Americans.[74] In

Table 3 Cytokine Gene Polymorphisms and GVHD Risk

Cytokine*	Chromosome	Polymorphism†	Study Population‡	Increased Acute GVHD	Increased Chronic GVHD	Reference
IFN-γ (IFNG)	12q14	Intron 1, Msat (CA)n	R (80)§	Recipient homozygous allele 3	—	56
			R (67)§	—	—	57
		+874, T/A	R (99), C (1)	—	—	58
IFNGR2	21q22	Arg64Gly (rs9808753)	R (67)§	—	—	57
IL-1A	2q14	−889 (rs1800587), C/T	R (115)	—	Donor T	59
			U (52)§ U (38)*¶	—	—	60
		Intron 6, 46 bp VNTR	R (115)	—	Donor allele 2 (1052 bp)	59
IL-1B	2q14	−511 (rs16944), T/C	R (993)§	—	—	61
			R (115)	—	—	59
			U (52)§, U (38)¶	—	—	60
			R (99)§	—	—	62
			R (160)§	—	—	63
		+3953 (rs1143634), T/C	R (993)§	—	—	61
			R (115)	—	—	59
			R (99)§	—	—	62
			R (160)§	Hepatic aGVHD with recipient T	—	63
IL-1RA (IL-1R1)	2q12	Intron 2, 86 bp VNTR	(107)§	Protective with donor allele 2	Recipient IL-1RA	64
			R(104)§	—	—	65
			R(115)	—	—	59
			U (52)§, U (38)¶	—	—	60
			R (99)§	Protective with donor allele 2	—	62
		Intron 2, G/A	R (993)§	—	—	61
IL-2	4q26	−330, (rs2069762), T/G	U (55)§, E (40)¶	Recipient G	—	66
IL-4	5q31	−590 (rs2243250), C/T	R (67)§	—	—	57
IL-4R	16p11	Ile50Val (rs1805010)	R (67)§	—	—	57
		Gln551Arg (Gln576Arg) (rs1801275)	R (67)§	—	—	57
IL-6	7p21	−174 (rs1800795), C/G	R (99), C(1)	—	Recipient GC or GG	58
			(107)§	—		64
			R (993)§	—	—	61
			R (104)§	—	—	65
			R (80)§	—	Recipient GG	56
			R (160)§	Donor G	Recipient GG —	63
IL-10	1q31	−3575, T/A	R (993)§	—	—	61
		−2763, C/A	R (993)§	—	—	61
		−1082 (rs1800896), A/G	(107)§	—	Recipient GG	64
			R (993)§	—	—	61
			R (144)§	—	—	67
			R (160)§	—	—	63
			U (120)§, U (62)*¶	—		68
		−1064 (IL10.G), MsaI (CA)n	R (49)§, U (13)§	—	Donor allele 13 or higher	69
			R (49)§	Recipients allele 12, 13, 14 or 15		70
			R (144)§	Recipient longer alleles (12–16)	—	67

Table 3 Continued

Cytokine*	Chromosome	Polymorphism†	Study Population‡	Increased Acute GVHD	Increased Chronic GVHD	Reference
			R (80)§	Recipient longer alleles (12–16)	—	56
			C (115)§	—		71
			U (120)§ U (62)¶	—		68
		−819 (rs1800871), C/T	R (104)§	—	—	65
			R (160)§	—	—	63
			R (993)§	—	—	61
			U (120)§, U (62)¶	—	—	68
		−592 (rs1800872), A/C	R (9093)§	Protective with recipient AA	—	61
			R (104)§	—	—	65
			R (160)§	—	—	63
			U (120)§, U (62)¶	—		68
		−571, A/C	R (67)*§	—	—	57
		−1064 CA, −1082, −819, −592" haplotype, R2 long allele)-GCC or R3GCC haplotypes	U (120)§, U (62)¶	—		68
		"−1082,−819,−592" haplotype, A-1082G, C-819T, A-592C	r (99), C (1)	Recipient GCC/GCC and donor non-GCC/GCC genotype	—	58
			R (993)§	Protective with recipient ATA/ATA		61
			R (104)§	—	—	65
			R (160)§	—	Recipient ATA haplotype	63
IL-18	11q22	"−137−607−656" haplotype, G-137C,C-607A, G-656T	U (157)	—	—	72
TGF-β (TGFB1)	19q13	Leu10Pro (rs1982073)	R (67)§	Donor Leu/Pro or Pro/Pro	—	57
		−509, C/T	R (67)§	—	—	57
TGF-β receptor (TGFBR2)	3p22	+1167, C/T, (Asn389Asn), (rs2228048)	R (67)§	Recipient CT or TT	—	57
TNF-α (TNF)	6p21	−308 (rs1800629), A/G	R (99), C (1)	—	—	58
			(107)§	—	—	64
			R (993)§			61
			R (49)§, U (13)§	Donor origin A	—	69
			R (49)§	—		70
			R (160)§	—	—	63
		−238 (rs361525), G/A	R (99), C (1)	—	—	58
			R (160)§	—	—	63
		−1031 (rs1799964), C/T	U (120)§, U (62)¶	—		68
		"−1031 (rs1799964), −863 (rs1800630), −857 (rs1799724)" (TNFA-U01 TCC, TNFA-U02 TCT, TNFA-U03 CAC, TNFA-U04 CCC)	U (444)§, U(7)¶	Donor and/or recipient U02 and U03		73

Table 3 Continued

Cytokine*	Chromosome	Polymorphism†	Study Population‡	Increased Acute GVHD	Increased Chronic GVHD	Reference
		+488, G/A	R (160)§	Recipient A	—	63
		TNFd, Msat (TC/GA)n	R (99), C (1)	—	—	58
			R (49)§	Recipient d3/d3		70
			R (144)§	—	—	67
			R (80)§	Recipient d3/d3	—	56
			C (115)§	—		71
			U (120)§, U (62)¶	—		68
		"−1031 −TNFd" halotype	U (120)§, U (62)¶	—		68
TNF-β (LTA)	6p21	+252 in the first intron (rs909253), (TNFn, NcoI RFLP), A/G,	R (99), C(1)	—	—	58
			(107)§	—	—	64
		TNFa, Msat (AC/GT)n	R (99), C(1)	—	—	58
		TNFb, Msat (TC/GA)n	R (99), C(1)	—	—	58
TNFRII (TNFRSF1B)	1p36	Met196Arg, (rs1061622)	R (104)§	Recipient MR or RR genotype	Donor RR	65
			U (44)§, U (7)¶	donor 196R		73

*HUGO nomenclature given in parenthesis if different.
†Known SNP rs number given in parenthesis; bp, base pair.
‡R, related; U, unrelated; C, cord blood.
§T replete.
¶T-cell deplete. Number of transplants indicated in parenthesis.

clinical studies, SNP variation has been shown to correlate with IL-10 production: for the IL-10 −1082 G/A SNP, the A allele is associated with lower in vitro IL10 production.[79] In most analyses, an inverse relationship between IL-10 levels and risk of acute GVHD is apparent, and supports the role of IL-10 as an anti-inflammatory cytokine.[80] In a prospective study of 84 allogeneic HSCT recipients, PBMC production of IL-10 was assayed using enzyme-linked immunosorbent assay (ELISA) methods prior to transplant and before initiation of the conditioning regimen.[81] High levels correlated with low incidence of GVHD and transplant-related mortality, consistent with a protective role for IL10. Among a subset of patients displaying high IL-10 production prior to conditioning, de novo release of TNF-α during conditioning was undetectable; in contrast, in patients with intermediate or low IL-10 production prior to conditioning, a TNF-α surge could be quantified. In an autologous transplant, patients with the IL-10 −592 A/C genotype or −592 A/A genotype had reduced incidence of GVHD, albeit with reduced levels of IL-10 mRNA in PBMC.[82]

Summary: Translating Genomic Data to Clinical Practice

GVHD remains a major cause of morbidity and mortality after alternative donor transplantation historically. The selection of prospective unrelated donors has been based on HLA matching for class I and II genes. Unmet needs include qualitative and quantitative measures of risk associated with HLA mismatching, information required in order to best address the needs of patients for whom a matched donor is not available. A better understanding of the role of NK cell–mediated cytotoxicity and especially the balance between T cell and NK cell allorecognition will provide additional options for donor selection, risk-assessment, and possibilities for post-grafting immunotherapy. More complete knowledge of the role of cytokine genes in modulating the severity of GVHD is important; recipient and donor polymorphisms for these genes will provide clinicians an additional tool for assessing risks and new avenues for the prevention and treatment of GVHD. The importance of structure in order to understand function requires a systematic approach, involving the examination of diverse populations in order to appreciate the full extent and nature of genetic variation, and application of these data to the analysis of clinical populations with careful attention to the transplant procedures and the nongenetic factors that also influence outcome.

References

1. Marsh SG: WHO Nomenclature Committee for Factors of the HLA System. Nomenclature for factors of the HLA System, update December 2004. Hum Immunol 66:329-330, 2005
2. Mickelson E, Petersdorf EW: Histocompatibility, in Blume KG, Forman SJ, Appelbaum FR (eds): Thomas' Hematopoietic Cell Transplantation (ed 3). Oxford, UK, Blackwell, 2004, pp31-42
3. Cornelissen JJ, Carston M, Kollman C, King R, Dekker AW, Lowenberg B, et al: Unrelated marrow transplantation for adult patients with poor-risk acute lymphoblastic leukemia: Strong graft-versus-leukemia effect and risk factors determining outcome. Blood 97:1572-1577, 2001
4. Morishima Y, Sasazuki T, Inoko H, Juji T, Akaza T, Yamamoto K, et al:

The clinical significance of human leukocyte antigen (HLA) allele compatibility in patients receiving a marrow transplant from serologically HLA-A, HLA-B and HLA-Dr matched unrelated donors. Blood 99:4200-4206, 2002
5. Petersdorf EW, Gooley TA, Anasetti C, Martin PJ, Smith AG, Mickelson E, et al: Optimizing outcome after unrelated marrow transplantation by comprehensive matching of HLA class I and II alleles in the donor and recipient. Blood 92:3515-3520, 1998
6. Sasazuki T, Juji T, Morishima Y, Kinukawa N, Kashiwabara H, Inoko H, et al: Effect of matching of class I HLA alleles on clinical outcome after transplantation of hematopoietic stem cells from an unrelated donor. N Engl J Med 339:1177-1185, 1998
7. Prezpiorka D, Saliba R, Cleary K, Fischer H, Tonai R, Fritsche H, et al: Tacrolimus does not abrogate the increased risk of acute graft-versus-host disease after unrelated-donor marrow transplantation with allelic mismatching at HLA-DRB1 and HLA-DQB1. Biol Blood Marrow Transplant 6:190-197, 2000
8. Ferrara GB, Bacigalupo A, Lamparelli T, Lanino E, Delfino L, Morabito A, et al: Bone marrow transplantation from unrelated donors: The impact of mismatches with substitutions at position 116 of the human leukocyte antigen class I heavy chain. Blood 98:3150-3155, 2001
9. Keever-Taylor CA, Bredeson C, Loberiza FR, Casper JT, Lawton C, Rizzo D, et al: Analysis of risk factors for the development of GVHD after T cell-depleted allogeneic BMT: Effect of HLA disparity, ABO incompatibility, and method of T-cell depletion. Biol Blood Marrow Transplant 7:620-630, 2001
10. Petersdorf EW, Gooley T, Malkki M, Anasetti C, Martin P, Woolfrey A, et al: The biological significance of HLA-DP gene variation in haematopoietic cell transplantation. Brit J Haematol 112:988-994, 2001
11. Petersdorf EW, Kollman C, Hurley CK, Dupont B, Nademanee A, Begovich AB, et al: Effect of HLA class II gene disparity on clinical outcome in unrelated donor hematopoietic cell transplantation for chronic myeloid leukemia: The US National Marrow Donor Program Experience. Blood 98:2922-2929, 2001
12. Schaffer M, Aldener-Cannavá A, Remberger M, Ringdén O, Olerup O: Roles of HLA-B, HLA-C and HLA-DPA1 incompatibilities in the outcome of unrelated stem-cell transplantation. Tissue Antigens 2:243-250, 2003
13. Shaw BE, Potter MN, Mayor NP, Pay AL, Smith C, Goldman JM, et al: The degree of matching at HLA-DPB1 predicts for acute graft-versus-host disease and disease relapse following haematopoietic stem cell transplantation. Bone Marrow Transplant 31:1001-1008, 2003
14. Caillat-Zucman S, Le Deist F, Haddad E, Gannagé M, Dal Cortivo L, Jabado N, et al: Impact of HLA matching on outcome of hematopoietic stem cell transplantation in children with inherited diseases: a single-center comparative analysis of genoidentical, haploidentical or unrelated donors. Bone Marrow Transplant 33:1089-1095, 2004
15. Flomenberg N, Baxter-Lowe LE, Confer D, Fernandez-Vina M, Filipovich A, Horowitz M, et al: Impact of HLA class I and class II high-resolution matching on outcomes of unrelated donor bone marrow transplantation: HLA-C mismatching is associated with a strong adverse effect on transplantation outcome. Blood 104:1923-1930, 2004
16. Gallardo D, Brunet S, Torres A, Alonso-Nieto M, Vallejo C, Jiménez A, et al: HLA-DPB1 mismatch in HLA-A-B-DRB1 identical sibling donor stem cell transplantation and acute graft-versus-host disease. Transplant 77:1107-1110, 2004
17. Petersdorf EW, Anasetti C, Martin PJ, Gooley T, Radich J, Malkki M, et al: Limits of HLA mismatching in unrelated hematopoietic cell transplantation. Blood 104:2976-2980, 2004
18. Petersdorf EW: Hematopoietic cell transplantation, in Blume KG, Forman SJ, Appelbaum FR (eds): Thomas' Hematopoietic Cell Transplantation (ed 3). Oxford, UK, Blackwell, 2004, pp 1132-1149
19. Drobyski WR, Klein J, Flomenberg N, Pietryga D, Vesole DH, Margolis DA, et al: Superior survival associated with transplantation of matched unrelated versus one-antigen-mismatched unrelated or highly leukocyte antigen-disparate haploidentical family donor marrow grafts for the treatment of hematologic malignancies: Establishing a treatment algorithm for recipients of alternative donor grafts. Blood 99:806-814, 2002
20. Kiehl MG, Kraut L, Schwerdtfeger R, Hertenstein B, Remberger M, Kroeger N, et al: Outcome of allogeneic hematopoietic stem-cell transplantation in adult patients with acute lymphoblastic leukemia: No difference in related compared with unrelated transplant in first complete remission. J Clin Oncol 22:2816-2825, 2004
21. Baker SK, Gurney JG, Ness KK, Bhatia R, Forman SJ, Francisco L, et al: Late effects in survivors of chronic myeloid leukemia treated with hematopoietic cell transplantation: Results from the Bone Marrow Transplant Survivor Study. Blood 104:1898-1906, 2004
22. Stewart BL, Storer B, Storek J, Deeg HJ, Storb R, Hansen JA, et al: Duration of immunosuppressive treatment for chronic graft-versus-host disease. Blood 104:3501-3506, 2004
23. Loiseau P, Espérou H, Busson M, Sghiri R, Tamouza R, Hilarius M, et al: DPB1 disparities contribute to severe GVHD and reduced patient survival after unrelated donor bone marrow transplantation. Bone Marrow Transplant 30:497-502, 2002
24. Zino E, Frumento G, Marktel S, Sormani MP, Ficara F, Di Terlizzi S, et al: A T-cell epitope encoded by a subset of HLA-DPB1 alleles determines nonpermissive mismatches for hematologic stem cell transplantation. Blood 103:1417-1424, 2004
25. Petersdorf EW, Gooley T, Malkki M, and Horowitz M for the International Histocompatibility Working Group in Hematopoietic Cell Transplantation: Impact of donor-recipient HLA matching on survival after myeloablative hematopoietic cell transplantation from unrelated donors, in Hansen J, Dupont B (eds): HLA 2004: Immunobiology of the Human MHC, Proceedings of the 13th International Histocompatibility Workshop and Conference. Seattle, WA: IHWG Press (in press)
26. Kaminski E, Hows J, Man S, Brookes P, Mackinnon S, Hughes T, et al: Prediction of graft versus host disease by frequency analysis of cytotoxic T cells after unrelated donor bone marrow transplantation. Transplantation 48:608-613, 1989
27. Niederwieser D, Maris M, Shizuru JA, Petersdorf E, Hegenbart U, Sandmaier BM, et al: Low-dose total body irradiation (TBI) and fludarabine followed by hematopoietic cell transplantation (HSCT) from HLA-matched or mismatched unrelated donors and postgrafting immunosuppression with cyclosporine and mycophenolate mofetil (MMF) can induce durable complete chimerism and sustained remissions in patients with hematological diseases. Blood 101:1620-1629, 2003
28. Ringdén O, Schaffer M, Le Blanc K, Persson U, Hauzenberger D, Abedi MR, et al: Which donor should be chosen for hematopoietic stem cell transplantation among unrelated HLA-A, -B, and –DRB1 genomically identical volunteers? Biol Blood Marrow Transplant 10:128-134, 2004
29. Dini G, Valsecchi M, Micalizzi C, Micalizzi C, Busca A, Balduzzi A, et al: Impact of marrow unrelated donor search duration on outcome of children with acute lymphoblastic leukemia in second remission. Bone Marrow Transplant 32:325-331, 2003
30. Barker JN, Krepski TP, DeFor TE, Davies SM, Wagner JE, Weisdorf DJ, et al: Searching for unrelated donor hematopoietic stem cells: Availability and speed of umbilical cord blood versus bone marrow. Biol Blood Marrow Transplant 8:257-260, 2002
31. Gluckman E, Broxmeyer HA, Auerbach AD, Friedman HS, Douglas GW, Devergie A, et al: Hematopoietic reconstitution in a patient with Fanconi's anemia by means of umbilical-cord blood from an HLA-identical sibling. N Engl J Med 321:1174-1178, 1989
32. Kurtzberg J, Laughlin M, Graham ML, Smith C, Olson JF, Halperin EC, et al: Placental blood as a source of hematopoietic stem cells for transplantation into unrelated recipients. N Engl J Med 335:157-166, 1996
33. Rubinstein P, Carrier C, Scaradavou A, Kurtzberg J, Adamson J, Migliaccio AR, et al: Outcomes among 562 recipients of placental-blood transplants from unrelated donors. N Engl J Med 339:1565-1577, 1998
34. Wagner JE, Barker JN, Defor TE, Baker KS, Blazar BR, Eide C, et al: Transplantation of unrelated donor umbilical cord blood in 102 patients with malignant and nonmalignant diseases: Influence of CD34 cell dose and HLA disparity on treatment-related mortality and survival. Blood 100:1611-1618, 2002
35. Laughlin MJ, Eapen M, Rubinstein P, Wagner JE, Zhang MJ, Champlin RE, et al: Outcomes after transplantation of cord blood or bone marrow

from unrelated donors in adults with leukemia. N Engl J Med 351:2265-2275, 2004
36. Rocha V, Labopin M, Sanz G, Arcese W, Schwerdtfeger R, Bosi A, et al: Transplants of umbilical-cord blood or bone marrow from unrelated donors in adults with acute leukemia. N Engl J Med 351:2276-2285, 2004
37. Gluckman E, Rocha V, Arcese W, Michel G, Sanz G, Chan KW, et al: Factors associated with outcomes of unrelated cord blood transplant: Guidelines for donor choice. Exp Hematol 32:397-407, 2004
38. Rubinstein P, Stevens CE: Placental blood for bone marrow replacement: The New York Blood Center's program and clinical results. Baillieres Best Pract Res Clin Haematol 13:565-584, 2000
39. Parham P: MHC class I molecules and KIRs in human history, health and survival. Nat Rev Immunol 5:201-214, 2005
40. Marsh SG, Parham P, Geraghty DE, Trowsdale J, Middleton D, Vilches C, et al: Killer-cell immunoglobulin-like receptor (KIR) nomenclature report, 2002. Immunogenetics 55:220-226, 2003
41. Hsu KC, Dupont B. Natural killer cell receptors: Regulating innate immune responses to hematologic malignancy. Semin Hematol 42:91-103, 2005
42. Trowsdale J, Barten R, Haude A, Steward C, Beck S, Wilson M, et al: The genomic context of natural killer receptor extended gene families. Immunol Rev 181:20-38, 2001
43. Ruggeri L, Capanni M, Urbani E, Perruccio K, Shlomchik WD, Tosti A, et al: Effectiveness of donor natural killer cell alloreactivity in mismatched hematopoietic transplants. Science 295:2097-2100, 2002
44. Aversa F, Tabilio A, Velardi A, Cunningham I, Terenzi A, Falzetti F, et al: Treatment of high-risk acute leukemia with T-cell-depleted stem cells from related donors with one fully mismatched HLA haplotype. N Engl J Med 339:1186-1193, 1998
45. Ruggeri L, Capanni M, Casucci M, Volpi I, Tosti A, Perruccio K, et al: Role of natural killer cell alloreactivity in HLA-mismatched hematopoietic stem cell transplantation. Blood 94:333-339, 1999
46. Beelen D, Ottinger H, Ferencik S, Elmaagacli A, Peceny R, Trenschel R, et al: Genotypic inhibitory killer immunoglobulin-like receptor ligand incompatibility enhances the long-term antileukemic effect of unmodified allogeneic hematopoietic stem cell transplantation in patients with myeloid leukemias. Blood 105:2594-2600, 2004
47. Giebel S, Locatelli F, Lamparelli T, Velardi A, Davies S, Frumento G, et al: Survival advantage with KIR ligand incompatibility in hematopoietic stem cell transplantation from unrelated donors. Blood 102:814-818, 2003
48. Davies SM, Ruggeri L, DeFor T, Wagner JE, Weisdorf DJ, Miller JS, et al: Evaluation of KIR ligand incompatibility in mismatched unrelated donor hematopoietic transplants. Killer immunoglobulin-like receptor. Blood 100:3825-3827, 2002.
49. Bornhauser M, Schwerdtfeger R, Martin H, Frank KH, Theuser C, Ehninger G, et al: Role of KIR ligand incompatibility in hematopoietic stem cell transplantation using unrelated donors. Blood 103:2860-2861, 2004
50. Bishara A, De Santis D, Witt CC, Brautbar C, Christiansen FT, Or R, et al: The beneficial role of inhibitory KIR genes of HLA class I NK epitopes in haploidentically mismatched stem cell allografts may be masked by residual donor-alloreactive T cells causing GVHD. Tissue Antigens 63:204-211, 2004
51. Farag S, Bacigalupo A, Dupont B, Caligiuri M, Nelson G, Miller J, et al: The effect of killer immunoglobulin-like receptor KIR ligand incompatibility on outcome of unrelated donor bone marrow transplantation UDT. Blood 104: 434, 2004
52. Leung W, Iyengar R, Turner V, Lang P, Bader P, Conn P, et al: Determinants of antileukemia effects of allogeneic NK cells. J Immunol 172: 644-650, 2004
53. Hsu K, Keever-Taylor C, Wilton A, Pinto C, Heller G, Arkun K, et al: Improved outcome in allogeneic hematopoietic stem cell transplantation in acute myelogenous leukemia (AML) predicted by donor KIR genotype and recipient HLA genotype in T-cell depleted HLA-identical sibling transplants. Blood 105:4878-4884, 2005
54. Hsu KC, Malkki M, Gooley TA, et al: Missing killer immunoglobulin-like receptor (KIR) ligand confers protection from relapse in recipients of unrelated hematopoietic cell transplantation (HSCT) for AML. Tandem ASBMT/CIBMTR Meetings, Keystone, CO, February 10-14, 2005 (abstr)
55. Ferrara JL: The cytokine modulation of acute graft-versus-host disease. Bone Marrow Transplant 21:S13-15, 1998 (suppl 3)
56. Cavet J, Dickinson AM, Norden J, Taylor PR, Jackson GH, Middleton PG, et al: Interferon-gamma and interleukin-6 gene polymorphisms associate with graft-versus-host disease in HLA-matched sibling bone marrow transplantation. Blood 98:1594-1600, 2001
57. Hattori H, Matsuzaki A, Suminoe A, Ihara K, Nagatoshi Y, Sakata N, et al: Polymorphisms of transforming growth factor-beta1 and transforming growth factor-beta1 type II receptor genes are associated with acute graft-versus-host disease in children with HLA-matched sibling bone marrow transplantation. Bone Marrow Transplant 30:665-671, 2002
58. Socie G, Loiseau P, Tamouza R, Janin A, Busson M, Gluckman E, et al: Both genetic and clinical factors predict the development of graft-versus-host disease after allogeneic hematopoietic stem cell transplantation. Transplantation 72:699-706, 2001
59. Cullup H, Dickinson AM, Cavet J, Jackson GH, Middleton PG: Polymorphisms of interleukin-1alpha constitute independent risk factors for chronic graft-versus-host disease after allogeneic bone marrow transplantation. Br J Haematol 122:778-787, 2003
60. MacMillan ML, Radloff GA, Defor TE, Weisdorf DJ, Davies SM: Interleukin-1 genotype and outcome of unrelated donor bone marrow transplantation. Br J Haematol 121:597-604, 2003
61. Lin MT, Storer B, Martin PJ, Tseng LH, Gooley T, Chen PJ, et al: Relation of an interleukin-10 promoter polymorphism to graft-versus-host disease and survival after hematopoietic-cell transplantation. N Engl J Med 349:2201-2210, 2003
62. Cullup H, Dickinson AM, Jackson GH, Taylor PR, Cavet J, Middleton PG: Donor interleukin 1 receptor antagonist genotype associated with acute graft-versus-host disease in human leucocyte antigen-matched sibling allogeneic transplants. Br J Haematol 113:807-813, 2001
63. Mullighan C, Heatley S, Doherty K, Szabo F, Grigg A, Hughes T, et al: HLA immunogenetic polymorphisms and the risk of complications after allogeneic hemopoietic stem-cell transplantation. Transplantation. 77:587-596, 2004
64. Rocha V, Franco RF, Porcher R, Bittencourt H, Silva WA Jr, Latouche A, et al: Host defense and inflammatory gene polymorphisms are associated with outcomes after HLA-identical sibling bone marrow transplantation. Blood 100:3908-3918, 2002
65. Stark GL, Dickinson AM, Jackson GH, Taylor PR, Proctor SJ, Middleton PG: Tumour necrosis factor receptor type II 196M/R genotype correlates with circulating soluble receptor levels in normal subjects and with graft-versus-host disease after sibling allogeneic bone marrow transplantation. Transplantation 76:1742-1749, 2003
66. MacMillan ML, Radloff GA, Kiffmeyer WR, DeFor TE, Weisdorf DJ, Davies SM: High-producer interleukin-2 genotype increases risk for acute graft-versus-host disease after unrelated donor bone marrow transplantation. Transplantation 76:1758-1762, 2003
67. Cavet J, Middleton PG, Segall M, Noreen H, Davies SM, Dickinson AM: Recipient tumor necrosis factor-alpha and interleukin-10 gene polymorphisms associate with early mortality and acute graft-versus-host disease severity in HLA-matched sibling bone marrow transplants. Blood 94:3941-3946, 1999
68. Keen LJ, Defor TE, Bidwell JL, Davies SM, Bradley BA, Hows JM: Interleukin-10 and tumor necrosis factor alpha region haplotypes predict transplant-related mortality after unrelated donor stem cell transplantation. Blood 103: 3599-3602, 2004
69. Takahashi H, Furukawa T, Hashimoto S, Suzuki N, Kuroha T, Yamazaki F, et al: Contribution of TNF-alpha and IL-10 gene polymorphisms to graft-versus-host disease following allo-hematopoietic stem cell transplantation. Bone Marrow Transplant 26:1317-1323, 2000
70. Middleton PG, Taylor PR, Jackson G, Proctor SJ, Dickinson AM: Cytokine gene polymorphisms associating with severe acute graft-versus-host disease in HLA-identical sibling transplants. Blood 92:3943-3948, 1998
71. Kogler G, Middleton PG, Wilke M, Rocha V, Esendam B, Enczmann J, et al: Recipient cytokine genotypes for TNF-alpha and IL-10 and the

minor histocompatibility antigens HY and CD31 codon 125 are not associated with occurrence or severity of acute GVHD in unrelated cord blood transplantation: A retrospective analysis. Transplantation 74: 1167-1175, 2002

72. Cardoso SM, Defor TE, Tilley LA, Bidwell JL, Weisdorf DJ, MacMillan ML: Patient interleukin-18 GCG haplotype associates with improved survival and decreased transplant-related mortality after unrelated-donor bone marrow transplantation. Br J Haematol 126:704-710, 2004
73. Ishikawa Y, Kashiwase K, Akaza T, Morishima Y, Inoko H, Sasazuki T, et al: Polymorphisms in TNFA and TNFR2 affect outcome of unrelated bone marrow transplantation. Bone Marrow Transplant 29:569-575, 2002
74. Delaney NL, Esquenazi V, Lucas DP, Zachary AA, Leffell MS: TNF-alpha, TGF-beta, IL-10, IL-6, and IFN-gamma alleles among African Americans and Cuban Americans. Report of the ASHI Minority Workshops: Part IV. Hum Immunol 65:1413-1419, 2004
75. Meenagh A, Williams F, Ross OA, Patterson C, Gorodezky C, Hammond M: Frequency of cytokine polymorphisms in populations from western Europe, Africa, Asia, the Middle East and South America. Hum Immunol 63:1055-1061, 2002
76. Udalova IA, Nedospasov SA, Webb GC, Chaplin DD, Turetskaya RL: Highly informative typing of the human TNF locus using six adjacent polymorphic markers. Genomics 16:180-186, 1993
77. Wilson AG, de Vries N, Pociot F, di Giovine FS, van der Putte LB, Duff GW: An allelic polymorphism within the human tumor necrosis factor alpha promoter region is strongly associated with HLA A1, B8, and DR3 alleles. J Exp Med 177:557-560, 1993
78. Schots R, Kaufman L, Van Riet I, Ben Othman T, De Waele M, Van Camp B, et al: Proinflammatory cytokines and their role in the development of major transplant-related complications in the early phase after allogeneic bone marrow transplantation. Leukemia 17:1150-1156, 2003
79. Turner DM, Williams DM, Sankaran D, Lazarus M, Sinnott PJ, Hutchinson IV: An investigation of polymorphism in the interleukin-10 gene promoter. Eur J Immunogenet 24:1-8, 1997
80. Takatsuka H, Takemoto Y, Okamoto T, Fujimori Y, Tamura S, Wada H, et al: Predicting the severity of graft-versus-host disease from interleukin-10 levels after bone marrow transplantation. Bone Marrow Transplant 24:1005-1007, 1999
81. Holler E, Roncarolo MG, Hintermeier-Knabe R, Eissner G, Ertl B, Schulz U, et al: Prognostic significance of increased IL-10 production in patients prior to allogeneic bone marrow transplantation. Bone Marrow Transplant 25:237-241, 2000
82. Miura Y, Thoburn CJ, Bright EC, Chen W, Nakao S, Hess AD: Cytokine and chemokine profiles in autologous graft-versus-host disease GVHD: interleukin 10 and interferon gamma may be critical mediators for the development of autologous GVHD. Blood 100:2650-2658, 2002

ELSEVIER

Seminars in
HEMATOLOGY

The Clinical Spectrum of Acute Graft-Versus-Host Disease

H. Joachim Deeg[a] and Joseph H. Antin[b]

Acute graft-versus-host disease (GVHD), initiated by the reaction of donor T lymphocytes against nonshared recipient antigens, typically leads to a clinical syndrome characterized by cutaneous eruptions and intestinal and hepatic dysfunction. These three organ systems are considered in the clinical grading of acute GVHD. However, other targets may be involved. With conventional transplant conditioning regimens and in vivo prophylaxis, GVHD becomes clinically manifest within 2 to 4 weeks. With reduced-intensity conditioning, the onset of acute GVHD may be delayed until 2 to 3 months after transplantation. Hyperacute GVHD may occur within a week of transplantation after severely human leukocyte antigen (HLA)-mismatched transplants or transplants without GVHD prophylaxis. There is no reliable laboratory test for acute GVHD, and the diagnosis is based on clinical assessment.
Semin Hematol 43:24-31 © 2006 Elsevier Inc. All rights reserved.

Graft-versus-host disease (GVHD), the clinical syndrome related to the reaction of donor-derived immunocompetent cells against patient tissues, remains the most frequent transplant-related complication. GVHD was first described under the term "secondary disease" in murine models of hemopoietic cell transplantation. Mice that had their marrow function ablated by total body irradiation[1] and were then given viable splenocytes from donors of a different strain—of a different tissue (histocompatibility) type—developed diarrhea, weight loss, skin break down, sparse fur, hunched posture, and odd gait. The syndrome was shown to be caused by immunocompetent cells from the donor.[2–4] Arguably, the first report of GVHD in humans was published in 1960 and was observed after marrow cells were used to treat survivors of a nuclear accident in Belgrade, Yugoslavia.[5]

The form of GVHD typically occurring early after transplantation is referred to as acute GVHD, while a later form with different clinical characteristics has been termed chronic GVHD. For practical purposes the two forms were distinguished by time of onset—less than 100 days after transplantation was considered acute, and more than 100 days chronic.[6] However, a clear distinction between acute and chronic forms of GVHD as originally described is no longer tenable. Observations in patients transplanted with reduced-intensity conditioning regimens or in patients receiving donor lymphocyte infusions (DLI) at various time intervals after transplantation indicate that manifestations of acute GVHD may appear several months after transplantation.[7] Conversely, GVHD with clinical and histologic characteristics of the "chronic" form can occur as early as 50 or 60 days after transplantation.[7,8] It has also been proposed to simply refer to life-threatening and non–life-threatening GVHD, regardless of the time of presentation.[9]

Description and Diagnosis

GVHD is characterized by a clinicopathologic syndrome involving the skin, liver, gastrointestinal tract, and possibly other organs. Any target can be affected alone or in combination with other organs. GVHD is a clinical diagnosis—there are no reliable laboratory tests that will confirm or refute its presence. Rather, the diagnosis of GVHD requires an interpretation of clinical and laboratory findings, recognizing that in some patients the differential diagnosis may be impossible to resolve. For instance, an elevated direct serum bilirubin is a relatively nonspecific abnormality, yet it is the principal criterion for the diagnosis of hepatic GVHD. In the absence of a liver biopsy, there is a considerable risk of mistakenly ascribing this finding to GVHD when it is actually related to an infection or other transplant-related toxicities. As it is often difficult to obtain an adequate tissue biopsy, the physician is left to use clinical judgment. Diarrhea may be

[a]Fred Hutchinson Cancer Research Center, Seattle WA.
[b]Dana-Farber Cancer Institute, Boston, MA.
Supported by Public Health Service Grants No. HL36444, CA18029, and CA15704.
Address correspondence to H. Joachim Deeg, MD, Fred Hutchinson Cancer Research Center, 1100 Fairview Ave N, D1-100, PO Box 19024, Seattle, WA 98109-1024. E-mail: jdeeg@fhcrc.org

doi:10.1053/j.seminhematol.2005.09.003

due to infections, related to conditioning, drug toxicity, or GVHD. Similarly, particularly with mild or limited skin rashes, it can be very difficult to distinguish GVHD from a drug eruption, even on histology.

A recent multicenter phase III trial used an independent committee to assess the presence and severity of GVHD. The incidence of GVHD as determined by investigators was substantially higher than the review committee could confirm.[10] Similarly, substantial interobserver variability in assigning GVHD severity grades was found.[11] Nevertheless, for an experienced clinician a combination of physical and laboratory findings in the appropriate context provides a working diagnosis of GVHD that is satisfactory to produce a meaningful prognostic scale.[12]

Time of Onset of GVHD

After high-intensity (conventional) conditioning, acute GVHD generally occurs within 14 to 35 days of stem cell infusion. The time of onset depends on the degree of histocompatibility, the number of donor T cells infused, and the prophylactic regimen for GVHD. A "hyperacute" form of GVHD may occur in patients with severe human leukocyte antigen (HLA) mismatches and in patients who receive T-cell–replete transplants without or with inadequate in vivo GVHD prophylaxis.[13] Hyperacute GVHD is manifested by fever, generalized erythroderma, desquamation, and often edema; the syndrome typically occurs about 1 week after stem cell infusion and may be rapidly fatal. In patients receiving more conventional (in vivo) GVHD prophylaxis, such as a combination of cyclosporine and methotrexate, the median onset of GVHD is 21 to 25 days after transplantation; however, after in vitro T-cell depletion of the graft the onset may be much later.[14] Thus, the findings of rash and diarrhea by 1 week after transplantation likely indicate hyperacute manifestations of GVHD if minimal or ineffective prophylaxis has been administered; the same kinetics are very unlikely with the use of calcineurin inhibitors or in vitro T-cell depletion of the stem cell inoculum. A less ominous combination of fever, rash, and fluid retention occurring in the first 1 to 2 weeks after stem cell infusion is the "engraftment syndrome." These manifestations may be seen with either allogeneic or autologous transplantation. While its pathophysiology is poorly understood, engraftment syndrome is thought to be secondary to a wave of cytokine production as the graft begins to function, and distinct from the "cytokine storm"[15] that is thought to contribute to acute GVHD in that there is no concomitant T-cell–mediated attack. Engraftment syndrome responds immediately to corticosteroids in most patients, and it typically presents earlier than does acute GVHD.[16] In autologous transplantation the differential diagnosis is of little relevance, but in allogeneic transplant recipients engraftment syndrome must be distinguished from hyperacute manifestations of GVHD. Prompt improvement following the administration of corticosteroids would argue in favor of engraftment syndrome, although some patients with GVHD will also respond.

Skin Manifestations

The most common manifestation of GVHD is a maculopapular, sometimes confluent, erythematous exanthema often involving palms and soles. Involvement of the palms is a particularly useful clinical hint, since drug eruptions are less likely to appear there. However, a painful, blistering acral erythema can be related to conditioning therapy (especially busulfan) and must be distinguished from acute GVHD. Acral erythema due to conditioning usually occurs in the second week and resembles a second-degree burn.[17] The greater sensitivity of skin on palms and soles to cytotoxic therapy may be due to higher cell proliferation rates there than for other parts of the integument less subject to abrasion. A GVHD rash may be asymptomatic, pruritic, or painful. GVHD typically starts on the upper body—shoulders, face, arms, behind the ears— in sun-exposed areas. A skin biopsy may help to substantiate the clinical diagnosis by suggesting causes other than GVHD, but it cannot itself prove the presence of GVHD. In its mildest manifestation, GVHD may involve less than one fourth of the body surface, but in its severest form, it can progress to whole-body erythema, gross bullae formation, and sloughing of the skin. Mild GVHD often responds to modest doses of corticosteroids (1 to 2 mg/kg per day) or other immunosuppressants. Severe GVHD can be difficult to distinguish from Stevens-Johnson syndrome or toxic epidermal necrolysis. In contrast to toxic epidermal necrolysis or Stevens-Johnson syndrome, severe acute GVHD usually does not involve the conjunctivae. The loss of integrity of the integument leads to a markedly increased risk of infection with normal skin flora such as *Stapylococcus aureus* and *Streptococcus epidermidis* as well as with Gram-negative rods and fungi. In severe GVHD, pain control, fluid and electrolyte replacement, metabolic support, and infection control are similar to the management of patients with severe burns—indeed for severe skin GVHD and desquamation, consultation with a burn specialist is advisable.

Mucositis was not part of the classic description of acute GVHD. However, if infection is excluded with appropriate cultures, mucosal lesions that fail to heal with hematologic recovery may signify mucosal (oral, conjunctival, and vaginal) GVHD.

Liver Involvement

Hepatic GVHD is graded on the basis of the total serum bilirubin level. In addition, alkaline phosphatase levels are usually elevated; abnormalities of transaminases are less consistent. Acute GVHD after DLI, longer after transplantation, may be more likely to take the form of "hepatitic" GVHD.[18] However, none of the routine serologic tests of liver injury are definitive, and only the total bilirubin level is considered in GVHD grading. Mild GVHD may result in only a three- to fourfold rise in serum bilirubin with or without transaminase elevations, while the most severely affected patients may have serum bilirubin levels of 10 to 20 mg/dL or higher and in extreme cases show loss of hepatic synthetic function. The lack of a specific test means that the diagnosis of hepatic

GVHD on clinical grounds alone may be quite tenuous. Drug toxicity, parenteral nutrition, hepatic veno-occlusive disease, infection, cholangitis lenta, cholelithiasis, acalculous cholecystitis, and other unrelated conditions can either coexist or be confused with hepatic GVHD. In contrast to veno-occlusive disease (sinusoidal obstruction syndrome), hepatic GVHD only rarely leads to weight gain, capsular pain, or ascites. Many infections can result in elevations of bilirubin. Infections with Gram-negative organisms may increase bilirubin, in the absence of specific hepatic invovlement. The presence of cytomegalovirus (CMV) may be particularly confusing, since CMV infection often occurs concomitantly with GVHD. Drugs such as cyclosporine and estrogens are some of the notorious hepatotoxins often utilized after stem cell transplantation.

Hepatic GVHD is more difficult to diagnose than is GVHD of the skin. Percutaneous liver biopsies are associated with potentially prohibitive risks. Transvenous biopsies have a lower morbidity, and, if results are unequivocal, they can alter the clinical diagnosis (and management) in almost 50% of patients.[19,20] However, a small biopsy sample may still cause diagnostic uncertainty. Nevertheless, most clinicians have had the experience of intensifying immunosuppression based on bilirubin elevations, only to find later that the liver dysfunction was due to infection or drug toxicity. Before embarking on augmented immunosuppressive therapy that increases the risk of infection, the diagnosis should be substantiated by obtaining liver tissue.

Intestinal Involvement

Involvement of the gut by GVHD may be manifested by nausea, anorexia, pain, and watery, secretory diarrhea. In severe cases there may be failure of intestinal function due to mucosal denudation, resulting in protein-losing enteropathy with hypoalbuminemia, bloody diarrhea, or frank ileus. The combination of major fluid losses through damaged skin and decreased hepatic synthetic function with massive diarrhea makes clinical management extremely difficult. Frequent evaluation of blood, urine, and stool electrolytes and careful input and output measurements are a necessity. Infection, conditioning-related toxicity, lactose intolerance, and nonspecific mucosal damage may either mimic gut GVHD or be present concurrently with GVHD, and substantially complicate management. In contrast to skin histopathology, the histology of rectal and gastric/duodenal mucosal biopsies is more specific and even pathognomonic, allowing therapy to be targeted more narrowly.[21–23]

Isolated gastric GVHD is common after stem cell transplantation. It must be distinguished from herpesvirus infection, candidiasis, and nonspecific inflammation.[21,24,25] Gastric or upper gastrointestinal GVHD can occur alone or with other organ involvement. Upper gastrointestinal GVHD is often the cause of otherwise unexplained nausea and vomiting. Esophagogastroduodenoscopy and mucosal biopsies usually lead to the correct diagnosis. GVHD of the upper intestinal tract is relatively sensitive to corticosteroid therapy administered systemically or orally in the form of a poorly absorbable formulation, such as beclomethasone.

Radiographic findings of intestinal GVHD are nonspecific but include increased bowel wall thickness and vascularity, and fluid-filled loops of bowel. Transit time may be extremely rapid, and Doppler studies may show increased arterial flow to the inflamed organ. Magnetic resonance imaging may show generalized increased bowel wall thickness associated with bowel-wall enhancement after administration of gadolinium.[26,27]

Other Organs

Whether GVHD affects organs other than the classic triad of skin, liver and gut has remained controversial. Numerous reports suggest additional organ manifestations. The most likely candidate is the lung (see Yanik and Cooke in this issue). Lung toxicity, including interstitial pneumonitis and diffuse alveolar hemorrhage, may occur in 20% to 60% of allogeneic transplant recipients, although in fewer autologous transplant recipients. Causes of pulmonary damage other than GVHD include engraftment syndrome (see below), infection, radiation pneumonitis, and chemotherapy-related toxicity (especially with methotrexate and busulfan). At least one retrospective analysis failed to link severe pulmonary complications to clinical acute GVHD.[28] Mortality due to pneumonia increases with the severity of GVHD, but this association does not necessarily imply that GVHD, as opposed to concurrent immunosuppressive therapy, is causative. A particular histopathologic syndrome of lymphocytic bronchitis has been attributed directly to GVHD,[29] although this identification has not been confirmed by others. The lungs are likely targets of GVHD because of their extensive reticuloendothelial system and direct exposure to the environment; mouse transplant models support this hypothesis. Other chronic post-hematopoietic stem cell transplant pulmonary syndromes, especially bronchiolitis obliterans, may represent manifestations of chronic GVHD.

Renal and urinary tract symptoms are common after transplantation but are generally attributed to the conditioning regimen, the use of immunosuppressive agents, or infection. There is no convincing evidence for a role of acute GVHD. Similarly, neurologic complications are common but most can be attributed to drug toxicity, infection, or vascular insults. Data on vasculitis of the central nervous system, possibly associated with GVHD, have been presented.[30,31]

Histopathology

Apoptosis of cells in the tissue layer responsible for proliferation and regeneration is a typical histologic feature of GVHD. In the skin, the dermoepidermal junction is most severely affected: there is epidermal and basal cell vacuolar degeneration, disorganization of epidermal cell maturation, eosinophilic body formation, and melanocyte incontinence.[32–35] Hepatic small bile ducts may show segmental disruption, injury to the periductular epithelium bile duct atypia, and cellular degeneration. Cholestasis may be present.[36,37] Mucosal ulcerations and crypt destruction are present in the intestinal tract; the bases of the crypts tend to be most severely affected. The colon, more frequently involved than is the ileum, shows crypt cell apoptosis and dropout with flattening of the villous architecture.[36–38] Typically, mononuclear cell infiltrates are subtle, and often surprisingly mild for the degree of clinical illness. The common features of gut and skin histology are the involvement of the stem cell layer of the organ, at the base of the crypts and the dermo-epidermal junction. Disruption of the stem cell layer results in a reduced ability to repopulate the damaged epithelium with the consequence of blister formation, loss of villi, and associated dysfunction.

Engraftment Syndrome

As noted above, a clinical entity relevant to discussion of acute GVHD is a constellation of fever, erythematous skin rash, and low-pressure pulmonary edema that may occur during neutrophil recovery. The combination of these manifestations may reflect the dysregulated production of inflammatory cytokines and cellular responses to these molecules, and has been termed engraftment or capillary leak syndrome.[39–41] Engraftment syndrome is most clearly recognized after autologous transplantation where, theoretically, GVHD should not occur. In allogeneic transplant recipients, distinction from acute GVHD is difficult. Engraftment syndrome occurs during early recovery of (donor-derived) blood cell counts, but there is no precise delineation of the offending cells and cytokines. Whether homeostatic proliferation of lymphocytes[42] contributes to the clinical picture is speculative. Engraftment syndrome may be associated with increased mortality, primarily from pulmonary failure but also (other) multi-organ dysfunction. Corticosteroid therapy may be effective, particularly for treatment of the lung.[16]

Differential Diagnosis

The differential diagnosis of cutaneous eruptions, diarrhea, and liver function abnormalities can be difficult to resolve. Skin rashes may reflect delayed reactions to the conditioning regimen, antibiotics, or infections. Histopathologic skin changes consistent with mild to moderate acute GVHD are mimicked by the effects of chemoradiotherapy and drug reactions.[43] Some diarrhea is expected after total body irradiation. Viral infections, especially with CMV and other herpes viruses, parasites, *Clostridium difficile*, nonspecific gastritis, and drug reactions can all mimic GVHD of the gut. Watery diarrhea may also occur for a day or two when narcotic analgesics are withdrawn. Liver dysfunction can be due to parenteral nutrition, veno-occlusive disease (sinusoidal obstruction syndrome), viral hepatitis, and drug-induced hepatitis (for example, due to cyclosporine, estrogens, or antifungal agents). Finally, it may be impossible to distinguish between multiple possible causes since the concurrent presence of infection and GVHD is the rule rather than the exception.[44–46]

Risk Factors for the Development of Acute GVHD

While in vitro predictive tests for GVHD have been described,[47–49], results have been difficult to reproduce,[50,51] and no assay has been widely adopted. Efforts to assign a GVHD risk based on donor or recipient polymorphisms of the CD31, CD54, interleukin (IL)-1 receptor antagonist, IL-10, IL-6, or tumor necrosis factor (TNF) genes (or their promoter regions) have not resulted in reliable models.[52–57]

The principle risk factor for the development of GVHD in humans is histoincompatibility between donor and patient. Functionally, histoincompatibility is most powerful when crossing major histocompatibility complex (MHC) barriers. Presumably, the development of GVHD in fully HLA-identical recipients of either family member or unrelated donor stem cells is due to differences in minor histocompatibility antigens. We are presently limited in our ability to assess these antigens. Male recipients express unique antigens encoded on the Y chromosome termed H-Y antigens. These H-Y antigens can be recognized as foreign by female donor cells in the context of HLA compatibility and trigger GVHD. The effect is most profound if the female donor has been allosensitized, generally by a prior pregnancy.[58–60] Other minor antigens include HA-1 and probably a multitude of MHC-restricted antigens that have not yet been identified.[59,61,62]

A high degree of donor T-cell chimerism, especially early after reduced-intensity conditioning regimens, is associated with an increased probability of acute GVHD, although it is not clear whether the high degree of chimerism is a risk factor for or a reflection of GVHD.[63]

Additional risk factors for the development of acute GVHD include older age of recipient, older age of donor, allosensitization of the donor (due to prior transfusions or pregnancy), disease stage, and conditioning regimen.[7,8,60,64–70] More controversial risk factors include certain HLA alleles,[67,71] prior splenectomy,[64,72] exposure to herpesviruses,[46] CD34 cell dose,[65] and ABO incompatibility.[73]

Staging and Grading of Acute GVHD

GVHD involvement of each organ is staged independently, and the composite score of liver, gut, and skin stage is considered in the (overall) GVHD grade. Pathologists have developed histologic grading systems to provide a semiquantitative estimate of severity. The histologic grade must not be confused with the clinical grade of GVHD. The original grading system was proposed by the Seattle group in 1974[6]; it was modified subsequently into a "consensus" system[74] (Table 1) and complemented by the International Bone Marrow Transplant Registry (IBMTR) GVHD severity index[12] (Table 2). This IBMTR system has been validated in a retrospective analysis, and severity as determined by this system is reflected in the incidence of transplant-related mortality. IBMTR levels A, B, C, and D roughly correspond to Glucksberg grades I, II, III, and IV, respectively.[11] If further clinical stud-

Table 1 Consensus grading of acute GVHD[74]

	Organ/Extent of Involvement		
	Skin	Liver	Intestinal Tract
Stage			
1	Rash on <25% of skin*	Bilirubin 2–3 mg/dL†	Diarrhea >500 mL/d‡ or persistent nausea§
2	Rash on 25–50% of skin	Bilirubin 3–6 mg/dL	Diarrhea >1,000 mL/d
3	Rash on >50% of skin	Bilirubin 6–15 mg/dL	Diarrhea >1,500 mL/d
4	Generalized erythroderma with bulla formation	Bilirubin >15 mg/dL	Severe abdominal pain with or without ileus
Grade			
0	None	None	None
I	Stage 1–2	None	None
II	Stage 3	or Stage 1	or Stage 1
III	—	Stage 2–3	or Stage 2–4
IV¶	Stage 4	or Stage 4	—

*Use the "rule of nines" to determine body surface area involvement.
†Range given as total bilirubin. Downgrade one stage if an additional cause of elevated bilirubin has been documented.
‡Volume of diarrhea applies to adults. For pediatric patients, the volume of diarrhea should be based on body surface area.
§Persistent nausea with histologic evidence of GVHD in the stomach or duodenum
¶Grade IV may also include lesser organ involvement but with extreme decrease in performance status

ies provide compelling evidence for manifestations of acute GVHD in other organs, such as the lungs, and for an impact of those organ manifestations on prognosis, these features may have to be considered in future grading systems.

The reason for the efforts that have been invested in GVHD grading is the establishment of a common basis for the conduct of clinical trials and, importantly, for prognosis. Mild to moderate GVHD (grades I or II [A or B]) is associated with little morbidity but is a significant risk factor for the development of subsequent chronic GVHD.[75] Grades III and IV (C and D) GVHD carry a grave prognosis: in grade IV GVHD (severity index D), mortality is 90% to 100%.

Syngeneic and Autologous GVHD

Occasionally, patients who have received autologous or syngeneic transplants will also develop a clinical syndrome that resembles GVHD, primarily manifest as a rash that usually responds promptly to corticosteroid therapy; a recent report suggested there may also be hepatic involvement.[76] The development of such a syndrome in the absence of an allogeneic barrier may be interpreted as evidence of a loss of tolerance to "self" that develops in the disrupted immune system. Hess and colleagues have proposed that infused T cells recognize MHC class II antigens in association with a peptide from the invariant chain (CLIP) (public determinants).[77,78] It is also possible that some cases of syngeneic GVHD reflected a mistaken assumption that the donor was syngeneic without the necessary molecular confirmation. An additional hypothesis was proposed by Nelson and colleagues, who showed that in some individuals maternal cells transmitted to them during their fetal development remain present throughout adult life.[79] In some instances, small numbers of HLA-incompatible cells (derived from the donor's mother) may be transmitted with HLA-identical transplants. Transplacentally transferred maternal cells may also play a role in the development of neonatal GVHD.[80]

Table 2 IBMTR Severity Index for Acute GVHD[12]

Index	Skin Stage		Gut Stage		Liver Stage
0	0		0		0
A	1	and	0	and	0
B	≤2		≤1	and/or	≤1*
	2	and	0	and	0
	≤2	and	≤2	and/or	≤2†
C	3	and	≤1	and	≤1
	≤3	and/or	≤3	and/or	≤3‡
D	≤4	and/or	≤4	and/or	≤4¶

*Either gut or liver = 1 but neither >1.
†Any organ = 2 but none >2.
‡Any organ = 3 but none >3.
¶Any organ = 4.

Transfusion-Associated GVHD

Most blood products administered to immunocompromised patients are now irradiated or at least leukocyte-depleted to avoid transfusion of viable alloreactive T cells. With most homologous blood products, MHC incompatibility between donor and recipient results in rapid clearance of transfused T cells by the recipient's immune system. However, occasionally transfusions from donors who are homozygous for one of the recipient's MHC haplotypes are not recognized as foreign by the recipient.[81] These cells can survive, "engraft," and then mount an immunologic attack against the unshared haplotype in the patient, resulting in transfusion-induced GVHD.[82,83] This syndrome of transfusion associated GVHD differs from GVHD occurring after transplantation in regards to its kinetics and its manifestations, as the recipient marrow is the major target. Since the number of stem cells in the offending blood product is inadequate, hematopoietic recovery from donor cells is impossible. Transfusion-associated GVHD is generally fatal due to refractory pancytopenia in addition to other organ involvement.

Summary and Conclusion

Acute GVHD is a complex clinical syndrome that occurs in a setting where the diagnosis may be difficult to establish. However, it is extremely important to recognize the disease, since the survival of patients may depend on the accuracy of the clinical diagnosis and prompt institution of therapy. It is not unusual for a patient with an elevated bilirubin to be treated aggressively with corticosteroids and to die of an opportunistic infection only to discover at postmortem examination that liver dysfunction was due to causes other than GVHD. There are no simple laboratory tests to facilitate the task. The diagnosis is left to clinical acumen, supported by tissue examination if possible.

References

1. Lorenz E, Uphoff D, Reid TR, et al: Modification of irradiation injury in mice and guinea pigs by bone marrow injections. J Natl Cancer Inst 12:197-201, 1951
2. Elkins WL: Cellular immunology and the pathogenesis of graft versus host reactions. Prog Allergy 15:78-187, 1971
3. van Bekkum DW, de Vries MJ: Radiation Chimaeras. London, UK, Logos Press, 1967
4. Billingham RE: The Biology of Graft-Versus-Host Reactions, The Harvey Lectures. New York, NY, Academic Press, 1966, pp 21-78
5. Mathé G, Jammet H, Pendic B, et al: Transfusions et greffes de moelle osseuse homologue chez des humains irradiés a haute dose accidentellement. Rev Franc Etudes Clin Biol 4:226-238, 1959
6. Glucksberg H, Storb R, Fefer A, et al: Clinical manifestations of graft-versus-host disease in human recipients of marrow from HL-A-matched sibling donors. Transplantation 18:295-304, 1974
7. Mielcarek M, Martin PJ, Leisenring W, et al: Graft-versus-host disease after nonmyeloablative versus conventional hematopoietic stem cell transplantation. Blood 102:756-762, 2003
8. Mielcarek M, Burroughs L, Leisenring W, et al: Prognostic relevance of "early-onset" graft-versus-host disease following nonmyeloablative hematopoietic cell transplantation. Br J Haematol 129:381-391, 2005
9. Flowers MED, Traina F, Storer B, et al: Serious graft-versus-host disease after hematopoietic cell transplantation following nonmyeloablative conditioning. Bone Marrow Transplant 35:277-282, 2005
10. Nash RA, Antin JH, Karanes C, et al: Phase 3 study comparing methotrexate and tacrolimus with methotrexate and CSP for prophylaxis of acute graft-versus-host disease after marrow transplantation from unrelated donors. Blood 96:2062-2068, 2000
11. Martin P, Nash R, Sanders J, et al: Reproducibility in retrospective grading of acute graft-versus-host disease after allogeneic marrow transplantation. Bone Marrow Transplant 21:273-279, 1998
12. Rowlings PA, Przepiorka D, Klein JP, et al: IBMTR Severity Index for grading acute graft-versus-host disease: Retrospective comparison with Glucksberg grade. Br J Haematol 97:855-864, 1997
13. Sullivan KM, Deeg HJ, Sanders J, et al: Hyperacute graft-v-host disease in patients not given immunosuppression after allogeneic marrow transplantation. Blood 67:1172-1175, 1986
14. Antin JH, Bierer BE, Smith BR, et al: Selective depletion of bone marrow T lymphocytes with anti-CD5 monoclonal antibodies: Effective prophylaxis for graft-versus-host disease in patients with hematologic malignancies. Blood 78:2139-2149, 1991
15. Antin JH, Ferrara JLM: Cytokine dysregulation and acute graft-versus-host disease. Blood 80:2964-2968, 1992
16. Spitzer TR: Engraftment syndrome following hematopoietic stem cell transplantation. Bone Marrow Transplant 27:893-898, 2001
17. Crider MK, Jansen J, Norins AL, et al: Chemotherapy-induced acral erythema in patients receiving bone marrow transplantation. Arch Dermatol 122:1023-1027, 1986
18. Akpek G, Boitnott JK, Lee LA, et al: Hepatitic variant of graft-versus-host disease after donor lymphocyte infusion. Blood 100:3903-3907, 2002
19. Shulman HM, Gooley T, Dudley MD, et al: Utility of transvenous liver biopsies and wedged hepatic venous pressure measurements in sixty marrow transplant recipients. Transplantation 59:1015-1022, 1995
20. Carreras E, Granena A, Navasa M, et al: Transjugular liver biopsy in BMT. Bone Marrow Transplant 11:21-26, 1993
21. Weisdorf DJ, Snover DC, Haake R, et al: Acute upper gastrointestinal graft-versus-host disease: Clinical significance and response to immunosuppressive therapy. Blood 76:624-629, 1990
22. Sale GE, Shulman HM, McDonald GB, et al: Gastrointestinal graft-versus-host disease in man. A clinicopathologic study of the rectal biopsy. Am J Surg Pathol 3:291-299, 1979
23. Kraus MD, Feran-Doza M, Garcia-Moliner ML, et al: Cytomegalovirus infection in the colon of bone marrow transplantation patients. Mod Pathol 11:29-36, 1998
24. Spencer GD, Hackman RC, McDonald GB, et al: A prospective study of unexplained nausea and vomiting after marrow transplantation. Transplantation 42:602-607, 1986
25. Wu D, Hockenbery DM, Brentnall TA, et al: Persistent nausea and anorexia after marrow transplantation: A prospective study of 78 patients. Transplantation 66:1319-1324, 1998
26. Klein SA, Martin H, Schreiber-Dietrich D, et al: A new approach to evaluating intestinal acute graft-versus-host disease by transabdominal sonography and colour Doppler imaging. Br J Haematol 115:929-934, 2001
27. Mentzel HJ, Kentouche K, Kosmehl H, et al: US and MRI of gastrointestinal graft-versus-host disease. Pediatr Radiol 32:195-198, 2002
28. Ho VT, Weller E, Lee SJ, et al: Prognostic factors for early severe pulmonary complications after hematopoietic stem cell transplantation. Biol Blood Marrow Transplant 7:223-229, 2001
29. Beschorner WE, Saral R, Hutchins GM, et al: Lymphocytic bronchitis associated with graft-versus-host disease in recipients of bone-marrow transplants. N Engl J Med 299:1030-1036, 1978
30. Padovan CS, Bise K, Hahn J, et al: Angiitis of the central nervous system after allogeneic bone marrow transplantation? Stroke 30:1651-1656, 1999
31. Takatsuka H, Okamoto T, Yamada S, et al: New imaging findings in a patient with central nervous system dysfunction after bone marrow transplantation. Acta Haematol 103:203-205, 2000
32. Lerner KG, Kao GF, Storb R, et al: Histopathology of graft-vs.-host reaction (GvHR) in human recipients of marrow from HL-A-matched sibling donors. Transplant Proc 6:367-371, 1974
33. Kohler S, Hendrickson MR, Chao NJ, et al: Value of skin biopsies in assessing prognosis and progression of acute graft-versus-host disease. Am J Surg Pathol 21:988-996, 1997
34. Zhou Y, Barnett MJ, Rivers JK: Clinical significance of skin biopsies in the diagnosis and management of graft-vs-host disease in early postallogeneic bone marrow transplantation. Arch Dermatol 136:717-721, 2000
35. Massi D, Franchi A, Pimpinelli N, et al: A reappraisal of the histopathologic criteria for the diagnosis of cutaneous allogeneic acute graft-vs-host disease. Am J Clin Pathol 112:791-800, 1999
36. Snover DC, Weisdorf SA, Ramsay NK, et al: Hepatic graft versus host disease: A study of the predictive value of liver biopsy in diagnosis. Hepatology 4:123-130, 1984
37. Shulman HM, Sharma P, Amos D, et al: A coded histologic study of hepatic graft-versus-host disease after human bone marrow transplantation. Hepatology 8:463-470, 1988
38. Atkinson K, Storb R, Prentice RL, et al: Analysis of late infections in 89

long-term survivors of bone marrow transplantation. Blood 53:720-731, 1979
39. Lee CK, Gingrich RD, Hohl RJ, et al: Engraftment syndrome in autologous bone marrow and peripheral stem cell transplantation. Bone Marrow Transplant 16:175-182, 1995
40. Ravoet C, Feremans W, Husson B, et al: Clinical evidence for an engraftment syndrome associated with early and steep neutrophil recovery after autologous blood stem cell transplantation. Bone Marrow Transplant 18:943-947, 1996
41. Cahill RA, Spitzer TR, Mazumder A: Marrow engraftment and clinical manifestations of capillary leak syndrome. Bone Marrow Transplant 18:177-184, 1996
42. Anderson BE, McNiff JM, Matte C, et al: Recipient CD4+ T cells that survive irradiation regulate chronic graft-versus-host disease. Blood 104:1565-1573, 2004
43. Sviland L, Pearson AD, Eastham EJ, et al: Histological features of skin and rectal biopsy specimens after autologous and allogeneic bone marrow transplantation. J Clin Pathol 41:148-154, 1988
44. Gleichmann E, Gleichmann H: Essential similarity between graft-versus-host disease and viral infections. Transplantation 22:399-401, 1976
45. Gratama JW, Stijnen T, Weiland HT, et al: Herpes-virus immunity and acute graft-versus-host disease. Lancet 741-743, 1987
46. Gratama JW, Sinnige LGF, Zwaan FE, et al: Marrow donor immunity to herpes simplex virus: Association with acute graft-versus-host disease. Exp Hematol 15:735-740, 1987
47. Sviland L, Dickinson AM: A human skin explant model for predicting graft-versus-host disease following bone marrow transplantation. J Clin Pathol 52:910-913, 1999
48. Vogelsang GB, Hess AD, Berkman AW, et al: An in vitro predictive test for graft versus host disease in patients with genotypic HLA-identical bone marrow transplants. N Engl J Med 313:645-650, 1985
49. Theobald M, Nierle T, Bunjes D, et al: Host-specific interleukin-2-secreting donor T-cell precursors as predictors of acute graft-versus-host disease in bone marrow transplantation between HLA-identical siblings. N Engl J Med 327:1613-1617, 1992
50. Dickinson AM, Sviland L, Wang XN, et al: Predicting graft-versus-host disease in HLA-identical bone marrow transplant: a comparison of T-cell frequency analysis and a human skin explant model. Transplantation 66:857-863, 1998
51. Wang XN, Taylor PR, Skinner R, et al: T-cell frequency analysis does not predict the incidence of graft-versus-host disease in HLA-matched sibling bone marrow transplantation. Transplantation 70:488-493, 2000
52. Nichols WC, Antin JH, Lunetta KL, et al: Polymorphism of adhesion molecule CD31 is not a significant risk factor for graft-versus-host disease. Blood 88:4429-4434, 1996
53. Dickinson AM, Cavet J, Cullup H, et al: GvHD risk assessment in hematopoietic stem cell transplantation: Role of cytokine gene polymorphisms and an in vitro human skin explant model. Hum Immunol 62:1266-1276, 2001
54. Rocha V, Franco RF, Porcher R, et al: Host defense and inflammatory gene polymorphisms are associated with outcomes after HLA-identical sibling bone marrow transplantation. Blood 100:3908-3918, 2002
55. Cullup H, Dickinson AM, Jackson GH, et al: Donor interleukin 1 receptor antagonist genotype associated with acute graft-versus-host disease in human leucocyte antigen-matched sibling allogeneic transplants. Br J Haematol 113:807-813, 2001
56. Takahashi H, Furukawa T, Hashimoto S, et al: Contribution of TNF-alpha and IL-10 gene polymorphisms to graft-versus-host disease following allo-hematopoietic stem cell transplantation. Bone Marrow Transplant 26:1317-1323, 2000
57. Lin M-T, Storer B, Martin PJ, et al: Relation of an interleukin-10 promoter polymorphism to graft-versus-host disease and survival after hematopoietic-cell transplantation. N Engl J Med 349:2201-2210, 2003
58. Rufer N, Wolpert E, Helg C, et al: HA-1 and the SMCY-derived peptide FIDSYICQV (H-Y) are immunodominant minor histocompatibility antigens after bone marrow transplantation. Transplantation 66:910-916, 1998
59. Goulmy E, Schipper J, Pool J, et al: Mismatches of minor histocompatibility antigens between HLA-identical donors and recipients and the development of graft-versus-host disease after bone marrow transplantation. N Engl J Med 334:281-285, 1996
60. Kollman C, Howe CWS, Anasetti C, et al: Donor characteristics as risk factors in recipients after transplantation of bone marrow from unrelated donors: the effect of donor age. Blood 98:2043-2051, 2001
61. Tseng L-H, Lin M-T, Hansen JA, et al: Correlation between disparity for the minor histocompatibility antigen HA-1 and the development of acute graft-versus-host disease after allogeneic marrow transplantation. Blood 94:2911-2914, 1999
62. Martin PJ: Increased disparity for minor histocompatibility antigens as a potential cause of increased GVHD risk in marrow transplantation from unrelated donors compared with related donors. Bone Marrow Transplant 8:217-223, 1991
63. Baron F, Baker JE, Storb R, et al: Kinetics of engraftment in patients with hematologic malignancies given allogeneic hematopoietic cell transplantation after nonmyeloablative conditioning. Blood 104:2254-2262, 2004
64. Hagglund H, Bostrom L, Remberger M, et al: Risk factors for acute graft-versus-host disease in 291 consecutive HLA-identical bone marrow transplant recipients. Bone Marrow Transplant 16: 747-753, 1995
65. Przepiorka D, Smith TL, Folloder J, et al: Risk factors for acute graft-versus-host disease after allogeneic blood stem cell transplantation. Blood 94:1465-1470, 1999
66. Nash RA, Pepe MS, Storb R, et al: Acute graft-versus-host disease: analysis of risk factors after allogeneic marrow transplantation and prophylaxis with cyclosporine and methotrexate. Blood 80:1838-1845, 1992
67. Bross DS, Tutschka PJ, Farmer ER, et al: Predictive factors for acute graft-versus-host disease in patients transplanted with HLA-identical bone marrow. Blood 63:1265-1270, 1984
68. Gale RP, Bortin MM, van Bekkum DW, et al: Risk factors for acute graft-versus-host disease. Br J Haematol 67:397-406, 1987
69. Weisdorf D, Hakke R, Blazar B, et al: Risk factors for acute graft-versus-host disease in histocompatible donor bone marrow transplantation. Transplantation 51:1197-1203, 1991
70. Nakai K, Mineishi S, Kami M, et al: Antithymocyte globulin affects the occurrence of acute and chronic graft-versus-host disease after a reduced-intensity conditioning regimen by modulating mixed chimerism induction and immune reconstitution. Transplantation 75:2135-2143, 2003
71. Storb R, Prentice RL, Hansen JA, et al: Association between HLA-B antigens and acute graft-versus-host disease. Lancet 2:816-819, 1983
72. Baughan AS, Worsley AM, McCarthy DM, et al: Haematological reconstitution and severity of graft-versus-host disease after bone marrow transplantation for chronic granulocytic leukaemia: The influence of previous splenectomy. Br J Haematol 56:445-454, 1984
73. Bacigalupo A, Van Lint MT, Occhini D, et al: ABO compatibility and acute graft-versus-host disease following allogeneic bone marrow transplantation. Transplantation 45:1091-1094, 1988
74. Przepiorka D, Weisdorf D, Martin P, et al: 1994 Consensus conference on acute GVHD grading. Bone Marrow Transplant 15:825-828, 1995
75. Anasetti C, Doney KC, Storb R, et al: Marrow transplantation for severe aplastic anemia: Long term outcome in fifty "untransfused" patients. Ann Intern Med 104:461-466, 1986
76. Saunders MD, Shulman HM, Murakami CS, et al: Bile duct apoptosis and cholestasis resembling acute graft-versus-host disease after autologous hematopoietic cell transplantation. Am J Surg Pathol 24:1004-1008, 2000
77. Hess AD, Bright EC, Thoburn C, et al: Specificity of effector T lymphocytes in autologous graft-versus-host disease: role of the major histocompatibility complex class II invariant chain peptide. Blood 89:2203-2209, 1997
78. Hess AD, Horwitz L, Beschorner WE, et al: Development of graft-vs.-host disease-like syndrome in cyclosporine-treated rats after syngeneic

bone marrow transplantation. I. Development of cytotoxic T lymphocytes with apparent polyclonal anti-Ia specificity, including autoreactivity. J Exp Med 161:718-730, 1985
79. Nelson JL: Microchimerism: Incidental byproduct of pregnancy or active participant in human health? Trends Mol Med 8:109-113, 2002
80. Adams KM, Holmberg LA, Leisenring W, et al: Risk factors for syngeneic graft-versus-host disease after adult hematopoietic cell transplantation. Blood 104:1894-1897, 2004
81. Juji T, Takahashi K, Shibata Y, et al: Post-transfusion graft-versus-host disease in immunocompetent patients after cardiac surgery in Japan. N Engl J Med 321:56, 1989 (letter)
82. Greenbaum BH: Transfusion-associated graft-versus-host disease: Historical perspectives, incidence, and current use of irradiated blood products. J Clin Oncol 9:1889-1902, 1991
83. Anderson KC, Weinstein HJ: Transfusion-associated graft-versus-host disease. N Engl J Med 323:315-321, 1990

ELSEVIER

Seminars in
HEMATOLOGY

Prophylaxis and Treatment of Acute Graft-Versus-Host Disease

Nelson J. Chao and Benny J. Chen

Acute graft-versus-host disease (GVHD) remains a major obstacle to successful allogeneic hematopoietic stem cell transplantation (HSCT). The ability to prevent GVHD—the application of successful prophylaxis—is crucial as treatment when prophylaxis fails or remains suboptimal. A calcineurin inhibitor in combination with methotrexate is still the mainstream regimen for prophylaxis of GVHD. Despite a steady increase in the repertoire of available drugs, corticosteroids remain the first-line therapy for patients who fail prevention and develop GVHD. Pan T-cell depletion studies suggest that success in prophylaxis and treatment of GVHD will depend on whether GVHD can be prevented without losing anti-malignancy and anti-infectious effects. Better understanding of the allogeneic response that is responsible for GVHD will facilitate the development of such an approach.
Semin Hematol 43:32-41

Graft-versus-host disease (GVHD) remains a major obstacle to successful allogeneic hematopoietic stem cell transplantation (HSCT), causing significant morbidity and mortality even when recipient and donor are matched at the major histocompatibility complex (MHC), termed human leukocyte antigen (HLA).[1] In its acute and chronic forms, GVHD has an important impact on survival and the recipient's quality of life.[2] The ability to prevent GVHD, the application of successful prophylaxis, is crucial as treatment when prophylaxis fails or remains suboptimal. An improving understanding of the pathophysiology of GVHD has led to rational approaches to both prophylaxis and therapy.

GVHD is a continuous process with afferent and efferent phases related to a "cytokine storm" that is triggered by the toxicity of the preparatory regimen with resultant tissue damage and endotoxemia.[3] Steps in this cascade present opportunities to block or attenuate the signals that lead to cytokine release, antigen presentation, costimulation, innate immunity signaling, T-cell activation, T-cell trafficking, recruitment and expansion of T cells and other possible effector cells, including both proinflammatory and regulatory cells.

Yet the presence of GVHD is not necessarily entirely negative[4]: GVHD is associated with a graft-versus-leukemia (GVL) or graft-versus-malignancy effect. GVHD and GVL are intricately related and difficult to separate. A significant portion of the curative potential of an allogeneic stem cell graft is directly related to the anti-malignancy effect of the donor T cells.[4] These initial observations have been validated by the results of donor lymphocyte infusions (DLIs) to treat the underlying disease in patients who have relapsed following allogeneic stem cell grafting.[5] The nonmyeloablative allogeneic stem cell approach is directly related to the ability to induce a chimeric state and GVL through donor cells. Thus, the goal of any approach for prophylaxis and treatment of GVHD is not only to effectively control GVHD but also to simultaneously preserve the anti-malignancy as well as anti-pathogen effects.

Overview

Pretransplant Phase

The stage for GVHD is set even before donor cells are infused. Perhaps the simplest maneuver is controlling the environment. Experimental data show a reduction in the incidence of GVHD following HSCT in gnotobiotic (germ-free) mice.[6] In clinical studies, gut decontamination and isolation in laminar air-flow rooms may decrease the incidence and severity of GVHD in selected allogeneic HSCT patients.[7]

The choice of conditioning (or preparative) regimen plays an important role in the development of GVHD.[8] Myeloablative regimens used to treat the patient's underlying disease and to immunosuppress the host result in multi-organ damage, especially to the gastrointestinal mucosa. Damaged or activated cells from recipient tissues secrete many inflamma-

Division of Cellular Therapy/Bone Marrow Transplantation, Department of Medicine and Immunology, Duke University Medical Center, Durham, NC.

Address correspondence to Nelson J. Chao, MD, Division of Cellular Therapy/BMT, Duke University Medical Center, 2400 Pratt St, Suite 1100, Box 3961, Durham, NC 27705. E-mail: chao0002@mc.duke.edu

 0037-1963/06/$-see front matter
doi:10.1053/j.seminhematol.2005.09.007

tory cytokines, such as interleukin-1 (IL-1), tumor necrosis factor-alpha (TNFα), granulocyte-macrophage colony-stimulating factor (GM-CSF), and interferon-gamma (IFN-γ).[8] Increased levels of these cytokines leads to increased expression of adhesion molecules and MHC molecules and to T-cell activation.[8] There is a correlation between the intensity of the conditioning regimen and GVHD in animal models and in human recipients of HSCT.[9,10] In some experimental and clinical studies, delaying the transfer of donor cells until well after conditioning results in a decreased risk of acute GVHD.[11,12] Therefore, one method for diminishing the severity and rate of acute GVHD is to reduce the intensity of the conditioning regimen, as in current nonmyeloablative regimens. For example, high doses of radiation and chemotherapy cause damage to the endothelial lining of the gut, allowing bacteria and lipopolysaccharides (LPS), a well-known stimulus for TNFα and other cytokines, to enter the circulation. Increased serum TNFα levels were found in patients who developed GVHD.[13] These signaling molecules are critical also in stimulating the innate immunity of the host. A monoclonal antibody (mAB) against endotoxin protected mice against GVHD,[14] while anti-TNFα mAB has some utility in treating patients with acute GVHD.[15] Experimental data suggest that keratinocyte-growth factor (KGF) may be protective against GVHD while preserving GVL.[16,17] The mechanism of action of KGF may be the prevention of mucosal damage and subsequent bacterial and LPS translocation from gut to circulation.

Another method of preventing GVHD by modification of the preparatory regimen is to include anti-thymocyte globulin (ATG); the intent is to decrease the incidence of graft rejection and possibly prevent GVHD. Results have varied.[18,19] Recent data in unrelated donor transplants[20] suggest that ATG is useful for the prevention of grades III to IV GVHD, but this benefit did not translate into lower treatment-related mortality because of increased infections. While survival was not different from that observed in patients not given ATG, the incidence of extensive chronic GVHD was markedly reduced and the quality of life improved in patients receiving ATG.

T-Cell Activation Phase

Most strategies of GVHD prophylaxis are aimed at the activation (induction)/expansion phase of donor T cells, critical for the induction of the disease. Following the infusion of allogeneic cells, immunologically competent donor T cells, via their T-cell receptors (TCRs), recognize foreign antigens presented by donor or host antigen-presenting cells (APC) in the context of the MHC. The APCs present foreign antigens as peptides bound to their MHC molecules, thereby initiating the first step in the immune response. The peptides bound to the same MHC are derived from various proteins and serve as minor histocompatibility antigens (miH) and as targets of the donor T cells.[21] Mismatches of miH antigens between donor and recipient in HLA-identical HSCT may be associated with significant GVHD.[22]

Donor T-cell activation requires multiple signaling events. Innate immunity likely plays a role in GVHD, considering the extent of gut toxicity in recipients of ablative regimens. While these signaling molecules have not been definitively linked with acute GVHD, they appear to be important in chronic GVHD. The adaptive immune response with its TCR–peptide–MHC interactions provides the first signal.[23] The second, a costimulatory signal, is provided by additional molecules on APCs and requires cell-to-cell contact.[24] The outcome of the first signal is regulated by the second signal, resulting either in complete activation, partial activation, or anergy, a long-lasting state of antigen-specific unresponsiveness. Several costimulatory molecules have been identified; B7-1 (CD80) and B7-2 (CD86) are the best characterized. CD28 and CTLA-4 are two T-cell surface receptors bound by B7 ligands. Normally, a signal from the TCR, a costimulatory signal from CD28, and an inhibitory signal from CTLA-4 determine the outcome of T-cell activation.[25,26] In the absence of a CD28 costimulatory signal, signaling through the TCR complex ultimately results in anergy. CTLA-4-Ig, a molecule created by fusion CTLA-4 with an immunoglobulin chain, blocks T-cell costimulation through the B7-CD28 signal pathway and thus induces a state of anergy.[24] One method for the prevention of GVHD would be the induction of a state of clonal anergy that is specific for host allogeneic antigens. In a clinical study of 12 patients who received one full haplotype-mismatched allogeneic HSCT, incubation of donor cells with CTLA-4-Ig was used to induce a state of anergy.[27] All patients successfully engrafted, and only three developed GVHD. These encouraging results need to be confirmed with larger numbers of patients.

Another molecule that may affect signaling through the CD28 molecule is sirolimus (rapamycin).[28] Sirolimus specifically inhibits the progression of cells from G1 into the S phase, and it may interfere with the signaling that is critical for the cyclin-cdk complex required for cellular proliferation. In human peripheral blood T cells, block of G1 may be related to an increase in a species of titratable inhibitor of G1 cyclin-cdk.[29,30] In addition to regulation of the cell cycle, sirolimus may also exert an effect in signal transduction pathways that mediate specific cytokine responses. For example, sirolimus has been shown to inhibit IL-1–driven IFN-γ production.[31] While signaling through the TCR is not affected, signaling through CD28 is inhibited by sirolimus[32]; CD28 signaling leads to a sustained downregulation of the inhibitor I kappa B (IkB). CD28-mediated downregulation of IkB alpha is prevented by sirolimus. Sirolimus' effects on the CD28 signaling pathway may be a mechanism of its action, distinct from that of other immunosuppressive drugs. Sirolimus also can selectively expand $CD4^+CD25^+$ regulatory T cells (Tregs).[33]

If a T cell engages its TCRs and receives a costimulatory signal, T-cell activation ensues. Activation is multi-step and involves calcium-dependent signal transduction pathways. Critical molecules in this pathway include calmodulin, calcineurin, and nuclear factor of activated T cells (NF-AT). The activation cascade following the first and second activation signals leads to calcium influx; calcium binds to calmodulin that in turn binds to calcineurin. The activated calcineurin triggers the dephosphorylation of the cytoplasmic unit of NF-AT. As a result, NF-AT translocates from the cytoplasm into the nucleus to form a competent transcriptional activator of the IL-2 gene. IL-2 is the critical survival and activation cytokine for T cells.

T-cell activation through the IL-2 pathway is prevented by cyclosporine or tacrolimus, which inhibit calcineurin. Both drugs, studied in phase III randomized trials, are effective in the prevention of acute GVHD. Usually, cyclosporine or tacrolimus is utilized in combination with methotrexate. The precise mechanism of action of methotrexate is unknown, although it likely acts as an anti-metabolite. Pharmacologic prophylaxis of GVHD with methotrexate was adopted early in the clinic after experiments in dogs showed that it decreased the incidence and severity of GVHD.[34] Various combinations of methotrexate, cyclosporine, FK 506, and glucocorticoids are widely used as GVHD prophylaxis. Pharmacologic GVHD prophylaxis is generally administered in the immediate post-transplant period, gradually tapered after 100 days, and stopped 6 to 12 months after transplantation (if no GVHD is present). The most utilized regimen is the combination of methotrexate and cyclosporine.[35]

Immunosuppression with pharmacologic agents such as cyclosporine or tacrolimus and methotrexate is more effective when drug combinations are used than with single agents.[35] There is a survival advantage for patients who receive a combination of cyclosporine and methotrexate compared to either drug alone.[36] Cyclosporine or tacrolimus is generally initiated from day −2; both are usually administered intravenously for the first several weeks, when patients are recovering from toxicities of the preparatory regimen. Because the oral mucosa and gastrointestinal tract are not healed, oral cyclosporine or tacrolimus may be difficult to tolerate and may be erratically absorbed. While these drugs are administered to achieve what are considered therapeutic target concentrations, no study to date has demonstrated a clear correlation of blood drug levels and GVHD prevention. Since both cyclosporine and tacrolimus can damage the kidneys, other nephrotoxic drugs should be avoided if possible so that the calcineurin inhibitors can be delivered at adequate doses. Use of leucovorin rescue following administration of methotrexate may be necessary in patients with severe side effects and has been advocated as a standard measure by some investigators, who have shown that such an approach does not increase the risk of GVHD.[37]

In several randomized studies comparing tacrolimus to cyclosporine,[38,39] tacrolimus was superior for the prophylaxis of acute GVHD but without a resulting survival advantage. In a large multicenter trial, 329 recipients of HLA-identical marrow transplants were randomized to receive a short course of methotrexate plus either tacrolimus or cyclosporine.[38] Although a significantly greater proportion of patients with advanced disease were randomized to tacrolimus, the incidence of grades II to IV acute GVHD was significantly lower in patients who received tacrolimus (32% *v* 44% with cyclosporine). This difference was largely due to a reduction in grade II disease. The incidence of chronic GVHD was similar in the two groups (56% and 49% respectively), but extensive chronic disease was more likely with cyclosporine. However, 2-year survival was lower with tacrolimus (41% *v* 50% with cyclosporine), as was overall survival (47% *v* 57% with cyclosporine). These differences were mostly due to poorer survival of patients with advanced disease (25% *v* 42% for tacrolimus and cyclosporine, respectively). A second clinical trial demonstrated similar results with less acute GVHD and a lower need for glucocorticoid therapy with tacrolimus than with cyclosporine (65% *v* 81%, respectively; $P = .019$),[39] but again no statistically significant difference in overall survival.

If there is no evidence of GVHD, cyclosporine or tacrolimus may be tapered at approximately day +90 and discontinued at 6 months in HLA-identical sibling transplants. In mismatched related or matched unrelated donor transplants, calcineurin inhibitors may need to be administered longer, sometimes even for years. A slower taper may be preferable in older patients to prevent the development of chronic GVHD. Patients must be carefully monitored during the taper for signs of incipient chronic GVHD.

Another potentially useful drug during this phase of T-cell activation is mycophenolate mofetil (MMF). MMF is a morpholinoethyl ester of mycophenolic acid (MPA). MMF inhibits the proliferation of T and B cells and the production of antibodies.[40] Purines are essential for the growth and survival of cells; T cells have two pathways to produce purines: de novo and salvage pathways. Activated lymphocytes are highly dependent on de novo synthesis while resting cells can utilize both pathways. For de novo synthesis, the ribose-phosphate portion of the purine nucleotide is derived from 5-phosphoribosyl-1-pyrophosphate, in turn a product of adenosine triphosphate and the sugar ribose-5-phosphate. Therefore, 5-phosphoribosyl-1-pyrophosphate is an essential intermediary in the synthesis of purines. Following T-cell stimulation, there is a brisk and sustained increase in 5-phosphoribosyl-1-pyrophosphate and guanosines and deoxyguanosines activate 5-phosphoribosyl-1-pyrophosphate synthetase.[41] Therefore depletion of guanosines would lead to a decrease in 5-phosphoribosyl-1-pyrophosphate synthetase and inhibition of the purine synthesis that is required for T-cell activation. MPA acts through the inhibition of inosine monophosphate dehydrogenase (IMPDH). This enzyme catalyzes oxidation of inosine monophosphate to xanthine monophosphate. Xanthine monophosphate is a required intermediate metabolite in the synthesis of guanosine triphosphate. The enzyme IMPDH is critical for the de novo biosynthesis of purine nucleotides, specifically guanosine monophosphate (GMP). Blockade of GMP synthesis leads to a negative feedback inhibition of 5-phosphoribosyl-1-pyrophosphate and prevention of T-cell activation. The therapeutic index of MMF depends on the lymphocyte reliance on de novo synthesis of purines, allowing for greater immunosuppressive activity with less toxicity.

Studies in a dog model of allogeneic transplantation showed the combination of MMF/cyclosporine to be highly effective in the prevention of host-versus-graft (rejection) and GVHD following a nonmyeloablative (reduced intensity) conditioning regimen.[42] Current studies suggest that post-transplant immunosuppression with MMF is useful in establishing donor chimerism.

Effector Phase

Once T cells are activated and begin to proliferate, they and associated immune cells release a variety of proinflammatory cytokines. Cytokines are important in various steps of the GVHD: in the initial stimulation of T cells but also in the maintenance of the efferent phase, when the disease manifests in toxicity to the skin, gut, and liver.[43] T cells driven by cross-linking of their TCR with the peptide bound to the MHC molecule divide and proliferate, developing into cytotoxic T cells that utilize both perforin and granzyme B to kill targets.[44] Nonspecific mechanisms to attenuate the inflammatory cascade, using histone deacetylase inhibitor suberoylanilide hydroxamic acid, also appear to reduce acute GVHD while preserving GVL.[45]

There are at least two types of T-helper (Th) cells, Th1 and Th2, classified based on the cytokines they produce and the cytokines to which they respond. Th1 cells produce IL-2 and IFN-γ; Th2 cells produce IL-4, IL-6, and IL-10. Th1 cells make and use IL-2 for their proliferation; Th2 cells produce IL-4 and require IL-1 or IL-4 for proliferation. A preponderance of Th1 cells could lead to activation of cytotoxic T lymphocytes (CTLs) and subsequent GVHD, compared to an abundance of Th2 cells, which promote a humoral response and prevention of GVHD.[45,46] Therefore, if donor T cells are driven by IL-10 toward a Th2 phenotype prior to their transfer into the host, alloreactivity may be modified and not cause GVHD. Allogeneic CD4^{+} T cells (activated in the presence of IL-10) show a state of long-term anergy.[47]

These laboratory conclusions have been supported by recent clinical studies.[48] Although the donor T-cell dose in the transplant inoculum is higher in allogeneic peripheral blood cells compared to nonmobilized marrow, use of this stem cell source did not result in an increased risk of acute GVHD, which may be attributable to donor progenitor cell mobilization with G-CSF, which polarizes donor T cells towards Th2.[49] There also is evidence that the function of CD14^{+} monocytes, which serve as APCs, is altered. While there is no increased risk of acute GVHD with allogeneic peripheral blood stem cell transplant, there is a tendency toward increased chronic GVHD.[50] Th1-type cytokines (such as IL-2 and IFN-γ) are invoked in inducing GVHD and thus deleterious, whereas Th2-type cytokines (IL-4 and IL-10) are considered suppressive and therefore protective of GVHD. The paradigm, however, may not be so simple in practice, and contradictory data also exist.[51]

As with most biologic processes, there are regulatory compensatory mechanisms in place to attenuate immune responses. Recent murine studies have identified subsets of T cells that act in a regulatory capacity to suppress the function of other T cells. The physiologic role of such Tregs is to dampen immune responses against viruses, tumors, and self-antigens.[52] There are several families of such Tregs; the naturally occurring Tregs that have been most studied belong to the CD4^{+} subset, constitutively express CD25^{hi}, and are Foxp3-positive. These Tregs exhibit a partially activated phenotype but are hypo-responsive to activation and proliferation stimuli. Naturally occurring Tregs are antigen-specific in that their generation and activation to effector function (the suppression of other T cells) require engagement of antigen and TCR signaling. After activation, suppression does not appear to be antigen-specific. Treg function is locally restricted, and they can inhibit both CD4^{+} and CD8^{+} T cells. In animal models, removal of Tregs has resulted in an increase in GVHD responses, whereas infusion of CD4^{+}CD25^{+} cells resulted in inhibition of GVHD.[53,54] These results suggest a potent immunomodulatory effect for such cells and raise the possibility that transfer of these cells in patients could be of clinical benefit. One area of concern however, is that the importance of Tregs is not limited to self-tolerance and the prevention of autoimmunity. Depletion of regulatory cells has led to increased tumor-specific immune responses and eradication of tumors in otherwise nonresponding animals.[55] Therefore, the addition of Tregs could possibly down modulate a GVL effect as well. Clinical trials are necessary to clarify the impact of these potential interactions.

Modulating T-Cell Response

Pan T-Cell Depletion

The sections above deal with T-cell–replete stem cell transplantation. Clearly, if T cells are not present, GVHD does not occur since GVHD is a T-cell–mediated disease.[56] In animal experiments and clinical trials, GVHD can be effectively prevented by vigorous depletion of T cells.[57] Patients who receive an adequately T-cell–depleted graft will not develop GVHD. However, nonspecific T-cell depletion results in an increase in the incidence of rejection, relapse, and a delay in immune recovery with a higher incidence of infectious complications.[57] These observations have led to the search for strategies that can selectively deplete GVHD-inducing T-cell subsets rather than total T cells (see below).

Removal of Alloreactive T Cells

The GVL effect may be mediated by both host histocompatibility antigen-specific T cells, which also mediate GVHD, and tumor antigen-specific T cells, which do not induce GVHD.[58] In principle, if tumor-specific antigens are different from the miH that cause GVHD, the GVL effect could be separated from GVHD. Elegant studies of TCR Vb chain usage suggest that predominantly oligoclonal T-cell responses are associated with GVHD.[59] Separation of GVHD and GVL could be accomplished by selectively depleting anti-host histocompatibility antigen-specific T cells (Fig 1). Several methods might specifically remove the allogeneic responsive T cells. In experimental models, host histocompatibility antigen-specific T cells activated by the host antigens ex vivo have been successfully depleted or tolerized, without impairing anti-leukemia or anti–third-party effect by targeting host-activated T cells.[27,60–64] Most strategies have used an antibody to target CD25.

We have utilized a photodynamic process, rhodamine dye

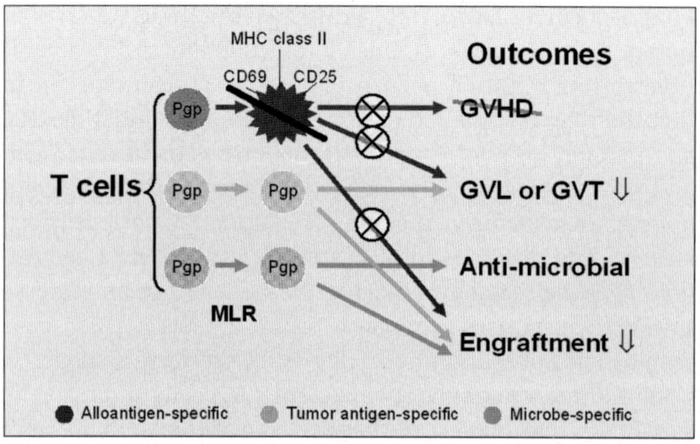

Figure 1 Activation-based alloreactive T-cell depletion for prevention of GVHD. MLR, mixed lymphocyte reaction; Pgp, P-glycoprotein 170; GVHD, graft-versus-host disease; GVL, graft-versus-leukemia; GVT, graft-versus-tumor.

and light, to selectively deplete donor anti-host histocompatibility antigen-specific T cells in order to reduce GVHD while preserving the GVL effect and anti–third-party responses.[65] Host-specific cytotoxic T cells as well as host-specific IFN-γ–secreting cells were significantly eliminated after this process of photodynamic purging, while third party-specific cells were mostly retained and tumor cell-specific cells were partly preserved. Selective depletion of host antigen-specific cytotoxic T cells and cytokine-producing cells explains how such a treatment of primed T cells prevented anti-same party GVHD; both GVL and anti–third-party effects are preserved. Allogeneic T cells stimulated by host antigens and then treated with rhodamine dye could provide both GVL and anti-pathogen immunity, either administered with hematopoietic stem cells or as a T-cell source for delayed lymphocyte infusion.[27] To preserve GVL without causing GVHD, responding T cells need to be activated exclusively by host histocompatibility antigens, without contamination from tumor antigens; host histocompatibility antigens and tumor-specific antigens would have to be unique. In the clinical setting dendritic cells (DCs) derived from bone marrow progenitor cells might serve as APCs; using DCs as APCs may minimize the contamination of tumor antigens in the culture. Similar results were obtained in human cells in vitro.[66]

Targeting of CD25 has been tested in phase I/II clinical trials in France[67] and by the National Institutes of Health.[68] T cells are activated by recipient cells derived from the peripheral blood and then treated with anti-CD25 immunotoxin to remove the activated cells. Patients are then grafted with $CD34^+$ cells plus the treated donor T cells. No immunosuppressant or only cyclosporine is used post-transplantation. The incidence and severity of GVHD was dramatically decreased; the French trial also demonstrated more rapid immune reconstitution. However, enhancement of GVL has yet to be proven in either protocol, which may be due to the relative small number of T cells infused.

Removal of Naive T Cells

Another potential manipulation of T cells would be directed at subpopulations of T cells that are primarily responsible for the induction of GVHD. Our laboratory has been interested in selecting T cells based on their naïve or memory phenotype.[69] Naive T cells ($CD62L^+$) are T cells that have never encountered antigens specific for their TCR. Memory/effector T cells (which can be either $CD62L^-$ or $CD62L^+$) are T cells that have previously been exposed to their corresponding antigens. If a donor T cell has not encountered host alloantigens, GVHD-inducing T cells should reside in the naive T-cell compartment. Since the donor has not encountered host alloantigen, the population of memory/effector T cells will not be host alloantigen-specific and therefore unable to induce GVHD. In vitro mixed lymphocyte culture studies demonstrate that the proliferative potential of the allogeneic cells was mainly in the naive cell population, as defined by the CD62L marker. When we separated the naïve phenotype from the memory phenotype cells, GVHD induction was robust in the naive phenotype in vivo whereas memory cells did not cause GVHD. Moreover, memory cells immunized against BCL1 (a leukemia/lymphoma cell) retained the ability to proliferate and to protect the animal against a challenge of tumor cells without causing GVHD in third-party recipients. Similar results were recently reported by other laboratories.[70–72] It may be possible to infuse selected memory cells, which would endow the recipient with cells incapable of causing GVHD while at the same time transferring the important memory cells protective against infectious agents. Antitumor effects could also be transferred through prior immunization against the tumor antigens, by post-transplant adoptive transfer of anti-tumor effector cells, or through active immunization.

Insertion of Suicide Genes

Another method of T-cell selection is to insert a specific marker gene that would allow T cells that have become activated to be selectively depleted should GVHD occur.[73] Donor lymphocytes transduced with the herpes simplex virus thymidine kinase (HSV-tk) gene can be infused into patients alone or as part of an initial graft. If GVHD should occur, treatment with ganciclovir would eliminate these cells. Eight patients who had relapsed or developed Epstein-Barr virus-induced lymphoma after T-cell–depleted HSCT were treated with donor lymphocytes transduced with the HSV-tk suicide gene; the transduced lymphocytes led to anti-tumor activity in five patients. When three patients developed GVHD, it was effectively controlled by treatment with ganciclovir, leading to elimination of the transduced cells. Thus genetic manipulation of donor lymphocytes can lead to the ability to remove undesired toxicity such as GVHD.

Minor Histocompatibility Antigen-Specific T Cells

T cells specific to some miHs mediate GVL effect without causing GVHD[74]; it seems that this separation of GVL effect from GVHD is due to a lower level of expression of the target miH on GVHD target organs as compared with hematopoietic cells. The efficacy of this strategy to mediate GVL needs to be tested in humans.

Allogeneic Natural Killer Cells

Another cellular component that may prevent GVHD is the natural killer (NK) cell. NK cells are innate immune lymphocytes critical to host defense against invading infectious pathogens and malignant transformation. NK cells act through elaboration of cytokines and cytolytic activity, which are regulated by specific receptors that recognize self antigens in the context of classical and non-classical HLA class I molecules.[75] Functionally, NK cells are an important source of innate immunoregulatory cytokines (IFN-γ, TNFα, GM-CSF) that play an important role in immune responses. Recent murine experiments in stem cell transplantation across MHC barriers suggest that NK cells facilitate engraftment while at the same time preventing GVHD.[76] In these mice, pretransplant infusion of alloreactive NK cells into the recipient eliminated the need for high-intensity conditioning and reduced the incidence of GVHD. NK cell alloreactivity could be exploited clinically to prevent GVHD. Recent studies from Perugia[76] have demonstrated remarkable activity of these NK cells in recipients of haploidentical HSCT. Patients with myeloid (but not lymphoid) leukemia had a marked difference in relapse if donor NK cells could function in the recipient (mismatched killer inhibitory receptors [KIRs]), compared to those who where matched (a setting in which NK cells would not be activated).

Natural Killer T Cells

Natural killer T (NKT) cells are a unique subset of T cells that share receptor structures with conventional T lymphocytes and NK cells.[77,78] NKT cells recognize glycolipid antigens presented by MHC class I-like CD1d. Upon activation, NKT cells secrete a large amount of IL-4 and promote a Th2 response. Infusion of NKT cells protects against lethal GVHD as demonstrated in a murine model[79]; IL-4 is required for the protection.

Treatment of Acute GVHD

In general, acute GVHD grade II or greater is an indication for treatment, but the timing of treatment varies between centers and may differ for subgroups of patients. Replacing cyclosporine with FK 506 has been suggested by some investigators for patients who fail to respond to cyclosporine, but in a careful analysis from Seattle, only two of 20 patients with resistant GVHD responded to this tactic.[80] Also, substituting FK 506 for cyclosporine did not improve microangiopathic hemolytic anemia but did benefit patients with cyclosporine-associated neurotoxicity.

Corticosteroids

Corticosteroids remain first-line therapy.[81] Their mechanism of action may be directly cytotoxic or a pro-apoptotic action on lymphocytes; however, there is evidence of an anti-inflammatory effect resulting in suppression of cytokine production[82] or modulation of adhesion molecules may also contribute to responses. Despite general acceptance of corticosteroids, a broad spectrum of drug doses and schedules has been employed.[83] Doses between 1 and 20 mg/kg/d of (methyl)-prednisolone have been administered. In a randomized trial comparing 2mg/kg versus 10mg/kg of methylprednisolone, there were minor advantages with regard to response rates for the high-dose regimen in young patients at the cost of a higher rate of infection.[84] Most widely used are initial doses of 2 mg/kg/d or 60 mg/m^2/d. Improvement of results of initial treatment must be a priority, as the response to corticosteroids has predicted long-term results in almost all trials reported: 50% to 60% of patients achieving stable responses to first-line treatment of GVHD survived, whereas long-term survival was only 5% to 30% in patients with corticosteroid-resistant GVHD.

In large retrospective series[85,86] as well as in prospective trials, 25% to 35% of patients have shown complete resolution of GVHD, and an additional 15% have experienced improvement. More rapid tapering may be equivalent to prolonged tapering for the end points of GVHD reactivation as well as long-term outcome.[87] Whether differences in tapering schedules or any distinct regimen translate into less severe long-term side effects of corticosteroid treatment (such as osteoporosis or osteonecrosis) remains uncertain. As the use of less intensive conditioning regimens allows an increasing number of older patients to be transplanted, the long-term effects of corticosteroid treatment have become more important.

Agents with potential therapeutic efficacy have been added to corticosteroids in treatment regimens: ricin A-conjugated anti-CD5 mABs,[88] anti-CD25 mAB,[89]or a murine mAB neutralizing TNFα (MAK195F).[82] While response rates tend to be higher, long-term survival was not significantly improved over that observed with corticosteroids alone. Agents such as etanercept are now being investigated at several institutions. Some recent pilot trials suggest that the addition of polyclonal ATGs might improve not only GVHD responses but also outcome. However, randomized studies[90] thus far have failed to show superiority.

Disappointing results with attempts aimed at improving the results of first treatment of GVHD might reflect the clinical heterogeneity of patients with regard to prognosis and subsequent severity of GVHD. Early predictive parameters allowing for identification of high versus standard risk GVHD might help to individualize first-line immunosuppressive therapy of GVHD. Broadly used surrogate parameters would be most useful. The Genova group recently suggested to use ATG pre-emptively in patients with elevated bilirubin and blood urea levels at day +7.[91] Transplant-related mortality was reduced as compared to historical controls; a prospective trial has been initiated. Any single molecule with a narrow target may be unlikely to successfully terminate an active immune response and combinations of these newer molecules may be necessary.

Also unresolved is whether GVHD manifestations should be treated in a more organ-specific manner. In animal models, different effector molecules were involved in skin versus gut and liver GVHD with a prominent role of TNFα in skin and gut GVHD and fas/fas-ligand (FasL) in liver GVHD.[92,93] Higher response rates of skin and gut GVHD as compared to liver GVHD with anti–TNFα treatment is consistent with this hypothesis. In contrast, intestinal biopsies in patients with gastrointestinal symptoms suggest that both TNFα and FasL are relevant in human gut GVHD.[94]

Treatment of Corticosteroid-Resistant GVHD

Clinically, two types of failure of corticosteroid treatment of acute GVHD can be distinguished: true steroid resistance, or progression of GVHD symptoms and manifestations in patients who are receiving full-dose corticosteroid treatment, and steroid dependence, or the re-occurrence (or flare) of GVHD during or after tapering of treatment. The prognosis of true steroid-resistant GVHD is worse than for steroid-dependent patients. A comparison of trials dealing with steroid-resistant GVHD is hampered by variable inclusion of both patient groups.

A variety of agents has been tested: MMF,[95] ATG,[96] and anti-CD3[97,98] anti–T-cell antibodies as well as more specific agents directed against activation or adhesion molecules (anti-CD25,[99] anti-CD147[100]) or cytokines. To date, none has clearly improved outcome in this difficult clinical situation.

Other Supportive Approaches

Infections are the main cause of death in patients with steroid-refractory acute GVHD, and careful surveillance and control of infections is mandatory during acute GVHD. Fungal infections, especially aspergillosis, are the leading complication. Prophylaxis and early aggressive treatment should be facilitated by the introduction of new azoles (voriconazole) or echinocandins (caspofungin, micafungin), which broaden therapeutic efficacy with acceptable toxicity.

A variety of further supplementary approaches have been suggested, such as to reduce large volumes of diarrhea by the use of octreotide.[101] Substitution of factor XIII had a positive impact on gastrointestinal bleeding in one series in 21 of 23 patients.[102] Milder intestinal GVHD might be controlled by addition of oral beclomethasone (or budesonide), as suggested in a randomized trial.[103,104] In skin GVHD, Fas-mediated apoptosis of keratinocytes is a major factor resulting in epidermolysis. Based on experience in patients with toxic epidermal necrolysis, treatment with high-dose immunoglobulins has been advocated.[105]

Conclusions

Although the repertoire of drugs to prevent and treat GVHD is increasing, true progress, especially in the treatment of steroid-refractory GVHD, has been limited. New drugs such as deoxyspergualin, anti-CD52 antibody, or agents blocking CD40:CD40L pathways, Th1 responses and transfer of regulatory T cells will strengthen the therapeutic armamentarium. However, qualitatively new strategies, such as risk-adapted first-line treatment or preemptive therapy, may more likely improve results; both require a better definition of predictive parameters. Endothelial cells have only recently been identified as important targets of GVHD,[106] and agents modulating endothelial activation have not been tested to date. The ability to prevent GVHD by selective depletion of alloreactive T cells potentially will allow maximal preservation of anti-malignancy as well as anti-infectious agent effects, because T-cell responses against tumor-specific antigens and pathogens are intact and T-cell numbers can be increased. Nevertheless, from lessons learned from the pan T-cell depletion trials, ultimate success in prophylaxis and treatment of GVHD will depend on whether GVHD can be prevented without losing critical anti-malignancy and anti-pathogen activities.

References

1. Vogelsang GB, Lee L, Bensen-Kennedy DM: Pathogenesis and treatment of graft-versus-host disease after bone marrow transplant. Annu Rev Med 54:29-52, 2003
2. Socie G, Stone JV, Wingard JR, et al: Long-term survival and late deaths after allogeneic bone marrow transplantation. Late Effects Working Committee of the International Bone Marrow Transplant Registry. N Engl J Med 341:14-21, 1999
3. Antin JH, Ferrara JL: Cytokine dysregulation and acute graft-versus-host disease. Blood 80:2964-2968, 1992
4. Horowitz MM, Gale RP, Sondel PM, et al: Graft-versus-leukemia reactions after bone marrow transplantation. Blood 75:555-562, 1990
5. Kolb HJ, Mittermuller J, Clemm C, et al: Donor leukocyte transfusions for treatment of recurrent chronic myelogenous leukemia in marrow transplant patients. Blood 76:2462-2465, 1990
6. van Bekkum DW, Roodenburg J, Heidt PJ, van der WD: Mitigation of secondary disease of allogeneic mouse radiation chimeras by modification of the intestinal microflora. J Natl Cancer Inst 52:401-404, 1974
7. Storb R, Prentice RL, Buckner CD, et al: Graft-versus-host disease and survival in patients with aplastic anemia treated by marrow grafts from HLA-identical siblings. Beneficial effect of a protective environment. N Engl J Med 308:302-307, 1983
8. Ferrara JL, Levy R, Chao NJ: Pathophysiologic mechanisms of acute graft-vs.-host disease. Biol Blood Marrow Transplant 5:347-356, 1999
9. Clift RA, Buckner CD, Appelbaum FR, et al: Allogeneic marrow transplantation in patients with acute myeloid leukemia in first remission: A randomized trial of two irradiation regimens. Blood 76:1867-1871, 1990
10. Hill GR, Teshima T, Gerbitz A, et al: Differential roles of IL-1 and TNF-alpha on graft-versus-host disease and graft versus leukemia. J Clin Invest 104:459-467, 1999
11. Johnson BD, Truitt RL: Delayed infusion of immunocompetent donor cells after bone marrow transplantation breaks graft-host tolerance allows for persistent antileukemic reactivity without severe graft-versus-host disease. Blood 85:3302-3312, 1995
12. Barrett AJ, Mavroudis D, Tisdale J, et al: T cell-depleted bone marrow transplantation and delayed T cell add-back to control acute GVHD and conserve a graft-versus-leukemia effect. Bone Marrow Transplant 21:543-551, 1998
13. Holler E, Kolb HJ, Moller A, et al: Increased serum levels of tumor necrosis factor alpha precede major complications of bone marrow transplantation. Blood 75:1011-1016, 1990
14. Shalaby MR, Fendly B, Sheehan KC, Schreiber RD, Ammann AJ: Prevention of the graft-versus-host reaction in newborn mice by antibodies to tumor necrosis factor-alpha. Transplantation 47:1057-1061, 1989
15. Piguet PF, Grau GE, Allet B, Vassalli P: Tumor necrosis factor/cachectin is an effector of skin and gut lesions of the acute phase of graft-vs.-host disease. J Exp Med 166:1280-1289, 1987
16. Panoskaltsis-Mortari A, Lacey DL, Vallera DA, Blazar BR: Keratinocyte growth factor administered before conditioning ameliorates graft-versus-host disease after allogeneic bone marrow transplantation in mice. Blood 92:3960-3967, 1998

17. Krijanovski OI, Hill GR, Cooke KR, et al: Keratinocyte growth factor separates graft-versus-leukemia effects from graft-versus-host disease. Blood 94:825-831, 1999
18. Bacigalupo A, Lamparelli T, Bruzzi P, et al: Antithymocyte globulin for graft-versus-host disease prophylaxis in transplants from unrelated donors: 2 randomized studies from Gruppo Italiano Trapianti Midollo Osseo (GITMO). Blood 98:2942-2947, 2001
19. Remberger M, Storer B, Ringden O, Anasetti C: Association between pretransplant Thymoglobulin and reduced non-relapse mortality rate after marrow transplantation from unrelated donors. Bone Marrow Transplant 29:391-397, 2002
20. Basara N, Baurmann H, Kolbe K, et al: Antithymocyte globulin for the prevention of graft-versus-host disease after unrelated hematopoietic stem cell transplantation for acute myeloid leukemia: Results from the multicenter German cooperative study group. Bone Marrow Transplant 35:1011-1018, 2005
21. den Haan JM, Sherman NE, Blokland E, et al: Identification of a graft versus host disease-associated human minor histocompatibility antigen. Science 268:1476-1480, 1995
22. Goulmy E, Schipper R, Pool J, et al: Mismatches of minor histocompatibility antigens between HLA-identical donors and recipients and the development of graft-versus-host disease after bone marrow transplantation. N Engl J Med 334:281-285, 1996
23. Sette A, Alexander J, Grey HM: Interaction of antigenic peptides with MHC and TCR molecules. Clin Immunol Immunopathol 76:S168-S171, 1995
24. Yang Y, Wilson JM: CD40 ligand-dependent T cell activation: Requirement of B7-CD28 signaling through CD40. Science 273:1862-1864, 1996
25. Green JM, Noel PJ, Sperling AI, et al: Absence of B7-dependent responses in CD28-deficient mice. Immunity 1:501-508, 1994
26. Freeman GJ, Gribben JG, Boussiotis VA, et al: Cloning of B7-2: A CTLA-4 counter-receptor that costimulates human T cell proliferation. Science 262:909-911, 1993
27. Guinan EC, Boussiotis VA, Neuberg D, et al: Transplantation of anergic histoincompatible bone marrow allografts. N Engl J Med 340: 1704-1714, 1999
28. Vezina C, Kudelski A, Sehgal SN: Rapamycin (AY-22,989), a new antifungal antibiotic. I. Taxonomy of the producing streptomycete and isolation of the active principle. J Antibiot (Tokyo) 28:721-726, 1975
29. Morice WG, Brunn GJ, Wiederrecht G, Siekierka JJ, Abraham RT: Rapamycin-induced inhibition of p34cdc2 kinase activation is associated with G1/S-phase growth arrest in T lymphocytes. J Biol Chem 268:3734-3738, 1993
30. Nourse J, Firpo E, Flanagan WM, et al: Interleukin-2-mediated elimination of the p27Kip1 cyclin-dependent kinase inhibitor prevented by rapamycin. Nature 372:570-573, 1994
31. Altmeyer A, Dumont FJ: Rapamycin inhibits IL-1-mediated interferon-gamma production in the YAC-1 T cell lymphoma. Cytokine 5:133-143, 1993
32. Lai JH, Tan TH: CD28 signaling causes a sustained down-regulation of I kappa B alpha which can be prevented by the immunosuppressant rapamycin. J Biol Chem 269:30077-30080, 1994
33. Battaglia M, Stabilini A, Roncarolo MG: Rapamycin selectively expands $CD4^+CD25^+FOXP3^+$ regulatory T cells. Blood 2005
34. Storb R, Epstein RB, Graham TC, Thomas ED: Methotrexate regimens for control of graft-versus-host disease in dogs with allogeneic marrow grafts. Transplantation 9:240-246, 1970
35. Storb R, Deeg HJ, Whitehead J, et al: Methotrexate and cyclosporine compared with cyclosporine alone for prophylaxis of acute graft versus host disease after marrow transplantation for leukemia. N Engl J Med 314:729-735, 1986
36. Ringden O, Klaesson S, Sundberg B, et al: Decreased incidence of graft-versus-host disease and improved survival with methotrexate combined with cyclosporin compared with monotherapy in recipients of bone marrow from donors other than HLA identical siblings. Bone Marrow Transplant 9:19-25, 1992
37. Nevill TJ, Tirgan MH, Deeg HJ, et al: Influence of post-methotrexate folinic acid rescue on regimen-related toxicity and graft-versus-host disease after allogeneic bone marrow transplantation. Bone Marrow Transplant 9:349-354, 1992
38. Ratanatharathorn V, Nash RA, Przepiorka D, et al: Phase III study comparing methotrexate and tacrolimus (prograf, FK506) with methotrexate and cyclosporine for graft-versus-host disease prophylaxis after HLA-identical sibling bone marrow transplantation. Blood 92: 2303-2314, 1998
39. Nash RA, Antin JH, Karanes C, et al: Phase 3 study comparing methotrexate and tacrolimus with methotrexate and cyclosporine for prophylaxis of acute graft-versus-host disease after marrow transplantation from unrelated donors. Blood 96:2062-2068, 2000
40. Suthanthiran M, Morris RE, Strom TB: Immunosuppressants: Cellular and molecular mechanisms of action. Am J Kidney Dis 28:159-172, 1996
41. Hovi T, Allison AC, Allsop J: Rapid increase of phosphoribosyl pyrophosphate concentration after mitogenic stimulation of lymphocytes. FEBS Lett 55:291-293, 1975
42. Storb R, Yu C, Wagner JL, et al: Stable mixed hematopoietic chimerism in DLA-identical littermate dogs given sublethal total body irradiation before and pharmacological immunosuppression after marrow transplantation. Blood 89:3048-3054, 1997
43. Ferrara JL, Deeg HJ: Graft-versus-host disease. N Engl J Med 324:667-674, 1991
44. Henkart PA, Sitkovsky MV: Cytotoxic lymphocytes. Two ways to kill target cells. Curr Biol 4:923-925, 1994
45. Mason DW: Subsets of T cells in the rat mediating lethal graft versus-host disease. Transplantation 32:222-226, 1981
46. Fong TA, Mosmann TR: Alloreactive murine $CD8^+$ T cell clones secrete the Th1 pattern of cytokines. J Immunol 144:1744-1752, 1990
47. Groux H, Bigler M, de Vries JE, Roncarolo MG: Interleukin-10 induces a long-term antigen-specific anergic state in human $CD4^+$ T cells. J Exp Med 184:19-29, 1996
48. Bensinger WI, Martin PJ, Storer B, et al: Transplantation of bone marrow as compared with peripheral-blood cells from HLA-identical relatives in patients with hematologic cancers. N Engl J Med 344:175-181, 2001
49. Mielcarek M, Graf L, Johnson G, Torok-Storb B: Production of interleukin-10 by granulocyte colony-stimulating factor-mobilized blood products: a mechanism for monocyte-mediated suppression of T-cell proliferation. Blood 92:215-222, 1998
50. Powles R, Mehta J, Kulkarni S, et al: Allogeneic blood and bone-marrow stem-cell transplantation in haematological malignant diseases: A randomised trial. Lancet 355:1231-1237, 2000
51. Yang YG, Dey BR, Sergio JJ, Pearson DA, Sykes M: Donor-derived interferon gamma is required for inhibition of acute graft-versus-host disease by interleukin 12. J Clin Invest 102:2126-2135, 1998
52. Shevach EM, McHugh RS, Piccirillo CA, Thornton AM: Control of T-cell activation by $CD4^+$ $CD25^+$ suppressor T cells. Immunol Rev 182:58-67, 2001
53. Taylor PA, Lees CJ, Blazar BR: The infusion of ex vivo activated and expanded CD4(+)CD25(+) immune regulatory cells inhibits graft-versus-host disease lethality. Blood 99:3493-3499, 2002
54. Edinger M, Hoffmann P, Ermann J, et al: $CD4^+CD25^+$ regulatory T cells preserve graft-versus-tumor activity while inhibiting graft-versus-host disease after bone marrow transplantation. Nat Med 9:1144-1150, 2003
55. Ghiringhelli F, Larmonier N, Schmitt E, et al: $CD4^+CD25^+$ regulatory T cells suppress tumor immunity but are sensitive to cyclophosphamide which allows immunotherapy of established tumors to be curative. Eur J Immunol 34:336-344, 2004
56. Korngold B, Sprent J: Lethal graft-versus-host disease after bone marrow transplantation across minor histocompatibility barriers in mice. Prevention by removing mature T cells from marrow. J Exp Med 148:1687-1698, 1978
57. Ho VT, Soiffer RJ: The history and future of T-cell depletion as graft-versus-host disease prophylaxis for allogeneic hematopoietic stem cell transplantation. Blood 98:3192-3204, 2001

58. Truitt RL, Johnson BD: Principles of graft-vs.-leukemia reactivity. Biol Blood Marrow Transplant 1:61-68, 1995
59. Michalek J, Collins RH, Durrani HP, et al: Definitive separation of graft-versus-leukemia- and graft-versus-host-specific $CD4^+$ T cells by virtue of their receptor beta loci sequences. Proc Natl Acad Sci U S A 100:1180-1184, 2003
60. Gribben JG, Guinan EC, Boussiotis VA, et al: Complete blockade of B7 family-mediated costimulation is necessary to induce human alloantigen-specific anergy: A method to ameliorate graft- versus-host disease and extend the donor pool. Blood 87:4887-4893, 1996
61. Blazar BR, Taylor PA, Noelle RJ, Vallera DA: CD4(+) T cells tolerized ex vivo to host alloantigen by anti-CD40 ligand (CD40L:CD154) antibody lose their graft-versus-host disease lethality capacity but retain nominal antigen responses. J Clin Invest 102:473-482, 1998
62. Zeller JC, Panoskaltsis-Mortari A, Murphy WJ, et al: Induction of $CD4^+$ T cell alloantigen-specific hyporesponsiveness by IL- 10 and TGF-beta. J Immunol 163:3684-3691, 1999
63. Cavazzana-Calvo M, Fromont C, Le Deist F, et al: Specific elimination of alloreactive T cells by an anti-interleukin-2 receptor B chain-specific immunotoxin. Transplantation 50:1-7, 1990
64. Solomon SR, Tran T, Carter CS, et al: Optimized clinical-scale culture conditions for ex vivo selective depletion of host-reactive donor lymphocytes: A strategy for GvHD prophylaxis in allogeneic PBSC transplantation. Cytotherapy 4:395-406, 2002
65. Chen BJ, Cui X, Liu C, Chao NJ: Prevention of graft-versus-host disease while preserving graft-versus-leukemia effect after selective depletion of host-reactive T cells by photodynamic cell purging process. Blood 99:3083-3088, 2002
66. Guimond M, Balassy A, Barrette M, et al: P-glycoprotein targeting: a unique strategy to selectively eliminate immunoreactive T cells. Blood 100:375-382, 2002
67. Andre-Schmutz I, Le Deist F, Hacein-Bey-Abina S, et al: Immune reconstitution without graft-versus-host disease after haemopoietic stem-cell transplantation: A phase 1/2 study. Lancet 360:130-137, 2002
68. Solomon SR, Tran T, Carter CS, et al: Selective depletion of alloreacting $CD25^+$ cells from stem cell allografts can reduce acute graft-versus-host disease following matched related donor transplantation. Blood 104:125A, 2004
69. Chen BJ, Cui XY, Sempowski GD, Liu CX, Chao NJ: Transfer of allogeneic CD62L(-) memory T cells without graft-versus-host disease. Blood 103:1534-1541, 2004
70. Anderson BE, McNiff J, Yan J, et al: Memory $CD4^+$ T cells do not induce graft-versus-host disease. J Clin Invest 112:101-108, 2003
71. Zhang Y, Joe G, Zhu J, et al: Dendritic cell-activated $CD44^{hi}CD8^+$ T cells are defective in mediating acute graft-versus-host disease but retain graft-versus-leukemia activity. Blood 103:3970-3978, 2004
72. Xystrakis E, Bernard I, Dejean AS, et al: Alloreactive CD4 T lymphocytes responsible for acute and chronic graft-versus-host disease are contained within the CD45RChigh but not the CD45RClow subset. Eur J Immunol 34:408-417, 2004
73. Bonini C, Ferrari G, Verzeletti S, et al: HSV-TK gene transfer into donor lymphocytes for control of allogeneic graft-versus-leukemia. Science 276:1719-1724, 1997
74. Fontaine P, Roy-Proulx G, Knafo L, et al: Adoptive transfer of minor histocompatibility antigen-specific T lymphocytes eradicates leukemia cells without causing graft-versus-host disease. Nat Med 7:789-794, 2001
75. Ruggeri L, Capanni M, Martelli MF, Velardi A: Cellular therapy: Exploiting NK cell alloreactivity in transplantation. Curr Opin Hematol 8:355-359, 2001
76. Ruggeri L, Capanni M, Urbani E, et al: Effectiveness of donor natural killer cell alloreactivity in mismatched hematopoietic transplants. Science 295:2097-2100, 2002
77. Bendelac A, Lantz O, Quimby ME, et al: CD1 recognition by mouse NK1+ T lymphocytes. Science 268:863-865, 1995
78. Porcelli SA: The CD1 family: A third lineage of antigen-presenting molecules. Adv Immunol 59:1-98, 1995
79. Zeng D, Lewis D, Dejbakhsh-Jones S, et al: Bone marrow NK1.1(-) and NK1.1(+) T cells reciprocally regulate acute graft versus host disease. J Exp Med 189:1073-1081, 1999
80. Furlong T, Storb R, Anasetti C, et al: Clinical outcome after conversion to FK 506 (tacrolimus) therapy for acute graft-versus-host disease resistant to cyclosporine or for cyclosporine-associated toxicities. Bone Marrow Transplant 26:985-991, 2000
81. Thomas E, Storb R, Clift RA, et al: Bone-marrow transplantation (first of two parts). N Engl J Med 292:832-843, 1975
82. Holler E, Kolb HJ, Wilmanns W: Treatment of GVHD—TNF-antibodies and related antagonists. Bone Marrow Transplant 12:S29-S31, 1993 (suppl 3)
83. Ruutu T, Hermans J, van Biezen A, et al: How should corticosteroids be used in the treatment of acute GVHD? EBMT Chronic Leukemia Working Party. European Group for Blood and Marrow Transplantation. Bone Marrow Transplant 22:614-615, 1998
84. Van Lint MT, Uderzo C, Locasciulli A, et al: Early treatment of acute graft-versus-host disease with high- or low-dose 6-methylprednisolone: A multicenter randomized trial from the Italian Group for Bone Marrow Transplantation. Blood 92:2288-2293, 1998
85. Martin PJ, Schoch G, Fisher L, et al: A retrospective analysis of therapy for acute graft-versus-host disease: Initial treatment. Blood 76:1464-1472, 1990
86. Weisdorf D, Haake R, Blazar B, et al: Treatment of moderate/severe acute graft-versus-host disease after allogeneic bone marrow transplantation: An analysis of clinical risk features and outcome. Blood 75:1024-1030, 1990
87. Hings IM, Filipovich AH, Miller WJ, et al: Prednisone therapy for acute graft-versus-host disease: Short- versus long-term treatment. A prospective randomized trial. Transplantation 56:577-580, 1993
88. Martin PJ, Nelson BJ, Appelbaum FR, et al: Evaluation of a CD5-specific immunotoxin for treatment of acute graft-versus-host disease after allogeneic marrow transplantation. Blood 88:824-830, 1996
89. Cahn JY, Bordigoni P, Tiberghien P, et al: Treatment of acute graft-versus-host disease with methylprednisolone and cyclosporine with or without an anti-interleukin-2 receptor monoclonal antibody. A multicenter phase III study. Transplantation 60:939-942, 1995
90. Cragg L, Blazar BR, Defor T, et al: A randomized trial comparing prednisone with antithymocyte globulin/prednisone as an initial systemic therapy for moderately severe acute graft-versus-host disease. Biol Blood Marrow Transplant 6:441-447, 2000
91. Bacigalupo A, Oneto R, Lamparelli T, et al: Pre-emptive therapy of acute graft-versus-host disease: A pilot study with antithymocyte globulin (ATG). Bone Marrow Transplant 28:1093-1096, 2001
92. Hattori K, Hirano T, Miyajima H, et al: Differential effects of anti-Fas ligand and anti-tumor necrosis factor alpha antibodies on acute graft-versus-host disease pathologies. Blood 91:4051-4055, 1998
93. Stuber E, Buschenfeld A, Von Freier A, Arendt T, Folsch UR: Intestinal crypt cell apoptosis in murine acute graft versus host disease is mediated by tumour necrosis factor alpha and not by the FasL-Fas interaction: Effect of pentoxifylline on the development of mucosal atrophy. Gut 45:229-235, 1999
94. Daneshpouy M, Socie G, Lemann M, et al: Activated eosinophils in upper gastrointestinal tract of patients with graft-versus-host disease. Blood 99:3033-3040, 2002
95. Basara N, Kiehl MG, Blau W, et al: Mycophenolate Mofetil in the treatment of acute and chronic GVHD in hematopoietic stem cell transplant patients: Four years of experience. Transplant Proc 33: 2121-2123, 2001
96. Doney KC, Weiden PL, Storb R, Thomas ED: Treatment of graft-versus-host disease in human allogeneic marrow graft recipients: A randomized trial comparing antithymocyte globulin and corticosteroids. Am J Hematol 11:1-8, 1981
97. Anasetti C, Martin PJ, Storb R, et al: Treatment of acute graft-versus-host disease with a nonmitogenic anti-CD3 monoclonal antibody. Transplantation 54:844-851, 1992
98. Carpenter PA, Appelbaum FR, Corey L, et al: A humanized non-FcR-binding anti-CD3 antibody, visilizumab, for treatment of steroid-refractory acute graft-versus-host disease. Blood 99:2712-2719, 2002

99. Lee SJ, Zahrieh D, Agura E, et al: Effect of up-front daclizumab when combined with steroids for the treatment of acute graft-versus-host disease: Results of a randomized trial. Blood 104:1559-1564, 2004
100. Deeg HJ, Blazar BR, Bolwell BJ, et al: Treatment of steroid-refractory acute graft-versus-host disease with anti-CD147 monoclonal antibody ABX-CBL. Blood 98:2052-2058, 2001
101. Ely P, Dunitz J, Rogosheske J, Weisdorf D: Use of a somatostatin analogue, octreotide acetate, in the management of acute gastrointestinal graft-versus-host disease. Am J Med 90:707-710, 1991
102. Grothaus-Pinke B, Gunzelmann S, Fauser AA, Kiehl MG: Factor XIII replacement in stem cell transplant (SCT) recipients with severe graft-versus-host disease of the bowel: Report of an initial experience. Transplantation 72:1456-1458, 2001
103. Bertz H, Afting M, Kreisel W, et al: Feasibility and response to budesonide as topical corticosteroid therapy for acute intestinal GVHD. Bone Marrow Transplant 24:1185-1189, 1999
104. McDonald GB, Bouvier M, Hockenbery DM, et al: Oral beclomethasone dipropionate for treatment of intestinal graft-versus-host disease: Arandomized, controlled trial. Gastroenterology 115: 28-35, 1998
105. French LE, Tschopp J: Fas-mediated cell death in toxic epidermal necrolysis and graft-versus-host disease: Potential for therapeutic inhibition. Schweiz Med Wochenschr 130:1656-1661, 2000
106. Biedermann BC, Sahner S, Gregor M, et al: Endothelial injury mediated by cytotoxic T lymphocytes and loss of microvessels in chronic graft versus host disease. Lancet 359:2078-2083, 2002

ELSEVIER

Seminars in
HEMATOLOGY

The Lung as a Target Organ of Graft-Versus-Host Disease

Gregory Yanik and Kenneth R. Cooke

Despite significant advances in critical care and transplantation medicine, non-infectious lung injury remains a major problem following allogeneic hematopoietic stem cell transplantation (HSCT) both in the immediate post-transplant period and in the months to years that follow. Historically, approximately 50% of all pneumonias seen after HSCT have been secondary to infection. Although non-infectious lung injury occasionally occurs following autologous transplants, the allogeneic setting greatly exacerbates toxicity acutely and chronically. Pulmonary injury is associated with significant morbidity and mortality and responds poorly to standard therapies. Insights generated using animal models suggest that the immunologic mechanisms contributing to lung inflammation after HSCT may be similar to those responsible for graft-versus-host disease (GVHD).
Semin Hematol 43:42-52

Diffuse lung injury is a major complication of hematopoietic stem cell transplantation (HSCT) that occurs in 25% to 55% of recipients and can account for approximately 50% of transplant-related mortality.[1–5] Historically, about half of all pneumonias seen after HSCT have been secondary to infection, but the judicious use of broad-spectrum antimicrobial prophylaxis in recent years has altered the balance of pulmonary complications from infectious to non-infectious causes.[6] Non-infectious lung injury can be either acute (termed idiopathic pneumonia syndrome, or IPS) or chronic depending on the time of onset after HSCT and the tempo of disease progression. Chronic lung injury (by definition, occurring in patients over 100 days post-transplant) is further subdivided into two types: obstructive and restrictive.[7–11] Each form of non-infectious lung injury is associated with significant morbidity and mortality and responds poorly to standard therapeutic approaches. A large body of experimental literature demonstrates that both types of lung injury after HSCT are immunologically mediated and share similar pathogenetic mechanisms with graft-versus-host disease (GVHD). This chapter will review the definitions, risk factors, and pathogeneses of non-infectious lung injury after allogeneic HSCT.

Department of Pediatrics, Division of Hematology/Oncology, Blood and Marrow Transplantation Program, University of Michigan Cancer Center, Ann Arbor, MI.

K.R.C. is an Amy Strelzer-Manasevit Scholar of the National Marrow Donor Program, a Fellow of the Robert Wood Johnson Minority Faculty Development Program, a Leukemia and Lymphoma Society Scholar in Clinical Research and the recipient of a Clinical Scientist Award in Translational Research from the Burroughs Wellcome Fund.

Address correspondence to Kenneth R. Cooke, MD, Assistant Professor of Pediatrics–Hematology/Oncology, University of Michigan Medical School, 1500 E Medical Center Dr, 6306 CCGC, Ann Arbor, MI 48109-0942. E-mail: krcooke@umich.edu

Acute Lung Injury: Idiopathic Pneumonia Syndrome

Definition, Clinical Course, and Spectrum of Disease

In 1993 a panel convened by the National Institutes of Health defined IPS as widespread alveolar injury following HSCT that occurs in the absence of an active lower respiratory tract infection and cardiogenic causes.[1] Diagnostic criteria of IPS include signs and symptoms of pneumonia, non-lobar radiographic infiltrates, abnormal pulmonary function, and the absence of infectious organisms as determined by bronchoalveolar lavage (BAL) or lung biopsy (Table 1).[1,2] Histopathologic findings associated with IPS include diffuse alveolar damage with hyaline membranes, lymphocytic bronchitis, and bronchiolitis obliterans organizing pneumonia (BOOP); however, the most frequently reported pattern is interstitial pneumonitis, a term used interchangeably with IPS.[3,12,13] The incidence of IPS in the first 120 days after allogeneic HSCT with myeloablative conditioning ranges between 3% and 15%.[1,3,4] The median time of onset for IPS was initially reported to be 6 to 7 weeks (range, 14 to 90 days) after the infusion of donor stem cells. Mortality rates ranged from 60% to 80% overall, and were greater than 95% for patients requiring mechanical ventilation.[1,3–6,14] In a recent publication

 0037-1963/06/$-see front matter
doi:10.1053/j.seminhematol.2005.09.004

Table 1 Definition of Idiopathic Pneumonia Syndrome

Evidence of widespread lung injury:
- (a) Multi-lobar infiltrates on chest radiograph or computed tomography.
- (b) Signs and symptoms of pneumonia (cough, dyspnea, rales).
- (c) Abnormal pulmonary physiology: increased alveolar to arterial oxygen gradient; or new or increased restrictive lung findings.

Absence of lower respiratory tract infection, based upon:
- (a) Bronchoalveolar lavage negative for bacterial pathogens and/or lack of improvement with broad spectrum antibiotics.
- (b) Bronchoalveolar lavage negative for pathogenic non-bacterial micro-organisms.
- (c) Transbronchial lung biopsy if condition permits.
- (d) Ideally, second confirmatory negative test for infection 2–14 days following the initial procedure.[1]

from the University of Michigan, the frequency of IPS after allogeneic HSCT ranged from 5% to 25%, depending on donor source and the degree of antigenic mismatch between donor and recipient.[15] In this series, day 100 mortality was 80%, and the median time from diagnosis of IPS to death was 13 days, despite aggressive treatment with high-dose corticosteroids and broad-spectrum antimicrobial therapy.[15]

The clinical spectrum of IPS encompasses various forms of pulmonary toxicity (Table 2). In one small subset of patients with IPS, diffuse alveolar hemorrhage (DAH) occurs. DAH generally develops in the immediate post-HSCT period and is characterized by progressive shortness of breath, cough, and hypoxemia with or without fever.[6,16,17] Progressively bloodier aliquots of BAL fluid have traditionally led to the diagnoses of DAH, but frank hemoptysis is rare.[16] Mortality from DAH is as high as 75%, despite treatment with high-dose (2 mg/kg to 1 g/m^2) corticosteroids, and death usually occurs within 3 weeks of diagnosis.[17]

Table 2 The Spectrum of Non-cardiogenic, Pulmonary Toxicity Defined by Idiopathic Pneumonia Syndrome

Interstitial pneumonitis (IP)
- Clinical symptoms: fever, cough, dyspnea, hypoxemia
- Onset: within first 6 months post transplant
- Etiology: infectious (ie, CMV, PCP) or non-infectious factors (chemo toxicity: BCNU, bleomycin, busulfan, MTX).
- Radiographic findings: bilateral interstitial infiltrates.

Bronchiolitis obliterans syndrome (BOS)
- Clinical symptoms: cough, dyspnea, wheezing, lack of fever.
- Pulmonary function testing: obstructive findings (diminished FEV_1, or FEV_1/FVC)
- Onset: 3–24 months post-transplant.
- Radiographic findings: hyperinflation. Otherwise typically normal.
- Computed tomography: bronchiectasis, centrilobular nodules, septal lines, ground glass appearance
- Histology: lymphocytic bronchitis. Bronchiolar inflammation with luminal obliteration.

Bronchiolitis obliterans organizing pneumonia (BOOP)
- Clinical symptoms: fever, dry cough, dyspnea
- Onset: 2–12 months post-transplant
- Radiographic findings: patchy airspace disease, ground glass appearance, nodular opacities
- Histology: peribronchiolar infiltration and fibrosis and the presence of intraluminal granulation tissue.

Diffuse alveolar hemorrhage (DAH)
- Clinical symptoms: progressive dyspnea, cough, rare hemoptysis
- Key finding: progressively bloodier aliquots of lavage fluid
- Onset: early, within first 100 days post transplant.
- Radiographic findings: diffuse infiltrates, central appearance initially noted.
- Histology: diffuse alveolar damage with alveolar hemorrhage

Peri-engraftment respiratory distress syndrome (PERDS)
- Clinical symptoms: fever, dyspnea, hypoxemia
- Onset: very early, within 5 to 7 days of engraftment, classically after autologous HSCT
- Radiographic findings: bilateral interstitial infiltrates

Delayed pulmonary toxicity syndrome (DPTS):
- Clinical symptoms: fever, dry cough, dyspnea
- Onset: late, months to years following autologous HSCT for breast cancer
- Responds to corticosteroid therapy

Non-cardiogenic capillary leak syndrome (CLS)
- Clinical symptoms: dyspnea, cough, weight gain, edema
- Onset: early, within first 30 days post transplant.
- Radiographic findings: bilateral perihilar infiltrates, pulmonary edema, pleural effusions

Abbreviations: CMV, cytomegalovirus; PCP, *Pneumocystis carinii* pneumonia;

Peri-engraftment respiratory distress syndrome (PERDS) and delayed pulmonary toxicity syndrome (DPTS) are also included within the definition of IPS.[6] PERDS and DPTS typically occur after autologous HSCT,[6] and both are characterized by fever, dyspnea, and hypoxemia.[18–20] By definition, PERDS appears within 5 days of engraftment, whereas the onset of DPTS may be delayed for months and is more common following conditioning regimens that contain cyclophosphamide, cisplatin, and bischloroethylinitrosurea (BCNU), as used in HSCT for breast cancer.[20] Although PERDS after autologous HSCT appears similar to IPS after allogeneic HSCT with respect to clinical presentation and time of onset, the two entities differ sharply in overall outcome.[21]

Risk Factors for IPS

Risk factors for IPS have included conditioning with total body irradiation (TBI), acute GVHD, older recipient age, and the use of methotrexate (MTX) for GVHD prophylaxis[4,12,22–24]; and the likelihood of developing IPS increases with the number of risk factors.[3] Recently, the cumulative incidence of IPS was found to be significantly lower after nonmyeloablative conditioning than observed following conventional conditioning[24]; however, once diagnosed, IPS progressed rapidly and was associated with a high mortality rate (75%) in both subsets of patients. Grades III to IV acute GVHD and patient age older than 40 years remained prognostic for IPS after adjusting for other risk factors, confirming previous reports. These results suggest that the intensity of HSCT conditioning plays an important role in the development of IPS, consistent with data generated from two murine HSCT models.[25,26]

Etiology of IPS

Potential etiologies for IPS include direct toxic effects of HSCT conditioning regimens, occult pulmonary infections, and the release of inflammatory cytokines that have also been implicated in other forms of pulmonary injury.[27–29] Other immunologic factors may be important, as suggested by the association of IPS and severe GVHD in several large series.[2–6] Acute GVHD often precedes IPS, suggesting a possible causal relationship.[4,12,30,31] The lung is not recognized as a classic target organ of GVHD, but the clinical association between lung injury and GVHD and the presence of pathologic lung changes in rodents with acute GVHD make this possibility intriguing.[26,32–35]

The role of GVHD and specifically alloreactive donor T lymphocytes in the pathogenesis of IPS remains controversial. Epithelial apoptosis is usually attributed to T-cell–mediated injury and is considered pathognomonic for acute GVHD. Although observed in the lungs of some patients with IPS,[13] epithelial apoptosis has not been consistently identified in allogeneic HSCT recipients with pulmonary dysfunction.[31,36,37] More recently described is a histologic spectrum of pulmonary GVHD that ranges from diffuse alveolar injury early after HSCT to cicatricial bronchiolitis obliterans (BrOb), a late and irreversible form of lung injury.[13] In this report, bronchitis/bronchiolitis with interstitial pneumonitis (BIP) was the most common finding.

Experimental IPS Following Allogeneic HSCT

Animal Models of Human Disease

Several laboratories have modeled the relationship between alloreactivity and IPS in rodents: animals with systemic GVHD consistently develop lung injury, whereas those receiving syngeneic HSCT do not (Fig 1).[32,34,38] Two major abnormalities emerge after allogeneic HSCT: a dense mononuclear cell infiltrate around both pulmonary vessels (Fig 1B) and bronchioles (Fig 1C) and an acute pneumonitis involving the interstitium and alveolar spaces (Fig 1D).[34] Both of these histopathologic patterns closely resemble those of the nonspecific, diffuse interstitial pneumonias seen in allogeneic HSCT recipients.[1,13,31] Lung histopathology is also associated with alterations in pulmonary function.[35,38] In one report, mice with IPS showed significant reductions in both dynamic compliance and airway conductance compared with syngeneic controls, reflecting changes expected from both the interstitial and peribronchial infiltrates, respectively.[35] Lung injury did not correlate with the severity of GVHD, consistent with clinical reports of IPS in allogeneic HSCT recipients whose signs and symptoms of GVHD were mild or absent.[7,15,39,40] Thus, mouse models of IPS reproduce histologic and functional changes observed during human disease.

The Pathophysiology of IPS

These experimental models support a shift away from the current paradigm of acute lung injury after HSCT representing an idiopathic clinical syndrome and toward a process in which the lung is susceptible to two distinct but interrelated pathways of immune-mediated injury following allogeneic HSCT: a T-cell axis and an inflammatory cytokine axis. These pathways involve aspects of the adaptive and the innate immune response, synergistic interactions between cells from the lymphoid and myeloid lineage, and the release of soluble inflammatory molecules (Fig 2). Although distinct, the pathways are inter-related; donor macrophages, primed by interferon-gamma (IFNγ) that is produced by activated T cells, are recruited to the lung where they are triggered by lipopolysaccharide (LPS) to secrete inflammatory cytokines like tumor necrosis factor-alpha (TNFα), resulting in enhanced chemokine expression, the recruitment of neutrophils to the lung, and increased tissue damage.

T lymphocyte axis. The lymphocyte activation pathway depends on interactions between donor T cells and host antigen-presenting cells (APCs). Donor-derived, IFNγ-producing T cells are subsequently recruited to the lung by specific chemokine receptor:ligand interactions,[41] and by engaging the TNFα and Fas-FasL cytotoxic pathways, contribute to the early pro-inflammatory events associated with lung injury that develops within the first weeks of HSCT.[35,38,42,43] Mature donor lymphocytes can continue to respond to host antigens and produce physiologically significant lung injury at later

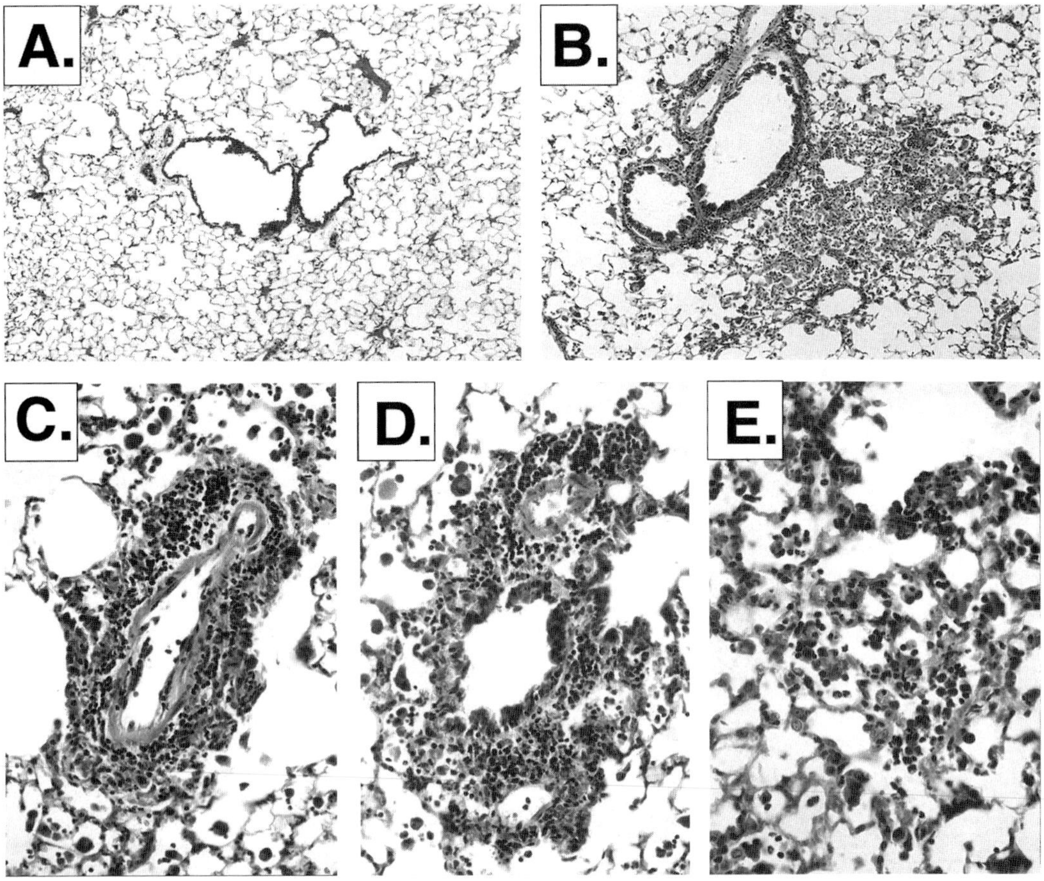

Figure 1 Histopathology of IPS. Following lethal irradiation, mice received hematopoietic HSCT from either allogeneic (major histocompatibility complex [MHC]-matched) or syngeneic donors. Lungs were harvested and prepared for microscopic analysis. At 6 weeks, lungs of mice receiving syngeneic HSCT maintain virtually normal histology (A), whereas allogeneic HSCT recipients develop significant lung histopathology (B–E). Two major abnormalities are apparent after allogeneic HSCT. First, dense mononuclear cell infiltrates are observed around both pulmonary vessels (C) and bronchioles (D). Second, an acute pneumonitis is present involving both the interstitial and alveolar spaces (E). The alveolar infiltrate is composed of macrophages, lymphocytes, epithelial cells and scattered polymorphonuclear cells within a fibrin matrix. Original magnification: 200× (A, B); 400× (C–E). Reproduced from Ferrara JLM, Cooke KR, and Deeg HJ: Graft-Versus-Host Disease. New York, NY, Marcel Dekker, 2005.

time points—even when systemic GVHD is mild or absent.[35] The precise mechanisms by which T cells interact with host antigens and cause injury remain unresolved but are likely to involve interactions with pulmonary APCs. Pulmonary dendritic cells (DCs) play a critical role in the initiation and regulation of immune responses in the lung, and they are important to both acute and chronic rejection of lung allografts.[44–47] Radio-resistant host DCs may persist longer in the lung than in other organs and thus sustain presentation of host antigens in that organ.[48]

Inflammatory cytokine axis. TNFα and LPS are important but not exclusive contributors to IPS; donor, non-lymphoid, accessory cells, including monocytes, macrophages, and neutrophils, are linked to this pathway of inflammatory release. TNFα levels are increased in both lung tissue and BAL fluid following allogeneic HSCT.[26,33,34,49,50] and strategies that block TNFα, either by neutralizing its effects or through the use of TNFα-deficient mice as HSCT donors, significantly reduce the severity of IPS.[43,49,50] In genetically altered mice, IPS is dependent on donor- rather than host-derived TNFα, and cytokine production from both donor accessory cells and T cells contributes to this toxicity.[43,51] Moreover, donor-derived TNFα is both a facilitator and effector of lung injury. TNFα secreted by donor T cells regulates the chemokine milieu in the lung within the first 2 weeks after HSCT, leading to the recruitment of monocytes and macrophages as lung injury progresses. The incomplete protection provided by abrogating the effects of TNFα after HSCT[32,49,52–55] suggests that other inflammatory and cellular mechanisms are important in the development of IPS.[38,56]

The release of inflammatory cytokines including TNFα following allogeneic HSCT is directly linked to endogenous LPS.[57] Translocation of LPS across a gut mucosa damaged early in the post-transplant period provides access to the systemic circulation, where the cellular activating effects of LPS contribute to GVHD target organ damage and dysfunction.[52,57–59] LPS also has a role in IPS. LPS levels are elevated in the BAL fluid of mice following allogeneic HSCT, and LPS

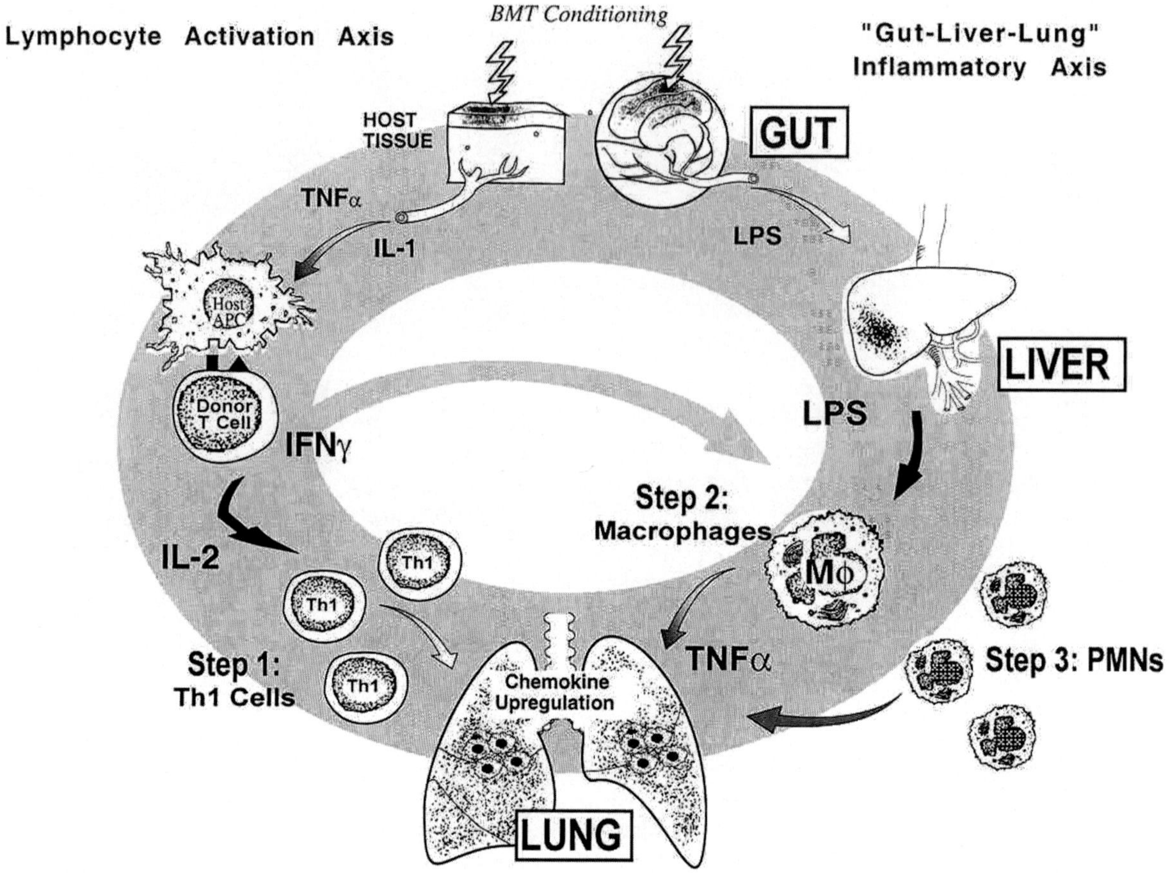

Figure 2 Pathophysiology of IPS after allogeneic HSCT. Data generated using murine HSCT models have been incorporated into a working hypothesis of IPS physiology. This schema postulates that the lung is susceptible to two distinct but inter-related pathways of immune mediated injury that occur along a T-lymphocyte activation axis and a "gut-liver-lung" axis of inflammation. Chemo-radiotherapy of HSCT conditioning causes TNFα and interleukin-1 (IL-1) release that enhance the ability of host APC to present alloantigens to mature donor T cells and upregulate chemokine expression in the lung. Once engaged, donor T cells become activated and secrete IFNγ and IL-2. IFNγ primes donor macrophages (Mϕ) and monocytes, whereas IL-2 facilitates T-cell activation and the generation of Th1 lymphocyte effectors that migrate to the lung early after HSCT in response to inflammatory chemokine gradients and contribute to pulmonary toxicity by Fas-FasL–mediated cell killing. The inflammatory axis focuses on the relationship between the cellular activating effects of LPS and the downstream production of TNFα as it occurs along a gut-liver-lung axis of inflammation. LPS enters the systemic circulation through gaps in the intestinal mucosa. The ability of systemic endotoxin to reach the alveolar space is related to the consequences of GVHD in other target organs, particularly the liver, which is pivotally located immediately downstream (via the splanchnic circulation) of the intestinal reservoir of Gram-negative bacteria and their toxic byproducts. Underlying liver damage from hepatic GVHD decreases the liver's capacity for LPS uptake and clearance, and allows passage of LPS into the pulmonary circulation. Donor macrophages primed by IFNγ are recruited to the lung where they are triggered by LPS to secrete inflammatory cytokines like TNFα resulting in enhanced chemokine expression, the recruitment of neutrophils to the lung and increased tissue damage.

stimulates the release of inflammatory cytokines that produce lung damage, including the development of alveolar hemorrhage in animals with advanced GVHD.[34,50] The role of donor accessory cell populations in the pathophysiology of IPS has been examined in HSCT donors which differ in their response to LPS because of a genetic mutation in the Toll-like receptor 4 (*Tlr 4*) gene[51] or the absence of CD14, a key cell surface receptor for the LPS–LPS-binding protein (LBP) complex.[60] In each case, a significant decrease in lung injury was observed in recipients of LPS-resistant compared to wild-type, LPS-sensitive donor cells. Results obtained using CD14-deficient donors are consistent with the report that monocytes recruited to an inflamed lung upregulate CD14 expression and show enhanced sensitivity to LPS stimulation,[61] and with the clinical observation that cytokine activation and components of the LPS-activating system including LBP and soluble CD14 is present in the BAL fluid of HSCT patients with IPS.[14]

Treatment Strategies for IPS

Current standard regimens for IPS include supportive care measures in conjunction with broad-spectrum antimicrobial agents, with or without intravenous corticosteroids (Table

Table 3 Therapies for IPS

Supportive therapy:
• Supplemental oxygen, mechanical ventilation
• Empiric broad spectrum antimicrobial agents pending culture results
• Management of iatrogenic fluid overload
• Continuous veno-venous hemofiltration (CVVH)
Immunosuppressive therapy:
• Corticosteroids (2 mg/kg/d)
• Investigational: cytokine inhibitors, including anti-TNF agents.

3).[5,15] Unfortunately, responses are limited and the mortality due to IPS remains high.[6] Advances in supportive care, such as the early institution of continuous veno-venous hemofiltration, may help to improve survival in some cases.[62] However, prospective studies addressing the treatment of IPS, including specifically the benefit of corticosteroids, are lacking in the literature. Recent reports from the University of Michigan and the Dana Farber Cancer Institute suggest that etanercept (Enbrel, Amgen Corp, Thousand Oaks, CA) might be useful in IPS.[15,63] Etanercept was administered subcutaneously in combination with systemic corticosteroids to a total of 18 patients with IPS, subcutaneously at a dose of 0.4 mg/kg twice weekly for a maximum of eight doses. Therapy was well tolerated. Thirteen of 18 patients were able to completely withdrawal from supplemental oxygen support within 28 days of therapy; survival at day 28 and day 56 (from the first etanercept dose) was 73% and 60%, respectively.[63] Based on these encouraging results, larger phase II and phase III trials are in development.

Chronic Obstructive Lung Disease and Restrictive Lung Disease Following HSCT

Definition, Clinical Course, and Risk Factors

Two forms of chronic pulmonary dysfunction are common in patients surviving greater than 100 days post-transplant: obstructive lung disease (OLD) and restrictive lung disease (RLD).[7,11,40,64,65] The incidence of both patterns of lung toxicity ranges from 20% to 50%, depending on donor source and time interval after HSCT.[7–11,64] Collagen deposition and the development of fibrosis either in the interstitial (RLD) or peri-bronchiolar space (OLD) are believed to contribute to abnormalities in pulmonary function testing (PFT). Though both exist as late-onset, non-infectious lung complications, RLD and OLD are distinguishable (Table 4). Restrictive changes are identified by reductions in forced vital capacity (FVC), total lung capacity (TLC), and diffusion capacity of the lung for carbon monoxide (DLCO), as measured by standard PFT.[6,8,11,40,64] In contrast, OLD is manifested on PFTs by a diminished forced expiratory volume (FEV_1) or FEV_1/FVC ratio, and, unlike restrictive disease, is clearly associated with chronic GVHD. OLD is a well-documented cause of morbidity after allogeneic HSCT,[40,65–68] with obstructive defects observed in approximately 15% to 25% of allogeneic HSCT recipients by day 180 post-transplant.[8,40,64]

Histologic features of RLD after HSCT are rarely described, although varying degrees of interstitial and alveolar inflammation and fibrosis, as seen in other forms of interstitial lung disease such as idiopathic pulmonary fibrosis (IPF), would be expected. An important exception is BOOP. Although reported in less than 2% of HSCT recipients, BOOP is associated with restrictive (rather than obstructive) PFTs.[6] Presenting symptoms of dry cough, shortness of breath, and fever are accompanied by radiographic findings of diffuse, peripheral, fluffy infiltrates, consistent with airspace consolidation.[69] Signature features on biopsy are patchy fibrosis; granulation tissue within alveolar spaces, alveolar ducts, and respiratory bronchioles; and the absence of infectious organisms.[69] The term BOOP should not be used interchangeably with BrOb or bronchiolitis obliterans syndrome (BOS) to describe a patient with chronic lung dysfunction after HSCT, although such usage is unfortunately widespread. The two disorders differ with respect to histopathology, pulmonary function characteristics, and most important, response to therapy; BOOP after HSCT is responsive to corticosteroids and in other settings may resolve spontaneously, whereas BrOb or BOS is not.[6,69]

BrOb remains the most common histologic pulmonary pattern in OLD following HSCT; small airway inflammation and fibrinous obliteration of the bronchiolar lumen are observed (Fig 3). Classically, BrOb is associated with a fixed obstructive defect on PFT, with diminished FEV_1 and FEV_1/FVC ratios.[7,70] Because OLD is rarely confirmed histopathologically, two phrases that identify affected patients are described: "obstructive bronchiolitis," functional airflow obstruction in patients with signs and symptoms of bronchial inflammation,[65] and BOS, the deterioration of graft function accompanying lung allograft rejection.

The lack of consistent terminology for OLD, along with variability in diagnostic criteria, has contributed to the wide variation in the reported incidence (from 6% to 20%) of this lung injury after HSCT.[6] The onset of OLD is later than for IPS and more insidious.[67] Respiratory symptoms may include cough, dyspnea, and wheezing, but many patients remain asymptomatic despite moderate to severe airway obstruction on PFTs.[40] Plain films of the chest are often unremarkable, with hyperinflation on end-expiratory films the primary radiographic feature. High-resolution computed tomography (CT) is required to optimally define the severity of disease. Chest CT findings range from normal early in the course of

Table 4 Clinical Factors in Obstructive Versus Restrictive Lung Disease

Clinical Factor	OLD	RLD
Onset	Late (3 to 12 mo)	Early (within 3 mo)
PFTs	Decreased FEV_1, FEV_1/FVC	Decreased FVC, TLC, DLCO
Chronic GVHD	Strong association	No association

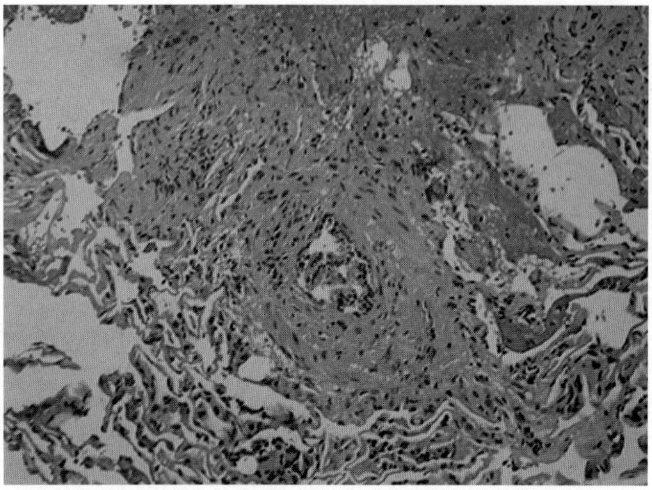

Figure 3 Histopathology of chronic obstructive pulmonary disease following allogeneic HSCT. The cicatricial form of obstructive lung disease/bronchiolitis obliterans is shown, with concentric, periluminal fibrous bands and obliteration of small airways (100×).

disease to extensive peribronchial inflammation (centrilobular nodules), bronchiectasis, and significant air trapping later.[7,71,72]

The clinical course of OLD varies from mild, with slow deterioration, to severe, with necrotizing bronchiolitis, a rapid decline in FEV_1, and a mortality rate of 25% to 50%.[7,9,10,39,67] Response to bronchodilator therapy is marginal since airflow obstruction tends to be fixed rather than reversible. Responses to immunosuppressive therapy (including various combinations of corticosteroids, cyclosporine, and azathioprine) are limited, typically resulting in preservation of remaining lung function rather than significant improvement; OLD developing more than 6 months post HSCT may show a more favorable response to therapy.[73] Since enhanced immunosuppression increases the risk of infection, the utility of such therapy is questionable when a clinical response is not apparent within the first weeks of treatment or when pulmonary dysfunction is chronic. Early detection of disease may be important[7,10,67]; a decrease of maximum mid-expiratory flow rates (MMFR) or high residual volume (RV) may be earlier indicators of BrOb than are changes in FEV_1.[10,39]

Risk factors for OLD are older donor age, the use of MTX for GVHD prophylaxis, the presence of esophageal dysfunction (with aspiration), employment of mismatched donors, and busulfan (rather than TBI) in HSCT conditioning regimens.[7,10,40,65,67,74] The development of OLD is strongly associated with chronic GVHD, particularly in patients with low serum IgG levels[67,75] and with chronic hepatic GVHD.[7] Recipients of human leukocyte antigen (HLA)-mismatched related donor or matched unrelated donor grafts have a much higher incidence of OLD than do patients receiving 6/6 HLA-matched related donor transplants (40% *v* 13%).[7]

The Pathogenesis of Obstructive Lung Disease and Restrictive Lung Disease

The pathophysiology of chronic lung injury after HSCT is poorly defined. There is a lack of correlative data obtained from afflicted HSCT recipients and a paucity of suitable HSCT animal models for either the restrictive or the obstructive form of chronic lung injury. The development of chronic lung disease likely involves an initial insult to lung parenchyma, followed by an ongoing inflammatory process involving interplay between recruited immune effector cells and the resident cells of the pulmonary vascular endothelium and interstitium. Mechanistic insights into OLD following HSCT have been derived from studies of lung allograft rejection. Data generated from both humans and mice support the hypothesis that the development of BrOb in this setting involves the secretion of inflammatory cytokines and chemokines, along with interactions between APCs and activated lymphocytes.[76,77]

A triphasic model of non-infectious lung injury after HSCT is proposed, in which alloantigen recognition is the inciting stimulus of the immune response (Fig 4). In phase I, an acute pneumonitis develops as a consequence of an allogeneic immune response, resulting in the sequential influx of lymphocytes, macrophages, and neutrophils into inflamed pulmonary parenchyma (Fig 4A). In phase II, persistence of an inflammatory signal in the setting of dysregulated repair mechanisms promotes the transition from acute to chronic injury. If the inciting injurious stimuli predominantly involves bronchiolar epithelial cells, phase II is associated with the concentric infiltration of lymphocytes and collagen deposition in the peri-bronchiolar areas, resulting in chronic bronchiolitis (Fig 4B). In contrast, if the principal target is the alveolar epithelium, leukocyte recruitment and matrix deposition during phase II are mainly confined to the interstitial space (Fig 4C); activated lymphocytes then migrate into the airway mucosa and contribute to epithelial injury. As chronic inflammation proceeds to phase III, lung fibroblasts increase dramatically in number and contribute to enhanced deposition of collagen and granulation tissue in and around bronchial structures, ultimately resulting in complete obliteration of small airways and fixed obstructive defects (Fig 4D). Fibroblast proliferation and intra-septal collagen deposition during phase III ultimately result in interstitial thickening, septal fibrosis, significant volume loss, and severe RLD (Fig 4E).

Clinical and experimental data suggest that the progression to a chronic, pro-fibrotic form of pulmonary toxicity involves the secretion of cytokines and chemokines,[26,78,79] and in this context, TNFα may be a central factor in the triphasic model. Strong evidence for a role of TNFα in the transition from acute to chronic lung injury comes from study of transgenic mice with targeted overexpression of TNFα in the lungs.[80] Early lung histopathology showed a lymphocytic infiltrate, similar to that seen in experimental IPS models,[32,34] whereas the histologic changes associated with more prolonged exposure to TNFα closely resembled those observed at later time points after HSCT.[13,26]

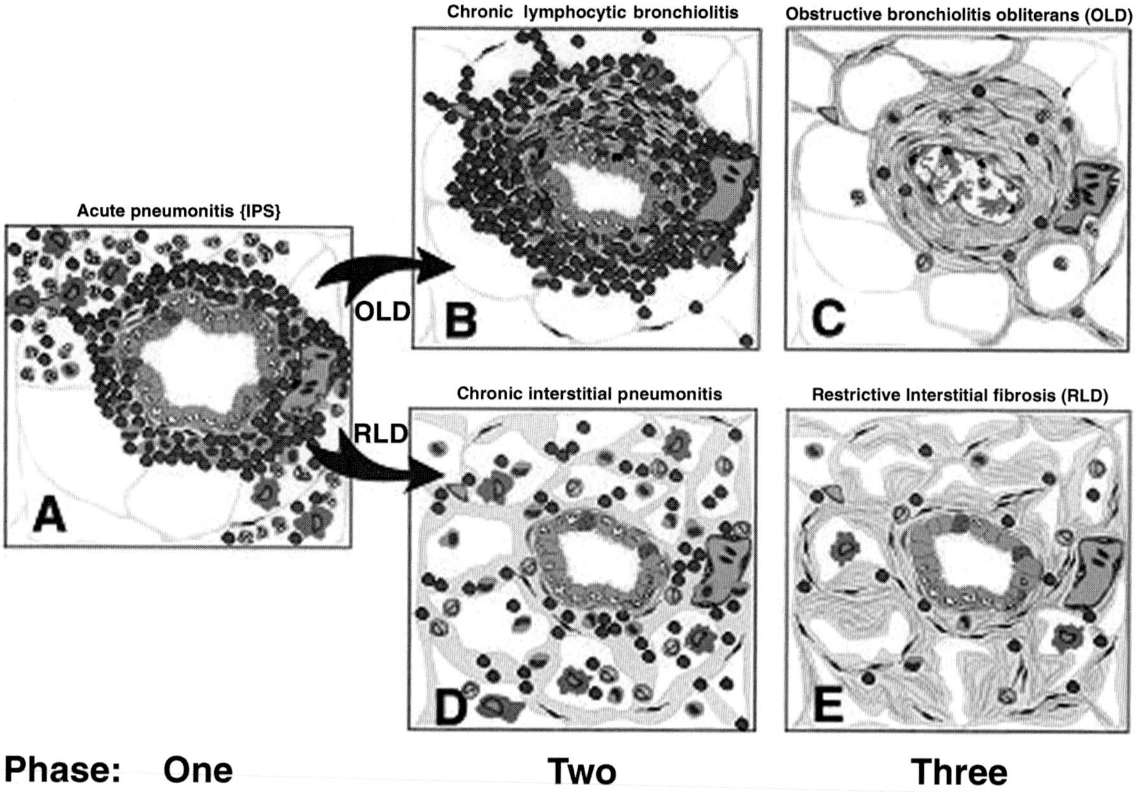

Figure 4 A triphasic model of both OLD and RLD following allogeneic HSCT. Immune-mediated injury to the lung after allogeneic HSCT can be conceptualized in three phases. In phase I, acute lung injury develops as a consequence of an allogeneic immune response and results in the sequential influx of lymphocytes, macrophages and neutrophils into an inflamed pulmonary parenchyma (A). Persistence of an inflammatory signal in the setting of dysregulated repair mechanisms promotes the transition from acute to chronic injury in phase II (B and D). As chronic inflammation proceeds to phase III, lung fibroblasts increase dramatically in number and contribute to the enhanced deposition of collagen and granulation tissue in and around bronchial structures, ultimately resulting in complete obliteration of small airways and fixed OLD (C). If, by contrast, the principal target of early damage is the alveolar epithelium, fibroblast proliferation and intra-septal collagen deposition ultimately results in interstitial fibrosis and RLD (E).

Treatment of Chronic Lung Injury After HSCT

The clear association between OLD and chronic GVHD has resulted in a general consensus that this form of lung damage is immunologically mediated. Thus "standard" therapy of OLD combines enhanced immunosuppression with supportive care, supplemental oxygen therapy, and broad-spectrum antimicrobial prophylaxis. Unfortunately, the response to multiple agents—corticosteroids, cyclosporine, tacrolimus, and azathioprine—is limited and tends to only occur early in the course of treatment.[10,39,67,75] Patients with more severe disease at the start of treatment have poor prognoses and high mortality rates, suggesting that early recognition of obstructive disease may be important.[10,39,67]

There are few published therapeutic trials for chronic lung injury after HSCT. In one study, the use of cyclosporine and MTX as GVHD prophylaxis prevented the development of OLD when compared to historical controls who received prednisone and MTX,[81] but results of prospective, randomized trials are not available. Three recently published case series exploited the anti-inflammatory effects of the macrolide antibiotic azithromycin to treat OLD in both allogeneic HSCT and lung allograft recipients. There was a beneficial effect in all studies of drug on pulmonary function when administered for 12 or more weeks.[82–84] The potential role for TNFα in the pathogenesis of both OLD and RLD implies that agents such as etanercept, which neutralize this protein, may have promise; several studies have demonstrated benefit of this drug in some HSCT patients with chronic lung injury.[85,86]

Conclusion

Non-infectious lung injury remains a major problem after allogeneic HSCT. Our understanding of the pathogenesis of lung injury in this context is limited by the absence of controlled clinical studies and the paucity of human data, but animal models have clearly shown immunologic mechanisms to be operative. Is the lung a target of GVHD? The weight of conceptual and experimental evidence favors this hypothesis. The lung is a rich source of histocompatibility antigens and professional APCs and is the site of complex immunologic networks of cytokine production and lymphocyte activation, both of which play a role in acute GVHD, directly contribute to acute lung injury in animal HSCT models, and have been identified in the BAL fluid of patients with IPS. Clinically, the major obstacle to accepting the lung as a GVHD target organ has been the lack of apoptotic epithelial injury. The unique aspects of epithelial anatomy in the lung may account for this discrepancy; the histopathologic repertoire of pulmonary damage is very limited due to the lack of stratification or layering of pulmonary epithelial cells as seen in the skin or intestine. The lung is clearly a target of chronic GVHD, but the pathogenesis and epidemiology of chronic lung injury remain ill defined. Similarities between the histopathologic features of BrOb seen with OLD after allogeneic HSCT and during lung allograft rejection, together with reports of improvement in lung function with immunosuppression, strongly support an immunologic mechanism. The case for the immune system in RLD is more tenuous and data from experimental allogeneic models remain scant. TNFα may be involved in both acute IPS and chronic lung disease of either the obstructive or restrictive type. Further research into mechanisms of injury after HSCT should improve our understanding of these disease processes and ultimately lead to successful therapies.

References

1. Clark J, Hansen J, Hertz M, Parkman R, Jensen L, Peavy H: NHLBI Workshop Summary: Idiopathic pneumonia syndrome after bone marrow transplantation. Am Rev Respir Dis 147:1601-1606, 1993
2. Crawford S, Hackman R: Clinical course of idiopathic pneumonia after bone marrow transplantation. Am Rev Respir Dis 147:1393-1400, 1993
3. Weiner RS, Mortimer MB, Gale RP, Gluckman E, Kay HEM, Kolb JJ, et al: Interstitial pneumonitis after bone marrow transplantation. Ann Intern Med 104:168-175, 1986
4. Crawford S, Longton G, Storb R: Acute graft versus host disease and the risks for idiopathic pneumonia after marrow transplantation for severe aplastic anemia. Bone Marrow Transplant 12:225-231, 1993
5. Kantrow SP, Hackman RC, Boeckh M, et al: Idiopathic pneumonia syndrome: Changing spectrum of lung injury after marrow transplantation. Transplantation 63:1079-1086, 1997
6. Afessa B, Litzow MR, Tefferi A: Bronchiolitis obliterans and other late onset non-infectious pulmonary complications in hematopoietic stem cell transplantation. Bone Marrow Transplant 28:425-434, 2001
7. Schultz KR, Green GJ, Wensley D, Sargent MA, Magee JF, Spinelli JJ, et al: Obstructive lung disease in children after allogeneic bone marrow transplantation. Blood 84:3212-3220, 1994
8. Crawford SW, Pepe M, Lin D, et al: Abnormalities of pulmonary function tests after marrow transplantation predict nonrelapse mortality. Am J Respir Crit Care Med 152:690-695, 1995
9. Sullivan K, Mori M, Sanders J, Siadak M, Witherspoon RP, Anasetti C, et al: Late complications of allogeneic and autologous bone marrow transplantation. Bone Marrow Transplant 10:127-134, 1992
10. Sanchez J, Torres A, Serrano J, Romain J, Martin C, Perula L, et al: Long term follow up of immunosuppressive treatment for obstructive airway disease after allogeneic bone marrow transplantation. Bone Marrow Transplant 20:403-408, 1997
11. Badier M, Guillot C, Delpierre S, et al: Pulmonary function changes 100 days and one year after bone marrow transplantation. Bone Marrow Transplant 12:457-461, 1993
12. Wingard JR, Mellits ED, Sostrin MB, Chen DY, Burns WH, Santos GW, et al: Interstitial pneumonitis after allogeneic bone marrow transplantation. Nine-year experience at a single institution. Medicine 67:175-186, 1988
13. Yousem SA: The histological spectrum of pulmonary graft-versus-host disease in bone marrow transplant recipients. Hum Pathol 26:668-675, 1995
14. Clark JG, Madtes DK, Martin TR, Hackman RC, Farrand AL, Crawford SW: Idiopathic pneumonia after bone marrow transplantation: Cytokine activation and lipopolysaccharide amplification in the bronchoalveolar compartment. Crit Care Med 27:1800-1806, 1999
15. Yanik G, Hellerstedt B, Custer J, Hutchinson R, Kwon D, Ferrara JL, et al: Etanercept (Enbrel) administration for idiopathic pneumonia syndrome after allogeneic hematopoietic stem cell transplantation. Biol Blood Marrow Transplant 8:395-400, 2002
16. Robbins RA, Linder J, Stahl MG, Thompson AB, Haire W, Kessinger A, et al: Diffuse alveolar hemorrhage in autologous bone marrow transplant recipients. Am J Med 87:511-518, 1989
17. Lewis ID, DeFor T, Weisdorf DJ: Increasing incidence of diffuse alveolar hemorrhage following allogeneic bone marrow transplantation: Cryptic etiology and uncertain therapy. Bone Marrow Transplant 26: 539-543, 2000
18. Capizzi SA, Kumar S, Huneke NE, Gertz MA, Inwards DJ, Litzow MR, et al: Peri-engraftment respiratory distress syndrome during autologous hematopoietic stem cell transplantation. Bone Marrow Transplant 27: 1299-1303, 2001
19. Wilczynski SW, Erasmus JJ, Petros WP, Vredenburgh JJ, Foltz RJ: Delayed pulmonary toxicity syndrome following high-dose chemotherapy and bone marrow transplantation for breast cancer. Am J Respir Crit Care Med 157:565-573, 1998
20. Bhalla KS, Wilczynski SW, Abushamaa AM, Petros WP, McDonald CS, Loftis JS, et al: Pulmonary toxicity of induction chemotherapy prior to standard or high-dose chemotherapy with autologous hematopoietic support. Am J Respir Crit Care Med 161:17-25, 2000
21. Cahill RA, Spitzer TR, Mazumder A: Marrow engraftment and clincial manifestations of capillary leak syndrome. Bone Marrow Transplant 18:177-184, 1996
22. Weiner RS, Horowitz MM, Gale RP, Dicke KA, van Bekkum DW, Masaoka T, et al: Risk factors for interstitial pneumonitis following bone marrow transplantation for severe aplastic anemia. Br J Haematol 71:535-543, 1989
23. Della Volpe A, Ferreri AJ, Annaloro C, Mangili P, Rosso A, Calandrino R, et al: Lethal pulmonary complications significantly correlate with individually assessed mean lung dose in patients with hematologic malignancies treated with total body irradiation. Int J Radiat Oncol Biol Phys 52:483-488, 2002
24. Fukuda T, Hackman RC, Guthrie KA, Sandmaier BM, Boeckh M, Maris MB, et al: Risks and outcomes of idiopathic pneumonia syndrome after nonmyeloablative and conventional conditioning regimens for allogeneic hematopoietic stem cell transplantation. Blood 102:2777-2785, 2003
25. Down JD, Mauch P, Warhol M, Neben S, Ferrara JLM: The effect of donor T lymphocytes and total-body irradiation on hemopoietic engraftment and pulmonary toxicity following experimental allogeneic bone marrow transplantation. Transplantation 54:802-808, 1992
26. Shankar G, Cohen DA: Idiopathic pneumonia syndrome after bone marrow transplantation: The role of pre-transplant radiation conditioning and local cytokine dysregulation in promoting lung inflammation and fibrosis. Int J Exp Pathol 82:101-113, 2001
27. Piguet P, Collart M, Grau G, Sappino A, Vassalli P: Requirement of tumour necrosis factor for development of silica-induced pulmonary fibrosis. Nature 344:245-247, 1990
28. Schmidt J, Pliver CN, Lepe-Zuniga JL, Green I, Gery I: Silica-stimulated monocytes release fibroblast proliferation factors identical to interleukin-1. A potential role for interleukin-1 in the pathogenesis of silicosis. J Clin Invest 73:1462-1472, 1984
29. Suter P, Suter S, Girardin E, Roux-Lombard P, Grau G, Dayer J: High bronchoalveolar levels of tumor necrosis factor and its inhibitors, interleukin-1, interferon, and elastase, in patients with adult respiratory distress syndrome after trauma, shock or sepsis. Am Rev Respir Dis 145:1016-1022, 1992
30. Bortin M, Ringden O, Horowitz M, Rozman C, Weiner R, Rimm A: Temporal relationships between the major complications of bone mar-

row transplantation for leukemia. Bone Marrow Transplant 4:339-344, 1989
31. Beschorner W, Saral R, Hutchins G, Tutschka P, Santos G: Lymphocytic bronchitis associated with graft versus host disease in recipients of bone marrow transplants. N Engl J Med 299:1030-1036, 1978
32. Piguet PF, Grau GE, Collart MA, et al: Pneumopathies of the graft-versus-host reaction. Alveolitis associated with an increased level of tumor necrosis factor MRNA and chronic interstitial pneumonitis. Lab Invest 61:37-45, 1989
33. Clark JG, Madtes DK, Hackman RC, Chen W, Cheever MA, Martin PJ: Lung injury induced by alloreactive Th1 cells is characterized by host-derived mononuclear cell inflammation and activation of alveolar macrophages. J Immunol 161:1913-1920, 1998
34. Cooke KR, Kobzik L, Martin TR, Brewer J, Delmonte J, Crawford JM, et al: An experimental model of idiopathic pneumonia syndrome after bone marrow transplantation. I. The roles of minor H antigens and endotoxin. Blood 88:3230-3239, 1996
35. Cooke KR, Krenger W, Hill GR, Martin T, Kobzik L, Brewer J, et al: Host reactive donor T cells are associated with lung injury after experimental allogeneic bone marrow transplantation. Blood 92:2571-2580, 1998
36. Hackman RC, Sale GE: Large airway inflammation as a possible manifestation of a pulmonary graft-versus-host reaction in bone marrow allograft recipients. Lab Invest 44:26A, 1981
37. Connor R, Ramsay N, McGlave P, Snover D, Kersey J, Burke B: Pulmonary pathology in bone marrow transplant recipients. Lab Invest 46:3, 1982
38. Panoskaltsis-Mortari A, Taylor PA, Yaegar TM, Wangensteen OD, Bitterman PB, Ingbar DH, et al: The critical early proinflammatory events associated with idiopathic pneumonia syndrome in irradiated murine allogenic recipients are due to donor T cell infusion and potentiated by cyclophoshamide. J Clin Invest 100:1015-1027, 1997
39. Curtis DJ, Smale A, Thien F, Schwarer AP, Szer J: Chronic airflow obstruction in long-term survivors of allogeneic bone marrow transplantation. Bone Marrow Transplant 16:169-173, 1995
40. Clark JG, Schwartz DA, Flournoy N, Sullivan KM, Crawford SW, Thomas ED: Risk factors for air-flow obstruction in recipients of bone marrow transplants. Ann Intern Med 107:648-656, 1987
41. Hildebrandt GC, Corrion LA, Olkiewicz KM, Lu B, Lowler K, Duffner UA, et al: Blockade of CXCR3 receptor:ligand interactions reduces leukocyte recruitment to the lung and the severity of experimental idiopathic pneumonia syndrome. J Immunol 173:2050-2059, 2004
42. Cooke K, Kobzik L, Teshima T, Lowler K, Clouthier S, Ferrara J: A role for Fas-Fas ligand but not perforin mediated cytolysis in the development of experimental idiopathic pneumonia syndrome. Blood 96:768a, 2000
43. Hildebrandt GC, Olkiewicz KM, Corrion LA, Chang Y, Clouthier SG, Liu C, et al: Donor-derived TNF-alpha regulates pulmonary chemokine expression and the development of idiopathic pneumonia syndrome after allogeneic bone marrow transplantation. Blood 104:586-593, 2004
44. Dupuis M, McDonald DM: Dendritic-cell regulation of lung immunity. Am J Respir Cell Mol Biol 17:284-286, 1997
45. Christensen PJ, Armstrong LR, Fak JJ, Chen GH, McDonald RA, Toews GB, et al: Regulation of rat pulmonary dendritic cell immunostimulatory activity by alveolar epithelial cell-derived granulocyte macrophage colony-stimulating factor. Am J Respir Cell Mol Biol 13:426-433, 1995
46. van Haarst JM, de Wit HJ, Drexhage HA, Hoogsteden HC: Distribution and immunophenotype of mononuclear and dendritic cells in the human lung. Am J Respir Cell Mol Biol 10:487-492, 1994
47. Yousem SA, Ray L, Paradis IL, Dauber JA, Griffith BP: Potential role of dendritic cells in bronchiolitis obliterans in heart-lung transplantation. Ann Thorac Surg 49:424-428, 1990
48. Holt PG, Haining S, Nelson DJ, Sedgwick JD: Origin and steady-state turnover of class II MHC-bearing dendritic cells in the epithelium of the conducting airways. J Immunol 153:256-261, 1994
49. Piguet PF, Grau GE, Allet B, Vassalli PJ: Tumor necrosis factor/cachectin is an effector of skin and gut lesions of the acute phase of graft-versus-host disease. J Exp Med 166:1280-1289, 1987
50. Cooke KR, Hill GR, Gerbitz A, Kobzik L, Martin TR, Crawford JM, et al: Tumor necrosis factor-alpha neutralization reduces lung injury after experimental allogeneic bone marrow transplantation. Transplantation 70:272-279, 2000
51. Cooke KR, Hill GR, Gerbitz A, Kobzik L, Martin TR, Crawford JM, et al: Hyporesponsiveness of donor cells to lipopolysaccharide stimulation reduces the severity of experimental idiopathic pneumonia syndrome: Potential role for a gut-lung axis of inflammation. J Immunol 165: 6612-6619, 2000
52. Cooke K, Hill G, Crawford J, Bungard D, Brinson Y, Delmonte J Jr., et al: Tumor necrosis factor-a production to lipopolysaccharide stimulation by donor cells predicts the severity of experimental acute graft versus host disease. J Clin Invest 102:1882-1891, 1998
53. Hattori K, Hirano T, Miyajima H, Yamakawa N, Tateno M, Oshimi K, et al: Differential effects of anti-Fas ligand and anti-tumor necrosis factor-a antibodies on acute graft-versus-host disease pathologies. Blood 91:4051-4055, 1998
54. Vallera DA, Taylor PA, Vannice JL, Panoskaltsis-Mortari A, Blazar BR: Interleukin-1 or tumor necrosis factor-alpha antagonists do not inhibit graft-versus-host disease induced across the major histocompatibility barrier in mice. Transplantation 60:1371-1374, 1995
55. Clark JG, Mandac JB, Dixon AE, Martin PJ, Hackman RC, Madtes DK: Neutralization of tumor necrosis factor-alpha action delays but does not prevent lung injury induced by alloreactive T helper 1 cells. Transplantation 70:39-43, 2000
56. Haddad I, Panoskaltsis-Mortari A, Ingbar D, Yang S, Milla C, Blazar B: High levels of peroxynitrite are generated in the lungs of irradiated mice given cyclophosphamide and allogeneic T cells: A potential mechanism of injury after marrow transplantation. Am J Respir Cell Mol Biol 20: 1125-1135, 1999
57. Hill G, Ferrara J: The primacy of the gastrointestinal tract as a target organ of acute graft-versus-host disease: Rationale for the use of cytokine shields in allogeneic bone marrow transplantation. Blood 95: 2754-2759, 2000
58. Cooke KR, Gerbitz A, Crawford JM, Teshima T, Hill GR, Tesolin A, et al: LPS antagonism reduces graft-versus-host disease and preserves graft-versus-leukemia activity after experimental bone marrow transplantation. J Clin Invest 107:1581-1589, 2001
59. Fegan C, Poynton CH, Whittaker JA: The gut mucosal barrier in bone marrow transplantation. Bone Marrow Transplant 5:373-377, 1990
60. Cooke KR, Olkiewicz K, Erickson N, Ferrara JL: The role of endotoxin and the innate immune response in the pathophysiology of acute graft versus host disease. J Endotoxin Res 8:441-448, 2002
61. Maus U, Herold S, Muth H, Maus R, Ermert L, Ermert M, et al: Monocytes recruited into the alveolar air space of mice show a monocytic phenotype but upregulate CD14. Am J Physiol Lung Cell Mol Physiol 280:L58-L68, 2001
62. DiCarlo JV, Alexander SR, Agarwal R, Schiffman JD: Continuous veno-venous hemofiltration may improve survival from acute respiratory distress syndrome after bone marrow transplantation or chemotherapy. J Pediatr Hematol Oncol 25:801-805, 2003
63. Yanik GA, Levine JE, Ferrara JLM, Uberti JP, Ho VT, Antin JH, et al: Survival following etantercept therapy for the treatment of idiopathic pneumonia syndrome following allogeneic stem cell transplantation. Blood 104:104a, 2004
64. Cerveri I, Fulgoni P, Giorgiani G, Zoia MC, Beccaria M, Tinelli C, et al: Lung function abnormalities after bone marrow transplantation in children: Has the trend recently changed? Chest 120:1900-1906, 2001
65. Ringden O, Remberger M, Ruutu T, Nikoskelainen J, Volin L, Vindelov L, et al: Increased risk of chronic graft-versus-host disease, obstructive bronchiolitis, and alopecia with busulfan versus total body irradiation: Long-term results of a randomized trial in allogeneic marrow recipients with leukemia. Blood 93:2196-2201, 1999
66. Ralph DD, Springmeyer SC, Sullivan KM, Hackman RC, Storb R, Thomas ED: Rapidly progressive air-flow obstruction in marrow transplant recipients. Possible association between obliterative bronchiolitis and chronic graft-versus-host disease. Am Rev Respir Dis 129:641-644, 1984
67. Clark JG, Crawford SW, Madtes DK, Sullivan KM: Obstructive lung

disease after allogeneic marrow transplantation. Clinical presentation and course. Ann Intern Med 111:368-376, 1989
68. Sullivan KM, Agura E, Anasetti C, Appelbaum F, Badger C, Bearman S, et al: Chronic graft-versus-host disease and other late complications of bone marrow transplantation. Semin Hematol 28:250-259, 1991
69. d'Alessandro MP, Kozakewich HP, Cooke KR, Taylor GA: Radiologic-pathologic conference of Children's Hospital Boston: New pulmonary nodules in a child undergoing treatment for a solid malignancy. Pediatr Radiol 26:19-21, 1996
70. King TE Jr: Overview of bronchiolitis. Clin Chest Med 14:607-610, 1993
71. Ooi GC, Peh WC, Ip M: High-resolution computed tomography of bronchiolitis obliterans syndrome after bone marrow transplantation. Respiration 65:187-191, 1998
72. Bankier AA, Van Muylem A, Knoop C, Estenne M, Gevenois PA: Bronchiolitis obliterans syndrome in heart-lung transplant recipients: Diagnosis with expiratory CT. Radiology 218:533-539, 2001
73. Dudek AZ, Mahaseth H, DeFor TE, Weisdorf DJ: Bronchiolitis obliterans in chronic graft-versus-host disease: Analysis of risk factors and treatment outcomes. Biol Blood Marrow Transplant 9:657-666, 2003
74. Beinert T, Dull T, Wolf K, Holler E, Vogelmeier C, Behr J, et al: Late pulmonary impairment following allogeneic bone marrow transplantation. Eur J Med Res 1:343-348, 1996
75. Holland HK, Wingard JR, Beschorner WE, Saral R, Santos GW: Bronchiolitis obliterans in bone marrow transplantation and its relationship to chronic graft-versus-host disease and low serum IgG. Blood 72:621-627, 1988
76. Belperio JA, DiGiovine B, Keane MP, Burdick MD, Ying Xue Y, Ross DJ, et al: Interleukin-1 receptor antagonist as a biomarker for bronchiolitis obliterans syndrome in lung transplant recipients. Transplantation 73: 591-599, 2002
77. Elssner A, Jaumann F, Dobmann S, Behr J, Schwaiblmair M, Reichenspurner H, , et al: Elevated levels of interleukin-8 and transforming growth factor-beta in bronchoalveolar lavage fluid from patients with bronchiolitis obliterans syndrome: Proinflammatory role of bronchial epithelial cells. Munich Lung Transplant Group. Transplantation 70:362-367, 2000
78. Coker R, Laurent G: Pulmonary fibrosis: Cytokines in the balance. Eur Respir J 11:1218-1221, 1998
79. Sime P, Marr R, Gauldie D, Xing Z, Hewlett B, Graham F, et al: Transfer of tumor necrosis factor-a to rat lung induces severe pulmonary inflammation and patchy interstitial fibrogenesis with induction of transforming growth factor-b1 and myofibroblasts. Am J Pathol 153:825-832, 1998
80. Miyazaki Y, Araki K, Vesin C, Garcia I, Kapanci Y, Whitsett J, et al: Expression of a tumor necrosis factor-a transgene in murine lung causes lymphocytic and fibrosing alveolitis. J Clin Invest 96:250-259, 1995
81. Payne L, Chan CK, Fyles G, Hyland RH, Bafundi P, Yueng M, et al: Cyclosporine as possible prophylaxis for obstructive airways disease after allogeneic bone marrow transplantation. Chest 104:114-118, 1993
82. Verleden GM, Dupont LJ: Azithromycin therapy for patients with bronchiolitis obliterans syndrome after lung transplantation. Transplantation 77:1465-1467, 2004
83. Gerhardt SG, McDyer JF, Girgis RE, Conte JV, Yang SC, Orens JB: Maintenance azithromycin therapy for bronchiolitis obliterans syndrome: Results of a pilot study. Am J Respir Crit Care Med 168:121-125, 2003
84. Khalid M, Al Saghir A, Saleemi S, Al Dammas S, Zeitouni M, Al Mobeireek A, et al: Azithromycin in bronchiolitis obliterans complicating bone marrow transplantation: A preliminary study. Eur Respir J 25: 490-493, 2005
85. Chiang KY, Abhyankar S, Bridges K, Godder K, Henslee-Downey JP: Recombinant human tumor necrosis factor receptor fusion protein as complementary treatment for chronic graft-versus-host disease. Transplantation 73:665-667, 2002
86. Yanik G, Uberti J, Ferrara JLM, White E, Hellerstedt B, Standiford T, et al: Etanercept for sub-acute lung injury following allogeneic stem cell transplantation. Blood 102:471a, 2003

ELSEVIER

Seminars in
HEMATOLOGY

Graft-Versus-Host Disease and Graft-Versus-Leukemia After Donor Leukocyte Infusion

David Porter[a] and John E. Levine[b]

Although dramatically effective for relapsed chronic myelogenous leukemia (CML), successful donor leukocyte infusion (DLI) remains limited primarily by inadequate responses for patients with diseases other than CML and by toxicity related to graft-versus-host disease (GVHD). Acute GVHD grades 2 to 4 follows 34% to 47% of infusions and chronic GVHD occurs in 33% to 61% of cases. Strategies to reduce the incidence and severity of GVHD while preserving the graft-versus-leukemia (GVL) effect, such as low-dose DLI, depletion of GVHD effector cells, and tumor-specific DLI, are reviewed.
Semin Hematol 43:53-61

It is now generally accepted that allogeneic hematopoietic stem cell transplantation (HSCT) is associated with an important graft-versus-leukemia (GVL) reaction mediated, at least in part, by donor T cells. Before the clinical application of donor leukocyte infusions (DLI) was used to induce a direct GVL reaction, the evidence for GVL activity in human transplantation was several important if indirect observations. In anecdotal reports, abrupt withdrawal of immunosuppression (or a flare of acute graft-versus-host disease [GVHD]) appeared to re-establish complete remission in some patients with relapsed leukemia.[1,2] Other data show that the risk of leukemic relapse is higher for recipients of syngeneic marrow grafts compared with recipients of allogeneic grafts,[3,4] and that GVHD may be protective against relapse after allogeneic HSCT.[3,5] Furthermore, while T-cell depletion of an allogeneic donor graft markedly limits GVHD, it increases the risk of relapse; in chronic myelogenous leukemia (CML), the incidence of relapse is as high as 50%, compared to 10% to 20% when unmanipulated donor marrow is transplanted.[3,6] However, the successful application of DLI for relapsed leukemia provided the first direct and indisputable demonstration of a GVL reaction in the clinical setting.[7-12]

[a]Department of Medicine, University of Pennsylvania Medical Center, Philadelphia, PA.

[b]Department of Pediatrics, University of Michigan Medical School, Ann Arbor, MI.

Address correspondence to John E. Levine, MD, Associate Professor of Pediatrics, University of Michigan Medical School, 1500 E Medical Center Dr, B1-207 CCGC, Ann Arbor, MI 48109-0914. E-mail: jelevine@umich.edu

DLI for CML

Given the convincing data that donor T cells were associated with potent GVL activity after allogeneic HSCT, it was logical to test the potential for DLI to induce a direct GVL reaction in patients with relapsed disease, independent of the initial transplant. One of the first published reports was from Kolb and colleagues, who treated three patients with relapsed CML after allogeneic HSCT with donor buffy coat cells from the original transplant donor: all three achieved a complete cytogenetic remission.[13] Over the next several years, many centers reported similar results using DLI for patients with CML who had relapsed after allogeneic HSCT.[9,14-16] DLI could induce complete remissions for the majority of patients in relapse of chronic-phase CML. Furthermore, the majority of patients also achieved a complete molecular response when assayed by polymerase chain reaction (PCR) techniques capable of detecting one CML cell in 1 million normal cells.[17]

Two large retrospective analyses further confirmed the potent GVL activity of DLI (Table 1).[7,8] These data are remarkably consistent with single-institution trials: 76% to 79% of patients treated with DLI for relapsed chronic-phase CML will achieve complete cytogenetic and molecular remission. DLI is most effective for patients with chronic-phase relapse but disappointing in accelerated phase or blast crisis relapse, in whom remissions were observed in only 12% to 28% of cases. In addition, even those patients with advanced-phase CML who respond to DLI are less likely to enjoy prolonged remissions[18,19]; relapses occur in up to 43% of,[18] and the rate may be higher with longer follow-up. In contrast, the majority of remissions are durable in patients treated for early-phase relapse

0037-1963/05/$-see front matter
doi:10.1053/j.seminhematol.2005.09.005

Table 1 Response Rates to Donor Leukocyte Infusions to Treat Relapse After Allogeneic Bone Marrow Transplantation

Disease	Response Rate
CML chronic phase	76% (28/37) (8)
	79% (53/67) (7)
CML advanced phase	28% (5/18) (8)
	12% (1/8) (7)
AML	15% (6/39) (8)
	29% (5/17) (7)
	36% (16/44) (12)*
ALL	18% (2/11) (8)
	0% (0/12) (7)
	13% (2/15) (11)
MDS	40% (2/5) (8)
	25% (1/4) (7)
NHL	0/6 (0%) (8)
Multiple myeloma	50% (2/4) (8)
	31% (4/13) (26)
	22% (6/27) (10)
	9% (2/22) (27)†

NOTE. Representative response rates are illustrated from either registry data or in some cases, larger series of DLI for a specific indication.

Abbreviations: AML, acute myelogenous leukemia; ALL, acute lymphocyte leukemia; MDS, myelodysplasia; NHL, non-Hodgkin's lymphoma; CML, chronic myelogenous leukemia.

*All patients were pretreated with chemotherapy by design of the protocol.

†A total of 25 patients were treated. An additional three patients achieved a complete response after treatment with chemotherapy before DLI.

of CML (hematologic, cytogenetic, or molecular relapse). In the North American retrospective analysis, long-term data were available from 39 patients in remission after DLI for CML.[20] Only five patients (13%) relapsed, including two of 32 (6%) recipients of DLI for early-phase relapse and three of seven (43%) recipients of DLI for advanced-phase relapse of CML. The probability of both event-free survival and overall survival was 73% at 3 years (Fig 1). The Hammersmith group also reported long-term outcomes for 66 recipients of DLI for relapsed CML; 44 patients achieved a molecular remission with DLI.[19] Four of these patients (9%) ultimately had recurrence of CML as documented by PCR analysis 15 to 87 weeks after remission. The probability of molecular remission at 3 years was 68% for the entire group. Again advanced-phase CML and a short duration of remission after transplant were poor prognostic factors for outcomes after DLI. Late relapses in both long-term follow-up studies raise the concern that the GVL effects provided by donor T cells might have limited durability.

DLI for Acute Leukemia

In contrast to excellent response rates for early-phase CML relapse, complete remissions after DLI are generally not seen in more than 20% to 25% of relapse in advanced hematologic malignancy and, for some diseases, responses are rare (Table 1), all suggesting that GVL activity from DLI has disease specificity. DLI for patients with acute myelogenous leukemia (AML) yields response rates between 15% and 29%,[7,8] and DLI for patients with acute lymphocytic leukemia (ALL) has generally been considered ineffective.[7] The poor outcomes for DLI in acute leukemia have not been explained. Leukemia cell growth outstripping the cytotoxicity rate of the donor leukocytes may partly explain the relatively low response rates. For example, when patients with advanced leukemia receive cytoreductive chemotherapy prior to DLI, complete remissions are more frequent. A compilation of 67 reported cases of acute leukemia demonstrated that 44 patients (AML 25/35, ALL 19/32) entered a complete remission, for an overall complete response rate of 66%,[8,21-23] and median disease-free survival (DFS) was 26 months. Because these studies were retrospective, selection and reporting bias may have influenced the results.

Levine et al reported results of a prospective study of 65 patients with hematologic relapse of advanced myeloid malignancy after human leukocyte antigen (HLA)-matched sibling HSCT, who were treated on a protocol of cytarabine-based chemotherapy, then granulocyte colony-stimulating factor (G-CSF)–primed DLIs.[12] Twenty-seven of 57 (47%) assessable patients entered a complete remission; overall survival at 2 years was 19%. Patients who recovered from chemotherapy and DLI in complete remission had 1- and 2-year survival rates of 51% and 41%, respectively, compared to a 1-year survival of only 5% in nonresponders. A post-transplant remission lasting more than 6 months before relapse was predictive of superior response and survival (Fig 2). Survival at 1 year for patients with relapse within 6 months of transplant was 10% compared to 44% for patients who relapsed more than 6 months from transplant ($P < .001$).[12]

Relapse rates for acute leukemia after DLI are high.[7,8] Porter et al reported long-term follow-up results for patients who achieved a complete remission following DLI.[24] Eleven of 27 (41%) patients, mainly with acute leukemia, in remission after DLI, relapsed at a median of 10 months from DLI (range,

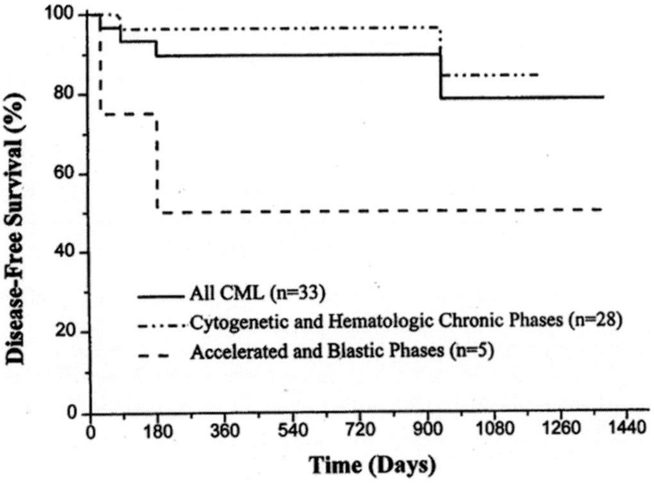

Figure 1 Disease-free survival after DLI for CML. Reprinted with permission from the American Society of Clinical Oncology.[20]

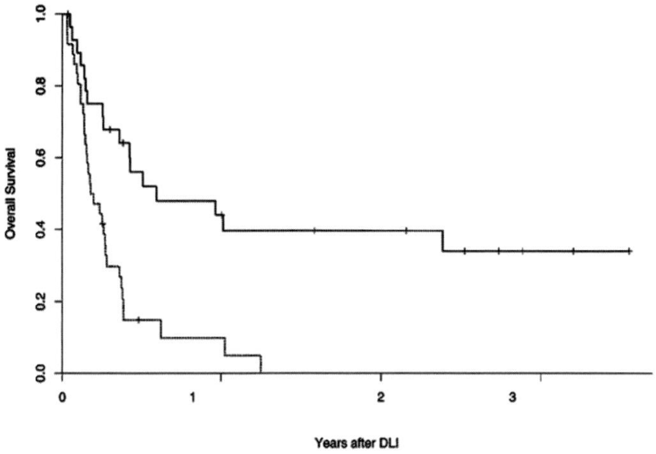

Figure 2 Survival after chemotherapy followed by DLI for AML; post-transplant remission greater than 6 months (solid line), post-transplant remission less than 6 months (dashed line). Reprinted with permission from the American Society of Clinical Oncology.[12]

1 to 37 months). Also affecting the durability of remission after DLI for acute leukemia has been the problem of extramedullary relapses, which have been reported in numerous sites, including some not usually considered sanctuary sites for leukemia.[23]

Optimal dosing of DLI for advanced leukemia has not been established, but two studies have suggested that a targeted DLI dose of 1×10^8 $CD3^+$ cells/kg of recipient body weight may be optimal.[12] In a Japanese protocol, the minimal dose of leukocytes associated with developing fatal GVHD was 7×10^7/kg of recipient body weight, indicative of the difficulty in separating therapeutic effect from toxicity.[12]

DLI for Myeloma, Hodgkin's Disease, and Non-Hodgkin's Lymphoma

Response rates and remission duration in patients with other diseases are less well defined. It is clear that a "graft-versus-myeloma" effect from DLI can induce remissions in some patients who relapse after allogeneic HSCT.[25] However, despite response rates of over 60%, complete responses have occurred in only 25% to 30% of patients and sustained remissions in 0% to 18%.[10,25-27] The North American multicenter analysis reported complete remissions in two of 22 patients who received DLI alone, but both relapsed 10 and 26 weeks after complete remission.[27] In addition to limited response rates, toxicity from DLI for myeloma is significant, with more than half the patients experiencing acute and chronic GVHD. A graft-versus-myeloma effect has been implicated in other settings, such as with the use of prophylactic DLI following T-cell–depleted HSCT[28] or reduced intensity conditioning.[29] These data suggest that DLI can generate a meaningful graft-versus-myeloma effect for some patients, but significant toxicity and relapse constrain its utility in this disease.

There are limited data on DLI in non-Hodgkin's lymphoma (NHL) and Hodgkin's lymphoma, but indirect evidence suggests both diseases are susceptible to GVL induction.[30,31] Although no responses in six patients with NHL were reported to the North American DLI registry,[8] other reports suggest DLI can induce a meaningful graft-versus-lymphoma reaction.[32-34] A graft-versus-Hodgkin's disease also appears to be generated using DLI in the setting of non-myeloablative allogeneic HSCT.[35]

Unrelated Donor Leukocyte Infusions

The use of matched unrelated donor (MUD) stem cell products for allogeneic HSCT is growing rapidly, and hence relapse after unrelated donor HSCT is an increasing problem. There is less information available about anticipated outcomes after unrelated DLI than for related donor DLI. Unrelated DLI might increase the severity and frequency of GVHD due to the higher degree of HLA disparity between recipient and donor; if unrelated DLI could provide similar, less, or even enhanced GVL activity compared to matched related DLI is unknown. While a number of reports include recipients of unrelated DLI,[7,8,11,19,36-38] in most cases, only limited numbers of patients were treated and data regarding the specific outcome after unrelated DLI are not always provided. Therefore, it has been difficult to draw conclusions about either the toxicity or efficacy of unrelated DLI.

Two large retrospective analyses suggested that unrelated DLI and related DLI result in similar outcomes, but both had small numbers of patients.[7,8] Two other studies focused primarily on the role of unrelated DLI for relapsed disease.[39] For relapsed CML, outcomes after related DLI in 18 patients were compared directly to outcomes for 12 recipients of unrelated DLI. A cytogenetic remission was achieved in 73% of related DLI recipients compared to in 64% of unrelated DLI recipients ($P = .71$). There was a trend toward more frequent grade II to IV acute GVHD after unrelated DLI (58% *v* 39%) that did not reach statistical significance ($P = .09$), possibly due to the small numbers of patients. The incidence of chronic GVHD was 49% for all patients and was not dependent on the donor source. The only factor associated with response was disease stage at the time of DLI, similar to other reports[7,8,40]; patients treated in cytogenetic or molecular relapse were seven times more likely to respond when compared to patients treated in hematologic relapse.

In a larger retrospective analysis, 58 recipients of unrelated DLI were identified through the National Marrow Donor Program database.[40] Patients received unrelated DLI for relapse of CML ($n = 25$), AML ($n = 23$), ALL ($n = 7$), or other diseases ($n = 3$). Donor and recipient were HLA-mismatched in at least 21% of cases. The median cell dose administered was 1.0×10^8 mononuclear cells (MNC)/kg. Several patients were in remission prior to DLI; for those patients with active disease at the time of DLI, complete remissions were achieved in 46% of patients with CML, 42% of patients with AML, and two of four patients with ALL. The incidence of grade II to IV acute GVHD was 25% and chronic GVHD occurred in 41% of patients, results consistent with data from large series of

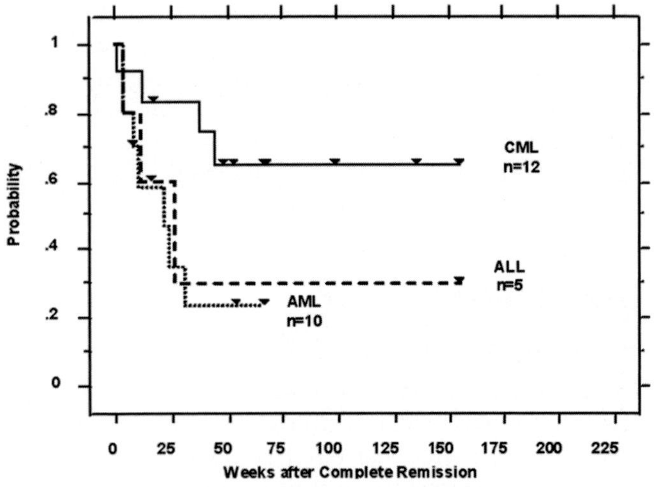

Figure 3 Disease-free survival after unrelated DLI for leukemia relapse. From: Porter et al, Treatment of relapsed leukemia after unrelated donor marrow transplantation with unrelated donor leukocyte infusions. *Blood* 2000;95:1214-1221. ©American Society of Hematology, used with permission.[40]

related DLI. The estimated probability of DFS for all recipients of DLI (regardless of remission status at the time of DLI) at 1 year after complete remission was 65% for CML, 23% for AML, and 30% for ALL (Fig 3). As anticipated, overall survival appeared superior for patients with early-phase relapse of CML compared with advanced-phase relapse. There was no association of mononuclear cell dose with GVHD, response, survival, or DFS. Only a longer time interval from transplant to relapse and of transplant to unrelated DLI was associated with improved survival and DFS, respectively. There also was no obvious association between acute and chronic GVHD and disease response, in contrast to several,[7,8,18] though not all,[41] related DLI studies.

GVHD After DLI

Acute and chronic GVHD have been the major direct complications from DLI. In retrospective and prospective studies, acute or chronic GVHD has been reported in 40% to 60% of evaluable patients (Table 2); usually GVHD has correlated with GVL activity and response.[7,8] In the North American analysis, over 90% of complete responders developed acute GVHD and 88% of responders developed chronic GVHD. Of 23 patients who did not experience GVHD, only three achieved a complete remission. In 92 patients who had no response, only 35% had acute GHVD and only 13% had chronic GVHD. In the European Group for Blood and Marrow Transplantation (EBMT) analysis, 41% of DLI recipients developed grade II to IV acute GVHD.[7] However, many patients who fail to respond to GVL induction will die shortly of progressive disease and not survive long enough to develop GVHD, particularly important for patients with acute leukemia. Some complete responses were seen in patients without any sign of GVHD, and a GVL effect in the absence of clinical GVHD provides important evidence for GVL activity separate from GVHD.

In general, GVHD that occurs after DLI has been mild to moderate and responsive to immunosuppressive therapy—important since the dose of T cells infused with DLI may be 10- to 100-fold higher than the T-cell dose administered at the time of transplant, and DLI is administered without additional immunosuppression. Indeed, at time of transplant, if immunosuppression were withheld or a similar dose of donor T cells were given as are used for DLI (to augment GVL), toxicity would be unacceptable.[42,43] Likely the effects of GVHD are more tolerable when separated from acute transplant toxicity: GVHD can be stimulated and exacerbated by the "cytokine storm" that accompanies transplantation. Tissue damage from the intensive conditioning regimen, infections, and other physiologic insults result in a cascade of events that ultimately augment the GVHD reaction.[44] When GVHD is induced independent of other transplant-related toxicity, it may be more manageable with immunosuppression. Nevertheless, in some cases DLI-induced GVHD may be quite severe; 20% to 35% of DLI recipients can be anticipated to develop grade III to IV acute GVHD (Table 2). Acute GVHD has contributed to death in almost 10% of patients.[18] Chronic GVHD occurs in 30% to 60% of recipients of unmanipulated DLI.

The clinical presentation of GVHD after DLI differs from GVHD post-myeloablative allogeneic HSCT. The onset of GVHD may be later after DLI; median time to onset of acute GVHD is approximately 32 to 42 days[8,45] compared to a median of 16 to 20 days following myeloablative T-replete transplantation.[46,47] Therefore, not only can the severity of GVHD be influenced by the use of intensive conditioning, the tissue damage and inflammatory cytokine release may influence the pace of GVHD development as well. That time to onset of acute GVHD is also delayed following reduced intensity transplantation supports this hypothesis.[48] The target organs of acute GVHD following DLI are the same as those involved after HSCT, but the clinical manifestations may vary. A hepatitic variant of liver GVHD, characterized by marked elevations of serum aminotransferase levels more than 10 times the upper limit of normal, was observed in 11 of 73 (15%) patients who received DLI at Johns Hopkins.[49] Characteristic skin, liver, and intestinal acute GVHD manifestations can be seen following DLI, but their frequency and severity have not been well characterized. Among 81 patients who received DLI for relapse, mixed chimerism, or prophylaxis following reduced intensity HSCT, skin, liver, and intestinal GVHD developed in 26%, 8%, and 14%, respectively.[50] Likewise, characteristic findings of chronic GVHD can be observed following DLI,[50] and occasionally both acute and chronic GVHD develop simultaneously.[51]

DLI After Reduced Intensity Transplantation

In recent years, reduced doses of conditioning chemotherapy have been employed in order to make HSCT safer, especially for patients with comorbidities or advanced age. When conditioning is minimal and GVHD has not already occurred, DLI is often required to either reverse mixed chimerism or to treat persistent disease.[50,52,53] GVHD after DLI in this setting

Table 2 The Occurrence of GVHD From Selected Series of Unmanipulated DLI to Treat Relapsed Malignancy

			Acute GVHD					
Reference	Diseases	N	Grade 0	Grade I	Grade II	Grade III–IV	Chronic GVHD	Comments
8	Various	125	40%	14%	24%	22%	61%	Non-relapse mortality 14% at 1 year
7	Various	135	41%	18%	NS	NS	NS	41% grade II–IV acute GVHD requiring treatment
40	Various	56	61%	4%	9%	25%	40%	Unrelated DLI only; treatment-related mortality 22%
67	Various	89	NS	NS	15%	19%	33%	DLI limited to centers from the Japanese Group for Marrow Transplant Registry
12	AML	65	43%	12%	17%	28%	36%	All patients pretreated with chemotherapy and received G-CSF–primed DLI; non-relapse mortality 23%
11	ALL	37	51%	3%	11%	35%	36%	Non-relapse mortality 28%; GVHD-related mortality, 2/36 (5%) of all death
19	CML (bulk-dose patients only)	28	37%	19%	19%	26%	41%	Recipients of escalating doses of DLI had significantly less GVHD
68	CML	30	NS	NS (53% grade 0–I)	17%	30%	49%	A trend (not statistically significant) toward higher acute GVHD in unrelated DLI recipients
27	Myeloma	25	48%	4%	24%	24%	52%	3 of 13 deaths (23%) treatment-related (1 GVHD and 1 infection)
69	Myeloma	54	43%	11%	26%	20%	47%	3 patients (5%) died of treatment-related toxicity (2 GVHD and 1 infection)

Abbreviations: AML, acute myelogenous leukemia; ALL, acute lymphocyte leukemia; CML, chronic myelogenous leukemia; NS, not stated.

develops in 19% to 45% of transplants, and chronic GVHD in 28% to 34%. In two studies of a combined 134 subjects who received DLI after reduced intensity transplantation, 37 (28%) patients developed acute GVHD, 15 (11%) developed grade 3 to 4 GVHD, and eight (6%) died from GVHD.[50,52] There was no statistically significant relationship between DLI dose and GVHD in either study. The clinical features of GVHD after DLI following reduced intensity HSCT are comparable to the GVHD that occurs after DLI is used to treat relapse following myeloablative HSCT. The similarity between GVHD after DLI in either setting suggests that the reduction of tissue damage associated with either no chemotherapy (as in DLI for relapse following prior myeloablative HSCT) or reduced dose chemotherapy (as in DLI after reduced intensity HSCT) may be the crucial common factor.

New Approaches to Minimize GVHD After DLI

Despite the dramatic achievements recorded with the use of DLI, high response rates are largely limited to CML, and success continues to be tempered by significant GVHD and other toxicity (Table 2). Several innovative approaches focus on minimizing GVHD to improve outcomes after DLI and cellular immunotherapy in general.

Low-Dose DLI and Dose Escalation

One approach that appears to minimize GVHD involves administration of low-dose DLI followed by dose escalation. In patients with early-phase relapse of CML, this strategy resulted in complete remissions in 86% of patients, and only one developed acute GVHD.[41] A retrospective analysis of 298 recipients of DLI also found an initial low T-cell dose ($\leq 2 \times 10^7$/ kg) was associated with less GVHD and improved survival, as compared to recipients of higher initial T-cell doses.[54] Treatment-related mortality at 3 years was 5% with the low initial dose as compared to 20% with the higher initial doses. The overall response rate was similar, regardless of the T-cell dose. An escalating dose strategy may not be practical for patients with relapse of less indolent diseases, since rapid disease progression may occur before an effective GVL response can be generated in many cases.

Why dose escalation of DLI minimizes GVHD is not clear. In some cases, there is likely an important effector to target cell ratio responsible for GVL induction; low doses of donor leukocytes may induce a GVL reaction against minimal numbers of leukemia cells but be insufficient to induce clinical GVHD. However, protection from GVHD using dose escalation of DLI may not simply be due to infusion of lower cell doses over time. When a dose escalation strategy was compared to infusions of similar T-cell doses given in one aliquot for relapsed CML, response rates were similar and the incidence of GVHD was lower using the dose escalation strategy.[19] Dose escalation may permit similar numbers of T cells to be delivered at progressively later times after the original transplant. T-cell infusions administered soon after transplant are more likely to induce severe GVHD than when infusions are delayed from the initial transplant.[2,55,56] A more intriguing explanation is that low doses of donor T cells may not be capable of inducing a GVL reaction if there is a significant leukemia cell burden, but they may result in generation of regulatory cells (or induction of anergy) that inhibits GVHD; only subsequent higher doses of DLI would suffice to overcome this effect and induce a GVH reaction. This possibility is supported by animal experiments showing that graft-versus-host tolerance could not be abrogated by the transfusion of lymphocytes from the marrow donor unless the donor was immunized against the recipient.[57] In transplanted dogs, donor lymphocytes did not produce GVHD if transfused more than 2 months after transplantation.[58] Similarly, delayed transfusion of donor lymphocytes improved the resistance of marrow-transplanted mice to leukemia, without producing GVHD.[56]

Depletion of GVHD Effector Cells

Preclinical and clinical evidence implicates $CD8^+$ T cells as primary mediators of GVHD. CD8 cell-depleted DLI has been used to treat relapsed CML after allogeneic HSCT,[37,51] and outcomes suggest that GVL activity can be retained with minimal GVHD; in small numbers of patients, the majority of responses have been sustained,[59] although the overall clinical impact of this approach will require direct comparison to unmanipulated DLI.

Inactivation of GVHD Effector Cells

Irradiated donor T cell DLI is based on the hypothesis that the cells would induce GVL effects at the time of infusion but could not proliferate in response to allo-antigens; preliminary data suggest that these cells do retain GVL activity and result in minimal GVHD.[60] Amotosalen-treated donor T cells, photochemically inactivated, have been tested as DLI in mice; these cells enhanced immune reconstitution, provided antiviral activity, and were protective against a leukemia challenge without causing GVHD,[61] suggesting that this novel approach separates clinical GVHD and GVL activity.[61]

Genetic Modification of Donor T Cells to Contain a Suicide Gene

A more specific method designed to limit GVHD without altering GVL reactivity has been the use of modified donor cells genetically engineered to contain a suicide gene. The best example has been the development of donor lymphocytes transduced with the herpes simplex thymidine kinase (*HSV-TK*) gene, rendering these cells sensitive to treatment with ganciclovir.[62] *HSV-TK* modified T cells induced complete remissions in patients with post-transplant lymphoproliferative disease. Acute GVHD that developed after DLI was treated with ganciclovir, with a decrease in the number and activity of allo-reactive cells and in the number of cells containing the *HSV-TK* gene.[63]

Tumor-Specific DLI

The most effective and efficient method of inducing GVL without GVHD would be to generate tumor-specific T cells. Leukemia-specific donor T cells have been isolated and expanded in vitro. Preliminary data in small numbers of patients suggest feasibility, and these cells can induce complete remission for relapsed CML with minimal toxicity.[64] Unfortunately, this approach is not only complicated and time-consuming, but tumor-reactive T-cell clones cannot be isolated in most patients.

Conclusions

The successes from DLI must be gratifying to those scientists who predicted in the 1950s and 1960s that allogeneic HSCT could transfer functional immunity capable of destroying leukemia cells.[65,66] In the past decade, it has become increasingly clear that this original hypothesis was not only correct but that the GVL effects of allogeneic cell therapy may be more potent, at least in some cases, than originally anticipated. DLI has provided a dramatic example of the potency of GVL, which can induce complete and sustained remissions in many patients even when all cytotoxic therapy has failed. Although DLI has been safer than alternative options like second allogeneic HSCT, that GVHD is a common complication resulting in significant morbidity and mortality is not surprising. However, in most cases, DLI can be given safely without GVHD prophylaxis, and observations regarding the timing and manifestations of GVHD after DLI, have all contributed to important inferences as to the factors necessary to initiate and sustain GVHD. The value of DLI in the clinic has also stimulated progress in the field of cellular immunotherapy with strategies to use selective T-cell subsets for GVL induction, gene-modified donor lymphocytes to regulate GVHD, donor T cells activated to enhance tumor cell killing, and development of tumor-specific donor lymphocytes for allogeneic cell therapy. The potential to harness the allogeneic GVL effect has led to a new paradigm in transplantation; less intensive nonmyeloablative conditioning therapy and allogeneic cell transplantation is now used as primary tumor immunotherapy, with exciting results. The ultimate goal is to determine how allogeneic immune cells can be used in specific adoptive immunotherapy against many different tumor types without inducing GVHD and other complications.

References

1. Odom L, August C, Githens J: Remission of relapsed leukaemia during a graft-versus-host reaction. A "graft-versus-leukaemia" reaction in man? Lancet 2:537-540, 1978
2. Sullivan K, Weiden P, Storb R: Influence of acute and chronic graft-versus-host disease on relapse and survival after bone marrow transplantation from HLA-identical siblings as treatment of acute and chronic leukemia. Blood 73:1720-1728, 1989
3. Horowitz MM, Gale RP, Sondel PM, et al: Graft-verus-leukemia reactions after bone marrow transplantation. Blood 75:555, -562, 1990
4. Gale R, Horowitz M, Ash R: Identical-twin bone marrow transplants for leukemia. Ann Intern Med 120:646-652, 1994
5. Weiden PL, Flournoy N, Sanders JE, Sullivan KM, Thomas ED, et al: Antileukemic effect of chronic graft-versus-host disease: Contribution to improved survival after allogeneic marrow transplantation. N Engl J Med 304:1529-1533, 1981
6. Goldman JM, Gale RP, Horowitz MM, Biggs JC, Champlin RE, Gluckman E, et al: Bone marrow transplantation for chronic myelogenous leukemia in chronic phase. Increased risk for relapse associated with T-cell depletion. Ann Intern Med 108:806-814, 1988
7. Kolb H-J, Schattenberg A, Goldman JM, Hertenstein B, Jacobsen N, Arcese W, et al: Graft-versus-leukemia effect of donor lymphocyte transfusions in marrow grafted patients. Blood 86:2041-2050, 1995
8. Collins RH, Jr, Shpilberg O, Drobyski WR, Porter DL, Giralt S, Champlin R, et al: Donor leukocyte infusions in 140 patients with relapsed malignancy after allogeneic bone marrow transplantation. J Clin Oncol 15:433-444, 1997
9. Porter D, Roth M, McGarigle C, Ferrara JL, Antin JH, et al: Induction of graft versus host disease as immunotherapy for relapsed chronic myeloid leukemia. N Engl J Med 330:100-106, 1994
10. Lokhorst HM, Schattenberg A, Cornelissen JJ, van Oers MH, Fibbe W, Russell I, et al: Donor lymphocyte infusions for relapsed multiple myeloma after allogeneic stem-cell transplantation: Predictive factors for response and long-term outcome. J Clin Oncol 18:3031-3037, 2000
11. Collins RH Jr, Goldstein S, Giralt S, Levine J, Porter D, Drobyski W, et al: Donor leukocyte infusions in acute lymphocytic leukemia. Bone Marrow Transplant 26:511-516, 2000
12. Levine JE, Braun T, Penza SL, Beatty P, Cornetta K, Martino R, et al: Prospective trial of chemotherapy and donor leukocyte infusions for relapse of advanced myeloid malignancies after allogeneic stem-cell transplantation. J Clin Oncol 20:405-412, 2002
13. Kolb H, Mittermuller J, Clemm C, Holler E, Ledderose G, Brehm G, et al: Donor leukocyte transfusions for treatment of recurrent chronic myelogenousleukemia in marrow transplant patients. Blood 76:2462-2465, 1990
14. Drobyski WR, Keever CA, Roth MS, Koethe S, Hanson G, McFadden P, et al: Salvage immunotherapy using donor leukocyte transfusions as treatment for relapse chronic myelogenous leukemia after allogeneic bone marrow transplantation: Efficacy and toxicity of a defined T-cell dose. Blood 82:2310-2318, 1993
15. Helg C, Roux E, Beris P, Cabrol C, Wacker P, Darbellay R, et al: Adoptive immunotherapy for recurrent CML after HSCT. Bone Marrow Transplant 12:125-129, 1993
16. Hertenstein B, Wiesneth M, Novotny J, Bunjes D, Stefanic M, Heinze B, et al: Interferon-alpha and donor buffy coat transfusions for treatment of relapsed chronic myeloid leukemia after allogeneic bone marrow transplantation. Transplantation 56:1114-1118, 1993
17. Roth MS, Antin JH, Bingham EL, Ginsburg D: Detection of Philadelphia chromosome-positive cells by the polymerase chain reaction following boe marrow transplant for chronic myelogenous leukemia. Blood 74: 882-885, 1989
18. Porter D, Antin J: Graft-versus-leukemia effect of allogeneic bone marrow transplantation and donor mononuclear cell infusions, in Winter J (ed): Blood Stem Cell Transplantation. Norwell, MA, Kluwer, 1997, pp 57-86
19. Dazzi F, Szydlo RM, Cross NC, Craddock C, Kaeda J, Kanfer E, et al: Durability of responses following donor lymphocyte infusions for patients who relapse after allogeneic stem cell transplantation for chronic myeloid leukemia. Blood 96:2712-2716, 2000
20. Porter DL, Connors JM, Van Deerlin VM, Duffy KM, McGarigle C, Saidman SL, et al: Graft-versus-tumor induction with donor leukocyte infusions as primary therapy for patients with malignancies. J Clin Oncol 17:1234-1243, 1999
21. Kolb HJ: Donor leukocyte transfusions for treatment of leukemic relapse after bone marrow transplantation. Immunology and Chronic Leukemia Working Parties. Vox Sang 74:321-329, 1998 (suppl 2)
22. Mandanas RA, Saez RA, Selby GB, Confer DL: G-CSF-mobilized donor leukocyte infusions as immunotherapy in acute leukemia relapsing after allogeneic marrow transplantation. J Hematother 7:449-456, 1998
23. Singhal S, Powles R, Kulkarni S, Treleaven J, Saso R, Mehta J, et al: Long-term follow-up of relapsed acute leukemia treated with immunotherapy after allogeneic transplantation: The inseparability of graft-versus-host disease and graft-versus-leukemia, and the problem of extramedullary relapse. Leuk Lymphoma 32:505-512, 1999
24. Akpek G, Zahurak ML, Piantadosi S, Margolis J, Doherty J, Davidson R, et al: Development of a prognostic model for grading chronic graft-versus-host disease. Blood 97:1219-1226, 2001
25. Tricot G, Vesole DH, Jagannath S, Hilton J, Munshi N, Barlogie B: Graft-versus-myeloma effect: Proof of principle. Blood 87:1196-1198, 1996
26. Lokhorst HM, Schattenberg A, Cornelissen JJ, Thomas LL, Verdonck LF: Donor leukocyte infusions are effective in relapsed multiple myeloma after allogeneic bone marrow transplantation. Blood 90:4206-4211, 1997
27. Salama M, Nevill T, Marcellus D, Parker P, Johnson M, Kirk A, et al: Donor leukocyte infusions for multiple myeloma. Bone Marrow Transplant 26:1179-1184, 2000

28. Alyea E, Weller E, Schlossman R, Canning C, Webb I, Doss D, et al: T-cell–depleted allogeneic bone marrow transplantation followed by donor lymphocyte infusion in patients with multiple myeloma: Induction of graft-versus-myeloma effect. Blood 98:934-939, 2001
29. Badros A, Barlogie B, Morris C, Desikan R, Martin SR, Munshi N, et al: High response rate in refractory and poor-risk multiple myeloma after allotransplantation using a nonmyeloablative conditioning regimen and donor lymphocyte infusions. Blood 97:2574-2579, 2001
30. Ratanatharathorn V, Uberti J, Karanes C, Abella E, Lum LG, Momin F, et al: Prospective comparative trial of autologous versus allogeneic bone marrow transplantation in patients with non-Hodgkin's lymphoma. Blood 84:1050-1055, 1994
31. Jones RJ, Ambinder RF, Piantadosi S, Santos GW: Evidence of a graft-versus-lymphoma effect associated with allogeneic bone marrow transplantation. Blood 77:649-653, 1991
32. Bernard M, Dauriac C, Drenou B, Leberre C, Branger B, Fauchet R, et al: Long-term follow-up of allogeneic bone marrow transplantation in patients with poor prognosis non-Hodgkin's lymphoma. Bone Marrow Transplant 23:329-333, 1999
33. Mandigers CM, Meijerink JP, Raemaekers JM, Schattenberg AV, Mensink EJ, et al: Graft-versus-lymphoma effect of donor leucocyte infusion shown by real-time quantitative PCR analysis of t(14;18). Lancet 352: 1522-1523, 1998
34. Robinson SP, Goldstone AH, Mackinnon S, Carella A, Russell N, de Elvira CR, et al: Chemoresistant or aggressive lymphoma predicts for a poor outcome following reduced-intensity allogeneic progenitor cell transplantation: An analysis from the Lymphoma Working Party of the European Group for Blood and Bone Marrow Transplantation. Blood 100:4310-4316, 2002
35. Porter DL, Stadtmauer EA, Lazarus HM: 'GVHD': Graft-versus-host disease or graft-versus-Hodgkin's disease? An old acronym with new meaning. Bone Marrow Transplant 31:739-746, 2003
36. Flowers ME, Leisenring W, Beach K, Riddell S, Radich JP, Higano CS, et al: Granulocyte colony-stimulating factor given to donors before apheresis does not prevent aplasia in patients treated with donor leukocyte infusion for recurrent chronic myeloid leukemia after bone marrow transplantation. Biol Blood Marrow Transplant 6:321-326, 2000
37. Giralt S, Hester J, Huh Y, Hirsch-Ginsberg C, Rondon G, Seong D, et al: CD8-depleted donor lymphocyte infusion as treatment for relapsed chronic myelogenous leukemia after allogeneic bone marrow transplantation. Blood 86:4337-4343, 1995
38. Mehta J, Powles R, Treleaven J, Horton C, Meller S, Pinkerton CR, et al: Outcome of acute leukemia relapsing after bone marrow transplantation: Utility of second transplants and adoptive immunotherapy. Bone Marrow Transplant 19:709-719, 1997
39. Leis J, Porter DL: Unrelated donor leukocyte infusions to treat relapse after unrelated donor bone marrow transplantation. Leuk Lymphoma 43:9-17, 2002
40. Porter DL, Collins RH Jr, Hardy C, Kernan NA, Drobyskin WR, Giralt S, et al: Treatment of relapsed leukemia after unrelated donor marrow transplantation with unrelated donor leukocyte infusions. Blood 95: 1214-1221, 2000
41. Mackinnon S, Papadopoulos E, Carabasi M, Reich L, Collins NH, Boulad F, et al: Adoptive immunotherapy evaluating escalating doses of donor leukocytes for relapse of chronic myeloid leukemia after bone marrow transplantation: Separation of graft-versus-leukemia responses from graft-versus-host disease. Blood 86:1261-1268, 1995
42. Elfenbein GG-PJ, Weiner R, Goedert T, Gross S: Consequences of no prophylaxis for acute graft-versus-host disease after HLA-identical bone marrow transplantation. Blood 70:305a, 1987 (suppl 1)
43. Sullivan K, Schulman H: Chronic graft-versus-host disease, obliterative bronchiolitis, and graft-versus-leukemia effect: Case histories. Transplant Proc 21:51-62, 1989
44. Antin JH, Ferrara JLM: Cytokine dysregulation and acute graft-versus-host disease. Blood 80:2964-2968, 1992
45. Porter D, Roth M, McGarigle C, et al: Induction of graft-vs-leukemia (GVL) reaction as therapy for relapsed leukemia after allogeneic bone marrow transplantation (HSCT). J Cell Biochem 18B:94a, 1994
46. Ratanatharathorn V, Nash RA, Przepiorka D, Devine SM, Klein JL, Weisdorf D, et al: Phase III study comparing methotrexate and tacrolimus (prograf, FK506) with methotrexate and cyclosporine for graft-versus-host disease prophylaxis after HLA-identical sibling bone marrow transplantation. Blood 92:2303-2314, 1998
47. Nash RA, Pepe MS, Storb R, Longton G, Pettinger M, Anasetti C, et al: Acute graft-versus-host disease analysis of risk factors after allogeneic marrow transpantation and prophylaxis with cyclosporine and methotrexate. Blood 80:1838-1845, 1992
48. Levine JE, Uberti JP, Ayash L, Reynolds C, Ferrara JL, Silver SM, et al: Lowered-intensity preparative regimen for allogeneic stem cell transplantation delays acute graft-versus-host disease but does not improve outcome for advanced hematologic malignancy. Biol Blood Marrow Transplant 9:189-197, 2003
49. Akpek G, Boitnott JK, Lee LA, Hallick JP, Torbenson M, Jacobsohn DA: Hepatitic variant of graft-versus-host disease after donor lymphocyte infusion. Blood 100:3903-3907, 2002
50. Marks DI, Lush R, Cavenagh J, Milligan DW, Schey S, Parker A, et al: The toxicity and efficacy of donor lymphocyte infusions given after reduced-intensity conditioning allogeneic stem cell transplantation. Blood 100:3108-3114, 2002
51. Alyea EP, Soiffer RJ, Canning C, Neuberg D, Schlossman R, Pickett C, et al: Toxicity and efficacy of defined doses of CD4(+) donor lymphocytes for treatment of relapse after allogeneic bone marrow transplant. Blood 91:3671-3680, 1998
52. Bethge WA, Hegenbart U, Stuart MJ, Storer BE, Maris MB, Flowers ME, et al: Adoptive immunotherapy with donor lymphocyte infusions after allogeneic hematopoietic cell transplantation following nonmyeloablative conditioning. Blood 103:790-795, 2004
53. Dey BR, McAfee S, Sackstein R, Colby C, Saidman S, Weymouth D, et al: Successful allogeneic stem cell transplantation with nonmyeloablative conditioning in patients with relapsed hematologic malignancy following autologous stem cell transplantation. Biol Blood Marrow Transplant 7:604-612, 2001
54. Guglielmi C, Arcese W, Dazzi F, Brand R, Bunjes D, Verdonck LF, et al: Donor lymphocyte infusion for relapsed chronic myelogenous leukemia: Prognostic relevance of the initial cell dose. Blood 100:397-405, 2002
55. Barrett AJ, Malkovska V: Graft-versus-leukemia: Understanding and using the alloimmune response to treat haematological malignancies. Br J Haematol 93:754-761, 1996
56. Johnson BD, Drobisky WD, Truitt RL: Delayed infusion of normal donor cells after MHC-matched bone marrow transplantation provides an anti-leukemia reaction without graft-versus-host disease. Bone Marrow Transplant 11:329, -336, 1993
57. Weiden P, Storb R, Tsoi M: Infusion of donor lymphocytes into stable canine radiation chimeras: Implications for mechanism of transplantation tolerance. J Immunol 116:1212-1219, 1978
58. Kolb HJ, Gunther W, Schumm M, Holler E, Wilmans W, Thierfelder S: Adoptive immunotherapy in canine chimeras. Transplantation 63:430-436, 1997
59. Shimoni A, Gajewski JA, Donato M, Martin T, O'Brien S, Talpaz M, et al: Long-term follow-up of recipients of CD8-depleted donor lymphocyte infusions for the treatment of chronic myelogenous leukemia relapsing after allogeneic progenitor cell transplantation. Biol Blood Marrow Transplant 7:568-575, 2001
60. Waller EK, Ship AM, Mittelstaedt S, Murray TW, Carter R, Kakhniashvili I, et al: Irradiated donor leukocytes promote engraftment of allogeneic bone marrow in major histocompatibility complex mismatched recipients without causing graft-versus-host disease. Blood 94:3222-3233, 1999
61. Truitt RL, Johnson BD, Hanke C, Talib S, Hearst JE: Photochemical treatment with S-59 psoralen and ultraviolet A light to control the fate of naive or primed T lymphocytes in vivo after allogeneic bone marrow transplantation. J Immunol 163:5145-5156, 1999
62. Servida P, Bordignon C: Gene therapy and apheresis. Int J Artif Organs 16:116-118, 1993 (suppl 5)
63. Bonini C, Ferrari G, Verzeletti S, Servida P, Zappone E, Ruggieri L, et al: HSV-TK gene transfer into donor lymphocytes for control of allogeneic graft-versus-leukemia. Science 276:1719-1724, 1997

64. Falkenburg JH, Wafelman AR, Joosten P, Smit WM, van Bergen CA, Bongaerts R, et al: Complete remission of accelerated phase chronic myeloid leukemia by treatment with leukemia-reactive cytotoxic T lymphocytes. Blood 94:1201-1208, 1999
65. Barnes D, Loutit J: Treatment of murine leukaemia with x-rays and homologous bone marrow. Br J Haematol 3:241-252, 1957
66. Mathe G, Amiel JL, Schwarzenberg L, Cattan L, Schneider M: Adoptive immunotherapy of acute leukemia: experimental and clinical results. Cancer Res 25:1525-1531, 1965
67. Shiobara S, Nakao S, Ueda M, Yamazaki H, Takahashi S, Asano S, et al: Donor leukocyte infusion for Japanese patients with relapsed leukemia after allogeneic bone marrow transplantation: Indications and dose escalation. Ther Apher 5:40-45, 2001
68. van Rhee F, Savage D, Blackwell J, Orchard K, Dazzi F, Lin F, et al: Adoptive immunotherapy for relapse of chronic myeloid leukemia after allogeneic bone marrow transplant: Equal efficacy of lymphocytes from sibling and matched unrelated donors. Bone Marrow Transplant 21: 1055-1061, 1998
69. Lokhorst HM, Wu K, Verdonck LF, Laterveer LL, van de Donk NW, van Oers MH, et al: The occurrence of graft-versus-host disease is the major predictive factor for response to donor lymphocyte infusions in multiple myeloma. Blood 103:4362-4364, 2004

ELSEVIER

Seminars in
HEMATOLOGY

$CD4^+CD25^+$ Regulatory T Cells and Graft-Versus-Host Disease

Petra Hoffmann and Matthias Edinger

Peripheral suppression of autoreactive T cells by specialized T-cell populations is one of several mechanisms ensuring self-tolerance within the adaptive immune system. Thymus-derived $CD4^+CD25^+$ T cells expressing the transcriptional repressor FOXP3 mediate such immunoregulatory functions and are pivotal for the prevention of autoimmunity. As peripheral tolerance induction is a prerequisite for successful treatment outcome after allogeneic hematopoietic stem cell transplantation (HSCT), the role of $CD4^+CD25^+$ T cells in transplantation models and clinical trials is now under investigation in many laboratories. Here we summarize recent results regarding protection from graft-versus-host disease (GVHD) by adoptively transferred $CD4^+CD25^+$ T cells in mice and discuss early findings from clinical studies in HSCT.
Semin Hematol 43:62–69

Mature donor T cells contained in stem cell grafts react to and attack host tissues, thereby causing graft-versus-host disease (GVHD). Since GVHD significantly contributes to treatment-related morbidity and mortality of allogeneic hematopoietic stem cell transplantation (HSCT), T-cell depletion of the graft seemed a promising strategy to improve treatment outcome. Such graft manipulations, however, resulted in increased rejection rates, impaired immune reconstitution, and a high risk for disease relapse in patients treated for hematologic malignancies, and thereby revealed the important contribution of transplanted donor T cells to treatment success.[1] Today, most transplants are performed with T-cell–replete grafts and pharmacologic immunosuppression is used to eliminate alloreactive donor T cells or to transiently block their effector function for prevention and treatment of GVHD. Nevertheless, the search for improved protocols that promote donor-host tolerance without loss of beneficial T-cell effects remains an important goal in allogeneic HSCT. The recent characterization of natural $CD4^+CD25^+$ regulatory T cells (Tregs) reinvigorated the concept of dominant regulation or suppression as a vital mechanism of peripheral T-cell tolerance, and several groups began to explore the role of Tregs in animal models of allogeneic HSCT. Here, we will briefly summarize the basic aspects of physiologic T-cell tolerance induction and then focus on the biology of $CD4^+CD25^+$ Tregs and their capacity to modulate alloresponses in experimental transplantation systems. Finally, we will discuss preliminary findings concerning the role of $CD4^+CD25^+$ Tregs in human stem cell transplantation.

T-Cell Tolerance

Discrimination of self from non-self is essential for the adaptive immune system to direct its powerful effector mechanisms against foreign pathogens and not its own normal tissues. Such discriminatory ability is acquired during the maturation of the immune system. The central maturation site for T cells is the thymus, where bone marrow-derived precursors differentiate via a $CD4^-CD8^-$ state into $CD4^+CD8^+$ (double-positive) thymocytes that express low levels of $\alpha\beta$-T-cell receptors (TCR). Only a small fraction of those cells (<5%) recognize self-MHC/peptide complexes presented by cortical epithelial cells and thereby receive a survival signal through their TCR (positive selection). The vast majority of double-positive thymocytes (>95%) do not react with self and die by neglect. Positive selection thus instructs T cells to respond exclusively to antigens presented by the major histocompatibility complex (MHC-restriction), which protects them from apoptosis not only in the thymus but also in the periphery, where repetitive recognition of self-MHC/peptide complexes is required for T-cell survival and homeostasis.[2] Depending on the type of the selecting MHC molecule (class I *v* class II), thymocytes further mature from their double-positive state into $CD4^+CD8^-$ or

Institute of Immunology and the Department of Hematology and Oncology, University Hospital Regensburg, Regensburg, Germany.
Address correspondence to Matthias Edinger, MD, Department of Hematology and Oncology, University Hospital Regensburg, Franz-Josef-Strauss-Allee 11, 93053 Regensburg, Germany. E-mail: matthias.edinger@klinik.uni-regensburg.de

 0037-1963/06/$-see front matter © 2006 Elsevier Inc. All rights reserved.
doi:10.1053/j.seminhematol.2005.09.006

$CD4^-CD8^+$ single-positive cells, which migrate from the thymic cortex to the medulla where they encounter bone marrow–derived antigen-presenting cells (APCs). These APCs ensure self-tolerance by inducing apoptosis (clonal deletion) in those single-positive thymocytes that express a TCR with high avidity for self-MHC/peptide complexes, while low to moderately reactive cells survive and are released to the periphery (negative selection). Thus, T-cell maturation in the thymus involves self-recognition as an initial selection step that risks generating auto-aggressive T-cell clones. Consequently, tolerance to self crucially depends on the subsequent deletion of those potentially harmful, auto-aggressive T-cell populations by negative selection. However, thymic deletion of autoreactive T cells is frequently incomplete, as evidenced by the occurrence of T-cell–mediated autoimmune diseases. On the other hand, autoreactive T cells are prevalent also in healthy individuals, suggesting that additional peripheral tolerance mechanisms compensate for the "leakiness" of central T-cell tolerance induction.[3] These mechanisms can be either deletional or nondeletional. Deletional mechanisms include activation-induced cell death (AICD) of autoreactive T-cell clones in peripheral lymphoid and non-lymphoid organs. Nondeletional mechanisms can be either intrinsic to the reactive T-cell population and result in altered or abrogated effector functions (anergy), or they can be mediated by other cell populations via dominant suppression. Although the important contribution of dominant suppression to the maintenance of peripheral T-cell tolerance has been shown convincingly in experimental systems, its detailed evaluation has been hampered by lack of phenotypic or molecular markers to identify the responsible cell populations. This obstacle has recently been overcome in parts by the description of naturally occurring $CD4^+CD25^+$ Tregs.[4]

$CD4^+CD25^+$ Regulatory T Cells

In mice, thymectomy at day 3 of life leads to an organ-specific autoimmune syndrome, which can be prevented by transfusion of peripheral $CD4^+$ T cells from syngeneic adult animals. Sakaguchi and colleagues demonstrated that the cells responsible for this effect constitutively express the alpha-chain of the interleukin-2 (IL-2) receptor, CD25.[5] The important role of $CD4^+CD25^+$ Treg-mediated suppression in protection from autoimmunity has been verified in multiple disease models.[4] In addition, the potency of Tregs to modulate immune responses to infectious pathogens,[6] tumors,[7] and allogeneic tissue[8] has been the focus of numerous studies.

$CD4^+CD25^+$ Tregs differ from nonregulatory or "conventional" T cells (T_{conv}), not only in their constitutive high intracellular expression of CTLA-4, but also in their preferential expression of other markers, including glucocorticoid-induced tumor necrosis factor (TNF) receptor family-related gene (*GITR*),[4] lymphocyte activation gene 3 (*LAG-3*),[9] and neuropilin.[10] None of these molecules unambiguously identifies Tregs, however, since subpopulations of nonregulatory T cells also express them under certain conditions, as for example after stimulation. This lack of a specific marker might now be overcome with the identification of the forkhead/winged helix transcription factor Foxp3, as described in more detail below.

The main functional characteristics of $CD4^+CD25^+$ Tregs in vitro are their hypoproliferation to standard T-cell stimulation and their potent suppression of both $CD4^+CD25^-$ and $CD8^+$ T cells.[4] Survival of $CD4^+CD25^+$ Tregs in vitro and in vivo depends on exogenous IL-2, since they themselves fail to undergo adequate chromatin remodelling in the IL-2 promoter region and to produce IL-2 (or any other pro-inflammatory cytokine) upon stimulation.[11] Tregs and conventional T cells also differ in their response to IL-2, in that signaling pathways supporting cell proliferation are blocked in Tregs, while the survival-promoting JAK/STAT5 pathway is intact.[12] Consequently, Tregs are virtually absent in IL-2- and IL-2R–deficient mice.[13] In contrast, they survive and proliferate substantially in vivo after transfer into wild-type lymphopenic animals or in response to their cognate antigen, and to a certain extent even under steady-state conditions in lymphocyte-replete animals, indicating that IL-2 in combination with other stimuli can overcome the anergic state these cells display in vitro.[14–16]

The molecular mechanism responsible for $CD4^+CD25^+$ Treg-mediated suppression is still not identified. To gain suppressive activity in vitro or in vivo, Tregs must be activated through their TCR. In vitro, their suppressive effect depends on cell contact, does not require secreted cytokines, and results in reduced activation, proliferation, and/or cytokine production of the targeted cells.[17] Membrane-bound transforming growth factor-beta (TGF-β)[18] and CTLA-4 have been proposed as mediators of suppressive function,[19,20] but mice deficient in CTLA-4 or TGF-β generate functionally active $CD4^+CD25^+$ Tregs. In vivo, Treg-mediated suppression appears to be much more complex, since cytokines irrelevant for their in vitro function clearly modulate their activity under these conditions. A role for IL-10 has been demonstrated in some but not all experimental disease models of Treg function.[4] Likewise, $CD8^+$ T cells expressing a dominant negative TGF-β receptor II do not respond to $CD4^+CD25^+$ Treg-mediated suppression in vivo.[21] Whether $CD4^+CD25^+$ Tregs themselves produce TGF-β or it is secreted in response to interaction with the suppressors by other cells like APC remains to be demonstrated.[22] Such encounters have been shown to result in down-modulation of MHC and costimulatory molecules on APCs,[23,24] as well as induction of indoleamine2,3-dioxygenase, which leads to increased tryptophan metabolism and thus decreased T-cell activation.[25] In summary, these observations suggest that $CD4^+CD25^+$ Tregs employ not one but several modes of suppression, depending on the local environment and their own activation status, and that they may act on more than one target cell population in vivo.

Treg biology advanced significantly with the identification of the forkhead/winged helix transcription factor Foxp3 as a key regulator of $CD4^+CD25^+$ Treg development and function.[22] The mutant mouse strain *scurfy* develops a lymphoproliferative disease and severe autoimmunity that results from a loss of function mutation in the *foxp3* gene.[26] Three independent research groups showed that Foxp3 is specifically expressed in CD4+CD25+ Tregs and that the adoptive transfer of wild-type (wt) CD4+CD25+ T cells rescues *scurfy* mice from disease.[27–29] Forced expression of Foxp3 partially reprograms peripheral CD4+CD25− T cells to become suppressor cells. These landmark studies revealed that Foxp3 is a non-redundant factor for both the generation and function of Tregs. In addition, they showed that autoimmunity in *scurfy* mice does not result from altered development or function of conventional T cells but from lack of peripheral suppression. Thus, Foxp3-expressing cells seem to represent a specialized suppressor T-cell lineage, as already predicted from the finding that cells with phenotypic, functional, and molecular characteristics of Tregs could be isolated from the thymus.[30,31]

The severe autoimmune syndrome in humans described by the acronym IPEX (immune dysregulation, polyendocrinopathy, enteropathy, X-linked) also results from mutations in FOXP3.[32] Affected boys suffer from multi-organ damage associated with an extensive expansion of autoreactive T cells and with the generation of humoral responses to self and otherwise non-immunogenic foreign antigens (manifest as food allergies). The similar immune pathologies observed in *scurfy* mice and IPEX patients, as well as their common mutations in the highly conserved *foxp3* gene, suggest that peripheral suppression mediated by Tregs is crucial for protection from autoimmunity also in humans. Consistent with these observations, a population of natural CD4+ Tregs has been identified in human blood, peripheral lymphoid organs, and thymus; these cells reside preferentially within the subpopulation expressing CD25 at high levels and show the same phenotypic, functional, and molecular characteristics as their murine counterparts, including preferential FOXP3 expression.[4,33,34] In contrast to these initial reports, low-level expression of Foxp3 and/or upregulation upon stimulation in T cells that are initially CD25− has now been observed in multiple studies.[22] Many investigators therefore suggest that peripheral T cells with regulatory capacity consist not only of thymus-derived suppressor cells, but also of cells generated de novo from non-regulatory T cells in the periphery. To further explore the relation between Foxp3 and CD25 expression, Rudensky and coworkers created GFP (green fluorescent protein)–Foxp3 knock-in mice: in these animals Foxp3 and CD25 expression in CD4+ T cells overlap largely but not completely, revealing a small number of Foxp3+ cells that reside within the CD4+CD25− T-cell pool. Upon polyclonal or antigen-specific stimulation Foxp3 induction was not observed in Foxp3− T cells, suggesting that peripheral de novo generation of Foxp3+ Tregs is at best a rare event and that the upregulation of Foxp3 mRNA and protein expression in the CD25− T-cell population occurs primarily in the few Foxp3+ cells already present in this T-cell pool.[35] Improved technologies for the detection of Foxp3 on a single cell level[33,36] will allow this issue to be addressed in detail also for stimulation conditions proposed to induce human Tregs in vitro.

Although the essential role of Foxp3 in the development and function of Tregs is now widely accepted, little is known of the induction of Foxp3 during Treg maturation in the thymus. The generation of Tregs is dependent on MHC class II expression on cortical epithelial cells[37] and a comparably strong avidity of TCRs for self-peptides (but weak enough to escape negative selection) leads to Foxp3 induction and in consequence to a preferential recognition of self-antigens by Tregs in the periphery.[38] Additional, yet unidentified signals provided by thymic epithelial cells, were also proposed.[39] Other cofactors required for sustained Treg generation and peripheral homeostasis include TGF-β, IL-2, and costimulatory signals via CD28.[22] Early experiments directed at identifying the immediate molecular targets of Foxp3 suggest that it physically interacts with nuclear factor kappa B (NF-κB) and nuclear factor of activated T cells (NF-AT), inhibiting the transcriptional activity of those factors and consequently, the production of cytokines, including IL-2, IL-4, interferon-γ, and TNF-α.[40] Thus, the important contribution of CD4+ CD25+Foxp3+ T cells to the maintenance of peripheral tolerance is now widely accepted, but their developmental pathway and their mechanism of suppression are still incompletely understood.

CD4+CD25+ Tregs in Murine Models of GVHD and Graft-Versus-Leukemia

In vitro, alloreactive T_{conv} cells show a proliferative response in mixed lymphocyte reactions (MLR). In contrast, CD4+ CD25+ Tregs do not proliferate when stimulated with MHC-mismatched APC but rather suppress the proliferation of CD4+CD25− or CD8+ T_{conv} cells in cocultures.[41,42] These findings have prompted investigators to study the potency of CD4+CD25+ Tregs to suppress alloresponses also in vivo.

Small numbers of donor T_{conv} cells induce acute GVHD when added to T-cell–depleted bone marrow (TCD-BM) and transplanted into lethally irradiated, MHC-mismatched mice. In contrast, cotransplantation of even large numbers of purified donor CD4+CD25+ Tregs with TCD-BM does not induce GVHD in such models.[42–44] Yet, transplanted CD4+ CD25+ Tregs are not simply inert, as they promote engraftment of allogeneic bone marrow and thus facilitate hematopoietic reconstitution as well as the development of sustained donor chimerism.[43,45–47] More important, when CD4+CD25+ Tregs are transplanted together with CD4+ CD25− or CD8+ T cells at high ratios (1:1 or 1:2), they prevent the induction of GVHD. Both unmanipulated and in vitro activated and expanded CD4+CD25+ Tregs are protective. Inhibition of GVHD is observed in partially and completely MHC-mismatched donor-recipient pairs, and the protective effect ranges from reduced body weight loss to prolonged mean survival time and even complete protection from otherwise lethal GVHD.[41,43,44,48–50] In transplant models with slow disease progression, protection can even be observed after delayed transfer of Tregs, suggesting that they can also ameliorate active GVHD.[43] In contrast to donor-type CD4+CD25+ Tregs, host-type Tregs are unable to prevent GVHD after transfer into lethally irradiated hosts.[41] Immunosuppressive cytokines derived from Tregs contribute to the protective effect in vivo, as IL-10 secretion by donor Tregs is required for full inhibition of lethal GVHD.[41] Protection from GVHD appears not solely the result of direct T-cell suppression but also involves effects of Tregs on other cells, such as donor- and/or host-type APC, as already demonstrated in vitro (see above). In addition, IL-10 secretion by $CD4^+CD25^+$ Tregs may induce a positive feedback loop, since IL-10–treated dendritic cells have been shown to promote the development of cytokine-secreting, adaptive Tregs.[51]

The ability of relatively small numbers of Tregs (below 1×10^6 cells/mouse) to protect animals from GVHD raises the question where they suppress alloreactive T_{conv} cells: in GVHD target organs or within lymphoid tissues. Several landmark studies revealed that secondary lymphoid organs, and in particular lymph nodes in proximity to GVHD target organs such as mesenteric lymph nodes and Peyer's patches, are the relevant sites for GVHD induction. Thus, it was shown that alloantigen presentation by BM–derived APC, but not on epithelial cells in GVHD target organs, is critical for GVHD induction.[52] Second, APC derived from the host, but not the donor, were shown to be necessary and sufficient for activation of alloreactive T_{conv} cells contained in the BM graft.[53] Although host-type APC, predominantly DC, can be found in almost all tissues, the most effective stimulation of donor T cells occurs within the supportive microenvironment of secondary lymphoid organs. Finally, Murai et al. showed that mice lacking Peyer's patches are resistant to GVHD induction.[54] Blockade of homing receptors for LN and PP, such as CD62L and $\alpha_4\beta_7$-integrin, prevented donor T-cell migration into these compartments and also resulted in reduced GVHD severity.[55] Similarly, effector/memory type donor T cells that do not express LN homing receptors such as CD62L and CCR7 at relevant levels were impaired in their ability to cause GVHD after allogeneic BMT.[56,57]

Since secondary lymphoid organs are the sites of donor T-cell priming by host APC, it seemed likely that protection from GVHD by co-transplanted donor Tregs might also occur at those sites. $CD4^+CD25^+$ Tregs, like T_{conv} cells, show a heterogeneous expression for the LN homing receptor CD62L.[58–60] *In vitro,* both, the $CD62L^+$ and the $CD62L^-$ subpopulation of $CD4^+CD25^+$ Tregs contain similar levels of Foxp3, do not release IL-2 in response to TCR triggering, and are equally suppressive after polyclonal or alloantigen-specific stimulation.[58,61] Thus, both populations meet the acknowledged criteria for Tregs. After allogeneic transplantation, however, only the $CD62L^+$ subpopulation of Tregs protects recipients from lethal GVHD.[58,60] This discrepancy can be explained by the different migratory and proliferative abilities of the two subpopulations, because transfer of $CD62L^-$ donor Tregs results in a significantly reduced Treg progeny in MLN as compared to transfer of $CD62L^+$ Tregs. Consequently, $CD62L^-$ Tregs restrict the expansion of conventional donor T cells at those sites to a much lesser extent resulting in much larger numbers of alloaggressive T cells in lymphoid as well as GVHD target organs early after transplantation.[58,60] These results indicate that host APC in secondary lymphoid organs efficiently activate not only potentially hazardous, alloreactive donor T_{conv} cells, but also protective donor-derived Tregs. Thus, Tregs acquire their suppressive activity in close proximity to their targets of suppression. The subsequent interaction impairs not only the expansion of T_{conv} cells, but also diminishes their capacity to migrate out of the LN into neighbouring tissue.[62] Nevertheless, some donor T_{conv} cells as well as Tregs can be detected in GVHD target organs. Since both populations are heterogeneous not only with respect to CD62L expression, but also with respect to other adhesion molecules and chemotactic receptors,[63–65] suppression of alloaggressive T_{conv} cells may also occur in peripheral tissues, although not with the same efficiency.

Mature T cells within the graft are detrimental due to GVHD induction, but they also mediate beneficial graft-versus-lymphoma/leukemia activity (GVL) in patients with hematopoietic malignancies. Broadly expressed major and/or minor histocompatibility antigens recognized in GVHD are also frequent targets for GVL, as evidenced by the reduced incidence of disease relapse in patients with GVHD and the often concomitant induction of disease regression and GVHD in patients treated with donor lymphocyte infusions (DLI) for relapse after HSCT.[66–68] Thus GVHD and GVL appear to be mediated by largely overlapping T-cell populations. Since hematopoietic malignancies are the main indication for HSCT, it was critical to determine whether donor $CD4^+CD25^+$ Tregs abrogate the GVL activity of donor T_{conv} cells.[43,44,47] In an animal study addressing this question, in vivo imaging methods were used to localize and quantify tumor cells in transplant recipients. The discrimination between GVHD-related and tumor-related mortality after transfer of the various donor T-cell subpopulations revealed that $CD4^+CD25^+$ Tregs did not mediate any GVL activity. Their cotransplantation with T_{conv} cells protected from GVHD also in these tumor-bearing hosts, thereby permitting the transfer of increased numbers of allogeneic T_{conv} cells. The GVL effect mediated by these T_{conv} cells was not abrogated by cotransplanted Tregs, as host-type leukemia and lymphoma were efficiently eradicated from infiltrated organs such as liver, spleen, lymph nodes, and bone marrow. These surprising findings could not be explained by the promotion of tumor-specific T-cell responses by Tregs, as tumor cytolysis in these MHC-disparate models depended on direct allorecognition, but not on tumor-specific priming, as extensively studied in vitro. Thus, maintained GVL activity in the absence of GVHD seemed to result from alterations of donor T-cell expansion or migration that differentially affected the two facets of the alloresponse. The proliferation of donor T_{conv} cells was inhibited up to 90% for the first seven days after HSCT when $CD4^+CD25^+$ Tregs were cotransplanted.[44] The remaining T_{conv} cells were not impaired in their functional activity, as demonstrated by successful tumor elimination in vivo as well as their unchanged cytokine secretion profile and cytotoxic potential after restimulation in vitro.[44] Thus, donor Tregs do not paralyze T_{conv} cell function but restrict the early and massive expansion of donor T_{conv} cells responsible for the progression of an alloresponse to clinical GVHD.[69,70] Since the elimination of tumor cells within the lympho-hematopoietic system does not depend on this same rapid donor T-cell expansion, GVL effects are retained.

Taken together, these in vitro and in vivo data suggest the following sequence of events: cotransplanted Tregs migrate into lymphoid organs and recognize alloantigen presented by host-type APC. Once activated, they gain suppressive activity and restrain the proliferation of T_{conv} cells. Although not substantially increased in number, alloreactive T_{conv} cells stimulated in the presence of Tregs maintain their effector functions. Since hematopoietic cells are the most sensitive targets of the alloresponse, donor T_{conv} cells exert their graft-versus-hematopoiesis effects, including GVL activity. Their restricted expansion, however, together with their impaired migratory capacity, prevents the accumulation of sufficient numbers of alloaggressive T cells in GVHD target tissues to reach the threshold required for the induction of clinical GVHD (Fig 1).

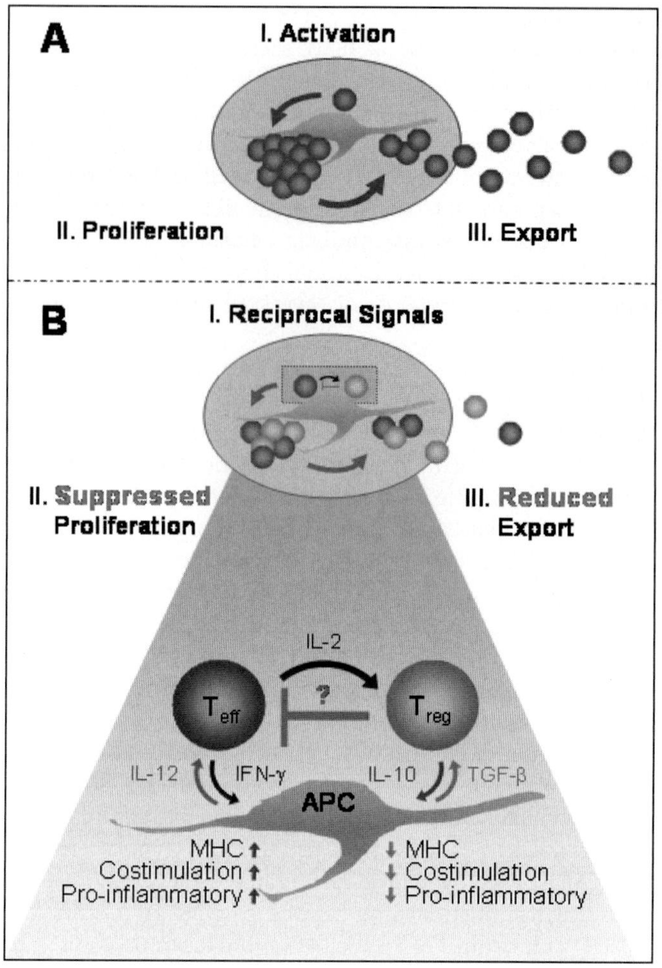

Figure 1 GVHD suppression as a result of reciprocal signaling between effector T cells (T_{eff}), regulatory T cells (T_{reg}) and antigen-presenting cells (APC). (A) Donor T cells migrate to secondary lymphoid organs after transplantation where they encounter alloantigen presented by host APCs. Following their activation and expansion, alloreactive T cells are exported in high numbers to potential GVHD target organs where they inflict damage. (B) Cotransplantation of donor regulatory T cells results in comigration of both T-cell populations into secondary lymphoid organs and their simultaneous activation by APCs. Upon activation T_{reg} cells acquire suppressive activity, which affects T_{eff} cell proliferation and migration both directly via a yet unknown, cell-contact dependent mechanism and indirectly via immunosuppressive cytokines such as IL-10, which lead to downregulation of MHC and costimulatory molecules on APCs, as well as secretion of suppressive instead of proinflammatory cytokines from these cells, such as TGF-β. Consequently, the export of alloreactive T_{eff} cells from lymph nodes is reduced to such an extent that threshold numbers required for the induction of clinical GVHD are no longer achieved within the target organs.

$CD4^+CD25^+$ Tregs in Clinical HSCT

The lethal autoimmune syndrome seen in IPEX patients proves that active suppression of autoaggressive T cells by specialized Tregs is required for the maintenance of self-tolerance in humans. By extrapolation, reconstitution of the Treg compartment probably contributes also to immune tolerance after allogeneic HSCT and thereby ameliorates or protects from GVHD. Results from a limited number of clinical studies comparing $CD4^+CD25^+$ T-cell numbers in peripheral blood of patients with and without GVHD are so far inconclusive. Thus, one study suggested a positive correlation between GVHD incidence and the number of $CD25^+$ T cells contained in the stem cell grafts. However, technical difficulties with phenotyping of previously frozen and banked stem cell samples did not permit differentiation of regulatory from activated nonregulatory T cells.[71] In a second study, Sanchez et al. examined the reconstitution of Tregs after HSCT and found no difference in the number of $CD4^+CD25^{high}$ T cells in patients either with or without acute GVHD, while patients with chronic GVHD showed a slight but still nonsignificant increase when compared to controls. Since these patients also had higher numbers of activated ($CD134^+$) T cells, it was proposed that the imbalance between effector T cells and Tregs results in impaired T-cell suppression.[72] Similarly, Clark et al. found increased numbers of $CD4^+CD25^{high}$ Tregs in patients with as compared to those without chronic GVHD and concluded that chronic GVHD does not result from a deficit in Tregs.[73] In the first study quantifying FOXP3 expression after HSCT to monitor Treg reconstitution, FOXP3 levels were reduced in mononuclear cells from patients with GVHD as compared to those without disease.[74] In addition, FOXP3 expression correlated with a marker for T cells newly emigrated from the thymus (T cell receptor gene rearrangement excision circles [TREC]). Based on this correlation, the authors suggested that thymic damage in GVHD results in Treg deficiency or, alternatively, that Tregs protect the thymus from donor T-cell-mediated attack during GVHD, thereby promoting improved immune reconstitution. Although such correlations do not prove causation, further evidence for donor Treg-mediated tolerance after HSCT was provided by another recent study that evaluated the combined treatment with an anti-CD25 immunotoxin and cyclosporine for the prevention of GVHD.[75] Contrary to the expected outcome, patients receiving this combination developed more severe GVHD than those receiving standard GVHD prophylaxis. In additional in vitro experiments, the authors showed that cyclosporine prohibited the upregulation of CD25 on alloreactive T cells (thereby protecting them from the toxin) while Tregs that constitutively express CD25 were thoroughly depleted by the toxin.

Several institutions have now initiated prospective clinical trials to quantitatively monitor the reconstitution of FOXP3 expressing cells after HSCT. Mere enumeration of such cells in peripheral blood is unlikely to be sufficient to elucidate the role of Tregs in the induction of tolerance. Changes in developmental or activation status, thymic selection, and distribution in peripheral tissues all may significantly affect their regulatory function in vivo. Such changes may be influenced by multiple variables within the HSCT process, including the intensity of the conditioning regimen, histocompatibility differences, the age and thymic function of recipients, concomitant drug therapy (especially immunosuppressives), and concurrent infections, among others. Therefore, guidelines for FOXP3 quantification and monitoring should be agreed on between different centers, since relevant factors for recovery will only be uncovered in multivariant analyses in large numbers of patients.

Based on results from animal models, the adoptive transfer of donor $CD4^+CD25^+$ Tregs appears a promising strategy for the prevention of GVHD in patients requiring allogeneic HSCT. Such trials require good manufacturing practice (GMP)-approved protocols for the isolation of Tregs from leukapheresis products of stem cell donors. The reagents needed for such isolation strategies will soon be widely available (Hoffmann et al, manuscript submitted). In our experience, efficient enrichment and isolation of human Tregs in clinically relevant numbers (1 to 3×10^6 cells per kg body weight) can be accomplished for engineering of stem cell grafts. Furthermore, recently described methods for the efficient in vitro expansion of Tregs should enable the generation of sufficient cell numbers for repetitive transfusions.[76–78] Such in vitro–expanded $CD4^+CD25^+$ Tregs show increased suppressive activity compared to freshly isolated cells and maintain expression of relevant lymph node homing receptors despite extensive in vitro proliferation.[76,77] These technologic advances, together with a revived appreciation of the essential role of peripheral suppression in T-cell homeostasis, have led to the first clinical trials exploring the tolerance-promoting potential of adoptively transferred donor Tregs in recipients of allogeneic stem cell grafts. Results from such trials will establish whether the potent protective effect of $CD4^+CD25^+$ Tregs, as seen in experimental systems, is operational and can be exploited also in clinical stem cell transplantation.

References

1. Ho VT, Soiffer RJ: The history and future of T-cell depletion as graft-versus-host disease prophylaxis for allogeneic hematopoietic stem cell transplantation. Blood 98:3192-3204, 2001
2. Sprent J, Kishimoto H: The thymus and negative selection. Immunol Rev 185:126-135, 2002
3. Wucherpfennig KW, Zhang J, Witek C, Matsui M, Modabber Y, Ota K, et al: Clonal expansion and persistence of human T cells specific for an immunodominant myelin basic protein peptide. J Immunol 152:5581-5592, 1994
4. Sakaguchi S: Naturally arising $CD4^+$ regulatory T cells for immunologic self-tolerance and negative control of immune responses. Annu Rev Immunol 22:531-562, 2004
5. Sakaguchi S, Sakaguchi N, Asano M, Itoh M, Toda M: Immunologic self-tolerance maintained by activated T cells expressing IL-2 receptor alpha-chains (CD25). Breakdown of a single mechanism of self-tolerance causes various autoimmune diseases. J Immunol 155:1151-1164, 1995
6. Belkaid Y, Rouse BT: Natural regulatory T cells in infectious disease. Nat Immunol 6:353-360, 2005
7. Terabe M, Berzofsky JA: Immunoregulatory T cells in tumor immunity. Curr Opin Immunol 16:157-162, 2004
8. Waldmann H, Graca L, Cobbold S, Adams E, Tone M, Tone Y: Regulatory T cells and organ transplantation. Semin Immunol 16:119-126, 2004
9. Huang CT, Workman CJ, Flies D, Pan X, Marson AL, Zhou G, et al: Role of LAG-3 in regulatory T cells. Immunity 21:503-513, 2004
10. Bruder D, Probst-Kepper M, Westendorf AM, Geffers R, Beissert S, Loser K, et al: Neuropilin-1: A surface marker of regulatory T cells. Eur J Immunol 34:623-630, 2004
11. Su L, Creusot RJ, Gallo EM, Chan SM, Utz PJ, Fathman CG, et al: Murine $CD4^+CD25^+$ regulatory T cells fail to undergo chromatin remodeling across the proximal promoter region of the IL-2 gene. J Immunol 173:4994-5001, 2004
12. Bensinger SJ, Walsh PT, Zhang J, Carroll M, Parsons R, Rathmell JC, et al: Distinct IL-2 receptor signaling pattern in $CD4^+CD25^+$ regulatory T cells. J Immunol 172:5287-5296, 2004
13. Malek TR, Bayer AL: Tolerance, not immunity, crucially depends on IL-2. Nat Rev Immunol 4:665-674, 2004
14. Annacker O, Burlen-Defranoux O, Pimenta-Araujo R, Cumano A, Bandeira A: Regulatory CD4 T cells control the size of the peripheral activated/memory CD4 T cell compartment. J Immunol 164:3573-3580, 2000
15. Fisson S, Darrasse-Jeze G, Litvinova E, Septier F, Klatzmann D, Liblau R, et al: Continuous activation of autoreactive $CD4^+$ $CD25^+$ regulatory T cells in the steady state. J Exp Med 198:737-746, 2003
16. Klein L, Khazaie K, von Boehmer H: In vivo dynamics of antigen-specific regulatory T cells not predicted from behavior in vitro. Proc Natl Acad Sci U S A 100:8886-8891, 2003
17. Shevach EM: $CD4^+$ $CD25^+$ suppressor T cells: More questions than answers. Nat Rev Immunol 2:389-400, 2002
18. Nakamura K, Kitani A, Strober W: Cell contact-dependent immunosuppression by $CD4(^+)CD25(^+)$ regulatory T cells is mediated by cell surface-bound transforming growth factor beta. J Exp Med 194:629-644, 2001
19. Birebent B, Lorho R, Lechartier H, de Guibert S, Alizadeh M, Vu N, et al: Suppressive properties of human $CD4^+CD25^+$ regulatory T cells are dependent on CTLA-4 expression. Eur J Immunol 34:3485-3496, 2004
20. Tang Q, Boden EK, Henriksen KJ, Bour-Jordan H, Bi M, Bluestone JA: Distinct roles of CTLA-4 and TGF-beta in $CD4^+CD25^+$ regulatory T cell function. Eur J Immunol 34:2996-3005, 2004
21. Chen ML, Pittet MJ, Gorelik L, Flavell RA, Weissleder R, von Boehmer H, et al: Regulatory T cells suppress tumor-specific CD8 T cell cytotoxicity through TGF-beta signals in vivo. Proc Natl Acad Sci U S A 102: 419-424, 2005
22. Fontenot JD, Rudensky AY: A well adapted regulatory contrivance: Regulatory T cell development and the forkhead family transcription factor Foxp3. Nat Immunol 6:331-337, 2005
23. Cederbom L, Hall H, Ivars F: $CD4^+CD25^+$ regulatory T cells down-regulate co-stimulatory molecules on antigen-presenting cells. Eur J Immunol 30:1538-1543, 2000
24. Misra N, Bayry J, Lacroix-Desmazes S, Kazatchkine MD, Kaveri SV: Cutting edge: Human $CD4^+CD25^+$ T cells restrain the maturation and

antigen-presenting function of dendritic cells. J Immunol 172:4676-4680, 2004
25. Fallarino F, Grohmann U, Hwang KW, Orabona C, Vacca C, Bianchi R, et al: Modulation of tryptophan catabolism by regulatory T cells. Nat Immunol 4:1206-1212, 2003
26. Brunkow ME, Jeffery EW, Hjerrild KA, Paeper B, Clark LB, Yasayko SA, et al: Disruption of a new forkhead/winged-helix protein, scurfin, results in the fatal lymphoproliferative disorder of the scurfy mouse. Nat Genet 27:68-73, 2001
27. Fontenot JD, Gavin MA, Rudensky AY: Foxp3 programs the development and function of $CD4^+CD25^+$ regulatory T cells. Nat Immunol 4:330-336, 2003
28. Khattri R, Cox T, Yasayko SA, Ramsdell F: An essential role for Scurfin in $CD4^+CD25^+$ T regulatory cells. Nat Immunol 4:337-342, 2003
29. Hori S, Nomura T, Sakaguchi S: Control of regulatory T cell development by the transcription factor Foxp3. Science 299:1057-1061, 2003
30. Annunziato F, Cosmi L, Liotta F, Lazzeri E, Manetti R, Vanini V, et al: Phenotype, localization, and mechanism of suppression of $CD4(^+)CD25(^+)$ human thymocytes. J Exp Med 196:379-387, 2002
31. Papiernik M, de Moraes ML, Pontoux C, Vasseur F, Penit C: Regulatory CD4 T cells: Expression of IL-2R alpha chain, resistance to clonal deletion and IL-2 dependency. Int Immunol 10:371-378, 1998
32. Sakaguchi S: Naturally arising Foxp3-expressing $CD25^+CD4^+$ regulatory T cells in immunological tolerance to self and non-self. Nat Immunol 6:345-352, 2005
33. Roncador G, Brown PJ, Maestre L, Hue S, Martinez-Torrecuadrada JL, Ling KL, et al: Analysis of FOXP3 protein expression in human $CD4(^+)CD25(^+)$ regulatory T cells at the single-cell level. Eur J Immunol 35:1681-1691, 2005
34. Baecher-Allan C, Viglietta V, Hafler DA: Human $CD4^+CD25^+$ regulatory T cells. Semin Immunol 16:89-98, 2004
35. Fontenot JD, Rasmussen JP, Williams LM, Dooley JL, Farr AG, Rudensky AY: Regulatory T cell lineage specification by the forkhead transcription factor foxp3. Immunity 22:329-341, 2005
36. Pop SM, Wong CP, Culton DA, Clarke SH, Tisch R: Single cell analysis shows decreasing FoxP3 and TGFbeta1 coexpressing $CD4^+CD25^+$ regulatory T cells during autoimmune diabetes. J Exp Med 201:1333-1346, 2005
37. Bensinger SJ, Bandeira A, Jordan MS, Caton AJ, Laufer TM: Major histocompatibility complex class II-positive cortical epithelium mediates the selection of $CD4(^+)25(^+)$ immunoregulatory T cells. J Exp Med 194:427-438, 2001
38. Jordan MS, Boesteanu A, Reed AJ, Petrone AL, Holenbeck AE, Lerman MA, et al: Thymic selection of $CD4^+CD25^+$ regulatory T cells induced by an agonist self-peptide. Nat Immunol 2:301-306, 2001
39. van Santen HM, Benoist C, Mathis D: Number of T reg cells that differentiate does not increase upon encounter of agonist ligand on thymic epithelial cells. J Exp Med 200:1221-1230, 2004
40. Bettelli E, Dastrange M, Oukka M: Foxp3 interacts with nuclear factor of activated T cells and NF-kappa B to repress cytokine gene expression and effector functions of T helper cells. Proc Natl Acad Sci U S A 102:5138-5143, 2005
41. Hoffmann P, Ermann J, Edinger M, Fathman CG, Strober S: Donor-type $CD4(^+)CD25(^+)$ regulatory T cells suppress lethal acute graft-versus-host disease after allogeneic bone marrow transplantation. J Exp Med 196:389-399, 2002
42. Taylor PA, Noelle RJ, Blazar BR: $CD4(^+)CD25(^+)$ immune regulatory cells are required for induction of tolerance to alloantigen via costimulatory blockade. J Exp Med 193:1311-1318, 2001
43. Jones SC, Murphy GF, Korngold R: Post-hematopoietic cell transplantation control of graft-versus-host disease by donor $CD4(^+)25(^+)$ T cells to allow an effective graft-versus-leukemia response. Biol Blood Marrow Transplant 9:243-256, 2003
44. Edinger M, Hoffmann P, Ermann J, Drago K, Fathman CG, Strober S, et al: $CD4^+CD25^+$ regulatory T cells preserve graft-versus-tumor activity while inhibiting graft-versus-host disease after bone marrow transplantation. Nat Med 9:1144-1150, 2003
45. Hanash AM, Levy RB: Donor $CD4^+CD25^+$ T cells promote engraftment and tolerance following MHC-mismatched hematopoietic cell transplantation. Blood 105:1828-1836, 2005
46. Joffre O, Gorsse N, Romagnoli P, Hudrisier D, Van Meerwijk JP: Induction of antigen-specific tolerance to bone marrow allografts with $CD4^+CD25^+$ T lymphocytes. Blood 103:4216-4221, 2004
47. Trenado A, Charlotte F, Fisson S, Yagello M, Klatzmann D, Salomon BL, et al: Recipient-type specific $CD4^+CD25^+$ regulatory T cells favor immune reconstitution and control graft-versus-host disease while maintaining graft-versus-leukemia. J Clin Invest 112:1688-1696, 2003
48. Cohen JL, Trenado A, Vasey D, Klatzmann D, Salomon BL: $CD4(^+)CD25(^+)$ immunoregulatory T Cells: New therapeutics for graft-versus-host disease. J Exp Med 196:401-406, 2002
49. Taylor PA, Lees CJ, Blazar BR: The infusion of ex vivo activated and expanded $CD4(^+)CD25(^+)$ immune regulatory cells inhibits graft-versus-host disease lethality. Blood 99:3493-3499, 2002
50. Xia G, Kovochich M, Truitt RL, Johnson BD: Tracking ex vivo-expanded $CD4^+CD25^+$ and $CD8^+CD25^+$ regulatory T cells after infusion to prevent donor lymphocyte infusion-induced lethal acute graft-versus-host disease. Biol Blood Marrow Transplant 10:748-760, 2004
51. Kubsch S, Graulich E, Knop J, Steinbrink K: Suppressor activity of anergic T cells induced by IL-10-treated human dendritic cells: association with IL-2- and CTLA-4-dependent G1 arrest of the cell cycle regulated by p27Kip1. Eur J Immunol 33:1988-1997, 2003
52. Teshima T, Ordemann R, Reddy P, Gagin S, Liu C, Cooke KR, et al: Acute graft-versus-host disease does not require alloantigen expression on host epithelium. Nat Med 8:575-581, 2002
53. Shlomchik WD, Couzens MS, Tang CB, McNiff J, Robert ME, Liu J, et al: Prevention of graft versus host disease by inactivation of host antigen-presenting cells. Science 285:412-415, 1999
54. Murai M, Yoneyama H, Ezaki T, Suematsu M, Terashima Y, Harada A, et al: Peyer's patch is the essential site in initiating murine acute and lethal graft-versus-host reaction. Nat Immunol 4:154-160, 2003
55. Li B, New JY, Tay YK, Goh E, Yap EH, Chan SH, et al: Delaying acute graft-versus-host disease in mouse bone marrow transplantation by treating donor cells with antibodies directed at L-selectin and alpha4-integrin prior to infusion. Scand J Immunol 59:464-468, 2004
56. Anderson BE, McNiff J, Yan J, Doyle H, Mamula M, Shlomchik MJ, et al: Memory $CD4^+$ T cells do not induce graft-versus-host disease. J Clin Invest 112:101-108, 2003
57. Chen BJ, Cui X, Sempowski GD, Liu C, Chao NJ: Transfer of allogeneic CD62L- memory T cells without graft-versus-host disease. Blood 103: 1534-1541, 2004
58. Ermann J, Hoffmann P, Edinger M, Dutt S, Blankenberg FG, Higgins JP, et al: Only the $CD62L^+$ subpopulation of $CD4^+CD25^+$ regulatory T cells protects from lethal acute GVHD. Blood 105:2220-2226, 2005
59. Szanya V, Ermann J, Taylor C, Holness C, Fathman CG: The subpopulation of $CD4^+CD25^+$ splenocytes that delays adoptive transfer of diabetes expresses L-selectin and high levels of CCR7. J Immunol 169: 2461-2465, 2002
60. Taylor PA, Panoskaltsis-Mortari A, Swedin JM, Lucas PJ, Gress RE, Levine BL, et al: L-Selectin(hi) but not the L-selectin(lo) $CD4^+25^+$ T-regulatory cells are potent inhibitors of GVHD and BM graft rejection. Blood 104:3804-3812, 2004
61. Thornton AM, Shevach EM: Suppressor effector function of $CD4^+CD25^+$ immunoregulatory T cells is antigen nonspecific. J Immunol 164:183-190, 2000
62. Sarween N, Chodos A, Raykundalia C, Khan M, Abbas AK, Walker LS: $CD4^+CD25^+$ cells controlling a pathogenic CD4 response inhibit cytokine differentiation, CXCR-3 expression, and tissue invasion. J Immunol 173:2942-2951, 2004
63. Huehn J, Siegmund K, Lehmann JC, Siewert C, Haubold U, Feuerer M, et al: Developmental stage, phenotype, and migration distinguish naive- and effector/memory-like $CD4^+$ regulatory T cells. J Exp Med 199:303-313, 2004
64. Iellem A, Mariani M, Lang R, Recalde H, Panina-Bordignon P, Sinigaglia F, et al: Unique chemotactic response profile and specific expression of chemokine receptors CCR4 and CCR8 by $CD4(^+)CD25(^+)$ regulatory T cells. J Exp Med 194:847-853, 2001
65. Sebastiani S, Allavena P, Albanesi C, Nasorri F, Bianchi G, Traidl C, et

al: Chemokine receptor expression and function in $CD4^+$ T lymphocytes with regulatory activity. J Immunol 166:996-1002, 2001

66. Kolb HJ, Mittermuller J, Clemm C, Holler E, Ledderose G, Brehm G, et al: Donor leukocyte transfusions for treatment of recurrent chronic myelogenous leukemia in marrow transplant patients. Blood 76:2462-2465, 1990
67. Raiola AM, Van Lint MT, Valbonesi M, Lamparelli T, Gualandi F, Occhini D, et al: Factors predicting response and graft-versus-host disease after donor lymphocyte infusions: A study on 593 infusions. Bone Marrow Transplant 31:687-693, 2003
68. Truitt RL, Johnson BD: Principles of graft-vs.-leukemia reactivity. Biol Blood Marrow Transplant 1:61-68, 1995
69. Sprent J, Schaefer M, Lo D, Korngold R: Properties of purified T cell subsets. II. In vivo responses to class I vs. class II H-2 differences. J Exp Med 163:998-1011, 1986
70. Ferrara JL: Pathogenesis of acute graft-versus-host disease: Cytokines and cellular effectors. J Hematother Stem Cell Res 9:299-306, 2000
71. Stanzani M, Martins SL, Saliba RM, St John LS, Bryan S, Couriel D, et al: CD25 expression on donor $CD4^+$ or $CD8^+$ T cells is associated with an increased risk for graft-versus-host disease after HLA-identical stem cell transplantation in humans. Blood 103:1140-1146, 2004
72. Sanchez J, Casano J, Alvarez MA, Roman-Gomez J, Martin C, Martinez F, et al: Kinetic of regulatory $CD25^{high}$ and activated $CD134^+$ (OX40) T lymphocytes during acute and chronic graft-versus-host disease after allogeneic bone marrow transplantation. Br J Haematol 126:697-703, 2004
73. Clark FJ, Gregg R, Piper K, Dunnion D, Freeman L, Griffiths M, et al: Chronic graft-versus-host disease is associated with increased numbers of peripheral blood $CD4^+$CD25high regulatory T cells. Blood 103: 2410-2416, 2004
74. Miura Y, Thoburn CJ, Bright EC, Phelps ML, Shin T, Matsui EC, et al: Association of Foxp3 regulatory gene expression with graft-versus-host disease. Blood 104:2187-2193, 2004
75. Martin PJ, Pei J, Gooley T, Anasetti C, Appelbaum FR, Deeg J, et al: Evaluation of a CD25-specific immunotoxin for prevention of graft-versus-host disease after unrelated marrow transplantation. Biol Blood Marrow Transplant 10:552-560, 2004
76. Godfrey WR, Ge YG, Spoden DJ, Levine BL, June CH, Blazar BR, et al: In vitro-expanded human $CD4(^+)CD25(^+)$ T-regulatory cells can markedly inhibit allogeneic dendritic cell-stimulated MLR cultures. Blood 104:453-461, 2004
77. Hoffmann P, Eder R, Kunz-Schughart LA, Andreesen R, Edinger M: Large-scale in vitro expansion of polyclonal human $CD4(^+)CD25^{high}$ regulatory T cells. Blood 104:895-903, 2004
78. Jiang S, Camara N, Lombardi G, Lechler RI: Induction of allopeptide-specific human $CD4^+CD25^+$ regulatory T cells ex vivo. Blood 102:2180-2186, 2003

ELSEVIER

Seminars in HEMATOLOGY

Diagnosis and Treatment of Chronic Graft-Versus-Host Disease

Andrew L. Gilman[a] and Jonathan Serody[b]

Chronic graft-versus-host disease (GVHD) is the major cause of non-relapse morbidity and mortality after hematopoietic stem cell transplant (HSCT). GVHD also is associated with a potent anti-leukemic effect. Chronic GVHD resembles autoimmune diseases and can likely affect any organ or tissue of the body. Skin, oral, liver, and lacrimal gland involvement are most common. The incidence and presentation have been in evolution as new stem cell sources and transplant approaches have been introduced. Although progress in the diagnosis and treatment of chronic GVHD has been limited for many years, there is renewed interest in this disorder. New prognostic scores and animal models of chronic GVHD have been developed. Large, multicenter phase III therapy and biology studies have been undertaken. The challenge for the future will be the discovery of targeted approaches that allow the anti-leukemic effect to be retained and for the reconstitution of normal immunity, thereby reducing infectious complications.
Semin Hematol 43:70-80

Chronic graft-versus-host disease (GVHD) is the major cause of non-relapse morbidity and mortality following allogeneic hematopoietic stem cell transplantation (HSCT). Chronic GVHD is also associated with a graft-versus-leukemia (GVL) effect and a reduced relapse rate. Unfortunately, little progress has been made in the understanding of the pathophysiology or outcome of chronic GVHD over the last 25 years.[1] There is currently an international effort sponsored by the National Institutes of Health to advance the conduct of clinical trials for chronic GVHD, which hopefully will improve outcomes in patients with this debilitating condition.

A major challenge in the understanding of chronic GVHD may be that it is a spectrum disorder. Although some manifestations, like skin, oral, liver, and lacrimal gland involvement, are common, the pattern of manifestations are protean and often occur in unique constellations. The pathophysiology underlying the various syndromes may differ depending on the clinical manifestations present. The lack of a homogeneous study population makes laboratory studies and clinical trials particularly vexing.

Excellent reviews of chronic GVHD are available as valuable resources.[1-4] Herein we discuss the presentation and management of chronic GVHD for clinical practice, and more briefly provide insights into its pathophysiology.

Diagnosis

Chronic GVHD historically has been considered to present more than 100 days after transplant. More recently, timing has been considered to be less important than the presence of typical symptoms and signs of chronic GVHD.[1] Diagnosis can also be complicated when acute and chronic GVHD coexist. The type of onset of chronic GVHD is described relative to acute GVHD. Progressive onset refers to chronic GVHD that develops prior to the resolution of acute GVHD. Quiescent or interrupted onset is when chronic GVHD develops after the resolution of acute GVHD. *De novo* onset refers to chronic GVHD that occurs in a patient who has not had acute GVHD. The most important presentation is progressive onset because it has a worse prognosis.[1] Patients who are receiving a significant dose of corticosteroids for the treatment of acute GVHD when chronic GVHD develops may have a similar poor outlook, despite the prior control of acute GVHD[5]; development of chronic GVHD in this situation would be analogous to progressive onset chronic GVHD.

An experienced clinician may be able to make a diagnosis of chronic GVHD based on classic manifestations such as lichenoid or sclerodermatous skin changes. If the findings are not typical, a tissue biopsy is warranted to aid the diagnosis and to determine if infection is present. Viral infections and

[a]Department of Pediatrics, University of North Carolina at Chapel Hill, Chapel Hill, NC.
[b]Department of Medicine, University of North Carolina at Chapel Hill, Chapel Hill, NC.
Address correspondence to Andrew Gilman, MD, University of North Carolina School of Medicine, 418 MacNider Hall, Chapel Hill, NC 27517. E-mail: agilman@med.unc.edu

 0037-1963/06/$-see front matter
doi:10.1053/j.seminhematol.2005.09.008

drug reactions can be diagnostic challenges even with biopsy.[6] Viral infections can coexist with chronic GVHD and trigger GVHD in some cases.[7] Differentiating drug reactions from chronic GVHD can be difficult because eosinophilia and the presence of eosinophils in tissue also occur in GVHD.[6,8] The typical histopathology of chronic GVHD may be less evident early in the presentation and in patients who are already receiving intensive immunosuppressive drugs. The lymphocytic infiltrate may only be perivascular and apoptosis infrequent.

The chronology of symptoms may be a clue to the diagnosis of chronic GVHD. Often, chronic GVHD will present during weaning or soon after stopping immunosuppression.[9] When a diagnosis of chronic GVHD is made, the patient should have a thorough evaluation for disease involvement: a complete skin examination, assessment of joint mobility, Schirmer's test for ocular dryness, pulmonary function tests, gynecologic exam, complete blood cell counts, liver function tests, and immunoglobulin levels. Assessment should be repeated periodically during treatment.[4]

Clinical Manifestations

Chronic GVHD resembles autoimmune diseases, including systemic lupus erythematosus (SLE), Sjogren's syndrome, lichen planus, scleroderma, and a number of other related disorders. Chronic GVHD can affect any organ or tissue of the body. Skin, oral, liver, and lacrimal gland involvement are most common. Other manifestations are much less frequent and are usually present in less than 10% to 20% of patients.[10] Chronic GVHD has been associated with almost all manifestations described in autoimmune diseases. Uncommon presentations are usually reported as case reports, and occasionally as case series. They may be underreported because of preconceived notions based on the original description of chronic GVHD, the reluctance to confirm some sites of involvement with biopsy (such as the cardiac conduction system and central nervous system), and because of concurrent viral infections may trigger a chronic GVHD exacerbation and can obscure the etiology. Some manifestations, including cardiac and renal involvement, may be more common in types of transplants that are associated with more immunologic reactivity, such as haplo-identical donor or non-myeloablative transplants. Clinical manifestations and related diagnostic testing are summarized in Table 1.

Skin/Hair/Nails

Skin manifestations can vary from macular erythema to papulosquamous lesions, as the earliest signs, to superficial and deep dermal fibrosis. The papules may be flesh-colored, erythematous, or purple; they are often polygonal, are typically flat on top, and may have a scale and be pruritic. The papular rash resembles lichen planus (Fig 1). The rash often has a reticulated pattern but no typical distribution. Occasionally the eruption will resemble eczema. A butterfly malar rash typical of systemic lupus erythematosis is sometimes seen. Chronic GVHD of the skin may develop from a typical acute GVHD erythematous rash, in which case the rash often develops a pebbly appearance and rough texture as it evolves. Also characteristic is involvement of the adnexal structures, hair follicles and sweat glands. As chronic GVHD of the skin progresses, there may be poikiloderma, with a multicolor appearance of the skin resulting from erythema, telangiectasias, atrophy, and dyspigmentation. Sclerosis of the dermis may be superficial (involving the upper dermis) or deep (involving the lower dermis and/or muscular fascia). The sclerotic changes may evolve from a lichen planus-like rash or occur without prior changes, and resemble the skin signs of scleroderma.[11] Superficial fibrosis is associated with thickening of the skin and changes in pigmentation. Deeper fibrosis causes hidebound, immovable skin that cannot be pinched. The skin may be fixed to underlying tissues. Minor abrasions may result in ulceration of the poorly vascularized tissue. Fibrosis over joints can result in contractures (Fig 2).

Chronic GVHD can also affect pigment cells in the skin, causing hyper- or hypopigmentation (vitiligo). Hyperpigmentation from chronic GVHD must be differentiated from post-inflammatory hyperpigmentation occuring at sites of resolved erythematous skin involvement. Sweat glands can be damaged, resulting in an inability to sweat and poor heat tolerance.[4] Chronic GVHD can damage hair follicles, causing loss of hair on the extremities and alopecia on the scalp. Hair may become thin and brittle. Growth of hair in previously affected areas may correlate with clinical improvement. Loss of pigment can result in premature graying of hair. Nails can have vertical ridging and be very fragile; onychodystrophy, degenerative changes or malformations of the nail, may occur. Hair loss and nail abnormalities can persist after skin changes have resolved.[4]

Eyes

Chronic GVHD causes inflammation and fibrosis of the lacrimal gland and results in decreased tear production. Patients may complain of dryness, burning, photophobia, or the sensation of a foreign object under the lids. Findings of conjunctivitis may be present, either due to dryness or to direct involvement by chronic GVHD. Corneal ulcerations may result from the severe dryness. Decreased tear production may be detected by a Schirmer's test; a value less than 5 mm or a value less than 10 mm with symptoms is consistent with dry eyes. Occasionally, patients will have excess tearing early in the course of the disease.[12]

Mouth

Chronic GVHD can damage the major and minor salivary glands, resulting in mouth dryness, mucosal and gingival irritation, and dental decay. Mucoceles (clear blisters) can develop at sites of minor salivary glands on the inner lower lip, soft palate, and buccal mucosa. Chronic GVHD can cause erythema, lichenoid changes, atrophy, and ulceration of the oral mucosa; erythema and lichenoid changes also occur on the tongue and gingiva. Lichenoid changes result from focal hyperkeratinization and appear as white striae or plaques (Fig 3). Patients may complain of pain, sometimes only with

Table 1 Clinical Manifestations and Diagnostic Testing

Organ	Signs, Symptoms, and Lab Tests	Diagnostic Testing
Skin	Erythematous or purple papular rash (lichenoid), may have scaling, may be pruritic	Skin biopsy
	Hyperpigmentation, hypopigmentation, poikiloderma (multiple colors)	
	Thickened, loss of elasticity, fixed, fragile (sclerodermatous)	
Hair/Nails	Thin, brittle hair; premature graying; alopecia	
	Vertical ridging, fragile nails	
Mouth	Erythema; white striae or plaques (lichenoid)	Buccal mucosal or labial biopsy
	Ulcers, pseudomembranes; mucoceles	
Eyes	Decreased tear production (may be increased early)	Schirmer's test for tear production
	Dryness, burning, foreign body sensation, photophobia	
	Conjunctivitis; corneal ulceration	
Liver	Increased bilirubin, alk phos, GGT; increased AST and ALT	Liver biopsy if only site of disease
Gastrointestinal tract	Difficulty and/or pain with swallowing; heartburn; retrosternal pain	Barium swallow; upper and lower endoscopy
	Weight loss; decreased appetite; nausea; emesis	Testing for malabsorption
	Diarrhea, abdominal pain	Testing for pancreatic insufficiency
Lungs	Cough, wheezing, dyspnea	Pulmonary functions tests including spirometry, lung volumes, and DLCO; high resolution CT scan with end inspiratory and end expiratory films
Musculoskeletal system	Arthralgias, arthritis; myalgias; weakness; contractures	CK, aldolase, EMG, ENG, muscle biopsy
	Pleural and pericardial effusions, ascites	Analysis of serosal fluid
Vulva/vagina	Erythema, white striae or plaques (lichenoid)	Gynecologic exam; biopsy
	Dryness, irritation, dyspareunia	
Heart	Bradycardia, chest pain	Electrocardigram, Holter, CK and lactate dehydrogenase isoenzymes, troponin
Renal	Proteinuria, edema	24-hour urine collection for protein; renal biopsy
Nervous system	Sensory and motor neuropathies	ENG
Blood	Immune thrombocytopenic purpura; autoimmune hemolytic anemia; eosinophilia	Coombs test; complete blood cell count
Immune system	Sepsis with encapsulated organisms; recurrent sinopulmonary infections; pneumocystis pneumonia; late cytomegalovirus; Herpes zoster	
	Lack of response to vaccinations	

Abbreviations: GGT, gamma-glutamyl transferase; DLCO, diffusion lung capacity for carbon monoxide; CK, creatine kinase; EMG, electromyography; ENG, electroneurography.

spicy or acidic foods, or a burning sensation with toothpaste. Ulcerations, sometimes with overlying pseudomembranes, typically appear along the bite line of the buccal mucosa (Fig 4). Manifestations of oral GVHD can resemble candida, herpes simplex virus, or cytomegalovirus infections, which are often present as secondary infections. Fibrosis of the oral mucosa is a late manifestation and can limit opening of the mouth.[13]

Liver

Chronic GVHD injures the bile duct epithelium and causes cholestasis. There is less correlation between bilirubin levels and outcome in chronic GVHD compared to acute GVHD.[9] Elevations of alkaline phosphatase and GGT are seen. Fibrosis and cirrhosis may occur. Hepatocyte effects may predominate, presenting as an acute hepatitis picture.[14]

Gastrointestinal Tract

Chronic GVHD can involve the upper and lower gastrointestinal tract. A classic manifestation is submucosal fibrosis of the esophagus, leading to poor motility and occasionally strictures and webs.[15] Desquamation and ulceration are uncommon. Patients may complain of difficulty and/or pain with swallowing, "heartburn," and retrosternal pain. Intestinal involvement can result in malabsorption and diarrhea; weight loss is not uncommon, from malabsorption, de-

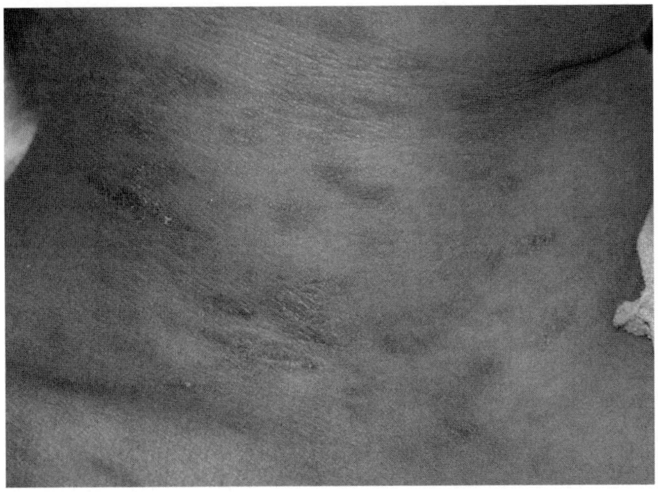

Figure 1 The lichen planus-like (lichenoid) rash of chronic GVHD typically consists of erythematous or purple, polygonal papules that are flat on top, with variable amount of scale.

creased oral intake, and an increased basal metabolic rate. Close attention should be paid to the patient's weight and nutritional status.[2] When immunosuppression is weaned, it can be difficult to differentiate a decline in body weight due to exacerbation of GVHD from the normal loss of increased fat stores during tapering of corticosteroids. Patients should be observed closely during this phase for signs of worsening GVHD.

Nausea, early satiety, diarrhea, and abdominal pain can be present in the setting of other typical chronic GVHD findings; whether these manifestations represent chronic GVHD or persistent or coexistent acute GVHD is unclear. In one study, many patients who were considered to have chronic GVHD of the gastrointestinal tract had acute GVHD or both acute and chronic GVHD; however, all had active disease.[16] Pancreatic insufficiency, which may be due to GVHD, is another cause of diarrhea and may respond to enzyme replacement.[17]

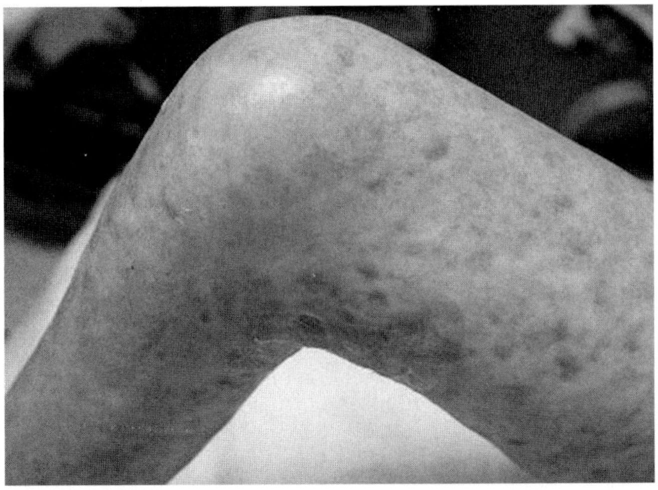

Figure 2 The skin is shiny and indurated due to sclerotic changes from chronic GVHD which resemble scleroderma. Poikiloderma is present with erythema, hyperpigmentation, and hypopigmented sclerosis. Ulcerations are present. The knee joint is fixed in this position.

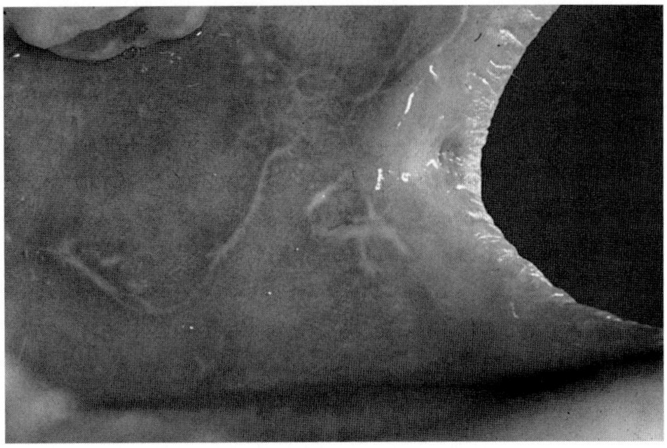

Figure 3 Lichenoid hyperkeratotic striae-like changes with varying degrees of patchy erythema. Photograph courtesy of Mark Schubert.

Lungs

Chronic GVHD is associated with airflow obstruction and bronchiolitis obliterans. In bronchiolitis obliterans, intimal proliferation and fibrosis obliterate the lumen of the small airways. Patients present with a cough, wheezing, and dyspnea on exertion.[18] Bronchiolitis obliterans may be triggered by a respiratory viral infection, perhaps due to stimulation of a dysregulated immune response. The diagnosis is based on findings of obstructive lung disease on pulmonary function tests. Chronic gastroesophageal reflux may exacerbate airflow obstruction. Bronchiolitis obliterans is typically associated with air trapping that may be detected by high resolution end-expiratory and end-inspiratory computed tomography (CT) scan.[18] CT scans can also be normal or show bronchiectasis in bronchiolitis obliterans. Lung biopsy is indicated in patients who have no other manifestations of chronic GVHD or when the diagnosis is unclear because clinical findings suggest other possible causes. Corticosteroids are the mainstay of treatment, and the addition of other immunosuppres-

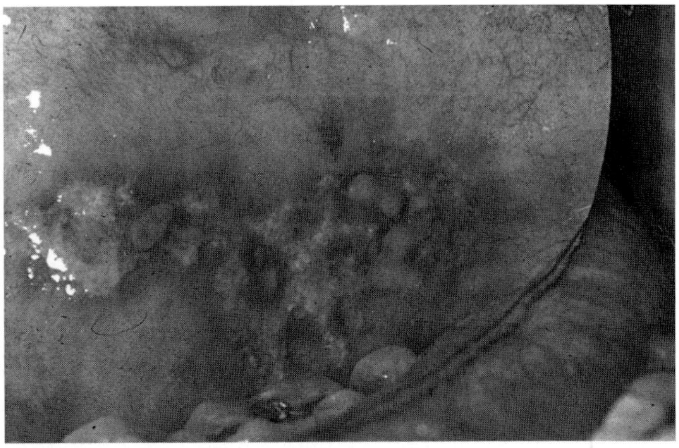

Figure 4 Lichenoid hyperkeratotic changes with areas of pseudomembranous ulcerations and intense erythema. Photograph courtesy of Mark Schubert.

sive or lympholytic agents did not appear to improve prognosis in a retrospective review.[19]

Chronic GVHD may also be a cause of bronchiolitis obliterans with organizing pneumonia (BOOP), restrictive lung disease, and lymphocytic pneumonitis, but these associations are less certain. BOOP typically presents with fever, cough, wheezing, and scattered pulmonary infiltrates.[20] An infectious etiology must be excluded. BOOP typically responds promptly to corticosteroids. Patients with chronic GVHD may also have chronic sinusitis, with or without infection.

Musculoskeletal system

Polymyositis, myasthenia gravis, serositis, arthralgia, arthritis, and fasciitis are manifestations of musculoskeletal involvement with chronic GVHD. Polymyositis occurred in 3% of patients in a large series, usually associated with an elevated creatine kinase (CK).[21] Tender muscles are typical, but a proximal myopathy may be the first development. Myasthenia gravis of GVHD is identical to the syndrome in sporadic cases.[22] Serositis causes multiple effusions, including pericardial and pleural effusions and ascites, and it is often associated with concurrent viral infections.[23] Arthralgia and arthritis resembling those in rheumatoid arthritis are occasionally seen. With fasciitis, inflammation and sclerosis of the fascia can cause contractures; although often associated with sclerosis of the skin, fasciitis can occur with normal-appearing, but fixed, overlying skin. Fasciitis often affects the forearms and legs. Muscle cramps of uncertain etiology can occur with chronic GVHD.[2]

Vulva/Vagina

Vulvar and vaginal manifestations resemble those of oral and esophageal GVHD: erythema, lichenoid changes, and vaginal strictures. Symptoms include dryness, burning, and dyspareunia.[24]

Heart

Cardiac manifestations, including bradycardia, coronary artery occlusion, and cardiomyolyis, have been reported; we recently reported a series of patients with cardiac involvement during acute GVHD or on a flare of chronic GVHD.[25]

Kidneys

Nephrotic syndrome in chronic GVHD resembles the proteinuria in a murine model of chronic GVHD. Membranous glomerulonephritis can also occur.[26]

Nervous System

Involvement of the brain was described in one case of chronic GVHD.[27] Central nervous system involvement similar to lupus cerebritis may be under-recognized because it would be difficult to distinguish depression and memory problems from chronic GVHD from side effects medications and prior irradiation and from the emotional impact of the disease itself. Peripheral neuropathies are uncommon in chronic GVHD.[28]

Hematologic System

Chronic GVHD can cause autoimmune cytopenias, eosinophilia, and bone marrow suppression. Immune thrombocytopenia (ITP) and autoimmune hemolytic anemia (AIHA) have been reported. AIHA may be more likely in the setting of increased human leukocyte antigen (HLA) disparity, after unrelated donor and mismatched related donor transplant.[29] Eosinophilia may be a marker of chronic GVHD.[8] Leukocytosis is occasionally seen.

Immune System

Chronic GVHD is both immunosuppressive and associated with autoimmunity. This paradoxical combination also occurs in congenital and acquired immunodeficiencies. The underlying mechanism may be Th2 T-lymphocyte predominance, with immunodeficiency mediated by interleukin-10 (IL-10) and production of auto-antibodies due to IL-4. Patients with chronic GVHD are at increased risk of infections.[30] The immunodeficiency and infectious complications are exacerbated by the immunosuppressive drugs used to treat chronic GVHD. Chronic GVHD also has been associated with auto-antibodies in addition to those against blood cells, although their role in producing disease is unclear.[31] Reports of benefit from rituximab (anti-CD20 or B cell antibody) in chronic GVHD, discussed below, suggest that auto-antibodies do contribute to at least some manifestations of chronic GVHD. Chronic GVHD is accompanied by functional asplenia and an increased susceptibility to infections with encapsulated bacteria.[32]

Pathophysiology

GVHD occurs as a result of the recognition by donor T cells of host (the transplant recipient) tissue antigens that differ from donor antigens. The immune response resembles the normal host defense against microbial pathogens. The manifestations of acute GVHD are an early acute inflammatory reaction, with T-lymphocyte stimulation and expansion and tissue damage mediated by effector cells and cytokines.[33] Chronic GVHD resembles the later immune/healing response characterized by collagen deposition, antibody production, and suppression of the acute inflammatory response when antigen persists. The similarities between chronic GVHD and a normal immune response make it difficult to use biologic markers for diagnosis or response.

The similarity between chronic GVHD and the later immune response has led to the hypothesis that at least some manifestations of chronic GVHD may be attributed to a Th2 (T-helper) lymphocyte predominance. Th2 cells produce cytokines, especially IL-4, that assist antibody production, IL-5, a growth factor for eosinophils, and IL-10, which causes immunosuppression. Although Th2 predominance has been observed in mouse models, its role in humans is less clear; as discussed above, the lack of a homogeneous patient population makes laboratory evaluation and interpretation more difficult. A further confounder is that acute and chronic GVHD can coexist. Possibly some patients have manifestations due to a Th1 predominance, others mainly due to Th2 cell activity, parallel to findings in different autoimmune disorders. Donor and recipient major and minor histocompatibility antigen differences, donor and recipient cytokine gene polymorphisms, and medications used to prevent and treat acute GVHD could influence the character of immune response. There are also similarities with inherited immunodeficiency disorders like Omenn's syndrome, which is characterized by a Th2 predominance, eosinophilia, and skin lesions resembling chronic GVHD.[34]

Chronic GVHD is probably due to both alloreactivity and autoreactivity. Alloreactivity creates the immunologic milieu and sustains chronic GVHD. Similarity between chronic GVHD and cyclosporine-induced autologous GVHD led to experiments in a murine model. In this model, autoreactive T lymphocytes escape normal intrathymic deletion and mediate chronic GVHD.[35] It is likely that at least some of the manifestations of chronic GVHD result from damage to the thymus by conditioning radiation and chemotherapy and by acute GVHD.

Animal models have also been used to examine the alloreactive component of chronic GVHD. Early experiments were better models for autoantibody manifestations of chronic GVHD. When donor (DBA/2) T cells were infused into unirradiated haploidentical F1 offspring recipients (DBA/2 × C57BL/6), the recipients developed chronic GVHD, manifested by Coombs' positive hemolytic anemia, anti-DNA antibodies, and proteinuria. Donor T cells were polarized toward a Th2 phenotype with production of IL-4 and IL-10.[36] More recent animal models generate sclerodermatous changes in the skin, typical of the fibrosis seen later in chronic GVHD. In a minor histocompatibility mismatch model, B.10.D2 T cells infused into irradiated BALB/c recipients caused chronic GVHD, characterized by skin thickening and lung fibrosis, without generation of autoantibodies or vascular injury.[37] Donor T cells appeared to activate donor and recipient monocytes in the skin, leading to the generation of transforming growth factor-β1 (TGF-β1) and fibrosis. Either donor or host antigen-presenting cells (APCs) could initiate chronic GVHD, and donor APCs were critical to the pathogenesis of chronic GVHD in the gastrointestinal tract, in contrast to an acute GVHD murine model in which residual host APCs were required.[38]

Unfortunately, murine lymphocyte profiles and chronic GVHD signs differ from those in humans, and it is not clear how much animal model data can be extrapolated to clinical disease. However, despite these limitations, there are several consistent features of chronic GVHD in animal models, which include a critical role for donor $CD4^+$ T cells and donor/recipient B cells in the pathogenesis of the disease. Recent results suggesting a role for rituximab (anti–B-cell antibody) in the treatment of chronic GVHD lends some credence to the predictive value of these animal models.[39]

Another mechanism, first suggested in the 1980s, is the presence of suppressor cells that cause the immunodeficiency associated with chronic GVHD.[40] More recently, the role of regulatory T cells (Tregs) has been evaluated. Multiple populations of suppressive or Tregs are present, which include thymic-derived $CD4^+/CD25^+$ Tregs, IL-10–secreting Tr1 cells, TGF-β–generating Th3 cells, and CD122-expressing $CD8^+$ T cells. $CD4^+/CD25^+$ Tregs have been reported to be increased in chronic GVHD.[41]

Treatment

A major decision to be made when chronic GVHD is diagnosed is the requirement for treatment, either topical or systemic therapy. A grading system for chronic GVHD was devised as a tool to determine who requires systemic treatment. This system divides chronic GVHD into limited or extensive disease. Patients with limited disease have localized skin and/or liver involvement, with the exception of more advanced liver histologies (chronic aggressive hepatitis, bridging necrosis, cirrhosis).[42] Other investigators have suggested that for localized, mild symptoms and signs, topical therapy is adequate.[1,4] Untreated extensive chronic GVHD has a high risk of severe morbidity and mortality, primarily due to immunodeficiency and infections, and to a lesser degree to organ failure.[43] Prompt diagnosis and initiation of treatment are important to limit the severity of chronic GVHD.

More recent recommendations to guide the introduction of more aggressive measures for chronic GVHD classify mild, localized findings, such as isolated oral or vaginal GVHD, as not requiring systemic therapy, provided that the patient is not receiving corticosteroid therapy at the time of diagnosis and that the platelet count is greater than 100,000/μL. Clinically extensive disease requiring systemic immunosuppression is defined as involvement of two organs by chronic GVHD. Significant localized disease, like localized sclerodermatous changes (morphea), also is treated systemically.[1]

There are also recent prognostic scores that can help with treatment decisions. Almost all analyses have found that progressive onset of chronic GVHD, thrombocytopenia (<100,000/μL), diffuse skin involvement, gastrointestinal involvement, and poor performance status predict worse outcomes.[1] An analysis of 151 patients showed that prognosis could be determined based on extent of skin disease, thrombocytopenia, and progressive onset[44]; the prognostic score was validated on other large data sets.[45] Another predictive system based on data from the International Bone Marrow Transplant Registry found Karnofsky performance score, diarrhea, weight loss, and cutaneous and oral involvement to be independent variables.[9]

The necessary intensity and duration of treatment are not well-established. The benefit of eradicating the manifestations of GVHD must be weighed against the complications of therapy. The duration of treatment must also assess the reversibility of some changes; for example, some damage, such as lacrimal gland destruction and obliteration of small airways, is irreversible regardless of GVHD activity with currently available therapies.

The frequency of corticosteroid-resistant or -dependent chronic GVHD and significant complications from steroids have encouraged the evaluation of other immunosuppressive medications. Many immunosuppressive drugs have shown activity for chronic GVHD, unsurprising for an immunolog-

Table 2 Summary of Selected Randomized Primary Therapy Trials

Treatment	No. of Evaluable Patients per Arm	Response rate (CR / CR + PR)	Reference	Comments
Prednisone *v* prednisone + azathioprine	63/63	33/62 *v* 37/64	46	All patients with platelet count > 100,000/μL and almost all with HLA-identical sibling donors; no difference in response; lower survival with azathioprine due to increased infection
Prednisone *v* prednisone + cyclosporine	145/142	No response rate given; need for secondary therapy: 17% *v* 11% (not significant)	47	All patients with platelet count > 100,000/μL and almost all with HLA-identical sibling donors; no difference in need for secondary therapy or 5-year survival
Prednisone + cyclosporine *v* prednisone + cyclosporine + thalidomide	24/27	55/73 *v* 50/85	64	Methylprednisolone 15 mg/kg weekly × 8 also given; no difference in response; closed early due to higher than predicted response rates

ically mediated disease. The majority of drugs and biologics in clinical practice were tested in phase II studies. However, the benefit of agents of salvage therapy cannot be extrapolated to their utility in newly diagnosed patients. Phase III studies that have been performed give caution to this practice. For example, despite the activity of azathioprine for chronic GVHD, it worsened outcome when combined with prednisone in newly diagnosed standard-risk patients.[46] A summary of randomized studies for newly-diagnosed chronic GVHD is provided in Table 2 and agents that have been evaluated for activity in chronic GVHD in Table 3.

Prednisone

Prednisone remains the standard therapy for chronic GVHD. Prednisone is usually initiated at 1 mg/kg per day for 2 weeks, during which time some response is typically seen. The dose is then tapered to 1 mg/kg every other day over 1 to 2 months, as tolerated, and then gradually reduced further. An early study of prednisone for chronic GVHD maintained patients on 1 mg/kg every other day until 9 months of therapy had been completed. Thirty-three percent of patients had a complete response (CR, defined as clinical and histological resolution of GVHD) and 29% a partial response (PR, clinical resolution but histological evidence of active GVHD). For high-risk patients with a platelet count of less than 100,000/μL, the CR rate was only 16% and the PR rate was 16%.[46] In a more recent study of prednisone alone, response rates were not reported but only 17% of patients needed secondary therapy; an earlier steroid taper was used, with a decrease to 0.5 mg/kg of prednisone every other day starting after 22 weeks and continuing until another taper after 40 weeks of therapy. The median duration of therapy was 2.2 years, which was similar to that reported in the earlier publication.[47] Common toxicities of corticosteroids include glucose intolerance, hypertension, cataracts, weight gain, fungal infections, and bone loss.

Cyclosporine

Cyclosporine, a calcineurin inhibitor, has activity for chronic GVHD. However, many patients are still receiving cyclosporine prophylaxis when chronic GVHD presents. A phase II study evaluated prednisone and cyclosporine for patients with a platelet count of less than 100,000/μL: the combination improved survival and response rates compared to historical patients treated only with prednisone.[48] A subsequent randomized trial of prednisone versus prednisone and cyclosporine for patients with a platelet count of greater than 100,000/μL failed to demonstrate a similar advantage. Survival without recurrent malignancy was lower in the two-drug arm ($P = .03$). The only benefit was that patients in the cyclosporine arm had less avascular necrosis.[47] These studies used alternate-day cyclosporine, and daily dosing of cyclosporine is now standard clinical practice.[49]

Thalidomide

Several studies have demonstrated activity of thalidomide for steroid-resistant chronic GVHD in adults and children. Despite the promising results with small numbers of patients, a large phase II study showed a low response rate and a high incidence of toxicities, including sedation, constipation, neuropathy, rash, and neutropenia.[50] A randomized phase III study of thalidomide in addition to prednisone and cyclosporine for newly diagnosed high-risk patients showed a high incidence of side effects that limited its usefulness.[51]

Mycophenolate Mofetil

There are several small studies of mycophenolate mofetil (MMF) for the treatment of steroid-resistant chronic GVHD

Table 3 Summary of Selected Reports of Options for Salvage Therapy (steroid-resistant or dependent disease)

Treatment	No. of Evaluable Patients	Response Rate	Reference	Comments
Cyclosporine (CSA)	21	CR 19%, PR 52%, 4-yr surv 67%	48	Alternate day CSA
Tacrolimus	39	CR 13% at 3 yr; 3-yr surv 64%	65	Prednisone/CSA failures
Mycophenolate mofetil (MMF)	15	CR 13%, PR 47%	52	Children only
	13	69% response rate (no details)	53	
Tacrolimus + MMF	26	CR 8%, PR 38%	66	Retrospective
Thalidomide	23	CR 30%, PR 48%, 2 yr survival 76%	67	
	38	CR 3%, PR 35%	68	
	13	CR 38%, PR 31%	69	Children only
	80	CR 11%, PR 9%	50	
Hydroxychloroquine	32	CR 9%, PR 41%	54	
Clofazimine	22	CR 0%, PR 55%	70	
Sirolimus	16	CR 12%, PR 82%	55	
Methylprednisolone, high-dose pulse	61	CR + PR 48%, 2-yr survival 81%	59	Retrospective
Pentostatin	16	CR 31%, additional 50% improved	58	
Etanercept	10	CR 10%, PR 50%	71	
Rituximab	10	5/10 improved	57	
PUVA	35	Skin response CR 41% / PR 38%	63	Retrospective
Prednisone + cyclosporine + azathioprine	16	CR 88%, PR 0%	60	
Photopheresis	32	Skin response CR 22%, PR 34%	72	Retrospective
	25	CR 0%, PR 64%	61	
	14	CR 28%, PR 36%	73	2/4 CR had limited chronic GVHD; children only

in adults and children. MMF is a prodrug of mycophenolic acid, which inhibits T-cell proliferation by blocking the activity of inosine monophosphate dehydrogenase. In 15 children with steroid-resistant chronic GVHD, responses to MMF were seen in gastrointestinal, oral, and nonsclerodermatous skin manifestations; thrombocytopenia also improved.[52] MMF in 13 adults produced responses of gastrointestinal, liver, and lichenoid and sclerodermatous skin GVHD.[53] There is currently a randomized phase III study of MMF added to prednisone and cyclosporine for newly diagnosed chronic GVHD (Martin P, personal communication).

Hydroxychloroquine

Hydroxychloroquine is an antimalarial that is widely used as a steroid-sparing agent for the treatment of rheumatoid arthritis and systemic lupus erythematosus. Hydroxychloroquine was active for steroid-resistant or -dependent chronic GVHD in a phase II study; skin, oral, and hepatic manifestations and thrombocytopenia often responded.[54] There was a recent randomized phase III study of hydroxychloroquine in addition to prednisone and cyclosporine for newly diagnosed chronic GVHD.

Sirolimus

Sirolimus, a natural macrolide that inhibits cytokine-driven signaling pathways in T cells, has been reported to have activity for chronic GVHD in a phase II trial for patients who had failed first-line or subsequent therapy; sirolimus improved skin, oral, ocular, and liver GVHD.[55]

Rituximab

Rituximab, a chimeric anti-CD20 monoclonal antibody, has demonstrated activity for post-transplant ITP and AIHA.[56] One small study demonstrated improvement of lichenoid and sclerodermatous skin manifestations, alopecia, and oral mucositis.[39] A recent phase II study of rituximab for chronic GVHD showed activity, mainly for skin and musculoskeletal manifestations.[57]

Pentostatin

Pentostatin is a purine nucleoside analogue that has been administered every other week for the treatment of chronic GVHD. In a recent report of 16 evaluable pediatric patients with refractory chronic GVHD, five (31%) had a CR and an additional eight had a "major" response.[58]

High-Dose Methylprednisolone

The use of methylprednisolone at 10 mg/kg/dose daily for 4 days for chronic GVHD has been reported; patients received broad infection prophylaxis following the steroid pulse. Significant benefits included skin softening, increased joint mobility, and improved performance score. The analysis is complicated by the fact that patients were started on a new immunosuppressive regimen following the steroid pulse.[59]

Multi-agent Approach

The use of a multi-agent approach including methylprednisolone, cyclosporine, and azathioprine has been used for initial or salvage treatments of patients with moderate to severe chronic GVHD. Cyclosporine was given daily, and methylprednisolone and azathioprine on alternating days. Cyclosporine and azathioprine were slowly tapered prior to reducing the methylprednisolone dose. The CR rates for initial and salvage therapy were high (94% and 88%, respectively). Of note, all the patients had been transplanted for thalassemia and almost all had HLA-identical donors; almost all had moderately severe chronic GVHD, graded according to a system unique to this report.[60]

Photopheresis

Extracorporeal photopheresis has produced promising results in phase II studies for chronic GVHD. The procedure involves leukapheresis to collect leukocytes, which are then incubated with UVADEX or 8-methoxypsoralen and then exposed to ultraviolet light; the leukocytes are then returned to the patient. Responses have consistently been reported for lichenoid and sclerodermatous skin disease, with some reports of improvement of GVHD involving the mouth, eyes, liver, lungs, and gastrointestinal tract.[61,62] A randomized phase III trial of extracorporeal photopheresis is in progress.

Local Treatments

Some manifestations of chronic GVHD can be treated locally, especially if they are isolated findings. Psoralen and UVA light (PUVA) therapy has good activity for lichenoid skin disease, less so for sclerodermatous disease.[63] Oral lesions can be treated with steroid rinses.[4] Pulmonary GVHD may benefit from inhaled steroids.[18]

Recommendations for Therapy

Primary systemic therapy should be based on known risk factors as described above. Patients with mild, localized disease can often be treated with topical therapy. Patients with more severe or extensive disease should receive prednisone and/or cyclosporine; a patient without thrombocytopenia transplanted from an HLA-identical donor probably does not require cyclosporine.

Unfortunately, there is no basis for comparison of the various salvage therapies. Patient populations often differ, with varying proportions of patients with lichenoid and sclerodermatous skin changes and with high-risk features like progressive onset and thrombocytopenia. A practical choice of treatment may be based on the severity of chronic GVHD and the inconvenience and cost of the therapy. For milder disease, the addition of oral drugs like sirolimus, hydroxychloroquine, MMF, clofazimine, and thalidomide is rational. For severe involvement, more expensive and involved therapies like extracorporeal photopheresis, rituximab, pentostatin, and high-dose methylprednisolone pulse therapy may be indicated. The results from one study suggested that the addition of weekly high-dose methylprednisolone to standard therapy was helpful.[64] For isolated lichenoid skin involvement, PUVA may be a good choice. Whenever possible, patients should be treated in clinical trials.

Supportive Care

Local Care

Physical therapy can help to reduce contractures. Deep tissue massage may benefit deep cutaneous sclerosis. Frequent use of preservative-free artificial tears and of preservative-free ointment at night can diminish symptoms and complications of dry eyes. Daily fluoride treatments and effective brushing and flossing can minimize tooth decay resulting from xerostomia (dry mouth).[4]

Infections

Chronic GVHD is associated with decreased splenic function, which may be irreversible. Therefore, patients are at risk for sepsis due to encapsulated bacteria, most seriously pneumococcal sepsis[32]; they should receive prophylaxis for pneumococcal disease, probably for at least 6 months after the end of immunosuppressive therapy, when recurrent chronic GVHD becomes unlikely. Patients with chronic GVHD are also at risk for *Pneumocystis carinii* pneumonia and should receive appropriate prophylaxis for at least the duration of immunosuppressive treatment and probably for at least 6 months more. Chronic GVHD increases the risk of late cytomegalovirus infection and herpes zoster. Patients receiving immunosuppression or with chronic GVHD should not be immunized with live virus vaccines.[9] Recommendations for infection prophylaxis and for immunizations for patients with chronic GVHD can be obtained at the Centers for Disease Control web site: http://www.cdc.gov/mmwr/preview/mmwrhtml/rr4910a1.htm.[2]

Nutrition

Patients with chronic GVHD often experience weight loss as a result of increased metabolic activity and decreased intestinal absorption. Close attention should be paid to nutritional status and protein and carbohydrate supplements provided as needed. Patients may also develop trace element deficiencies due to malabsorption.[2]

Sun Block

Activation of chronic GVHD by sun exposure is well described. Patients should minimize their time in direct sunlight; in the sun, they should apply sun block of at least SPF 30 liberally and often.[4]

Conclusions

Chronic GVHD remains a common complication of allogeneic HSCT. Chronic GVHD correlates with graft-versus-leukemia and a decreased risk of relapse. Unfortunately, GVHD increases transplant-related mortality, mainly as a result of infectious complications, and has a negative impact on quality of life. A challenge for the future will be the discovery of approaches that can target the cause of chronic GVHD rather than inducing global immunosuppression. Reconstitution of normal immunity will be crucial to reducing infectious complications. A better understanding of the pathophysiology of chronic GVHD remains critical to providing more specific therapy and to facilitating immune recovery. Only broad participation in well-conducted, randomized phase III trials will advance our understanding of the biology underlying the benefits and detriments of chronic GVHD, ultimately impacting on post-transplant survival and quality of life.

Acknowledgment

This review is dedicated to the memory of John Skelley, PA-C. He was a superb individual who was very dedicated to the transplant care of children and adults.

References

1. Lee SJ, Vogelsang G, Flowers ME: Chronic graft-versus-host disease. Biol Blood Marrow Transplant 9:215-233, 2003
2. Higman MA, Vogelsang GB: Chronic graft versus host disease. Br J Haematol 125:435-454, 2004
3. Ratanatharathorn V, Ayash L, Lazarus HM, Fu J, Uberti JP: Chronic graft-versus-host disease: clinical manifestation and therapy. Bone Marrow Transplant 28:121-129, 2001
4. Vogelsang GB: How I treat chronic graft-versus-host disease. Blood 97:1196-1201, 2001
5. Stewart BL, Storer B, Storek J, Deeg HJ, Storb R, Hansen JA, et al: Duration of immunosuppressive treatment for chronic graft-versus-host disease. Blood 104:3501-3506, 2004
6. Nghiem P: The "drug vs graft-vs-host disease" conundrum gets tougher, but there is an answer: The challenge to dermatologists. Arch Dermatol 137:75-76, 2001
7. Holler E: Cytokines, viruses, and graft-versus-host disease. Curr Opin Hematol 9:479-484, 2002
8. Jacobsohn DA, Schechter T, Seshadri R, Thormann K, Duerst R, Kletzel M: Eosinophilia correlates with the presence or development of chronic graft-versus-host disease in children. Transplantation 77:1096-1100, 2004
9. Sullivan KM, Mori M, Sanders J, Siadak M, Witherspoon RP, Anasetti C, et al: Late complications of allogeneic and autologous marrow transplantation. Bone Marrow Transplant 10:127-134, 1992 (suppl 1)
10. Lee SJ, Klein JP, Barrett AJ, Ringden O, Antin JH, Cahn JY, et al: Severity of chronic graft-versus-host disease: association with treatment-related mortality and relapse. Blood 100:406-414, 2002
11. Shulman HM, Sale GE, Lerner KG, Barker EA, Weiden PL, Sullivan K, et al: Chronic cutaneous graft-versus-host disease in man. Am J Pathol 91:545-570, 1978
12. Jack MK, Jack GM, Sale GE, Shulman HM, Sullivan KM: Ocular manifestations of graft-v-host disease. Arch Ophthalmol 101:1080-1084, 1983
13. Schubert MM, Sullivan KM, Morton TH, Izutsu KT, Peterson DE, Flournoy N, et al: Oral manifestations of chronic graft-v-host disease. Arch Intern Med 144:1591-1595, 1984
14. Strasser SI, Shulman HM, Flowers ME, Reddy R, Margolis DA, Prumbaum M, et al: Chronic graft-versus-host disease of the liver: Presentation as an acute hepatitis. Hepatology 32:1265-1271, 2000
15. McDonald GB, Sullivan KM, Schuffler MD, Shulman HM, Thomas ED: Esophageal abnormalities in chronic graft-versus-host disease in humans. Gastroenterology 80:914-921, 1981
16. Akpek G, Chinratanalab W, Lee LA, Torbenson M, Hallick JP, Anders V, et al: Gastrointestinal involvement in chronic graft-versus-host disease: A clinicopathologic study. Biol Blood Marrow Transplant 9:46-51, 2003
17. Akpek G, Valladares JL, Lee L, Margolis J, Vogelsang G B: Pancreatic insufficiency in patients with chronic graft-versus-host disease. Bone Marrow Transplant 27:163-166, 2001
18. Schultz KR, Green GJ, Wensley D, Sargent MA, Magee JF, Spinelli JJ, et al: Obstructive lung disease in children after allogeneic bone marrow transplantation. Blood 84:3212-3220, 1994
19. Dudek AZ, Mahaseth H, DeFor TE, Weisdorf DJ: Bronchiolitis obliterans in chronic graft-versus-host disease: Analysis of risk factors and treatment outcomes. Biol Blood Marrow Transplant 9:657-666, 2003
20. Schwarer AP, Hughes JM, Trotman-Dickenson B, Krausz T, Goldman JM: A chronic pulmonary syndrome associated with graft-versus-host disease after allogeneic marrow transplantation. Transplantation 54: 1002-1008, 1992
21. Parker P, Chao NJ, Ben-Ezra J, Slatkin N, Openshaw H, Niland JC, Linker CA, et al: Polymyositis as a manifestation of chronic graft-versus-host disease. Medicine (Baltimore) 75: 279-285, 1996
22. Bolger GB, Sullivan KM, Spence AM, Appelbaum FR, Johnston R, Sanders JE, et al: Myasthenia gravis after allogeneic bone marrow transplantation: Relationship to chronic graft-versus-host disease. Neurology 36:1087-1091, 1986
23. Seber A, Khan SP, Kersey JH: Unexplained effusions: Association with allogeneic bone marrow transplantation and acute or chronic graft-versus-host disease. Bone Marrow Transplant 17:207-211, 1996
24. Spiryda LB, Laufer MR, Soiffer RJ, Antin JA: Graft-versus-host disease of the vulva and/or vagina: Diagnosis and treatment. Biol Blood Marrow Transplant 9:760-765, 2003
25. Rackley C, Schultz KR, Goldman FD, Chan KW, Serrano A, Hulse JE, et al: Cardiac manifestations of graft-versus-host disease. Biol Blood Marrow Transplant 11:773-780, 2005
26. Barbara JA, Thomas AC, Smith PS, Gillis D, Ho JO, Woodroffe AJ: Membranous nephropathy with graft-versus-host disease in a bone marrow transplant recipient. Clin Nephrol 37:115-118, 1992
27. Rouah E, Gruber R, Shearer W, Armstrong D, Hawkins EP: Graft-versus-host disease in the central nervous system. A real entity? Am J Clin Pathol 89:543-546, 1988
28. Greenspan A, Deeg HJ, Cottler-Fox M, Sirdofski M, Spitzer TR, Kattah J: Incapacitating peripheral neuropathy as a manifestation of chronic graft-versus-host disease. Bone Marrow Transplant 5:349-352, 1990
29. O'Brien TA, Eastlund T, Peters C, Neglia JP, Defor T, Ramsay NK, et al: Autoimmune haemolytic anaemia complicating haematopoietic cell transplantation in paediatric patients: High incidence and significant mortality in unrelated donor transplants for non-malignant diseases. Br J Haematol 127:67-75, 2004
30. Atkinson K, Farewell V, Storb R, Tsoi MS, Sullivan KM, Witherspoon RP, et al: Analysis of late infections after human bone marrow transplantation: Role of genotypic nonidentity between marrow donor and recipient and of nonspecific suppressor cells in patients with chronic graft-versus-host disease. Blood 60:714-720, 1982
31. Quaranta S, Shulman H, Ahmed A, Shoenfeld Y, Peter J, McDonald GB, et al: Autoantibodies in human chronic graft-versus-host disease after hematopoietic cell transplantation. Clin Immunol 91:106-116, 1999
32. Kulkarni S, Powles R, Treleaven J, Riley U, Singhal S, Horton C, et al: Chronic graft versus host disease is associated with long-term risk for pneumococcal infections in recipients of bone marrow transplants. Blood 95:3683-3686, 2000
33. Ferrara JL, Deeg HJ: Graft-versus-host disease. N Engl J Med 324:667-674, 1991
34. Romagnani S, Parronchi P, D'Elios MM, Romagnani P, Annunziato F, Piccinni MP, et al: An update on human Th1 and Th2 cells. Int Arch Allergy Immunol 113:153-156, 1997
35. Hess A, Thoburn C, Chen W, Horwitz L: Autoreactive T-cell subsets in acute and chronic syngeneic graft-versus-host disease. Transplant Proc 33:1754-1756, 2001
36. De Wit D, Van Mechelen M, Zanin C, Doutrelepont JM, Velu T, Gerard C, et al: Preferential activation of Th2 cells in chronic graft-versus-host reaction. J Immunol 150:361-366, 1993
37. McCormick LL, Zhang Y, Tootell E, Gilliam AC: Anti-TGF-beta treatment prevents skin and lung fibrosis in murine sclerodermatous graft-versus-host disease: A model for human scleroderma. J Immunol 163: 5693-5699, 1999
38. Anderson BE, McNiff JM, Jain D, Blazar BR, Shlomchik WD, Shlomchik MJ: Distinct roles for donor- and host-derived antigen-presenting cells and costimulatory molecules in murine chronic graft-versus-host disease: Requirements depend on target organ. Blood 105:2227-2234, 2005
39. Canninga-van Dijk MR, van der Straaten HM, Fijnheer R, Sanders CJ, van

den Tweel JG, Verdonck LF: Anti-CD20 monoclonal antibody treatment in 6 patients with therapy-refractory chronic graft-versus-host disease. Blood 104:2603-2606, 2004

40. Tsoi MS, Storb R, Dobbs S, Santos E, Thomas ED: Specific suppressor cells and immune response to host antigens in long-term human allogeneic marrow recipients: Implications for the mechanisms of graft-host tolerance and chronic graft-versus-host disease. Transplant Proc 13:237-240, 1981
41. Clark FJ, Gregg R, Piper K, Dunnion D, Freeman L, Griffiths M, et al: Chronic graft-versus-host disease is associated with increased numbers of peripheral blood $CD4^{+}CD25^{high}$ regulatory T cells. Blood 103: 2410-2416, 2004
42. Sullivan KM, Shulman HM, Storb R, Weiden PL, Witherspoon RP, McDonald GB, et al: Chronic graft-versus-host disease in 52 patients: Adverse natural course and successful treatment with combination immunosuppression. Blood 57:267-276, 1981
43. Shulman HM, Sullivan KM, Weiden PL, McDonald GB, Striker GE, Sale GE, et al: Chronic graft-versus-host syndrome in man. A long-term clinicopathologic study of 20 Seattle patients. Am J Med 69:204-217, 1980
44. Akpek G, Zahurak ML, Piantadosi S, Margolis J, Doherty J, Davidson R,et al: Development of a prognostic model for grading chronic graft-versus-host disease. Blood 97:1219-1226, 2001
45. Akpek G, Lee SJ, Flowers ME, Pavletic SZ, Arora M, Lee S, et al: Performance of a new clinical grading system for chronic graft-versus-host disease: A multicenter study. Blood 102:802-809, 2003
46. Sullivan KM, Witherspoon RP, Storb R, Weiden P, Flournoy N, Dahlberg S, et al: Prednisone and azathioprine compared with prednisone and placebo for treatment of chronic graft-v-host disease: Prognostic influence of prolonged thrombocytopenia after allogeneic marrow transplantation. Blood 72:546-554, 1988
47. Koc S, Leisenring W, Flowers ME, Anasetti C, Deeg HJ, Nash RA, Sanders JE, et al: Therapy for chronic graft-versus-host disease: A randomized trial comparing cyclosporine plus prednisone versus prednisone alone. Blood 100:48-51, 2002
48. Sullivan KM, Witherspoon RP, Storb R, Deeg HJ, Dahlberg S, Sanders JE, et al: Alternating-day cyclosporine and prednisone for treatment of high-risk chronic graft-v-host disease. Blood 72:555-561, 1988
49. Flowers ME, Lee S, Vogelsang G: An update on how to treat chronic GVHD. Blood 102:2312, 2003 (letter)
50. Parker PM, Chao N, Nademanee A, O'Donnell MR, Schmidt GM, Snyder DS, et al: Thalidomide as salvage therapy for chronic graft-versus-host disease. Blood 86:3604-3609, 1995
51. Koc S, Leisenring W, Flowers ME, Anasetti C, Deeg HJ, Nash RA, et al: Thalidomide for treatment of patients with chronic graft-versus-host disease. Blood 96:3995-3996, 2000
52. Busca A, Saroglia EM, Lanino E, Manfredini L, Uderzo C, Nicolini B, et al: Mycophenolate mofetil (MMF) as therapy for refractory chronic GVHD (cGVHD) in children receiving bone marrow transplantation. Bone Marrow Transplant 25:1067-1071, 2000
53. Baudard M, Vincent A, Moreau P, Kergueris MF, Harousseau JL, Milpied N: Mycophenolate mofetil for the treatment of acute and chronic GVHD is effective and well tolerated but induces a high risk of infectious complications: A series of 21 BM or PBSC transplant patients. Bone Marrow Transplant 30:287-295, 2002
54. Gilman AL, Chan KW, Mogul A, Morris C, Goldman FD, Boyer M, et al: Hydroxychloroquine for the treatment of chronic graft-versus-host disease. Biol Blood Marrow Transplant 6:327-334, 2000
55. Johnston LJ, Brown J, Shizuru JA, Stockerl-Goldstein KE, Stuart MJ, Blume KG, et al: Rapamycin (sirolimus) for treatment of chronic graft-versus-host disease. Biol Blood Marrow Transplant 11:47-55, 2005
56. Raj K, Narayanan S, Augustson B, Ho A, Mehta P, Duncan N, et al: Rituximab is effective in the management of refractory autoimmune cytopenias occurring after allogeneic stem cell transplantation. Bone Marrow Transplant 35:299-301, 2005
57. Cutler C, Miklos D, Lee SJ, Woo SBNT, Bienfang D, Klickstein L, et al: Rituximab therapy for steroid-refractory chronic GVHD: Safety and efficacy analysis. Blood 104:619a, 2004
58. Jacobsohn DA, Browning B, Thormann K, Higman M, Phelps ML, Chen AR,et al: Pentostatin: Efficacy in refractory chronic GVHD in children. Blood 104:619a, 2004
59. Akpek G, Lee SM, Anders V, Vogelsang GB: A high-dose pulse steroid regimen for controlling active chronic graft-versus-host disease. Biol Blood Marrow Transplant 7:495-502, 2001
60. Gaziev D, Lucarelli G, Polchi P, Angelucci E, Galimberti M, Giardini C, et al: A three or more drug combination as effective therapy for moderate or severe chronic graft-versus-host disease. Bone Marrow Transplant 27:45-51, 2001
61. Foss FM, Divenuti GM, Chin K, Sprague K, Grodman H, Klein A, et al: Prospective study of extracorporeal photopheresis in steroid-refractory or steroid-resistant extensive chronic graft-versus-host disease: Analysis of response and survival incorporating prognostic factors. Bone Marrow Transplant 35:1187-1193, 2005
62. Seaton ED, Szydlo RM, Kanfer E, Apperley JF, Russell-Jones R: Influence of extracorporeal photopheresis on clinical and laboratory parameters in chronic graft-versus-host disease and analysis of predictors of response. Blood 102:1217-1223, 2003
63. Vogelsang GB, Wolff D, Altomonte V, Farmer E, Morison WL, Corio R, et al: Treatment of chronic graft-versus-host disease with ultraviolet irradiation and psoralen (PUVA). Bone Marrow Transplant 17:1061-1067, 1996
64. Arora M, Wagner JE, Davies SM, Blazar BR, Defor T, Enright H, et al: Randomized clinical trial of thalidomide, cyclosporine, and prednisone versus cyclosporine and prednisone as initial therapy for chronic graft-versus-host disease. Biol Blood Marrow Transplant 7:265-273, 2001
65. Carnevale-Schianca F, Martin P, Sullivan K, Flowers M, Gooley T, Anasetti C, et al: Changing from cyclosporine to tacrolimus as salvage therapy for chronic graft-versus-host disease. Biol Blood Marrow Transplant 6:613-620, 2000
66. Mookerjee B, Altomonte V, Vogelsang G: Salvage therapy for refractory chronic graft-versus-host disease with mycophenolate mofetil and tacrolimus. Bone Marrow Transplant 24:517-520, 1999
67. Vogelsang GB, Farmer ER, Hess AD, Altamonte V, Beschorner WE, Jabs DA, et al: Thalidomide for the treatment of chronic graft-versus-host disease. N Engl J Med 326:1055-1058, 1992
68. Browne PV, Weisdorf DJ, DeFor T, Miller WJ, Davies SM, Filipovich A, et al: Response to thalidomide therapy in refractory chronic graft-versus-host disease. Bone Marrow Transplant 26:865-869, 2000
69. Rovelli A, Arrigo C, Nesi F, Balduzzi A, Nicolini B, Locasciulli A, et al: The role of thalidomide in the treatment of refractory chronic graft-versus-host disease following bone marrow transplantation in children. Bone Marrow Transplant 21:577-581, 1998
70. Lee SJ, Wegner SA, McGarigle CJ, Bierer BE, Antin JH: Treatment of chronic graft-versus-host disease with clofazimine. Blood 89:2298-2302, 1997
71. Chiang KY, Abhyankar S, Bridges K, Godder K, Henslee-Downey JP: Recombinant human tumor necrosis factor receptor fusion protein as complementary treatment for chronic graft-versus-host disease. Transplantation 73:665-667, 2002
72. Apisarnthanarax N, Donato M, Korbling M, Couriel D, Gajewski J, Giralt S, et al: Extracorporeal photopheresis therapy in the management of steroid-refractory or steroid-dependent cutaneous chronic graft-versus-host disease after allogeneic stem cell transplantation: feasibility and results. Bone Marrow Transplant 31:459-465, 2003
73. Salvaneschi L, Perotti C, Zecca M, Bernuzzi S, Viarengo G, Giorgiani G, et al: Extracorporeal photochemotherapy for treatment of acute and chronic GVHD in childhood. Transfusion 41:1299-1305, 2001

Vol 43, No 1, Suppl 1 January 2006

Supplement to

Seminars in HEMATOLOGY

Neal S. Young · Photis Beris
Editors

8th Novo Nordisk Symposium on Haemostasis Management and Novo Nordisk-sponsored symposia at the [illegible] Congress of the International Society on Thrombosis and Haemostasis

Gilbert C. White II
Guest Editor

W.B. Saunders

Seminars in HEMATOLOGY

Neal S. Young · Photis Beris
Editors

Peter A. Miescher, *Founding Editor* Ernst R. Jaffé, *Co-Editor Emeritus*

Editorial correspondence should be addressed to Photis Beris, MD, Division d'Hématologie, Hôpital Cantonal Universitaire, 25 rue Micheli-du-Crest, 1211 Geneve 14, Switzerland, or Neal S. Young, MD, 4400 17th Street, NW, Washington, DC 20011.

Business correspondence (subscriptions, change of address) should be addressed to the Publisher, Elsevier, 6277 Sea Harbor Dr, Orlando, FL 32887-4800; Email elspcs@elsevier.com.

Change of address notices, including both the old and new addresses of the subscriber, should be sent at least one month in advance.

Customer Service: 1-800-654-2452; outside the United States and Canada, (407) 345-4000.

Yearly subscription rates: United States and possessions: individual, $169.00; institution, $267.00; single issues, $81.00. All other countries: individual, $239.00; institution, $339.00; single issues, $81.00. Student and resident: United States and possessions, and Canada: $85.00; all other countries: $122.00. To receive student/resident rate, orders must be accompanied by name of affiliated institution, date of term, and the *signature* of program/residency coordinator on institution letterhead. Orders will be billed at individual rate until proof of status is received. Current prices are in effect for back volumes and back issues. Single issues, both current and back, exist in limited quantities and are offered for sale subject to availability. Back issues sold in conjunction with a subscription are on a prorated basis. Prices are subject to change without notice. *Checks* should be made payable to Elsevier and sent to *Seminars in Hematology*, Elsevier, Periodicals Department, PO Box 628239, Orlando, FL 32862-8239.

The contents of *Seminars in Hematology* are indexed in *Index Medicus* and *MEDLINE, Current Contents/Clinical Medicine, Current Contents/Life Sciences,* Science Citation Index, and *EMBASE/* Excerpta Medica.

The *Seminars in Hematology* home page is located at *www.seminhematol.org.*

W.B. Saunders **Philadelphia, PA**

Seminars in HEMATOLOGY

Vol 43, No 1, Supplement 1, January 2006

8th Novo Nordisk Symposium on Haemostasis Management and Novo Nordisk-sponsored symposia at the XXth Congress of the International Society on Thrombosis and Haemostasis

Gilbert C. White II
Guest Editor

Introduction S1
Gilbert C. White II

8th Novo Nordisk Symposium on Haemostasis Management
Papers

Impact of Choice of Treatment for Bleeding Episodes on Inhibitor Outcome in Patients With Mild/Moderate Hemophilia A and Inhibitors S3
Roseline d'Oiron, F. Volot, J. Reynaud, K. Peerlinck, J. Goudemand, C. Guérois, C. Rothschild, H. Chambost, A. Borel-Derlon, V. Roussel-Robert, A. Marquès-Verdier, A. Lienhart, A.M. Berthier, P. Moreau, and T. Lambert, for the MHAI Study Group

Inhibitors to Factor XI in Patients With Severe Factor XI Deficiency S10
Ophira Salomon, Ariella Zivelin, Tami Livnat, and Uri Seligsohn

Update on Liver Disease in Hemophilia Patients S13
Craig M. Kessler

Pathogenesis of Hemophilic Arthropathy S18
W. Keith Hoots

Surgery in Hemophilia. The General View: Patient Selection, Timing, and Preoperative Assessment S23
Jørgen Ingerslev and Ivan Hvid

Functional Assessment of Arthropathy—An International Perspective S27
Pradeep M. Poonnoose and Alok Srivastava

Glanzmann's Thrombasthenia Treatment: A Prospective Observational Registry on the Use of Recombinant Human Activated Factor VII and Other Hemostatic Agents S33
Man-Chiu Poon, Rainer Zotz, Giovanni Di Minno, Zvika S. Abrams, Jens B. Knudsen, and Yves Laurian

Congenital and Acquired Platelet Disorders: Current Dilemmas and Treatment Strategies S37
Gilbert C. White II

Steps Towards an Effective Treatment Strategy in Congenital Factor VII Deficiency S42
Guglielmo Mariani, Mario Lapecorella, and Alberto Dolce

Acquired von Willebrand Syndrome: An Underdiagnosed and Misdiagnosed Bleeding Complication in Patients With Lymphoproliferative and Myeloproliferative Disorders S48
Augusto B. Federici

Massive Transfusion Coagulopathy S59
Jerrold H. Levy

Assessing Efficacy and Therapeutic Claims in Emerging Indications for Recombinant Factor VIIa: Regulatory Perspectives S64
Albert Farrugia

Ultra-early Hemostatic Therapy for Acute Intracerebral Hemorrhage S70
Stephan A. Mayer and Fred Rincon

New Anti-thrombotic Agents: Emphasis on Hemorrhagic Complications and Their Management S77
Heng Joo Ng and Mark A. Crowther

Milestones in Hemophilia and Concepts in Future Clinical Trial Design S84
Jeanne M. Lusher

Abstracts

The Incidence of Factor VII and Factor IX Inhibitors in the Hemophilia Population of the UK and Their Effect on Subsequent Mortality, 1977–99 S88
Sarah C. Darby, David M. Keeling, Rosemary J.D. Spooner, Sau Wan Kan, Paul L.F. Giangrande, Peter W. Collins, Frank G.H. Hill, and Charles R.M. Hay

Intensive Exposure to FVII May Be a Risk Factor for Inhibitor Development in Mild Hemophilia A S89
Manuel D. Carcao

Acquired Hemophilia S90
Peter Collins

Recombinant Activated Factor VII in Severe Trauma S91
Bruno Riou

Excluded Abstracts S93

XXth Congress of the International Society on Thrombosis and Haemostasis

Papers

The Platelet: Form and Function — S94
John H. Hartwig

Advances in Gene Therapy Using Factor VIIa in Hemophilia — S101
Paris Margaritis and Katherine A. High

Mechanism of Action of Recombinant Activated Factor VII: An Update — S105
Ulla Hedner

High-Dose Recombinant Factor VIIa Therapy in Hemophilia Patients With Inhibitors — S108
Gili Kenet

Haemostasis Award Winner

Protein S Multimers Are Generated In Vitro and Affect Protein S Structure-Function Analyses — S111
Kristin M. Seré, George M. Willems, Jan Rosing, and Tilman M. Hackeng

Abstracts

Dynamics of Thrombus Formation — S121
Bruce Furie

Recombinant Factor VIIa and COAT Platelets — S122
Marianne Kjalke and Rasmus Rojkjaer

Excluded Abstracts — S123

Seminars in HEMATOLOGY

8th Novo Nordisk Symposium on Haemostasis Management
Copenhagen, Denmark
May 11-13, 2005
and
Novo Nordisk-sponsored symposia at the XXth Congress of the International Society on Thrombosis and Haemostasis
Sydney, Australia
August 7 and August 10, 2005

Gilbert C. White II

Guest Editor

This supplement was made possible by an unrestricted educational grant from Novo Nordisk A/S, Bagsvaerd, Denmark.

The opinions or views expressed in this professional education supplement are those of the authors and do not necessarily reflect the opinions or recommendations of Novo Nordisk.

The guest editors, authors, and publisher have tried to ensure that recommended measures and drug dosages discussed in this supplement are accurate and conform to the standards that prevailed at the time of publication. The reader is advised, however, to check the product information available for any product discussed in this supplement to be familiar with any changes in the dosage schedule, techniques of use, or contraindications. Because of the uniqueness of each patient, physicians should use this information only as a general guide in determining the best treatment for each patient. For approved product information, consult the manufacturer's prescribing information.

This supplement has been developed in collaboration with Jens Bjerre Knudsen of Novo Nordisk A/S.

ELSEVIER

Seminars in
HEMATOLOGY

Volume 43, Number 1, Supplement 1 **January 2006**

Introduction

This supplement brings together the proceedings from three Novo Nordisk-sponsored symposia held during 2005, and reflects the varied and stimulating array of topics discussed by the world's leading scientists and clinicians at these internationally renowned meetings.

The 8th Novo Nordisk Symposium on Haemostasis Management was held in Copenhagen, Denmark, on May 11–13, 2005. This biennial symposium has long been a platform for the sharing and exchange of knowledge in the field of hemostasis research, combining new scientific discoveries with the latest clinical experience. This year's program was no exception, focusing on four key areas in the management of hemostasis: the biology of inhibitor development, the hemophilic joint, the management of rare bleeding disorders, and the treatment of patients with critical bleeding.

Despite advances in our understanding of factor VIII and factor IX inhibitor development in hemophilia patients, it remains one of the most serious complications of treatment. David Keeling, Manuel Carcao, and Roseline d'Oiron provided timely updates of recent studies and data collection surveys conducted to increase our understanding of inhibitors in hemophilia, while Ophira Salomon and Peter Collins explored inhibitor development in severe factor XI deficiency and acquired hemophilia, respectively. The session then moved away from inhibitors, with a presentation from Craig Kessler focusing on the management of those hemophilia patients who have also become infected with the hepatitis C virus through the use of contaminated blood products.

The second session discussed new and important insights into the pathogenesis of hemophilic arthropathy. Keith Hoots highlighted the role of iron as a critical player in the development of hemophilic arthropathy, and described how similarities between this condition and rheumatoid arthritis have opened new avenues of investigation into the pathogenesis of the hemophilic joint. Human parvovirus B19 has also been implicated in the development of acute arthritis in hemophilia patients, as discussed by Michael Soucie. Orthopedic surgery to correct chronic hemophilic arthropathy was the subject of a presentation from Jørgen Ingerslev, and the session concluded with Alok Srivastava's review of the scoring systems currently available for the assessment of musculoskeletal function in hemophilia patients.

Session 3 turned the spotlight on rare bleeding disorders. In 2004, recombinant activated factor VII (rFVIIa; NovoSeven®, Novo Nordisk, Bagsvaerd, Denmark) received European approval for use in patients with FVII deficiency and Glanzmann's thrombasthenia (GT) refractory to platelet transfusion. Man-Chiu Poon presented an update on a postmarketing registry for the collection of data on rFVIIa use in GT, and Guglielmo Mariani described an online registry for the assessment of various treatment options—including rFVIIa—in FVII deficiency. Gilbert White discussed current dilemmas and treatment strategies in congenital and acquired platelet disorders, and Augusto Federici looked at the clinical impact and management of acquired von Willebrand syndrome.

Recent years have witnessed increased exploration of rFVIIa use in nonhemophilic patients with critical bleeding, and the final session of the meeting examined some of these emerging indications. Jerrold Levy reviewed the pathogenesis of massive transfusion coagulopathy in trauma victims, and Bruno Riou described how the benefits of rFVIIa therapy in such patients may include not only control of hemorrhage, but also reduced transfusion requirements and a subsequent decrease in transfusion-related morbidity and mortality. Stephan Mayer provided an overview of a recent clinical trial in which this agent was found to be of significant benefit in preventing early hematoma growth in patients with intracerebral hemorrhage, and Mark Crowther examined the efficacy of rFVIIa in reversing the effects of novel anticoagulants such as rNAPc2, fondaparinux, idraparinux, and argatroban. Regulatory issues surrounding the use and approval of rFVIIa in new and emerging indications were discussed by Albert Farrugia, and an update on the safety profile of rFVIIa was presented by Stephanie Seremetis. The final presentation of the meeting was given by Jeanne Lusher, whose informative and timely review of the history of medical care in patients with bleeding disorders highlighted just how far clinical and scientific research has evolved over recent decades.

The first of two Novo Nordisk-sponsored symposia at the XXth Congress of the International Society on Thrombosis and Haemostasis (ISTH), entitled *New Insights into the Biology*

Address correspondence to Dr G.C. White, Blood Research Institute, 8727 Watertown Plank Rd, Milwaukee, WI 53226. E-mail: gcwhite@bcsew.edu

doi:10.1053/j.seminhematol.2005.11.005

of Thrombus Formation, took place in Sydney, Australia, on August 7, 2005. This symposium moved away from the clinical arena to discuss recent scientific advances in our understanding of hemostatic and thrombotic disorders. Over the last few years, the previously simplistic view of thrombus formation has evolved into a greater understanding of the highly complex interactions involved. This meeting reviewed the scientific advances that have re-shaped our knowledge of these processes, and examined some of the techniques and modeling systems used to explore the various aspects of coagulation and related physiological systems.

Bruce Furie opened the meeting with a review of studies utilizing intravital, confocal, widefield microscopy imaging systems to visualize real-time thrombus formation following vessel wall injury in mouse models. John Hartwig explored new insights into the form and function of the platelet, while Marianne Kjalke discussed a single subpopulation of highly procoagulant COAT (collagen- and thrombin-activated) platelets, which preferentially retain rFVIIa on their surfaces thus ensuring that enhanced thrombin generation is localized to the site of vessel damage. Finally, Emrys Kirkman presented data from recent studies that demonstrate a beneficial effect of rFVIIa on blood loss and survival in a porcine model of severe uncontrolled bleeding from a major artery.

The second Novo Nordisk-sponsored symposium at the XXth Congress of the ISTH, *Advances in the Therapy of Haemophilia*, was held on August 10, 2005 and focused on current and future treatment options for hemophilia patients. Tremendous advances in the management of bleeds in inhibitor patients have contributed to a greatly improved quality of life for these individuals, and parallel research into gene therapy offers hope for future treatments and even a permanent cure.

Katherine High provided a fascinating overview of the current status of gene therapy research in animal models, and discussed preliminary data assessing the feasibility of FVIIa gene transfer as a possible treatment for hemophilia. Following Ulla Hedner's update on the mechanism of action of rFVIIa in clot formation, Gili Kenet presented a comparison of standard vs higher bolus dosing of rFVIIa in inhibitor patients. The last presentation of the day was given by Kristin Seré, winner of the 2005 Novo Nordisk Haemostasis Award. This annual grant is presented to a young investigator in recognition of their original contribution to research leading to an improved understanding of the mode of action or therapeutic potential of rFVIIa. Dr Seré described a previously unrecognized mechanism in which protein S enhances the inhibition of tissue factor (TF)/FVIIa-catalyzed FX activation by tissue factor pathway inhibitor (TFPI). This observation changes previous concepts of TF activity, and demonstrates that protein S and TFPI act in concert to inhibit TF/FVIIa-mediated coagulation.

The data presented at all three symposia reflect the dynamic nature of hemostasis research, and demonstrate how new scientific developments lead to constantly evolving clinical breakthroughs in the care and management of patients with bleeding disorders. In particular, the exploration of new therapeutic indications for rFVIIa continues to provide exciting and important discoveries, and has helped to save the lives of many patients with severe bleeding and otherwise limited treatment options. The success of rFVIIa to date, and its ever-increasing promise as a highly effective hemostatic agent, could not have been achieved without the hard work and dedication of many people within both Novo Nordisk and the international medical community: the clinicians, scientists, patients, and numerous others who have all contributed to recent developments and ongoing research.

Gilbert C. White II
Blood Research Institute, Milwaukee, WI

ELSEVIER

Seminars in
HEMATOLOGY

8th Novo Nordisk Symposium on Haemostasis Management Papers

Impact of Choice of Treatment for Bleeding Episodes on Inhibitor Outcome in Patients With Mild/Moderate Hemophilia A and Inhibitors

Roseline d'Oiron[a,d], F. Volot[b], J. Reynaud[c], K. Peerlinck[d], J. Goudemand[e], C. Guérois[f], C. Rothschild[g], H. Chambost[h], A. Borel-Derlon[i], V. Roussel-Robert[j], A. Marquès-Verdier[k], A. Lienhart[l], A.M. Berthier[m], P. Moreau[n], and T. Lambert[a], for the MHAI Study Group

Patients with mild/moderate hemophilia A (MHA) may develop inhibitors to factor VIII (FVIII). In this condition, FVIII clotting activity (FVIII:C) baseline levels may remain stable for some patients, but may be reduced to less than 0.01 U/mL for others. Several risk factors for the development of inhibitors in MHA have been proposed. Genetic factors, such as mutations in the FVIII gene, may play a central role; however, other influences, such as intensive treatment with FVIII products, may also be important. Optimal treatment regimens have yet to be determined, not only for the eradication of inhibitors, but also for the management or surgical prophylaxis of hemorrhages associated with this condition. Several treatment options for the control of bleeding in patients with MHA and inhibitors (MHAI) are currently available, and the choice of therapeutic strategy should be given careful consideration; some treatments may produce an anamnestic response, thus delaying the return to FVIII:C baseline levels and adversely affecting the duration of the severe bleeding phenotype. To increase our knowledge of MHAI, a retrospective collection of data is currently being performed among hemophilia centers in France and Belgium. Based on five examples of patients with MHAI collated from preliminary study data, we illustrate the impact on inhibitor outcome of the therapeutic choices used to treat bleeding episodes in these patients.
Semin Hematol 43(suppl 1):S3-S9

Patients with mild/moderate hemophilia A (MHA) can develop antibodies (inhibitors) to factor VIII (FVIII), which may lead to an increased frequency or severity of bleeding episodes. The first observation of MHA with inhibitors (MHAI) was described by Beck et al in 1969.[1] The presence of inhibitors in patients with MHA has subsequently been considered as uncommon, and only one large cohort of such patients (N = 26)[2] has been reported to date. The incidence of inhibitors in patients with MHA, as described in small surveys, has been found to be highly variable (0% to 29%).[3,4] However, more consistent results (2.7% to 13%) have been obtained in studies including larger numbers of patients.[5–7] In the cohort of 26 patients with MHAI described by Hay et al,[2] an annual incidence of 0.84 per 1000 patients per year for MHA was reported, compared with 3.5 per year for patients with severe hemophilia A. However, the reported incidence may increase if measured only among those patients who are exposed to FVIII, rather than among all patients with MHA.[8] Increases in the number of anecdotal cases of MHAI report-

[a]Hemophilia Center, APHP Bicêtre University Hospital, Le Kremlin-Bicêtre, France. Hemophilia Centers—University Hospitals of
[b]Dijon (France),
[c]St-Etienne (France),
[d]Center for Molecular and Vascular Biology, University of Leuven, Leuven, Belgium,
[e]Lille (France),
[f]Tours (France),
[g]Paris Necker (France),
[h]Marseille (France),
[i]Caen (France),
[j]Paris Cochin (France),
[k]Clermont-Ferrand (France),
[l]Lyon (France),
[m]Rennes (France),
[n]Le Mans (France).
See Appendix for list of MHAI Study Group investigators.
Address correspondence to Roseline d'Oiron, MD, Hemophilia Center, Hôpital Bicêtre, 78 avenue du Général Leclerc, 94275 Le Kremlin-Bicêtre Cedex, France. E-mail: roseline.doiron@bct.ap-hop-paris.fr

0037-1963/06/$-see front matter
doi:10.1053/j.seminhematol.2005.11.002

ed[3,8–28] raise the possibility of an association with current methods of treatment, including increased use of FVIII products. Alternatively, as the development of inhibitors has become an increasingly recognized concern,[29] the apparent increase in the number of cases may be a consequence of such an awareness coupled with improved follow-up of patients with MHA.

In patients with MHAI, the severity of the bleeding phenotype is related to the FVIII epitopes that are recognized by the inhibitors during the anti-FVIII response. In this article, the term "endogenous FVIII" will be used to define the mutated (variant, self, autologous) FVIII of the patient with MHA, and the term "exogenous FVIII" will be dedicated to the nonmutated (wild-type, non-self, allogeneic) FVIII, either plasma-derived or recombinant, that is administered as treatment. Antibodies that inhibit exogenous FVIII, but which exert minimal or no inhibition of endogenous FVIII, have been described.[21,30] In such cases, endogenous FVIII may still be detectable and effective in preventing spontaneous bleeds, as in patients who have MHA without inhibitors. However, treatment with exogenous FVIII may be ineffective and may induce an anamnestic response.[30] Alternatively, other patients with MHAI exhibit a more generalized response in which both exogenous and endogenous FVIII are inhibited, which may result in baseline FVIII clotting activity (FVIII:C) levels of less than 0.01 IU/mL.[27] Such patients generally present with unusual and spontaneous bleeds, as seen in patients with severe hemophilia A. A bleeding pattern reminiscent of acquired hemophilia is often observed, and the inhibitors frequently exhibit a type 2 kinetic profile.

Not only may inhibitors have different epitope specificity, but different outcomes in relation to these can also be apparent. Patients with MHAI may have low (defined as ≤5 Bethesda Units [BU]) or high (>5 BU) inhibitor titers when tested in vitro against exogenous FVIII.[31] Inhibitors may disappear spontaneously, or they may be lost after immune tolerance induction (ITI) or treatment with immunomodulatory drugs. Some low inhibitors, known as transient inhibitors, disappear within 12 months of their initial detection despite repeated FVIII use.[32] In other patients, inhibitors may persist at low or high titers. Indeed, in the cohort of patients with MHAI described by Hay et al,[2] 38% of patients demonstrated persistent inhibitors over a median period of 99 months' follow-up. Further challenge with FVIII or an activated prothrombin complex concentrate (aPCC) may induce inhibitor recurrence at low or high titers.

As with the development of inhibitors in severe hemophilia A, several risk factors for the development of inhibitors in MHA have been proposed; genetic factors may play a central role, although environmental influences can also be involved.[33] Data from the internet-based Hemophilia A Mutation, Search, Test and Resource (HAMSTeRS) database[34] demonstrate that missense mutations are the most frequent type of mutation found in patients with MHA. The incidence of inhibitors related to missense mutations is comparable between MHA and severe hemophilia A (4.3%); however, missense mutations in the C1 and C2 domains of the FVIII protein are associated with a fourfold increase in the risk of inhibitor formation.[6] Moreover, specific mutations appear to confer an increased risk of inhibitor development. A missense mutation in the C1 domain of the FVIII light chain (Arg[2150] to His) in patients with mild hemophilia A and antibodies to FVIII has been described.[18,21,25] This mutation results in reduced FVIII binding to von Willebrand factor and alters a B-cell epitope in the FVIII C1 domain.[35,36] In the HAMSTeRS database,[34] updated in August 2005, this mutation has been found to be associated with an 18.8% (10/53 patients) incidence of inhibitor development. The Trp[2229] to Cys mutation in the FVIII C2 domain may also be associated with an increased risk of inhibitor formation, as incidences of 39% (7/18) and 42% (8/19) have been reported by Hay et al[2] and in the HAMSTeRS database,[34] respectively. An Arg[593] to Cys missense mutation in the FVIII A2 domain[15,27,30,37] has also been found to be related to inhibitor formation. In a group of patients with mild hemophilia A caused by this mutation, the cumulative inhibitor incidence was 14% over 22 years.[38] In the HAMSTeRS database,[34] this mutation is associated with an incidence of inhibitor development of 16.2% (6/37 patients). Knobe et al[15] have reported that the Arg[593] amino acid residue in the FVIII protein is part of a strictly conserved sequence from man, pig, and mouse, suggesting a structural role for this region. Arg[593] is solvent-exposed and involved in electrostatic molecular interactions. Mutation of this residue may therefore induce a conformational change in the FVIII protein, and may have a potential role in altering FVIII immunogenicity. Other mutations in the FVIII gene have also been described in patients with MHAI. However, the role of each FVIII mutation in inhibitor formation is still difficult to assess, as very few centers undertake the genotyping of MHA patients on a systematic basis. The role of human leukocyte antigen (HLA) with regard to inhibitor formation in patients with severe hemophilia is described as a weak determinant, or not conclusive.[39,40] This role is poorly documented for patients with MHA. Bril et al[38] have suggested that, in patients with mild hemophilia A and the Arg[593] to Cys mutation, inhibitor development is not linked to the HLA class II profile. Further studies in large cohorts of MHA patients are warranted to provide more information about the role of HLA in inhibitor development.

Patients with MHA may have a familial predisposition to develop inhibitors. In the cohort of patients with MHAI described by Hay et al,[2] 41% of treated family members had a history of FVIII inhibitors. Data from the Malmö International Brother Study (MIBS), which recruited siblings with hemophilia, have provided further evidence that familial history appears to be a high risk factor for inhibitor development.[41] However, most of the hemophilia A brother pairs included in this study were severely affected patients. Again, further data are required before the role of familial factors in inhibitor formation can be fully assessed in MHA patients.

Despite the strong genetic predisposition for the development of inhibitors, MIBS data have recorded monozygotic twins with discordant inhibitor status.[41] This demonstrates that other factors also play a role in inhibitor development. Treatment with FVIII replacement therapy may be influential in such circumstances. Increases in the dose or duration of

FVIII treatment, and administration of the agent by continuous infusion (often in the context of surgery) may all affect the risk of inhibitor development in patients with MHA.[8,29] The type of FVIII concentrate with which patients are treated may also play a role.[24]

Other influential factors may include concomitant vaccinations and clinical factors such as the occurrence of intracranial bleeds, subcutaneous diffusion of infused FVIII, inflammatory diseases, and infections. However, such associations are difficult to confirm without performing appropriate case-control studies.

A range of therapeutic options that may help to eradicate inhibitors is currently available, although these options are not well defined for patients with MHAI. ITI has been implemented in some instances[2,8,27,42]; however, ITI seems less successful in patients with MHA than in those with severe hemophilia A. Other options include the administration of immunomodulatory drugs, such as corticosteroids and/or cyclophosphamide.[23] Recently, use of the anti-CD20 monoclonal antibody, rituximab, has also been described.[43] The decision not to administer any specific treatment is also a viable option.[2]

A variety of treatments can also be used to treat the bleeding episodes associated with MHAI, including desmopressin (DDAVP), FVIII concentrates, FEIBA (Baxter Corp, Deerfield, IL),[23] and recombinant activated factor VII (rFVIIa; NovoSeven®, Novo Nordisk, Bagsvaerd, Denmark).[16,23,30]

Optimum treatment regimens for the eradication of inhibitors and for the management of bleeding episodes during and after the inhibitor phase have yet to be determined. In order to increase knowledge and improve understanding of MHAI, a retrospective collection of data is currently being performed in France and Belgium. The methodology of this study is presented briefly below. Based on examples of five typical patients with MHAI collated from preliminary study data, we discuss the impact of the therapeutic choices used to treat bleeding episodes on inhibitor outcome. Of course, specific treatment for the eradication of inhibitors may also influence inhibitor outcome, but this will not be discussed here.

Methods

To facilitate the collection of data for this study, forms were sent to investigators practising in hemophilia centers. If an investigator could identify at least one patient with MHAI, it was requested that the forms were completed. The following data were recorded for each patient: family history of MHA and/or MHAI; basal FVIII:C level; age at diagnosis of MHA, first FVIII treatment, and inhibitor diagnosis; response to DDAVP (if assessed); and FVIII genotype (if available).

A range of data pertaining to therapy prior to inhibitor diagnosis was also collected. This included the following details: the type of FVIII concentrates (plasma-derived or recombinant) with which a patient had previously been treated; whether this therapy had been administered as bolus doses or by continuous infusion; the number of cumulative exposure days (CED) to FVIII therapy; and whether or not a patient had a history of intensive use of FVIII therapy (defined as use of the treatment for more than 4 consecutive days, or prophylaxis every other day for 10 days or more) for bleeds or surgical prophylaxis. The clinical circumstances affecting the patient prior to the inhibitor diagnosis (ie, an intracranial bleed, subcutaneous diffusion, inflammation or infection, surgery, vaccination, associated autoimmune disease) were also recorded, as was the manner in which the inhibitor had been discovered (ie, as a consequence of the inefficacy of FVIII therapy, after a specific inhibitor test following FVIII treatment, or following an unusual bleed).

After inhibitors had been diagnosed in a patient, the inhibitor titer at diagnosis was recorded, together with the maximum historical titer and the corresponding baseline FVIII:C levels. Any specific treatment for inhibitor eradication was noted, as was the nature of therapy used for the treatment of bleeds. Outcomes in relation to inhibitor titers and baseline FVIII:C levels were recorded, particularly when patients were rechallenged with FVIII-containing products (FVIII concentrates or aPCC) or DDAVP.

Patients

Patient 1

The first patient was 10 years old when he was diagnosed with moderate hemophilia A and received his first infusion of plasma-derived FVIII concentrate. His baseline FVIII:C level was 0.03 to 0.07 IU/mL. The patient had type II diabetes mellitus and hepatitis C virus (HCV)-related cirrhosis. His human immunodeficiency virus (HIV) status was negative. Desmopressin testing was contraindicated for cardiovascular reasons.

Before inhibitor discovery, the patient had received a total of 101 CED to FVIII therapy, including 61 with plasma-derived products, mostly for recurrent left knee hemarthroses. Recombinant FVIII had first been used 6 years before the appearance of inhibitors and he had received intensive treatment with this over a 7-day period to treat a gastrointestinal bleed. Anti-FVIII inhibitors were not discovered until 17 months after this treatment, as a consequence of a dental extraction during which FVIII therapy failed to prevent bleeding and a low recovery of infused FVIII was apparent. Increased doses of FVIII enabled the bleed to be arrested.

Retrospective analysis of frozen plasma samples collected 1 month after the gastrointestinal bleed and just prior to the dental procedure revealed inhibitor titers of 159 and 2.3 BU, respectively. No change in the FVIII:C baseline level was observed in either of these samples.

Two months after the inhibitor diagnosis, a peak of 28 BU was reached; there was no modification of the baseline endogenous FVIII:C. After a rapid decrease of the inhibitor during the following year, the inhibitor titer remained stable and persistent (between 2 and 4 BU) over the next 2 years. No specific treatment for inhibitor eradication was given. Three episodes were successfully treated using rFVIIa during this period—two minor bleeds and one total knee replacement. Despite the patient's endogenous FVIII:C baseline level increasing to 0.20 IU/mL during the inflammatory state in the postoperative period for the total knee replacement, no thrombotic events occurred either during or after the rFVIIa treatment.

Patient 2

In patient 2, diagnosis of moderate hemophilia A, first introduction of FVIII, and inhibitor detection occurred at the ages of 51, 52, and 57 years, respectively. The FVIII:C baseline level was 0.03 to 0.04 IU/mL and DDAVP testing showed no response. The patient was seronegative for HIV and HCV. Before the inhibitor diagnosis, he received a total of 7 CED with plasma-derived FVIII. An inhibitor titer of 18 BU and undetectable FVIII:C were discovered when an unusual spontaneous bleed occurred 3 months after the patient had received 2 days of FVIII treatment for a dental procedure. After a decrease of the inhibitor titer from 18 to 5 BU within 6 weeks, a tongue hematoma was treated using FEIBA for 1 day. The treatment was effective, but anamnesis subsequently occurred, with the inhibitor titer increasing to 20 BU during the following month. ITI was attempted 2 weeks later, while the inhibitor was spontaneously declining, but was prematurely interrupted after 6 weeks. The reintroduction of FVIII for the ITI produced further anamnesis, with a peak inhibitor titer of 35 BU after 2 months. Rechallenge with FVIII therapy was not attempted again after the ITI interruption. The patient was treated with corticosteroids and cyclophosphamide for 3 months, while receiving concomitant immune tolerance therapy. However, this treatment combination did not prevent further recurrence of inhibitor from 4 BU to 8 BU after the patient received 5 days of FEIBA therapy for a dental extraction 8 months after the end of ITI. The inhibitor finally disappeared spontaneously within 29 months, at which time the endogenous FVIII:C level became detectable at 0.01 IU/mL. Return to the FVIII:C baseline level of 0.03 IU/mL occurred gradually over the next 30 months.

Patient 3

Patient 3 was diagnosed with moderate hemophilia A aged 1 year. He first received FVIII at the age of 10 years, and was 53 years old when inhibitor development was reported. His FVIII:C baseline level was 0.02 IU/mL. He was seronegative for HIV and HCV. Before inhibitor discovery, he received a total of 37 CED to FVIII therapy: 12 with plasma-derived FVIII, and 25 with intense recombinant FVIII treatment for a surgical procedure. The presence of inhibitor was suspected, as very high doses of FVIII were required to achieve adequate postoperative FVIII:C levels over the subsequent 39 days. Endogenous FVIII was still detectable after interruption of treatment with exogenous FVIII. The maximum recorded inhibitor titer was 0.6 BU, and the inhibitor disappeared without specific treatment within 3 months. A muscle bleed occurred 1 month after disappearance of the inhibitor, and the patient received further treatment with FVIII. This led to the recurrence of a low-titer inhibitor and an endogenous FVIII:C value of less than 0.01 IU/mL. Immune tolerance induction was initiated, and continued for a 7-month period. Several spontaneous bleeds were subsequently treated successfully using rFVIIa during the ITI. The inhibitor disappeared and endogenous FVIII:C became detectable within 7 and 9 months after the start of ITI, respectively.

Patient 4

Patient 4[20] was diagnosed with MHA aged 5 years, and a FVIII:C baseline value of 0.09 IU/mL was apparent at this time. The patient had a FVIII genotype exhibiting an Arg^{2150} to His mutation. He was seronegative for HIV but seropositive for HCV. Age at first treatment was unknown, and he had received a very low number of FVIII treatments prior to being given 10 days of intensive therapy with plasma-derived FVIII to cover surgery for a total hip replacement when he was 39 years old. The subsequent development of a high-titer inhibitor led to the manifestation of a severe bleeding phenotype, with a FVIII:C of less than 0.01 IU/mL. No replacement therapy was given during this time. Nineteen years later, FVIII therapy was used to treat an intracranial hemorrhage. A high-titer inhibitor recurred, peaking at 350 BU. The inhibitor was directed only against exogenous FVIII, as the patient's endogenous FVIII:C levels remained stable. No specific treatment for inhibitor eradication was given. As one dose of FVIII failed to increase FVIII:C activity, DDAVP was given prior to surgical removal of an infected hip prosthesis. The patient's response to DDAVP was excellent, with FVIII:C reaching 0.40 to 0.97 IU/mL; however, the half-life of the FVIII released after DDAVP treatment was very short (2.5 hours). The postoperative period was successfully covered by rFVIIa. Thirty-three months after the FVIII treatment, the inhibitor had decreased slowly to 14 BU, and FVIII:C values of 0.08 to 0.28 IU/mL were apparent. During this period, five bleeding episodes were successfully treated with DDAVP. No subsequent retreatment with FVIII was attempted.

Patient 5

This patient was 18 months old when he was diagnosed with MHA and received FVIII for the first time. Inhibitor development was recorded when the patient was 10 years old. FVIII:C baseline values of between 0.10 and 0.15 IU/mL were recorded. The patient's response to DDAVP showed a sixfold increase of FVIII:C values, but a short half-life (3 hours). The patient's FVIII genotype showed an Arg^{2159} to Cys mutation, and he was seronegative for HIV and HCV. Before the appearance of inhibitor, the patient had received a total of 22 CED of plasma-derived FVIII and 7 CED of recombinant FVIII. Recombinant FVIII had first been used 7 months prior to inhibitor development. The FVIII treatment had been given sporadically and no history of intense exposure to FVIII had been recorded. The presence of an inhibitor was suspected when the patient exhibited a poor response to FVIII administered to arrest a joint bleed, 6 weeks after the last infusion of FVIII. Additional doses of FVIII were successful in stopping the bleed. A low-titer (1.4 BU) inhibitor was subsequently found, but there was no decrease in the level of endogenous FVIII:C. Despite frequent on-demand use of FVIII concentrates during 93 months of follow-up after the inhibitor diagnosis, the inhibitor disappeared 1 month after its appearance, without specific treatment being given, and it did not recur. During the follow-up period, 10 other mild bleeding episodes were successfully treated with DDAVP.

Discussion

The results from the patients described in this study illustrate several important points with regard to the treatment of patients with MHAI.

Need for Specific Inhibitor Assays and Regular Follow-up

Inhibitor assays may help to avoid the consequences that may otherwise arise as a result of failing to detect the presence of inhibitors in patients with MHA. Regular specific inhibitor assays, particularly after intensive exposure to FVIII, are therefore needed. Indeed, in recent years, improvements in the follow-up of MHA patients may have contributed to the increased incidence of MHAI that is now being reported. Baseline measurements of FVIII:C alone are not sufficient to evaluate potential tolerance to treatment with exogenous FVIII. This point is emphasized by the case of patient 1, who had detectable endogenous FVIII when inhibitor occurrence was suspected; specific testing was therefore required to detect the inhibitor. In this patient, adequate testing prior to the dental procedure would have permitted therapy with FVIII to be avoided in favor of a more effective method of treatment. This could have prevented both the postoperative bleeding and the anamnestic response. Fortunately, the postoperative bleeding was not life-threatening and the anamnestic response was not directed against self FVIII, and so it did not lead to a dramatic change in the bleeding phenotype.

Risk of Anamnesis and Changes in Bleeding Phenotype in Relation to the Treatment of Bleeding Episodes

To treat bleeding episodes, or to prevent bleeding in surgical settings, rFVIIa does not present an intrinsic risk of inducing anamnesis. Consequently, in patients with MHAI, use of this agent may help to reduce the duration of the presence of the inhibitor and/or the duration of a severe bleeding phenotype before undetectable endogenous FVIII:C levels become $\geq$0.01 IU/mL. Avoiding therapy with FVIII or aPCCs containing low levels of FVIII has been found to be a valuable strategy for the treatment of MHAI.[23] Johanessen et al[44] have reported that such an approach results in a significant decline in inhibitor level in severe hemophilia A patients with high-responding inhibitors, although titers for low responders remained unchanged, regardless of the treatment that these patients received. If bypassing agents prove ineffective in preventing or stopping a bleed in patients with a low-titer inhibitor, high-dose FVIII treatment may enable the inhibitor to be overwhelmed, providing effective and valuable hemostasis for at least a few days.

In patient 1, the absence of additional treatment with FVIII-containing products after the dental procedure is likely to have contributed to the ultimate decrease of the inhibitor titer to less than 5 BU. The lack of further FVIII treatment may also have avoided the risk of the patient's bleeding phenotype changing from mild to severe, as could have been the case if an anamnestic response directed against endogenous FVIII had occurred. Patient 3 was less fortunate in this regard, as the anamnesis was combined with a more generalized immune response against both endogenous and exogenous FVIII, with spontaneous bleeds subsequently occurring. Conversely, the immune response in patient 4 was initially directed against both endogenous and exogenous FVIII but was restricted to exogenous FVIII when the inhibitor recurred. In patient 2, the anamnestic responses after FVIII and aPCC treatments increased the duration of inhibitor persistence and the subsequent high risk of bleeding, delaying normalization of the patient's FVIII:C baseline level.

In contrast, some patients with transient inhibitors, such as patient 5, may remain tolerant to FVIII therapy without exhibiting further anamnesis. This may permit retreatment with FVIII concentrates on several occasions. However, in the absence of any criteria to predict whether or not a patient with MHAI will respond to rechallenge with FVIII-containing products, the choice of therapy for treatment of bleeds should take into account the possibility of anamnesis of inhibitor, and should consider the likely efficacy of available products in the light of a patient's history and the type of bleed.

DDAVP

It is possible that, in recent years, clinicians may have increased their use of FVIII and not considered therapy with DDAVP for the treatment of mild bleeds or suitable surgical procedures, and this may have contributed to an increased incidence of MHAI. Appropriate use of DDAVP (ie, in mild bleeds or invasive procedures with a low risk of bleeding) may avoid the use of FVIII therapy, thereby preventing the formation and/or recurrence of inhibitors in some patients. However, the wide spectrum of response to DDAVP observed in different patients emphasizes the need for preliminary testing of the drug before it is used to treat a bleed. In the absence of any contraindications, and when the patient is of sufficient age (usually after 4 years old), DDAVP testing should be performed in all patients with mild and even moderate hemophilia A, and both the FVIII:C level at peak and the released FVIII:C half-life should be assessed. Physicians should ensure that the patient's fluid intake is restricted to limit the risk of DDAVP-induced hyponatremia and concurrent clinical complications. When DDAVP is used for the treatment of a bleed or to cover an invasive procedure, the clinical efficacy of the drug, together with the patient's FVIII:C level, must be followed carefully to enable a switch to standard FVIII treatment if necessary. This is particularly important, as DDAVP treatment carries a risk of tachyphylaxis.

It is noteworthy that MHA patients, such as patient 4, in whom the Arg^{2150} to His mutation results in impaired FVIII binding to von Willebrand factor,[35] can present with FVIII:C baseline levels as low as 0.02 IU/mL. This may be a consequence of the lack of protection of FVIII from clearance or proteolytic inactivation, as is also seen in type 2N von Willebrand disease. However, such patients frequently exhibit an unexpectedly high response to DDAVP,[21,25] rendering the agent suitable for some therapeutic use. Given the propensity of patients carrying this mutation to develop inhibitors following FVIII infusion (ie, 18.8% in the HAMSTeRS database), the possibility of DDAVP treatment is particularly interesting in these individuals.

Safety of Bypassing Agents

When considering the use of bypassing agents, such as rFVIIa or FEIBA, it is necessary to be aware of the potential risk of thrombosis in patients with detectable FVIII:C levels. An acute myocardial infarction that complicated therapy with a prothrombin complex concentrate was described in one MHAI child.[45] Even if this type of product is no longer used, this report emphasizes the need for caution when aPCC or rFVIIa is used in MHAI. Particular attention should be paid to those patients with mild hemophilia A who initially present with undetectable FVIII:C and whose endogenous FVIII:C levels increase during recovery. However, in this regard, available reports[16,21,23,25,29] suggest that the overall efficacy and tolerance of bypassing agents for the treatment of patients with MHAI appears to be good. These results have been confirmed for the patients (1–4) described here.

Conclusion

Optimal treatment regimens have yet to be determined not only for the eradication of inhibitors in MHA patients, but also for the management or surgical prophylaxis of hemorrhages associated with this condition. Although several treatment options for the control of bleeding episodes are currently available (FVIII, aPCC, rFVIIa, DDAVP), the choice of therapeutic strategy is difficult; inappropriate treatment may produce an anamnestic response, thus delaying normalization of FVIII:C levels and adversely affecting the clinical severity of the bleeding phenotype. In this regard, regular inhibitor testing of patients with MHA, particularly after FVIII exposure, should help in choosing an adequate treatment. Furthermore, as the patient history is often insufficiently extensive, it is rarely possible to evaluate the risk of anamnesis prior to treatment. In the absence of reliable criteria that can be used to predict the immunologic response following rechallenge with FVIII-containing products in MHAI patients, the type of treatment administered should be given careful consideration. Further understanding of these issues is expected from the analysis of the ongoing data collection conducted by the MHAI Study Group.

Acknowledgment

The authors thank Dr Yves Laurian (Department of Hematology, APHP-Hôpital Jean Verdier, Bondy; and Paris XIII-University, Bobigny, France) for critical review of the manuscript.

Appendix

The MHAI Study Group consists of the following centers (in order of number of analyzed forms) and investigators: Lille, France (Goudemand J, Wibaut B); Paris-Bicêtre, France (Lambert T, Rafowicz A, d'Oiron R); Marseille, France (Chambost H); Tours, France (Guérois C); Paris-Necker, France (Rothschild C, Torchet MF); Caen, France (Borel-Derlon A, Gautier P); Clermont-Ferrand, France (Marquès-Verdier A, Chaleteix C); Leuven, Belgium (Peerlinck K); Paris-Cochin, France (Stieltjes N, Robert-Roussel V); Le Mans, France (Moreau P); Lyon, France (Lienhart A); Bordeaux, France (Guérin V, Ferrer AM); Dijon, France (Volot F, Dutrillaux F); Le Chesnay, France (Peynet J); Montpellier, France (Navarro R); Nantes, France (Fressinaud E); Rennes, France (Berthier AM, Coatmelec B); Rouen, France (Borg JY); St-Etienne, France (Reynaud J, Berger C); Ajaccio, France (Lecomte B); Amiens, France (Voyer AL, Diéval J, Pautard B); Bayonne, France (Bauduer F); Besançon, France (Bertrand MA); Brest, France (Pan-Petesch B); Brussels, Belgium (Efira A); Brussels, Belgium (Hermans C); Poitiers, France (Macchi L, Alcalay M); Reims, France (Pouzol P); Gent, Belgium (Hunninck K).

Departments of Molecular Biology involved in FVIII genotyping: Paris-Bicêtre, France (J.M. Lavergne, B. Guillet), and Lyon, France (C. Vinciguerra).

References

1. Beck P, Giddings JC, Bloom AL: Inhibitor of factor VIII in mild hemophilia. Br J Haematol 17:283-288, 1969
2. Hay CRM, Ludlam CA, Colvin BT, Hill FGH, Preston FE, Wasseem N, et al: Factor VIII inhibitors in mild and moderate-severity haemophilia A. Thromb Haemost 79:762-766, 1998
3. Ören H, Yaprak I, Irken G: Factor VIII inhibitors in patients with hemophilia A. Acta Haematol 102:42-46, 1999
4. Colvin BT, Hay CRM, Hill FG, Preston FE: The incidence of factor VIII inhibitors in the United Kingdom, 1990-93. Br J Haematol 89:908-910, 1995
5. Ehrenforth S, Kreuz W, Scharrer I, Linde R, Funk M, Gungor T, et al: Incidence of development of factor VIII and factor IX inhibitors in haemophiliacs. Lancet 339:594-598, 1992
6. Oldenburg J, El-Maarri O, Schwaab R: Inhibitor development in correlation to factor VIII genotypes. Haemophilia 8:23-29, 2002
7. Lusher JM, Arkin S, Abildgaard CF, Schwartz RS: Recombinant factor VIII for the treatment of previously untreated patients with hemophilia A. Safety, efficacy, and development of inhibitors. Kogenate Previously Untreated Patient Study Group. N Engl J Med 328:453-459, 1993
8. Sharathkumar A, Lillicrap D, Blanchette VS, Kern M, Leggo J, Stain AM, et al: Intensive exposure to factor VIII is a risk for inhibitor development in mild hemophilia A. J Thromb Haemost 1:1228-1236, 2003
9. Bauduer F, Ducout L, Bendriss P, Falaises B, Lavergne JM: Mild haemophilia A discovered in a previously multi-operated 73-year-old man: Characterization of a new mutation. Haemophilia 7:419-421, 2001
10. Bovill EG, Burns SL, Golden EA: Factor VIII antibody in a patient with mild haemophilia. Br J Haematol 61:323-328, 1985
11. Capel P, Toppet M, van Remoortel E, Fondu P: Factor VIII inhibitor in mild haemophilia. Br J Haematol 62:786-787, 1986
12. Crowell EB: A factor VIII inhibitor in a mild hemophiliac. Am J Med Sci 260:261-263, 1970
13. Fijnvandraat K, Turenhout EAM, van den Brink EN, ten Cate JW, van Mourik JA, Peters M, et al: The missense mutation $Arg^{593}\rightarrow Cys$ is related to antibody formation in a patient with mild hemophilia A. Blood 89:4371-4377, 1997
14. Kesteven PJ, Holland LJ, Lawrie AS, Savidge GF: Inhibitor to factor VIII in mild haemophilia. Thromb Haemost 52:50-52, 1984

15. Knobe KE, Villoutreix BO, Tengborn LI, Petrini P, Ljung RC: Factor VIII inhibitors in two families with mild haemophilia A: Structural analysis of the mutations. Haemostasis 30:268-279, 2000
16. Leebeek FWG, Kappers-Klunne MC, Jie KSG: Effective and safe use of recombinant factor VIIa (NovoSeven®) in elderly mild haemophilia A patients with high-titre antibodies against factor VIII. Haemophilia 10: 250-253, 2004
17. Lechner K, Ludwig E, Niessner H, Thaler E: Factor VIII inhibitor in a patient with mild hemophilia A. Hemostasis 1:261-270, 1972
18. Liu ML, Nakaya S, Thompson AR: Non-inversion factor VIII mutations in 80 hemophilia A families including 24 with alloimmune responses. Thromb Haemost 87:273-276, 2002
19. Lowe G, Forbes CD: Inhibitor to factor VIII in mild haemophilia. Thromb Haemost 53:159, 1985
20. Peerlinck K, Arnout J, Jacquemin M, Gilles JG, Lavend'homme R, Kreson K, et al: A patient with mild hemophilia and a high titer antifactor VIII antibody against exogenous factor VIII only: Clinical features, surgical management and partial characterization of the inhibitor. Blood 90:36a, 1997 (suppl 1)
21. Peerlinck K, Jacquemin MG, Arnout J, Hoylaerts MF, Gilles JGG, Lavend'homme R, et al: Antifactor VIII antibody inhibiting allogeneic but not autologous factor VIII in patients with mild hemophilia A. Blood 93:2267-2273, 1999
22. Puetz JJ, Bouhasin JD: High-titre factor VIII inhibitor in two children with mild haemophilia A. Haemophilia 7:215-219, 2001
23. Robbins D, Kulkarni R, Gera R, Scott-Emuakpor AB, Bosma K, Penner JA: Successful treatment of high titer inhibitors in mild hemophilia A with avoidance of factor VIII and immunosuppressive therapy. Am J Hematol 68:184-188, 2001
24. Roussel-Robert V, Torchet MF, Legrand F, Rothschild C, Stieltjes N: Factor VIII inhibitors development following introduction of B-domain-deleted recombinant factor VIII in four hemophilia A previously treated patients. J Thromb Haemost 1:2450-2541, 2003
25. Santagostino E, Gringeri A, Tagliavacca L, Mannucci PM: Inhibitors to factor VIII in a family with mild hemophilia: molecular characterization and response to factor VIII and desmopressin. Thromb Haemost 74: 619-621, 1995
26. Suzuki T, Arai M, Miyasaka S, Watanabe J, Sugimura D, Amano K, et al: Factor VIII inhibitor developed in a 60-year-old patient with mild hemophilia A after surgery for colon cancer. Int J Hematol 62:127-132, 1995
27. Thompson AR, Murphy MEP, Liu ML, Saenko EL, Healey JF, Lollar P, et al: Loss of tolerance to exogenous and endogenous factor VIII in a mild hemophilia A patient with an Arg^{593} to Cys mutation. Blood 90:1902-1910, 1997
28. Yee TT, Pasi KJ, Lilley PA, Lee CA: Factor VIII inhibitors in haemophiliacs: A single-centre experience over 34 years, 1964-97. Br J Haematol 104:909-914, 1999
29. White B, Cotter M, Byrne M, O'Shea E, Smith OP: High responding factor VIII inhibitors in mild haemophilia—Is there a link with recent changes in clinical practice? Haemophilia 6:113-115, 2000
30. van den Brink EN, Timmermans SM, Turenhout EA, Bank CM, Fijnvandraat K, Voorberg J, et al: Longitudinal analysis of factor VIII inhibitors in a previously untreated mild haemophilia A patient with an $Arg^{593}\rightarrow$Cys substitution. Thromb Haemost 81:723-726, 1999
31. White GC II, Rosendaal F, Aledort LM, Lusher JM, Rothschild C, Ingerslev J, on behalf of the Factor VIII and Factor IX Subcommittee: Classification of inhibitors. Scientific Subcommittees on Factor VIII and Factor IX of the Scientific and Standardization Committee of the International Society on Thrombosis and Haemostasis, Minutes and Annual report 2000, http://www.med.unc.edu/isth/SSC/communications/factor8and9/defhem.pdf
32. Gill J: Proposal to refine the low response inhibitor definition. Scientific Subcommittees on Factor VIII and Factor IX of the Scientific and Standardization Committee of the International Society on Thrombosis and Haemostasis, Minutes and Annual report 2004, http://www.med.unc.edu/isth
33. Oldenburg J, Schroder J, Hermann Brackmann H, Muller-Reible C, Schwaab R, Tuddenham E: Environmental and genetic factors influencing inhibitor development. Semin Hematol 41:82-88, 2004 (suppl 1)
34. Kemball-Cook G, Tuddenham EG, Wacey AI: The factor VIII structure and mutation resource site: HAMSTeRS version 4. Nucleic Acids Res 26:216-219, 1998
35. Jacquemin M, Benhida A, Peerlinck K, Desqueper B, Vander Elst L, Lavend'homme R, et al: A human antibody directed to the factor VIII domain inhibits factor VIII cofactor activity and binding to von Willebrand factor. Blood 95:156-163, 2000
36. Jacquemin M, Lavend'homme R, Benhida A, Vanzieleghem B, d'Oiron R, Lavergne JM, et al: A novel cause of mild/moderate hemophilia A: mutations scattered in the factor VIII C1 domain reduce factor VIII binding to von Willebrand factor. Blood 96:958-965, 2000
37. Bril WS, Turenhout EAM, Kaijen PHP, van den Brink EN, Koopman MMW, Peters M, et al: Analysis of factor VIII inhibitors in a haemophilia A patient with an $Arg^{593}\rightarrow$Cys mutation using phage display. Br J Haematol 119:393-396, 2002
38. Bril WS, MacLean PE, Kaijen PHP, van den Brink EN, Lardy NM, Fijnvandraat K, et al: HLA class II genotype and factor VIII inhibitors in mild hemophilia A patients with an Arg^{593} to Cys mutation. Haemophilia 10:509-514, 2004
39. Hay CR, Ollier W, Pepper L, Cumming A, Keeney S, Goodeve AC, et al: HLA class II profile: A weak determinant of factor VIII inhibitor development in severe hemophilia A. Thromb Haemost 77:234-237, 1997
40. Oldenburg J, Picard JK, Schwaab R, Brackmann HH, Tuddenham EG, Simpson E: HLA genotype of patients with severe haemophilia A due to intron 22 inversion with and without inhibitors of factor VIII. Thromb Haemost 77:238-242, 1997
41. Astermark J, Berntorp E, White GC, Kroner BL, The MIBS Study Group: The Malmö International Brother Study (MIBS): Further support for genetic predisposition to inhibitor development. Haemophilia 7:267-272, 2001
42. Vlot AJ, Wittebol S, Strengers PF, Turenhout EA, Voorberg J, van den Berg HM, et al: Factor VIII inhibitor in a patient with mild haemophilia A and an $Asn^{618}\rightarrow$Ser mutation responsive to immune tolerance induction and cyclophosphamide. Br J Haematol 117:136-140, 2002
43. Wiestner A, Cho HJ, Asch AS, Michells MA, Zeller JA, Peerschke EIB: Rituximab in the treatment of acquired factor VIII inhibitors. Blood 100:3426-3428, 2002
44. Johannessen M, Andreasen RB, Nordfang O: Decline of factor VIII and factor IX inhibitors during long-term treatment with NovoSeven. Blood Coagul Fibrinolysis 11:239-242, 2000
45. Karayalcin G, Goldberg B, Cherrick I, Kurer C, Bierman F, Lanzkowsky P: Acute myocardial infarction complicating prothrombin complex concentrate therapy in an 8-year-old boy with hemophilia A and factor VIII inhibitor. Am J Pediatr Hematol Oncol 15:416-419, 1993

Seminars in
HEMATOLOGY

Inhibitors to Factor XI in Patients With Severe Factor XI Deficiency

Ophira Salomon, Ariella Zivelin, Tami Livnat, and Uri Seligsohn

Factor XI (FXI) deficiency is a rare bleeding disorder that may arise from any of a number of missense, nonsense, splice site, insertion, and deletion mutations within the FXI gene. Severely affected patients are at considerable risk of developing inhibitors to FXI and, although spontaneous bleeding is uncommon in such patients, bleeding after surgery or trauma can be severe. As treatment with fresh frozen plasma (FFP) or FXI concentrates is ineffective in patients with inhibitors, other therapies must be sought. Traditionally, such patients have been treated with various agents and methods, including plasma exchange, cyclophosphamide, intravenous immunoglobulin, and prothrombin complex concentrates. However, emerging data indicate that recombinant activated factor VII (rFVIIa; NovoSeven®, Novo Nordisk, Bagsvaerd, Denmark) may also be effective in FXI deficiency with inhibitors. Further work is required to determine the optimal dosing schedules of the agent in this indication.
Semin Hematol 43(suppl 1):S10-S12

Factor XI (FXI) is a homodimeric serine protease. It is activated by the thrombin generated by the tissue factor pathway, when both FXI and thrombin bind to glycoprotein Ibα on the activated platelet surface.[1] FXI then activates factor IX (FIX), and this leads to further thrombin generation. The continuous generation of thrombin by this mechanism, even after clot formation, results in activation of thrombin-activatable fibrinolysis inhibitor (TAFI), which stabilizes the fibrin clot.[2]

Mutations in the FXI gene can result in FXI deficiency, which is inherited as an autosomal recessive trait. In individuals who are homozygous or have compound heterozygosity for mutations, the deficiency is manifested by FXI levels of $\leq$15 U/dL; in heterozygotes, the FXI level is intermediate between that of patients with a severe FXI deficiency and that of normal subjects.[3] Patients with a severe FXI deficiency do not usually bleed spontaneously. However, they are prone to bleeding following surgery or trauma, particularly when tissues rich in fibrinolytic activators—such as the nasal or oral mucosa, or the urinary tract—are involved.[4] Although patients with a severe FXI deficiency have an injury-related bleeding tendency, heterozygotes with partial FXI deficiency do not usually bleed unless an additional hemostatic defect is present, or unless the mutation causing the deficiency exerts a dominant negative effect.[5]

Currently, 86 mutations in the FXI gene have been described in patients with FXI deficiency. A partial list of these mutations can be found in the International Society on Thrombosis and Haemostasis (ISTH) database of mutations causing rare bleeding disorders (*http://www.med.unc.edu/isth/mutations-databases/Factor_XI.htm*). Missense, nonsense, splice site, insertion, and deletion mutations have all been found, with the various mutations located throughout the gene. Mutations leading to severe forms of the disease can cause impaired protein production, secretion, or dimerization; intracellular trapping of heterodimeric FXI; or synthesis of a dysfunctional protein (cross-reactive material positive variants).

FXI Inhibitors

Several cases of severe FXI deficiency and inhibitors to FXI have been described. These inhibitors are polyclonal and of the immunoglobulin G type. Characterization shows that they act on different epitopes of FXI.[6] The inhibitors can impair binding to high-molecular-weight kininogen or factor XIIa, impair the activation of FXI by thrombin or FXIIa, and diminish the activation of FIX by FXIa.[6-9] The absence of activated partial thromboplastin time (aPTT) correction following mixing of patient and control plasma usually leads to

Amalia Biron Research Institute of Thrombosis and Hemostasis, Chaim Sheba Medical Center, Tel Hashomer and Sackler Faculty of Medicine, Tel Aviv University, Tel Aviv, Israel
Address correspondence to Ophira Salomon, MD, Senior Hematologist, Amalia Biron Research Institute of Thrombosis and Hemostasis, Chaim Sheba Medical Center, Tel Hashomer and Sackler Faculty of Medicine, Tel Aviv University, 52621 Israel. E-mail: ophiras@sheba.health.gov.il

 0037-1963/06/$-see front matter
doi:10.1053/j.seminhematol.2005.11.018

Table 1 Countries in Which Patients Lacking FXI Antigen and Activity Have Been Identified

Country	Mutation in Homozygous State	Reference
France	Gln88stop	Quelin et al (2004)[10]
Israel, UK, USA	Glu117stop	Asakai et al (1991)[3] Salomon et al (2003)[6]
Italy	Cys118stop	Zadra et al (2004)[11]
Japan	Gln263stop	Sato et al (2000)[12]
	Trp501stop	Iijima et al (2000)[13]
Portugal	nt1075delA*	Ventura et al (2000)[14]
UK	Cys128stop	Bolton-Maggs et al (2004)[15]

Abbreviation: FXI, factor XI.
*Antigen level not reported.

the identification of an inhibitor, and this can subsequently be quantified using the Bethesda method.

Patients with severe FXI deficiency who develop inhibitors do not usually bleed spontaneously. However, bleeding following surgical procedures can be severe. The presence of an inhibitor is usually suspected when treatment with fresh frozen plasma (FFP) or FXI concentrates fails to be hemostatically effective, or when normal plasma fails to correct a prolonged aPTT.

In a recent study, we assessed the prevalence of inhibitors in patients with severe FXI deficiency.[6] Of 118 unrelated Israeli patients examined, seven had an inhibitor to FXI. All seven of these patients had undetectable levels of FXI in their plasma, and all had been exposed to blood products in the past. They were all homozygous for the Glu117stop mutation (type II mutation), and comprised one third of the total of 21 patients who were found to have this genotype. Inhibitors were not found in any of the other plasma-exposed patients with severe FXI deficiency caused by homozygosity for Phe283Leu mutation (type III mutation) (14 patients) or compound heterozygosity for type II/III mutations (27 patients). DNA samples from a further five patients with an inhibitor to FXI were sent to our institute from the United States and the United Kingdom, and these patients were all identified as type II homozygotes. Also, a patient from western France with a homozygous Gln88stop mutation and less than 1 U/dL of FXI activity developed an inhibitor following exposure to FXI concentrates.[10] These observations suggest that patients harboring mutations that cause severe FXI deficiency (listed at: *http://www.med.unc.edu/isth/mutations-databases/Factor_XI.htm*) are prone to the development of an inhibitor.

Table 1 lists some of the countries in which non-Jewish patients with mutations causing lack of FXI have been described.[3,6,10-15] Class II subtypes of human leukocyte antigen (HLA) DRB1* and DQB1*, which have been found to be weak determinants of inhibitor formation in hemophilia A,[16] have not been associated with the development of FXI inhibitors.[6]

Treatment of Patients With FXI Inhibitors

Patients with an inhibitor to FXI should receive neither FFP nor FXI concentrates. If patients with severe FXI deficiency (<1 U/dL) and a history of exposure to FXI are scheduled to undergo surgery, it is essential to test for the presence of an inhibitor to FXI. In the past, these patients were treated with Auto-Factor IX, cyclophosphamide and intravenous immunoglobulin,[17], plasma exchange,[17] FEIBA (Baxter Corp, Ontario, Canada), or Autoplex (Baxter Healthcare Corp, Glendale, CA).[18]

Recent data suggest that patients can also be treated successfully with recombinant activated factor VII (rFVIIa; NovoSeven®, Novo Nordisk, Bagsvaerd, Denmark). In 1990, Hedner[19] described the first use of rFVIIa in a FXI-deficient patient and, since that time, a number of authors have reported effective hemostatic treatment of severe FXI deficiency and inhibitors using this agent[20-23] (Table 2). However, the optimal dose has yet to be determined. As shown in Table 2, the reported doses of rFVIIa used in FXI-deficient patients undergoing surgery have varied among procedures, as the dosages have been determined by the institutions at which surgery was performed. One patient with FXI deficiency and an inhibitor developed an anterior wall myocardial infarction when continuous infusion of rFVIIa was administered for vitrectomy; however, a high dose was

Table 2 Treatment With rFVIIa in Patients With Severe FXI Deficiency and an Inhibitor

Authors	FXI level	Inhibitor (Bethesda units)	Dose of rFVIIa	Surgical Procedure
Hedner et al (1990)[19]	Unavailable	Unavailable	60 μg/kg every 3 h for 3 days	Successful orchidectomy
Billon et al (2001)[20]	5 U/dL	38	30 μg/kg before procedure and 4 h later	Uneventful thoracocentesis
Lawler et al (2002)[21]	<1 U/dL	48	90 μg/kg followed by continuous infusion of 20 μg/kg/h for 18 h	Uneventful cataract extraction
Bern et al (2005)[22]	0–2 U/dL	2.2	90 μg/kg every 2 h for 5 doses	Successful repair of anterior cruciate ligament
Salomon et al (2003)[23]	<1 U/dL	5	80 μg/kg/h continuous infusion for 36 h	Vitrectomy complicated by acute myocardial infarction

Abbreviations: FXI, factor XI; rFVIIa, recombinant activated factor VII.

administered (80 μg/kg/h for 36 hours).[23] We recently observed that relatively low concentrations of rFVIIa corrected in vitro thrombin generation in plasma from patients with severe FXI deficiency and an inhibitor.[24] Consequently, it is possible that patients with an inhibitor to FXI may benefit from infusions of rFVIIa at doses that are lower than those required for patients with severe hemophilia A or B and inhibitors.

References

1. Baglia FA, Shrimpton CN, Emsley J, Kitagawa K, Ruggeri ZM, Lopez JA, et al: Factor XI interacts with leucine-rich repeats of glycoprotein Ibα on the activated platelet. J Biol Chem 279:49323-49329, 2004
2. von dem Borne PAK, Meijers JCM, Bouma BN: Feedback activation of factor XI by thrombin in plasma results in additional formation of thrombin that protects fibrin clots from fibrinolysis. Blood 86:3035-3042, 1995
3. Asakai R, Chung DW, Davie EW, Seligsohn U: Factor XI deficiency in Ashkenazi Jews in Israel. N Engl J Med 325:153-158, 1991
4. Seligsohn U: Factor XI deficiency. Thromb Haemost 70:68-71, 1993
5. Kravtsov DV, Wu W, Meijers JCM, Sun MF, Blinder MA, Dang TP, et al: Dominant factor XI deficiency caused by mutations in the factor XI catalytic domain. Blood 104:128-134, 2004
6. Salomon O, Zivelin A, Livnat T, Dardik R, Loewenthal R, Avishai O, et al: Prevalence, causes, and characterization of factor XI inhibitors in patients with inherited factor XI deficiency. Blood 101:4783-4788, 2003
7. Stern DM, Nossel HL, Owen J: Acquired antibody to factor XI in a patient with congenital factor XI deficiency. J Clin Invest 69:1270-1276, 1982
8. De La Cadena RA, Baglia FA, Johnson CA, Wenk RE, Amernick R, Walsh PN, et al: Naturally occurring human antibodies against two distinct functional domains in the heavy chain of FXI/FXIa. Blood 72: 1748-1754, 1988
9. Goldsmith GH Jr, Silverman P: Inhibitors of plasma thromboplastin antecedent (factor XI): Studies on mechanism of inhibition. J Lab Clin Med 106:279-285, 1985
10. Quelin F, Trossaert M, Sigaud M, Mazancourt PD, Fressinaud E: Molecular basis of severe factor XI deficiency in seven families from the West of France. Seven novel mutations, including an ancient Q88X mutation. J Thromb Haemost 2:71-76, 2004
11. Zadra G, Asselta R, Malcovati M, Santagostino E, Peyvandi F, Mannucci PM, et al: Molecular genetic analysis of severe coagulation factor XI deficiency in six Italian patients. Haematologica 89:1332-1340, 2004
12. Sato E, Kawamata N, Kato A, Oshimi K: A novel mutation that leads to a congenital factor XI deficiency in a Japanese family. Am J Hematol 63:165-169, 2000
13. Iijima K, Udagawa A, Kawasaki H, Murakami F, Shimomura T, Ikawa S: A factor XI deficiency associated with a nonsense mutation (Trp501stop) in the catalytic domain. Br J Haematol 111:556-558, 2000
14. Ventura C, Santos AI, Tavares A, Gago T, Lavinha J, McVey JH, et al: Molecular genetic analysis of factor XI deficiency: Identification of five novel gene alterations and the origin of type II mutation in Portuguese families. Thromb Haemost 84:833-840, 2000
15. Bolton-Maggs PH, Peretz H, Butler R, Mountford R, Keeney S, Zacharski L, et al: A common ancestral mutation (C128X) occurring in 11 non-Jewish families from the UK with factor XI deficiency. J Thromb Haemost 2:918-924, 2004
16. Hay CR, Ollier W, Pepper L, Cumming A, Keeney S, Goodeve AC, et al: HLA class II profile: A weak determinant of factor VIII inhibitor development in severe haemophilia A. UKHCDO Inhibitor Working Party. Thromb Haemost 77:234-237, 1997
17. Teruya J, Styler M: Management of factor XI inhibitor for cardiac intervention: Successful treatment with immunosuppressive therapy and plasma exchange. Haemophilia 6:158-161, 2000
18. Connelly NR, Brull SJ: Anesthetic management of a patient with factor XI deficiency and factor XI inhibitor undergoing a cesarean section. Anesth Analg 76:1365-1366, 1993
19. Hedner U: Factor VIIa in the treatment of haemophilia. Blood Coag Fibrinolysis 1:307-317, 1990
20. Billon S, Le Niger C, Escoffre-Barbe M, Vicariot M, Abgrall JF: The use of recombinant factor VIIa (NovoSeven) in a patient with a factor XI deficiency and circulating anticoagulant. Blood Coagul Fibrinolysis 12: 551-553, 2001
21. Lawler P, White B. Pye S, Hermans C, Riddell A, Costello C, et al: Successful use of recombinant factor VIIa in a patient with inhibitor secondary to severe factor XI deficiency. Hemophilia 8:145-148, 2002
22. Bern MM, Sahud M, Zhukov O, Qu K, Mitchell W Jr: Treatment of factor XI inhibitor using recombinant activated factor VIIa. Haemophilia 11:20-25, 2005
23. Salomon O, Steinberg DM, Dardik R, Rosenberg N, Zivelin A, Tamarin I, et al: Inherited factor XI deficiency confers no protection against acute myocardial infarction. J Thromb Haemost 1:658-661, 2003
24. Livnat O, Salomon O, Zivelin A, Seligsohn U: The severely impaired thrombin generation in 5 patients with severe factor XI deficiency and inhibitors is corrected in vitro by recombinant VIIa. Thromb Haemost 89, 2003 (abstr 1188)

Seminars in
HEMATOLOGY

Update on Liver Disease in Hemophilia Patients

Craig M. Kessler

Prior to the introduction of viral inactivation techniques in the mid-1980s, the vast majority of patients with hemophilia who received plasma-derived clotting factor concentrates were exposed to and infected with the hepatitis C virus (HCV), a lipid-enveloped bloodborne pathogen. Hemophilia patients may also have been co-infected with the human immunodeficiency virus (HIV) after receiving contaminated blood products. HCV mono-infection has a very slow progression, but patients with hemophilia who are co-infected with HCV and HIV can exhibit a comparatively rapid progression of liver disease. Potential complications of chronic HCV infection are subsequent cirrhosis with hepatic failure and the ultimate onset of hepatocellular carcinoma. The treatment of either of these may involve orthotopic liver transplantation. Liver biopsy and morphologic evaluation of tissue remain the current "gold standard" by which the severity of HCV-induced liver disease can be reliably assessed. Although there has been a reluctance to perform invasive percutaneous liver biopsies in patients with hemophilia, available evidence suggests that they appear to be safe and they certainly provide greater specificity and sensitivity than radiographic techniques such as computerized tomography or magnetic resonance imaging. Treatment of HCV-infected patients is targeted towards preventing the progression of early cirrhosis and end-stage liver disease. The current standard of care for individuals with hemophilia has generally been considered to be the combination of standard interferon-alpha (IFN-α) with ribavirin for at least 6 months. Data concerning the use of PEGylated IFN, substituting for standard IFN-α, are now emerging, although relatively little of this information relates specifically to hemophilia patients with liver disease. Nevertheless, the favorable data from large non-hemophilia-related HCV disease with early cirrhosis have been extrapolated to the hemophilia scenario, and there has been no evidence in the limited number of hemophiliacs treated in this way to refute this conclusion.
Semin Hematol 43(suppl 1):S13-S17

Prior to the introduction of viral inactivation techniques in the mid-1980s, the majority of patients with hemophilia who received infusions of plasma-derived clotting factor concentrates became infected with the hepatitis C virus (HCV).[1,2] In such patients, HCV infections are predominantly attributable to genotypes 1, 2, and 3, with genotypes 1 and 3 tending to exhibit a higher prevalence than genotype 2.[3,4] The HCV genotypes with which hemophilia patients have been infected are likely to reflect the prior exposures of the donors to the plasma pool in northern Europe and the United States, from whom the plasma had been obtained.[5]

Franchini et al[6] have shown that approximately 14% of HCV-infected hemophilia patients may clear the virus naturally and spontaneously. Their data also confirm the slow progression of HCV mono-infection, although more advanced liver disease is associated with HCV genotype 1 and increased patient age.[6] Co-infection with the human immunodeficiency virus (HIV) can also occur as a result of receiving contaminated blood products,[7] is implicated in the significantly accelerated rate of developing end-stage liver disease,[8] and is associated with higher mortality than HCV mono-infection alone.[4]

Hepatocellular Carcinoma

One of the most morbid potential complications of long-term HCV infection is the onset of hepatocellular carcinoma (HCC), which is invariably associated with liver cirrhosis. The crude rate of HCC in patients with hemophilia may be 30 times greater than in individuals who do not have this coagulopathy.[9] A study by Santagostino et al[10] has reported the overall incidence of HCC in HCV-infected hemophilia patients to be 239 per 100,000 per year. Mulitivariate analysis

Lombardi Comprehensive Cancer Center, Georgetown University Medical Center, Washington, DC.
Address correspondence to Craig M. Kessler, MD, Chief, Division of Hematology–Oncology, Lombardi Comprehensive Cancer Center, Georgetown University Medical Center, 3800 Reservoir Rd NW, Washington, DC 20007. E-mail: kesslerc@gunet.georgetown.edu

0037-1963/06/$-see front matter
doi:10.1053/j.seminhematol.2005.11.021

has shown the risk of HCC to be increased by almost 13-fold in patients with an alcohol intake of greater than 80 g/d. In addition, serum alpha-fetoprotein (AFP) levels greater than 11 ng/mL are associated with an increased risk of HCC development by around 15-fold.[10] Tradati et al[11] had previously shown that the prognosis and median survival of HCC in hemophilia patients were greater in individuals with serum AFP less than 11 ng/mL compared with those with levels above this value.

Hemophilia patients with end-stage liver disease or HCC may be successfully treated by orthotopic liver transplantation.[12] In patients who receive a liver transplant, there may be a spontaneous reduction in HCV viral load over time.[13] However, it is critical that patients who are co-infected with HCV and HIV remain on highly active antiretroviral therapy (HAART). Furthermore, Ashrani et al[14] have suggested that the transplanted liver may be able to induce immune tolerance. They described a successful liver transplant in a patient with severe hemophilia A, complicated by a high-titer factor VIII (FVIII) alloantibody inhibitor, HCV with early cirrhosis, and HCC. After a modest anamnestic response of the inhibitor titer after FVIII replacement therapy in the early postoperative period, immunologic tolerance to FVIII, reestablishment of normal FVIII recovery and circulating survival levels (t1/2), and eradication of the alloantibody inhibitor were subsequently observed.

Liver Biopsies in Hemophilia Patients With HCV

There is lively debate surrounding the usefulness and safety of liver biopsies in hemophilia patients with hepatitis C. Liver biopsies are the only way to reliably assess the severity of liver disease, particularly with regard to the degree of fibrosis that may be present on the retrieved tissue specimen. The histology of the liver is important with regard to both prognosis and treatment strategies in patients with HCV. However, there may be a reluctance to perform invasive liver biopsies in HCV patients with hemophilia due to concerns relating to the potential risks of bleeding. Several publications have described the utility and safety of performing liver biopsies in patients with congenital bleeding disorders.[15-27] The available data indicate that morbidity and deaths related to bleeding complications from the invasive procedure are very uncommon if care is focused on appropriate clotting factor replacement. Overall, the literature suggests that liver biopsies can be safely performed in patients with hemophilia. Both transjugular and percutaneous biopsies appear to be safe, but there remains a lack of data comparing these two procedures in terms of safety, cost-effectiveness and the optimal hemostatic regimen that should be employed.

Some physicians may favor transjugular over percutaneous liver biopsies. Although the transjugular approach was originally regarded as being more likely to yield specimens of inadequate quality and was criticized for the possibility that fibrosis and inflammation may be unevenly distributed and therefore missed as a result of sampling error, these problems tend not to occur in practice. As interventional radiologists become more facile with the technique, the tissue yield and the representation of the pathology in the specimen are adequate. Transjugular biopsies have several advantages over the percutaneous technique, including: a reduced duration of patient monitoring; a potential decrease in the amount of clotting factor that is required; and the possibility of obtaining additional prognostic information whilst performing the biopsy. Sinusoidal and portal vein pressures may be measured during transjugular biopsies, and these measurements can provide evidence of the progression of liver disease prior to the appearance of histologically detectable cirrhosis. The procedure also affords the opportunity to insert stents, which may provide patients with protection against future problems relating to portal hypertension. Information from liver biopsies, whether percutaneous or transjugular, can validate the utility of non-invasive surrogate markers of disease severity.

Stieltjes et al[28] have recently described results from a study in which transjugular liver biopsies were performed on patients with hemophilia or other congenital bleeding disorders who were infected with HCV. Liver histology was found to be significantly worse in patients who had been infected with HCV for more than 20 years ($P = .04$). No significant difference in liver histology was apparent between patients who were co-infected with HIV and those who were not ($P = .19$). It was also reported that patients infected with HCV genotype 1 did not have significantly different liver histology from those with other HCV genotypes ($P = .93$). The biopsies in one-third of the patients showed minimal histological changes, and consequently systemic anti-HCV treatment was not proposed in these cases. Avoiding unnecessary therapy based on the results of liver biopsies demonstrates one benefit arising from their use.

Surrogate Markers of Disease Progression

There have been a number of attempts to use surrogate markers of disease progression to avoid the need for liver biopsies in patients with hemophilia and HCV infection. Unfortunately, none of these have proven to be uniformly sensitive or specific. Zhang et al[29] assessed $CD4^+$ or $CD8^+$ T lymphocytes in hemophilia patients with hepatitis C and found no association between either cleared or chronic HCV states and altered levels of these lymphocyte subsets. Reduced numbers of $CD19^+$ B cells have been detected in hemophilia patients with high-level chronic HCV viremia, compared with patients in whom the HCV infection has cleared.[29] However, these are not considered to be adequate surrogate markers of disease progression.

Although it has been suggested that a homozygous 32-base deletion in the CCR5 chemokine receptor gene (CCR5-Δ32) may be an adverse host factor in HCV hepatitis,[30] Zhang et al[31] have shown that the increased frequency of this genotype in HCV-infected, HIV-uninfected hemophilia patients is a result of the protective effect of this genotype against HIV infection. Therefore, although the homozygous CCR5-Δ32 genotype is an excellent surrogate marker for HIV, it does not correlate well with HCV disease progression.

Biochemical markers of liver fibrosis and necroinflammatory features have also been studied in patients with HCV.[32] Consequently, the FibroTest (Biopredictive, Paris, France) and the ActiTest (Biopredictive) have been recommended as alternatives to liver biopsies to assess liver injury arising from chronic hepatitis C infection.[33] The FibroTest measures α_2-macroglobulin, haptoglobulin, apolipoprotein A1, γ-glutamyl transpeptidase, and total bilirubin. The ActiTest measures the five variables included in the FibroTest, together with alanine aminotransferase. Use of these tests allows estimations of both the stage of fibrosis (FibroTest) and the degree of necroinflammatory activity (ActiTest) associated with the liver disease. The utility of these markers in hemophilia patients infected with HCV remains to be determined.

Treatment of HCV Infection

Treatment of HCV-infected patients is targeted towards preventing cirrhosis and end-stage liver disease. The current standard of care is generally considered to be the combination of standard interferon-alpha (IFN-α) with ribavirin. This has been shown to be twice as effective as the use of IFN-α alone.[5] The duration of therapy that patients receive should be determined by the HCV genotype with which they are infected, together with their level of viremia. For patients with HCV genotype 1 and a high level of viremia ($>2 \times 10^6$ copies/mL), 12 months of treatment is recommended. Six months' therapy may be appropriate for patients with genotype 1 and a low level of viremia ($<2 \times 10^6$ copies/mL), and for patients with HCV genotypes 2 or 3.[5]

The attachment of polyethylene glycol (PEG) to IFN molecules, to produce PEGylated IFN, prolongs the drug's half-life in plasma, thereby producing a protracted effect. PEGylated IFN is an emerging therapy and data concerning the use of PEGylated IFN and ribavirin are now starting to be generated. Relatively little of this information relates specifically to hemophilia patients, however, although some data are provided by the Second Multicenter Hemophilia Cohort Study (MHCS-II).[34]

The MHCS-II cooperative study involves 52 centers in North America, South America and Europe, which have enrolled patients with hemophilia and laboratory evidence of HCV or HIV-1 infection.[34] Their results indicate that, during 2001–2003, 30% of the surviving patients from the active HIV era who were seropositive for HCV were also co-infected with HIV. Furthermore, 4.6% of them also carried the hepatitis B virus (HBV). In these co-infected patients, major complications were more likely to be associated with liver failure and bleeding than with opportunistic infections. The natural history of HIV/HCV co-infected individuals could be altered by HAART. The majority of the HIV-positive patients were negative for HIV RNA and most had $CD4^+$ counts greater than 200 cells/μL, although HAART was only used for the treatment of 59% of these patients. Combined treatment with PEGylated interferon and ribavirin resulted in more than 50% of HIV-negative patients achieving sustained clearance of HCV.

In general, data from hemophilia patients co-infected with HIV and HCV are limited, making it difficult to ascertain the long-term effects of this therapy in a large enough cohort to satisfy biostatistical powering. Consequently, it has been both informative and necessary to extrapolate results from treatment of non-hemophilia cohorts to the hemophilia patient population. For instance, Carrat et al[35] have described a randomized controlled trial studying the effects of PEGylated IFN-α2b and ribavirin with standard IFN-α2b and ribavirin in the treatment of non-hemophilic HIV/HCV co-infected patients. PEGylated IFN-α2b (1.5 μg/kg) was administered as a weekly subcutaneous injection. Standard IFN-α2b (3 million units) was given via subcutaneous injection three times each week. All patients received oral ribavirin (400 mg twice daily). Treatment was continued for 48 weeks. Sustained virologic responses, as defined by undetectable serum HCV RNA at week 72, were found in 27% of all patients who were treated with PEGylated IFN-α2b, compared with 20% of those who received the standard therapy (P = .047). Analyzing the results according to HCV genotype, each IFN-α product cleared HCV to a greater degree in patients with genotypes 2, 3, or 5 (44% for PEGylated IFN-α2b *v* 43% for standard IFN-α2b; P = .88), but both IFN-α products were considerably less beneficial for genotypes 1 and 4 (17% *v* 6% for the PEGylated and standard therapies, respectively; P = .006). Importantly, PEGylated IFN-α2b appeared more efficient in clearing the more resistant HCV genotypes 1 and 4.

A recently published retrospective analysis of hemophilia patients who received IFN-α and ribavirin for the treatment of chronic hepatitis C has suggested this treatment combination may also result in decreased overall use of clotting factor replacement therapy.[36] Many hemophilia patients who have end-stage liver disease actually have an increased use of clotting factor concentrate, and so these results are particularly interesting, but remain to be validated by others.

Other Treatment Approaches

New approaches to the treatment of HCV include the addition of amantadine to the PEGylated IFN and ribavirin combination. Amantadine has activity against flaviviridae viruses, such as influenza,[37,38] and may also be effective against HCV, which is also a member of this family of viruses. In a randomized controlled trial of treatment-naïve patients with chronic hepatitis C, Mangia et al[39] showed that 48 weeks of therapy with amantadine, PEGylated IFN-α2a and ribavirin produced a greater rate of sustained virologic response (defined as undetectable HCV RNA after 24 weeks of untreated follow-up) than treatment with either the conventional IFN-α2a and ribavirin combination alone, or triple therapy with amantadine, conventional IFN-α2a and ribavirin.

The production of ribavirin analogs (eg, Barnard[40]) is also receiving consideration, as is the use of serine protease inhibitors (eg, Hinrichsen et al[41]), which can target various aspects of the genomic structure of the HCV virus.

Recombinant Activated Factor VII and Liver Disease

Recombinant activated factor VII (rFVIIa; NovoSeven®, Novo Nordisk, Bagsvaerd, Denmark) may be expected to ameliorate severe factor VII deficiency caused by end-stage liver disease. A single dose of rFVIIa (5 μg/kg) has been reported to correct coagulopathy prior to biopsy in cirrhotic patients.[42] Perioperative use of the agent in liver transplantation has also been described.[43] However, recently published results from two placebo-controlled, randomized trials in liver transplant patients did not confirm that the prophylactic administration of rFVIIa reduced the transfusion requirements for red blood cells when compared with placebo.[44,45] Further studies of rFVIIa in this indication are required.

Conclusions

Treatment options for hemophilia patients infected with HCV are influenced by results obtained from patients with liver disease who do not have such coagulopathy. Additional considerations have to be taken into account when treating patients with hemophilia. Studies such as the MHCS-II provide valuable data specific for this patient population, and knowledge of new therapeutic choices is now beginning to emerge.

References

1. Morfini M, Mannucci PM, Ciavarella N, Schiavoni M, Gringeri A, Rafanelli D, et al: Prevalence of infection with hepatitis C virus among Italian hemophiliacs before and after the introduction of virally inactivated clotting factor concentrates: A retrospective evaluation. Vox Sang 67:178-182, 1994
2. Brettler DB, Alter HJ, Dienstag JL, Forsberg AD, Levine PH: Prevalence of hepatitis C virus antibody in a cohort of hemophilia patients. Blood 76:254-256, 1990
3. Eyster ME, Sherman KE, Goedert JJ, Katsoulidou A, Hatzakis A: Prevalence and changes in hepatitis C virus genotype among multitransfused persons with haemophilia. The Multicenter Hemophilia Cohort Study. J Infect Dis 179:1062-1069, 1999
4. Yee TT, Griffioen A, Sabin CA, Dusheiko G, Lee CA: The natural history of HCV in a cohort of haemophiliac patients infected between 1961 and 1985. Gut 47:845-851, 2000
5. Lee C, Dusheiko G: The natural history and antiviral treatment of hepatitis C in haemophilia. Haemophilia 8:322-329, 2002
6. Franchini M, Rossetti G, Tagliaferri A, Capra F, de Maria E, Pattacini C, et al: The natural history of chronic hepatitis C in a cohort of HIV-negative Italian patients with hereditary bleeding disorders. Blood 98: 1836-1841, 2001
7. Kroner BL, Rosenberg PS, Aledort LM, Alvord WG, Goedert JJ: HIV-1 infection incidence among persons with hemophilia in the United States and western Europe, 1978–1990. Multicenter Hemophilia Cohort Study. J Acquir Immune Defic Syndr 7:279-286, 1994
8. Ragni MV, Belle SH: Impact of human immunodeficiency virus infection on progression to end-stage liver disease in individuals with haemophilia and hepatitis C virus infection. J Infect Dis 183:1112-1115, 2001
9. Colombo M, Mannucci PM, Brettler DB, Girolami A, Lian ECY, Rodeghiero F, et al: Hepatocellular carcinoma in hemophilia. Am J Hematol 37:243-246, 1991
10. Santagostino E, Colombo M, Rivi M, Rumi MG, Rocino A, Linari S, et al: Study Group of the Association of Italian Hemophilia Centers. A 6-month versus a 12-month surveillance for hepatocellular carcinoma in 559 hemophiliacs infected with the hepatitis C virus. Blood 102: 78-82, 2003
11. Tradati F, Colombo M, Mannucci PM, Rumi MG, De Fazio C, Gamba G, et al: A prospective multicenter study of hepatocellular carcinoma in Italian hemophiliacs with chronic hepatitis C. The Study Group of the Association of Italian Hemophilia Centers. Blood 91:1173-1177, 1998
12. Gordon FH, Mistry PK, Sabin CA, Lee CA: Outcome of orthotopic liver transplantation in patients with haemophilia. Gut 42:744-749, 1998
13. Sugawara Y, Ohkubo T, Makuuchi M, Kimura S, Morisawa Y, Tachikawa N, et al: Living-donor liver transplantation in an HIV-positive patient with hemophilia. Transplantation 74:1655-1656, 2002
14. Ashrani AA, Reding MT, Shet A, Osip J, Humar A, Lake JR, et al: Successful liver transplantation in a patient with severe haemophilia A and a high-titre factor VIII inhibitor. Haemophilia 10:735-737, 2004
15. Aledort LM, Levine PH, Hilgartner M, Blatt P, Spero JA, Goldberg JD, et al: A study of liver biopsies and liver disease among hemophiliacs. Blood 66:367-372, 1985
16. Ahmed MM, Mutimer DJ, Elias E, Linin J, Garrido M, Hubscher S, et al: A combined management protocol for patients with coagulation disorders infected with hepatitis C virus. Br J Haematol 95:383-388, 1996
17. Hanley JP, Jarvis LM, Andrews J, Dennis R, Lee R, Simmonds P, et al: Investigation of chronic hepatitis C infection in individuals with haemophilia: assessment of invasive and non-invasive methods. Br J Haematol 94:159-165, 1996
18. Makris M, Preston FE, Rosendaal FR, Underwood JC, Rice KM, Triger DR: The natural history of chronic hepatitis C in haemophiliacs. Br J Haematol 94:746-752, 1996
19. Gupta R, Druy EM, Kessler CM: Safety and potential usefulness of liver biopsy in HIV-seropositive haemophiliacs employing a transjugular venous approach. Haemophilia 3:201-204, 1997
20. Wong VS, Baglin T, Beacham E, Wight DD, Petrik J, Alexander GJ: The role for liver biopsy in haemophiliacs infected with the hepatitis C virus. Br J Haematol 97:343-347, 1997
21. Fukuda Y, Nakano I, Katano Y, Toyoda H, Imoto M, Takamatsu J, et al: Assessment and treatment of liver disease in Japanese haemophilia patients. Haemophilia 4:595-600, 1998
22. Venkataramani A, Behling C, Rond R, Glass C, Lyche K: Liver biopsies in adult hemophiliacs with hepatitis C: A United States center's experience. Am J Gastroenterol 95:2374-2376, 2000
23. McMahon C, Pilkington R, Shea EO, Kelleher D, Smith OP: Liver biopsy in Irish hepatitis C-infected patients with inherited bleeding disorders. Br J Haematol 109:354-359, 2000
24. Lethagen S, Widell A, Berntorp E, Verbaan H, Lindgren S: Clinical spectrum of hepatitis C-related liver disease and response to treatment with interferon and ribavirin in haemophilia or von Willebrand disease. Br J Haematol 113:87-93, 2001
25. DiMichele DM, Mirani G, Wilfredo Canchis P, Trost DW, Talal AH: Transjugular liver biopsy is safe and diagnostic for patients with congenital bleeding disorders and hepatitis C infection. Haemophilia 9:613-618, 2003
26. Shin JL, Teitel J, Swain MG, Bain VG, Adams PC, Croitoru K, et al: Virology and Immunology Committee of the Association of Hemophilia Clinic Directors of Canada. A Canadian multicentre retrospective study evaluating transjugular liver biopsy in patients with congenital bleeding disorders and hepatitis C: Is it safe and useful? Am J Hematol 78:85-93, 2005
27. Theodore D, Fried MW, Kleiner DE, Kroner BL, Goedert JJ, Eyster ME, et al: Liver biopsy in patients with inherited disorders of coagulation and chronic hepatitis C. Haemophilia 10:413-421, 2004
28. Stieltjes N, Ounnoughene N, Sava E, Paugy P, Roussel-Robert V, Rosenberg AR, et al: Interest of transjugular liver biopsy in adult patients with haemophilia or other congenital bleeding disorders infected with hepatitis C virus. Br J Haematol 125:769-776, 2004
29. Zhang M, O'Brien TR, Kopp WC, Goedert JJ: Lymphocyte subsets in hemophilic patients with hepatitis C virus infection with or without human immunodeficiency virus co-infection: A nested cross-sectional study. BMC Blood Disord 5:2, 2005
30. Woitas RP, Ahlenstiel G, Iwan A, Rockstroh JK, Brackmann HH, Kupfer B, et al: Frequency of the HIV-protective CC chemokine receptor

5-Δ32/Δ32 genotype is increased in hepatitis C. Gastroenterology 122:1721-1728, 2002

31. Zhang M, Goedert JJ, O'Brien TR: High frequency of CCR5-Δ32 homozygosity in HCV-infected, HIV-1-uninfected hemophiliacs results from resistance to HIV-1. Gastroenterology 124:867-868, 2003
32. Imbert-Bismut F, Ratziu V, Pieroni L, Charlotte F, Benhamou Y, Poynard T, MULTIVIRC Group: Biochemical markers of liver fibrosis in patients with hepatitis C infection: A prospective study. Lancet 357: 1069-1075, 2001
33. Poynard T, Imbert-Bismut F, Munteanu M, Messous D, Myers RP, Thabut D, et al: Overview of the diagnostic value of biochemical markers of liver fibrosis (FibroTest, HCV FibroSure) and necrosis (ActiTest) in patients with chronic hepatitis C. Comp Hepatol 3:8, 2004
34. Goedert JJ, Brown DL, Hoots K, Sherman KE: Human immunodeficiency and hepatitis virus infections and their associated conditions and treatments among people with haemophilia. Haemophilia 10:205-210, 2004 (suppl 4)
35. Carrat F, Bani-Sadr F, Pol S, Rosenthal E, Lunel-Fabiani F, Benzekri A, et al: ANRS HCO2 RIBAVIC Study Team. Pegylated interferon alfa-2b vs standard interferon alfa-2b, plus ribavirin, for chronic hepatitis C in HIV-infected patients: A randomized controlled trial. JAMA 292:2839-2848, 2004
36. Honda T, Toyoda H, Hayashi K, Katano Y, Yano M, Nakano I, et al: Ribavirin and use of clotting factors in patients with hemophilia and chronic hepatitis C. JAMA 293:1190-1192, 2005
37. De Clercq E: Antiviral drugs: current state of the art. J Clin Virol 22: 73-89, 2001
38. Dolin R, Reichman RC, Madore HP, Maynard R, Linton PN, Webber-Jones J: A controlled trial of amantadine and rimantadine in the prophylaxis of influenza A infection. N Engl J Med 307:580-584, 1982
39. Mangia A, Ricci GL, Persico M, Minerva N, Carretta V, Bacca D, et al: A randomized controlled trial of pegylated interferon α-2a (40 KD) or interferon α-2a plus ribavirin and amantadine vs interferon α-2a and ribavirin in treatment-naive patients with chronic hepatitis C. J Virol Hepat 12:292-299, 2005
40. Barnard D: Viramidine (Ribapharm). Curr Opin Invest Drugs 3:1585-1589, 2002
41. Hinrichsen H, Benhamou Y, Wedemeyer H, Reiser M, Sentjens RE, Calleja JL, et al: Short-term antiviral efficacy of BILN 2061, a hepatitis C virus serine protease inhibitor, in hepatitis C genotype 1 patients. Gastroenterology 127:1347-1355, 2004
42. Carvalho A, Leitao J, Louro E, Maia R, Geraldes C, Ventura C, et al: Small dose of recombinant factor VIIa (rFVIIa) to perform percutaneous liver biopsies in cirrhotic patients. Rev Esp Enferm Dig 94: 280-285, 2002
43. Jureczko L, Kolacz M, Trzebicki J, Szyszko G, Pacholczyk M, Lagiewska B, et al: Perioperative use of recombinant activated factor VII in liver transplantation. Ann Transplant 8:40-42, 2003
44. Lodge JP, Jonas S, Jones RM, Olausson M, Mir-Pollard J, Soefelt S, et al: Efficacy and safety of repeated perioperative doses of recombinant factor VIIa in liver transplantation. Liver Transpl 11:973-979, 2005
45. Planinsic RM, van den Meer J, Testa G, Grande L, Candela A, Porte RJ, et al: Safety and efficacy of a single bolus administration of recombinant factor VIIa in liver transplantation due to chronic liver disease. Liver Transpl 11:895-900, 2005

ELSEVIER

Seminars in
HEMATOLOGY

Pathogenesis of Hemophilic Arthropathy

W. Keith Hoots

Intra-articular bleeding is the most common clinical manifestation of hemophilia, and can adversely affect joints and lead to arthropathy. Affected joints are associated with changes to the synovium, bone, cartilage and blood vessels. Iron plays a critical role in the pathogenesis of this condition, and may exert its effects through a variety of different mechanisms. Hemophilic arthropathy shares some injury characteristics with rheumatoid arthritis, although the degree of analogy is a matter of some debate. The influences of the mechanisms underlying joint inflammation are better understood for rheumatoid arthritis than for hemophilia, and it is hoped that this knowledge can be used to provide a more comprehensive knowledge of the pathological process of hemophilic arthropathy. This, in turn, may enable novel targets for therapeutic intervention to be identified.
Semin Hematol 43(suppl 1):S18-S22

Intra-articular bleeding (hemarthrosis) is the most common clinical manifestation of hemophilia.[1] Recurrent hemarthrosis can lead to synovitis, which is a persistent inflammatory disorder. In the traditional view of chronic hemophilic synovitis, hydrolytic enzymes are released in response to bleeding into the joint.[2] Together with elevated levels of prostaglandins, these enzymes play a role in maintaining an inflammatory response in the synovium. Recurrent stimulation of the synovium produces hypertrophy with villus formation and increased vascularity, and this hypertrophic synovium can be characterized by the presence of chronic inflammatory cells.[3] In these circumstances, the synovium has an invasive and destructive interface (pannus) with bone and cartilage. In young patients with hemophilia, the subsequent inflammatory reaction can result in epiphyseal overgrowth.[3] Radiological changes to the affected joints may be observed, and these characterize hemophilic arthropathy. Atrophy occurs as a consequence of effects on the synovium, bone, cartilage, and blood vessels. Iron plays a critical role in the pathogenesis of this condition.

Gulf States Hemophilia and Thrombophilia Center, Houston; University of Texas Medical School at Houston; and University of Texas—M.D. Anderson Cancer Center, Houston, TX.

Address correspondence to W. Keith Hoots, MD, Gulf States Hemophilia and Thrombophilia Center, 6655 Travis St, Suite 400, Houston, TX 77030. E-mail: keith.hoots@uth.tmc.edu

Use of Data From Rheumatoid Arthritis to Understand the Pathogenesis of Hemophilic Arthropathy

Patients with rheumatoid arthritis (RA) experience an inflammatory reaction in affected joints, and more data have been published with regard to the inflammatory response in the joints of patients with RA than for the same response in hemophilic arthropathy. Consequently, it may be informative to consider information that has been produced from the study of RA in relation to patients with hemophilia. However, before attempting to understand the pathogenesis of hemophilic arthropathy using such data, it is appropriate to consider whether the conditions are sufficiently analogous to warrant exploring common biological pathways.

Both conditions exhibit upregulation of inflammatory cytokines as a hallmark of synovitis[4,5] and, as in patients with hemophilia, evidence of focal bone erosions (cystic changes, bone remodeling) can be associated with RA.[5,6] Cell-derived microparticles can be found in the inflamed joints of patients with hemophilic arthropathy, as they can in patients with RA.[7] In addition, evidence of synovial cell transformation has been described in both conditions.[8,9]

There are also histopathologic correlates between joint disease in hemophilia and RA. In patients with both hemophilic synovitis[10–12] (Fig 1) and RA,[13,14] synovial deposition of iron (siderosomes) may be apparent. Evidence has shown that iron deposits may affect the inflammatory response in RA.[15,16] Morris et al[11] have described the presence of both

 0037-1963/06/$-see front matter
doi:10.1053/j.seminhematol.2005.11.026

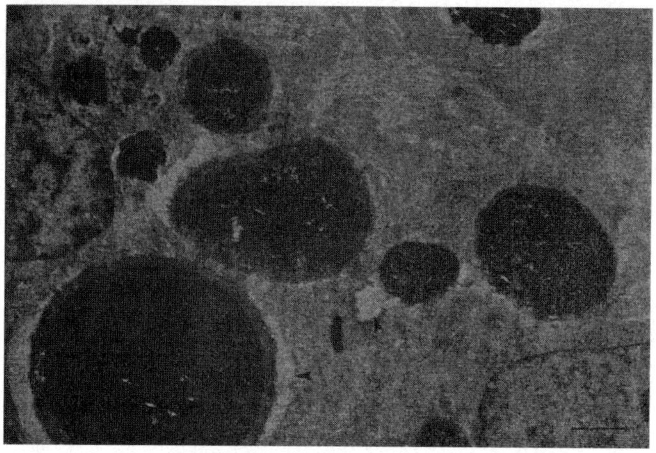

Figure 1 Electron micrograph of siderosomes in deep synovial macrophages from a case of hemophilic synovitis.[12] Scale line = 2 μm. Reproduced with permission from Morris et al.[12] © 1986, the BMJ Publishing Group.

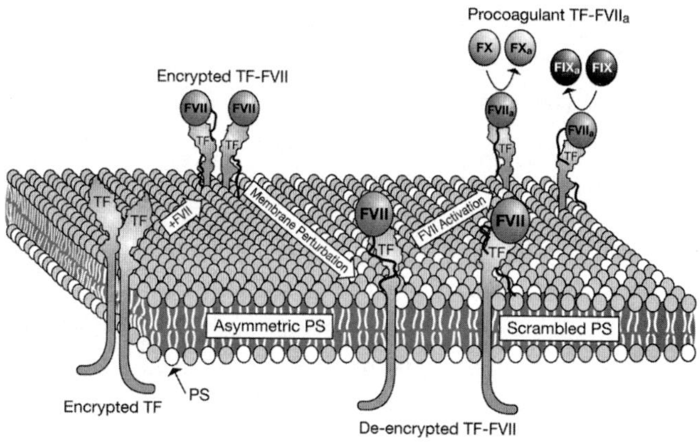

Figure 2 Proposed model showing de-encryption of tissue factor (TF) on the cell surface.[19] Encrypted TF molecules exhibit homodimerization, whilst de-encrypted molecules exist as monomers. FIX, factor IX; FIXa, activated factor IX; FVII, factor VII; FVIIa, activated factor VII; FX, factor X; FXa, activated factor X; PS, phosphatidylserine. Reproduced with permission.[19] © 2001, Schattauer.

pure iron and iron-saturated ferritin in hemophilic synovial membranes, and have suggested that the presence of iron-saturated ferritin may promote lipid peroxidation, thereby increasing or perpetuating inflammation in such patients. Roosendaal et al[4] reported that, in hemosideritic synovial tissue from patients with hemophilia, increased iron deposition was associated with increased catabolic activity when compared with normal tissue. Although the inflammatory changes in such tissue are mild compared with RA, in vitro production of catabolic agents such as interleukin (IL)-1, IL-6 and tumor necrosis factor alpha (TNFα) is comparable between the two conditions.[4] In vitro evidence suggests that whole blood may have a directly harmful effect on cartilage, irreversibly inhibiting the synthesis of proteoglycan.[17] Cartilage damage, as a consequence of hemarthrosis, may therefore occur in patients with hemophilia and RA.

There are also clear arguments against using rheumatoid arthropathy as the pathogenetic surrogate of hemophilic arthropathy. Changes in both conditions are inflammatory, but these are particularly degenerative in hemophilia when compared with RA. Blood-associated iron is the sine qua non for the arthropathy that hemophilia patients can experience, and although iron is involved in the arthropathy of RA, its role may be less important. The proinflammatory, tissue-destructive cytokines associated with arthropathy appear transiently following bleeding in patients with hemophilia; in RA, these cytokines remain present unless they are downregulated therapeutically. Nevertheless, in both conditions, red blood cell–macrophage interactions induce the production of IL-1β and activation of chondrocytes to produce H_2O_2, which, in the presence of iron, induces chondrocyte apoptosis.[18]

Joint Bleeds in Hemophilia

One intriguing issue for physicians involved with the treatment of hemophilia relates to why the hemophilic joint is so predisposed to bleed spontaneously, particularly in patients with pristine joints. It is possible that certain biological properties of the joint may account for this. Leukocyte-derived microparticles are present in synovial fluid, and these are able to induce coagulation activity via the factor VII (FVII)-dependent pathway.[7] Tissue factor (TF) is the receptor and cofactor for FVII/activated FVII (FVIIa). However, the majority of cell-surface TF is normally "encrypted"; it does not express full activity and become fully activated until it is "de-encrypted" by some form of cellular perturbation.[19] In a study of patients with RA, Berckmans et al[7] have reported synovial microparticles to be associated with the activation of coagulation in inflamed arthritic joints. Mechanisms of de-encryption appear to be both phosphatidylserine (PS)-dependent and PS-independent. In one such mechanism, it is proposed that encrypted TF molecules exhibit homo-dimerization, while de-encrypted molecules exist as monomers[19] (Fig 2). When the TF-FVIIa complex assembles on cell surfaces, limited proteolysis of factors IX and X initiates coagulation and ultimately leads to thrombin generation.

There may be, however, another reason why the joints of patients with hemophilia are predisposed to bleed. Brinckmann et al[20] have shown that expression of endogenous tissue factor pathway inhibitor (TFPI) is higher in cloned human synovial cells than in cloned human chondrocytes. As TFPI regulates the TF-FVIIa complex, upregulation of TFPI may downregulate clotting ability, thus leading to a hemorrhagic tendency.

Synovial Changes

In patients with RA, expression of the Myc oncoprotein has been found to be associated with synovial hypercellularity.[21] Wen et al[8] subsequently considered the role of the c-*myc* proto-oncogene in hemophilic synovitis. In vitro experiments using a primary human synovial fibroblast cell (HSFC) line showed that iron, in the form of ferric citrate, increased HSFC proliferation in a dose-dependent fashion; ferric citrate also enhanced c-*myc* expression compared with a sodium

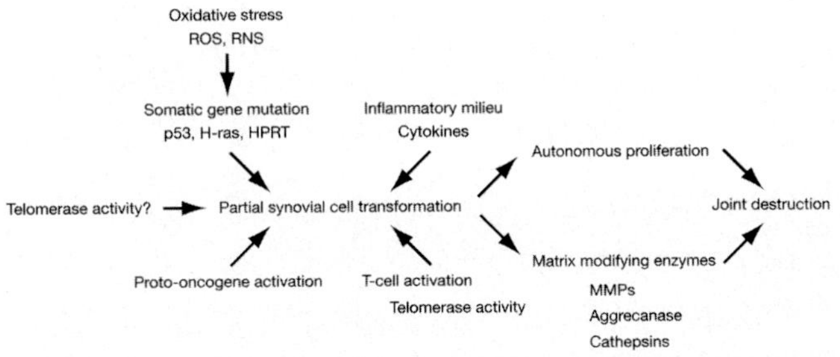

Figure 3 Proposed schema for the role of synoviocyte transformation in rheumatoid arthritis.[9] MMPs, matrix metalloproteinases; RNS, reactive nitrogen species; ROS, reactive oxygen species. Reprinted from Yamanishi et al.[9] © 2001, with permission from Elsevier.

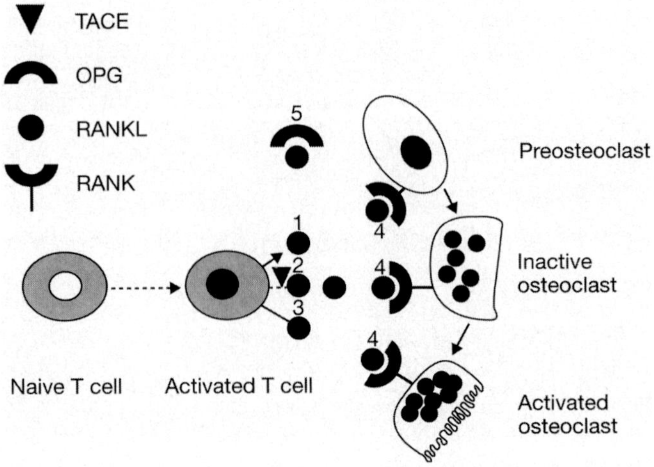

Figure 4 Roles of receptor activator of nuclear factor κB ligand (RANKL), receptor activator of nuclear factor κB (RANK) and osteoprotegerin (OPG) in osteoclast regulation[24]. Activated T lymphocytes express a primary soluble form (1) and a cellular form (3) of RANKL. The cellular form of RANKL is post-translationally cleaved by the protease tumor necrosis factor α-converting enzyme-like protease (TACE) to produce a secondary soluble ectodomain form of RANKL (2). All 3 RANKL variants bind to and activate RANK on the osteoclast surface (4) to induce osteoclast formation, survival, fusion, and activation, and to inhibit osteoclast apoptosis. This expands the pool of osteoclasts that are capable of resorbing bone and cartilage. OPG represents a decoy receptor that blocks RANK–RANKL interactions. Reprinted from Hofbauer et al.[24] © 2001, John Wiley & Sons, Inc. Reprinted with permission from Wiley-Liss Inc., a subsidiary of John Wiley & Sons, Inc.

citrate control. Consequently, aberrant expression of c-*myc* may underlie iron-induced proliferative changes in hemophilic synovitis. However, these changes may be reversed by ceramide. C_2-ceramide inhibits both iron-induced proliferation of HSFCs and c-*myc* expression,[8] and has also been shown to induce apoptosis of HSFCs.[8] Not only can iron upregulate c-*myc* activity in HSFCs,[8] but in vitro experiments have also shown that it can induce the expression of the *mdm2* oncogene in synovial cells.[22] Such changes may result in apoptosis being blocked in inflamed, iron-laden synoviocytes. In addition, iron catalyzes oxidative radical reactions[15]; synovial cells contain increased reactive oxygen/nitrogen species, which may cause somatic mutations.[23]

Such data suggest that the presence of blood in the joint can lead to cellular changes that may be associated with transformation. Indeed, many of the features of transformation have been described in RA synovial tissue or cells. These include anchorage-independent growth, loss of contact inhibition, oncogene activation, and somatic gene mutation.[9] This is not, however, true malignancy, and the term "partial transformation" may be appropriate in this circumstance.[9] A proposed schema to illustrate the role of synoviocyte transformation in RA has been advanced by Yamanishi and Firestein[9] (Fig 3). A variety of mechanisms are involved here, with the ultimate outcome being joint destruction. Although the details of such a scheme are less well known with regard to hemophilic arthropathy, research in this area is ongoing.

Bone Remodeling

Much of the data relating to the bone remodeling that occurs in response to inflammation in arthropathy has been limited to RA; little work has been done in the context of hemophilia. In patients with RA, osteoclasts are the key mediators of bone loss.[24] The receptor activator of nuclear factor κB ligand (RANKL) is a key cytokine that affects osteoclasts. The receptor for this ligand, receptor activator of nuclear factor κB (RANK) is expressed on osteoclasts and dendritic cells. Osteoprotegerin (OPG) is a soluble decoy receptor for RANKL that is produced by a variety of tissues and cell types. Both RANKL and OPG are members of the TNF family of receptors.

In vitro experiments have shown that RANKL can stimulate the differentiation, proliferation, fusion, and activation of osteoclasts, and suppress apoptosis.[24] Consequently, RANKL may act to increase the number of functionally active osteoclasts, with subsequent enhancement of bone resorption (Fig 4). In mice, disruption of the RANKL gene leads to severe osteopetrosis.[25] The effects of RANKL can be inhibited by OPG.[26]

The RANKL–RANK–OPG system provides a link between bone metabolism and the immune system.[24] RANKL–RANK interactions are involved with pre-B cell and pre-T cell development and maturation in the bone marrow and thymus. They also have a role in interactions between mature dendritic cells and T cells. The RANK:OPG ratio may be modulated in response to various cytokines,[27] and this can affect bone resorption. Proposed sites of action of cytokines and growth factors relevant to the regulation of bone resorption are shown in Fig 5. It should be noted that several of these mediators can act at more than one site. Not only can IL-1 and TNFα enhance the formation of osteoclasts, but they may also induce apoptosis of osteoblasts,[28] thereby retarding re-ossification of lytic bone sites. As OPG can abrogate the effects of RANKL, OPG therapy might be beneficial in patients with RA.[29] If this were to be successfully implemented, similar treatment may also prove valuable to patients with hemophilic arthropathy.

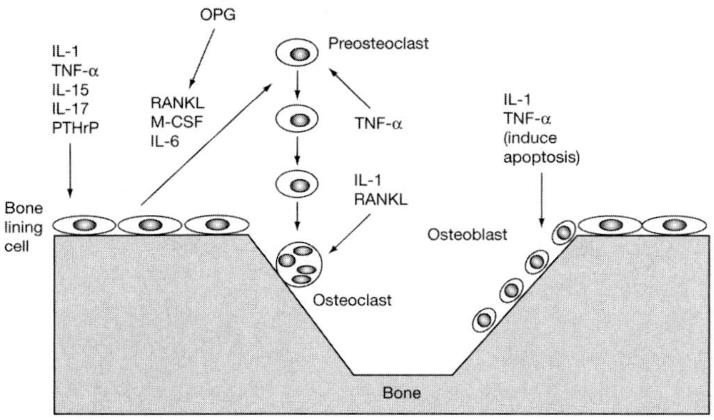

Figure 5 The proposed sites of action of cytokines and growth factors involved in the regulation of bone resorption.[6] Interleukin-1 (IL-1), tumor necrosis factor α (TNFα), interleukin-15 (IL-15), interleukin-17 (IL-17), and parathyroid hormone related peptide (PTHrP) enhance osteoclast formation by stimulating production of receptor activator of nuclear factor κB ligand (RANKL), interleukin-6 (IL-6), and monocyte/macrophage-colony stimulating factor (M-CSF) from bone-lining cells. Osteoprotegerin (OPG) is a soluble decoy receptor that binds RANKL, blocking its osteoclast-inducing activity. TNFα also acts directly on osteoclast precursors to induce their differentiation into osteoclasts. IL-1 and RANKL act directly on osteoclasts to increase their resorbing activity. IL-1 and TNFα may also contribute to bone loss by inducing osteoblast apoptosis. Reprinted with permission from Goldring et al.[6]

Cartilage

Cartilage formation is dependent on aggrecan, the chondroitin sulfate proteoglycan, which creates the cartilaginous surface that allows movement of joints. Multiple aggrecans bind to hyaluronic acid (via a "link protein") to form multimers that provide articular cartilage with frictionless motion. Aggrecan is very abundant in cartilage and also plays a critical role in providing compressibility of the joint. Although bone is continuously remodeled, the turnover of cartilage is relatively limited and damaged tissue has a restricted capability for repair. Chondrocytes are responsible for this process, providing mediators that can degrade damaged matrix material to enable subsequent repair. Chondrocytes also synthesize the extracellular matrix of articular cartilage.

In RA, cartilage destruction proceeds by two independent mechanisms—one indirect and one direct.[5] In the indirect method of cartilage loss, chondrocyte function is disrupted by pannus-derived cytokines and other mediators (such as IL-1 and TNFα). The chondrocytes are subsequently induced to release products that degrade the cartilage. The direct method of cartilage destruction occurs when products (such as matrix metalloproteinases and cathepsins) that can degrade the cartilage matrix are produced by the synovium.

Angiogenesis

An increase in vasculature is associated with the invasive and destructive processes that can occur in the joints of patients. Vascular endothelial growth factor (VEGF) plays a key role here.[30] Ballara et al[31] have shown that, in patients with early RA, there is a significant correlation between concentrations of serum VEGF measured at presentation and the development of joint damage 1 year later. Expression of synovial VEGF may be modulated by TNFα.[32] Acharya et al[33] have recently described the first direct evidence implicating angiogenesis in the development of hemophilic synovitis. Patients who had joint disease as a consequence of hemophilia exhibited significantly increased concentrations of plasma VEGF compared with healthy controls and individuals with bleeding disorders that did not result in joint disease. Levels of matrix metalloproteinase-9, another proangiogenic factor, were also elevated in patients with hemophilic joint disease compared with the other two groups.

Conclusions

Hemophilic arthropathy occurs as a result of changes to the synovium, bone, cartilage and blood vessels associated with affected joints. Iron has a critical role in the pathogenesis of such changes, and may be involved in a variety of different pathways. Hemophilic arthropathy shares some injury characteristics with rheumatoid arthropathy, although the degree of analogy is a matter of some debate. The mechanisms underlying joint inflammation are better understood for RA than for hemophilia, and it is hoped that increased knowledge of the changes associated with RA might provide new avenues of investigation into the pathogenesis of hemophilic arthropathy. This, in turn, may allow the identification of possible targets for novel therapeutic intervention.

References

1. Rodriguez-Merchan EC: Pathogenesis, early diagnosis, and prophylaxis for chronic hemophilic synovitis. Clin Orthop Relat Res 343:6-11, 1997
2. Arnold WD, Hilgartner MW: Hemophilic arthropathy. Current concepts of pathogenesis and management. J Bone Joint Surg Am 59:287-305, 1977
3. Rodriguez-Merchan EC: Pathogenesis of musculoskeletal complications of haemophilia, in Rodriguez-Merchan EC, Lee CA (eds): Inhibitors in patients with haemophilia. Oxford, UK, Blackwell, 2002, pp 115-119
4. Roosendaal G, Vianen ME, Wenting MJ, van Rinsum AC, van den Berg HM, Lafeber FP, et al: Iron deposits and catabolic properties of synovial tissue from patients with haemophilia. J Bone Joint Surg Br 80:540-545, 1998
5. Goldring SR: Pathogenesis of bone and cartilage destruction in rheumatoid arthritis. Rheumatology (Oxford) 42:11-16, 2003 (suppl 2)
6. Goldring SR: Pathogenesis of bone erosions in rheumatoid arthritis. Curr Opin Rheumatol 14:406-410, 2002
7. Berckmans RJ, Nieuwland R, Tak PP, Boing AN, Romijn FP, Kraan MC, et al: Cell-derived microparticles in synovial fluid from inflamed arthritic joints support coagulation exclusively via a factor VII-independent mechanism. Arthritis Rheum 46:2857-2866, 2002
8. Wen F-Q, Jabbar AA, Chen Y-X, Kazarian T, Patel DA, Valentino LA: c-*myc* proto-oncogene expression in hemophilic synovitis: In vitro studies of the effects of iron and ceramide. Blood 100:912-916, 2002
9. Yamanishi Y, Firestein GS: Pathogenesis of rheumatoid arthritis: The role of synoviocytes. Rheum Dis Clin North Am 27:355-371, 2001
10. Stein H, Duthie RB: The pathogenesis of chronic haemophilic arthropathy. J Bone Joint Surg Br 63B:601-609, 1981
11. Morris CJ, Wainwright AC, Steven MM, Blake DR: The nature of iron deposits in haemophilic synovitis. An immunochemical, ultrastruc-

tural and X-ray microanalytical study. Virchows Arch A Pathol Anat Histopathol 404:75-85, 1984
12. Morris CJ, Blake DR, Wainwright AC, Steven MM: Relationship between iron deposits and tissue damage in the synovium: an ultrastructural study. Ann Rheum Dis 45:21-26, 1986
13. Muirden KD, Senator GB: Iron in the synovial membrane in rheumatoid arthritis and other joint diseases. Ann Rheum Dis 27:38-48, 1968
14. Ogilvie-Harris DJ, Fornaiser VL: Synovial iron deposition in osteoarthritis and rheumatoid arthritis. J Rheumatol 7:30-36, 1980
15. Blake DR, Hall ND, Bacon PA, Dieppe PA, Halliwell B, Gutteridge JM: The importance of iron in rheumatoid disease. Lancet 8256:1142-1144, 1981
16. Blake DR, Gallagher PJ, Potter AR, Bell MJ, Bacon PA: The effect of synovial iron on the progression of rheumatoid disease. A histologic assessment of patients with early rheumatoid synovitis. Arthritis Rheum 27:495-501, 1984
17. Roosendaal G, Vianen ME, van den Berg HM, Lafeber FP, Bijlsma JW: Cartilage damage as a result of hemarthrosis in a human in vitro model. J Rheumatol 24:1350-1354, 1997
18. Roosendaal G: Deleterious effects of a short exposure of joint cartilage to blood: A mechanism of blood-induced arthropathy. Presented at The Joint Workshop: The Haemophilic Joint Under the Microscope, Toronto, Canada, November 12-13, 2004
19. Key NS, Bach RR: Tissue factor as a therapeutic target. Thromb Haemost 85:375-376, 2001
20. Brinkmann T, Kahnert H, Prohaska W, Nordfang O, Kleesiek K: Synthesis of tissue factor pathway inhibitor in human synovial cells and chondrocytes makes joints the predilected site of bleeding in haemophiliacs. Eur J Clin Chem Clin Biochem 32:313-317, 1994
21. Roivainen A, Söderström K-O, Pirală L, Aro H, Kortekangas P, Merilahti-Palo R, et al: Oncoprotein expression in human synovial tissue: An immunohistochemical study of different types of arthritis. Br J Rheumatol 35:933-942, 1996
22. Hakobyan N, Kazarian T, Jabbar AA, Jabbar KJ, Valentino LA: Pathobiology of hemophilic synovitis I: Overexpression of mdm2 oncogene. Blood 104:2060-2064, 2004
23. Tak PP, Zvaifler NJ, Green DR, Firestein GS: Rheumatoid arthritis and p53: How oxidative stress might alter the course of inflammatory diseases. Immunol Today 21:78-82, 2000
24. Hofbauer LC, Heufelder AE: The role of osteoprotegerin and receptor activator of nuclear factor κB ligand in the pathogenesis and treatment of rheumatoid arthritis. Arthritis Rheum 44:253-259, 2001
25. Kong YY, Yoshida H, Sarosi I, Tan HL, Timms E, Capparelli C, et al: OPGL is a key regulator of osteoclastogenesis, lymphocyte development and lymph-node organogenesis. Nature 397:315-323, 1999
26. Wong BR, Josien R, Choi Y: TRANCE is a TNF family member that regulates dendritic cell and osteoclast function. J Leukoc Biol 65:715-724, 1999
27. Hofbauer LC, Khosla S, Lacey DL, Dunstan CR, Lacey DL, Boyle WJ, et al: The roles of osteoprotegerin and osteoprotegerin ligand in the paracrine regulation of bone resorption. J Bone Miner Res 15:2-12, 2000
28. Tsuboi M, Kawakami A, Nakashima T, Matsuoka N, Urayama S, Kawabe Y, et al: Tumor necrosis factor-α and interleukin-1β increase the Fas-mediated apoptosis of human osteoblasts. J Lab Clin Med 134:222-231, 1999
29. Saidenberg-Kermanac'h N, Cohen-Solal M, Bessis N, De Vernejoul MC, Boissier MC: Role for osteoprotegerin in rheumatoid inflammation. Joint Bone Spine 71:9-13, 2004
30. Afuwape AO, Kiriakidis S, Paleolog EM: The role of the angiogenic molecule VEGF in the pathogenesis of rheumatoid arthritis. Histol Histopathol 17:961-972, 2002
31. Ballara SC, Taylor PC, Reusch P, Marmé D, Feldmann M, Maini RN, et al: Raised serum vascular endothelial growth factor levels are associated with destructive change in inflammatory arthritis. Arthritis Rheum 44:2055-2064, 2001
32. Paleolog EM, Young S, Stark AC, McCloskey RV, Feldmann M, Maini RN: Modulation of angiogenic vascular endothelial growth factor by tumor necrosis factor α and interleukin-1 in rheumatoid arthritis. Arthritis Rheum 41:1258-1265, 1998
33. Acharya SS, MacDonald DD, DiMichele DM, Hilgartner MW, Greninger DA, Goldberg I, et al: A role for angiogenesis in hemophilic synovitis. Blood 104:16a, 2004 (abstr 42)

ELSEVIER

Seminars in
HEMATOLOGY

Surgery in Hemophilia. The General View: Patient Selection, Timing, and Preoperative Assessment

Jørgen Ingerslev and Ivan Hvid

Although often overlooked, the life of the patient with severe hemophilia is characterized by both intermittent and chronic pain. Bleeds into joints and muscles cause extensive pressure on sensory nerves and, following recurrent bleeds, joint destruction, and synovial reaction is accompanied by constant pains that are frequently mistaken for further bleeding. The orthopedic surgeon may break the vicious cycle of chronic synovitis by excising inflamed and hypertrophic synovium or severely damaged cartilage and adjacent bone ends, and implanting an artificial joint. Numerous technical solutions are now available and orthopedic surgery is increasingly on offer to those hemophilia patients who, since childhood, have been victims of insufficiently treated bleeds because no or limited treatment was available, and because the concept of prophylaxis had not yet been developed. Nonetheless, orthopedic surgery in patients with hemophilia requires much more effort and planning than surgery in non-hemophilic patients. In this overview, we will address issues related to surgery in hemophilic patients, as well as some practical issues related to the timing of surgery, preoperative testing, perioperative hemostasis, and patient rehabilitation.
Semin Hematol 43(suppl 1):S23-S26

Just a few decades ago, surgical interventions in patients with hemophilia were regarded as difficult and associated with great risks; this was particularly the case in abdominal surgery. Major issues included the lack of sufficient replacement factor concentrate, the risk of hemolytic complications associated with use of the relatively impure concentrates available, uncontrolled bleeding, transmission of blood-borne infectious agents, postoperative infections, and problems with wound healing. Today, substitution factor concentrates are abundantly available and are characterized by high purity, few or no red cell alloagglutinin antibodies, and a high degree of viral safety. Irrespective of these advances, the relative fragility of the hemophilic clot, which may undergo premature fibrinolysis causing re-bleeding, delayed wound healing, and thus impaired outcome, is a challenge to surgical intervention in the hemophilic patient. Due to the high costs of surgery and the associated replacement therapy, as well as the relative risk of untoward complications, indications should be stringently defined prior to any surgical intervention in patients with hemophilia.

When planning surgery in the hemophilic patient, the type of procedure selected is an important consideration. Recently developed, low-cost management programs for dental surgery have considerably helped to improve dental health status in people with hemophilia and, nowadays, oral surgical procedures are commonplace in most countries. Indeed, any type of surgery available to patients with a normal bleeding pattern may now be offered to hemophilic patients. Thus, elective procedures, such as appendectomies, herniotomies, cholecystectomies, and even coronary artery bypass grafting, are technically manageable in hemophilic patients and are associated with a low frequency of bleeding problems. Even acute surgical interventions are not uncommon in these patients.

Orthopedic surgery has an important role in adult hemophilia patients who, during childhood, had no or limited access to effective hemostatic agents. Joint and bone surgery occurs predominately in the elderly. Inadequately treated hemophilia is a painful disorder causing discomfort to the patient during bleeding episodes and pain when recurrent bleeds lead to synovial inflammation. When recurrent hem-

Centre for Haemophilia and Thrombosis, and Department of Orthopaedic Surgery, University Hospital Aarhus, Aarhus N, Denmark.
Address correspondence to Jørgen Ingerslev, DMSc, Centre for Haemophilia and Thrombosis, University Hospital, Aarhus/Skejby, Brendstrupgaardsvej 100, DK-8200, Aarhus N, Denmark. E-mail: Ingerslev@ki.au.dk

0037-1963/06/$-see front matter
doi:10.1053/j.seminhematol.2005.11.024

arthrosis eventually converts the bleeding joint into chronic arthropathy, the patient's physical range of motion and ability to mobilize is painfully restricted.

The orthopedic surgeon can offer the disabled patient a wide range of options for the relief of chronic pain. These include surgical synovectomies, which can be very helpful in the early stages of joint degeneration. When arthropathy is severe, arthroplasties of various kinds, such as replacement of knees and hips, may be feasible. Recent advances in artificial joint manufacture have provided joint replacement technologies for ankles, shoulders, and elbows.

The optimal timing of orthopedic surgery during the lifetime of the hemophilic patient is a matter of some controversy. While some surgeons delay surgery until joint destruction is advanced, others believe that the patient should have access to joint replacements while still relatively young and in good physical shape with strong muscles and an active life. These issues, together with some of the practical considerations of orthopedic surgery in the hemophilia patient, will be addressed in this overview.

Rehabilitation Surgery—Who Are the Users?

In contrast with elderly hemophilia patients, for whom treatment options in childhood were severely limited, the young child of today has many therapies available, which avail a bright outlook for their future health. Easy access to treatment with concentrate at appropriate dosages, including early home treatment of bleeds, is essential for an on-demand treatment program. Although medical evidence by highest standards has not been found to favor prophylactic treatment programs, the very positive and convincing results emanating from the strict use of such programs are widely recognized in countries where prophylaxis has been used for two or more decades.[1-3] Not only does the patient who underwent strict prophylactic treatment during his growth period present in good physical condition, as witnessed by low joint scores; he is also much less likely to require surgery, particularly orthopedic interventions.[4] In countries where strict prophylactic administration of factor concentrates was initiated more than 25 years ago, the population of hemophilia patients can be strikingly divided by age, with the physical capabilities of the under-25s dramatically better than those of more advanced age. Although we are still not encouraged to conclude that, in the longer term, orthopedic surgery will not be needed by people with hemophilia, we have good reasons to believe that the physical health of the younger generation of patients will be better than anything seen before. Indeed, in today's hemophilia setting, it is the elderly who are the major consumers of orthopedic surgery.

Which Type of Surgery?

More than 75% of bleeds in patients with severe hemophilia are joint bleeds; the remaining 25% of episodes include muscle hematomas and other bleeds. This bleeding pattern explains why joint hemorrhage is the major cause of devastating pain and disabling joint destruction in people with hemophilia. The task of the orthopedic surgeon is to relieve pain and, hopefully, to restore some of the lost joint function.

The list of surgical interventions available to hemophilic patients is rapidly growing. Only a few years ago the choice was limited to surgical "cleaning" of inflamed and neovascularized synovium by careful "open" or arthroscopic procedures. The options have widened to include joint replacement of knees and hips as well as fusion of painful ankle joints, and a large variety of joint replacements are offered today. During the last decade, joint replacement of ankles, elbows, and shoulders has become technically manageable and increasingly practiced in many centers. In addition, alignment osteotomy and tendon release and lengthening are procedures often provided to improve joint mobility.

How Far Can We Go Without Surgery?

Before consulting the orthopedic surgeon, a thorough evaluation of the patient's joint problems is advisable. Secondary prophylaxis over a 2-month period, where factor concentrate in doses ranging from 25 IU/kg to 40 IU/kg is administered three times per week or every 2 days (every 3 days in patients with hemophilia B), serves two important purposes. If the problem of painful motion and joint swelling is due to unresolved recurrent bleeding or chronic synovitis, the patient may recover in a month or two with this regimen. If there are no signs of resolution, and if supplementary investigations such as ultrasound, x-ray, or magnetic resonance imaging point to a diagnosis of chronic synovitis or end-stage joint destruction, then chemical synoviorthesis or a surgical procedure may be required.

Is Surgery Advisable?

From information on outcomes of orthopedic hemophilia surgery extracted from the literature, it is quite obvious that opinions amongst our orthopedic surgeon colleagues are quite mixed, particularly in relation to joint replacements, ranging from deep pessimism to a very optimistic approach. Concerns relate to deep infection, bleeding, and loosening of the replaced joint. Since surgical procedural techniques in hemophilia have not been challenged with controlled randomized clinical trials, outcome data will, to a large extent, depend on local skills and traditions developed in hemophilia patients and those with simple osteoarthritis. Likewise, selection of an artificial joint from the numerous types available on the market, and decisions on whether to use bone cement, are matters for individual consideration.

Timing of Surgery

The timing of surgery during the life of the hemophilic person is a matter of some controversy. While there is general agreement that advanced surgery, particularly joint replace-

Table 1 Preoperative Screening Program Before Major Hemophilic Surgery

Platelets	
	Count
	Aggregation with agonists (collagen and adenosine diphosphate)
Plasma clotting tests	
	Activated partial thromboplastin time
	Prothrombin time
	Factor VIII/factor IX
	Inhibitor test
	Fibrinogen
Response recording	
	Recovery of factor VIII/factor IX after a dose of around 30 IU/kg to 50 IU/kg bodyweight

ment, has no place in children and young patients during their growth period, the tendency towards a more aggressive approach to surgery in younger patients is based on the rationale that the patient deserves optimal physical health while young and while the musculature is still in a good condition. Furthermore, young persons are generally more easily rehabilitated after orthopedic surgery than older patients. The more demanding social and professional life of youth also favors the early correction of joint disease. These factors have contributed to the tendency towards early orthopedic intervention, and the focus of such procedures has shifted from the relief of pain towards the correction of functional disability.

Patient Compliance

When the issue of surgery is first raised, the patient should be aware that his personal commitment to active engagement with the rehabilitation training program is critical to outcome. He should also be informed that there is no guarantee for significant postsurgical improvement in joint range of motion, even with an optimal surgical procedure. Patients receiving a new joint should be informed about the limited long-term durability of prostheses and the risk of both joint loosening and bone shaft fractures, should excessive strain be applied to the new joint.

Preparing for Surgery

The patient's hemostatic functions should be screened prior to surgery. Laboratory tests monitored by the authors prior to all major orthopedic procedures in hemophilic patients are given in Table 1. It is important that an inhibitor test be performed no earlier than 2 months before surgery, and that an in vivo response assessment is performed to test the recovery of a standardized dose of the factor concentrate selected for substitution during surgery. Data obtained from these tests can be used to plan the substitution program during and after surgery. Blood chemistry data should minimally include platelet count, platelet function, prothrombin time, and fibrinogen levels. Thromboprophylaxis should be administered according to local guidelines for hemophilia surgery. In addition, the patient's blood group should be determined and the presence of irregular antibodies screened for. If a plasma-derived concentrate is used in patients with a non-O blood group, the alloagglutinin titer of the batch used should be obtained from the manufacturer.

Based on the response (recovery), a substitution program should be outlined, giving exact information on the number of units of coagulation factor to be used and the timing of concentrate infusion during surgery and the entire post-operative period. Both the administration schedule and sufficient bottles of concentrate should be brought to the surgical ward prior to surgery. In our clinic, the patient is provided with a copy of the substitution plan.

The substitution schedule should also provide information about the need for prophylactic treatment during the rehabilitation training program both in hospital and at home. Monitoring of factor VIII (FVIII) or factor IX (FIX) should be done immediately after the first preoperative infusion of concentrate, and at least once daily for the first 3 to 5 postoperative days. If a dosing program based on bolus injections is selected, the trough value in the postoperative period should not go below 50 IU/dL during the first 3 to 4 days. For regimens with continuous infusion, a similar target level of FVIII or FIX is desirable during that same time period, but infusion rates may be reduced from day 5. Concentrate costs may therefore be lowered with continuous infusion. Samples may be collected at any time during stable constant infusion delivery.

The Patient With Inhibitors to Factor VIII or IX

The patient with hemophilia complicated by inhibitors will need particular attention during any orthopedic procedure. The preoperative laboratory screening should follow the principles outlined in Table 1. However, the efficacy of bypassing agents, such as FEIBA (Baxter Corp, Deerfield, IL) and recombinant activated factor VII (rFVIIa; NovoSeven®, Novo Nordisk, Bagsvaerd, Denmark), varies among patients, and assessment of response cannot be made in the usual way. In the authors' laboratory, in vivo and ex vivo investigations of response to bypassing agents are performed using a thrombelastograph.[5] In contrast with hemophilic patients without inhibitors, the inhibitor patient has not been documented in larger clinical trials of orthopedic surgery, and so information is primarily based on single cases and reports documenting small patient populations.

In practice, activated prothrombin complex concentrate (FEIBA) doses of approximately 200 U/kg per 24 hours are administered as 3 doses per 24 hours during the first 3 days after surgery; thereafter the dose is reduced to 100 to 150 U/kg per 24 hours.[6] When used during orthopedic surgery, rFVIIa 90 to 100 μg/kg is administered every 2 hours during the first 36 to 48 hours, after which the intervals between doses are gradually prolonged.[7]

Mobilization and Training

An issue of particular interest and a frequent point of discussion is the timing of patient mobilization, including the use of constant passive movement machines, during the postoperative period. The contradictory points relate to a rough balance between the benefit of an increased range of motion achieved by early mobilization of the newly operated joint, versus avoidance of post-operative bleeding and prevention of long-term loss of motion achieved by immobilization of the same joint. The pros and cons of each argument are multiple and relate primarily to local experience. Most surgical departments tend to select the same postoperative training program for hemophilic patients as is used for non-hemophilic patients. When planning postoperative activities, however, they should take into account the reduced robustness of the blood clot, which is characteristic of hemophilia. Definitively secured hemostasis is achieved from around day 7 to 8, at which time rehabilitation training is considered safe for all patients. During rehabilitation training, the patient will receive concentrate before each exercise session for a minimum of 3 to 4 weeks.

Conclusions

Orthopedic surgery in hemophilic patients is truly a collective effort, involving not only the surgeon but also collaboration with the comprehensive hemophilia center to address serious considerations, such as patient age, hematologic status, and type of procedure likely to be most beneficial to the patient. The preoperative assessment of hemostasis and the patient's response to infusion should be scrutinized well before the planned procedure. Similarly, well in advance of surgery, the patient should be made aware of the need for personal commitment to rehabilitation training so that maintenance—or even improvement—of joint and muscle function can be ensured.

References

1. Nilsson IM, Berntorp E, Löfqvist T, Pettersson H: Twenty-five years' experience of prophylactic treatment in severe haemophilia A and B. J Intern Med 232:25-32, 1992
2. Petrini P, Lindvall N, Egberg N, Blombäck M: Prophylaxis with factor concentrates in preventing hemophilic arthropathy. Am J Paediatr Hematol Oncol 13:280-287, 1991
3. Fischer K, van der Bom JG, Molho P, Negrier C, Mauser-Bunschoten EP, Roosendaal G, et al: Prophylactic versus on-demand treatment strategies for severe haemophilia: A comparison of costs and long-term outcome. Haemophilia 8:745-752, 2002
4. Steen Carlsson K, Höjgård S, Glomstein A, Lethagen S, Schulman S, Tengborn L, et al: On-demand vs. prophylactic treatment for severe haemophilia in Norway and Sweden: Differences in treatment characteristics and outcome. Haemophilia 9:555-566, 2003
5. Sørensen B, Ingerslev J: Whole blood clot formation phenotypes in haemophilia A and rare coagulation disorders. Patterns of response to recombinant factor VIIa. J Thromb Haemost 2:102-110, 2004
6. Tjønnfjord GE, Brinch L, Gedde-Dahl T, Brosstad FR: Activated prothrombin complex concentrate (FEIBA) treatment during surgery in patients with inhibitors to FVIII/IX. Haemophilia 10:174-178, 2004
7. Ingerslev J: Efficacy and safety of recombinant factor VIIa in the prophylaxis of bleeding in various surgical procedures in hemophilic patients with factor VIII and factor IX inhibitors. Semin Thromb Hemost 26:425-432, 2000

ELSEVIER

Seminars in
HEMATOLOGY

Functional Assessment of Arthropathy—An International Perspective

Pradeep M. Poonnoose[a] and Alok Srivastava[b]

Treatment of hemophilia aims to minimize structural damage to joints and maximize patients' functional independence and quality of life. From an orthopedic perspective, treatment efficacy can be judged by quantifying the extent of musculoskeletal damage. Joint scores—both clinical and radiologic—have traditionally been measured in patients with hemophilia. However, such scores may lack the sensitivity to detect early changes in the hemophilic joint, and this has prompted the development of more sensitive measures. In addition, scores based on the status of individual joints do not consider the impact of arthropathy on overall musculoskeletal function. It would prove valuable to understand the implications of small differences in clinical/radiologic scores in terms of overall musculoskeletal function and patients' quality of life. The development of functional scores such as the Functional Independence Score for Haemophilia (FISH) and the Haemophilia Activities List (HAL), along with the quality-of-life (QoL) measurement tools, have helped to provide a more comprehensive assessment of health in hemophilia. Such improved understanding should assist with the development of contextually relevant guidelines for the management of hemophilia.
Semin Hematol 43(suppl 1):S27-S32

Musculoskeletal dysfunction in hemophilia arises as a consequence of damage to joints and soft tissue caused by repeated bleeding. Therapy has been designed to treat, and indeed prevent, such bleeding. From an orthopedic perspective, treatment efficacy has been judged by quantifying the extent of musculoskeletal damage. This has traditionally been measured using both clinical and radiologic joint scores.[1,2] Long-term musculoskeletal outcome has been assessed using these scores, and has been correlated with the intensity of factor replacement therapy.[3-7]

There are, however, limitations to this approach. For instance, the clinical scoring system has never been validated, and both clinical and radiologic scores lack the sensitivity to detect early changes to the hemophilic joint.[8] Consequently, attention has been given to the development of more sensitive measures for clinical and radiologic assessments.[8-12] Another limitation associated with the currently used scores is that they are based on the status of individual joints rather than on the impact of changes on the overall musculoskeletal function of the individual.[13,14] Awareness of this limitation is important when evaluating the clinical significance of differences in the scores, and when correlating the scores with treatment protocols reported in the literature. Rather than relying on joint scores alone, joint health in hemophilia should be evaluated comprehensively using the standards set by the International Classification of Functioning, Disability, and Health (ICF).[13]

Musculoskeletal Outcome: Traditional Assessment Methods

Radiologic Scores

Jordon, in 1958, and later De Palma, in 1967, described the characteristic X-ray abnormalities seen in hemophilic arthropathy.[15] De Palma proposed four classes of joint destruction based on a combination of roentgenographic and clinical manifestations.[15] In 1977, Arnold and Hilgartner refined this classification into five stages.[16] Wood proposed a radiologic classification in 1969, but several parameters he described pertained to soft tissue changes seen in the acute stage of hemarthrosis.[17] In 1980, Pettersson created a scoring system based on the degree of joint destruction, as assessed by ra-

[a]Department of Orthopaedics, Christian Medical College, Vellore, India.
[b]Department of Haematology, Christian Medical College, Vellore, India.
Supported in part by the FLUID Research grant from the Christian Medical College, Vellore, India, and a grant received from the Bayer Haemophilia Awards Program.
Address correspondence to Alok Srivastava, MD, Professor of Medicine, Department of Haematology, Christian Medical College, Vellore 632004, India. E-mail: aloks@cmcvellore.ac.in

0037-1963/06/$-see front matter
doi:10.1053/j.seminhematol.2005.11.022

diologic changes seen in the six most commonly affected joints (ie, the knee, elbow, and ankle joints).[1] This was incorporated into the first joint-scoring system endorsed by the World Federation of Hemophilia (WFH)[2,18]—a system that has now become the standard for long-term outcome measurement in hemophilia.

The introduction of higher doses of primary prophylaxis enabled joints to be maintained at a stage where no radiologic changes could be detected.[3,4] As more patients maintained scores of zero (normal joints), conventional radiographs were deemed insensitive to early changes in the hemophilic joint. Consequently, scoring systems based on magnetic resonance imaging (MRI) were developed. These could detect changes to the joint before they were apparent in x-rays. Changes observed by MRI were first described in 1986 by Kulkarni et al,[19] and several other reports of MRI use soon followed. The Denver scale,[9] the European scale used by the Pediatric Network for Hemophilia Management (PedNet),[10] and the scale currently being developed by the International Prophylaxis Study Group (IPSG)[8] are all examples of scores based on MRI changes. These scoring systems will be important in assessing minimal joint arthropathy. However, the implications of minor changes in MRI/radiologic scores in terms of individual joint function and overall long-term musculoskeletal functional ability remain to be determined.

Physical Examination Scores

Although x-rays are widely available, and although the Pettersson score is reproducible,[20] the utility of x ray evaluation is limited because of the risk of radiation to young children. In addition, x-ray evaluation rarely reflects changes that occur in joint function as a result of therapeutic interventions, such as physiotherapy or surgical procedures.[12,21] Range of motion (ROM) has been the most commonly used physical outcome measure for evaluating the effects of intervention on joint health.[22-24] As more medical and surgical methods to improve function have become available, it has been necessary to develop an instrument to compare physical outcome measures across different populations of patients with hemophilia. With this in mind, the WFH developed the Physical Examination (PE) Scale. This scoring system, first described in 1985,[2,18] evaluates ROM, flexion deformity, swelling, crepitus, wasting, instability, and axial deformity in the six major joints. However, this scale was adopted and recommended for routine use at a time when most hemophilia patients in Western countries used much lower quantities of replacement therapy than they do now. In the Orthopaedic Outcome Study, reported in 1994, 90% of patients with hemophilia demonstrated changes in their joints, as assessed by radiologic and physical examination scores.[5] As larger quantities of factor concentrates were used for replacement therapy, and as the frequency of bleeding was reduced with the use of primary prophylaxis, more joints maintained zero (normal) scores on the WFH PE Scale.[25] In addition to this lack of sensitivity, the original WFH score has several other shortcomings. For instance, it does not take into account the normal physiologic changes that occur in children (ie, changes in hyper-extensibility, axial deformity, and muscle bulk differences between dominant and nondominant limbs).[12] Furthermore, the score does not assess strength—an important function that affects physical activity.

These observations have provided the impetus to develop new scoring systems with improved sensitivity and the ability to detect earlier deterioration in joint function. One such system involves the Colorado PE instruments (full and half point), described by Manco-Johnson et al.[11,12] Development of this scale involved modification of the WFH PE score (addition of one grade) to make it more sensitive in the areas of swelling, muscle atrophy, crepitus, ROM, and flexion contracture. Evaluations of gait and strength were also added, with strength being assessed using functional (rather than confrontational) tests. The same group also described the Young Child Scale,[11,12] in which pain is assessed using the Wong Baker Faces Pain Scale. The PedNet group have also introduced another tool based on the WFH PE score (the Stockholm instrument) in an attempt to increase the sensitivity of physical assessment.[26] These scores have been further modified by the IPSG to produce the Hemophilia Joint Health Score (HJHS), the initial validity of which has been assessed in 8 pediatric patients.[8] The inter-observer coefficient (as assessed by scoring the patients on 2 consecutive days) was 0.83, and the reliability of the test was found to be excellent. However, the instrument needs to be re-evaluated in a larger number of patients from different populations. It is also necessary to determine the extent to which each item in the score correlates with the structural/functional status of the joint.

An effective physical examination measure should reflect not only the changes seen in joint structure, but also the individual's disability. To evaluate items in a scoring system, it is necessary to assess how each item correlates with both structural changes in the joint (x-ray/MRI score) and an individual's functional independence. The weight given to each item should be based on the extent to which it affects structure/function; for example, it should be decided whether swelling in the knee joint should be scored the same as a flexion deformity of 90 degrees. An additional consideration is that similar changes in different joints affect functional independence to different extents. In the knee joint, a lack of full extension is disabling, whereas a lack of full flexion is more disabling in the elbow. A person with a 15-degree loss of extension at the elbow may not have any disability, but a person with full extension and a flexion limitation to 90 degrees at this joint would find it extremely difficult to eat and perform activities of daily living with the upper limb. If a physical examination score is to reflect disability, the scoring system should incorporate these factors.

While some items on assessment scores (such as ROM and strength) may reflect function and structure, others (such as crepitus and swelling) may involve changes in the joint that do not necessarily correlate with either disability or the severity of hemophilia. However, it is necessary to account for such structural differences, even if they do not impact di-

Table 1 Clinical Characteristics, Treatment Details, and Musculoskeletal Outcome in Patients With Severe Hemophilia

	Sweden		The Netherlands			India
	Group 1*	Group 2*	1980†	1990†	2000†	2004‡
Age (yr)	21–35	13–20	20.3 (15–25)	19.4 (15–25)	19.2 (15–25)	19 (15–26)
No.	25	19	45	46	44	30
Clinical score	5.1 (0–15)	1.2 (0–7)	NA	NA	NA	11 (0–26)
Pettersson's score	18 (0–41)	4.8 (0–22)	17 (11.5–33.8)	17 (7–27)	8 (0–16)	18 (0–48)
% with Pettersson's score of zero	NR	NR	4	10	32	3
Annual clotting factor usage (IU/kg/yr)	400–3,300	1,600–5,400	855 (411–1,121)	1,319 (769–1,667)	2,036 (1,554–2,425)	25–150

Abbreviations: NA, not available; NR, not reported.
Adapted with permission from Fischer et al,[28] Blackwell Publishing.
*Values are means (ranges). From Nilsson et al.[6]
†Values are medians (interquartile ranges).
‡Clinical and radiological score values are medians (ranges); age is mean value.

rectly on function, as they are pathological features of the diseased joint.

Musculoskeletal Outcome: Correlation With Factor Replacement Therapy

In most Western countries, treatment for hemophilia has focused on preventing joint arthropathy by administering high-dose factor replacement.[3-6] Aledort expounded that the key to joint preservation was to reduce the incidence of joint bleeds through full-time primary prophylaxis,[5] and a study by Astermark emphasized the importance of starting prophylaxis at an early age.[7] In the Netherlands, where hemophilic children are given primary prophylaxis with intravenous factors from the age of 1 year, radiologic and clinical joint scores are significantly lower than those of similar French patients treated primarily with an on-demand strategy.[4] In addition, Fischer et al studied the effect of intermediate and high-dose prophylactic treatment on joint arthropathy. It was reported that patients in a high-dose prophylaxis group had fewer joint bleeds than those in a group receiving an intermediate dose (median 0.3 per year *v* 3.3 per year, respectively) and more joints with a radiologic score of zero (69% *v* 32%, respectively).[27] It would be interesting to study radiologic and clinical scores in relation to the dosage of factor used, and to determine the implications of minor differences in these scores with regard to function and quality of life (QoL). Objective functional outcome measures could be a valuable adjunct to determine the impact of high-dose therapy, and to analyze its cost/benefit ratio.

Comparison of data from Sweden and the Netherlands with those from India produces some interesting results.[28] The median radiologic score in an Indian cohort of patients with hemophilia was 18 (range, 0 to 48), which is similar to the scores seen in the other two countries two decades ago, despite a wide variation in factor usage (400 to 3,300 U/kg/yr in Sweden and 25 to 150 U/kg/yr in India) (Table 1). This observation seems to indicate that eventual joint arthropathy may not be influenced by the amount of factor consumed, as originally suggested by Aledort.[5] It could also imply that present outcome measures are not sensitive enough. Despite similar radiologic joint scores in the three countries, there may be significant differences in the functional ability of these patients. Therefore, it is necessary to evaluate the effect of hemarthrosis not only on a single joint, but also on musculoskeletal function as a whole.

Musculoskeletal Outcome: The Concept of Overall Function

Global assessment of joint health should not only include changes in joint architecture and joint function, but should also evaluate how these changes affect both the patient's ability to perform activities and the patient's QoL. Such an assessment is in line with the principles of the ICF[29] (Fig 1).

According to the ICF, evaluation of disability and health should focus on two areas. The first of these covers "*components of functioning and disability*" and consists of *body structures and functions, activities,* and *participation. Body structures* are parts of the body such as organs, limbs, and their components. *Body functions* are defined as the physiological functions of these systems, such as ROM, strength, and instability. *Activities* involve executing tasks or actions, and a range of activities that can be performed by the individual are cov-

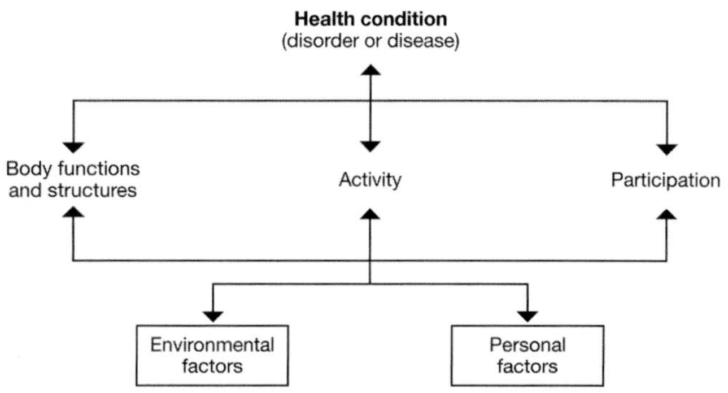

Figure 1 Interactions between the components of the International Classification of Functioning, Disability, and Health.[29]

ered. *Participation* is defined as involvement in a life situation, such as sport, leisure, work, or social events. The ICF provides a single list of *activities* and *participation* in nine domains. According to their needs and purposes, investigators can designate some domains as *activities* and others as *participation*, without overlap; alternatively, they can designate all domains to be potentially both *activities* and *participation*, and use qualifiers to differentiate the data. The components of the list can be affected by *contextual factors*, which represent a person's background, and include both *environmental* and *personal* factors. *Environmental factors* comprise the physical, social, and attitudinal environment in which an individual lives and conducts day-to-day activities. These factors are either barriers to, or facilitators of, functioning. They include social attitudes, architectural characteristics, and social and legal structures, as well as climate and terrain. *Personal factors* include aspects of an individual's life that are not necessarily part of the health condition or health status, such as age, sex, and indigenous status. The concept of *QoL* is complex, and embraces many characteristics of the social and physical environment, as well as the health and internal state of the individual.[29]

Table 2 Functional Independence Score in Haemophilia[41]

Self-care	Transfer	Locomotion
Eating and grooming	Chair	Walking
Bathing	Squatting	Step climbing
Dressing		

Scores in each area range from 1–4:
1: The subject is unable to perform the activity, or needs complete assistance to perform the activity.
2: The subject needs partial assistance/aids/modified instruments/a modified environment to perform the activity.
3: The subject is able to perform the activity without aids or assistance, but with slight discomfort. He is unable to perform the activity like healthy peers.
4: The subject is able to perform the activity without any difficulty, like healthy peers.

Reproduced with permission from Poonnoose et al,[41] Blackwell Publishing.

Musculoskeletal Outcome: Assessment of Functional Independence in Hemophilia

Several validated outcome instruments are available to assess functional independence in patients with musculoskeletal conditions.[30-38] Some of these measure patients' general health status, while others measure outcomes specific to an organ or disease condition. Several of the instruments have been used to assess patients with hemophilia. The Short Form of the Medical Outcomes Study (SF36)[30-32] and the Sickness Impact Profile (SIP)[33,34] do not refer to any specific disease, but provide information relating to general health. The Western Ontario McMaster Questionnaire (WOMAC)[35,36] was originally designed to be used in patients with osteoarthritis, while the Stanford Health Assessment Questionnaire (HAQ)[37] and the Childhood Health Assessment Questionnaire (CHAQ)[25,38] are used primarily for patients with juvenile rheumatoid arthritis. In one review, De Kleijn et al identified 12 clinimetric instruments that have been used to assess the impact of hemophilia on the patient's ability to perform activities.[39] None were specific for hemophilia, nor were they validated for use in this condition. They were all based on the subjective assessment of disability, and none were performance-based. More recently, van Genderen et al developed the Hemophilia Activities List (HAL), a self-assessment questionnaire that assesses disability in hemophilia patients.[40] This is a disease-specific, self-rated questionnaire based on the ICF classification. It is a subjective assessment of disability, and is therefore language-dependent. As the HAL was validated on patients with an average age of approximately 40 years, its applicability in children needs to be assessed. The applicability of the questionnaire in different cultures also remains to be determined.

Studies evaluating outcomes in individuals from different cultural backgrounds would require a performance-based assessment tool and validated, translated versions of subjective scores such as the HAL—or, better still, a combination of both subjective and objective scores. We have developed a performance-based score for this purpose—the Functional Independence Score in Haemophilia (FISH). This provides an objective assessment of different aspects of a patient's functional ability.[41] Hemophilia patients and their therapists were asked to list activities that could be affected by hemophilia, and these were categorized according to the ICF. Activities that were considered unsafe to perform were excluded from the assessment. Other activities that could not be assessed objectively in the clinic, such as participation in education and employment, and the use of transport, were also excluded. The final assessment included seven activities (eating, grooming, dressing, chair transfer, squatting, walking, and step climbing) that were graded from 1 to 4 according to the amount of assistance required to perform them (Table 2). Each activity and level of independence was clearly defined to reduce inter-observer variance. Initial psychometric evaluation has shown good internal consistency (Cronbach's alpha 0.83). The FISH has a good correlation with the HAQ, but only moderate correlation with the radiologic and WFH PE scores. The reliability and responsiveness of the FISH, together with its correlation to other functional scores, are currently being assessed, as is its applicability in different cultural settings.

The Pettersson score has shown good correlation with the severity of hemophilia, the duration of the disease, and the number of hemarthroses.[1,12,42] Several studies appear to suggest that there is also a good correlation between bleeding frequency and disability.[5,37] The correlation between the WFH PE score and functional independence, as measured by a patient's ability to perform activities, needs to be further evaluated with appropriate instruments. In osteoarthritis, it has been observed that there is poor correlation between functional independence and those structural changes in the joint that can be detected by x-rays.[43] It is likely that the same holds true for patients with hemophilia. In our study with the FISH, where a large number of patients had significantly damaged joints, we found that radiologic scores correlated only moderately with functional independence.[41] Many patients with hemophilia appear to function reasonably well despite having severe arthropathy, using a limited ROM.[37,44]

Musculoskeletal Outcome: Assessment of Participation and QoL

Although the FISH provides an objective measure of a patient's ability to perform activities, it does not study the effect of hemarthrosis on a patient's ability to participate in social activities. Days missed from work, and the ability to engage in sports/physical activities, are not assessed. These activities affect QoL and are measured using other scoring systems like the SF36,[30-32,45] the Arthritis Impact Measurement Scale (AIMS),[46] and the EuroQoL Five-Dimension Questionnaire (EQ–5D).[32,47] More recently, hemophilia-specific scores, such as the Haemo-QoL,[48] the Canadian Health Outcomes–Kids Life Assessment Tool (CHO-KLAT),[49] the Hemofilia QoL,[50] and the Hemolatin-QoL,[51] have been developed and studied in the different populations. The use of these tools will need to be evaluated in a range of cultures before any of them can be accepted as a universal assessment tool in hemophilia. As QoL questionnaires are cumulative outcome measures, giving little insight into the problems that give rise to a diminished QoL score, they may not be helpful in targeting interventions.[40] Nevertheless, evaluating the effect of repeated hemarthroses on the QoL of patients with hemophilia is an important aspect of outcome measurement that needs further assessment.

Concluding Remarks

The aims of treatment in hemophilia are to minimize structural damage and maximize functional independence and QoL. While a radiologic score of zero may be construed as ideal, the level of factor support required to achieve this may not be feasible in most parts of the world. We need to document long-term musculoskeletal structural and functional outcomes at different dosing regimens.[28] It would be helpful to understand the implications of small but statistically significant differences in radiologic/clinical scores in terms of overall musculoskeletal function and QoL. Such data should assist the development of contextually relevant guidelines for the management of hemophilia.

References

1. Pettersson H, Ahlberg A, Nilsson IM: A radiologic classification of hemophilic arthropathy. Clin Orthop Relat Res 149:153-159, 1980
2. Pettersson H, Gilbert MS: Classification of the hemophilic arthropathy, in Pettersson H, Gilbert MS (eds): Diagnostic imaging in hemophilia. New York, NY, Springer-Verlag, 1985, pp 56-68
3. Lofqvist T, Nilsson IM, Berntorp E, Pettersson H: Haemophilia prophylaxis in young patients—A long-term follow-up. J Intern Med 241:395-400, 1997
4. Fischer K, van der Bom JG, Molho P, Negrier C, Mauser-Bunschoten EP, Roosendaal G, et al: Prophylactic versus on-demand treatment strategies for severe haemophilia: A comparison of costs and long-term outcome. Haemophilia 8:745-752, 2002
5. Aledort LM, Haschmeyer RH, Pettersson H, Orthopaedic Outcome Study Group: A longitudinal study of orthopaedic outcomes for severe factor-VIII-deficient haemophiliacs. J Intern Med 236:391-399, 1994
6. Nilsson IM, Berntorp E, Lofqvist T, Pettersson H: Twenty-five years' experience of prophylactic treatment in severe haemophilia A and B. J Intern Med 232:25-32, 1992
7. Astermark J, Petrini P, Tengborn L, Schulman S, Ljung R, Berntop E: Primary prophylaxis in severe haemophilia should be started at an early age but can be individualized. Br J Haematol 105:1109-1113, 1999
8. Manco-Johnson MJ, Pettersson H, Petrini P, Babyn PS, Bergstrom B-M, Bradley C-S, et al: Physical therapy and imaging outcome measures in a haemophilia population treated with factor prophylaxis: current status and future directions. Haemophilia 10:88-93, 2004 (suppl 4)
9. Nuss R, Kilcoyne RF, Geraghty S, Shroyer AL, Rosky JW, Mawhinney S, et al: MRI findings in haemophilic joints treated with radiosynoviorthesis with development of an MRI scale of joint damage. Haemophilia 6:162-169, 2000
10. Lundin B, Pettersson H, Ljung R: A new magnetic resonance imaging scoring method for assessment of haemophilic arthropathy. Haemophilia 10:383-389, 2004
11. Manco-Johnson MJ, Nuss R, Funk S, Murphy J: Joint evaluation instruments for children and adults with haemophilia. Haemophilia 6:649-657, 2000
12. Manco-Johnson MJ, Funk S: Joint evaluation instruments in haemophilia, in Rodriguez-Merchan EC (ed): The Haemophilic Joints. New Perspectives. Oxford, UK, Blackwell Publishing, 2003, pp 45-55
13. De Kleijn P, Heijnen L, Roosendaal G, Mauser-Bunschoten EP, Fischer K, Van Den Berg HM, et al: Towards a new WFH standard for assessment of health status in hemophilia patients. Haemophilia 6:402, 2000 (abstr)
14. De Kleijn P, Gilbert M, Roosendaal G, Poonnoose P, Narayan PM, Tahir N: Functional recovery after bleeding episodes in haemophilia. Haemophilia 10:157-160, 2004 (suppl 4)
15. DePalma AF: Hemophilic arthropathy. Clin Orthop Relat Res 52:145-165, 1967
16. Arnold WD, Hilgartner MW: Haemophilic arthropathy. Current concepts of pathogenesis and management. J Bone Joint Surg Am 59:287-305, 1977
17. Wood K, Omer A, Shaw MT: Haemophilic arthropathy. A combined radiological and clinical study. Br J Radiol 42:498-505, 1969
18. Rodriguez-Merchan EC, de la Corte H: Musculoskeletal outcomes research in haemophilia, in Rodriguez-Merchan EC (ed): The Haemophilic Joints. New Perspectives. Oxford, UK, Blackwell, 2003, pp 36-44
19. Kulkarni MV, Drolshagen LF, Kaye JJ, Green NE, Burks DD, Janco RL, et al: MR imaging of hemophilic arthropathy. J Comput Assist Tomogr 10:445-449, 1986
20. Erlemann R, Rosenthal H, Walthers EM, Almeida P, Calleja R: Reproducibility of the Pettersson scoring system. An interobserver study. Acta Radiol 30:147-151, 1989
21. Hamel J, Pohlmann H, Schramm W: Radiological evaluation of chronic hemophilic arthropathy by the Pettersson score: Problems in correlation in adult patients. Skeletal Radiol 17:32-36, 1988
22. Aronstam A, Wassef M, Hamad Z, McLellan DS: The effect of bleeding patterns on the response of haemophilic haemarthrosis to different doses of factor VIII. Clin Lab Haematol 3:107-112, 1981
23. Ekert H, Moorehead M, Williamson G: Home treatment of haemophilia. A follow-up study. Med J Aust 2:21-23, 1981
24. Rodriguez-Merchan EC: Therapeutic options in the management of articular contractures in haemophiliacs. Haemophilia 5:5-9, 1999 (suppl 1)
25. Schoenmakers MAGC, Gulmans VAM, Helders PJM, Van Den Berg HM: Motor performance and disability in Dutch children with haemo-

philia: A comparison with their healthy peers. Haemophilia 7:293-298, 2001

26. Hill F, Ljung R, European Paediatric Network for Haemophilia Management: Third and Fourth Workshops of the European Paediatric Network for Haemophilia Management. Haemophilia 9:223-228, 2003
27. Fischer K, Astermark J, Van der Bom JG, Ljung R, Berntop E, Grobbee DE, et al: Prophylactic treatment for severe haemophilia: Comparison of an intermediate-dose to a high-dose regimen. Haemophilia 8:753-760, 2003
28. Fischer K, Van Den Berg HM, Thomas R, Kumar S, Poonnoose P, Viswabandya A, et al: Dose and outcome of care in haemophilia—How do we define cost-effectiveness? Haemophilia 10:216-220, 2004 (suppl 4)
29. ICIDH-2: International Classification of Functioning and Disability, Beta-2 draft, Full Version. Geneva, Switzerland, World Health Organization, 1999, pp 1-214
30. Molho P, Rolland N, Lebrun T, Dirat G, Courpied JP, Croughs T, et al: Epidemiological survey of the orthopaedic status of severe haemophilia A and B patients in France. Haemophilia 6:23-32, 2000
31. Aznar JA, Magallón M, Querol F, Gorina E, Tusell JM: The orthopaedic status of severe haemophiliacs in Spain. Haemophilia 6:170-176, 2000
32. Miners AH, Sabin CA, Tolley KH, Jenkinson C, Kind P, Lee C: Assessing health-related quality-of-life in individuals with haemophilia. Haemophilia 5:378-385, 1999
33. De Joode E, Van Meeteren NLU, Van Den Berg HM, De Kleijn P, Helders PJM: Validity of health status measurements with the Dutch Arthritis Impact Measurement Scale 2 in individuals with severe haemophilia. Haemophilia 7:190-197, 2001
34. Bergner M, Bobbitt RA, Kressel S, Pollard WE, Gilson BS, Morris JR: The sickness impact profile: Conceptual formulation and methodology for the development of a health status measure. Int J Health Serv 6:393-415, 1976
35. Schick M, Stucki G, Rodriguez M, Meili EO, Huber E, Michel BA, et al: Haemophilic arthropathy: assessment of quality of life after total knee arthroplasty. Clin Rheumatol 18:468-472, 1999
36. Bellamy N, Buchanan WW, Goldsmith CH, Campbell J, Stitt LW: Validation study of WOMAC: A health status instrument for measuring clinically important patient-relevant outcomes to antirheumatic therapy in patients with osteoarthritis of the hip or knee. J Rheumatol 15:1833-1840, 1988
37. Solovieva S: Clinical severity of disease, functional disability and health-related quality of life. Three-year follow-up study of 150 Finnish patients with coagulation disorders. Haemophilia 7:53-63, 2001
38. Singh G, Athreya BH, Fries JF, Goldsmith DP: Measurement of health status in children with juvenile rheumatoid arthritis. Arthritis Rheum 37:1761-1769, 1994
39. De Kleijn P, Heijnen L, Van Meeteren NLU: Clinimetric instruments to assess functional health status in patients with haemophilia: a literature review. Haemophilia 8:419-427, 2002
40. Van Genderen FR, Van Meeteren NLU, Van Der Bom JG, Heijnen L, De Kleijn P, Van Den Berg HM, et al: Functional consequences of haemophilia in adults: The development of the Haemophilia Activities List. Haemophilia 10:565-571, 2004
41. Poonnoose PM, Manigandan C, Thomas R, Shyamkumar NK, Kavitha ML, Bhattacharji S, et al: Functional Independence Score in Haemophilia (FISH): A new performance-based instrument to measure disability. Haemophilia 11:598-602, 2005
42. Klukowska A, Czyrny Z, Laguna P, Brzewski M, Serafin-Krol MA, Rokicka-Milewska R: Correlation between clinical, radiological, and ultrasonographical image of knee joints in children with haemophilia. Haemophilia 7:286-292, 2001
43. Bruyere O, Honore A, Rovati LC, Giacovelli G, Henrotin YE, Seidel L, et al: Radiologic features poorly predict clinical outcomes in knee osteoarthritis. Scand J Rhuematol 31:13-16, 2002
44. Heeg M, Meyer K, Smid WM, Van Horn JR, Van Der Meer J: Total knee and hip arthroplasty in haemophilic patients. Haemophilia 4:747-751, 1998
45. Fischer K, Bom JG, Mauser-Bunschoten EP, Roosendal G, Berg HM: Effects of haemophilic arthropathy on health-related quality of life and socio-economic parameters. Haemophilia 11:43-48, 2005
46. Tanaka S, Hachisuka K, Okazaki T, Shirahata A, Ogata H: Health status and satisfaction of asymptomatic HIV-positive haemophiliacs in Kyushu, Japan. Haemophilia 5:56-62, 1999
47. Trippoli S, Vaiani M, Linari S, Longo G, Morfini M, Messori A: Multivariate analysis of factors influencing quality of life and utility in patients with haemophilia. Haematologica 86:722-728, 2001
48. von Mackensen S, Bullinger M: Haemo-QoL Group: Development and testing of an instrument to assess the Quality of Life of Children with Haemophilia in Europe (Haemo-QoL). Haemophilia 10:17-25, 2004 (suppl 1)
49. Young NL, Bradley CS, Blanchette V, Wakefield CD, Barnard D, Wu JK, McCusker PJ: Development of a health-related quality of life measure for boys with haemophilia: The Canadian Haemophilia Outcomes—Kids Life Assessment Tool (CHO–KLAT). Haemophilia 10:34-43, 2004 (suppl 1)
50. Arranz P, Remor E, Quintana M, Villar A, Díaz JL, Morena M, et al: Development of a new disease-specific quality-of-life questionnaire to adults living with haemophilia. Haemophilia 10:376-382, 2004
51. Remor E, Young NL, von Mackensen S, Lopatina EG. Disease-specific quality-of-life measurement tools for haemophilia patients. Haemophilia 10:30-34, 2004 (suppl 4)

ELSEVIER

Seminars in HEMATOLOGY

Glanzmann's Thrombasthenia Treatment: A Prospective Observational Registry on the Use of Recombinant Human Activated Factor VII and Other Hemostatic Agents

Man-Chiu Poon[a], Rainer Zotz[b], Giovanni Di Minno[c], Zvika S. Abrams[d], Jens B. Knudsen[d], and Yves Laurian[e]

Glanzmann's thrombasthenia (GT) is a rare congenital bleeding disorder caused by deficiency or dysfunction of platelet surface glycoprotein (GP) IIb/IIIa receptor. Platelet transfusion is the standard treatment for bleeding that remains non-responsive to conservative measures, and for surgical coverage. Platelet transfusions, however, may result in the development of antibodies to GPIIb/IIIa and/or human leukocyte antigen (HLA), rendering further transfusions ineffective. Recombinant human activated factor VII (rFVIIa; NovoSeven®/Niastase® [Canada], Novo Nordisk, Bagsvaerd, Denmark) has documented efficacy in GT patients, and is approved in the European Union for the treatment of GT patients with platelet antibodies and platelet refractoriness. However, there are insufficient data to determine the optimal rFVIIa regimen (eg, for major surgery) or to allow thorough safety evaluation (eg, thrombotic risk). A post-marketing, prospective, observational, multinational registry has been developed to collect data on the efficacy and safety of rFVIIa in the treatment and prevention of bleeding in GT patients with platelet antibodies or platelet refractoriness. Patients treated with other hemostatic agents or rFVIIa to avoid the development of antibodies against GPIIb/IIIa will also be reported. Standardized data will be collected using a customized internet-based (www.glanzmann-reg.org) data collection tool. Data collection will begin in 2005 and continue for up to 6 years. Patients of all ages from any country are eligible for inclusion.
Semin Hematol 43(suppl 1):S33-S36

Glanzmann's thrombasthenia (GT) is a rare, congenital bleeding disorder characterized by platelet dysfunction, which results from a quantitative or qualitative defect of the platelet membrane glycoprotein (GP) IIb/IIIa (α_{IIb}-β_3) complex.[1,2] Clinical manifestations start in childhood and include easy bruising, epistaxis, gingival bleeding, menorrhagia and, less frequently, gastrointestinal bleeding, hematuria, hemarthrosis, muscle hematoma, and central nervous system bleeding.[1] Bleeding complications are also frequent after dental extraction, surgery, and delivery.[1] The bleeding tendency in GT patients is highly variable: some patients remain asymptomatic, whereas others experience severe bleeding episodes. When bleeding does not respond to local measures, hemostatic agents such as fibrin glue and/or antifibrinolytic drugs may be administered. Platelet transfusion is currently the standard treatment for bleeding that remains nonresponsive to conservative measures; however, repeated transfusions may result in the development of antibodies against GPIIb/IIIa and/or human leukocyte antigen (HLA), resulting in refractoriness to further platelet transfusion.[1,3] Blood products also carry other risks, including infections[4] and allergic reactions. Finally, platelet concentrates, especially those prepared from single-donor apheresis and/or HLA-compatible donors, may not always be readily available.

[a]University of Calgary, Southern Alberta Hemophilia Clinic, Calgary Health Region, and Canadian Blood Services, Calgary, Canada.
[b]Heinrich-Heine-Universität, Düsseldorf, Germany.
[c]Universita' degli Studi di Napoli Federico II, IRCCS "Casa Sollievo della Sofferenza" S. Giovanni Rotondo, Italy.
[d]Novo Nordisk A/S, Bagsvaerd, Denmark.
[e]AP-HP & UFR Medicine Paris XIII, Paris, France.
Address correspondence to Man-Chiu Poon, MD, University of Calgary, Foothills Hospital, 1403 29th Street NW, Calgary, Alberta, Canada T2N 2T9. E-mail: mcpoon@ucalgary.ca

0037-1963/06/$-see front matter
doi:10.1053/j.seminhematol.2005.11.009

Use of rFVIIa in GT Patients: Data From an International Registry on Recombinant Factor VIIa and Congenital Platelet Disorders

A relatively large international survey has documented the efficacy of recombinant activated factor VII (rFVIIa; NovoSeven®/Niastase® [Canada]; Novo Nordisk, Bagsvaerd, Denmark) in treating GT patients with a wide range of bleeding episodes, or in providing prophylaxis for those undergoing invasive surgical procedures.[5] The International Registry on Recombinant Factor VIIa and Congenital Platelet Disorders (coordinators: Dr M-C. Poon, Calgary, Canada and Dr R. d'Oiron, Paris, France) was started in 1999, with wide participation from 49 centers in 17 countries, providing data that include some previously published cases.[6-12] The survey evaluated rFVIIa treatment of 108 bleeding episodes and 34 surgical procedures in 59 patients.[5] There were 24 males and 35 females, aged 1 to 72 years (median, 22 years), including 27 children (aged 15 years or younger). The majority of patients (39 of 49 known) had severe disease (type 1, <5% GPIIb/IIIa), and 35 patients had platelet antibodies (to GPIIb/IIIa and/or HLA) and/or platelet refractoriness.

Of the 34 surgical procedures covered (9 major, 25 minor), there were 29 successes, 2 recurrent bleeds, and 3 that were not evaluable due to confounding by concurrent platelet transfusion. Thus, the intention-to-treat success rate for surgical procedures was 85%, and the success rate of the evaluable episodes was 94%.

Of 108 bleeding episodes assessed (17 gastrointestinal bleeds, 45 nosebleeds, 29 oropharyngeal bleeds, and 17 miscellaneous bleeds), 76 were considered severe and 32 moderate. Following treatment with rFVIIa, 77 bleeding episodes were successfully controlled, although eight recurred within 48 hours (resulting in 69 successful treatments overall). A further 26 bleeding episodes did not respond to rFVIIa therapy and were therefore declared failures, with patients switching to alternative treatments. A total of five bleeding episodes could not be evaluated due to the concurrent administration of platelet transfusions. The intention-to-treat success rate for bleeding episodes was therefore 64%, while the success rate for evaluable episodes was 67%. Of the 80 bleeding episodes in which the time of bleeding cessation was known, 58 (73%) were stopped within 6 hours of the first dose of rFVIIa.

Several other observations were also made.[5] For instance, when given as bolus injections, rFVIIa appears to be a safe and mostly effective alternative to platelet transfusion for the treatment and prevention of bleeding in GT patients, particularly for those with anti-platelet antibodies and/or refractoriness to platelet transfusions. No serious adverse events directly related to rFVIIa treatment were observed using this method of administration. Indeed, only two serious adverse events directly related to rFVIIa treatment were observed, and both occurred after prolonged continuous infusion of rFVIIa at relatively high doses in conjunction with antifibrinolytic drugs. The first was a clot in the renal pelvis/ureter following a gynecologic procedure, whilst the second was a thromboembolism after a bowel resection.

Furthermore, the success rate for evaluable severe bleeding episodes treated with bolus doses of rFVIIa at ≥80 μg/kg at intervals of ≤2.5 hours for at least 3 doses was significantly higher (24/31, 77%) than that achieved with less "optimal" bolus dose regimens (18/33, 55%) or continuous infusion (1/7, 14%) ($P = .010$). Recurrence of bleeding may be prevented by providing one to two maintenance dose(s) after bleeding has stopped. The proportion of episodes given maintenance doses was higher for those that stopped without recurrence than for those that did recur (36/62 *v* 1/8 bleeding episodes, respectively; $P = .022$).

Finally, continuous infusion was found to be effective in preventing bleeding during invasive surgical procedures in 6/6 cases, although the total amount of rFVIIa used was not reduced when compared with bolus injections. Continuous infusion, however, was not effective in treating bleeding episodes. The majority (6/7) of continuous infusions for bleeding episodes were unsuccessful, even though the total amount of rFVIIa administered was higher than that used for bolus injections.

Although the survey did not collect data to assess the timing of treatment, the observations of Almeida et al[11] suggest that treatment for bleeding episodes should be given as early as possible. They found good or excellent responses in 10 of 14 episodes (71%) treated within 12 hours of bleeding onset, but in only two of 11 (18%) treated after 12 hours.

Several unresolved issues are raised by this survey. For instance, the data are insufficient to allow determination of the optimal rFVIIa regimen for surgical coverage in these patients. In addition, although some preliminary suggestions for the optimal rFVIIa regimen in bleeding episodes can be derived from the analysis, confirmation from larger studies will be required. There are also insufficient data to evaluate the safety of rFVIIa in GT patients, particularly with regard to the incidence of thromboembolic events.

Treatment of GT: A Prospective Observational Registry

Rationale

In 2004, the European Medical Evaluation Agency (EMEA) approved the use of rFVIIa in European Union (EU) countries for the treatment of bleeding episodes and for surgical coverage in GT patients with anti-platelet antibodies (to GPIIb/IIIa and/or HLA) and past/present history of platelet refractoriness. The manufacturer (Novo Nordisk, Bagsvaerd, Denmark) was required to conduct a post-marketing study on the safety and efficacy of rFVIIa in GT patients for up to 6 years, reporting to the EMEA every 6 months. Wide participation in this post-marketing surveillance study will allow sufficient data to be gathered in order to address currently unresolved issues, including the optimal treatment regimen and the safety of treatment in this patient population. GT is a rare disorder, and the need for treatment with systemic hemostatic agents is uncommon; large numbers of patients, treated over long periods of time, are therefore required. This is particularly important for safety evaluation, as has been shown for drugs for common diseases, where significant post-marketing complications and risks have been recognized only after long periods of use in a large patient population.[13]

Protocol Planning and Development

The planning and development of this rFVIIa post-marketing surveillance study were based on input from an international expert panel that included Drs M-C. Poon (Canada), Y. Laurian (France), R. Zotz (Germany), and G. Di Minno (Italy), with the assistance of Covance, a contract clinical research organization, and support from Novo Nordisk.

Objectives

The primary objective of the study is to evaluate the efficacy and safety (particularly with regard to thromboembolic events) of rFVIIa treatment for surgical coverage or treatment of bleeding episodes in GT patients with platelet antibodies (to GPIIb/IIIa and/or HLA) and past or present history of platelet refractoriness. The secondary objective is to describe the safety and efficacy of systemic hemostatic agents (including rFVIIa and platelets, with or without antifibrinolytics or other agents) in GT patients with or without platelet antibodies and/or platelet refractoriness in a real clinical setting. Thus, the study will allow comparison of the efficacy and safety of rFVIIa and other treatment modalities in GT patients experiencing bleeding episodes or undergoing surgery, whether or not platelet antibodies or platelet refractoriness are present.

Patient Eligibility

Patients must have been diagnosed with congenital Glanzmann's thrombasthenia (GT), as defined by platelet aggregometry and/or GPIIb/IIIa quantitation and/or molecular studies or other recognized assays.

Informed consent, where this is required by the local Research Ethics Board, must be obtained from patients. Templates for subject information and informed consent forms can be found at www.glanzmann-reg.org.

Patients must be receiving rFVIIa or other systematic hemostatic agent(s) (eg, platelets, desmopressin [DDAVP]), with or without antifibrinolytics, for the treatment of bleeding episodes or for surgical coverage, when considered necessary by the treating physicians.

As an international study, patients from any country are eligible. The recruitment is not confined to EU countries.

Patient Exclusion

Patients with acquired thrombasthenia of any etiology are excluded.

Protocol Contents

The following information will be collected during the study:

- Admission status, including anonymous patient identification, patient height and weight at the time of treatment, and treatment location (hospital, clinic/emergency department, home).
- Patient demographics.
- Clinical history, ie, past history of bleeding and type/location of bleeding; GT diagnosis and severity; antibody status; platelet refractoriness; previous treatment modalities; and past major illnesses, including hepatitis virus infection and hepatic, renal, and rheumatologic disorders.
- Current treatment report for bleeding episodes and surgical coverage using rFVIIa, including cause and type of bleeding or type of invasive procedures, details of rFVIIa treatment (dosage, schedule, etc), use of other concomitant hemostatic agents and relevant medications, description of post-treatment complications, and efficacy evaluation. If platelets were used, information on the source of platelets (eg, single or random donors) and whether they were HLA-matched is also collected.
- Current treatment report for bleeding episodes and surgical coverage using alternative hemostatic agents where rFVIIa is not used. Details similar to those described above are collected.
- Details of any re-bleeding, including signs, location, intensity, and timing after treatment starts and after last rFVIIa dose.
- Laboratory monitoring methods and other details, where available.
- Details of any adverse events, including arterial and venous thromboembolic events, allergic reactions and disseminated intravascular coagulation. The seriousness of the event, timing of the event in relationship to treatment, medication used before occurrence of the event, treatment of the event, and outcome will also be assessed. In case of death, evaluation of whether the death was related to a complication of bleeding or treatment will be required, and the findings of post-mortem examination (if performed) will be analyzed.

Protocol Design

This international, multicenter study will be organized and conducted as follows.

An internet-based, standardized data collection tool (www.glanzmann-reg.org) will be used. Paper data collection forms can also be downloaded from the website for manual completion and submission. The website also contains a help manual.

Covance, a contract research organization, will host the website and manage and validate the submitted data. This will be conducted in a way that meets data safety/security and confidentiality requirements.

Recruitment will begin in 2005 and continue for up to 6 years from the time at which the first patient is enrolled, and the study will end in 2011.

The data and documents will be retained by Novo Nordisk for the duration of rFVIIa being in the market and for a minimum of 20 years. Retention by the investigators will be conducted in accordance with local regulations.

Publication Policy

For publications based on analysis of data submitted to this surveillance study, the author list will include members of the expert panel and investigators submitting the greatest number of treatment episodes. The number of authors included will be based on the number allowable by the chosen journal. All investigators submitting data will be appropriately acknowledged in the publication.

Conclusions

This post-marketing surveillance study has been developed as a requirement for the EU approval of rFVIIa for the treatment of bleeding episodes and the provision of surgical prophylaxis in GT patients with platelet antibodies and platelet refractoriness. The study is international and multicenter in nature, and is not confined to EU patients. It will include treatment data not only on rFVIIa, but also on other systemic hemostatic agents used in real-life clinical settings. It is hoped that there will be wide participation to provide sufficient data on a large number of patients, thus facilitating the development of general treatment guidelines for bleeding and surgical coverage in GT patients. Data submission is internet-based (*www.glanzmann-reg.org*), with paper forms for manual completion and submission also available from the website. Any data on GT patients that would have been submitted to the International Registry on Recombinant Factor VIIa and Congenital Platelet Disorders will now be submitted to this post-marketing surveillance study instead.

Acknowledgments

We wish to thank all the investigators who have submitted data to the International Registry on Recombinant Factor VIIa and Congenital Platelet Disorders, thus helping to develop the present post-marketing study protocol. The list of these investigators appears in the paper reporting the results of data analysis from this registry.[5] We also wish to thank Novo Nordisk A/S for assistance in the planning and development of the post-marketing study protocol.

References

1. George JN, Caen JP, Nurden AT: Glanzmann's thrombasthenia: The spectrum of clinical disease. Blood 75:1383-1395, 1990
2. Nurden AT: Inherited abnormalities of platelets. Thromb Haemost 82: 468-480, 1999
3. Levy-Toledano S, Tobelem G, Legrand C, Bredoux R, Degos L, Nurden A, et al: Acquired IgG antibody occurring in a thrombasthenic patient: Its effect on human platelet function. Blood 51:1065-1071, 1978
4. Vrielink H, Reesink HW: Transfusion-transmissible infections. Curr Opin Hematol 5:396-405, 1998
5. Poon MC, d'Oiron R, Von Depka M, Khair K, Negrier C, Karafoulidou A, et al: Prophylactic and therapeutic recombinant factor VIIa administration to patients with Glanzmann's thrombasthenia: Results of an international survey. J Thromb Haemost 2:1096-1103, 2004
6. Tengborn L, Petruson B: A patient with Glanzmann thrombasthenia and epistaxis successfully treated with recombinant factor VIIa. Thromb Haemost 75:981-982, 1996 (letter)
7. Poon M-C, Demers C, Jobin F, Wu JW: Recombinant factor VIIa is effective for bleeding and surgery in patients with Glanzmann thrombasthenia. Blood 94:3951-3953, 1999
8. Musso R, Cultrera D, Russo M, Giuffrida G, Venturino L, Ferlito C, et al: Recombinant activated factor VII as haemostatic agent in Glanzmann's thrombasthenia. Thromb Haemost 82:621, 1999 (suppl, abstr)
9. Robinson KL, Savoia H, Street AM: Thrombotic complications in two patients receiving NovoSeven. Haemophilia 6:349, 2000 (abstr)
10. d'Oiron R, Menart C, Trzeciak MC, Nurden P, Fressinaud E, Dreyfus M, et al: Use of recombinant factor VIIa in 3 patients with inherited type I Glanzmann's thrombasthenia undergoing invasive procedures. Thromb Haemost 83:644-647, 2000
11. Almeida AM, Khair K, Hann I, Liesner R: The use of recombinant factor VIIa in children with inherited platelet function disorders. Br J Haematol 121:477-481, 2003
12. Devecioglu O, Unuvar A, Anak S, Bilge I, Ander H, Ziylan O: Pyelolithotomy in a patient with Glanzmann thrombasthenia and antiglycoprotein IIb/IIIa antibodies: the shortest possible duration of treatment with recombinant activated factor VII and platelet transfusions. Turk J Pediatr 45:64-66, 2003
13. Okie S: Safety in numbers—Monitoring risk in approved drugs. N Engl J Med 352:1173-1176, 2005

ELSEVIER

Seminars in
HEMATOLOGY

Congenital and Acquired Platelet Disorders: Current Dilemmas and Treatment Strategies

Gilbert C. White II

Platelets are important for primary hemostasis. When a blood vessel is damaged, platelets adhere to exposed subendothelial connective tissue and form a hemostatic plug. Formation of the plug is contingent upon a series of processes, with adhesion, activation, and aggregation all being involved. Patients with quantitative platelet disorders have reduced numbers of platelets. Patients with qualitative disorders have platelets that exhibit abnormal functioning. Defects that impair function can affect platelet receptors, secretory responses, or intracellular signaling pathways. Examples of qualitative platelet disorders include Glanzmann's thrombasthenia (GT) and Bernard-Soulier syndrome (BSS). The treatment of platelet disorders is primarily with platelet concentrates. However, in patients with abnormalities of their platelet surface receptors, platelet transfusion may provoke an immune response. Recombinant factor VIIa (rFVIIa) may provide hemostatically effective therapy in such patients.
Semin Hematol 43(suppl 1):S37-S41

Platelets are important for primary hemostasis. They are produced by megakaryocytes in the bone marrow and have a complex anucleate structure. Under normal conditions, platelets circulate in blood vessels as inactive cells. However, hemostatic stress causes rapid activation of platelets, enabling the cells to perform their unique function in the process of blood clotting. In this regard, platelets are perfectly adapted to their role, being inactive when they are not needed but able to respond very quickly when a blood vessel is damaged. As a consequence of their ability to be rapidly activated, platelets are a good model of signal transduction. A variety of pathways are involved in the signal transduction, and abnormalities of these pathways can result in the manifestation of clinical disorders. This article will briefly consider platelet structure and function, mention some of the clinical problems that can be associated with platelet abnormalities, and conclude with reference to treatment for affected patients.

Platelet Structure and Function

Platelet Structure

Platelets are surrounded by a typical plasma membrane, in which a number of proteins are embedded that endow the cell with its ability to respond to environmental changes. Glycoproteins act as receptors for substances that trigger platelet activation, and as substrates for platelet adhesion and clumping reactions. Transport proteins regulate platelet volume and intracellular concentrations of divalent cations. In addition, membrane phospholipids provide a surface for reactions involving coagulation proteins and supply the initial substrate for the production of thromboxane A_2 (TXA_2) via platelet enzymes (see below). Signals from the platelet surface are translated into intracellular signals via the proteins and lipid domains that are part of the platelet membrane. At various places, the plasma membrane is invaginated, forming a surface-connected canalicular system that extends into the platelet interior. This canalicular system is important for the ingress of materials that platelets accumulate (eg, fibrinogen, and possibly other coagulation factors), and is also involved in the egress of the contents of platelet granules—the secretory response.

A number of contractile proteins are also present in platelets. A microtubule bundle is present in the marginal rim of the platelet, and contractile proteins, such as actin, are found within the cytoplasm. When platelets are activated, the microtubule bundle contracts, repositioning the intracellular contents. The contractile system facilitates changes in shape and enables platelets to form pseudopodial extensions.

Several types of granules are found within platelets. The most easily identifiable of these are the δ- (or dense) granules. These contain nucleotides, serotonin, and calcium. The most numerous granules are the α-granules, which contain vari-

Blood Research Institute, Milwaukee, WI.
Address correspondence to G.C. White, MD, Blood Research Institute, 8727 Watertown Plank Rd, Milwaukee, WI 53226. E-mail: gcwhite@bcsew.edu

0037-1963/06/$-see front matter
doi:10.1053/j.seminhematol.2005.11.011

ous clotting factor proteins, such as fibrinogen and factor V (FV), platelet-derived growth factor (PDGF), platelet factor 4, and β-thromboglobulin, together with some other proteins. Lysosomal granules are also present; these contain a variety of enzymes.

Platelets also have a dense tubular system (DTS)—derived from the smooth endoplasmic reticulum found in the parent megakaryocyte—in which calcium for the triggering of contractile events is concentrated.

Platelet Function

Platelets normally reside on the edge of blood vessels and tend to move along the vessel wall. When a blood vessel is damaged, subendothelial connective tissue, such as collagen, becomes exposed and platelets rolling along the surface of the damaged vessel adhere to this and form a hemostatic plug. Formation of the plug is contingent upon a series of processes; platelet adhesion, platelet activation—during which the cell undergoes morphological changes and some of its contents are released—and platelet aggregation are all involved.

Activation of the blood coagulation system is coordinated with the formation of the primary platelet plug, and secondary hemostasis results in the generation of thrombin and formation of the fibrin net.

Platelet Adhesion

Platelet adhesion to subendothelial tissue is mediated by glycoprotein (GP) receptors on the platelet surface. Most of these promote the interaction of platelets with collagen, but fibronectin and other proteins in the subendothelial connective tissue may also be involved. The initial interaction between platelets and the subendothelial matrix involves von Willebrand factor (vWF). Under conditions of high shear stress, vWF binds simultaneously to collagen and GPIb,[1] which is part of the platelet GPIb-V-IX complex. However, this interaction alone is not sufficiently stable to allow the assembly of a platelet thrombus, and more stable binding to collagen also takes place, with GPIa-IIa, also known as $\alpha_2\beta_1$ integrin, being involved here.[2] Additional collagen binding occurs via a multiprotein complex containing GPVI and the Fc receptor γ-chain (FcRγ).[3] GPIV is also a receptor for collagen.[4] GPIc-IIa interacts with fibronectin.[5]

Platelet Activation

Platelets undergo morphological changes upon activation. Platelet shape changes from a disk to a spiny sphere with multiple pseudopodial extensions. The platelet membrane becomes rearranged, with exposure of negatively charged phospholipids that facilitate the interaction with coagulation proteins to form the tenase and prothrombinase complexes. The contents of the platelet granules are secreted through the surface-connected canalicular system, with adenosine diphosphate (ADP), fibrinogen, and FV appearing on the platelet surface and in the milieu immediately surrounding the platelet. PDGF is secreted and leads to smooth muscle proliferation. Repeated secretion of PDGF resulting from recurrent episodes of platelet activation increases smooth muscle proliferation and initiates atherosclerosis.[6] Platelet factor 3 is also expressed after platelet activation. Small pieces of the platelet are able to bud off to form circulating microparticles.

Platelet–agonist interactions result in the production or release of a variety of intracellular messenger molecules that facilitate these reactions. Phosphoinositides are generated from membrane inositol phospholipids through the action of phospholipases. Two products of these reactions, inositol 1,4,5-triphosphate (IP_3) and diacylglyceride, are known to play important roles in platelet function. IP_3 is a calcium ionophore that promotes the release of calcium from the DTS and increases intracellular calcium after platelets are activated. Diacylglyceride is able to activate protein kinase C, a phosphorylating enzyme, which is then able to activate proteins in other pathways thought to be important in platelet activation. Protein kinase C also catalyzes pleckstrin phosphorylation.

During platelet activation, arachidonic acid is also liberated from membrane phospholipids by phospholipases. The arachidonic acid is metabolized by cyclooxygenase-1 (COX-1) into prostaglandin G_2, and this is subsequently converted into prostaglandin H_2.[7] Thromboxane synthase then processes prostaglandin H_2, resulting in the formation of TXA_2. TXA_2 enhances platelet aggregation and recruitment of platelets to the primary hemostatic plug.[8] Aspirin irreversibly acetylates COX-1,[9] which is a central enzyme in the conversion of membrane phospholipids to TXA_2.

Calcium is an important second messenger in platelets. Sarco-endoplasmic reticulum-type calcium pumps (SERCA) in the plasma membrane transport calcium into the platelet. Cyclic adenosine monophosphate (cAMP) facilitates the transport of calcium from the cytosol into the DTS. The release of calcium from the DTS is facilitated by IP_3. The calcium pumps involved have been identified, cloned, and sequenced.[10,11] Increased cytosolic concentrations of calcium activate gelsolin, which initially breaks down actin microfilaments early in platelet activation before they repolymerize to form pseudopods. Activation by calcium of the calmodulin-regulated myosin light chain kinase phosphorylates the myosin light chain, which then activates the actin-associated myosin adenosine triphosphatase (ATPase) activity and leads to contraction of myosin along actin filaments. This creates a contractile wave inside the platelet that contributes to changes in shape and pseudopod formation.

Platelet Secretion

When platelets are activated, the contents of the platelet granules are released and participate in various processes. ADP, released from platelet-dense granules, activates additional platelets, increasing the size of the platelet plug. Serotonin, also released from dense granules, causes vascular constriction. At the same time, changes occur in the platelet membrane that facilitate humoral coagulation.

Platelet Aggregation

The final step in the function of platelets in hemostasis is the interaction of one platelet with another—platelet aggregation—mediated by the $\alpha_{IIb}\beta_3$ integrin (GPIIb-IIIa) on the platelet surface. As a consequence of platelet activation, the short cytoplasmic domains of the GPIIb-IIIa receptor react with intracellular components of the platelet to induce a conformational change in the extracellular domain of the receptor. The conformational change enables the receptor to bind to fibrinogen, as well as vWF, fibronectin, and thrombospondin.[12] Platelet aggregation ensues, with these adhesive proteins forming bridges between the platelets.

Platelet Disorders

Quantitative Platelet Disorders

Disorders of platelets may be qualitative or quantitative, congenital or acquired. Patients with quantitative disorders have reduced numbers of platelets, with the function being proportional to the platelet number. Characteristic quantitative abnormalities include primary bone marrow disorders (in which patients have reduced platelet production by megakaryocyte precursors), hypersplenism, immunological platelet disorders, and other causes of platelet destruction. Aplastic anemia, leukemia, myeloma, and vitamin B_{12} or folate deficiency are all primary bone marrow disorders associated with decreased platelet production. Hypersplenism causes thrombocytopenia by increased sequestration of platelets in the spleen. Idiopathic thrombocytopenic purpura, neonatal alloimmune thrombocytopenic purpura, and drug-induced thrombocytopenias are all examples of immune thrombocytopenias. Diffuse intravascular coagulation and cardiac valvular abnormalities are other causes of platelet destruction.

Qualitative Platelet Disorders

Patients with qualitative platelet disorders have normal numbers of platelets, but their platelets exhibit abnormal function. Such disorders occur less frequently than quantitative disorders and prove more difficult to diagnose definitively. They may have a variety of causes, including defects in platelet receptors, secretory responses, or intracellular signaling pathways.

Among the first defects in platelets to be identified at a molecular level were those that affected the membrane proteins. Defects in the GPIIb-IIIa receptor give rise to Glanzmann's thrombasthenia (GT). Patients with this condition have normal platelet adhesion to regions of damaged endothelium but binding of fibrinogen is adversely affected. This inhibits platelet aggregation, and recruitment of platelets into the primary hemostatic plug is defective.

Several hundred cases of GT are probably now documented. In a study reviewing data from published reports for 113 patients with this condition, the average age at the time of reporting was 20 years.[13] The relatively young age of the patients was considered to reflect the facts that diagnosis of the condition has become established and most adults experience minimal symptoms. In this cohort of patients, 60 (53%) were female, which is consistent with the condition having an autosomal mode of inheritance. Glanzmann's thrombasthenia tends to be concentrated within ethnic groups; consanguinity may permit expression of the autosomal recessive genetic traits responsible for the condition. The most common forms of bleeding experienced by these patients are purpura, epistaxis, gingival hemorrhage and menorrhagia. Indeed, bleeding at menarche is a particular risk and this can be of a severity that warrants blood transfusion. Spontaneous, unprovoked bleeding is uncommon. Platelet transfusion in patients with GT often results in the development of antibodies directed at the functional epitopes of GPIIb-IIIa, which precludes further treatment with platelets.

Mutations in the GPIb-V-IX receptor that affect its ability to bind vWF can result in Bernard-Soulier syndrome (BSS). In patients with this condition, platelet adhesion to the subendothelium of damaged blood vessels is impaired. The GPIb-V-IX complex comprises four subunits: GPIbα, GPIbβ, GPV, and GPIX. Each of the subunits is encoded by a separate gene and a variety of mutations have been described.

Although BSS is a major bleeding disorder, it is an extremely rare disease. In a recent comprehensive review, López and colleagues[14] reported that, in the most intensively studied populations (Europe, North America, and Japan), a prevalence of less than one in 1 million may be estimated from the literature, although misdiagnosis and under-reporting may result in this being an underestimate. This review described 88 patients with BSS, 47 of whom were female. Although this is a relatively small sample, it suggests that there is no gender preference for the condition, as may be expected in a disorder with an autosomal mode of inheritance.[14] Clinical manifestations of BSS include frequent episodes of epistaxis and gingival/cutaneous bleeding. Trauma-associated hemorrhage may also be observed.

Other receptor abnormalities can also occur. Gain-of-function mutations in the GPIb-V-IX receptor can give rise to platelet-type (or pseudo) von Willebrand disease, in which platelets exhibit spontaneous binding to vWF. Reduced platelet adhesion may also result from defects in the GPIc-IIa receptor. Defects in collagen signal transduction can occur as a consequence of a defective GPVI receptor, and impaired binding to collagen may be evident if abnormalities in the GPIa-IIa receptor are present.

Hypercoagulable states may be associated with integrin mutations. The $Pl^{A1/A2}$ polymorphism of GPIIIa has been investigated with regard to coronary risk, and it has been reported that Pl^{A2} has a significant (but weak) association with overall cardiovascular disease in the general population.[15] Kritzik et al[16] have reported that the level of expression of $\alpha_2\beta_1$ integrin on the platelet surface is associated with polymorphisms in the α_2 gene; three alleles, defined by eight polymorphisms, have been described. One of these alleles has been associated with increased expression of $\alpha_2\beta_1$ and the others produced lower levels of the receptor. A threefold difference in the levels of $\alpha_2\beta_1$ expression was apparent. In vitro studies demonstrated that at high shear (1,500/s) the rate of attachment of platelets to collagen in whole blood was proportional to the $\alpha_2\beta_1$ receptor density.[16] If these differences were translated into effects on platelet function in vivo, increased expression of $\alpha_2\beta_1$ may result in an increased risk of thrombosis.

Abnormalities of platelet granules have also been described. These are structurally identifiable in many cases. In gray platelet syndrome (GPS), which is a mild bleeding disorder exhibiting autosomal recessive inheritance, platelets appear characteristically gray after Romanovsky staining. Immunoelectron microscopy shows that normal α-granules are absent[17]; they are replaced by vacuoles. However, it appears that the granule-limiting membranes are present and their protein components are normally expressed[18]; P-selectin is also present. Patients with GPS may have a defect affecting the storage or packaging of the α-granules.[19] The early onset of myelofibrosis in the bone marrow is a feature of most patients with GPS. Myelofibrosis may be a consequence of extracellular leakage of α-granule proteins.[20] Quebec syndrome is also associated with an α-granule defect. Abnormalities in δ-granules may be associated with Hermansky-Pudlak syndrome, Chediak-Higashi syndrome, or Wiskott-Aldrich syndrome. Patients in whom both α- and δ-granules are affected may have $\alpha\delta$-storage pool disease.

Acquired drug-induced qualitative platelet disorders, such as that caused by aspirin use, affect secretory responses of platelets. In addition, congenital defects in COX-1 and thromboxane synthesis may occur and these can give rise to abnormalities of platelet secretion. Hirata et al[21] have identified an arginine to leucine mutation at codon 60 in the TXA_2 receptor, which is part of the transmembrane domain. This mutation impairs both phospholipase C (PLC) activation[21] and adenylyl cyclase activation.[22] The defect results in platelet aggregation responses that resemble those seen after aspirin ingestion by control donors.

Treatment of Platelet Disorders

The treatment of platelet disorders is primarily with platelet concentrates. These are effective in patients who have thrombocytopenia, and in some instances of platelet metabolic abnormality. However, platelet concentrates are less effective in patients with GT and BSS. As these patients have abnormalities of their platelet surface receptors, proteins associated with the transfused platelets are recognized as foreign, and antibodies are produced. In patients with GT, the antibodies are directed against GPIIb-IIIa. In BSS patients, the antibodies are most commonly targeted towards GPIb, although GPIX or GPV may also provoke an immune response. However, recombinant factor VIIa (rFVIIa; NovoSeven®, Novo Nordisk, Bagsvaerd, Denmark) is able to bypass these platelet defects and may provide hemostatically effective therapy in patients with platelet disorders.[23,24] Indeed, the agent has recently been approved in the European Union for use in GT refractory to platelet transfusion. The precise means by which rFVIIa exerts its efficacy in such patients has yet to be elucidated. Recombinant FVIIa may improve thrombin generation through direct binding to activated platelets.[25] In some instances, the agent has been shown to induce, at least partly, thrombin-activatable fibrinolysis inhibitor-dependent downregulation of fibrinolysis.[26] Consequently, it is possible that rFVIIa may reduce fibrinolysis in patients with GT and BSS, and promote hemostasis.

Conclusion

Patients may have platelet disorders that are quantitative, whereby they have reduced numbers of platelets, or qualitative, in which platelets exhibit abnormal functioning. The treatment of platelet disorders is primarily with platelet concentrates. However, in patients with defects in their platelet surface receptors, platelet transfusion may provoke an immune response and therapy with rFVIIa may be hemostatically effective.

References

1. Alevriadou BR, Moake JL, Turner NA, Ruggeri ZM, Folie BJ, Phillips MD, et al: Real-time analysis of shear-dependent thrombus formation and its blockade by inhibitors of von Willebrand factor binding to platelets. Blood 81:1263-1276, 1993
2. Santoro SA, Zutter MM: The alpha2beta1 integrin: A collagen receptor on platelets and other cells. Thromb Haemost 74:813-821, 1995
3. Tsuji M, Ezumi Y, Arai M, Takayama H: A novel association of Fc receptor γ-chain with glycoprotein VI and their co-expression as a collagen receptor in human platelets. J Biol Chem 272:23528-23531, 1997
4. Tandon NN, Kralisz U, Jamieson GA: Identification of glycoprotein IV (CD36) as a primary receptor for platelet-collagen adhesion. J Biol Chem 264:7576-7583, 1989
5. Piotrowicz RS, Orchekowski RP, Nugent DJ, Yamada KY, Kunicki TJ: Glycoprotein Ic-IIa functions as an activation-independent fibronectin receptor on human platelets. J Cell Biol 106:1359-1364, 1988
6. White GC II: Platelet physiology and function. Blood Coagul Fibrinolysis 11:S53, 2000 (suppl 1)
7. Smith W, Garavito RM, DeWitt DL: Prostaglandin endoperoxide H synthases (cyclooxygenases)-1 and -2. J Biol Chem 271:33157-33160, 1996
8. Fitzgerald GA: Mechanisms of platelet activation: Thromboxane A_2 as an amplifying signal for other agonists. Am J Cardiol 68:11B-15B, 1991
9. Roth GJ, Stanford N, Majerus PW: Acetylation of prostaglandin synthase by aspirin. Proc Natl Acad Sci U S A 72:3073-3076, 1975
10. Papp B, Enyedi A, Kovacs T, Sarkadi B, Wuytack F, Thastrup O, et al: Demonstration of two forms of calcium pumps by thapsigargin inhibition and radioimmunoblotting in platelet membrane vesicles. J Biol Chem 266:14593-14596, 1991
11. Dode L, Wuytack F, Kools PFJ, Baba-Aissa F, Raeymaekers L, Brik F, et al: cDNA cloning, expression and chromosomal localization of the human sarco/endoplasmic reticulum CA^{2+}-ATPase 3 gene. Biochem J 318:689-699, 1996
12. Woodside DG, Liu S, Ginsberg MH: Integrin activation. Thromb Haemost 86:316-323, 2001
13. George JN, Caen JP, Nurden AT: Glanzmann's thrombasthenia: The spectrum of clinical disease. Blood 75:1383-1395, 1990
14. López JA, Andrews RK, Afshar-Khargan V, Berndt MC: Bernard-Soulier syndrome. Blood 91:4397-4418, 1998
15. Di Castelnuovo A, de Gaetano G, Donati MB, Iacoviello L: Platelet glycoprotein receptor IIIa polymorphism PLA1/PLA2 and coronary risk: A meta-analysis. Thromb Haemost 85:626-633, 2001
16. Kritzik M, Savage B, Nugent DJ, Santoso S, Ruggeri ZM, Kunicki TJ: Nucleotide polymorphisms in the α_2 gene define multiple alleles that are associated with differences in platelet $\alpha_2\beta_1$ density. Blood 92:2382-2388, 1998
17. Cramer EM, Vainchenker W, Vinci G, Guichard J, Breton-Gorius J: Gray platelet syndrome: Immunoelectron microscopic localization of fibrinogen and von Willebrand factor in platelets and megakaryocytes. Blood 66:1309-1316, 1985
18. Rosa JP, George JN, Bainton DF, Nurden AT, Caen JP, McEver RP: Gray

platelet syndrome: Demonstration of α-granule membranes that can fuse with the cell surface. J Clin Invest 80:1138-1146, 1987
19. Drouin A, Favier R, Massé J-M, Debili N, Schmitt A, Elbim C, et al: Newly recognized cellular abnormalities in the gray platelet syndrome. Blood 98:1382-1391, 2001
20. Schmitt A, Jouault H, Guichard J, Wendling F, Drouin A, Cramer EM: Pathologic interaction between megakaryocytes and polymorphonuclear leukocytes in myelofibrosis. Blood 96:1342-1347, 2000
21. Hirata T, Kakizuka A, Ushikubi F, Fuse I, Okuma M, Narumiya S: Arg^{60} to Leu mutation of the human thromboxane A_2 receptor in a dominantly inherited bleeding disorder. J Clin Invest 94:1662-1667, 1994
22. Hirata T, Ushikubi F, Kakizuka A, Okuma M, Narumiya S: Two thromboxane A_2 receptor isoforms in human platelets. Opposite coupling to adenylyl cyclase with different sensitivity to Arg^{60} to Leu mutation. J Clin Invest 97:949-956, 1996
23. Poon M-C, D'Oiron R, Von Depka M, Khair K, Négrier C, Karafoulidou A, et al: Prophylactic and therapeutic recombinant factor VIIa administration to patients with Glanzmann's thrombasthenia: Results of an international survey. J Thromb Haemost 2:1096-1103, 2004
24. Levi M, Peters M, Büller HR: Efficacy and safety of recombinant factor VIIa for treatment of severe bleeding: A systematic review. Crit Care Med 33:883-890, 2005
25. Monroe DM, Hoffman M, Oliver JA, Roberts HR: Platelet activity of high-dose factor VIIa is independent of tissue factor. Br J Haematol 99:542-547, 1997
26. Antovic JP, Antovic A: Does recombinant factor VIIa, apart from overall hemostasis, regulate TAFI dependent fibrinolysis? In vitro analysis using overall hemostasis potential (OHP) assay. Thromb Haemost 90: 620-627, 2003

ELSEVIER

Seminars in
HEMATOLOGY

Steps Towards an Effective Treatment Strategy in Congenital Factor VII Deficiency

Guglielmo Mariani,[a] Mario Lapecorella,[b] and Alberto Dolce[c]

Congenital factor VII (FVII) deficiency is a consequence of a genetic polymorphism that can produce a wide spectrum of disease severity. Mildly affected patients may experience increased bleeding after surgery, trauma or mucosal bleeding, while spontaneous and life-threatening bleeding occurs in patients who are severely affected. Replacement therapy is the mainstay of treatment for patients with FVII deficiency. This has traditionally been achieved using fresh frozen plasma (FFP), prothrombin complex concentrates (PCCs), or plasma-derived FVII concentrates. However, recombinant activated FVII is now widely used for therapy in these patients. As cases of FVII deficiency tend to be encountered infrequently in most centers, no consolidated evidence-based therapeutic regimens have evolved and the side effects of the available treatments have not been comprehensively evaluated. Consequently, an online registry, the Seven Treatment Evaluation Registry (STER) has been set up. This is a prospective study that aims to evaluate the efficacy and safety of the different therapeutic options with which FVII-deficient patients may be treated. Recruitment of patients into the study is currently underway.
Semin Hematol 43(suppl 1):S42-S47

Congenital factor VII (FVII) deficiency is a rare bleeding disorder affecting both male and female patients.[1] In mildly affected individuals, the disorder is characterized by increased bleeding after surgery and trauma and/or by skin and mucous membrane bleeds; in severely affected patients, spontaneous, severe, and life-threatening bleeding occurs most frequently.[1-4] Correlation between FVII coagulation activity (FVII:C) and bleeding tendency is poor.[1,4] Although asymptomatic subjects with FVII:C levels of $< 1\%$ have consistently been reported,[1,2,4,5] severe bleeding episodes occur most often in homozygous or double heterozygous individuals with FVII:C levels of $< 2\%$ of normal.[5]

Diagnosis of FVII deficiency is not as straightforward as may be inferred from analyzing severe cases alone. Only around half of patients (51%) are diagnosed at disease presentation or within 6 months of their first symptoms; other patients are diagnosed after a variable delay, which may sometimes last for several years.[5] However, severe cases of FVII deficiency are most frequently diagnosed during childhood.[3,5]

As the heterogeneity of the clinical picture is a striking feature of the disease, and because FVII:C cannot be used to reliably classify disease severity, management should be based on clinical data. To create groups of patients with a similar bleeding risk, we have recently proposed a disease severity classification based on the timing and mode of disease presentation (Table 1 and Fig 1), which incorporates residual FVII function and disease zygosity.[5] Accordingly, accurate records of bleeding history are essential for disease management. Our classification is useful to assess and improve therapeutic strategies in homogeneous groups of patients with FVII deficiency.

Clinical Issues Useful for Treatment

As mentioned above, the most severe cases of FVII deficiency are diagnosed during childhood. Hemorrhages underlying this early disease onset can occur in the gastrointestinal tract or central nervous system (Fig 1), with prevalences of 14% and 5%, respectively. Taken together, these are the most frequent bleeds in the first 6 months of life (65% and 70% of cases, respectively).[5] Hemarthrosis, another common presenting symptom (18.5% of cases), can arise when infants

[a]L'Aquila University Medical School, Department of Medicine and Public Health, L'Aquila, Italy.
[b]Hematology Unit, Ospedale S. Salvatore, L'Aquila, Italy.
[c]Department of Economic Development, Sicily Region, Palermo, Italy.
Address correspondence to Guglielmo Mariani, Full Professor of Hematology, Universita degli Studi de L'Aquila, Ematologia Dipartimento di Medicina Internae Sanita Pubblica, Largo Tommasi 1, Coppito, 67100 L'Aquila, Italy. E-mail: gmariani@cc.univaq.it

 0037-1963/06/$-see front matter
doi:10.1053/j.seminhematol.2005.11.017

Table 1 Severity Classification for FVII Deficiency

Class of Severity	Clinical Phenotype
Severe	CNS bleeding and/or GI bleeding and/or hemarthrosis with or without other bleeding symptoms
Moderate	Three or more bleeding symptoms (CNS bleeding, GI bleeding, or hemarthrosis excluded)
Mild	One or two symptoms (CNS bleeding, GI bleeding, or hemarthrosis excluded)

Abbreviations: CNS, central nervous system; FVII, factor VII; GI, gastrointestinal.
Reproduced with permission from Mariani G, et al.[5]

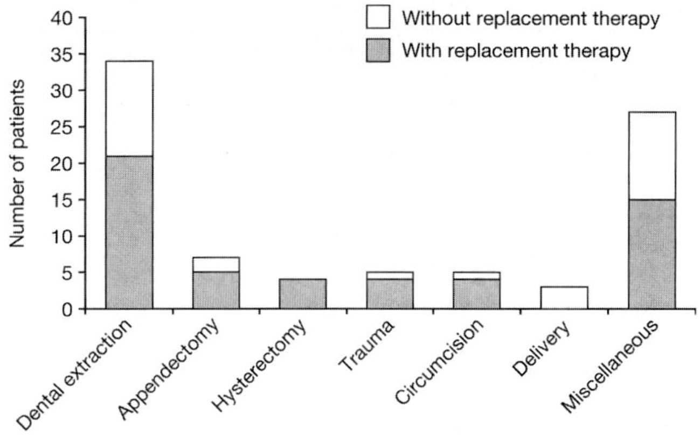

Figure 2 Postoperative bleeding in factor VII deficiency, in relation to replacement therapy.

start to crawl or walk (Fig 1). When this symptom occurs frequently, it can be considered as the hallmark for a severe clotting defect with very low FVII:C levels (median, 1%; range, 0.9% to 3%).[5] Early presentation of these life-threatening or disabling symptoms provides an important argument in favor of early and aggressive disease management. In addition, long-term prophylaxis should be considered.[5]

Another important feature of this disease is the excess of symptomatic female patients. In the International Registry on Congenital Factor VII Deficiency (IRF7) database, symptomatic females are more prevalent (56%) than symptomatic males. This is due partly to the frequency of menorrhagia among females of fertile age (60%), and partly to a higher prevalence of easy bruising and gum bleeding among women.[5] The prevalence of iron-deficient anemia among females with menorrhagia is very high and this points towards the need for hemostatic screening in women with excessive blood loss, particularly when invasive procedures are planned. In addition, short courses of prophylaxis during menses should be considered, especially when refractoriness/side effects to the contraceptive pill are observed.

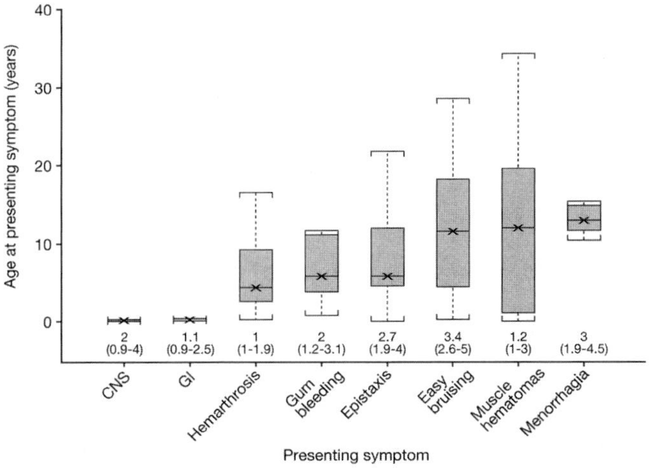

Figure 1 Ranking of symptoms by age at presentation. The gray area in the box and whisker plot comprises 50% of the cases (25th–75th percentile). × represents the median values of age; caps denote extreme values. The values under the boxes denote median factor VII coagulation activity values (confidence intervals in brackets). CNS, central nervous system; GI, gastrointestinal. Reproduced with permission from Mariani G, et al.[5]

Postoperative bleeding is a frequent symptom (25% of cases) in the IRF7 database,[5] with a significant proportion of patients bleeding despite the administration of replacement therapy (Fig 2). These data emphasize that management of FVII deficiency, in terms of substitution therapy and treatment schedules, is not yet optimal. Replacement therapy for surgery is also a debatable issue: the need for such treatment has been questioned, at least in asymptomatic subjects, regardless of FVII:C levels.[6]

Treatment of FVII Deficiency

Unlike other rare clotting factor disorders, the treatment of congenital FVII deficiency does afford some therapeutic options (Table 2).[7] Replacement therapy with FVII is the mainstay of treatment, and such therapy is characterized by features that are specific to this hemorrhagic disorder, ie, (1) the very short half life of FVII, which is apparent for both the zymogen and the active form, and which is independent of the dose[8-10]; (2) the recovery of FVII, which is similar to that of factor IX (FIX); and (3) the clearance of FVII, which is fast in adults[9] and even faster in children.[9-11] The minimum protective FVII levels appear to be about 9% to 12%. To maintain these trough levels, a repeated administration schedule (two to four times per day) is often required, especially for post-surgical treatment.

FVII replacement has traditionally been achieved with fresh frozen plasma (FFP), prothrombin complex concentrates (PCCs), or plasma-derived FVII concentrates.[7,12] However, plasma-derived products are associated with a risk, albeit very small, of blood-borne pathogen transmission. In addition, FFP may cause circulatory overload, particularly if repeated administration is needed, i.e. in the surgical setting. Administration of PCCs results in an unwanted increase in other vitamin K-dependent factors and is associated with both arterial and venous thrombosis.[13] Therapy with recombinant activated FVII (rFVIIa; NovoSeven®, Novo Nordisk, Bagsvaerd, Denmark) is now widely used for the treatment of

Table 2 Treatments Available for Congenital FVII Deficiency

Treatment	Potency (IU/mL)	Advantages	Disadvantages
FFP (VA)	1	Cheap; readily available	Limited efficacy; unsuitable for surgery; risk of circulatory overload
PCCs (VA)	5–10	Suitable for surgery	Concentrations of other vitamin K-dependent factors are higher than that of FVII; presence of activated factors; risk of thrombosis
Plasma-derived FVII (VA)	20–40	Effective; suitable for surgery	Concentrations of other vitamin K-dependent factors are higher than that of FVII; risk of thrombosis
rFVIIa	>25,000	Very effective in low doses; no risk of viral transmission	Cost per treatment is high, but affordable

Abbreviations: FFP, fresh frozen plasma; FVII, factor VII; rFVIIa, recombinant activated factor VII; PCCs, prothrombin complex concentrates; VA, virus attenuated.
Adapted with permission from Mariani G, et al.[7] Blackwell Publishing.

FVII deficiency, but no clear-cut information on optimal dosages and treatment schedules is currently available.[7,14-16]

Initially approved for use in hemophilia with inhibitors, rFVIIa has recently received approval in the European Union to treat bleeding in patients with congenital FVII deficiency or patients with Glanzmann's thrombasthenia who are refractory to platelet transfusions. The rationale behind the use of rFVIIa in congenital FVII deficiency is based on the fact that the agent provides only the missing protein in a low-volume preparation, and is devoid of other human proteins and potential blood-borne pathogens. The main advantage of therapy is that rFVIIa is the physiological replacement protein in FVII deficiency and, as a consequence of the very low levels found in normal individuals (1% of FVII:C, 0.1 nmol/L or 4 ng/mL), low-dose substitution therapy can be performed.

rFVIIa in the Treatment of FVII Deficiency: Compassionate- and Emergency-Use Programs and Independent Reports

The treatment of congenital FVII deficiency with rFVIIa has recently been reviewed.[17] In compassionate- and emergency-use programs, the amount of data collected was limited, but the data that are available provide convincing evidence of the efficacy of rFVIIa in both children and adults with FVII deficiency.

A summary of the use of rFVIIa in compassionate- and emergency-use programs is provided in Table 3. rFVIIa was effective in 62/69 (90%) of the treatment episodes. This level of efficacy is similar to that observed for recombinant factor VIII in patients with hemophilia A. Other reports describe efficacy rates of 76% to 100% for rFVIIa in FVII deficiency.[18-20] In compassionate- and emergency-use programs, patients with FVII deficiency were generally treated with rFVIIa after the failure of other therapy, and dosing regimens varied widely among the patients. This is a serious drawback with regard to efficacy evaluation, as these programs selected patients with the most severe problems.

Independent reports have described the use of rFVIIa in 26 treatment episodes in 20 patients with congenital FVII deficiency (Table 4). An overall efficacy rate similar to that of the compassionate-use study was apparent. Surgical coverage was the most frequent reason for using rFVIIa, and all reported procedures were completed without excessive bleeding. Acute bleeding episodes were also treated with rFVIIa, and all resolved satisfactorily without drug-related complications. The successful use of rFVIIa was reported in two cesarean sections and one vaginal birth.[17] Other reports have described the use of rFVIIa in children as prophylaxis for intracerebral hemorrhage (ICH), recurrent epistaxis, menorrhagia, and hemarthrosis.[17] The prophylactic dosing regimens were in the range of 15 to 90 μg/kg by bolus injection, administered from twice daily to twice weekly for up to 2 years.

In general, the recommended dose of 15 to 30 μg/kg rFVIIa every 4 to 6 hours appears to be effective in maintaining hemostasis during bleeding episodes or surgery in FVII-deficient patients. The same conclusions were drawn in the first published analysis of the compassionate-use programs.[21] Brummel Ziedins et al[22] recently indicated that a low FVIIa replacement dose in individuals with severe FVII deficiency can achieve hemostasis in the nonbleeding state; 23 μg/kg of rFVIIa was shown to induce "normal" FVIIa concentrations

Table 3 Summary of rFVIIa Therapy in Compassionate- and Emergency-Use Programs

	Surgery	CNS	Joint	Other	Total
Effective	25	11	20	6	62
Partially effective	0	2	0	1	3
Ineffective	0	1	0	0	1
Other	1	0	0	2	3
Overall effectiveness	25/26 (96%)		37/43 (86%)		62/69 (90%)

Abbreviations: CNS, central nervous system; rFVIIa, recombinant activated factor VII.

Table 4 Independent Published Reports From 1995 to 2003 Describing the use of rFVIIa in FVII Deficiency (overall efficacy 89%)[17]

Treatment Episode	No. of Episodes (patients)	Age Range (yr)	rFVIIa Dosing Regimen
Surgery	11 (8)	13–85	11–40 μg/kg; 2.5 μg/kg/h CI
Acute bleeding	5 (4)	0–55	25–80 μg/kg; 5 μg/kg/h CI
Childbirth	3 (3)	22–30	20–50 μg/kg; 1.7–3.3 μg/kg/h CI
Prophylaxis	7 (7)	0–15	15–90 μg/kg (twice daily to twice weekly)

Abbreviations: CI, continuous infusion; rFVIIa, recombinant activated factor VII.

in vivo (0.3 to 0.7 nmol/L, equivalent to 1 to 4 ng of FVIIa), a correction that lasted for about 6 hours. This experimental finding is in line with those of Mariani et al,[21] who analyzed rFVIIa efficacy in FVII-deficient patients from the compassionate- and emergency-use studies and found that an average dose of 20 μg/kg normalized the international normalized ratio (INR).

As FVII zymogen competes with FVIIa for binding to tissue factor to initiate blood coagulation,[9,22] the dose used in treating FVII-deficient patients could be altered according to the concentration of the FVII zymogen (presence/absence of FVIIAg).[22]

Side Effects of Replacement Therapy

As mentioned above, plasma derivatives such as those outlined in Table 2 may carry a residual risk of transmitting blood-borne pathogens, although this risk is actually very small. The most relevant side effects of replacement therapy in FVII deficiency are thrombosis and the development of inhibitory antibodies to FVII; these complications do not appear to be related to any specific treatment. However, apparently spontaneous thromboembolic events have been reported in patients with FVII deficiency in the absence of treatment.[13] In addition, thromboembolic episodes have been reported in surgical patients with FVII deficiency.[13] Surgery is a well-known and powerful triggering factor for thrombosis, and replacement therapies (FFP, PCCs, or plasma-derived FVII concentrates) may contribute to the problem by producing unnecessarily high levels of FVII and other activated and nonactivated factors (FIX/FIXa, FX/FXa, FIIa). This suggests that replacement therapy should ideally be carried out using a pure FVII concentrate in controlled dosages.

There also exist reports of thrombosis in FVII-deficient patients receiving treatment with rFVIIa. Analysis of 11 such patients, together with nine previously unreported cases, suggests that none of the thrombotic episodes were related to the use of rFVIIa.[13] However, this remains to be confirmed. A subsequently referred case of FVII deficiency and thrombosis was also unrelated to the use of rFVIIa. Despite high FVII:C levels observed immediately after infusion of rFVIIa, no thromboembolic complications have been reported with the use of rFVIIa in the compassionate- and emergency-use programs, or in the literature. However, three thromboembolic events in FVII-deficient patients who received rFVIIa were spontaneously reported to Novo Nordisk before rFVIIa was approved for use in FVII deficiency (two arterial thrombotic events and one pulmonary embolism).[17] It is not known whether these patients had severe FVII deficiency, and at least two of the cases involved doses of rFVIIa that were higher than the recommended dose (90 μg/kg followed by 40 μg/kg in one case, and two doses of 50 μg/kg in another).

Recently, a comparative analysis of thromboembolic events in patients treated with either factor VIII bypassing agents or rFVIIa has been published, based on the MedWatch program of the US Food and Drug Administration.[23] However, the data collated in this report do not provide information on clinical settings or treatment schedules, and trauma patients are compared with patients with hemophilia or other hemorrhagic disorders, both congenital and acquired.[23,24] At present, there are too few data to draw any firm conclusions as to the risk of thrombosis in FVII-deficient patients treated with rFVIIa. Until further data become available, the potential risk of thrombosis should be taken into account when evaluating the need for, and the dose of, substitution therapy, particularly for patients undergoing surgery.

There has been no systematic testing for FVII alloantibody development in patients with FVII deficiency who have received rFVIIa. To date, three such instances of FVII alloantibody development have been identified. One case was described in an independently published report, and two cases were from the compassionate- and emergency-use programs, in which 13 patients were tested for antibody formation.[25-27] All three patients had previously been exposed to plasma-derived FVII, and it therefore remains uncertain whether rFVIIa was responsible for the alloantibody development. Little is known about the kinetic features of these alloantibodies. There are currently insufficient data on substitution therapy in FVII deficiency to draw any conclusions regarding the risk of clinically significant alloantibody formation.

Based on these limited data, it is clear that prospective studies on the occurrence of therapy-related side effects are needed.

The Seven Treatment Evaluation Registry

The IRF7 Study Group was set up, as an informal group, in 1999. A worldwide collection of data relating to patients with congenital FVII deficiency was subsequently implemented, totaling 515 cases.[5] For 313 of these cases, analysis included full molecular characterization. The resulting database included 41 primary and 18 derived variables for each patient, 22 of which pertained to clinical data.

From the outset, it was apparent that disease management was a major issue,[5] as shown by the high prevalence of post-surgical bleeding even in patients receiving replacement therapy (Fig 2). This may be related to the varied therapies used—not only in terms of treatment materials, but also with regard to dosages and schedules. Thrombotic events were another issue.[13,23] Furthermore, none of the IRF7 centers had a method of assaying inhibitors to FVII.

Consequently, we were prompted to create a registry—the Seven Treatment Evaluation Registry (STER)—to collate data on the treatment of patients with FVII deficiency, including therapy-related side effects. This prospective observational study intends to elucidate the efficacy and safety of the currently available treatment modalities for spontaneous bleeds, surgical coverage, and prophylaxis. This should enable evidence-based knowledge of the treatment of patients with FVII deficiency to be obtained, as this has been an area of medicine where treatment decisions have been based more on personal clinical experience than on consolidated clinical evidence.

The primary objectives of the STER are: (1) to describe treatment modalities for bleeding episodes in a well-defined, international cohort of FVII-deficient patients; (2) to study the occurrence of antibodies/inhibitors to FVII; (3) to evaluate the occurrence of thrombotic complications; (4) to describe, and consider the effectiveness of, short-term prophylactic schedules in relation to elective surgical procedures; (5) to describe long-term schedules of prophylaxis; and (6) to evaluate the efficacy and safety of the available therapeutic tools in real-life clinical settings.

The secondary objectives involve: (1) evaluation and comparison of the in vivo recovery of FVII after the administration of different types of substitution therapy; and (2) assessment of the specificity and sensitivity of a new method for assaying inhibitors to FVII in a large cohort of FVII-deficient patients (with different gene mutations) treated with different methods. Inhibitor testing will be carried out in a centralized fashion, using a method specifically developed for measuring antibodies to FVII.[25]

The STER uses a specifically created online registry. When treating physicians have obtained clearance from the Review Board and received a password from the system administrator, they can report case information electronically by accessing a secured website (*https://www.IRF7therapy.org*, or, preferably, *www.targetseven.org*). Patient files on the website can be accessed only by the enrolling physicians, system administrators and the laboratory that is performing the inhibitor assay. The database security has been set up in accordance with the standard requirements for safety and security described in the Minimum Security Requirements (MSR) for hosting documents. When centralized inhibitor testing has been performed, the information will be entered into the patient's file, and the case will be validated.

The STER has the following main sections: (a) patient demographics and clinical characterization; (b) treatment of "spontaneous" bleeding episodes; (c) prophylaxis; (d) surgical interventions (including delivery); (e) adverse events. Physicians will enter data into either section b, c, or d, depending on the case involved. Treatment with the following types of substitution therapy will be considered: (1) virus-inactivated plasma; (2) FPP; (3) PCCs; (4) plasma-derived FVII concentrate; and (5) rFVIIa. Fig 3 shows flow charts relating to the main clinical features of the study.

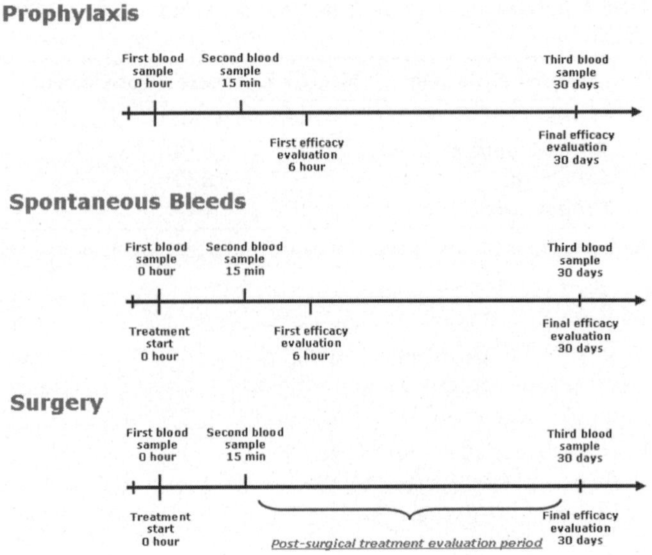

Figure 3 Flow charts for the Seven Treatment Evaluation Registry (STER) study.

Details of the registry (both the protocol and other documents) can be found at *www.targetseven.org*, from where a demonstration and the Center Enrolment Form can also be accessed. A complimentary hard copy of the protocol is available upon request (*assister@targetseven.org*).

Summary

FVII deficiency is a consequence of genetic polymorphisms that can produce a wide spectrum of disease severity. Unlike hemophilia, the clinical severity of patients with FVII deficiency cannot be predicted by residual levels of the affected factor and, therefore, management strategies in these patients should be based mostly on clinical information (eg, bleeding history).[5] We have proposed a scale of severity classification, and this is useful in enabling clinicians to select an appropriate treatment strategy.

Replacement therapy is the mainstay of treatment in FVII deficiency. However, there are no guidelines or evidence-based data concerning optimal schedules or dosages. As cases of FVII deficiency are encountered infrequently in most centers, no consolidated, evidence-based practice has evolved, and it has proven difficult to comprehensively evaluate side effects of treatment. Several cases of thrombosis (approximately 20 in 40 years) have been described; some of these cases may have been spontaneous, whereas others were clearly related to therapy and/or surgery. Inhibitory antibodies to FVII are encountered very infrequently; screening for these rarely takes place and no standard methods of screening are available.

Consequently, the IRF7 Study Group has proposed a prospective study in which details from carefully characterized patients are recorded. Any replacement therapy can be used (from plasma to rFVIIa), and a strictly defined methodology for the screening of side effects has been set up. The study is based on an online registry (STER), and it is planned to collate information from at least 200 cases. As agreed with the European Agency for the Evaluation of Medicinal Products (EMEA), data from cases treated with rFVIIa will provide the core of pharmaco-surveillance data for this drug in patients with FVII deficiency. The data are property of the IRF7 Study Group and, apart from a commitment to reporting the rFVIIa-treated cases to the EMEA, they will be analyzed and reported autonomously.

By September 2005, 56 centers from 19 countries worldwide had applied to take part in the study, and the first patients had been enrolled. To obtain both data from patients with a broad array of genetic mutations, and information relating to a comprehensive range of clinical variations and management strategies, we aim to involve a total of around 80 to 100 centers.

Acknowledgment

We wish to thank the members of the IRF7 Study Group (listed in Mariani et al[5]) for the data, and members of the Steering Committee for their suggestions and continuous support.

References

1. Mariani G, Dolce A: Congenital factor VII deficiency, in Lee C, Berntorp E, Hoots K (eds): Textbook of Hemophilia. Malden, MA, Blackwell, 2005, p 311
2. Peyvandi F, Mannucci PM, Asti D, Abdoullahi M, Di Rocco N, Sharifian R: Clinical manifestations in 28 Italian and Iranian patients with severe factor VII deficiency. Haemophilia 3:242-246, 1997
3. Ragni MV, Lewis JH, Spero JA, Hasiba U: Factor VII deficiency. Am J Hematol 10:79-88, 1981
4. Mariani G, Mazzucconi MG: Factor VII congenital deficiency. Clinical picture and classification of the variants. Haemostasis 13:169-177, 1983
5. Mariani G, Herrmann F, Dolce A, Batorova A, Etro D, Peyvandi F, et al: Clinical phenotypes and factor VII genotype in congenital factor VII deficiency. Thromb Haemost 93:481-487, 2005
6. Giansily-Blaizot M, Biron-Andreani C, Aguilar-Martinez P, de Moerloose P, Briquel ME, Goudemand J, et al: Inherited factor VII deficiency and surgery: Clinical data are the best criteria to predict the risk of bleeding. Br J Haematol 117:172-175, 2002
7. Mariani G, Dolce A, Marchetti G, Bernardi F: Clinical picture and management of congenital factor VII deficiency. Haemophilia 10:180-183, 2004 (suppl 4)
8. Mariani G, Mannucci PM, Mazzucconi MG, Capitanio A: Treatment of congenital factor VII deficiency with a new concentrate. Thromb Haemost 39:675-682, 1978
9. Berrettini M, Mariani G, Schiavoni M, Rocino A, Di Paolantonio T, Longo G, et al: Pharmacokinetic evaluation of recombinant, activated factor VII in patients with inherited factor deficiency. Haematologica 86:640-645, 2001
10. Erhardtsen E: Pharmacokinetics of recombinant activated factor VII (rFVIIa). Semin Thromb Hemost 26:385-391, 2000
11. Villar A, Aronis S, Morfini M, Santagostino E, Auerswald G, Thomsen HF, et al: Pharmacokinetics of activated recombinant coagulation factor VII (NovoSeven) in children vs. adults with haemophilia A. Haemophilia 10:352-359, 2004
12. Ingerslev J, Kristensen HL: Clinical picture and treatment strategies in factor VII deficiency. Haemophilia 4:689-696, 1998
13. Mariani G, Herrmann FH, Schulman S, Batorova A, Wulff K, Etro D, et al: Thrombosis in inherited factor VII deficiency. J Thromb Haemost 1:2153-2158, 2003
14. Eskandari N, Feldman N, Greenspoon JS: Factor VII deficiency in pregnancy treated with recombinant factor VIIa. Obstet Gynecol 99:935-937, 2002
15. Perry DJ: Factor VII deficiency. Br J Haematol 118:689-700, 2002
16. United Kingdom Haemophilia Centre Doctors' Organisation (UKHCDO): Guidelines on the selection and use of therapeutic products to treat haemophilia and other hereditary bleeding disorders. Haemophilia 9:1-23, 2003
17. Mariani G, Konkle BA, Ingerslev J: Congenital factor VII deficiency: Therapy with recombinant activated factor VII. A critical appraisal. Haemophilia (in press)
18. Berry EW, Teague L, Pitcher L, Ockelford P: NovoSeven® prophylaxis for severe FVII deficiency. Abstract from the Free-Paper Session and the Poster Session presented at the 6th Novo Nordisk Symposium on Treatment of Bleeding and Thrombotic Disorders, Copenhagen, Denmark, May 3-4, 2001
19. Mathijssen NCJ, Masereeuw R, Verbeek K, Lavergne JM, Costa J-M, van Heerde WL, et al: Prophylactic effect of recombinant factor VIIa in factor VII deficient patients. Br J Haematol 125:494-499, 2004
20. Muleo G, Santoro R, Iannaccaro P, Papaleo G, Elia L, Leo F, et al: rFVIIa in congenital FVII deficiency. Thromb Res 91:S86, 1998 (suppl 1, abstr 169)
21. Mariani G, Testa MG, Di Paolantonio T, Molskov Bech R, Hedner U: Use of recombinant, activated factor VII in the treatment of congenital factor VII deficiencies. Vox Sang 77:131-136, 1999
22. Brummel Ziedins K, Rivard GE, Pouliot RL, Butenas S, Gissel M, Parhami-Seren B, et al: Factor VIIa replacement therapy in factor VII deficiency. J Thromb Haemost 2:1735-1744, 2004
23. Aledort LM: Comparative thrombotic event incidence after infusion of recombinant factor VIIa versus factor VIII bypass activity. J Thromb Haemost 2:1700-1708, 2004
24. Hay CRM. Thrombosis and recombinant factor VIIa (commentary). J Thromb Haemost 2:1698-1699, 2004
25. Ingerslev J, Christiansen K, Sørensen B: Inhibitors to factor VII in severe factor VII deficiency: Detection and course of inhibitory response. J Thromb Haemost 3:799-800, 2005
26. Bergmann F, Scharrer I: Transient factor VII inhibitor after replacement therapy with recombinant FVIIa (rFVIIa) in a child with FVII deficiency. Bone Marrow Transplant 92:104, 1998 (suppl 1, abstr 3430)
27. Nicolaisen EM: Antigenicity of activated recombinant factor VII followed through nine years of clinical experience. Blood Coagul Fibrinolysis 9:S119-S123, 1998 (suppl 1)

ELSEVIER

Seminars in
HEMATOLOGY

Acquired von Willebrand Syndrome: An Underdiagnosed and Misdiagnosed Bleeding Complication in Patients With Lymphoproliferative and Myeloproliferative Disorders

Augusto B. Federici

Acquired von Willebrand syndrome (AVWS) is a rare bleeding disorder with laboratory findings similar to those for congenital von Willebrand disease (VWD). Unlike the congenital disease, AVWS usually occurs in individuals with no personal or family history of bleeding. The prevalence of AVWS in the general population is unknown because data from large prospective studies of this syndrome are not available. Although AVWS is particularly frequent in lymphoproliferative or myeloproliferative disorders, it can also be associated with solid tumors, immunologic and cardiovascular disorders, and other miscellaneous conditions. Diagnosis of AVWS is based on assays measuring the activity of von Willebrand factor (VWF). This tends to be abnormally low, but factor VIII (FVIII) coagulant activity can sometimes be normal. FVIII/VWF inhibiting activity is found in only a minority of cases. Bleeding episodes in patients with AVWS are mostly of the mucocutaneous type and can be managed with desmopressin, plasma-derived FVIII/VWF concentrates, and intravenous immunoglobulin (IVIg). Recombinant activated factor VII can be useful in patients unresponsive to standard therapy. An updated version of the International Registry on AVWS, recently available online, will provide more information on this rare, but underdiagnosed and misdiagnosed, disorder.
Semin Hematol 43(suppl 1):S48-S58

Acquired von Willebrand syndrome (AVWS) is a rare bleeding disorder similar to inherited von Willebrand disease (VWD) in terms of laboratory findings and clinical severity. It is characterized by a prolonged bleeding time (BT) and variably low plasma levels of factor VIII (FVIII) and von Willebrand factor (VWF). The syndrome usually occurs in individuals with no personal or family history of bleeding. Data from large prospective studies are not available, and the actual prevalence of AVWS in the general population is therefore unknown. Mohri et al reported a prevalence of approximately 10% in 260 patients with hematological disorders studied by a single institution.[1] The majority of information pertaining to the clinical and laboratory features of the syndrome, as well as on different therapeutic approaches, has been derived from retrospective studies. Since the original description of AVWS in 1968, in a patient with systemic lupus erythematosus (SLE),[2] more than 300 cases of AVWS have been reported. Several review articles have been published,[3-11] and data from an International Registry on AVWS are also available.[12]

Angelo Bianchi Bonomi Hemophilia and Thrombosis Center, Department of Internal Medicine and Dermatology, IRCCS Foundation Maggiore Policlinico Hospital, Mangiagalli, Regina Elena and University of Milan, Milan, Italy.

Supported in part by the Explorative Action on International Registry on AVWS grant given to A.B.F. by the University of Milan. Most of the data on the diagnosis and management of AVWS are updated from the International Registry on AVWS, and have been previously published on behalf of the Scientific Standardization Subcommittee (SSC) on VWF of the International Society on Thrombosis and Haemostasis (ISTH).

Address correspondence to Augusto B. Federici, MD, Angelo Bianchi Bonomi Hemophilia and Thrombosis Center, Department of Internal Medicine and Dermatology, IRCCS Foundation Maggiore Policlinico Hospital, Mangiagalli, Regina Elena and University of Milan, Via Pace 9, 20122 Milano, Italy. E-mail: augusto.federici@unimi.it

Pathophysiology and Classification

VWF is synthesized normally in most AVWS patients,[12,13] but not in those with hypothyroidism, who characteristically exhibit decreased VWF synthesis or release.[5-12] In patients

 0037-1963/06/$-see front matter
doi:10.1053/j.seminhematol.2005.11.003

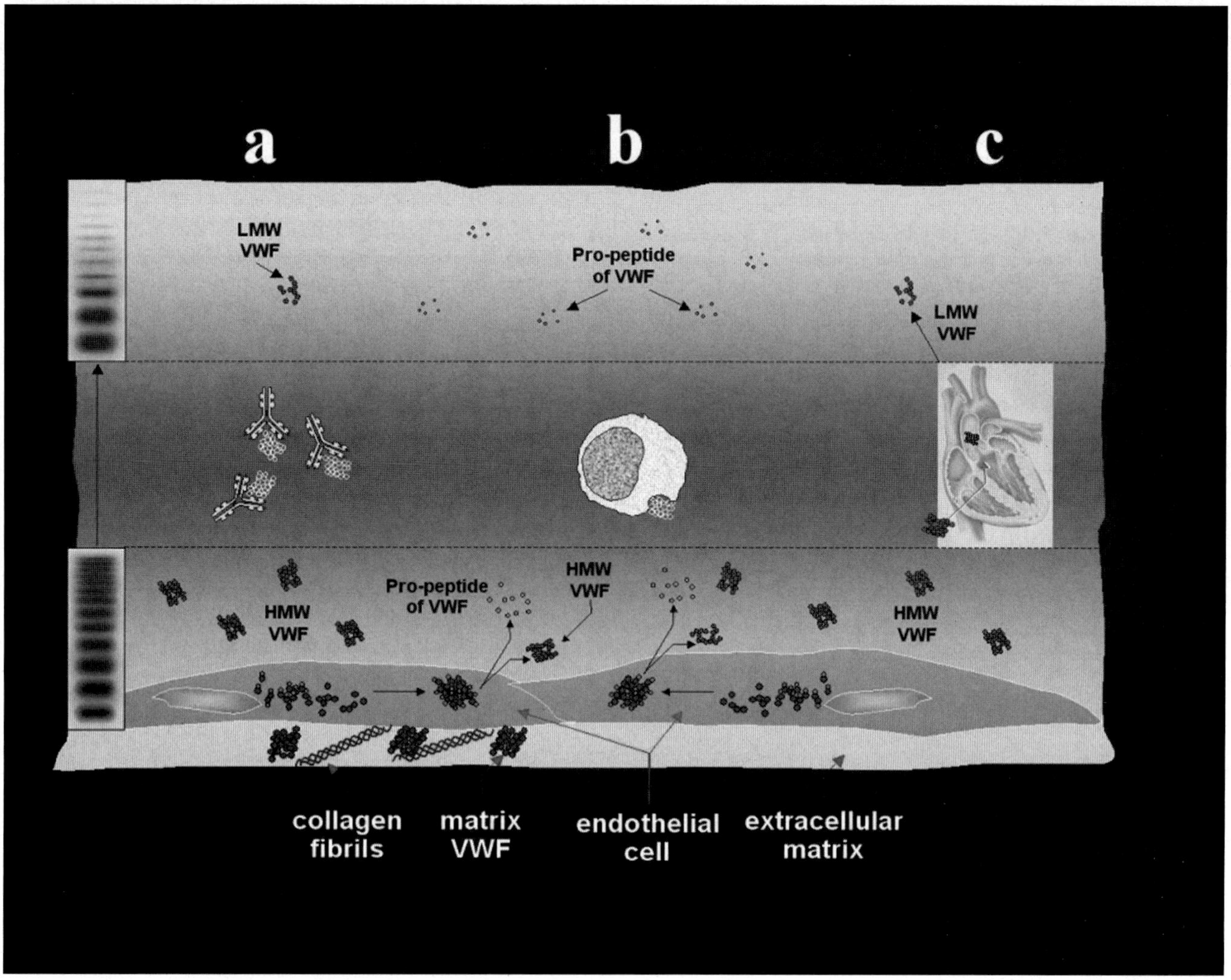

Figure 1 Pictorial representation of the three main pathogenetic mechanisms causing acquired von Willebrand Syndrome (AVWS). *Lower panel:* Normal von Willebrand factor (VWF) biosynthesis and release from endothelial cells. Note that all the high-molecular-weight multimers (HMW VWF) are present in the released VWF after the cleavage of VWF propeptide, which can be found in the circulation in equal amounts to native VWF. *Middle panel:* The three main mechanisms causing AVWS: (a) specific or nonspecific autoantibodies that inactivate VWF. These autoantibodies form circulating immune complexes with VWF and are cleared, together with VWF, by Fc-bearing cells; (b) absorption of VWF onto malignant cell clones; (c) loss of HMW VWF multimers under conditions of high shear stress occurring in heart valve abnormalities. *Upper panel:* The effects of these three mechanisms on VWF structure and function. In the case of autoantibodies (mechanism a), the entire native VWF normally secreted from the endothelial cells is usually removed from the circulation, resulting in very low concentrations of both VWF activity and antigen, but normal levels of VWF propeptide. When malignant cell clones (mechanism b) and conditions of high shear stress (mechanism c) cause AVWS, preferential removal of HMW VWF multimers occurs, resulting in reduced VWF activity with relatively normal VWF concentrations.

with normal synthesis of VWF, low levels of this factor result from its accelerated removal from the plasma by three main pathogenetic mechanisms (Fig 1): (a) specific or nonspecific autoantibodies that form circulating immune complexes with, and inactivate, VWF (these complexes are cleared by Fc-bearing cells); (b) absorption of VWF onto malignant cell clones; and (c) loss of high-molecular-weight (HMW) VWF multimers under conditions of high shear stress.

In patients with autoantibodies (mechanism a), the entire native VWF, normally secreted from the endothelial cells, is usually removed from the circulation; this results in very low concentrations of both VWF activity and VWF antigen (VWF:Ag), but normal levels of VWF propeptide are maintained.[14] When malignant cell clones (mechanism b) and conditions of high shear stress (mechanism c) cause AVWS, preferential removal of HMW VWF multimers occurs. This results in reduced VWF activity with relatively normal VWF concentrations (Fig 1).

An additional mechanism to be considered is the increased proteolytic degradation of VWF, which occurs in several clinical conditions characterized by the presence of circulating proteases.[15,16] This results in reduced VWF activity with rel-

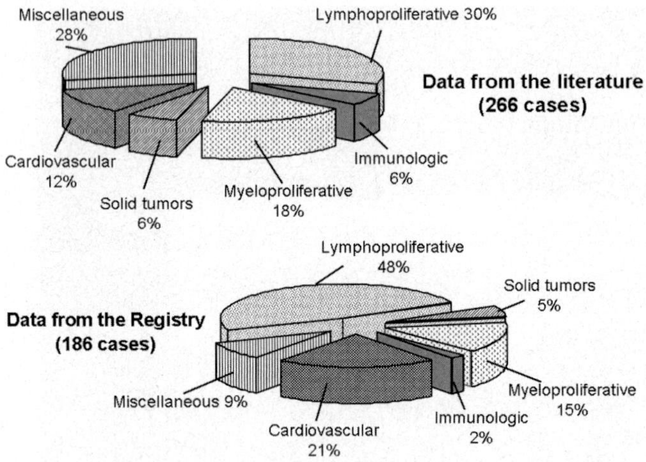

Figure 2 Distribution of the underlying disorders associated with acquired von Willebrand syndrome (AVWS): comparison between data from the literature and data obtained from the International Registry on AVWS. Note that a higher incidence of lymphoproliferative and cardiovascular disorders is observed in the data obtained from the registry (see also Tables 1 and 2).

atively normal VWF concentrations. Compared with acquired hemophilia, which is always due to autoantibodies against FVIII, the pathogenetic mechanisms underlying AVWS are more heterogeneous. None of the proposed mechanisms appear to be disease-specific, and the same mechanism can be responsible for AVWS in different underlying disorders that are known to be associated with the syndrome. In both recent reviews and the International Registry on AVWS, six categories of underlying disorders have been reported to occur frequently in patients with AVWS: lymphoproliferative and myeloproliferative disorders; solid tumors; immunologic and cardiovascular disorders; and miscellaneous conditions.[5-12] Taken together, lymphoproliferative and myeloproliferative disorders appear to be most frequently associated with AVWS in both the literature and the registry, accounting for 48% to 63% of cases (Fig 2).

General Diagnosis of AVWS

Diagnosis of AVWS is usually based on the laboratory parameters typical for VWD in the absence of a family history of bleeding. BT, VWF ristocetin cofactor activity (VWF:RCo), or collagen-binding assay (VWF:CB) in plasma compared with VWF:Ag, ristocetin-induced platelet agglutination, multimeric analysis in plasma and platelets, and VWF propeptide (formerly known as VWF antigen II) have all been used to identify patients with AVWS.[12,14] Testing for anti-FVIII/VWF antibodies should always be performed, because the presence of these inhibitors is clinically significant.[1] Testing for these antibodies can be carried out by measuring VWF activity after mixing experiments involving patient plasma and normal plasma incubated at 37°C for 1 to 4 hours. Some solid-phase tests have also been proposed by different authors.[17] Recently, an assay to test for anti-VWF antibodies using a sandwich enzyme-linked immunosorbent assay (ELISA) has been described.[18] In this assay, normal exogenous VWF is bound to the ELISA plate; plasma from a patient with AVWS is added, incubated, and then washed. If IgG or IgM auto-antibodies against VWF are present in the patient plasma, they remain bound to the exogenous VWF and can subsequently be revealed by horseradish peroxidase anti-human IgG or IgM antibodies. The sensitivity of this assay is promising, but its specificity in screening for autoantibodies against VWF should be tested further in multicenter studies.

A diagnostic flow chart, which can be used in cases of excessive bleeding or before surgery in patients with underlying disorders known to be associated with AVWS, is shown in Fig 3.

General Management of AVWS

There are three treatment goals in AVWS: to control current bleeding episodes; to prevent bleeding when an invasive procedure is necessary; and, when possible, to control the underlying disease. In several disorders associated with AVWS, surgery,[19-28] chemotherapy,[29-32] radiotherapy,[33] or discontinuation of the responsible drugs[34,35] can sometimes control the underlying disease, with resolution of the bleeding diathesis and normalization of the laboratory parameters. In one patient with AVWS and lymphoma, prolonged BT and low plasma VWF levels were normalized when remission of lymphoma was obtained after chemotherapy; the lymphoma subsequently relapsed, together with the features of AVWS.[30]

Unfortunately, in some cases of AVWS, the underlying disorders cannot be identified. In others, such as AVWS associated with a monoclonal gammopathy of undetermined significance (MGUS), the underlying disease is usually not treated. Hence, in such cases, the best approach to stop

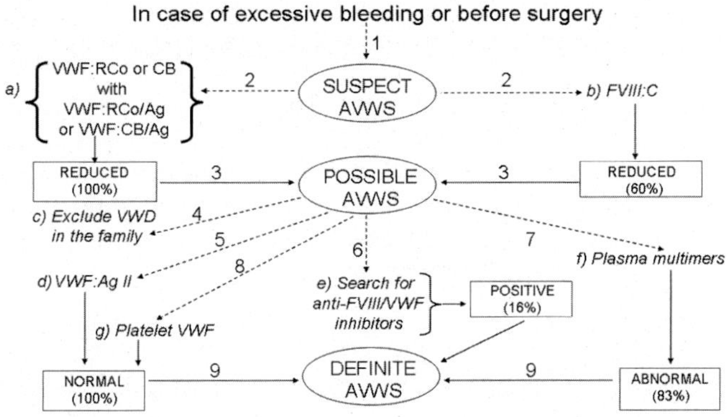

Figure 3 Diagnostic flow chart for patients with underlying disorders known to be associated with acquired von Willebrand syndrome (AVWS). Ag, antigen; CB, collagen-binding assay; FVIII, factor VIII; FVIII:C, FVIII coagulant activity; VWD, von Willebrand disease; VWF, von Willebrand factor; VWF:RCo, VWF ristocetin cofactor activity. Reprinted with permission from Federici AB, Rand JH, Bucciarelli P, Budde U, van Genderen PJ, Mohri H, et al: Subcommittee on von Willebrand Factor: Acquired von Willebrand syndrome: Data from an international registry. Thromb Haemost 84: 345-349, 2000.

bleeding episodes and/or to prevent bleeding during surgery must be identified.[36]

A variety of therapeutic approaches have been used to treat patients with AVWS, including desmopressin (DDAVP), FVIII/VWF concentrates, high-dose intravenous immunoglobulin (IVIg), plasmapheresis, corticosteroids, and immunosuppressive drugs.[8] Desmopressin, FVIII/VWF concentrates, and high-dose IVIg have been tested prospectively in 10 patients with AVWS associated with MGUS, with particular attention to the short- and long-term administration of IVIg.[36] In this small therapeutic trial, DDAVP and FVIII/VWF concentrates induced only a short-lasting correction of the acquired VWF defects, because the auto-antibodies against VWF were able to rapidly remove the high levels of both endogenous VWF, released by DDAVP (Fig 4), and exogenous VWF, provided by FVIII/VWF concentrates (Haemate-P; ZLB Behring, Marburg, Germany [Fig 5]). In the same trial, it was shown that two single daily IVIg infusions (short-term therapy) were more effective than DDAVP and FVIII/VWF concentrates, because they induced a prompt and sustained increase of FVIII/VWF activity and shortening of the BT in patients with AVWS associated with IgG–MGUS, with a correction of VWF multimeric structure (Fig 6). As plasma-derived commercial preparations of IVIg contain human IgG, and only trace amounts of IgA, this therapeutic approach cannot induce any changes of FVIII/VWF activity in cases of AVWS associated with IgM–MGUS (Fig 7).

The therapeutic doses of IVIg for AVWS are 1 g/kg/d for 2 days or 0.4 g/kg/d for 5 days, as proposed for other autoimmune disorders, such as immune thrombocytopenic purpura.[37] As IVIg usually requires 24 to 48 hours to normalize plasma FVIII/VWF activity (Fig 6), DDAVP or FVIII/VWF concentrates can be given together with IVIg to achieve normal hemostasis immediately in cases of emergency bleeding or surgery.[38]

Repeated doses of IVIg given every 21 days (long-term therapy) can produce consistent responses in FVIII/VWF measurements, but high doses seem critical for IVIg effects (Fig 8). Following a loading dose of 1 g/kg for two doses in two patients with AVWS associated with IgG–MGUS and severe recurrent gastrointestinal bleeding, repeated single infusions of IVIg (1 g/kg) were effective in improving FVIII/VWF activity, with a return to baseline levels in about 3 weeks. Lower doses (0.5 g/kg) were attempted, but these did not achieve the same effects on laboratory measurements: transient improvement of these parameters was again achieved when a dose of 1 g/kg was administered.[36] The mechanisms by which IVIg exerts its effect are not completely understood: it can prevent the clearance of the inhibitor–VWF complex from the circulation by blocking Fc receptors, but other mechanisms, such as those reported for other clinical conditions,[39] cannot be excluded.

Recombinant activated factor VII (rFVIIa; NovoSeven®, Novo Nordisk; Bagsvaerd, Denmark) is another useful therapeutic approach. This agent has been successfully used when bleeding associated with AVWS has been unresponsive to standard therapy.[40]

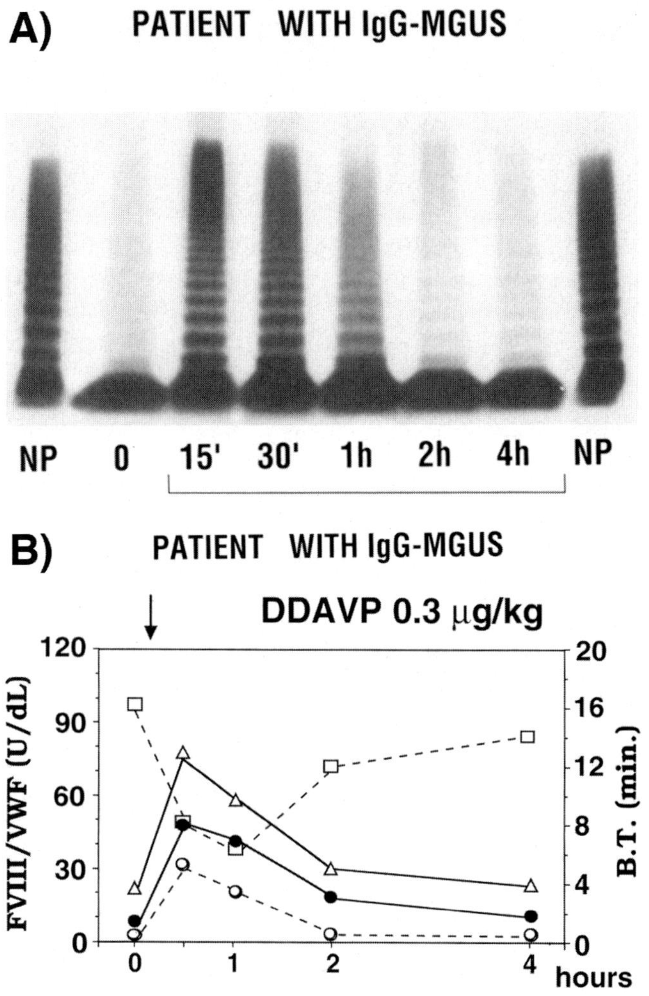

Figure 4 The effects of a standard dose (0.3 μg/kg) of desmopressin (DDAVP) in patients with acquired von Willebrand syndrome (AVWS) associated with IgG–monoclonal gammopathy of uncertain significance (IgG–MGUS). (A) The multimeric pattern of von Willebrand factor (VWF) as shown by low–intermediate resolution sodium dodecyl sulfate (SDS)–1.2% low gelling temperature (LGT) agarose gels compared with normal plasma (NP) before and 15 min, 30 min, 1, 2, and 4 h after DDAVP administration. Note that a progressive increase of all the high-molecular-weight multimers is apparent up to 1 h after DDAVP administration, but the multimers then disappear to produce a pattern similar to baseline. (B) Bleeding time (BT, □), factor VIII (FVIII) levels (△), VWF antigen levels (●), and VWF ristocetin cofactor activity (○) before and after DDAVP administration. Note that BT shortened and FVIII/VWF activity normalized within 1 h, but values returned to baseline after 2.4 h. This figure was originally published in *Blood*.[36] © The American Society of Hematology.

AVWS in Lymphoproliferative Disorders

MGUS is the condition most frequently associated with AVWS.[8-12] The first case was described by Ingram et al in 1971.[41] According to data from the International Registry on AWVS, this disorder can be also associated with multiple myeloma (9%), Waldenstrom macroglobulinemina (9%), non-Hodgkin's lymphomas (4%), and chronic lymphocytic

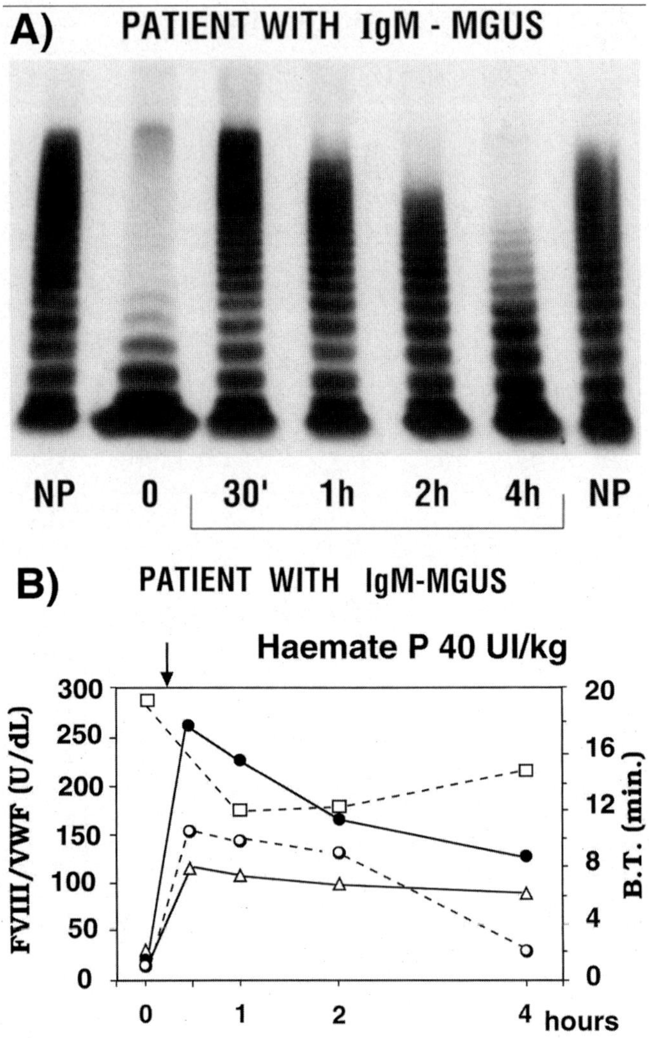

Figure 5 The effects of a standard dose of an intermediate-purity factor VIII/von Willebrand factor (FVIII/VWF) concentrate (Haemate-P; 40 FVIII U/kg) in patients with acquired von Willebrand syndrome associated with IgM–monoclonal gammopathy of uncertain significance (IgM–MGUS). (A) The multimeric pattern of VWF as shown by low–intermediate resolution sodium dodecyl sulfate–1.2% LGT agarose gels compared with normal plasma (NP) before and 30 min, 1, 2, and 4 h after FVIII/VWF concentrate administration. Note that a progressive increase of all the high-molecular-weight multimers is apparent up to 30 min after the administration, but these then progressively disappear. (B) Bleeding time (BT, □), factor VIII (FVIII) levels (△), VWF antigen (●), and VWF ristocetin cofactor activity (VWF:RCo, ○) before and after FVIII/VWF concentrate administration. Note that, up to 2 h after administration, BT shortened without reaching normal values and FVIII/VWF activity normalized. At 4 h, VWF:RCo values were similar to baseline. This figure was originally published in *Blood*.[36] © The American Society of Hematology.

leukemia (3%). The registry also contains a single case report of AVWS with acute lymphocytic leukemia.[12] AVWS associated with lymphoproliferative disorders is slightly more frequent (63%) in adult males (median age, 64 years) than in females (Table 1). The majority of patients (55%) were alive at the time of enrollment in the registry, suggesting that, in these disorders, AVWS may mirror the relatively indolent course of the underlying disorder.[12] AVWS was accompanied by bleeding symptoms in the majority of patients (87%); in asymptomatic patients (13%), the syndrome was diagnosed on the basis of laboratory abnormalities.

The main laboratory findings for those patients in the registry who have AVWS associated with lymphoproliferative disorders are shown in Table 1. BT was often prolonged, with

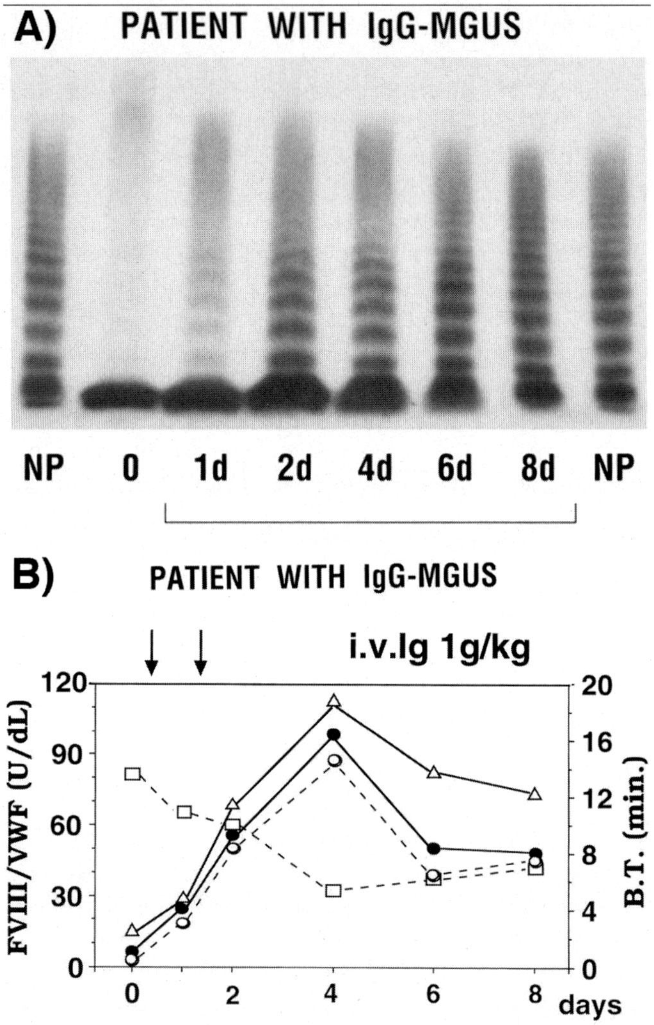

Figure 6 The effects of a standard dose (1 g/kg daily for 2 days) of intravenous immunoglobulin (IVIg) in patients with acquired von Willebrand syndrome (AVWS) associated with IgG–monoclonal gammopathy of uncertain significance (IgG–MGUS).(A) The multimeric pattern of von Willebrand factor (VWF) as shown by low–intermediate resolution sodium dodecyl sulfate–1.2% LGT agarose gels compared with normal plasma (NP) before and 1, 2, 4, 6, and 8 days after IVIg administration. Note that a progressive increase of all the high-molecular-weight multimers is apparent until 4 days after IVIg administration, and these multimers remain constant until at least day 8. (B) Bleeding time (BT, □) and factor VIII (FVIII) levels (△), VWF antigen levels (●),and VWF ristocetin cofactor activity (○) before and after IVIg administration. Note that BT shortened and FVIII/VWF activity normalized progressively, with a delay of approximately 2 days, and remained within normal ranges for at least 8 days. This figure was originally published in *Blood*.[36] © The American Society of Hematology.

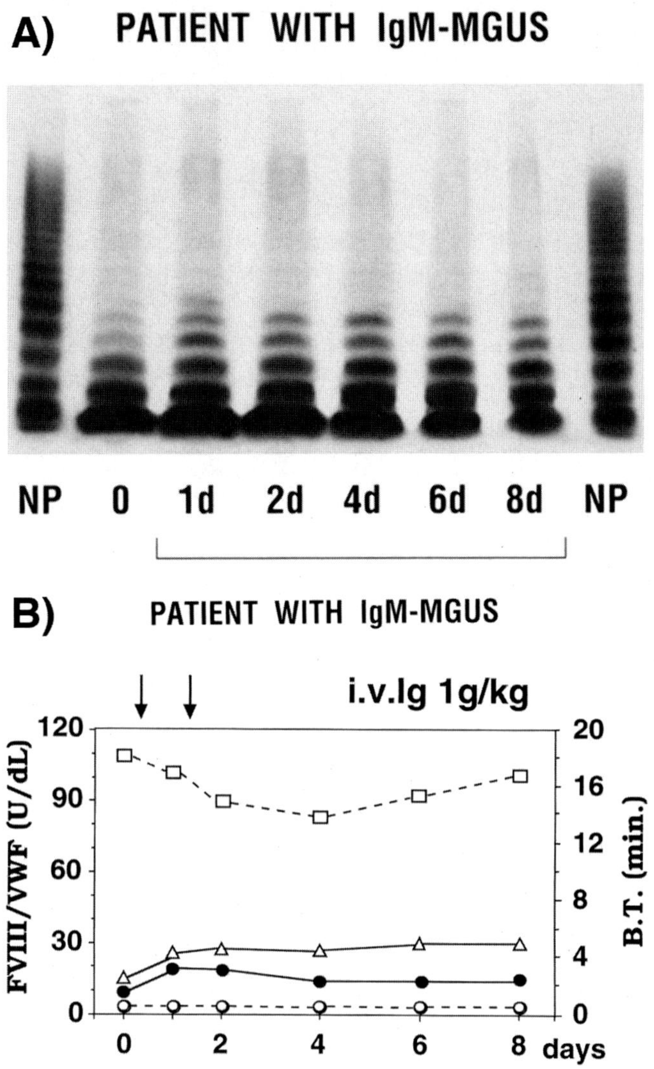

Figure 7 The effects of a standard dose (1 g/kg daily for 2 days) of intravenous immunoglobulin (IVIg) in patients with acquired von Willebrand syndrome (AVWS) associated with IgM–monoclonal gammopathy of uncertain significance (IgM–MGUS). (A) The multimeric pattern of von Willebrand factor (VWF) as shown by low–intermediate resolution sodium dodecyl sulfate–1.2% LGT agarose gels compared with normal plasma (NP) before and 1, 2, 4, 6, and 8 days following IVIg administration. Note that no significant changes are observed in these patients. (B) Bleeding time (BT, □) and factor VIII (FVIII) levels (△), VWF antigen levels (●), and VWF ristocetin cofactor activity (○) before and after IVIg administration. Note that BT is apparently shortened, but FVIII/VWF activity did not change significantly. This figure was originally published in *Blood*.[36] © The American Society of Hematology.

a median value of 15 minutes and a wide range (3 to >30 minutes). The slight prolongation of activated partial thromboplastin time (aPTT; expressed as a ratio) was consistent with the mildly reduced levels of FVIII:C, which were reduced in many patients but were normal in some cases. VWF:Ag was generally reduced, with a median value of 17 U/dL, although a wide range was observed (4 to 80 U/dL). Assays for VWF activity, measured either in terms of VWF: RCo or by VWF:CB, appeared to be the most sensitive for the diagnosis of the VWF defect in AVWS, with a median value of 8 U/dL for both assays (range, 3 to 45 U/dL). The calculated ratio of VWF:RCo or VWF:CB to VWF:Ag was 0.57. Only 5/186 (3%) patients in the registry were tested for VWF propeptide. In all tested patients with MGUS, levels of VWF propeptide were normal (median, 75; range, 60 to 121) in the presence of reduced VWF:Ag. Plasma VWF multimers were analyzed in approximately two-thirds of the patients, and the larger multimers were missing in the majority of cases tested (76%). VWF was measured in platelets in only 12/89 cases (13%), and was found to be normal. The methods most often used to search for inhibitory activity against FVIII/VWF were based on the measurement of FVIII/VWF properties in plasma after mixing patient plasma with normal plasma. This assay was carried out for 80/89 (90%) cases reported, but inhibitory activity was found in only a minority of cases (10/89, 11%). The prevalence of anti-FVIII/VWF activity found in the registry is similar to that reported in the literature (38/226, 14%).

Several therapeutic approaches were used for the treatment of AVWS associated with lymphoproliferative conditions in patients reported to the registry (Table 2). Desmopressin was administered in 59/89 cases (66%), and successfully controlled bleeding in 26 (44%) of these by restoring normal levels of FVIII/VWF in plasma. Desmopressin is relatively inexpensive and carries no risk of blood-borne infections. However, its usefulness in AVWS is limited by the short half-life of the endogenous FVIII/VWF that is released. A DDAVP infusion test, measuring BT and FVIII/VWF pre-

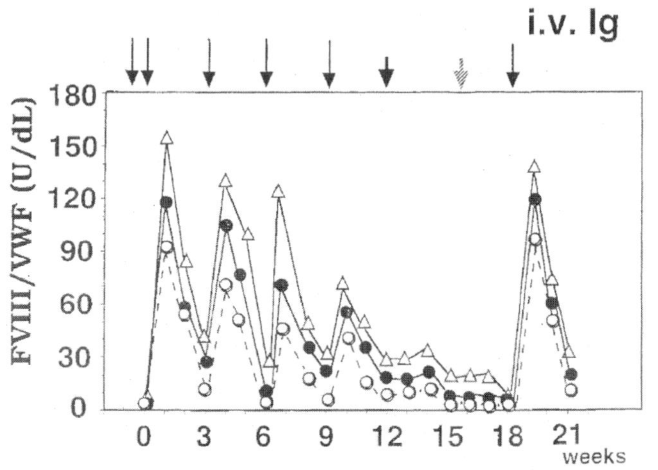

Figure 8 Representative example of long-term intravenous immunoglobulin (IVIg) therapy in a patient with acquired von Willebrand syndrome associated with IgM–monoclonal gammopathy of uncertain significance. Factor VIII/von Willebrand factor (FVIII/VWF) measurements (FVIII, △ ; VWF antigen, ●; VWF ristocetin cofactor activity, ○) before and at various times after repeated infusions of high-dose IVIg. Arrows at the top indicate the infusion of different doses of IVIg: 1g/kg, solid long arrow; 0.75 g/kg, solid short arrow; 0.5 g/kg, hatched short arrow. Note that the response of FVIII/VWF measurements is consistent when 1g/kg IVIg is used, but lower when the dosage is tapered. This figure was originally published in *Blood*.[36] ©The American Society of Hematology.

Table 1 Main Features of 186 Cases of AVWS Reported in the International Registry on Acquired von Willebrand syndrome

	Associated Disorders						
	Lymphoproliferative	Myeloproliferative	Solid Tumors	Immunologic	CV	Misc	Total
No. of cases (%)	89 (48)	29 (15)	9 (5)	4 (2)	39 (21)	16 (9)	186 (100)
Sex (% of male)	63	35	45	20	57	36	53
Age at onset (yr) (range)	64 (28–96)	45 (27–72)	62 (26–93)	52 (40–58)	68 (2–85)	44 (6–75)	62 (2–96)
Still alive (%)	55	24	67	80	57	73	53
Bleeders (%)	87	48	75	60	77	57	72
Bleeding time (min) (range)	15 (3–>30)	11 (3–22)	20 (5–20)	5 (3–8)	14 (5–>30)	20 (10–>30)	15 (3–>30)
aPTT (patient/normal ratio) (range)	1.4 (1–2.5)	1.0 (1–1.37)	1.0 (0.9–1.7)	1.2 (0.86–1.89)	1.37 (1.2–1.7)	1.2 (1.2–1.7)	1.3 (0.9–2.5)
Mean FVIII:C (U/dL) (range)	20 (4–92)	45 (16–75)	23 (12–83)	112 (33–191)	28 (3–185)	33 (3–191)	25 (3–191)
VWF:Ag (U/dL) (range)	17 (4–80)	70 (20–404)	20 (5–59)	39 (14–91)	113 (8–3000)	94 (10–221)	33 (4–404)
VWF:RCo or VWF:CB (U/dL) (range)	8 (3–45)	39 (3–130)	10 (4–32)	26 (10–40)	60 (3–150)	6 (3–150)	20 (3–150)
VWF:RCo/Ag or VWF: CB/Ag ratio (range)	0.57 (0.08–1.5)	0.52 (0.11–1.40)	0.69 (0.1–1.5)	0.53 (0.23–1.22)	0.47 (0.13–1.57)	0.58 (0.31–1.23)	0.5 (0.08–1.5)
VWF:propeptide (range)	75 (60–121)	NT	NT	NT	NT	NT	NC
Lack of HMW multimers (%)	76	86	96	80	80	70	83
Positive anti-FVIII/ VWF (%)	12	0	22	42	0	9	7

NOTE. Values are medians unless otherwise stated.

Abbreviations: Ag, antigen; aPTT, activated partial thromboplastin time; AVWS, acquired von Willebrand syndrome; CB, collagen-binding assay; CV, cardiovascular; FVIII, factor VIII; FVIII:C, FVIII coagulant activity; HMW, high molecular weight; Misc, miscellaneous; RCo, ristocetin cofactor activity; VWF, von Willebrand factor.

Reprinted with permission from Federici AB, et al. Acquired von Willebrand syndrome. Data from an International Registry On behalf of the Subcommittee on von Willebrand Factor. Thromb Haemost 84:345–349, 2000.

Table 2 Different Therapeutic Approaches in 186 Cases of AVWS Reported in the International Registry of Acquired von Willebrand Syndrome

	Associated Disorders						
	Lymphoproliferative	Myeloproliferative	Solid Tumors	Immunologic	CV	Misc	Total
No. of cases (%)	89 (48)	29 (15)	9 (5)	4 (2)	39 (21)	16 (9)	186 (100)
DDAVP	26/59	3/14	3/4	1/3	3/30	2/9	38/119 (32%)
FVIII/VWF concentrate	28/56	2/14	6/6	—	4/30	2/9	42/115 (37%)
IV immunoglobulin	18/48	—	2/2	1/2	0/10	0/1	21/63 (33%)
Plasmapheresis	6/30	—	—	—	0/2	—	6/32 (19%)
Corticosteroids	10/31	—	0/1	—	2/25	0/6	12/63 (19%)
Immunosuppressive agents or chemotherapy	17/47	5/14	1/2	—	—	0/3	23/66 (35%)

NOTE. Multiple treatment approaches are used in some patients. Values describe number of treated patients who responded to therapy.
Abbreviations: CV, cardiovascular; DDAVP, desmopressin; FVIII, factor VIII; IV, intravenous; Misc, miscellaneous; VWF, von Willebrand factor.
Reprinted with permission from Federici AB et al. Acquired von Willebrand syndrome: Data from an International Registry. On behalf of the Subcommittee on von Willebrand Factor. Thromb Haemost 84:345–349, 2000.

and post-infusion, is advisable for every new diagnosis of AVWS.[36]

FVIII/VWF concentrates were used to treat 56/89 (63%) patients with AVWS associated with lymhoproliferative disorders in the registry, and were clinically effective in 28 (50%) cases. High-dose IVIg was administered to 48/89 (54%) patients; this was effective in only 18 (37%) cases, and mainly in those with MGUS (15/18). It has been proposed that IVIg is more effective in AVWS cases characterized by the presence of anti-FVIII/VWF activity. Although prospective data are not available, data in the registry show that 13/21 (62%) AVWS patients responsive to IVIg had anti-FVIII/VWF activity. Due to the high cost of this treatment, IVIg should be reserved for AVWS patients unresponsive to DDAVP and FVIII/VWF concentrates, and for cases with anti-FVIII/VWF inhibitors.[12]

Plasmapheresis or extracorporeal immunoadsorption were used to treat 30/89 (34%) cases of AVWS associated with lymphoproliferative disorders, and these procedures were effective in 6/30 (20%) cases. A total of 31/89 (35%) cases were given corticosteroids, which were effective in 10/31 (32%) instances. In 17/47 (36%) patients who were receiving immunosuppressive agents and chemotherapy for their lymphoproliferative disorders, a beneficial effect of this therapy on AVWS was observed.

In addition to this registry data, the literature also contains one recent report describing successful use of rFVIIa in a patient with bleeding associated with AVWS and IgG–MGUS. Prior to the administration of rFVIIa, bleeding had remained unresponsive to various treatments, including DDAVP, FVIII/VWF concentrates, and IVIg.[40]

AVWS in Myeloproliferative Disorders

The first case of AVWS in a myeloproliferative disorder was described by Duran-Saurez et al in a patient with chronic granulocytic leukemia.[29] Clinical and laboratory features of AVWS associated with essential thrombocythemia have been extensively evaluated by the work of Budde and Michiels,[4,10,11,32,42,43] who demonstrated that the clinical syndrome and recurrent bleeding are associated with very high platelet counts, and that reduction of the platelet count is associated with a decrease in the frequency of bleeding episodes.[32,42]

Mohri et al reported a prevalence of 11.6% (17/147) for cases of AVWS associated with myeloproliferative disorders,[1] which is similar to other values observed in the literature and in the International Registry on AVWS.[12] In the registry, the associated myeloproliferative disorders are essential thrombocythemia (11%), chronic granulocytic leukemia (3%), myelofibrosis (1%), and polycythemia vera (1%). Among patients reported to the registry, AVWS associated with myeloproliferative disorders was observed more frequently (65%) in adult women (≥45 years) than in men (Table 1). Only 24% of the cases were still in follow-up at the time of enrollment in the registry, as most of the patients had been lost to observation or had died. Laboratory investigations were performed in response to bleeding symptoms in only 48% of cases. VWF:Ag levels were low in only a few patients (mean, 70 U/dL). As VWF:RCo or VWF:CB levels were always lower than VWF:Ag, the RCo/Ag or CB/Ag ratios were always lower than 0.7 (mean, 0.52). There was an absence of larger multimers in most cases (86%), which is in agreement with previously reported data showing a significant loss of HMW multimers and increased VWF proteolysis in myeloproliferative disorders.[42,43] Anti-FVIII/VWF activity was measured in only a few cases, and no inhibitory activity was found.

Desmopressin was administered to 14/29 (48%) of the patients in the registry and was effective in 3/14 (21%), while FVIII/VWF concentrates were used in 14/29 (48%) and effective in only 2/14 (14%) cases (Table 2). The use of IVIg, plasmapheresis or corticosteroids to treat patients with myeloproliferative disorders was not reported in any of the registry cases. Immunosuppressive agents or chemotherapy were used in 14/29 (48%) cases, correcting AVWS abnormalities in 5/14 (36%) patients.

AVWS in Patients With Solid Tumors

AVWS was first associated with solid tumors in a patient with nephroblastoma or Wilm's tumor.[19] Additional cases were subsequently reported.[20] Data in the registry showed that 75% of the cases were investigated as a result of excessive bleeding in response to minor trauma and surgery. Evidence for anti-FVIII/VWF antibodies was found in 22% of cases. There was an absence of HMW multimers, together with low VWF:RCo/Ag and VWF:CB/Ag ratios and low FVIII:C levels (Table 1). In addition to surgical removal of the tumor, all therapeutic approaches (DDAVP, FVIII/VWF concentrates, IVIg) were highly effective in these patients (Table 2).

AVWS in Immunologic Disorders

The first description of an association between AVWS and immunologic disorders was reported in 1968 in a patient with SLE.[2] Several other cases have subsequently been recorded, as recently reviewed by Michiels et al.[10] Available data from the literature and the International Registry on AVWS indicate that these disorders affect more females than males. Several cases have been found to be asymptomatic, while others have mild or moderate bleeding symptoms. BT and FVIII:C levels have been reported to be relatively normal, with decreased levels of VWF:RCo. Multimeric analysis of VWF in the cases evaluated has generally shown a type 2 pattern.

The response to DDAVP was apparently good in one case of the five that have been described in the literature.[10] The response to FVIII/VWF concentrates was not always determined, although slight recovery and a very short half-life have been observed in some cases. The response to IVIg was observed for two patients with AVWS associated with SLE: one of these showed a transient correction of FVIII/VWF activity lasting for a few weeks, suggesting that there is an immune-mediated etiology of AVWS in SLE. Unfortunately, there are no data concerning the relationship between the relatively high percentages of anti-FVIII/VWF antibodies found in this group of patients and the responses to IVIg because only a small number of patients received this treatment.[10]

In the literature, therapy with prednisolone (30 to 40 mg or 1 to 2 mg/kg daily) has been reported as effective in several cases of AVWS associated with SLE. In a few cases, concomitant prednisolone and cyclophosphamide (single intravenous doses of 700 mg/m^2) therapy induced complete correction of both FVIII:C and VWF levels.[10]

AVWS and Cardiovascular Disorders

Cardiovascular disorders are also frequently associated with AVWS, as reported in both the literature (12%) and the registry (21%) (Fig 2). Gill et al were the first to describe the loss of large VWF multimers from the plasma of patients with congenital cardiac defects.[44] Other authors subsequently reported similar abnormalities in patients with multiple congenital and cardiac defects.[11,45,46] Recently, a type 2A-like AVWS was described in a study of 50 consecutive patients with aortic stenosis, 42 of whom underwent valve replacement.[28] VWF abnormalities were present in most patients and correlated significantly with the severity of valve stenosis.

In valvular abnormalities, the underlying mechanism of AVWS relates to the high shear rate of flowing blood, which induces degradation of large VWF multimers in plasma. Most patients are diagnosed following excessive bleeding before or during surgery. In these patients, BT may be prolonged and FVIII:C reduced. With the relative loss of HMW VWF multimers, VWF:RCo or VWF:CB are always lower than VWF:Ag. Attempts to reduce the bleeding tendency using such therapeutic approaches as DDAVP, FVIII/VWF concentrates, or IVIg are seldom effective. Repair of cardiac defects by cardiac surgery usually corrects the typical abnormalities of AVWS.[11,27] However, in one study, the hemostatic abnormalities tended to recur at 6 months, especially when there was a mismatch between patient and prosthesis.[28]

Miscellaneous Disorders

AVWS has been described in association with drugs, including repeated administration of hydroxyethyl starch,[34,47] valproic acid,[48] griseofulvin,[49] and ciprofloxacin.[35,50] The syndrome has also been reported in association with hydatid disease of the spleen, although splenectomy normalized FVIII/VWF activity.[21] In addition, AVWS has been described in association with Epstein-Barr virus infection.[51] Associations between AVMS and infective colitis and sarcoidosis have also been reported in the International Registry on AVWS.[12]

AVWS has been also described in other systemic diseases, including hypothyroidism,[52] in which some patients remain asymptomatic while others presented with mild-to-moderate bleeding symptoms. Two such cases have been reported in the registry, with FVIII/VWF activity levels similar to those described in the literature.[10] No anti-FVIII/VWF antibodies were identified in these two patients, and both responded well to DDAVP. FVIII/VWF abnormalities suggestive of AVWS have also been reported in uremia,[53] hemoglobinopathies,[54] and teleangiectasia.[55] The VWF defects in these conditions were corrected by DDAVP or FVIII/VWF concentrates.

Several cases of AVWS without any associated conditions or known etiologies have been reported in the literature.[5-12] Responses to DDAVP and IVIg were not tested in six of seven cases. One patient, with AVWS and anti-FVIII/VWF antibodies, responded poorly to DDAVP and FVIII/VWF concentrates: only IVIg was effective in correcting the VWF defects.

Conclusions and Perspectives

Available data from the literature and the International Registry indicate that AVWS occurs in association with a variety of underlying disorders, most frequently in lymphoproliferative and myeloproliferative disorders, although the actual prevalence in clinical practice has not been determined. AVWS is remarkably heterogeneous and its basic mechanisms remain undefined in many cases. Functional assays of VWF in patients' plasma are essential for making a firm diagnosis of AVWS. While assays for anti-FVIII/VWF activity should be performed to identify patients with inhibitors, these tests are often negative. The use of more sensitive and specific assays should be encouraged to determine the role of anti-VWF autoantibodies in AVWS. Management of bleeding in AVWS relies mainly on DDAVP, FVIII/VWF concentrates, and high-dose IVIg, but no single drug is effective for all AVWS cases. As bleeding episodes are sometimes life-threatening and require prolonged hospitalization with the infusion of large doses of blood products, the organization of large, prospective, multicenter studies in patients with lymphoproliferative and myeloproliferative disorders is needed. An updated version of the International Registry on AVWS (www.intreavws.com) has been organized to promote direct registration of new cases. This aims to gain a better understanding of the basic mechanisms of AVWS (through the use of new assays), the limits of standard therapies, and the efficacy of novel and experimental therapeutic approaches.

Acknowledgment

The author wishes to thank all the members of the ISTH SSC on VWF who participated in this registry and contributed to the preparation of the guidelines for diagnosis and therapy of AVWS.[12] Many of the results on AVWS have been also presented, in part, at several international meetings, and are derived from previous original and review articles published by ABF during the last 7 years. The author acknowledges the work of Dr Luigi Flaminio Ghilardini, who prepared the figures reported in this article.

References

1. Mohri H, Motomura S, Kanamori H, Matsuzaki M, Watanabe S, Maruta A, et al: Clinical significance of inhibitors in acquired von Willebrand syndrome. Blood 91:3623-3629, 1998
2. Simone JV, Cornet JA, Abildgaard CF: Acquired von Willebrand's syndrome in systemic lupus erythematosus. Blood 31:806-812, 1968
3. Jakway JL: Acquired von Willebrand's disease. Hematol Oncol Clin North Am 6:1409-1419, 1992
4. van Genderen PJJ, Leenknegt H, Michiels JJ, Budde U: Acquired von Willebrand disease in myeloproliferative disorders. Leuk Lymphoma 22:79-82, 1996 (suppl 1)
5. Rinder MR, Richard RE, Rinder HM: Acquired von Willebrand's disease: A concise review. Am J Hematol 54:139-145, 1997
6. Tefferi A, Nichols WL: Acquired von Willebrand disease: Concise review of occurrence, diagnosis, pathogenesis and treatment. Am J Med 103:536-540, 1997
7. Nitu-Whalley IC, Lee CA: Acquired von Willebrand syndrome—Report of 10 cases and review of the literature. Haemophilia 5:318-326, 1999
8. Federici AB: Therapeutic approaches to acquired von Willebrand syndrome. Expert Opin Invest Drugs 9:347-354, 2000
9. Veyradier A, Jenkins CS, Fressinaud E, Meyer D: Acquired von Willebrand syndrome: From pathophysiology to management. Thromb Haemost 84:175-182, 2000
10. Michiels JJ, Budde U, van der Planken M, van Vliet HH, Schroyens W, Berneman Z: Acquired von Willebrand syndromes: Clinical features, aetiology, pathophysiology, classification and management. Best Pract Res Clin Hematol 14:401-436, 2001
11. Budde U, Bergmann F, Michiels: Acquired von Willebrand syndrome: experience from 2 years in a single laboratory compared with data from the literature and an international registry. Semin Thromb Hemost 28:227-238, 2002
12. Federici AB, Rand JH, Bucciarelli P, Budde U, van Genderen PJ, Mohri H, et al: Subcommittee on von Willebrand Factor: Acquired von Willebrand syndrome: Data from an international registry. Thromb Haemost 84:345-349, 2000
13. Mannucci PM, Lombardi R, Bader R, Horellou MH, Finazzi G, Besana C, et al: Studies of the pathophysiology of acquired von Willebrand's disease in seven patients with lymphoproliferative disorders or benign monoclonal gammopathies. Blood 64:614-621, 1984
14. van Genderen PJJ, Boertjes RC, van Mourik JA: Quantitative analysis of von Willebrand factor and its propeptide in plasma in acquired von Willebrand syndrome. Thromb Haemost 80:495-498, 1998
15. Federici AB, Berkowitz SD, Zimmerman TS, Mannucci PM: Proteolysis of von Willebrand factor after thrombolytic therapy in patients with acute myocardial infarction. Blood 79:38-44, 1992
16. Federici AB, Berkowitz SD, Lattuada A, Mannucci PM: Degradation of von Willebrand factor in patients with acquired clinical conditions in which there is heightened proteolysis. Blood 81:720-725, 1993
17. Mannucci PM, Federici AB: Antibodies to von Willebrand factor in von Willebrand disease, in Aledort LM, Hoyer LW, Reisner HM, White GC II (eds): Inhibitors to Coagulation Factors. New York, Plenum Press, 1995, pp 87-92
18. Siaka C, Rugeri L, Caron C, Goudemand J: A new ELISA assay for diagnosis of acquired von Willebrand Syndrome. Haemophilia 9:303-308, 2003
19. Noronha PA, Hruby MA, Maurer HS: Acquired von Willebrand disease in a patient with Wilms tumor. J Pediatr 95:997-999, 1979
20. Scott JP, Montgomery RR, Tubergen DG, Hays T. Acquired von Willebrand's disease in association with Wilm's tumor: Regression following treatment. Blood 58:665-669, 1981
21. Richard C, Sedano MC, Cuadrado MA, Recio M, Hermosa V, Zubizarreta A: Acquired von Willebrand's syndrome associated with hydatid disease of the spleen—Disappearance after splenectomy. Thromb Haemost 52:90-93, 1984
22. Cappell MS, Lebwohl O: Cessation of recurrent bleeding from gastrointestinal angiodysplasia after aortic valve replacement. Ann Intern Med 105:54-57, 1986
23. Weinstein M, Ware JA, Troll JH, Salzman EW: Changes in von Willebrand factor during cardiac surgery: Effect of desmopressin acetate. Blood 71:1648-1655, 1988
24. Coppes MJ, Zandvoort SWH, Sparling CR, Poon AO, Weitzman S, Blanchette VS: Acquired von Willebrand disease in Wilms' tumor patients. J Clin Oncol 10:422-427, 1992
25. Facon T, Caron C, Courtin P, Wurtz A, Deghaye M, Bauters F, et al: Acquired type II von Willebrand's disease associated with adrenal cortical carcinoma. Br J Haematol 80:488-494, 1992
26. Anderson RP, McGrath K, Street A: Reversal of aortic stenosis, bleeding gastrointestinal angiodysplasia, and von Willebrand syndrome by aortic valve replacement. Lancet 347:689-690, 1996
27. Pareti FI, Lattuada A, Bressi C, Zanobini M, Sala A, Steffan A, et al: Proteolysis of von Willebrand factor and shear stress-induced platelet aggregation in patients with aortic valve stenosis. Circulation 102: 1290-1295, 2000
28. Vincentelli A, Susen S, Le Tourneau T, Six I, Fabre O, Juthier F, et al:

Acquired von Willebrand syndrome in aortic stenosis. N Engl J Med. 349:343-349, 2003
29. Duran-Saurez JR, Pico M, Zuazu J, Cortes M, Monasterio J, Tringiner J: Acquired von Willebrand's disease caused by a chronic granulocytic leukemia. Br J Haematol 48:173-175, 1981
30. Tran-Thang C, Mannucci PM, Schneider P, Federici AB, Bachmann F: Profound alterations of the multimeric structure of von Willebrand factor in a patient with malignant lymphoma. Br J Haematol 61:307-314, 1985
31. Murakawa M, Okamura T, Tsutsumi K, Tanoguchi S, Kamura T, Shibuya T, et al: Acquired von Willebrand's disease in association with essential thrombocythemia: Regression following treatment. Acta Haematol 87:83-87, 1992
32. Budde U, van Genderen PJJ: Acquired von Willebrand disease in patients with high platelet counts. Semin Thromb Hemost 23:425-431, 1997
33. Joist JH, Cowan JF, Zimmerman TS: Acquired von Willebrand's disease. Evidence for a quantitative and qualitative factor VIII disorder. N Engl J Med 298:988-991, 1978
34. Dalrymple-Hay M, Aitchison R, Collins R, Sekhar M, Colvin B: Hydroxyethyl starch induced acquired von Willebrand's disease. Clin Lab Haematol 14:209-211, 1992
35. Castaman G, Lattuada A, Mannucci PM, Rodeghiero F: Characterization of two cases of acquired transitory von Willebrand syndrome with ciprofloxacin: Evidence for heightened proteolysis of von Willebrand factor. Am J Hematol 49:83-86, 1995
36. Federici AB, Stabile F, Castaman G, Canciani MT, Mannucci PM: Treatment of acquired von Willebrand syndrome in patients with monoclonal gammopathy of uncertain significance: comparison of three different therapeutic approaches. Blood 92:2707-2711, 1998
37. Imbach PA, Kuhne T, Hollander G: Immunologic aspects in the pathogenesis and treatment of immune thrombocytopenic purpura in children. Curr Opin Pediatr 9:35-40, 1997
38. van Genderen PJJ, Terpstra W, Michiels JJ, Kapteijn L, van Vliet HH: High-dose intravenous immunoglobin delays clearance of von Willebrand factor in acquired von Willebrand disease. Thromb Haemost 73:891-892, 1995
39. Kazatchkine MD, Kaveri SV: Immunomodulation of autoimmune and inflammatory diseases with intravenous immune globulin. N Engl J Med 345:747-755, 2001
40. Friederich PW, Wever PC, Briet E, Doorenbos CJ, Levi M: Successful treatment with recombinant factor VIIa of therapy-resistant severe bleeding in a patient with acquired von Willebrand disease. Am J Hematol 66:292-294, 2001
41. Ingram GIC, Kingston PJ, Leslie J, Bowie EJW: Four cases of acquired von Willebrand's syndrome. Br J Haematol 21:189-199, 1971
42. Budde U, Schaefer G, Mueller N, Egli H, Dent J, Ruggeri Z, et al: Acquired von Willebrand's disease in the myeloproliferative syndrome. Blood 64:981-985, 1984
43. Budde U, Dent JA, Berkowitz SD, Ruggeri ZM, Zimmerman TS: Subunit composition of plasma von Willebrand factor in patients with the myeloproliferative syndrome. Blood 68:1213-1217, 1986
44. Gill JC, Wilson AD, Endres-Brooks J, Montgomery RR: Loss of the largest von Willebrand factor multimers from the plasma of patients with congenital cardiac defects. Blood 67:758-761, 1986
45. Pickering NJ, Brody JI, Barrett MJ: von Willebrand syndromes and mitral-valve prolapse: Linked mesenchymal dysplasias. N Engl J Med 305:131-134, 1981
46. Rauch R, Budde U, Koch A, Girisch M, Hofbeck M: Acquired von Willebrand syndrome in children with patent ductus arteriosus. Heart 8:87-88, 2002
47. Strauss RG, Stump DC, Henriksen RA: Hydroxyethyl starch accentuates von Willebrand's disease. Transfusion 25:235-237, 1985
48. Kreuz W, Linde R, Funk M, Meyer-Schrod R, Foll E, Nowak-Gottl U, et al: Induction of von Willebrand disease type I by valproic acid. Lancet 335:1350-1351, 1990
49. Conrad ME, Latour LF: Acquired von Willebrand's disease, IgE polyclonal gammopathy and griseofulvin therapy. Am J Hematol 41:143-144, 1992
50. Castaman G, Rodeghiero F: Acquired transitory von Willebrand syndrome with ciprofloxacin. Lancet 343:492, 1994
51. Kinoshita S, Yoshioka K, Kasahara M, Takamiya O: Acquired von Willebrand disease after Epstein-Barr virus infection. J Pediatr 119:595-598, 1991
52. Rogers JS II, Shane SR, Jencks FS: Factor VIII activity and thyroid function. Ann Intern Med 97:713-716, 1982
53. Mannucci PM, Remuzzi G, Pusineri F, Lombardi R, Valsecchi C, Mecca G, et al: Deamino-8-D-arginine vasopressin shortens the bleeding time in uremia. N Engl J Med 308:8-12, 1983
54. Brody JI, Levison SP, Jung CJ: Sickle cell trait and hematuria associated with von Willebrand syndromes. Ann Intern Med 86:529-533, 1977
55. McGrath KM, Johnson CA, Stuart JJ: Acquired von Willebrand disease associated with an inhibitor to factor VIII antigen and gastrointestinal telangiectasia. Am J Med 67:693-696, 1979

Seminars in
HEMATOLOGY

Massive Transfusion Coagulopathy

Jerrold H. Levy

Coagulopathy following massive transfusion is a consequence of post-traumatic and surgical hemorrhage. Bleeding following massive transfusion can occur due to hypothermia, dilutional coagulopathy, platelet dysfunction, fibrinolysis, or hypofibrinogenemia. Transfusion of 15 to 20 units of blood products causes dilutional thrombocytopenia, and both antiplatelet agents (eg, clopidogrel [Plavix®, Sanofi, Bridgewater, NJ]) and hemostatic inhibitors (eg, low-molecular-weight heparins, pentasaccharides, and direct thrombin inhibitors) are contributing factors to bleeding. Tests for platelet dysfunction are not readily available. Excessive fibrinolysis and low fibrinogen are also causes of bleeding in these patients. Currently, however, there are several agents that have been reported to be effective for the prophylaxis of hemorrhage in surgical patients, including aprotinin for cardiac surgery, orthopedic surgery, and hepatic transplantation, and the off-label use of recombinant activated factor VII (NovoSeven®, Novo Nordisk, Bagsvaerd, Denmark) as rescue therapy for life-threatening hemorrhage.
Semin Hematol 43(suppl 1):S59-S63

Uncontrolled bleeding is a clinical problem commonly faced by hematologists, emergency medicine physicians, surgeons, anesthesiologists, and other healthcare professionals involved in the management of trauma and surgical patients. Such clinical situations often necessitate the massive transfusion of blood and blood products. Many other factors may also trigger a complex coagulopathy that further compromises the efficacy of subsequent hemostatic treatments. Patients undergoing massive transfusion—commonly defined as replacing at least one blood volume in 24 hours—will develop defective hemostasis that can be attributed to both the transfusion strategy and the trauma itself.[1]

There are three major components of hemostasis—the vasculature, coagulation proteins, and platelets—that interact in dynamic ways. Hemostasis is initially dependent on the normal response to damage to the vascular endothelium, which has a fundamental role in homeostatic mechanisms due to its potent anticoagulant and anti-inflammatory effects. When the vasculature is damaged by surgery or trauma, the integrity of the endothelium is compromised, leading to a change from anticoagulant and anti-inflammatory to procoagulant and pro-inflammatory effects. A major consequence of systemic endothelial dysfunction sometimes associated with trauma is disseminated intravascular coagulation (DIC), a complex syndrome of systemic and excess coagulation that is most frequently caused by sepsis.[1,2]

Department of Anesthesiology, Emory University School of Medicine, Cardiothoracic Anesthesiology and Critical Care, Emory Healthcare, Atlanta, GA.
Address correspondence to Jerrold H. Levy, MD, Professor of Anesthesiology, Department of Anesthesiology, Emory University School of Medicine, Cardiothoracic Anesthesiology and Critical Care, Emory Healthcare, Atlanta, GA 30322. E-mail: Jerrold.Levy@emoryhealthcare.org

Disseminated Intravascular Coagulation

The loss of vascular protection through endothelial injury can induce the expression of tissue factor (TF), which, as well as contributing to normal hemostasis, has a prominent procoagulant role in DIC.[2] This release of TF leads to fibrin deposition in the microvasculature and a microangiopathic hemolytic anemia, in which red blood cells become fragmented as a consequence of circulating through damaged vasculature and a fibrin meshwork. Microcirculatory disturbances eventually result in apoptosis and necrosis of parenchymal cells, leading to multiple organ dysfunction syndrome or multiple organ failure.[3] DIC related to trauma or other situations where there is extensive endothelial injury produces TF activation and subsequent generation of thrombin. The fact that such thrombin generation is not regulated by multiple systemic and local thrombin regulatory mechanisms contributes to the coagulopathy state characterized by DIC.

The hemostatic signature of DIC—low platelets, low fibrinogen, prolonged prothrombin time (PT), prolonged partial thromboplastin time (PTT), elevated D-dimers, and low antithrombin (AT)—is seen after almost every procedure in-

0037-1963/06/$-see front matter
doi:10.1053/j.seminhematol.2005.11.019

volving cardiopulmonary bypass (CPB), because dilutional coagulopathy is created. Levels of AT as low as 30% have been measured in patients undergoing CPB.[4] Both laboratory parameters and clinical signs should be taken into account when diagnosing DIC.

Pathophysiology of Hemostatic Abnormalities With Trauma

Hemostatic abnormalities associated with trauma can develop as a result of depletion of hemostatic factors through blood loss, tissue injury, and/or consumption of factors. Volume resuscitation with crystalloids, colloids, and red blood cells (RBCs), or the use of cell salvage systems following blood loss, can lead to dilutional coagulopathy, which reduces the levels of hemostatic factors. The hemostatic balance between anticoagulant and procoagulant activity may be lost due to tissue injury following trauma (including head trauma), tissue hypoxia/acidosis, burns/sepsis or other physical events (eg, intraoperative suction, reinfusion of debris).

Other mechanisms leading to post-traumatic hemostatic defects include hypothermia, in which coagulation reactions are decreased, platelet function is compromised, and plasmin/thrombin-mediated factor consumption is increased. Adding to this is impaired platelet function due to increased fibrinogen degradation products (FDP) and D-dimer levels, or the use of plasma expanders (particularly hydroxyethyl starch [HES]). Other important considerations include anemia-related factors, ie, decreased RBC adenosine diphosphate and decreased platelet diffusivity, and the effects of acidemia, which may include hypocalcemia with massive transfusions.

Causes of Bleeding After Massive Transfusion Coagulopathy

Predicting the risk of a patient developing coagulopathy following massive transfusion requires careful consideration of additional medications the patient was receiving. For instance, factors such as whether the patient has received antiplatelet agents (eg, aspirin, clopidogrel) are important. In surgical patients, there may be an opportunity to administer prophylactic agents to reduce blood loss and thus prevent or limit the need for blood transfusions, and this is particularly relevant in cardiac surgical patients. Following CPB, platelet dysfunction occurs.[5] The presence of endotoxin in the blood may also influence the course of coagulopathy as it has potent pro-inflammatory actions, upregulating adhesion molecules in the vascular endothelium, increasing levels of neutrophils and platelets, and inducing platelet–neutrophil adherence. Although these various conditions may affect the progression and management of massive transfusion coagulopathy, the actual causes of bleeding after massive transfusion are most frequently considered to be hypothermia, dilutional coagulopathy (>1 to 1.5 blood volumes), platelet dysfunction, fibrinolysis, and low fibrinogen levels. Each of these factors will be discussed in turn.

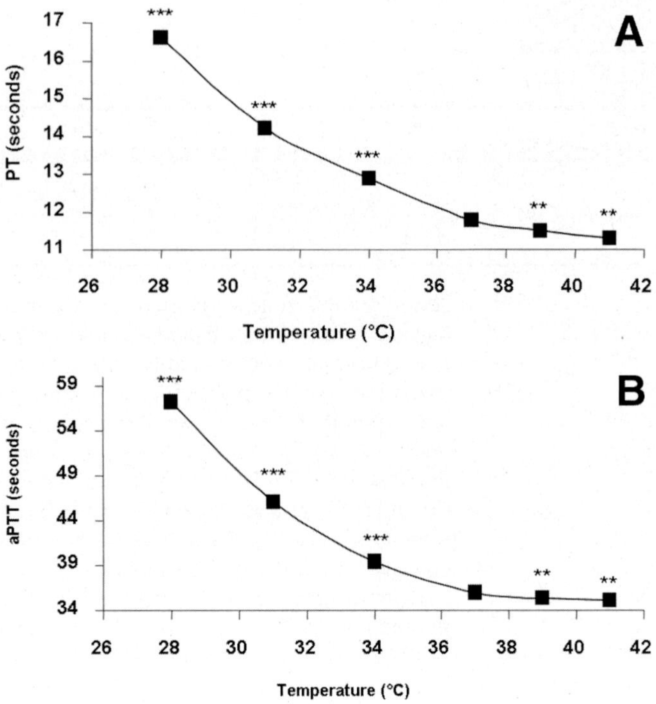

Figure 1 Hypothermia leads to prolongation of (A) prothrombin time (PT) and (B) activated partial thromboplastin time (aPTT). $^{**}P < .01$ compared with mean at 37°C; $^{***}P < .001$ compared with mean at 37°C or any other temperature.[6] Reprinted with permission.[6] Rohrer MJ et al: Effect of hypothermia on the coagulation cascade. Crit Care Med 20:1402-1405, 1992

Hypothermia

Hypothermia (usually considered to be a temperature of <34°C) is a complex syndrome that has several consequences. Hemostasis is an enzymatic process, and is therefore cooled and slowed down by reduced body temperatures. Hypothermia also causes reversible platelet dysfunction, increases fibrinolysis, and reduces the production of coagulation factors.[1,6] In addition, PT and activated PTT (aPTT) were found to be significantly prolonged when measured in samples of pooled normal plasma at temperatures of 34°C or less when compared with measurements at 37°C (Fig 1).[6] One of the problems faced by clinicians is that blood taken from a patient whose temperature is less than 34°C will be tested at 37°C, so the influence of hypothermia on their bleeding status may be overlooked. However, the effects of reduced temperature are clinically meaningful and hypothermia is an important contributor to coagulopathy in trauma patients. Maintenance of normal body temperature is therefore important for minimizing blood loss in trauma patients and during surgery,[1] and there are new devices that can be used for warming post-traumatic, surgical, and other hypothermic patients.

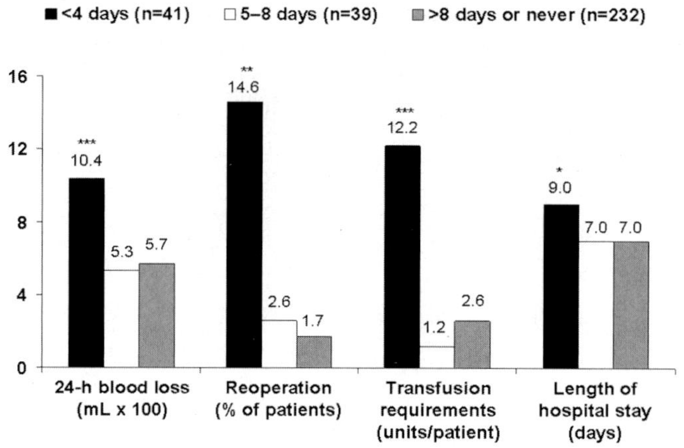

Figure 2 Administration of clopidogrel within 4 days of coronary artery bypass grafting leads to greater blood loss, reoperation, transfusion requirements and duration of hospitalization. ***$P < .001$, **$P < .01$, *$P < .05$ *v* groups receiving clopidogrel within 5 to 8 days or more than 8 days previously (or never).[8]

Dilutional Coagulopathy

Dilutional coagulopathy is one of the most common causes of bleeding after massive transfusion. Over 30 years ago, Miller et al[7] described the coagulation defects associated with massive transfusions in 21 acutely traumatized soldiers. They found that dilutional coagulopathy occurred after transfusion of 20 to 25 units of stored whole blood treated with acid-citrate dextrose (ACD), and that platelet deficiency appeared to be the main cause of the bleeding tendency. This deficiency was attributed to diminished platelet levels in ACD blood. Importantly, the results showed that the mean platelet counts paralleled the predicted platelet counts derived from a standard washout equation, further supporting a dilutional basis for the thrombocytopenia. Transfusion of approximately 15 to 20 units of blood creates a 1 to 1.5 dilution of the blood volume, with the platelet count falling to a critical level (approximately 20,000 to 30,000 mm^3) at which spontaneous bleeding can occur.

Platelet Dysfunction

Platelet dysfunction can also cause excessive bleeding. The increasing use of the platelet inhibitor, clopidogrel (Plavix, Sanofi, Bridgewater, NJ), is a cause of growing concern in clinical medicine—most individuals with atherosclerotic vascular disease, a coronary stent, peripheral vascular disease or cerebrovascular disease will receive clopidogrel, with high use in the elderly population. One study evaluated outcomes of 312 patients who received the drug within 4 days, 5 to 8 days, or more than 8 days (or never) prior to undergoing coronary artery bypass grafting (CABG).[8] Those who received clopidogrel within 4 days of the procedure experienced significantly greater blood loss (Fig 2), and a significantly higher proportion required transfusion compared with patients who received clopidogrel within 5 to 8 days or more than 8 days previously (75.6% *v* 35.9% and 42.2%, respectively; $P < .001$). Similarly, the mean total transfusion requirements, proportion of patients requiring reoperation for bleeding, and the median length of hospital stay were significantly greater in the group who received clopidogrel within 4 days (Fig 2). Other studies of clopidogrel have reported similar results.[9-11]

The use of other hemostatic inhibitors such as low-molecular-weight heparins, warfarin, pentasaccharide (fondaparinux) or newer thrombin inhibitors (eg, ximelagatran) may also be contributing factors. A complicating issue when attempting to identify platelet dysfunction is the lack of point-of-care platelet function testing. Platelet count provides no indication of platelet dysfunction and bleeding times have been shown to have no predictive value for surgical bleeding.[12] Even the Platelet Function Analyzer (PFA-100, Dade Behring, Inc, Deerfield, IL), a relatively new in vitro bleeding test that is sensitive to abnormalities of platelet function, has not been sufficiently studied to determine whether it can accurately predict bleeding. Recent experimental research into developing new testing techniques has focused on specific, clopidogrel-related testing using P2Y12 receptor whole blood aggregometry. However, the difficulty with many of these platelet function assays is that dilutional thrombocytopenia affects the measurements.

When platelet dysfunction has been identified or suspected, platelets are transfused. However, side effects need to be considered, and can include anaphylactic shock and hypersensitivity reactions such as transfusion-related acute lung injury [TRALI]. Analysis of a database of phase III clinical trials of aprotinin compared adverse outcome data (N = 1,720) from patients who received perioperative platelets with those who did not during CABG surgery.[13] Platelet transfusions were associated with an increased risk of serious adverse events, including stroke and death. Platelet transfusions were also associated with longer hospital stays, longer surgical procedures, more re-operations for bleeding, more RBC transfusions, and postoperative infection.

Fibrinolysis

Under normal circumstances, fibrinolysis occurs in association with hemostasis, but excessive fibrinolysis can cause bleeding. Fibrinolysis is initiated by multiple mechanisms, including tissue plasminogen activator (tPA) released in response to vascular endothelial damage,[14] stress responses,[15] and multiple other mechanisms. Plasmin degrades fibrinogen and von Willebrand's factor (vWF), cleaves receptors from platelets (glycoprotein Ib), and creates degradation products that bind glycoprotein IIb/IIIa receptors, thus interfering with platelet function. Plasmin is also generated by contact activation,[16] in which kallikrein plays the central role in addition to being involved in processes such as white cell chemotaxis and chemokinesis.[17] Rinder et al[18] showed that contact activation led to the cleaving of glycoprotein Ib receptors from platelets, and that the generation of FDP resulted in the creation of multimers that bind with glycoprotein IIb/IIIa receptors to prevent platelet–fibrinogen cross-linking, similar to the effects of the glycoprotein IIb/IIIa receptor inhibitor, abciximab.[19] These alterations in fibrinolysis adversely affect platelet function.

Low Fibrinogen

Fibrinogen, an acute-phase reactant protein, is the main plasma protein coagulation factor,[20] and normal fibrinogen levels are currently estimated to fall within the range of 175 to 400 mg/dL.[21] Genetic defects of fibrinogen resulting in structural abnormalities that alter protein function (dysfibrinogenemia) can increase the risk of bleeding or thrombosis, or sometimes a combination of these effects.[22] Increased levels of fibrinogen produce hypercoagulability and can compensate for platelet dysfunction. For example, in the late stages of pregnancy, the normal physiological response is hypercoagulability to reduce the risk of bleeding complications during birth.[23] Although benign dilutional thrombocytopenia often develops, with a platelet count of 80,000 to 150,000 mm^3, fibrinogen levels increase to 400 to 500 mg/dL. During delivery, a systemic hemostatic state develops with consumption of platelets and coagulation factors (including fibrinogen) to allow clotting to occur; hemostasis then normalizes within 4 to 6 weeks postpartum.

If fibrinogen levels fall to 80 to 100 mg/dL or lower, PT and PTT can be affected. These changes may not be corrected by transfusion of fresh frozen plasma (FFP), which is likely to contain insufficient fibrinogen, but cryoprecipitate can be used as it has the advantage of also containing vWF. A major problem with managing bleeding is that most transfusion algorithms only recommend initiating treatment when fibrinogen levels are less than 100 mg/dL, and it may be difficult to reverse the effects of such low levels of this vital component of hemostatic function.

Preventative Strategies for Bleeding

Surgery allows the potential use of prophylaxis for hemostatic activation and inflammatory responses. Aprotinin, a broad-spectrum protease inhibitor, and the most potent plasmin inhibitor available, has been studied extensively in cardiac surgery, orthopedic surgery, liver transplantation, and other procedures.[24-28] Aprotinin inhibits a whole series of proteases (eg, myeloperoxidase), as well as kallikrein, and probably modulates thrombin-mediated PAR1 receptor activation. In a multicenter, double-blind, placebo-controlled trial, the safety and dose-related efficacy of aprotinin were examined in 287 patients undergoing repeat CABG surgery.[29] It was shown that fewer patients receiving high-dose (54%; $P < .001$), low-dose (53%; $P < .001$) or pump-prime-only aprotinin prior to surgery (74%; $P = .125$) required transfusions of any blood products when compared with those receiving placebo (85%), and that all doses of aprotinin were associated with significant reductions in the number of units of blood products required, the total number of blood-product exposures and the rate of post-operative thoracic drainage during the first 6 hours (Fig 3). Total thoracic drainage volume was significantly reduced by 47% and 38.5% in the high- and low-dose aprotinin groups, respectively, compared with placebo ($P \leq .001$). However, administration of

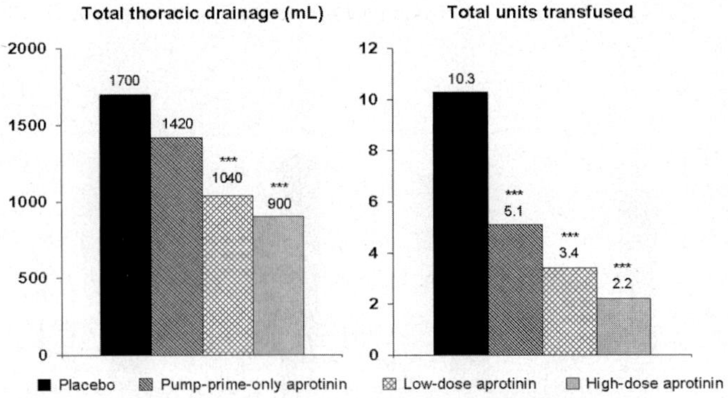

Figure 3 Aprotinin reduces transfusion requirements and thoracic drainage volume in patients undergoing repeat coronary artery bypass grafting. $***P \leq .001$ v placebo.[29]

aprotinin during surgery, when bleeding had already begun, produced no detectable haemostatic efficacy.

Lysine analogues, such as epsilon aminocaproic acid (EACA) and tranexamic acid, are other commonly used agents for bleeding prophylaxis in hemophilia and a number of other clinical situations.[30,31] Unlike currently approved pharmacologic agents, these drugs have not undergone rigorous safety testing.[32] Modulating kallikrein may also be an appropriate target for the prevention of bleeding, and a recombinant plasma kallikrein inhibitor is currently being studied in angioedema.[33]

Other agents, including the off-label use of recombinant activated factor VII (rFVIIa, NovoSeven®, Novo Nordisk, Bagsvaerd, Denmark), have the potential to be used as prophylaxis to modulate hemostatic function in high-risk surgical procedures that involve extensive tissue injury.[34] For example, rFVIIa has already demonstrated effectiveness in treating excessive bleeding during cardiac surgery,[35-40] and a recent study showed that rFVIIa had beneficial effects in patients requiring massive transfusion and with coagulopathy refractory to conventional treatments.[41] Earlier intervention with such agents presents a promising new perspective for preventing hemorrhagic complications during surgery and other clinical situations.

Summary

Coagulopathy following massive transfusions is a complex, multicellular, multifactorial clinical problem. When evaluating the causes of coagulopathy in this setting, preexisting pharmacotherapy with agents such as clopidogrel, low-molecular-weight heparins, pentasaccharides, or anticoagulants needs to be considered. The roles of hypothermia, dilutional coagulopathy, platelet dysfunction and fibrinolysis should also be taken into account. Evaluation of fibrinogen levels should form an element of all transfusion algorithms, especially in those for patients with excessive bleeding. Correlating hemostatic tests with bleeding using transfusion algorithms needs to be considered following massive transfusions. Current evidence suggests that prevention of massive bleeding and associated complications may be possible with pharmacological agents, including aprotinin and rFVIIa, and further studies are underway to assess the applicability and efficacy of these approaches.

References

1. Hardy JF, De Moerloose P, Samama M, Groupe d'interet en Hemostase Perioperatoire: Massive transfusion and coagulopathy: pathophysiology and implications for clinical management. Can J Anaesth 51:293-310, 2004
2. Toh CH, Dennis M: Disseminated intravascular coagulation: old disease, new hope. BMJ 327:974-977, 2003
3. Keel M, Trentz O: Pathophysiology of polytrauma. Injury 36:691-709, 2005
4. Levy JH, Despotis GJ, Szlam F, Olson P, Meeker D, Weisinger A: Recombinant human transgenic antithrombin in cardiac surgery: A dose-finding study. Anesthesiology 96:1095-1102, 2002
5. Rinder CS, Bohnert J, Rinder HM, Mitchell J, Ault K, Hillman R: Platelet activation and aggregation during cardiopulmonary bypass. Anesthesiology 75:388-393, 1991
6. Rohrer MJ, Natale AM: Effect of hypothermia on the coagulation cascade. Crit Care Med 20:1402-1405, 1992
7. Miller RD, Robbins TO, Tong MJ, Barton SL: Coagulation defects associated with massive blood transfusions. Ann Surg 174:794-801, 1971
8. Chu MW, Wilson SR, Novick RJ, Stitt LW, Quantz MA: Does clopidogrel increase blood loss following coronary artery bypass surgery? Ann Thorac Surg 78:1536-1541, 2004
9. van der Linden J, Lindvall G, Sartipy U: Aprotinin decreases postoperative bleeding and number of transfusions in patients on clopidogrel undergoing coronary artery bypass graft surgery: A double-blind, placebo-controlled, randomized clinical trial. Circulation 112:I276-80, 2005 (suppl 9)
10. Hongo RH, Ley J, Dick SE, Yee RR: The effect of clopidogrel in combination with aspirin when given before coronary artery bypass grafting. J Am Coll Cardiol 40:231-237, 2002
11. Yende S, Wunderink RG: Effect of clopidogrel on bleeding after coronary artery bypass surgery. Crit Care Med 29:2271-2275, 2001
12. Lind SE: The bleeding time does not predict surgical bleeding. Blood 77:2547-2552, 1991
13. Spiess BD, Royston D, Levy JH, Fitch J, Dietrich W, Body S, et al: Platelet transfusions during coronary artery bypass graft surgery are associated with serious adverse outcomes. Transfusion 44:1143-1148, 2004
14. Loskutoff DJ, Curriden SA: The fibrinolytic system of the vessel wall and its role in the control of thrombosis. Ann N Y Acad Sci 598:238-247, 1990
15. Shinohara M, Kurokawa H, Yoshihara Y, Kokubu S, Kusano T, Horie K, et al: Responses to surgical stress in blood coagulation and fibrinolysis, platelet counts and thromboxane B2 after esophageal cancer operation. Rinsho Byori 45:179-184, 1997
16. Motta G, Rojkjaer R, Hasan AA, Cines DB, Schmaier AH: High molecular weight kininogen regulates prekallikrein assembly and activation on endothelial cells: A novel mechanism for contact activation. Blood 91:516-528, 1998
17. Becker EL: Stimulated neutrophil locomotion: chemokinesis and chemotaxis. Arch Pathol Lab Med 101:509-513, 1977
18. Rinder CS, Mathew JP, Rinder HM, Bonan J, Ault KA, Smith BR: Modulation of platelet surface adhesion receptors during cardiopulmonary bypass. Anesthesiology 75:563-570, 1991
19. Collet JP, Montalescot G, Lesty C, Soria J, Mishal Z, Thomas D, et al: Disaggregation of in vitro preformed platelet-rich clots by abciximab increases fibrin exposure and promotes fibrinolysis. Arterioscler Thromb Vasc Biol 21:142-148, 2001
20. Lowe GD, Rumley A, Mackie IJ: Plasma fibrinogen. Ann Clin Biochem 41:430-440, 2004
21. Kratz A, Lewandrowski KB: Case records of the Massachusetts General Hospital. Weekly clinicopathological exercises. Normal reference laboratory values. N Engl J Med 339:1063-1072, 1998
22. Meyer M: Molecular biology of haemostasis: Fibrinogen, factor XIII. Hamostaseologie 24:108-115, 2004
23. Hellgren M: Hemostasis during normal pregnancy and puerperium. Semin Thromb Hemost 29:125-130, 2003
24. Kokoszka A, Kuflik P, Bitan F, Casden A, Neuwirth M: Evidence-based review of the role of aprotinin in blood conservation during orthopaedic surgery. J Bone Joint Surg Am 87:1129-1136, 2005
25. Kinzel V, Shakespeare D, Derbyshire D: The effect of aprotinin on blood loss in bilateral total knee arthroplasty. Knee 12:107-111, 2005
26. Levy JH: Efficacy and safety of aprotinin in cardiac surgery. Orthopedics 27:s659-s662, 2004 (suppl 6)
27. Sedrakyan A, Treasure T, Elefteriades JA: Effect of aprotinin on clinical outcomes in coronary artery bypass graft surgery: A systematic review and meta-analysis of randomized clinical trials. J Thorac Cardiovasc Surg 128:442-448, 2004
28. Xia VW, Steadman RH: Antifibrinolytics in orthotopic liver transplantation: Current status and controversies. Liver Transpl 11:10-18, 2005
29. Levy JH, Pifarre R, Schaff HV, Horrow JC, Albus R, Spiess B, et al: A multicenter, double-blind, placebo-controlled trial of aprotinin for reducing blood loss and the requirement for donor-blood transfusion in patients undergoing repeat coronary artery bypass grafting. Circulation 92:2236-2244, 1995
30. Levi MM, Vink R, de Jonge E: Management of bleeding disorders by prohemostatic therapy. Int J Hematol 76:139-144, 2002 (suppl 2)
31. Dunn CJ, Goa KL: Tranexamic acid: A review of its use in surgery and other indications. Drugs 57:1005-1032, 1999
32. Dobkowski WB, Murkin JM: A risk-benefit assessment of aprotinin in cardiac surgical procedures. Drug Saf 18:21-41, 1998
33. Tanaka KA, Szlam F, Katori N, Vega JD, Levy JH: Evaluation of a novel kallikrein inhibitor on hemostatic activation in vitro. Thromb Res 113:333-339, 2004
34. Levi M, Peters M, Buller HR: Efficacy and safety of recombinant factor VIIa for treatment of severe bleeding: A systematic review. Crit Care Med 33:883-890, 2005
35. von Heymann C, Hotz H, Konertz W, Kox WJ, Spies C: Successful treatment of refractory bleeding with recombinant factor VIIa after redo coronary artery bypass graft surgery. J Cardiothorac Vasc Anesth 16:615-616, 2002
36. Hendriks HG, van der Maaten JM, de Wolf J, Waterbolk TW, Slooff MJ, van der Meer J: An effective treatment of severe intractable bleeding after valve repair by one single dose of activated recombinant factor VII. Anesth Analg 93:287-289, 2001
37. Kastrup M, von Heymann C, Hotz H, Konertz WF, Ziemer S, Kox WJ, et al: Recombinant factor VIIa after aortic valve replacement in a patient with osteogenesis imperfecta. Ann Thorac Surg 74:910-912, 2002
38. Tanaka KA, Waly AA, Cooper WA, Levy JH: Treatment of excessive bleeding in Jehovah's Witness patients after cardiac surgery with recombinant factor VIIa (NovoSeven). Anesthesiology 98:1513-1515, 2003
39. Stratmann G, Russell IA, Merrick SH: Use of recombinant factor VIIa as a rescue treatment for intractable bleeding following repeat aortic arch repair. Ann Thorac Surg 76:2094-2097, 2003
40. Halkos ME, Levy JH, Chen E, Reddy VS, Lattouf OM, Guyton RA et al: Early experience with activated recombinant factor VII for intractable hemorrhage after cardiovascular surgery. Ann Thorac Surg 79:1303-1306, 2005
41. Gowers CJ, Parr MJ: Recombinant activated factor VIIa use in massive transfusion and coagulopathy unresponsive to conventional therapy. Anaesth Intensive Care 33:196-200, 2005

ELSEVIER

Seminars in
HEMATOLOGY

Assessing Efficacy and Therapeutic Claims in Emerging Indications for Recombinant Factor VIIa: Regulatory Perspectives

Albert Farrugia

When compared with the evidence-based, cost-effectiveness criteria underpinning most government reimbursement schemes in the social market economies, the three regulatory hurdles of safety, quality and efficacy are probably of modest impact in influencing increased usage of recombinant activated factor VII (rFVIIa; NovoSeven®, Novo Nordisk, Bagsvaerd, Denmark). Nevertheless, efficacy claims must be supported if regulatory approval is to be granted for the wider range of indications that have been proposed for rFVIIa. With the refinement of clinical trial designs over the past 40 years, the randomized controlled trial (RCT) has assumed the role of gold standard, providing the highest level of evidence for therapeutic efficacy. However, it is incorrect to assume that regulatory authorities give sole credence to RCTs in assessing claims. It is noteworthy that the indications already accepted for rFVIIa by international regulatory authorities—including the treatment of inhibitors to factor VIII and factor IX, substitution for FVII deficiency, and treatment of Glanzmann's thrombasthenia—were supported not by RCTs but by studies conventionally considered to provide modest evidence levels. Therefore, the use of studies other than RCTs for the more recently proposed indications for rFVIIa in a range of conditions requiring hemostatic correction is perfectly feasible. What regulators expect are well-conducted and well-described studies adhering to principles of good clinical practice, which can be scrutinized for evidence of clinical efficacy and which are based on the initially proven principle for the drug. This paper discusses the regulatory history of rFVIIa in the major regulatory authorities and assesses the route needed to support claims being made in the mainstream literature. Recent episodes where post-market events have forced regulators to be more than usually cautious will be used as examples to suggest possible pitfalls to the extension of approved claims for rFVIIa. The major paths for enhancing access for indications in small patient numbers, where RCTs are even more difficult to perform, will be described and their use for possible extension of rFVIIa indications will be discussed.
Semin Hematol 43(suppl 1):S64-S69 © 2006 Elsevier Inc. All rights reserved.

Introduction—The Role of Therapeutic Product Regulation in Healthcare Decision Making

Therapeutic product regulators are charged through law with approving market access on the basis of safety, quality, and efficacy. However, increasing demands on public healthcare budgets are causing policy makers to incorporate cost-effectiveness assessments even into regulatory decision making (see, for example, Schedule 4 in the National Blood Agreement between the nine governments of the Australian federation, specifying the process whereby new proposals, including those resulting from mandatory regulatory measures, are assessed against evidence-based and cost-effectiveness criteria. Available at: www.nba.gov.au). The statutory link between regulatory and policy/funding decision making that exists within the bureaucratic framework of many healthcare delivery systems lends itself to such scrutiny. Approval by the relevant regulatory authority, a pre-requisite for most public and insurance-based drug reimbursement schemes, provides another example of the growing linkage between supposedly independent criteria for cost and safety, quality, and efficacy. Therefore, for new therapies, access to the market is governed by the four barriers of safety, quality,

Therapeutic Goods Administration, Woden, Australia.
Address correspondence to Albert Farrugia, PhD, Senior Principal Research Scientist and Head, Blood and Tissues Unit, Office of Devices, Blood and Tissues, Therapeutic Goods Administration, PO Box 100, Woden, ACT, Australia 2606. E-mail: albert.farrugia@health.gov.au

 0037-1963/06/$-see front matter © 2006 Elsevier Inc. All rights reserved.
doi:10.1053/j.seminhematol.2005.11.013

efficacy (the supposed brief of regulators), and cost-effectiveness or reimbursement (the domain of policy and funding decision makers). Irrespective of the degree of linkage that has evolved around these supposedly independent areas of public policy, regulatory approval remains a crucial prelude to significant penetration of the market.

The incipient tensions in these interactions are standard consequences of the dynamics underpinning most of public care and healthcare policy in the Western economies: the competing demands of electoral populism and evidence-based interventions shape the delivery of increasingly expensive health measures. The imperatives of getting the government of the day re-elected, while still delivering necessary microeconomic reform and improved population health outcomes, constitute the basic dynamics of public health policy. The selective exploitation of public conceptions (and misconceptions), along with intensive market research into the values and moods of core groups of influential electors, sits uneasily but unavoidably alongside the demands of the research-based evidence that seeks value for resources with equity through defined health outcomes.[1] Regulators are not immune to these tensions, and the link between market approval and public/private reimbursement for therapies such as new drugs inevitably results in pressures over and above those exerted by issues of safety and efficacy. Public perceptions that regulators have been remiss in their mission of assuring product safety, leading to substantial levels of patient harm,[2] augment these tensions, as the effects of "politically" driven and accelerated regulatory processes come home to roost. These factors need to be kept in mind when considering the regulatory authorities' perspective on emerging and expensive drugs, as exemplified by the case of recombinant activated factor VII (rFVIIa; NovoSeven®, Novo Nordisk, Bagsvaerd, Denmark).

Evidence-Based Medicine in Public Health and Regulation

All public service delivery systems are trying to manage the tension between demand, capacity, and cost. They are seeking to improve performance and value for money, while assuaging the demands of the populist imperative. Hence, they are asking questions about how to evaluate performance. Evidence-based medicine (EBM) is a structuralized concept that has arisen not only as a result of these tensions, but also from clinicians' need to objectively assess and utilize the increasingly complex and expensive interventions of modern therapeutics. The development and principles of EBM have been reviewed elsewhere.[3] EBM initially focused on the best research evidence that was relevant to the clinical issue under review, although more traditional determinants of clinical practice have recently been incorporated into this concept. Furthermore, EBM now recognizes the role of patient preferences and societal issues in making therapeutic choices.

The primary tool of EBM is the gradation of the levels of scientific evidence that are applied to the assessment of therapeutic interventions.[4] The hierarchy of levels of evidence has also evolved, and a recent proposed example is shown in Table 1.[5] On this basis, the randomized clinical trial (RCT) provides the foundation of the highest level of EBM. RCTs are controlled clinical experiments in which patients are allocated by the investigators to receive, or not to receive, the treatment under study. If randomization is used, all the trial participants are equally likely to be allocated to either the treatment or the control arm. If blinding is used, the investigators are unaware of the treatment allocations. Double-blind RCTs, in which the participants are also unaware of the treatment allocations, are meant to exclude the possibility of bias in study design and execution, and to obviate the role of confounding factors in trial interpretation, as explained by Vamvakas.[4]

Table 1 Hierarchy of Strength of Evidence Concerning Efficacy of Therapeutic Interventions

1. N of 1 randomized trial
2. Systematic reviews of randomized trials
3. Single randomized controlled trial
4. Systematic reviews of observational studies
5. Single observational studies
6. Physiological studies
7. Unsystematic clinical observations

Reproduced with permission, JAMA 284:1290-1296, 2000.[5]

Therefore, as specifically designed experimental studies, RCTs are different from observational studies of ongoing therapeutic intervention. Observational studies may be subject to the effects of bias and confounding, which would weaken the evidence base of any conclusion. Sacks et al[6] have shown that, for six different interventions, historically controlled observational trials consistently overestimated the therapeutic effect when compared with RCTs. However, McKee et al[7] found different outcomes when analyzing 18 papers in which a single intervention was evaluated by both methods. Whilst summarizing why observational studies are still important in the hierarchy of evidence assessment, these authors argue in favor of considering observational and experimental—RCT—studies as complementary tools in the overall assessment of evidence. Furthermore, Padkin et al[8] highlight the problems in assessing the generalizability and applicability of an RCT to mainstream clinical practice. Indeed, they argue for the use of large-scale and high-quality databases of observational studies in order to supplement and validate conclusions derived from RCTs.

These synergies are insufficiently appreciated in many public policy environments, where the problems posed by the need for RCTs are frequently exploited in order to obviate consideration of emerging and sometimes promising interventions, primarily because of cost considerations. The ethical and practical difficulties posed by conducting trials of serious conditions, sometimes involving small numbers of patients and using a modality that gives readily observable and dramatic effects,[9] have contributed to the development of modified approaches to trial design and data analyses using sequential testing to enable data examination at a series of interim points.[10] Studies of trials employing this sequential approach have been published,[11–13] and its inclusion in the Food and Drug Administration (FDA)'s Guidelines for "Statistical Principles for Clinical Trials"[14] demonstrates an acknowledgment from regulatory authorities. This is encouraging in the context of rFVIIa, the subject of this review.

Recombinant Activated Factor VII in Clinical Practice

The development of rFVIIa as a treatment modality for securing hemostasis in patients with hemophilia and inhibitors to factor VIII or IX has been extensively reviewed.[15] As a recombinant product free of the risk of transmitting human blood-borne pathogens, many clinicians prefer rFVIIa to activated (plasma-derived) prothrombin complex concentrates (aPCCs) for the treatment of this condition.

A review from the Cochrane Collaboration[16] comments on the lack of RCTs comparing the two treatment modalities, and promotes such a trial to generate the required evidence. The relative cost-effectiveness of rFVIIa and aPCCs has also been a matter of debate.[17,18] The level of evidence accruable from extensive observational studies was sufficient for regulatory authorities to grant market authorization for rFVIIa in the absence of RCTs, despite the reservations expressed in the FDA's Summary Basis for Approval.[19] Since initial authorization for the treatment of hemophilia with inhibitors, the European Medicines Agency (EMEA) has extended the range of indications to include acquired hemophilia, factor VII deficiency and Glanzmann's thrombasthenia (GT) refractory to platelet transfusion. All of these approvals were granted on the basis of observational studies. Scrutiny of the EMEA's European Public Assessment Report (EPAR) for rFVIIa in GT shows that the authority requested re-submission of the data from the manufacturer in order to exclude patients not covered by the requested indication. This resulted in further reduction of an already small patient population, but still resulted in approval after the claimed level of efficacy was shown to be unchanged. The EMEA also requested the establishment of a post-marketing registry for the use of rFVIIa in the treatment of patients with GT.[20]

The approval of indications for rFVIIa demonstrates the willingness of authorities to accept well-conducted observational studies in the absence of level I evidence of efficacy. Recent statements from the FDA,[21] among others, show that regulators will not allow what they consider to be unsubstantiated claims for this (or any) agent to pass unchallenged. This is of particular importance for rFVIIa, where the number of proposed indications is rapidly expanding.

Emerging Indications for rFVIIa—Regulatory Perspectives

The mechanism of the therapeutic action of rFVIIa is still under investigation. However, laboratory studies indicate that, at pharmacologic (supraphysiologic) levels, the drug can generate thrombin on activated platelet surfaces independently of coagulation factors VIII and IX. The activation of platelets depends on the generation of thrombin through the activation of factor X (FX) following tissue factor exposure through vessel injury. Once this is achieved, a substantial "thrombin burst" results from the tissue factor-independent generation of factor Xa through pharmacologic amounts of rFVIIa.[22] The ability of rFVIIa to bypass many of the conventionally accepted principles of blood clotting, together with its apparent efficacy in treating hemophilia with inhibitors and GT, led to its designation as a putative "universal hemostatic agent."[23] This somewhat unfortunate concept does not take into account that the actions of rFVIIa in hemostasis may be disease specific, as shown by its apparently different effect on fibrinolysis in hemophilia and cirrhotic bleeding.[24,25] Furthermore, this model for the mechanism of action of rFVIIa does not fully explain the apparent efficacy of the drug in thrombocytopenia and other thrombocytopathic conditions, as stated by the EMEA in its EPAR for rFVIIa.[26] The attraction of a hemostatic agent whose action is immediate, short lasting, and localized to the site of vascular injury—all features of rFVIIa—is undeniable. Following the publication of a case report describing the control of bleeding in severe trauma, a plethora of such reports have described the successful use of rFVIIa in a wide range of clinical situations involving hemostatic challenge.[27]

Until agencies approve rFVIIa use in these situations, however, its use in these "emerging" indications is off-label and generally unsupported by the reimbursement processes that rely on regulatory approval. Such approval is unlikely to be granted in the absence of higher levels of evidence than those provided by the case reports that form the majority of studies reporting these indications. It is worth noting that many of the investigator-authored reports on these indications emphatically encourage the performance of prospective RCTs to confirm the observational studies. The limitations of observational studies, and their cited tendency to overestimate therapeutic effect, have also been exemplified with rFVIIa. An open-label study that indicated a reduction in blood loss following rFVIIa therapy in patients undergoing orthotopic liver transplantation (OLT)[28] was not confirmed by a multicenter RCT for the same indication.[29] (Unfortunately, the RCT is limited to a relatively inaccessible abstract, compared with the full publication status of the open-label study.) The heterogeneity of clinical disease states that constitute apparently similar groupings such as "bleeding in liver disease," "bleeding from trauma," etc, is highlighted by the contrasting outcomes of RCTs for patients given rFVIIa while undergoing laparoscopic liver biopsy[30] and OLT.[29] As these issues have gained appreciation from the drug's manufacturer and the clinical community, RCTs have been initiated to assess further the possible therapeutic benefits of rFVIIa suggested by observational studies.

Emerging Indications for rFVIIa—Recently Reported and Ongoing Trials

One RCT has shown that rFVIIa decreases perioperative blood loss and transfusion requirements in patients undergoing retropubic prostatectomy.[31] A cost analysis has indicated savings when using rFVIIa for this indication in the institution that performed the study.[32] However, this finding is sensitive to the unit costs of red cells and rFVIIa, which vary between different markets; such costs therefore need to be considered by each institution interested in assessing the cost benefits of using rFVIIa. The possible infectious hazards of red cell transfusion must also be considered in view of the safety of blood in the markets likely to be able to afford rFVIIa.[33]

Recombinant FVIIa reverses the anticoagulant effect of the FX inhibitor fondaparinux[34] and, to date, is the only proposed antidote for this agent. However, there are currently no trials investigating rFVIIa in patients with fondaparinux-related bleeding, and a recent study showed that rFVIIa does not completely reverse the inhibitory effects of fondaparinux on thrombin generation.[35] These observations increase the caution of regulators, who will require studies of efficacy before approving the use of rFVIIa for this indication. Other trials assessing rFVIIa use for reversing the effects of anticoagulant drugs are ongoing.[36]

The recently published RCT for the use of rFVIIa in acute intracerebral hemorrhage (ICH)[37] is described as a dose-ranging proof-of-concept (phase 2B) trial, and will subsequently be extended to a larger, multi-center, phase 3 study. Although the primary outcome—the decrease in the volume of ICH—was significant only for the highest dose (160 μg/kg body weight), the investigators and study sponsors elected to use the dose of 80 μg/kg body weight for the phase 3 study.[38] Analysis by the investigators indicated an optimal risk-benefit profile for this dose, taking into account the thromboembolic events encountered during the trial. These events were small in number and severity, but sufficient to cause the study's overseeing safety board to require the exclusion of any patients with a history of thromboembolic or vaso-occlusive disease. This will clearly restrict regulator approval of various indications until more evidence is available. However, this study not only represents an important milestone in the evidence base for rFVIIa as a hemostatic agent, but is also a valuable contribution towards the treatment of ICH, a leading cause of neurological disability and death.[39]

A major area of activity in the use of rFVIIa has been the treatment of intractable hemorrhage from trauma. The difficulties in assigning historical controls in observational studies led a major investigational group to conclude that "*Prospective trials of FVIIa in patients with traumatic coagulopathy are strongly indicated.*"[40] A multicenter RCT of rFVIIa as an adjunctive treatment for the control of bleeding in patients with severe blunt or penetrating trauma has recently been reported in the literature.[41] Following retrospective exclusion of patients who died in the initial 48-hour period following rFVIIa administration, the investigators reported several benefits in the treated group, including a decrease in transfusion requirements, multi-organ system failure, and acute respiratory distress syndrome, but no difference in mortality. The statistical "propriety" of excluding patients who were in the initially recruited population after the data had been analyzed must be called into question, and this study appears to be a typical example where sequential analysis would have benefited the study design and, possibly, the outcome. Clearly, the heterogeneous nature of the putative indication makes this particular area of rFVIIa investigation extremely challenging, and regulators are justifiably inclined to consider mortality a relevant clinical endpoint. Additional studies on more narrowly specified patient groups would appear to be in order; in the interim, the excellent guidelines published by one of the most experienced investigational groups[42] should give structure and credibility to further observational studies. Such studies are probably essential if this important area is to achieve regulatory and financial support for its inclusion into therapeutics.

Regulatory Considerations When Approaching a Study Design

Certain therapeutic areas in which rFVIIa use appeared promising have failed to acquire the level of evidence available from RCTs, probably because the study design received inadequate consideration. This problem may have been exacerbated by the current lack of consensus on the drug's mechanism of action, and an accompanying adherence to the "universality" concept. For example, preliminary studies on non-bleeding cirrhotic patients indicated that rFVIIa corrected laboratory markers of abnormal coagulation, suggesting that a clinical hemostatic effect might be observable in bleeding patients.[43] An RCT on such patients failed to find such an effect overall; however, when patients with milder disease were excluded, exploratory data analysis suggested that patients with more advanced disease showed a trend towards receiving benefit. Patients with the most advanced disease state were excluded from entry into the study.[44] It is easy to be wise after the event, but this study provides a basis for further work targeting specific groups of cirrhotic patients—a concept that investigators may well keep in mind, rather than attempting to capture all the patients within a putative indication.

Another area where reflection may result in better study design and therapeutic outcomes concerns the designation of appropriate endpoints. For example, the use of multi-organ system failure (MOSF) as an efficacy, rather than a safety, endpoint should be considered in studies using severely ill patients, such as those with trauma. Clearly, while doubts on its safety in relation to thromboembolic events persist in the minds of investigators and their overseeing bodies, MOSF is a legitimate safety indicator. This emphasizes the need for more work on the putative mechanism of rFVIIa, as investigators continue to propose dosage regimens that exceed by several-fold the amounts predicted from laboratory studies, thus accentuating the possible thromboembolic hazards in regulators' minds.

Conclusions

Recombinant FVIIa has established itself as the treatment of choice for hemophilia with inhibitors, a major complication of this disease. Its potent hemostatic profile has stimulated investigation into a wide range of hemostatic problems, with varying results. While some of the proposed uses for rFVIIa are now approaching the status of high-level, evidence-based indications, more trials are needed for most of these emerging areas. The results from such trials will hopefully improve therapeutic practice as well as enhance our understanding of the mechanism of rFVIIa. While some indications are difficult to capture through mainstream RCTs, supplemental methodologies, such as sequential analyses, are available and suitable for these investigations. Importantly, these approaches are endorsed by the regulators, whose decisions will continue to be considered crucial by the reimbursement bodies charged with funding this expensive but interesting and promising drug.

References

1. Gray A: Evidence-based policies and indicator systems: From profane arithmetic to a sacred geometry? Third International Inter-disciplinary Evidence-Based Policies and Indicator Systems Conference, July 2001. Available at: http://www.cemcentre.org/eb2003/Forward%20by%20Andrew%20Gray%20WITHOUT%20SHADING.doc
2. News Target network: FDA fails to protect public from dangerous drugs. http://www.newstarget.com/002325.html. Accessed 21/07/05
3. Centre for Evidence-Based Medicine: Evidence-Based Medicine: What it is and what it isn't. http://www.cebm.net/ebm_is_isnt.asp. Accessed 21/07/05
4. Vamvakas EC: Evidence-based practice of transfusion medicine: Is it possible and what do the words mean? Transfus Med Rev 18:267-278, 2004
5. Guyatt GH, Haynes RB, Jaeschke RZ, Cook DJ, Green L, Naylor CD, et al: Users' Guides to the Medical Literature: XXV. Evidence-based medicine: principles for applying the Users' Guides to patient care. Evidence-Based Medicine Working Group. JAMA 284:1290-1296, 2000
6. Sacks H, Chalmers TC, Smith H: Randomized versus historical controls for clinical trials. Am J Med 72:233-240, 1982
7. McKee M, Britton A, Black N, McPherson K, Sanderson C, Bain C: Methods in health service research. Interpreting the evidence: Choosing between randomised and non-randomised studies. BMJ 319:312-315, 1999
8. Padkin A, Rowan K, Black N: Using high quality clinical databases to complement the results of randomised controlled trials: The case of recombinant human activated protein C. BMJ 323:923-926, 2001
9. Everitt BS, Pickles A: Statistical aspects of the design and analysis of clinical trials. World Scientific Publishing, 2004. Available at: http://www.worldscibooks.com/lifesci/p321.html. Accessed 28/07/05
10. Todd S, Whitehead A, Stallard N, Whitehead J. Interim analyses and sequential designs in phase III studies. Br J Clin Pharmacol 51:394-399, 2001
11. Montaner JS, Lawson LM, Levitt N, Belzberg A, Schechter MT, Ruedy J: Corticosteroids prevent early deterioration in patients with moderately severe Pneumocystis carinii pneumonia and the acquired immunodeficiency syndrome (AIDS). Ann Intern Med 113:14-20, 1990
12. Whitehead J: Sequential designs for pharmaceutical clinical trials. Pharm Med 6:179-191, 1992
13. Moss AJ, Hall WJ, Cannom DS, Daubert JP, Higgins SL, Klein H, et al: Improved survival with an implanted defibrillator in patients with coronary disease at high risk for ventricular arrhythmia. Multicenter Automatic Defibrillator Implantation Trial Investigators. N Engl J Med 335:1933-1940, 1996
14. Food and Drug Administration: International Conference on Harmonisation; Guidance on Statistical Principles for Clinical Trials. http://www.fda.gov/cber/gdlns/ichclinical.pdf. Accessed 21/07/05
15. Ingerslev J: Efficacy and safety of recombinant factor VIIa in the prophylaxis of bleeding in various surgical procedures in hemophilic patients with factor VIII and factor IX inhibitors. Semin Thromb Hemost 26:425-432, 2000
16. Hind D, Lloyd-Jones M, Makris M, Paisley S: Recombinant Factor VIIa concentrate versus plasma derived concentrates for the treatment of acute bleeding episodes in people with Haemophilia A and inhibitors. Cochrane Database Syst Rev CD004449, 2004. http://www.mrw.interscience.wiley.com/cochrane/clsysrev/articles/CD004449/pdf_fs.html. Accessed 21/07/05
17. Odeyemi IAO, Guest JF: Modelling the economic impact of recombinant activated factor VII compared to activated prothrombin-complex concentrate in the home treatment of a mild to moderate bleed in adults with inhibitors to clotting Factors VIII and IX in the UK. J Med Econ 5:119-133, 2002
18. Putnam KG, Bohn RL, Ewenstein BM, Winkelmayer WC, Avorn J: A cost minimization model for the treatment of minor bleeding episodes in patients with haemophilia A and high-titre inhibitors. Haemophilia 11:261-269, 2005
19. Center for Biologics Evaluation and Research: Summary Basis for Approval—NovoSeven. Available at: http://www.fda.gov/cber/sba/viianov032599S.pdf. Accessed 21/07/05
20. European Medicines Agency: Scientific discussion to the European Public Assessment Report for NovoSeven. http://www.emea.eu.int/humandocs/PDFs/EPAR/Novoseven/072995en6.pdf. Accessed 22/09/05
21. Center for Biologics Evaluation and Research: Warning letter on NovoSeven claims 9 August 2004. On http://www.fda.gov/foi/warning_letters/g4906d.pdf. Accessed 21/07/05
22. Hoffman M, Monroe DM 3rd, Roberts HR: Activated factor VII activates factors IX and X on the surface of activated platelets: thoughts on the mechanism of action of high-dose activated factor VII. Blood Coagul Fibrinolysis 9:S61-S65, 1998 (suppl 1)
23. Hedner U: NovoSeven as a universal haemostatic agent. Blood Coagul Fibrinolysis 11:S107-S111, 2000 (suppl 1)
24. Lisman T, Mosnier LO, Lambert T, Mauser-Bunschoten EP, Meijers JC, Nieuwenhuis HK, et al: Inhibition of fibrinolysis by recombinant factor VIIa in plasma from patients with severe hemophilia A. Blood 99:175-179, 2002
25. Lisman T, Leebeek FW, Meijer K, Van Der Meer J, Nieuwenhuis HK, De Groot PG: Recombinant factor VIIa improves clot formation but not fibrinolytic potential in patients with cirrhosis and during liver transplantation. Hepatology 35:616-621, 2002
26. European Medicines Agency: Scientific discussion to the European Public Assessment Report for NovoSeven. http://www.fda.gov/cber/sba/viianov032599S.pdf. Accessed 21/07/05
27. Roberts HR, Monroe DM, White GC: The use of recombinant factor VIIa in the treatment of bleeding disorders. Blood 104:3858-3864, 2004
28. Hendriks HG, Meijer K, de Wolf JT, Klompmaker IJ, Porte RJ, de Kam PJ, et al: Reduced transfusion requirements by recombinant factor VIIa in orthotopic liver transplantation: a pilot study. Transplantation 71: 402-405, 2001
29. Planinsic RM, van der Meer J, Testa G, Grande L, Candela A, Porte RJ, et al: Safety and efficacy of a single bolus administration of recombinant factor VIIa in liver transplantation due to chronic liver disease. Liver Transplant 11:895-900, 2005
30. Jeffers L, Chalasani N, Balart L, Pyrsopoulos N, Erhardtsen E: Safety and efficacy of recombinant factor VIIa in patients with liver disease undergoing laparoscopic liver biopsy. Gastroenterology 123:118-126, 2002
31. Friederich PW, Henny CP, Messelink EJ, Geerdink MG, Keller T, Kurth KH, et al: Effect of recombinant activated factor VII on perioperative blood loss in patients undergoing retropubic prostatectomy: A double-blind placebo-controlled randomised trial. Lancet 361:201-205, 2003
32. Odeyemi IAO, Friedrich PW, Levi M: Economic impact of recombinant activated factor VII in the control of bleeds associated with abdominal prostatectomy. J Med Econ 7:107-115, 2004
33. Stramer SL, Glynn SA, Kleinman SH, Strong DM, Caglioti S, Wright DJ, National Heart, Lung, and Blood Institute Nucleic Acid Test Study Group, et al: Detection of HIV-1 and HCV infections among antibody-

negative blood donors by nucleic acid-amplification testing. N Engl J Med 351:760-768, 2004

34. Bijsterveld NR, Moons AH, Boekholdt SM, van Aken BE, Fennema H, Peters RJ, et al: Ability of recombinant factor VIIa to reverse the anticoagulant effect of the pentasaccharide fondaparinux in healthy volunteers. Circulation 106:2550-2554, 2002
35. Gerotziafas GT, Depasse F, Chakroun T, Samama MM, Elalamy I: Recombinant factor VIIa partially reverses the inhibitory effect of fondaparinux on thrombin generation after tissue factor activation in platelet rich plasma and whole blood. Thromb Haemost 91:531-537, 2004
36. Erhardtsen E: Ongoing NovoSeven trials. Intensive Care Med 28:S248-S255, 2002 (suppl 2)
37. Mayer SA, Brun NC, Begtrup K, Broderick J, Davis S, Diringer MN, Recombinant Activated Factor VII Intracerebral Hemorrhage Trial Investigators, et al: Recombinant activated factor VII for acute intracerebral hemorrhage. N Engl J Med 352:777-785, 2005
38. Brun NC: Personal communication, 2005
39. Brown DL, Morgenstern LB: Stopping the bleeding in intracerebral hemorrhage. N Engl J Med 352:828-830, 2005
40. Dutton RP, McCunn M, Hyder M, D'Angelo M, O'Connor J, Hess JR, et al: Factor VIIa for correction of traumatic coagulopathy. J Trauma 57: 709-718, 2004
41. Boffard KD, Riou B, Warren B, Choong PI, Rizoli S, Rossaint R, Novo-Seven Trauma Study Group, et al: Recombinant factor VIIa as adjunctive therapy for bleeding control in severely injured trauma patients: Two parallel randomized, placebo-controlled, double-blind clinical trials. J Trauma 59:8-18, 2005
42. Martinowitz U, Michaelson M, The Israeli Multidisciplinary rFVIIa Task Force: Guidelines for the use of recombinant activated factor VII (rFVIIa) in uncontrolled bleeding: A report by the Israeli Multidisciplinary rFVIIa Task Force. J Thromb Haemost 3:640-648, 2005
43. Bernstein DE, Jeffers L, Erhardtsen E, Reddy KR, Glazer S, Squiban P, et al: Recombinant FVIIa corrects prothrombin time in cirrhotic patients: A preliminary study. Gastroenterology 113:1930-1937, 1997
44. Bosch J, Thabut D, Bendtsen F, D'Amico G, Albillos A, Gonzalez Abraldes J, European Study Group on rFVIIa in UGI Haemorrhage, et al: Recombinant factor VIIa for upper gastrointestinal bleeding in patients with cirrhosis: A randomized, double-blind trial. Gastroenterology 127:1123-1130, 2004

ELSEVIER

Seminars in
HEMATOLOGY

Ultra-early Hemostatic Therapy for Acute Intracerebral Hemorrhage

Stephan A. Mayer and Fred Rincon

Intracerebral hemorrhage (ICH) is the least treatable form of stroke, and causes high mortality, severe disability, and a staggering economic burden. ICH accounts for 15% of stroke cases in the United States and Europe, and up to 30% in Asian populations. Computed tomography-based studies suggest that ICH growth within the first few hours of onset is common, and the principal cause of early neurological deterioration. Hematoma volume is also a well-established predictor of 30-day mortality. Intervention with ultra-early hemostatic therapy could minimize or prevent this early dynamic bleeding process, and might improve outcome. Recombinant activated factor VII (rFVIIa; NovoSeven®, Novo Nordisk, Bagsvaerd, Denmark) is approved for the treatment of bleeding in patients with hemophilia and inhibitors, but it may also promote hemostasis in patients with normal coagulation by acting locally at the bleeding site without activation of systemic coagulation. In a randomized, double-blind, placebo-controlled trial of 399 ICH patients treated with a single dose of 40, 80, or 160 μg/kg of rFVIIa or placebo within 4 hours of onset, subsequent hematoma growth was reduced by approximately 50% with rFVIIa. This was associated with a significant reduction (38%) in mortality, and improved functional outcomes among survivors. A phase III trial comparing 20 and 80 μg/kg rFVIIa with placebo is now in progress to confirm these results.
Semin Hematol 43(suppl 1):S70-S76

Stroke, in all its forms (ischemic, hemorrhagic, and subarachnoid hemorrhage), is the third most common cause of death in the United States[1] and the second most common cause of mortality worldwide.[2,3] Stroke leads to devastating disability, particularly among elderly individuals.[4] Loss of patient work-hours, extended hospitalization, and staggering rehabilitation and chronic-care costs make stroke a major public health problem that generates annual losses of up to $40 billion in the United States alone.[5]

Intracerebral hemorrhage (ICH) is responsible for approximately 15% of stroke cases in the United States and Europe, and for 20% to 30% of cases in Asian populations. Already notorious as the least treatable form of stroke, ICH is also associated with higher mortality and greater disability than either ischemic stroke or subarachnoid hemorrhage.[6] Data from the United States in 1997 indicated that, from an estimated 37,000 patients presenting with ICH in that year, 35% to 52% died within 1 month, 10% were living independently after 1 month, and only 20% were independent at 6 months.[7] This disturbing picture represents a prime target for therapeutic improvement.

A unique risk factor profile accompanies ICH. Hypertension, particularly if untreated, is the most important risk factor for ICH,[4,8,9] being present in around 50% to 70% of cases.[10] Conversely, risk factors for ischemic stroke, such as diabetes mellitus, coronary artery disease, and history of transient ischemic attack (TIA), appear to be less important in ICH. The elderly are especially at risk for ICH: incidence is very low among individuals under 45 years of age, but increases dramatically in those older than 65 years.[6,11] Other risk factors include low cholesterol levels, oral anticoagulants, and excessive alcohol abuse.[6,12]

Early Hematoma Growth in ICH

New insights into the pathophysiology of ICH have recently emerged and have drastically changed our understanding of this disease. What was formerly considered to be a simple and rapid bleeding event is now understood to be a dynamic and complex process that involves several distinct phases. Initially, it was thought that the bleeding associated with ICH was completed within minutes of the ictus, and that the sub-

Neurological Intensive Care Unit, Columbia-Presbyterian Medical Center, New York, NY.

Address correspondence to Stephan A Mayer, MD, Division of Critical Care Neurology, Neurological Institute, 710 W 168th St, Box 39, New York, NY 10032. E-mail: sam14@columbia.edu

 0037-1963/06/$-see front matter
doi:10.1053/j.seminhematol.2005.11.020

Table 1 Hematoma Growth (%) in Patients With ICH: Data From One Prospective and Three Retrospective Studies

	Prospective	Retrospective		
Interval From ICH Onset to CT (h)	Brott et al 1997[18] (n = 103)	Fujitsu et al 1990[16] (n = 107)	Fujii et al 1998[21] (n = 627)	Kazui et al 1996[17] (n = 204)
0–3	38	NA	18	36
3.1–6.0	NA	NA	8	16
0–6	NA	21	17	29
6.1–24.0	NA	NA	2	19

Abbreviations: CT, computed tomography; ICH, intracerebral hemorrhage; NA, not available.
Reprinted with permission. Mayer SA: Ultra-early hemostatic therapy for intracerebral hemorrhage. Stroke 34:224–229, 2003.

sequent neurological derangement observed during the first day after the bleed could be attributed to cerebral edema and mass effect around the hemorrhage.[13] However, more recent data from pathological studies, computed tomography (CT) analysis, and clinical observations suggest that early hematoma growth occurs as a result of "ultra-early re-bleeding" into congested and damaged areas around the hematoma.

In the late 1980s, several retrospective studies using CT scan analyses of small numbers of non-coagulopathic patients[14,15] first described the phenomenon of early hematoma growth. More recently, retrospective studies and a single pro spective report involving larger patient populations (N = 103 to 627) have provided further support for the occurrence of this early phenomenon.[16-19] In these studies, 18% to 30% of patients scanned within 3 hours of ICH onset had early hematoma growth, as confirmed by subsequent CT scans (Table 1). Interestingly, the highest rate of early hematoma growth was seen in the single prospective study; the investigators concluded that the true frequency of hematoma growth must have been higher than the observed rate, because clinical deterioration and immediate surgical intervention precluded the performance of follow-up scans in some individuals.[18]

Early hematoma growth has been linked to poor clinical outcomes[18-21] and higher mortality rates when compared with no growth.[17,19] Similarly, significantly greater deterioration in the Glasgow Coma Scale (GCS) and National Institutes of Health Stroke Scales (NIHSS) has been reported among patients with documented hematoma growth on 1-hour follow-up CT scans, versus those without growth.[18]

Pathophysiology of Early Hematoma Growth in ICH

Precise understanding of the pathophysiology of early hematoma growth has proved difficult to achieve, as there are no accurate animal models available to mimic the dynamic processes involved in human ICH. The notion that ultra-early re-bleeding continues at the site of a single ruptured lenticulostriate artery or arteriole has been a matter of intense debate. Evidence from studies employing histopathology, CT analysis, single-photon emission computed tomography (SPECT), and both conventional and CT angiography (CTA), suggests that secondary multifocal bleeding into the tissue at the periphery of an existing clot is more likely to occur in those cases of early hematoma enlargement than in those without. Analyses of brain tissue have indicated the presence of micro- and macroscopic bleeds in the area surrounding the fatal hemorrhage, perhaps representing ruptured arterioles or venules.[22] Other studies employing simultaneous CT and SPECT analysis have shown that, in some cases, early ICH growth relates to secondary bleeding into ischemic, congested, perilesional tissue around the periphery of the existing clot (Fig 1).[23]

The association between early hematoma growth and irregular clot morphology, which may reflect multifocal bleeding,[19,20] has been reported by several studies. In one report, the incidence of hematoma growth was greater in patients with irregularly shaped hematomas than in patients with round hematomas, and it was postulated that the irregular shape might indicate bleeding from multiple arterioles.[20] In one study involving CTA immediately after ICH, the presence of active contrast extravasation into the hematoma was associated with subsequent hematoma enlargement[24] and increased mortality[25] in 30% to 46% of patients. Finally, simultaneous bleeding from multiple lenticulostriate arteries has been demonstrated angiographically immediately after ICH.[26,27]

The evidence provided by these observations suggests that early hematoma growth results from bleeding into a congested layer of tissue that forms acutely at the periphery of the hematoma.[28] Possible contributing factors include: (1) increased local tissue pressure leading to mechanical injury; (2) reduced cerebral blood flow; (3) plasma protease induction; and (4) secondary inflammation related to clotting proteins and end-blood products. However, the relative importance of these factors in the early hours after ICH is unclear.[29-32] One theory is that a form of "congestive" ischemia, which is associated with vascular congestion and increase in local tissue pressure, occurs in the brain tissue surrounding the hematoma. This phenomenon may be similar to that seen after venous infarctions from isolated cortical vein or dural sinus thrombosis. All these mechanisms, coupled with regional mechanical and ischemic tissue damage and the possibility of a local coagulopathic environment, may worsen secondary bleeding from venules and arterioles.

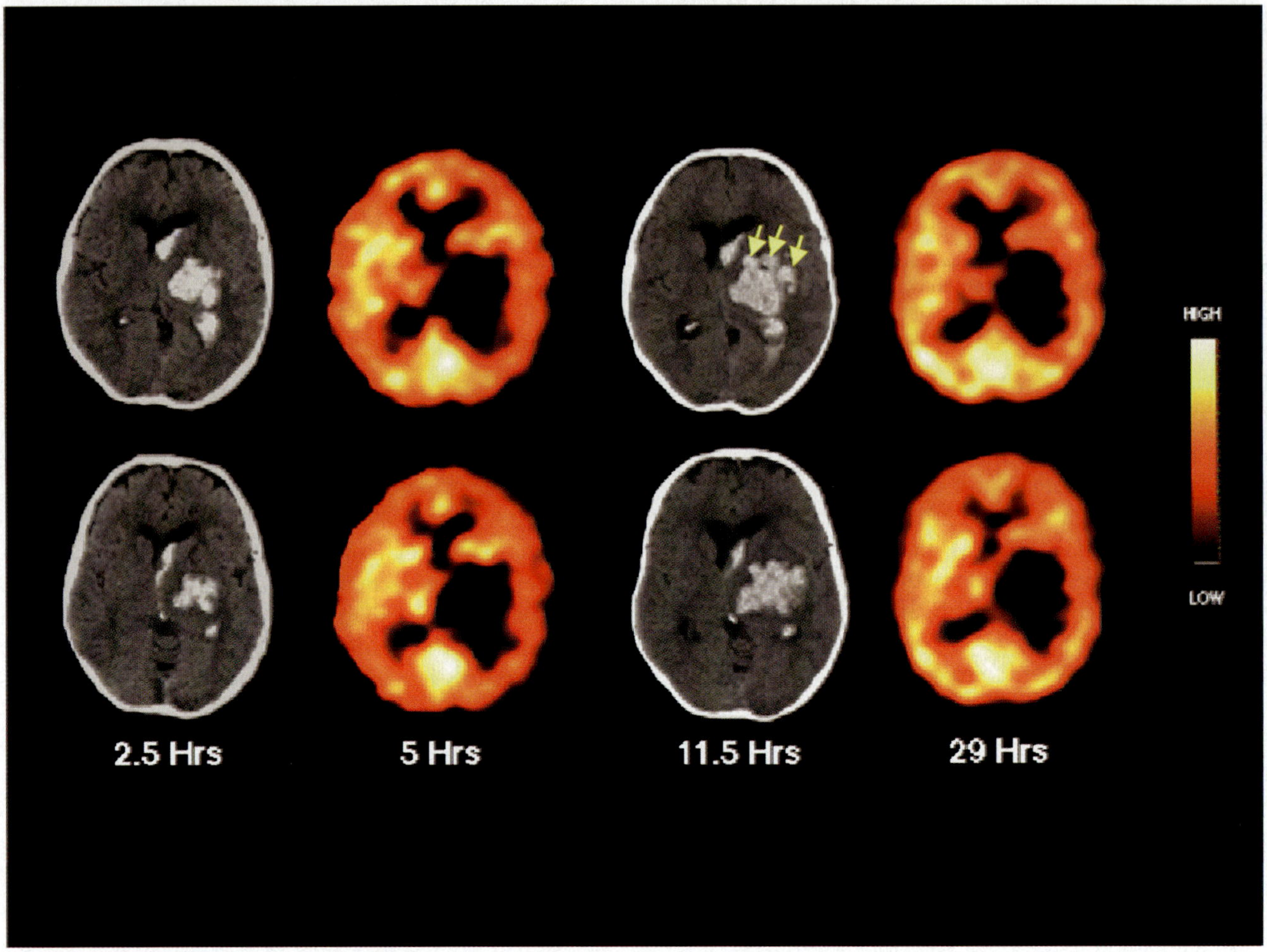

Figure 1 Early hematoma growth in a 71-year-old woman with left putaminal hemorrhage. The intracerebral hemorrhage volume increased by 80%, from 15 mL at 2.5 h to 26 mL at 11.5 hours. Concurrent single-photon emission computed tomography images indicate that the enlargement resulted from the addition of discrete hemorrhages within the no-flow zone around the existing clot (yellow arrows). Reprinted with permission.[23] Mayer SA, et al: Perilesional blood flow and edema formation in acute intracerebral hemorrhage: A SPECT study. Stroke 29:1791-1798, 1998.

Current Therapies for ICH

Recent advances in the treatment of ischemic stroke and subarachnoid hemorrhage present a stark contrast to the lack of effective, evidence-based therapies for ICH. The current management of ICH is primarily supportive (blood pressure control, intracranial pressure monitoring, fluid administration, body temperature maintenance, and prevention of seizures), and outcomes remain poor. Although a small number of randomized clinical trials of surgical or medical interventions in ICH have been published,[7] no conclusive beneficial effects have been found. Such interventions include, among others, surgical evacuation of the hematoma,[33] and the use of corticosteroids or glycerol.[34] In an American Heart Association call to perform well-designed and well-executed studies to investigate new treatments for ICH, it was hypothesized that ultra-early interventions will be critical for the effective treatment of ICH.[7]

A New Therapeutic Approach for ICH

Ultra-early Hemostatic Therapy

To be effective, hemostatic therapy must be given early after the onset of symptoms of ICH. By extrapolating prospective data from patients scanned within 3 hours of onset,[18] and by assuming that ultra-early re-bleeding occurs at something between a linear and an exponential rate during the 60 minutes after scanning, then substantial hematoma enlargement would be expected to occur in 10%, 17% or 21% of patients after a 15-, 30-, or 45-minute treatment delay, respectively, following the baseline scan—even if the intervention is completely successful (Fig 2). Underlying this principle is the fact that the only consistently identified predictor of early hematoma growth is the interval between the onset of symptoms and the performance of a CT scan: the earlier the first scan is obtained, the more likely subsequent bleeding will be de-

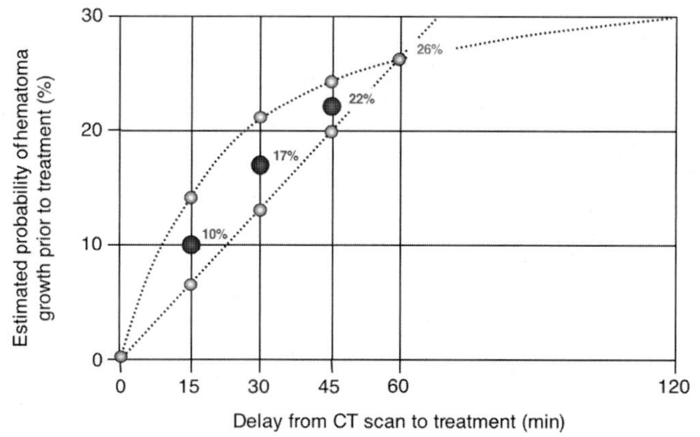

Figure 2 Estimated effect of the interval between computed tomography (CT) scan and treatment on the probability of interval hematoma expansion when the initial CT scan is performed within 3 hours of onset of intracerebral hemorrhage. Reprinted with permission. Mayer SA: Ultra-early hemostatic therapy for intracerebral hemorrhage. Stroke 34:224-229, 2003.

tected on a follow-up scan.[17,20] As a corollary, hematoma growth occurs in only 5% of patients who are initially scanned after 6 hours of symptom onset.[17,20]

Ultra-early hemostatic therapy may have the potential to halt both early and late (≥12 hours after ICH onset) neurological deterioration, which occurs as a result of perihematomal edema and mass effect. Prevention of late neurological deterioration might be crucial: in a study involving 46 patients with ICH initially scanned 13 hours after onset, approximately 33% experienced late neurological deterioration. This deterioration, which was highly associated with subsequent mortality, could be predicted by ICH volume.[35] This suggests that perilesional edema related to large, established hemorrhages is the main cause of late neurological deterioration after ICH.

However, ultra-early hemostatic therapy is, as yet, a novel approach to treating ICH. When administered alone or in conjunction with surgical or neuroprotective intervention, such ultra-early hemostatic therapy may have the potential to become the standard of care for ICH, revolutionizing the treatment of this condition in the emergency room and intensive care unit. If effective, it may become the counterpart to tissue plasminogen activator in the management of acute ischemic stroke.

Potential Agents for Ultra-early Hemostatic Therapy in ICH

Ideally, an ultra-early hemostatic medication that inhibits fibrinolysis and activates coagulation at the local level, allowing fast and effective hemostasis without systemic adverse effects, would be the preferred agent in ICH patients. Several agents may potentially be used for this purpose.

Tranexamic Acid and ϵ-Aminocaproic Acid

These synthetic lysine analogues have proven anti-fibrinolytic activity in humans,[36] and exert their effect by blocking the lysine-binding site of the plasminogen molecule and displacing plasminogen from fibrin. Tranexamic acid has a longer half-life and is sevenfold more potent than ϵ-aminocaproic acid. Both agents inhibit fibrinolysis and act as effective clot stabilizers, but they do not activate coagulation, thrombin generation, or clot formation. They are effective in treating bleeding disorders, including primary menorrhagia,[37] upper gastrointestinal bleeding,[38] and mucosal bleeding in patients with thrombocytopenia or other coagulation disorders.[39,40]

Aprotinin

Aprotinin exerts its anti-fibrinolytic effect by the inhibition of serine proteases, such as trypsin, chymotrypsin, plasmin, and kallikrein. Coagulation is inhibited by the indirect interruption of factor XII formation, which, in turn, is caused by the agent's inhibitory effects on plasma and tissue kallikrein. It has been demonstrated that aprotinin reduces blood loss during surgical procedures, including cardiac surgery[41] and orthotopic liver transplantation.[42] Aprotinin has no effect on platelet function.

Factor VIIa

Coagulation factor VII (FVII) is a naturally occurring initiator of hemostasis, and its activated form (FVIIa) triggers the extrinsic coagulation pathway. Recombinant FVIIa (rFVIIa; NovoSeven®, Novo Nordisk, Bagsvaerd, Denmark) is a genetically engineered protein produced in cultured baby hamster kidney cells, and is nearly identical to human plasma-derived FVIIa in structure and function. Recombinant FVIIa acts by binding to the surface of activated platelets, where it generates FXa and thus allows partial restoration of platelet-surface thrombin generation.[43] This agent was developed for the treatment of spontaneous and surgical bleeds in patients with hemophilia A or B and inhibitors to factors VIII or IX, respectively.[44] In 1999, a report of its successful use to control what was deemed to be a lethal hemorrhage after an abdominal gunshot wound in a young soldier with no preexisting coagulopathy prompted exploration of other uses of rFVIIa.[45] Through its action of enhancing local hemostasis after binding to exposed tissue factor, rFVIIa has recently been shown to be an effective initiator of hemostasis in patients with a normal coagulation system.[46,47] Moreover, in one study of hemophilic patients with central nervous system hemorrhages, cessation of bleeding occurred in 84% of bleeding episodes after administration of 80 to 100 μg/kg rFVIIa. Only one patient died, and there were no adverse events related to rFVIIa administration.[48]

When compared with the use of blood products, treatment with rFVIIa decreases the risk of viral transmission and has virtually no risk of transfusion reactions, fluid overload, human leukocyte antigen (HLA) antibody formation and anaphylaxis. The theoretical lack of systemic adverse effects, together with its rapid action at the site of bleeding and short half-life of 2.5 hours, suggest that rFVIIa may be an ideal agent for intervention during the high-risk stage of ICH. Hence, a recent randomized, placebo-controlled, dose-rang-

Table 2 ICH Volumes From the rFVIIa ICH Trial[49]

ICH Volume	Placebo (N = 96)	rFVIIa 40 μg/kg (N = 108)	rFVIIa 80 μg/kg (N = 92)	rFVIIa 160 μg/kg (N = 103)	rFVIIa Combined (N = 303)
At baseline (mL)	24 ± 22	22 ± 22	23 ± 24	26 ± 30	24 ± 26
At 24 hours (mL)	32 ± 29	26 ± 29	28 ± 31	28 ± 32	27 ± 30
Estimated mean relative increase from baseline, % (98.3% CI)	29 (16–44)	16 (4–28)	14 (2–27)	11 (0–23)	14 (7–21)
P value, *v* placebo	—	.07	.05	.02*	.01*
Estimated mean absolute increase from baseline, mL (98.3% CI)	8.7 (4.9–12.4)	5.4 (1.7–9.0)	4.2 (0.3–8.0)	2.9 (−0.8–6.6)	4.2 (2.0–6.3)
P value, *v* placebo	—	.13	.04	.008*	.01*

NOTE. Values are means ± SD. For estimated mean differences, 98.3% CIs are derived from a generalized linear mixed model with the patient and the reader as random effects and baseline ICH volume, time from onset to CT, and time from CT to treatment as fixed effects.

Abbreviations: CI, confidence interval; ICH, intracerebral hemorrhage; rFVIIa, recombinant activated factor VII.

Reprinted with permission [49]. Mayer SA, et al: Recombinant activated factor VII for acute intracerebral hemorrhage. N Engl J Med 352:777–785, 2005. Adapted with permission, 2005.

*The comparison was statistically significant according to the prespecified Bonferroni-corrected threshold of $P = 0.0167$.

ing study was conducted to assess the use of rFVIIa in non-coagulopathic patients with ICH.[49] A summary of this study, and of the significance of the observed outcomes, is presented below.

The rFVIIa ICH Trial

This international, multicenter, randomized, double-blind, placebo-controlled, parallel-group, dose-ranging study sought to determine the ability of rFVIIa to limit ongoing bleeding, reduce hematoma growth, and improve outcomes in patients with ICH.

Methods. Three randomly assigned, single doses of rFVIIa (40, 80, and 160 μg/kg), administered intravenously over 1-2 minutes, were compared with placebo. Patients with spontaneous ICH diagnosed by CT scan within 3 hours of symptom onset were enrolled. Their allocated treatment was then administered within one hour of the baseline CT scan. The primary outcome measure was the mean percentage change in ICH volume between baseline and 24 hours, as determined by CT scan. Additionally, clinical outcomes at 3 months were determined using the following assessment instruments: the modified Rankin Scale (mRS), the Barthel Index, the Extended GCS, and the NIHSS. The main safety outcome measure was the frequency of thromboembolic serious adverse events (SAEs) at 90 days.

Results. In total, 399 patients (61% male, mean age 66 years, mostly Caucasian) were randomized to one of the treatment arms: placebo (N = 96) or rFVIIa 40 μg/kg (N = 108), 80 μg/kg (N = 92), or 160 μg/kg (N = 103). The ICH volume at baseline (mean, 24 mL; range, 0.4 to 153 mL) was similar in each treatment group (Table 2). The mean interval from symptom onset to baseline CT scan was 114 ± 35 minutes; the mean interval from CT scan to treatment was 54 ± 21 minutes, and mean onset-to-needle time was 167 ± 32 minutes.

The mean percentage increase in ICH volume was 29% following placebo treatment, versus 16%, 14%, and 11% in the rFVIIa 40, 80, and 160 μg/kg groups, respectively (combined treatment effect, $P = .01$) (Table 2). The difference between the rFVIIa 160 μg/kg dose group and placebo was statistically significant ($P = .02$). A similar pattern emerged for the absolute mean change in ICH volume from baseline to 24 hours, which was significantly reduced with rFVIIa treatment versus placebo ($P = .01$) (Table 2). Mean absolute growth in ICH volume was reduced by 3.3, 4.5, and 5.8 mL with rFVIIa 40 μg/kg ($P = .13$), rFVIIa 80 μg/kg ($P = .04$), and rFVIIa 160 μg/kg ($P = .008$), respectively, when compared with placebo. When administered within 3 hours of symptom onset, the hemostatic effect of rFVIIa treatment was more pronounced. In this subgroup of patients (N = 269), the mean percentage increase in ICH volume was 34% in the placebo group versus 13% in rFVIIa-treated patients ($P = .004$), and the absolute increase in ICH volume was 10.7 versus 4.4 mL, respectively ($P = .009$).

Mortality at 3 months was 29% in the placebo group, versus 18% in all rFVIIa treatment groups combined. Furthermore, all 4 global outcome scale assessments at 3 months showed more favorable outcomes following intervention with rFVIIa than with placebo. For 90-day mRS and NIHSS outcome assessments, all dose levels of rFVIIa provided significantly better measurements than placebo. Similarly, for the Barthel Index, comparisons were significantly in favor of rFVIIa 80 and 160 μg/kg, versus placebo. These results indicate that treatment with rFVIIa more than doubled patients' odds of improving by one level on the mRS, and decreased the proportion of patients who died or became disabled from 69% in the placebo group to 53% with rFVIIa treatment.

Thromboembolic SAEs occurred in 2% of patients receiving placebo versus 6%, 4%, and 10% of patients receiving rFVIIa 40, 80, and 160 μg/kg, respectively ($P = .12$). The frequencies of arterial thromboembolic SAEs in the treatment groups were 6%, 2%, and 8% in the rFVIIa 40, 80, and 160 μg/kg groups, respectively, versus 0% in the placebo group (overall $P = .01$). These SAEs included seven myocardial ischemic events and nine cases of cerebral infarction that occurred within 3 days of dosing. However, fatal or disabling thromboembolic SAEs that were considered possibly or probably related to treatment occurred in 2% of patients receiving placebo and in 2% of rFVIIa-treated patients.

Summary. When administered within 4 hours of ICH onset, rFVIIa significantly reduced subsequent hemorrhage growth and improved patients' clinical outcome, despite a non-significant increase in the frequency of thromboembolic SAEs. A reduction in ICH volume of approximately 5 mL was evident 24 hours after rFVIIa administration; this translated to a reduction of 11 mL in total lesion volume at 72 hours, and an absolute reduction of 16% in the risk of death or severe disability at 3 months when compared with placebo, as assessed by the mRS. A dose-response effect was evident for reduction of hemorrhage growth; the smallest effect occurred with rFVIIa 40 μg/kg and the most substantial effect with 160 μg/kg. Overall, mortality was reduced by 38% with rFVIIa treatment. Timing of administration appears to be critical, as treatment within 3 hours of symptom onset provided the best outcomes. These results are supportive of ultra-early hemostatic therapy with rFVIIa; they are also consistent with the view that active bleeding occurs in a large proportion of patients within the first few hours of ICH onset, before rapidly diminishing. However, additional research is needed to help identify those patients at risk for thromboembolic complications, to define the optimal dose and therapeutic window, and to assess the role of rFVIIa for the coagulopathic patient with ICH.[50]

Conclusion

Based on the lack of effective treatments and the significant morbidity and mortality generated by ICH, new therapies for this disease are desperately needed. The results of the prospective, randomized, controlled phase IIB trial of rFVIIa in ICH are encouraging, and further support the concept of ultra-early hemostatic therapy as a feasible biological therapeutic intervention to limit ongoing bleeding and early hematoma growth. A phase III trial (the FAST Trial) of 675 ICH patients, comparing doses of 20 and 80 μg/kg rFVIIa with placebo, is currently underway. The main outcome measure of this trial is the proportion of patients classified as dead or severely disabled at 90 days on the mRS. If the results of the phase IIB trial are confirmed, the FAST trial might help to establish the first effective emergency intervention for ICH.

References

1. National Vital Statistics Report 2002. Available at: http://www.cdc.gov/nchs/data/nvsr/nvsr53/nvsr53_05acc.pdf2002
2. Barnett HJ, Eliasziw M, Meldrum HE: Evidence based cardiology: Prevention of ischaemic stroke. BMJ 318:1539-1543, 1999
3. Gorelick PB, Sacco RL, Smith DB, Alberts M, Mustone-Alexander L, Rader D, et al: Prevention of a first stroke: A review of guidelines and a multidisciplinary consensus statement from the National Stroke Association. JAMA 281:1112-1120, 1999
4. Foulkes MA, Wolf PA, Price TR, Mohr JP, Hier DB: The Stroke Data Bank: Design, methods, and baseline characteristics. Stroke 19:547-554, 1988
5. Meister J, Levy D: Stroke: A case review. Clin Excell Nurse Pract 4:212-215, 2000
6. Sacco RL, Mayer SA: Epidemiology of intracerebral hemorrhage, in Feldmann E (ed): Intracerebral Hemorrhage. Armonk, NY, Futura, 1994, pp 3-23
7. Broderick JP, Adams HP Jr, Barsan W, Feinberg W, Feldmann E, Grotta J: Guidelines for the management of spontaneous intracerebral hemorrhage: A statement for healthcare professionals from a special writing group of the Stroke Council, American Heart Association. Stroke 30: 905-915, 1999
8. Weisberg LA, Stazio A, Shamsnia M, Elliott D: Nontraumatic parenchymal brain hemorrhages. Medicine (Baltimore) 69:277-295, 1990
9. Broderick J, Brott T, Tomsick T, Huster G: Importance of hypertension in lobar hemorrhages. Neurology 42:181, 1992 (abstr)
10. Wityk RJ, Caplan LR: Hypertensive intracerebral hemorrhage. Epidemiology and clinical pathology. Neurosurg Clin N Am 3:521-532, 1992
11. Bonita R: Epidemiology of stroke. Lancet 339:342-344, 1992
12. Segal AZ, Chiu RI, Eggleston-Sexton PM, Beiser A, Greenberg SM: Low cholesterol as a risk factor for primary intracerebral hemorrhage: A case-control study. Neuroepidemiology 18:185-193, 1999
13. Kase C, Mohr JP: General features of intracerebral hemorrhage, in Barnett H, Stein B, Mohr JP (eds): Stroke: Pathophysiology, Diagnosis and Management. New York, NY, Churchill Livingstone, 1986, pp 497-523
14. Chen ST, Chen SD, Hsu CY, Hogan EL: Progression of hypertensive intracerebral hemorrhage. Neurology 39:1509-1514, 1989
15. Broderick JP, Brott TG, Tomsick T, Barsan W, Spilker J: Ultra-early evaluation of intracerebral hemorrhage. J Neurosurg 72:195-199, 1990
16. Fujitsu K, Muramoto M, Ikeda Y, Inada Y, Kim I, Kuwabara T: Indications for surgical treatment of putaminal hemorrhage. Comparative study based on serial CT and time-course analysis. J Neurosurg 73:518-525, 1990
17. Kazui S, Naritomi H, Yamamoto H, Sawada T, Yamaguchi T: Enlargement of spontaneous intracerebral hemorrhage. Incidence and time course. Stroke 27:1783-1787, 1996
18. Brott T, Broderick J, Kothari R, Barsan W, Tomsick T, Sauerbeck L, et al: Early hemorrhage growth in patients with intracerebral hemorrhage. Stroke 28:1-5, 1997
19. Cheung RT: Predictors of hematoma growth? Stroke 29:2442-2443, 1998
20. Fujii Y, Tanaka R, Takeuchi S, Koike T, Minakawa T, Sasaki O, et al: Hematoma enlargement in spontaneous intracerebral hemorrhage. J Neurosurg 80:51-57, 1994
21. Fujii Y, Takeuchi S, Sasaki O, Minakawa T, Tanaka R: Multivariate analysis of predictors of hematoma enlargement in spontaneous intracerebral hemorrhage. Stroke 29:1160-1166, 1998
22. Fisher CM: Pathological observations in hypertensive cerebral hemorrhage. J Neuropathol Exp Neurol 30:536-550, 1971
23. Mayer SA, Lignelli A, Fink ME, Kessler DB, Thomas CE, Swarup R, et al: Perilesional blood flow and edema formation in acute intracerebral hemorrhage: A SPECT study. Stroke 29:1791-1798, 1998
24. Murai Y, Takagi R, Ikeda Y, Yamamoto Y, Teramoto A. Three-dimensional computerized tomography angiography in patients with hyperacute intracerebral hemorrhage. J Neurosurg 91:424-431, 1999
25. Becker KJ, Baxter AB, Bybee HM, Tirschwell DL, Abouelsaad T, Cohen WA: Extravasation of radiographic contrast is an independent predictor of death in primary intracerebral hemorrhage. Stroke 30:2025-2032, 1999
26. Mizukami M, Araki G, Mihara H, Tomita T, Fujinaga R: Arteriographically visualized extravasation in hypertensive intracerebral hemorrhage. Report of seven cases. Stroke 3:527-37, 1972
27. Komiyama M, Yasui T, Tamura K, Nagata Y, Fu Y, Yagura H: Simultaneous bleeding from multiple lenticulostriate arteries in hypertensive intracerebral haemorrhage. Neuroradiology 37:129-30, 1995
28. Takasugi S, Ueda S, Matsumoto K: Chronological changes in spontaneous intracerebral hematoma—An experimental and clinical study. Stroke 16:651-658, 1985
29. Yang GY, Betz AL, Chenevert TL, Brunberg JA, Hoff JT: Experimental intracerebral hemorrhage: relationship between brain edema, blood flow, and blood-brain barrier permeability in rats. J Neurosurg 81:93-102, 1994

30. Wagner KR, Xi G, Hua Y, Kleinholz M, de Courten-Myers GM, Myers RE, et al: Lobar intracerebral hemorrhage model in pigs: Rapid edema development in perihematomal white matter. Stroke 27:490-497, 1996
31. Lee KR, Colon GP, Betz AL, Keep RF, Kim S, Hoff JT: Edema from intracerebral hemorrhage: the role of thrombin. J Neurosurg 84:91-96, 1996
32. Rosenberg GA, Navratil M: Metalloproteinase inhibition blocks edema in intracerebral hemorrhage in the rat. Neurology 48:921-926, 1997
33. Hankey GJ, Hon C: Surgery for primary intracerebral hemorrhage: Is it safe and effective? A systematic review of case series and randomized trials. Stroke 28:2126-2132, 1997
34. Yu YL, Kumana CR, Lauder IJ, Cheung YK, Chan FL, Kou M, et al: Treatment of acute cerebral hemorrhage with intravenous glycerol. A double-blind, placebo-controlled, randomized trial. Stroke 23:967-971, 1992
35. Mayer SA, Sacco RL, Shi T, Mohr JP: Neurologic deterioration in non-comatose patients with supratentorial intracerebral hemorrhage. Neurology 44:1379-1384, 1994
36. Mannucci PM: Hemostatic drugs. N Engl J Med 339:245-253, 1998
37. Bonnar J, Sheppard BL: Treatment of menorrhagia during menstruation: Randomised controlled trial of ethamsylate, mefenamic acid, and tranexamic acid. BMJ 313:579-582, 1996
38. Henry DA, O'Connell DL: Effects of fibrinolytic inhibitors on mortality from upper gastrointestinal haemorrhage. BMJ 298:1142-1146, 1989
39. Walsh PN, Rizza CR, Matthews JM, Eipe J, Kernoff PB, Coles MD, et al: Epsilon-Aminocaproic acid therapy for dental extractions in haemophilia and Christmas disease: A double blind controlled trial. Br J Haematol 20:463-475, 1971
40. Forbes CD, Barr RD, Reid G, Thomson C, Prentice CR, McNicol GP, et al: Tranexamic acid in control of haemorrhage after dental extraction in haemophilia and Christmas disease. BMJ 2:311-313, 1972
41. Royston D, Bidstrup BP, Taylor KM, Sapsford RN: Effect of aprotinin on need for blood transfusion after repeat open-heart surgery. Lancet 2:1289-1291, 1987
42. Neuhaus P, Bechstein WO, Lefebre B, Blumhardt G, Slama K: Effect of aprotinin on intraoperative bleeding and fibrinolysis in liver transplantation. Lancet 2:924-925, 1989
43. Monroe DM, Hoffman M, Oliver JA, Roberts HR: Platelet activity of high-dose factor VIIa is independent of tissue factor. Br J Haematol 99:542-547, 1997
44. Key NS, Aledort LM, Beardsley D, Cooper HA, Davignon G, Ewenstein BM, et al: Home treatment of mild to moderate bleeding episodes using recombinant factor VIIa (Novoseven) in haemophiliacs with inhibitors. Thromb Haemost 80:912-918, 1998
45. Kenet G, Walden R, Eldad A, Martinowitz U: Treatment of traumatic bleeding with recombinant factor VIIa. Lancet 354:1879, 1999
46. Hedner U: Recombinant activated factor VII as a universal haemostatic agent. Blood Coagul Fibrinolysis 9:S147-S152, 1998 (suppl 1)
47. Hedner U, Ingerslev J: Clinical use of recombinant FVIIa (rFVIIa). Transfus Sci 19:163-176, 1998
48. Rice KM, Savidge GF: NovoSeven (recombinant factor VIIa) in central nervous systems bleeds. Haemostasis 26:131-134, 1996 (suppl 1)
49. Mayer SA, Brun NC, Begtrup K, Broderick J, Davis S, Diringer MN, et al: Recombinant activated factor VII for acute intracerebral hemorrhage. N Engl J Med 352:777-785, 2005
50. Fewel ME, Park P: The emerging role of recombinant activated factor VII in neurocritical care. Neurocrit Care 1:19-30, 2004

ELSEVIER

Seminars in
HEMATOLOGY

New Anti-thrombotic Agents: Emphasis on Hemorrhagic Complications and Their Management

Heng Joo Ng[a] and Mark A. Crowther[b]

Our advanced knowledge of coagulation has led to the synthesis of novel procoagulant substances, such as recombinant activated factor VII (rFVIIa; NovoSeven®, Novo Nordisk, Bagsvaerd, Denmark). Similarly, in-depth understanding of the interaction between anticoagulant proteins and their natural inhibitors has led to the synthesis of various novel anticoagulants. Novel anticoagulants are characterized by highly specific coagulation-inhibiting activities and, frequently, a complete lack of effective antidotes. This lack of antidotes is particularly important in the case of novel inhibitors with extended half-lives; for example, idraparinux may produce effective anticoagulation for as long as one week after subcutaneous administration. As novel anticoagulants complete licensing evaluations and are used in clinical practice, the likelihood of anticoagulant-associated hemorrhage will increase. This will require physicians to have an understanding of the mechanism of action of these anticoagulants, and to have an advanced degree of knowledge of the potential specific and nonspecific inhibitors of these anticoagulant agents. This paper will briefly review the biochemistry of coagulation, focusing on the complexes inhibited by currently available and novel anticoagulants. Specific and nonspecific prohemostatic agents will be reviewed and discussed. The ability of nonspecific procoagulant agents (particularly rFVIIa) to reverse the effects of novel anticoagulants will also be reviewed.
Semin Hematol 43(suppl 1):S77-S83

Vascular occlusion as a result of pathological thrombus formation and embolization remains a leading cause of both mortality and morbidity. Occlusion of blood flow causes structural damage to the involved blood vessels, ischemia and infarcts of downstream tissues, and impairment of pulmonary gaseous exchange. Anticoagulation is effective in reducing the risk of venous and some forms of arterial thromboembolism, and is the mainstay of primary and secondary prevention strategies.[1-4] For the past 60 years, the heparins and warfarin have been the principal anticoagulants in day-to-day clinical use. These agents are inexpensive, widely available, easily monitored and very effective.[5,6] However, these agents are difficult to use due to their narrow therapeutic windows and extensive interactions with other drugs and dietary components. As a result, these agents need frequent monitoring and dose adjustment. Furthermore, all anticoagulants carry a significant risk of bleeding. These limitations have fuelled the development of newer anticoagulants in an effort to produce treatments that are safer or more effective.[7]

[a]Department of Haematology, Singapore General Hospital, Singapore.
[b]St Joseph's Hospital, Hamilton, Ontario, Canada.
Address correspondence to Mark A. Crowther, Room L208 St Joseph's Hospital, 50 Charlton Ave E, Hamilton, Ontario, Canada L8N 4A6. E-mail: crowthrm@mcmaster.ca

New Anticoagulants: Concepts and Classification

Our understanding of the coagulation cascade has advanced greatly in the last 25 years, resulting in a clear understanding of the molecular mechanism of thrombosis. This understanding has led to the refinement of older anticoagulants, such as the development of low-molecular-weight heparins (LMWH) from unfractionated heparins. It has also fostered the development of potent new anticoagulants that are designed to inhibit specific components of the coagulation cascade.[7,8]

Anticoagulants that are currently in use, or in advanced phases of development, can be broadly classified as outlined in Table 1. Newer anticoagulants are designed to specifically inhibit the following targets: (1) the activated factor VII (FVIIa)/tissue factor (TF) pathway; (2) activated factors IX (FIXa) and X (FXa); (3) activated factors V (FVa) and VIII (FVIIIa); and (4) thrombin. Since they inhibit coagulation, bleeding is an inevitable consequence of these new anticoagulants, regardless of their mode of action. Bleeding may occur either within the usual therapeutic window or as a result of overdosing. Although these agents are all associated with a theoretical risk of bleeding, the actual risk cannot be

0037-1963/06/$-see front matter
doi:10.1053/j.seminhematol.2005.11.023

Table 1 Classification of Parenteral and Oral Anticoagulation by Mode of Action

Parenteral
Antithrombin-dependent
• Heparin, low-molecular-weight heparin
• Fondaparinux, Idraparinux
Other cofactor-dependent
• Danaparoid
Antithrombin-independent
• Hirudin/argatroban/melagatran
• Other low-molecular-weight inhibitors
• IIb/IIIa inhibitors
Oral
Vitamin K antagonists
Other
• Ximelagatran and others
• Other low-molecular-weight inhibitors

accurately defined until post-marketing surveillance and experience with exposure of many patients becomes available. Interestingly, while the bleeding risks of heparin and warfarin use are widely known, effective antidotes that reverse their anticoagulant effects during bleeding episodes are available. Thus, the considerable mortality and morbidity associated with bleeding can be successfully reduced. Most new agents do not have antidotes; thus, their reversal strategies remain ill-defined and largely untested.[9]

This paper will discuss the mechanism of action and utility of these new anticoagulants, with an emphasis on their bleeding risks and currently available strategies for their reversal.

Inhibitors of the FVIIa/TF Pathway

Tissue factor pathway inhibitor (TFPI) and nematode anticoagulant peptide (NAPc2) are two novel, potent anticoagulants with a highly specific mechanism of action against the FVIIa/TF pathway (Fig 1).

TFPI and Tifacogin

TFPI is a naturally occurring inhibitor of the FVIIa/TF complex, and therefore prevents the initiation of coagulation. In experimental animal models of sepsis, TFPI attenuates coagulopathy and improves survival. Based on these observations, recombinant TFPI (tifacogin) has been compared with placebo in phase II[10] and phase III[11] studies in patients with severe sepsis. In the latter study, tifacogin did not prolong survival when compared with placebo. Its activity as an in vivo anticoagulant was, however, confirmed by the observation that patients who received tifacogin had more bleeding than those who received placebo (6.5% *v* 4.8%, respectively). Reversal strategies for bleeding have not been defined, but tifacogin has a short half-life once infusion is discontinued.

NAPc2 and rNAPc2

Originally isolated from the canine hookworm, *Ancylostoma caninum*,[12] NAPc2 is now available in its recombinant form, rNAPc2. It prevents the initiation of coagulation by binding to FX and FXa, and then inhibiting FVIIa within the FVIIa/TF complex.[13] There is minimal prolongation of prothrombin time (PT) and it has no effect on activated partial thromboplastin time (aPTT) at therapeutic plasma levels.[14] Recombinant NAPc2 has a half-life of 50 hours after subcutaneous injections. Its prophylactic use in orthopedic surgery and cardiac interventions has been studied: a dose of 3 μg/kg given 1 hour after surgery, and every second day thereafter for four doses, was effective for the prevention of deep vein thrombosis (DVT) in patients undergoing knee arthroplasty. Doses beyond 7.5 μg/kg were associated with a high rate of bleeding in patients undergoing elective coronary angioplasty.[15]

There is currently no antidote for rNAPc2. This has raised concerns about the management of bleeding complications, in view of its long half-life. In addition to supportive measures, recombinant activated factor VII (rFVIIa; NovoSeven®, Novo Nordisk, Bagsvaerd, Denmark) may be effective in reversing its anticoagulant activity. Recombinant FVIIa induces a transient procoagulant state and has been shown in healthy volunteers to reverse the biochemical effects of rNAPc2.[16] However, its use to treat bleeding associated with this anticoagulant agent has not been reported.

Inhibitors of FXa

Available inhibitors of FXa act indirectly by catalyzing the activity of antithrombin, which inhibits FXa. Unfractionated heparin and LMWH are both nonspecific inhibitors of FXa, with significant inhibitory activity against thrombin and other activated clotting factors. Newer anticoagulants in this class, such as fondaparinux and idraparinux, are synthetic and act specifically against FXa. Direct inhibitors of FXa, which bind directly to the active site of FXa, are currently undergoing clinical evaluation.

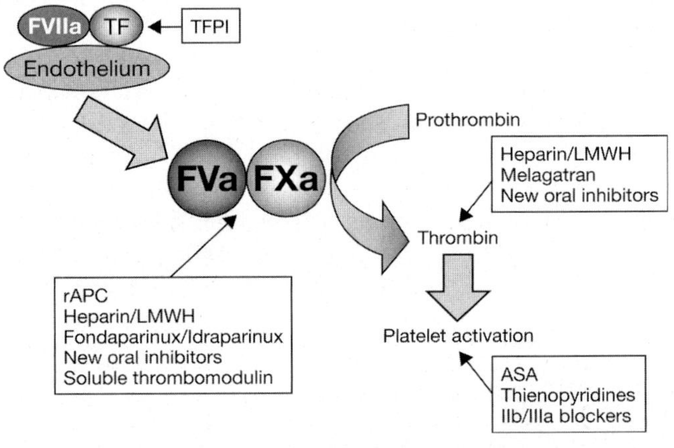

Figure 1 Schematic diagram demonstrating the sites of actions of various anticoagulants. ASA, aspirin; LMWH, low-molecular-weight heparin; rAPC, recombinant activated protein C; TF, tissue factor; TFPI, tissue factor pathway inhibitor; FVIIa, activated factor VII; FVa, activated factor V; FXa, activated factor X.

Fondaparinux

Fondaparinux is a synthetic analog of the antithrombin-binding domains of heparin and LMWH, which exist as a pentasaccharide sequence. It binds to antithrombin and enhances its activity against FXa, but not that against thrombin.[17] Administered subcutaneously, it has a half-life of 17 hours, which allows for once-daily dosing. Fondaparinux has been approved in some countries for use as thromboprophylaxis in high-risk orthopedic surgery and for the treatment of both acute DVT and acute pulmonary embolism (PE). In comparison with standard forms of prophylaxis in patients undergoing hip or knee arthroplasty, four large trials have demonstrated the superior efficacy of fondaparinux.[18] It has also been found to be at least as effective and safe as LMWH and unfractionated heparin for the initial treatment of venous thromboembolism (VTE).[19,20]

Currently, there are no specific antidotes available for fondaparinux. Protamine does not reverse the effects of this agent. If uncontrolled bleeding does occur, rFVIIa may be considered as a potential reversing agent. In vitro studies have shown that rFVIIa accelerates thrombin generation in the presence of inhibitory concentrations of fondaparinux, but does not completely reverse its inhibitory effects.[21] In healthy volunteers given fondaparinux, rFVIIa has been shown to reverse its effects (as measured by coagulation tests)[22] and normalize coagulation times and thrombin generation.[23] Another potential reversal agent is heparinase I, which has been shown to degrade and inactivate fondaparinux in vitro.[24] It is important to note that fondaparinux bio-accumulates in patients with renal insufficiency.

Idraparinux

This is a chemically modified variant of fondaparinux that binds antithrombin with very high affinity, producing a complex that has a half-life similar to that of antithrombin.[25] It is currently in late-phase clinical trials that are examining its use in the treatment of acute VTE, with promising results. Its exceptionally long half-life means that idraparinux produces therapeutic anticoagulation for about a week after its administration, allowing weekly dosing. This has raised concerns about its reversal in the event of unwanted anticoagulant effect or excessive bleeding. In a study of healthy volunteers, rFVIIa administered at 3 hours and 7 days after idraparinux was found to normalize coagulation parameters, suggesting that it may produce a transient reversal of the anticoagulant effect.[26] In contrast to its efficacy as an antidote against fondaparinux, heparinase I does not neutralize idraparinux activity.[24] Protamine does not reverse the effects of idraparinux.

DX-9065a, Razaxaban, and Other Direct FXa Inhibitors

Unlike indirect FXa inhibitors, direct inhibitors not only inhibit free FXa but also inactivate FXa bound to platelets within the prothrombinase complex.

DX-9065a is one such direct, selective, reversible, small-molecule FXa inhibitor.[27] Initial experience with this drug given as continuous infusion for percutaneous angiograms and acute coronary syndromes suggests very low bleeding rates.[28,29] Reversal strategies have not been defined.

Another agent is razaxaban, a small-molecule, orally administered, direct FXa inhibitor with demonstrated efficacy as thromboprophylaxis in orthopedic surgery when compared with enoxaparin.[30] At the lowest effective dose tested, it has low rates of bleeding similar to those observed with enoxaparin, but has no known antidote. Other oral direct FXa inhibitors are also currently in development.

Inhibitors of FVa and FVIIIa

Activated Protein C

Activated protein C (APC) modulates thrombin generation and propagation of coagulation by inactivating FVa and FVIIIa.[31] Drotrecogin alfa, its recombinant form (rAPC), was compared with placebo in a phase III study involving 1,690 patients with severe sepsis, and was found to reduce mortality by 6% at 28 days.[32] In this study, rAPC increased the risk of major bleeding from 2% to 3.5%. It is currently licensed for use in patients with severe sepsis. The short half-life of rAPC after discontinuation of infusion precludes the need for any specific reversal strategies, and it has no known antidote. When considering the use of this product, nuisance or minor bleeding (such as bleeding from arterial puncture sites and in nasogastric drainage) should not be a contraindication for its use in qualifying patients.

Soluble Thrombomodulin

Soluble thrombomodulin, a recombinant analog of thrombomodulin, exerts its anticoagulant effect by binding to thrombin and converting it into a potent activator of protein C. APC inhibits coagulation by proteolytically inactivating FVa and FVIIIa.[33] Soluble thrombomodulin has a half-life of 2 to 3 days after subcutaneous injections, and has been evaluated in a phase II study of patients undergoing hip surgery.[34] Major bleeding occurred in 1.4% and 6.3% of patients receiving the low or high dose of thrombomodulin, respectively. There is currently no known antidote for this agent.

Inhibitors of Thrombin

Thrombin is the target of many established and novel anticoagulants. Heparin and its derivatives are indirect thrombin inhibitors requiring antithrombin for their anticoagulant effect. Danaparoid inhibits thrombin by catalyzing the activity not only of thrombin, but also of chondroitin sulfate and dermatan sulfate. Direct thrombin inhibitors, on the other hand, bind directly to thrombin and block its interaction with substrates.

Hirudin and Lepirudin

Hirudin and its variants are direct thrombin inhibitors originally isolated from the medicinal leech, *Hirudo medicinalis*. Hirudins are currently manufactured using recombinant technology. Lepirudin (the most commonly available variant) has a half-life of 60 minutes when given in the intravenous form and 120 minutes after subcutaneous injection.[8] It is monitored using the aPTT or ecarin clotting time (ECT). Hirudin and its derivatives have been evaluated for acute coronary syndromes and the treatment and prevention of VTE, but it is currently indicated only for the treatment of patients with suspected heparin-induced thrombocytopenia.[35,36] Rapid renal clearance accounts for its short half-life, which precludes the need for urgent reversal in patients with normal renal function; in patients with impaired renal function, hirudin (and its derivatives) may bio-accumulate.[37,38] There is no known antidote for the anticoagulant effect of lepirudin. Dialysis with selected membranes may, however, be effective in removing this agent. There is limited experience with the use of rFVIIa in the treatment of hirudin-associated bleeding, although experimental models suggest that it might be partially effective in controlling bleeding associated with high hirudin levels.[39]

Bivalirudin

Bivalirudin, an analog of hirudin, is also a direct thrombin inhibitor, but has a shorter half-life of 25 minutes. It is rapidly cleared via a combination of renal and proteolytic mechanisms.[40] Bivalirudin is an alternative to heparin in patients undergoing percutaneous coronary angioplasty[41] and has been studied as an adjunct to thrombolytic therapy.[42] It has also been used as an alternative to heparin in patients with heparin-induced thrombocytopenia undergoing cardiopulmonary bypass surgery.[43] Its short half-life means that reversal strategies are likely to be unnecessary.

Argatroban

Argatroban is a competitive inhibitor of thrombin with a half-life of 45 minutes, licensed for the treatment of heparin-induced thrombocytopenia.[44] As it is metabolized in the liver, it will bio-accumulate if administered at standard doses to patients with impaired hepatic function.[8] There is currently no known antidote for argatroban. Preliminary studies on whole blood suggest that rFVIIa may reverse at least some of its anticoagulant effect; however, as is the case with other novel anticoagulants, rFVIIa has not been used to reverse the effects of argatroban in the clinical setting.

Ximelagatran and Melagatran

Ximelagatran is a prodrug of melagatran and the first orally available direct thrombin inhibitor.[45] It is well absorbed from the gastrointestinal tract and is rapidly converted to melagatran. It provides a predictable anticoagulant effect with no interactions with food or other drugs, and has a half-life of 4 to 5 hours. Monitoring is not required, but dose adjustment is advised in patients with renal impairment.[45] The agent has been evaluated for initial and long-term treatment of VTE,[46,47] thromboprophylaxis in high-risk orthopedic patients,[48-51] and prevention of embolic events in nonvalvular atrial fibrillation.[52,53]

There is currently no antidote for ximelagatran. In studies of healthy volunteers, rFVIIa did not reverse the anticoagulant effect of high doses of melagatran.[54] However, the short half-life of ximelagatran makes reversal unnecessary in most instances. This drug has not been commercially approved in North America but is licensed as Exanta (AstraZeneca, Macclesfield, UK) in selected jurisdictions for orthopedic prophylaxis.

Dabigatran

This orally active direct thrombin inhibitor is in the early phases of development. Administered as its prodrug, dabigatran etixilate,[55] it has a half-life of 12 hours with mainly renal elimination. It is being evaluated in early phase studies for the prevention and treatment of VTE and atrial fibrillation.

General Management of Anticoagulant-Associated Bleeding

The primary complication of anticoagulant therapy is bleeding, which can cause both morbidity and mortality. For example, in a recent meta-analysis of 33 studies involving 4,374 patient-years of oral anticoagulant therapy, the case-fatality rate of major bleeding was 13.4% (95% confidence interval [CI], 9.4% to 17.4%) and the rate of intracranial bleeding was 1.15 per 100 patient-years (CI, 1.14 to 1.16 per 100 patient-years). The risk of bleeding declines with the duration of anticoagulation: patients who had received anticoagulant therapy for more than 3 months had a case-fatality rate of 9.1% (CI, 2.5% to 21.7%), and the rate of intracranial bleeding was 0.65 per 100 patient-years (CI, 0.63% to 0.68 per 100 patient-years).[56] Since the risk of death is so high, any bleeding episode in an anticoagulated patient must be treated as potentially serious. The actual severity of an individual event should be determined by the type and location of bleeding, presence of co-morbidities, concomitant medications (such as platelet inhibitors), and the dose and type of anticoagulants. Bleeding episodes may be classified as nuisance, minor, and major.

Bruises, menorrhagia, and minor epistaxis are considered to be nuisance bleeding, and are the most commonly observed complications of anticoagulant therapy. They rarely require dose modification or specific interventions, and are usually of no medical significance, being treated with local measures. However, persistent nuisance bleeding may be a marker for imminent and more serious bleeding. Minor bleeding includes epistaxis requiring nasal packing, hematochezia without hemodynamic compromise, and most forms of postsurgical bleeding. While non–life-threatening, minor bleeding episodes usually require some form of medical intervention, along with changes to anticoagulant dose and frequency.

Major bleeding, by definition, requires a significant medical intervention (such as transfusion, endoscopy, or surgery), will routinely result in the suspension or discontinuation of anticoagulants, and may cause long-term morbidity or death.

The bleeding patient should be carefully assessed and

should receive interventions appropriate to the severity of their bleeding. Initially, it can be difficult to determine the right quantum of interventions, and the severity of bleeding episodes is routinely overestimated. Basic principals should prevail, however, and the first priority should be to monitor the patient and to provide hemodynamic stability with crystalloid resuscitation while further assessment and specific diagnostic plans are determined. Mechanical causes of bleeding should be identified and addressed; this may require surgical or endoscopic evaluation. Anticoagulant therapy should be stopped; in critically ill patients, the anticoagulant should be removed from the patient's bedside to avoid inadvertent bolus dosing. The activity of the coagulation cascade should be immediately and frequently assessed; this measurement should include both nonspecific (aPTT, PT/international normalized ratio [INR], fibrinogen) and specific (eg, drug levels or ECT, where appropriate) measures. Transfusion of fresh frozen plasma or cryoprecipitate should only be given if there is specific evidence of a relevant factor deficiency, as prophylactic transfusions have no proven benefit. Furthermore, transfusion will delay other needed prohemostatic therapies and may falsely reassure healthcare providers. Red blood cell transfusion should only be provided to patients with clear and imminent fatal bleeding, or to patients with documented symptomatic anemia. Other measures, such as rewarming in hypothermic patients and calcium administration to patients with proven hypocalcemia, may be required to control hemorrhage.

Nonspecific prohemostatic agents such as desmopressin acetate (DDAVP), which cause release of von Willebrand factor and other prohemostatic agents from the endothelium, may be considered. Fibrinolytic inhibitors, such as tranexamic acid and ϵ-aminocaproic acid, are highly effective at controlling some forms of bleeding and may be particularly useful in selected clinical settings (eg, when used as a mouthwash in patients with dental or gingival bleeding). Intravenous estrogen appears to have a benefit in certain patients, including those with significant vaginal bleeding and those with bleeding in the setting of uremia.

In the presence of major bleeding, specific antidotes should be administered when available. Bleeding caused by the anticoagulant effects of heparin and LMWH should be reversed with protamine, though there is incomplete reversal for the latter.[57] Plasma or coagulation factor concentrates (if given at the correct dose) will reverse the anticoagulant effect of warfarin. Vitamin K should be given concomitantly in such cases.

In instances of life-threatening bleeding, where conventional measures have failed or are unavailable, other nonspecific prohemostatic agents such as rFVIIa and prothrombin complex concentrates should be considered. However, the strength of the recommendations for the use of these agents is poor; thus, widespread use of rFVIIa to treat anticoagulant-associated bleeding is based on a combination of case reports and the absence of alternative therapies that might be effective.

rFVIIa and Anticoagulant Reversal

rFVIIa has been shown to initiate hemostasis at sites of bleeding because it can directly activate thrombin on the surface of platelets.[58] Its success in the treatment of bleeding episodes among hemophiliacs with inhibitors has led to its use for the control of bleeding in various and diverse clinical situations. rFVIIa has also been used extensively to treat warfarin-associated bleeding; in this setting, it has been shown to correct the INR in healthy volunteers, and case series suggest that it effectively stops bleeding in patients receiving warfarin.[59] Experience of rFVIIa use in treating hemorrhage caused by LMWH therapy is mainly anecdotal. rFVIIa has been considered as a potential reversal agent for most of the newer anticoagulants, as discussed in the earlier sections of this paper. Reports of efficacy, however, are derived mainly from laboratory experiments or from healthy volunteers. Recommendations for the widespread use of rFVIIa in the setting of major or life-threatening hemorrhage associated with other anticoagulants must await publication of clinical trials, as there are currently few or no reports of efficacy in the clinical setting.

Conclusion

New anticoagulants are being developed in an effort to improve the efficacy, and overcome the limitations, of heparin and warfarin, the current standard anticoagulants. Hemorrhage will invariably be a complication of all anticoagulants, and we recommend that reversal strategies be developed in concert with the clinical evaluation of these novel agents. Such strategies will, however, be validated only through use in patients with major or life-threatening bleeding. Irrespective of the type of anticoagulant and the type of bleeding, basic clinical concepts to secure hemostasis should prevail.

References

1. Buller HR, Agnelli G, Hull RD, Hyers TM, Prins MH, Raskob GE: Antithrombotic therapy for venous thromboembolic disease: The Seventh ACCP Conference on Antithrombotic and Thrombolytic Therapy. Chest 126:401S-428S, 2004 (suppl 3)
2. Geerts WH, Pineo GF, Heit JA, Bergqvist D, Lassen MR, Colwell CW, Ray JG: Prevention of venous thromboembolism: The Seventh ACCP Conference on Antithrombotic and Thrombolytic Therapy. Chest 126: 338S-400S, 2004 (suppl 3)
3. Singer DE, Albers GW, Dalen JE, Go AS, Halperin JL, Manning WJ: Antithrombotic therapy in atrial fibrillation: The Seventh ACCP Conference on Antithrombotic and Thrombolytic Therapy. Chest 126: 429S-456S, 2004 (suppl 3)
4. Salem DN, Stein PD, Al-Ahmad A, Bussey HI, Horstkotte D, Miller N, Pauker SG: Antithrombotic therapy in valvular heart disease—Native and prosthetic: The Seventh ACCP Conference on Antithrombotic and Thrombolytic Therapy. Chest 126:457S-482S, 2004 (suppl 3)
5. Hirsh J: Oral anticoagulant drugs. N Engl J Med 324:1865-1875, 1991
6. Hirsh J: Heparin. N Engl J Med 324 :1565-1574, 1991
7. Hirsh J, O'Donnell M, Weitz JI: New anticoagulants. Blood 105:453-463, 2005
8. Weitz JI, Crowther M: Direct thrombin inhibitors. Thromb Res 106: V275-V284, 2002

9. Warkentin TE, Crowther MA: Reversing anticoagulants both old and new. Can J Anaesth 49:S11-S25, 2002
10. Abraham E, Reinhart K, Svoboda P, Seibert A, Olthoff D, Dal Nogare A, et al: Assessment of the safety of recombinant tissue factor pathway inhibitor in patients with severe sepsis: A multicenter, randomized, placebo-controlled, single-blind, dose escalation study. Crit Care Med 29:2081-2089, 2001
11. Abraham E, Reinhart K, Opal S, Demeyer I, Doig C, Rodriguez AL, et al: Efficacy and safety of tifacogin (recombinant tissue factor pathway inhibitor) in severe sepsis: A randomized controlled trial. JAMA 290:238-247, 2003
12. Cappello M, Vlasuk GP, Bergum PW, Huang S, Hotez PJ: Ancylostoma caninum anticoagulant peptide: A hookworm-derived inhibitor of human coagulation factor Xa. Proc Natl Acad Sci U S A 92:6152-6156, 1995
13. Bergum PW, Cruikshank A, Maki SL, Kelly CR, Ruf W, Vlasuk GP: Role of zymogen and activated factor X as scaffolds for the inhibition of the blood coagulation factor VIIa-tissue factor complex by recombinant nematode anticoagulant protein c2. J Biol Chem 276:10063-10071, 2001
14. Lee A, Agnelli G, Buller H, Ginsberg J, Heit J, Rote W, et al: Dose-response study of recombinant factor VIIa/tissue factor inhibitor recombinant nematode anticoagulant protein c2 in prevention of postoperative venous thromboembolism in patients undergoing total knee replacement. Circulation 104:74-78, 2001
15. Moons AH, Peters RJ, Bijsterveld NR, Piek JJ, Prins MH, Vlasuk GP, et al: Recombinant nematode anticoagulant protein c2, an inhibitor of the tissue factor/factor VIIa complex, in patients undergoing elective coronary angioplasty. J Am Coll Cardiol 41:2147-2153, 2003
16. Friederich PW, Levi M, Bauer KA, Vlasuk GP, Rote WE, Breederveld D, et al: Ability of recombinant factor VIIa to generate thrombin during inhibition of tissue factor in human subjects. Circulation 103:2555-2559, 2001
17. Boneu B, Necciari J, Cariou R, Sie P, Gabaig AM, Kieffer G, et al: Pharmacokinetics and tolerance of the natural pentasaccharide (SR90107/Org31540) with high affinity to antithrombin III in man. Thromb Haemost 74:1468-1473, 1995
18. Turpie AG, Bauer KA, Eriksson BI, Lassen MR: Fondaparinux vs enoxaparin for the prevention of venous thromboembolism in major orthopedic surgery: A meta-analysis of 4 randomized double-blind studies. Arch Intern Med 162:1833-1840, 2002
19. Buller HR, Davidson BL, Decousus H, Gallus A, Gent M, Piovella F, et al: Subcutaneous fondaparinux versus intravenous unfractionated heparin in the initial treatment of pulmonary embolism. N Engl J Med 349:1695-1702, 2003
20. Buller HR, Davidson BL, Decousus H, Gallus A, Gent M, Piovella F, et al: Fondaparinux or enoxaparin for the initial treatment of symptomatic deep venous thrombosis: A randomized trial. Ann Intern Med 140:867-873, 2004
21. Gerotziafas GT, Depasse F, Chakroun T, Samama MM, Elalamy I: Recombinant factor VIIa partially reverses the inhibitory effect of fondaparinux on thrombin generation after tissue factor activation in platelet rich plasma and whole blood. Thromb Haemost 91:531-537, 2004
22. Lisman T, Bijsterveld NR, Adelmeijer J, Meijers JC, Levi M, Nieuwenhuis HK, et al: Recombinant factor VIIa reverses the in vitro and ex vivo anticoagulant and profibrinolytic effects of fondaparinux. J Thromb Haemost 1:2368-2373, 2003
23. Bijsterveld NR, Moons AH, Boekholdt SM, van Aken BE, Fennema H, Peters RJ, et al: Ability of recombinant factor VIIa to reverse the anticoagulant effect of the pentasaccharide fondaparinux in healthy volunteers. Circulation 106:2550-2554, 2002
24. Daud AN, Ahsan A, Iqbal O, Walenga JM, Silver PJ, Ahmad S, et al: Synthetic heparin pentasaccharide depolymerization by heparinase I: Molecular and biological implications. Clin Appl Thromb Hemost 7:58-64, 2001
25. Herbert JM, Herault JP, Bernat A, van Amsterdam RG, Lormeau JC, Petitou M, et al: Biochemical and pharmacological properties of SANORG 34006, a potent and long-acting synthetic pentasaccharide. Blood 91:4197-4205, 1998
26. Bijsterveld NR, Vink R, van Aken BE, Fennema H, Peters RJ, Meijers JC, et al: Recombinant factor VIIa reverses the anticoagulant effect of the long-acting pentasaccharide idraparinux in healthy volunteers. Br J Haematol 124:653-658, 2004
27. Rezaie AR: DX-9065a inhibition of factor Xa and the prothrombinase complex: Mechanism of inhibition and comparison with therapeutic heparins. Thromb Haemost 89:112-121, 2003
28. Alexander JH, Dyke CK, Yang H, Becker RC, Hasselblad V, Zillman LA, The XaNADU-PCI PILOT Investigators, et al: Initial experience with factor-Xa inhibition in percutaneous coronary intervention: The XaNADU-PCI Pilot. J Thromb Haemost 2:234-241, 2004
29. Alexander JH, Yang H, Becker RC, Kodama K, Goodman S, Dyke CK, et al: First experience with direct, selective factor Xa inhibition in patients with non-ST-elevation acute coronary syndromes: Results of the XaNADU-ACS Trial. J Thromb Haemost 3:439-447, 2005
30. Lassen MR, Davidson BL, Gallus AS, Pineo G, Ansell J, Deitchman D: A phase II randomized, double-blind, five-arm, parallel-group, dose-response study of a new oral directly-acting factor Xa inhibitor, razaxaban, for the prevention of deep vein thrombosis in knee replacement surgery. Blood 102:41, 2003 (abstr)
31. Esmon C: The protein C pathway. Crit Care Med 28:S44-S48, 2000 (suppl 9)
32. Bernard GR, Vincent JL, Laterre PF, LaRosa SP, Dhainaut JF, Lopez-Rodriguez A, et al: Recombinant human protein C Worldwide Evaluation in Severe Sepsis (PROWESS) study group. Efficacy and safety of recombinant human activated protein C for severe sepsis. N Engl J Med 344:699-709, 2001
33. Parkinson JF, Grinnell BW, Moore RE, Hoskins J, Vlahos CJ, Bang NU: Stable expression of a secretable deletion mutant of recombinant human thrombomodulin in mammalian cells. J Biol Chem 265:12602-12610, 1990
34. Kearon C, Comp P, Douketis J, Royds R, Yamada K, Gent M: Dose-response study of recombinant human soluble thrombomodulin (ART-123) in the prevention of venous thromboembolism after total hip replacement. J Thromb Haemost 3:962-968, 2005
35. Greinacher A, Volpel H, Janssens U, Hach-Wunderle V, Kemkes-Matthes B, Eichler P, et al: Recombinant hirudin (lepirudin) provides safe and effective anticoagulation in patients with heparin-induced thrombocytopenia: a prospective study. Circulation 99:73-80, 1999
36. Greinacher A, Janssens U, Berg G, Bock M, Kwasny H, Kemkes-Matthes B, et al: Lepirudin (recombinant hirudin) for parenteral anticoagulation in patients with heparin-induced thrombocytopenia. Circulation 100:587-593, 1999
37. Lefevre G, Duval M, Gauron S, Brookman LJ, Rolan PE, Morris TM, et al: Effect of renal impairment on the pharmacokinetics and pharmacodynamics of desirudin. Clin Pharmacol Ther 62:50-59, 1997
38. Nowak G, Bucha E, Goock T, Thieler H, Markwardt F: Pharmacology of r-hirudin in renal impairment. Thromb Res 66:707-715, 1992
39. Fareed J, Walenga JM, Pifarre R, Hoppensteadt D, Koza M: Some objective considerations for the neutralization of the anticoagulant actions of recombinant hirudin. Haemostasis 21:64-72, 1991 (suppl 1)
40. Fox I, Dawson A, Loynds P, Eisner J, Findlen K, Levin E, et al: Anticoagulant activity of Hirulog, a direct thrombin inhibitor, in humans. Thromb Haemost 69:157-163, 1993
41. Bittl JA, Strony J, Brinker JA, Ahmed WH, Meckel CR, Chaitman BR, et al: Treatment with bivalirudin (Hirulog) as compared with heparin during coronary angioplasty for unstable or postinfarction angina. Hirulog Angioplasty Study Investigators. N Engl J Med 333:764-769, 1995
42. White H: Thrombin-specific anticoagulation with bivalirudin versus heparin in patients receiving fibrinolytic therapy for acute myocardial infarction: the HERO-2 randomised trial. Lancet 358:1855-1863, 2001
43. Vasquez JC, Vichiendilokkul A, Mahmood S, Baciewicz FA Jr: Anticoagulation with bivalirudin during cardiopulmonary bypass in cardiac surgery. Ann Thorac Surg 74:2177-2179, 2002
44. Lewis BE, Wallis DE, Leya F, Hursting MJ, Kelton JG, Argatroban-915 Investigators: Argatroban anticoagulation in patients with heparin-induced thrombocytopenia. Arch Intern Med 163:1849-1856, 2003
45. Gustafsson D, Nystrom J, Carlsson S, Bredberg U, Eriksson U,

Gyzander E, et al: The direct thrombin inhibitor melagatran and its oral prodrug H 376/95: Intestinal absorption properties, biochemical and pharmacodynamic effects. Thromb Res 101:171-181, 2001
46. Eriksson H, Wahlander K, Gustafsson D, Welin LT, Frison L, Schulman S, Thrive Investigators: A randomized, controlled, dose-guiding study of the oral direct thrombin inhibitor ximelagatran compared with standard therapy for the treatment of acute deep vein thrombosis: THRIVE I. J Thromb Haemost 1:41-47, 2003
47. Schulman S, Wahlander K, Lundstrom T, Clason SB, Eriksson H: Secondary prevention of venous thromboembolism with the oral direct thrombin inhibitor ximelagatran. N Engl J Med 349:1713-1721, 2003
48. Colwell CW, Berkowitz SD, Davidson BL, Lotke PA, Ginsberg JS, Lieberman JR, et al: Comparison of ximelagatran, an oral direct thrombin inhibitor, with enoxaparin for the prevention of venous thromboembolism following total hip replacement. A randomized, double-blind study. J Thromb Haemost 1:2119-2130, 2003
49. Eriksson BI, Agnelli G, Cohen AT, Dahl OE, Lassen MR, Mouret P, et al. for the EXPRESS Study Group: The direct thrombin inhibitor melagatran followed by oral ximelagatran compared with enoxaparin for the prevention of venous thromboembolism after total hip or knee replacement: the EXPRESS study. J Thromb Haemost 1:2490-2496, 2003
50. Eriksson BI, Lindbratt S, Kalebo P, Bylock A, Frison L, Welin L, et al: METHRO II: Dose-response study of the novel oral, direct thrombin inhibitor, H 376/95 and its subcutaneous formulation, melagatran, compared with dalteparin as thromboembolic prophylaxis after total hip or total knee replacement. Haemostasis 30:183, 2000 (abstr) (suppl 1)
51. Eriksson BI, Bergqvist D, Kalebo P, Dahl OE, Lindbratt S, Bylock A, et al: Melagatran for thrombin inhibition in orthopaedic surgery. Ximelagatran and melagatran compared with dalteparin for prevention of venous thromboembolism after total hip or knee replacement: The METHRO II randomised trial. Lancet 360:1441-1447, 2002
52. Olsson SB: Stroke prevention with the oral direct thrombin inhibitor ximelagatran compared with warfarin in patients with nonvalvular atrial fibrillation (SPORTIF III): Randomised controlled trial. Lancet 362:1691-1698, 2003
53. Petersen P, Grind M, Adler J, SPORTIF II Investigators: Ximelagatran versus warfarin for stroke prevention in patients with nonvalvular atrial fibrillation. SPORTIF II: A dose-guiding, tolerability, and safety study. J Am Coll Cardiol 41:1445-1451, 2003
54. Wolzt M, Levi M, Sarich TC, Bostrom SL, Eriksson UG, Eriksson-Lepkowska M, et al: Effect of recombinant factor VIIa on melagatran-induced inhibition of thrombin generation and platelet activation in healthy volunteers. Thromb Haemost 91:1090-1096, 2004
55. Eriksson BI, Dahl OE, Buller HR, Hettiarachchi R, Rosencher N, Bravo ML, et al: A new oral direct thrombin inhibitor, dabigatran etexilate, compared with enoxaparin for prevention of thromboembolic events following total hip or knee replacement: The BISTRO II randomized trial. J Thromb Haemost 3:103-111, 2005
56. Linkins LA, Choi PT, Douketis JD: Clinical impact of bleeding in patients taking oral anticoagulant therapy for venous thromboembolism: A meta-analysis. Ann Intern Med 139:893-900, 2003
57. Crowther MA, Berry LR, Monagle PT, Chan AK: Mechanisms responsible for the failure of protamine to inactivate low-molecular-weight heparin. Br J Haematol 116:178-186, 2002
58. Monroe DM, Hoffman M, Oliver JA, Roberts HR: Platelet activity of high-dose factor VIIa is independent of tissue factor. Br J Haematol 99:542-547, 1997
59. Levi M, Peters M, Buller HR: Efficacy and safety of recombinant factor VIIa for treatment of severe bleeding: A systematic review. Crit Care Med 33:883-890,2005

ELSEVIER

Seminars in
HEMATOLOGY

Milestones in Hemophilia and Concepts in Future Clinical Trial Design

Jeanne M. Lusher

Hemophilia has long been documented as a bleeding disorder that afflicts males from early childhood. While some early societies set guidelines or laws to protect affected children, true advances in the understanding of the underlying deficiency and in the treatment of hemophilia have been relatively recent and continue today. This paper presents some of the key milestones that mark the path to current knowledge on hemophilia. Given that further studies are needed to explore issues such as optimal treatment and dosage, particularly in patients with inhibitors to factor VIII or factor IX, this paper also considers potential pitfalls in the design and conduct of clinical trials in hemophilia and suggests how careful forward planning may help to avoid them.
Semin Hematol 43(suppl 1):S84-S87

Milestones From the Talmud to the Present Day

The earliest written references to the disorder we now know as hemophilia appeared during the 12th century AD in the Talmud, an authoritative record of Jewish customs, laws, stories, and ethics. The Talmudian philosopher, Maimonides, wrote in the *Mishneh Torah*, the first recording of Jewish oral law, that if a woman's first two sons died as the result of circumcision, the third son should not be circumcised at the proper time (8th day of life).[1,2] Undoubtedly, the most renowned family to have hemophilia was that of Queen Victoria, in whom the mutation is supposed to have arisen spontaneously. In the mid 1800s, she and Prince Albert had two daughters, Alice and Beatrice, who were carriers of the disorder, and a son, Leopold, with hemophilia. Descendants of Alice married into the Royal Houses of Russia and Germany, while a descendant of Beatrice married into the Spanish royal family, thus passing "Queen Victoria's gene" to the Royal Houses of Europe.[3,4]

It was not until 1893 that Sir Almroth Wright in the United Kingdom documented the existence of an abnormal prolongation of coagulation in capillary vessels of persons with hemophilia[5]; in 1946, American pathologist Dr Kenneth Brinkhous recorded that this defect in coagulation occurred in the plasma component of blood.[6] Research carried out by Brinkhous also showed that factor VIII (FVIII) is completely or partly missing in people with hemophilia. Shortly after these discoveries, Brinkhous and Graham established the first hemophilic dog colony at the University of North Carolina at Chapel Hill, thus providing an excellent animal model for hemophilia.[7]

Another milestone in the understanding and treatment of hemophilia occurred in the mid 1960s, when Dr Judith Graham Pool discovered—almost by accident—a simple way of producing cryoprecipitate (a cold insoluble precipitate derived from frozen plasma that had been thawed in the cold and containing at least half of the plasma's original FVIII activity).[8] Almost overnight this method became routinely used to produce cryoprecipitate for treating persons with hemophilia A—indeed, almost any blood bank drawing donors could produce cryoprecipitate simply by placing the bags of plasma into ethanol and dry ice and then allowing them to thaw in a refrigerator. Cryoprecipitates were used to treat bleeds in persons with hemophilia A from the late 1960s to the mid 1970s (and, in some instances, considerably beyond this time). They were usually given in a clinic or hospital setting and provided much higher levels of FVIII to the recipient than had been possible with fresh frozen plasma, which had previously been the standard treatment for bleeds.

In the late 1960s and early 1970s, pharmaceutical companies developed methods for mass-producing plasma-derived FVIII and factor IX (FIX) concentrates. Units of plasma from several thousand donors (40,000 to 60,000 or more) were combined to create a plasma pool, which provided the starting material for a single batch of intermediate-purity, freeze-dried, plasma-derived FVIII or FIX concentrate. Until the

Division of Hematology/Oncology, Children's Hospital of Michigan, Detroit, MI.
Address correspondence to Jeanne M. Lusher, Professor of Hematology, Department of Hematology/Oncology, Children's Hospital of Michigan, 3901 Beaubien St, Detroit, MI 48201. E-mail: jlusher@med.wayne.edu

 0037-1963/06/$-see front matter
doi:10.1053/j.seminhematol.2005.11.008

mid 1980s, virucidal methods were not employed to eradicate contamination by blood-borne viruses, such as hepatitis viruses or the human immunodeficiency virus (HIV). While the availability of FVIII and FIX concentrates greatly enhanced treatment options—particularly home treatment, which allowed more rapid treatment of bleeding episodes, much less time lost from work or school, and a greater feeling of independence—it soon became apparent that there was a price to be paid for their use. Not only did the majority of recipients develop hepatitis B,[9] and "non-A, non-B hepatitis" (now known as hepatitis C), but in 1981 the first cases of acquired immune deficiency syndrome (AIDS) occurred in persons with hemophilia who had received plasma-derived FVIII concentrates.[10] From 1981 to 1986, the number of newly diagnosed cases of AIDS continued to escalate in the hemophilia population. From 1983 to 1986, and primarily in response to the increased incidence of these often deadly blood-borne diseases, pharmaceutical companies introduced better testing methods for screening blood donors, and developed and introduced viral attenuation methods such as dry heat, pasteurization, and solvent-detergent treatment of concentrate. Since 1987, as a result of these measures, there have been no new cases of AIDS in North American hemophilic patients. The development and use of recombinant vaccines for the prevention of hepatitis A and hepatitis B, as well as the mandatory use of "universal precautions" in the late 1980s, were also extremely helpful in preventing new hepatitis A and B infections, as well as some cases of human immunodeficiency virus (HIV) infection. By 1990, an assay for hepatitis C antibody was licensed and routine screening of donors began.[11]

Following effective lobbying by the National Hemophilia Foundation, another milestone in the history of hemophilia occurred in 1975 with the passage of the "Public Law 94-63" in the United States. This law authorized monetary appropriations for grants to hemophilia treatment centers (HTCs) offering comprehensive hemophilia care. These measures resulted in the establishment of a national network of HTCs providing not only diagnosis and clotting factor concentrates for persons with hemophilia, but also education, home treatment training, physical therapy, social work services, access to dental treatment by persons experienced in hemophilia care, and genetic counseling. While the amount of federal funding was by no means large, it did provide status to the center and the impetus to obtain extra funds for the additional services needed. As new needs arose, such as the need for AIDS testing, counseling, and treatment in the 1980s, HTC staff obtained the necessary expertise and established liaisons with other health care providers in the disciplines involved, such as hepatologists and infectious disease specialists.

In the late 1980s, the immunopurification of FVIII and FIX using monoclonal antibodies yielded highly purified concentrates, permitting the administration of smaller infusion volumes. Two further major milestones in hemophilia treatment were the cloning of FIX in 1982[12] and the cloning of FVIII in 1984.[13] In an amazingly short period of time, scale up, purification, and standardization of recombinant FVIII (rFVIII) had been accomplished, with clinical trials beginning in 1987 and licensure of the first rFVIII preparation, Recombinate (Baxter Healthcare Corp, Hyland Division, Glendale, CA) following in 1992. Five years later, the rFIX product, BeneFIX (Wyeth Pharmaceuticals, Collegeville, PA) was also licensed. Newer, and presumably safer "next generation" rFVIII preparations, formulated with sucrose rather than with human serum albumin, were licensed by 2000, and a smaller, B-domain–deleted rFVIII preparation, ReFacto (Wyeth Pharmaceuticals) is now available. Further attempts to generate so-called "designer molecules," with longer half-lives or the ability to promote hemostasis in hemophilics with inhibitors to FVIII, are being explored.

A number of studies conducted between the late 1980s and 2004 uncovered the important fact that approximately 30% of patients with severe hemophilia A develop inhibitor antibodies to FVIII,[14–16] while 1% to 2% of those with severe hemophilia B develop inhibitors to FIX.[17] These landmark studies also demonstrated that, while some of the FVIII inhibitors are transient, others persist, making treatment of bleeding episodes difficult and costly. Documented risk factors for inhibitor development include severity of hemophilia, the particular mutation in the individual's FVIII or FIX gene, family history of an inhibitor in a close relative with hemophilia, ethnicity, and number of exposure days to FVIII or FIX. Despite many published studies aimed at determining the best ways to manage patients with persisting, "high responder" inhibitors, there are still many unanswered questions regarding the best product to use, dose, dosing interval, etc, for particular types of bleeding episodes. Thus, there is still a need for additional well-designed clinical studies in these areas.

Since the initial report of clinical efficacy of recombinant activated factor VII (rFVIIa; NovoSeven®, Novo Nordisk, Bagsvaerd, Denmark) in a patient with hemophilia A and a high-titer inhibitor who underwent open synovectomy,[18] numerous other hemophilia patients have also received rFVIIa for the treatment of bleeding episodes and for surgical coverage. However, the optimal dose and dosage schedule of rFVIIa for various types of bleeding have yet to be determined.

Consideration of Potential Pitfalls in the Design and Conduct of Clinical Trials

In designing and conducting a meaningful clinical trial in patients with hemophilia, a number of issues must be addressed (Table 1). First and foremost, the aim of the trial should be unambiguously specified. For instance, in a study of rFVIIa administered as a treatment for hemophilic patients with "high responder" inhibitors, should the aim of the study be to determine which of three dosages is most effective in controlling acute hemarthroses, or to determine the most effective dosing interval in a particular type of bleed, or to

Table 1 Considerations in the Design and Conduct of Clinical Trials

Aim of trial
Which types of bleeding should be considered (acute hemarthroses, intramuscular bleeding, other)?
Statistical considerations (involve a statistician early!)
Number of subjects needed?
Number of evaluable bleeding episodes?
How will responses be assessed? Subjectively? Objectively? Both?
Will a Data Safety Monitoring Board be set up during the trial?

compare the efficacy of rFVIIa versus a bypassing agent, such as FEIBA-VH (Baxter Healthcare, Deerfield, IL), in controlling a particular type of bleed?

Since patients with hemophilia are subject to different types of bleeding episodes, it is important to decide which types of bleeds should be evaluated in the trial. If major surgical bleeding is to be evaluated, what level of bleeding should be considered as "major"? Or will evaluations be based on acute hemarthroses, or intramuscular bleeding, or both? Will "target joints" be included and, if so, how will baseline assessments of joint bleeds or intramuscular hemorrhage be made? If joint range of motion is to be determined by goniometry, it must be predetermined who will ensure the accuracy of these measurements. Also, what will be considered as an improvement in joint mobility (eg, increase of 10% or 30% in range of motion)? Will this percentage vary according to the joint examined? In addition, such factors as the time interval between onset of the bleed and first treatment must be assessed and, if subjective assessments are included, it needs to be decided whether analgesics will be permitted. Statistician input is required to predetermine the number of subjects to be enrolled in the trial, how many evaluable bleeding episodes are required, and whether this number is realistic in terms of study duration. Time points for evaluation of drug efficacy in arresting bleeding must also be predetermined; time points may range from 1 to several hours or days, depending on the trial endpoint and the aspects of bleeding and rebleeding to be evaluated.

Other study considerations involve methodology; for example, if the trial compares two treatment regimens in a double-blind, randomized, cross-over design, how will the study products be blinded? Unless the subject is in a Clinical Trials Unit, blinding may prove difficult to achieve. Not all HTCs have a Clinical Trials Unit available, and not all subjects are willing to be admitted to one.

If one is to conduct a trial from which meaningful, reliable conclusions can be drawn, one must also be aware of the trial's limitations. An important limitation of any trial is inherent in the statistical method employed. For example, if one wishes to determine the "equivalence" of two products, one must formulate a hypothesis of equivalence. In planning a randomized, controlled trial, one should estimate the null position and decide what difference should be detected. With help and input from a statistician, one should then determine the sample size needed to demonstrate such a difference, if one exists. When determined by such prior planning, the sample size may be much larger than the investigators had in mind! If the required sample size is beyond practical limits, one may have to admit a higher α or β risk, and/or settle for a larger Δ required for discrimination.[19]

Other practical considerations include the facts that many potential subjects live far from the HTC and that many patients are receiving home treatment (self infusion or infusion of clotting factor concentrate by a caregiver). Under these circumstances, patients may be reluctant to participate in a clinical trial that requires frequent trips to the HTC. If they do travel to the HTC for initial assessment of a bleeding episode, many hours may elapse from the onset of the bleed until the time of treatment, resulting in a poorer response to the study product and jeopardy to the joint involved. Alternatively, if the bleed is assessed and treated at home, joint range-of-motion measurements are usually less accurate and may be improperly recorded. In the case of young children, the caregiver at home may have difficulty in determining the child's subjective improvement at a certain time point.

In summary, many potential pitfalls exist in designing and conducting clinical trials in persons with hemophilia. However, many of these can be circumvented by careful planning. It is extremely important to involve a good statistician early in the planning stage. In addition, one should identify the aim(s) of the study, methods and times of assessment of response, the study endpoint, sample size, and whether or not the latter is realistic. With careful planning and supervision, proper patient recruitment and retention in the study, it is not impossible to get good, meaningful data!

References

1. Mishneh Torah, Hilkhot Micah 1:18
2. Rosner F: Moses Maimonides (1135-1204). Ann Intern Med 62:372-375, 1965
3. Potts DM, Potts WTW: Queen Victoria's Gene. Haemophilia and the Royal Family. Stroud, Gloucestershire, UK, Alan Sutton, 1995
4. McKusick VA: The royal hemophilia. Sci Am 213:88-95, 1965
5. Wright AE: On the method of determining the condition of blood coagulability for clinical and experimental purposes, and on the effect of the administration of calcium salts in haemophilia and actual or threatened haemorrhage. BMJ 2:223-225, 1893
6. Brinkhous KM: Clotting defect in haemophilia: Deficiency in a plasma factor required for platelet utilisation. Proc Soc Exp Biol Med 66:117-120, 1947
7. Smith N: A History of the National Hemophilia Foundation. New York, NY, National Hemophilia Foundation, 1984
8. Pool JG, Hershgold EJ, Pappenheim AR: High-potency antihemophilic factor concentrate prepared from cryoglobulin precipitate. Nature 203: 312, 1964
9. Mannucci PM, Capitanio A, Del Ninno E, Columbo M, Pareti F, Ruggeri ZM: Asymptomatic liver disease in haemophiliacs. J Clin Pathol 28: 620-624, 1975
10. Centers for Disease Control (CDC): Pneumocystis carinii pneumonia among persons with hemophilia A. MMWR Morb Mortal Wkly Rep 31:365-367, 1982
11. Donahue JG, Munoz A, Ness PM, Brown DE Jr, Yawn DH, McAllister HA Jr, et al: The declining risk of post-transfusion hepatitis C virus infection. N Engl J Med 327:369-373, 1992
12. Anson DS, Choo KH, Rees DJ, Giannelli F, Gould K, Huddelston JA, et

al: The gene structure of human anti-haemophilic factor IX. EMBO J 3:1053-1060, 1984

13. Gitschier J, Wood WI, Goralka TM, Wion KL, Chen EY, Eaton DH, et al: Characterization of the human factor VIII gene. Nature 312: 826-830, 1984
14. Lusher JM: Natural history of inhibitor development in children with severe hemophilia A treated with factor VIII products, in Lee CA, Berntorp EE, Hoots WK (eds): Textbook of Haemophilia. Oxford, UK, Blackwell, 2005, pp 34-38
15. DiMichele D: Inhibitors to factor VIII—Epidemiology and treatment, in Lee CA, Berntorp EE, Hoots WK (eds): Textbook of Haemophilia. Oxford, UK, Blackwell, 2005, pp 64-70
16. Scharrer I, Bray GL, Neutzling O: Incidence of inhibitors in haemophilia A patients: A review of recent studies of recombinant and plasma-derived factor VIII concentrates. Haemophilia 5:145-154, 1999
17. Warrier I: Inhibitors in hemophilia B, in Lee CA, Berntorp EE, Hoots WK (eds): Textbook of Haemophilia. Oxford, UK, Blackwell, 2005, pp 97-100
18. Hedner U, Glazer S, Pingel K, Alberts KA, Blomback M, Schulman S, et al: Successful use of recombinant factor VIIa in patient with severe haemophilia A during synovectomy. Lancet 2:1193, 1988
19. Lee MC, Lusher JM: The problem of therapeutic equivalence with paired qualitative data: An example from a clinical trial using haemophiliacs with an inhibitor to factor VIII. Stat Med 10:433-441, 1991

ELSEVIER

Seminars in
HEMATOLOGY

Abstracts

The Incidence of Factor VIII and Factor IX Inhibitors in the Hemophilia Population of the UK and Their Effect on Subsequent Mortality, 1977–99[1]*

Sarah C. Darby, David M. Keeling, Rosemary J.D. Spooner, Sau Wan Kan, Paul L.F. Giangrande, Peter W. Collins, Frank G.H. Hill, and Charles R.M. Hay

Background: Previous studies of the development of inhibitors and their impact on mortality have been small.

Objectives: To examine the development of inhibitors in people with hemophilia in the UK and their effect on subsequent mortality.

Patients: 6078 males with hemophilia A and 1172 males with hemophilia B registered in the UK Haemophilia Centre Doctors' Organisation database, 1977–98.

Results: In severe hemophilia A inhibitors developed at rates of 34.4, 5.2 and 3.8 per 1000 years at ages <5, 5–14 and 15+ years; cumulative risks at ages 5 and 75 were 16% and 36%. In hemophilia A the rate of inhibitor development decreased during 1977–90, but increased during the 1990s. In severe hemophilia B inhibitors developed at rates of 13.3 and 0.2 per 1000 years at ages <5 and 5+ and cumulative risks at ages 5 and 75 were 6% and 8%. With HIV, inhibitor development did not increase mortality. In severe hemophilia without HIV, inhibitor development doubled mortality during 1977–92, but during 1993–99 mortality was identical with and without inhibitors. In severe hemophilia without HIV but with inhibitors, mortality from causes involving bleeding decreased during 1977–99 ($P = .001$) as did mortality involving intracranial hemorrhage ($P = .007$).

Conclusions: These data provide estimates of the rate of inhibitor development in hemophilia A and hemophilia B, and they show that the rate of inhibitor development has varied over time, although the reasons for this remain unclear. They also show that in severe hemophilia the substantial increase in mortality previously associated with inhibitors is no longer present.

*Please note that this abstract has been reproduced in its entirety from Darby SC et al. J Thromb Haemost 2004;2:1047-1054, with permission from Blackwell Publishing.

UK Haemophilia Centre Doctors' Organisation.

Address correspondence to Professor F.G.H. Hill, Chairman, UK Haemophilia Centre Doctors' Organisation, Department of Clinical and Laboratory Haematology, The Birmingham Children's Hospital, Steelhouse Lane, Birmingham B4 6NH, United Kingdom. E-mail: frank.hill@bhamchildrens.wmids.nhs.uk

Reference

1. Darby SC, Keeling DM, Spooner RJ, Wan Kan S, Giangrande PL, Collins PW, et al: The incidence of factor VIII and factor IX inhibitors in the hemophilia population of the UK and their effect on subsequent mortality, 1977-99. J Thromb Haemost 2:1047-1054, 2004

 0037-1963/06/$-see front matter Published by Elsevier Inc.
doi:10.1053/j.seminhematol.2005.12.004

ELSEVIER

Seminars in
HEMATOLOGY

Intensive Exposure to Factor VIII May Be a Risk Factor for Inhibitor Development in Mild Hemophilia A

Manuel D. Carcao

In mild hemophilia A (MHA; median baseline factor VIII activity [FVIII:C] level >5%), the development of inhibitors is an infrequently reported complication (3% to 13%). Little is known about the risk factors for inhibitor development in MHA, particularly with regard to the role of factor VIII (FVIII) exposure (the amount and intensity of exposure, and the context in which exposure occurs). Recent case reports and small case series, usually involving adults, implicate intense exposure—particularly by continuous infusion (CI) in inhibitor development in MHA.

Our group at The Hospital for Sick Children in Toronto, Canada, undertook a review of FVIII exposure and inhibitor development in a population of boys (n = 54; age, 0 to 18 years) with MHA who were treated at our institution from 1996 to 2001. All 54 boys were prospectively followed with yearly inhibitor screening. Twenty-nine of these 54 boys (54%) had been exposed to FVIII at some time during their childhood. Mean age at initial exposure to any FVIII was 5.4 years (range, 5 days to 16.3 years).

For the 29 FVIII-exposed boys, the mean number of cumulative exposure days (an exposure day [ED] being defined as a day in which a patient receives at least one dose of FVIII regardless of the amount or method of administration, ie, bolus infusion [BI] *v* CI) was 16.3 days (range, 1 to 46 days). Of 16 boys who received an intense exposure to FVIII (defined as receiving FVIII daily for ≥6 consecutive days), seven received exposure by CI and 9 by BI. Four of the seven boys (57%) exposed to a CI developed inhibitors (high titer in three). These patients developed a severe and unusual bleeding pattern reminiscent of that seen in acquired hemophilia. None of the other boys with MHA, including the nine boys exposed to daily BI (≥6 consecutive days), developed inhibitors ($P = .02$ by Fisher's exact test), suggesting that CI of FVIII may be associated with an increased risk of inhibitor development.

The mechanism and incidence of inhibitor development in MHA following intense FVIII exposure is not known. Recently, some hemophilia treatment centers have recommended against the use of CI in MHA patients. Given the potential benefits of CI, it may be premature to cease using this modality of treatment in patients with MHA.

Based on our single-center experience, we are in the process of evaluating all MHA patients in Canada to determine the incidence of inhibitor development in such patients following intense exposure (including CI) to FVIII. Conceivably, there may be a group of MHA patients at high risk of developing inhibitors in the setting of CI and other intense exposures to FVIII. For such patients, consideration may need to be given to alternatives to intense FVIII exposure in the context of management of bleeds or surgical bleeding prophylaxis.

Division of Hematology/Oncology, Department of Pediatrics, The Hospital for Sick Children, Toronto, Canada.

Address correspondence to Dr Manuel D. Carcao, Division of Haematology/Oncology, Hospital for Sick Children, Toronto, ON, Canada, M5G 1X8. E-mail: manuel.carcao@sickkids.ca

doi:10.1053/j.seminhematol.2005.12.001

ELSEVIER

Seminars in
HEMATOLOGY

Acquired Hemophilia

Peter Collins

Acquired hemophilia is a bleeding disorder caused by an autoantibody directed against a coagulation factor, usually factor VIII (FVIII). The incidence is about 1.5 per million per year and increases with age. The clinical presentation is of a bleeding disorder in a person with no previous history of hemostatic symptoms. The phenotype is variable and unpredictable ranging from mild bruising to fatal bleeding. Typical features include: spontaneous bleeding unrelated to FVIII level, superficial bruising, muscle bleeds, hematuria, postpartum hemorrhage, and gastrointestinal bleeding. Hemarthroses are less common. Mortality is reported to be as high as 20% in some series.[1]

Diagnosis is confirmed by the finding of a prolonged activated partial thromboplastin time which does not correct with normal plasma (although the action of the inhibitor may be delayed). The FVIII level is low. The inhibitor titer should be measured by the Bethesda assay but, due to the often complex kinetics, inhibitor titers are difficult to interpret and it is usual to report the dilution nearest to 50% inactivation after 2 hours.

Management should be undertaken at a center experienced in acquired hemophilia and involves controlling the bleeding, eradication of the inhibitor, and treating any underlying cause. Eradication of the inhibitor is usually attempted with a combination of steroids and cytotoxics (often cyclophosphamide or azathioprine). Results are variable and are all from single center cohorts apart from one study which randomized patients who had failed to respond to an initial 3 weeks of prednisolone to prednisolone, cyclophosphamide or a combination of the two. The study does not have sufficient subjects randomized to allow firm conclusions to be drawn.[2] A meta-analysis of single center cohorts suggests that whilst steroids and cyclophosphamide leads to more patients achieving remission, disease-free survival is similar with both treatments.[3] Mortality and morbidity related to immunosuppression in elderly patients is an important treatment consideration. Recent uncontrolled data have shown that rituximab can induce remission in patients with acquired hemophilia at similar rates to those reported for other immunosuppressive agents.[4]

There are a number of options for the treatment of bleeding episodes. Measured FVIII levels may not equate to haemostatic efficacy in vivo and if FVIII is used to treat patients close clinical observation is required and FVIII levels and inhibitor titers must be monitored regularly. Recombinant activated factor VII (rFVIIa; NovoSeven®, Novo Nordisk, Bagsvaerd, Denmark) has been shown to have good efficacy as first line therapy and after other treatment options have failed.[5] Activated prothrombin complex concentrates are widely used and good efficacy has been reported.[6] A short-term rise in FVIII may be seen with desmopressin (DDAVP) in patients with low titer inhibitors. Unresolved issues included the incidence, clinical phenotype, and response to immunosuppression. These issues are currently being addressed in a UK-wide surveillance study. A European collaborative study has been initiated with reporting of patients through an internet link (*www.eachregistry.org*); this study is ongoing and will hopefully provide more knowledge on the management of bleeds and immunosuppression.

University Hospital of Wales, Cardiff, Wales.
Address correspondence to Peter Collins, MD, University Hospital of Wales, Heath Park, Cardiff, Wales CF14 4XW. E-mail: peter.collins@cardiffandvale.wales.nhs.uk

References

1. Green D, Lechner K: A survey of 215 non-hemophilic patients with inhibitors to factor VIII. Thromb Haemost 45:200-203, 1981
2. Green D, Rademaker AW, Briet E: A prospective, randomised trial of prednisolone and cyclophosphamide in the treatment of patients with factor VIII autoantibodies. Thromb Haemost 70:753-757, 1993
3. Delgado J, Jimenez-Yuste V, Hernandez-Navarro F, Villar A: Acquired haemophilia: review and meta-analysis focused on therapy and prognostic factors. Br J Haematol 121:21-35, 2003
4. Stasi R, Brunetti M, Stipa E, Amadori S: Selective B-cell depletion with rituximab for the treatment of patients with acquired hemophilia. Blood 103:4424-4428, 2004
5. Hay CRM, Negrier C, Ludlam CA: The treatment of bleeding in acquired haemophilia with recombinant factor VIIa: A multicentre study. Thromb Haemost 78:1463-1467, 1997
6. Sallah S: Treatment of acquired haemophilia with factor eight inhibitor bypassing activity. Haemophilia 10:169-173, 2004

doi:10.1053/j.seminhematol.2005.11.012

ELSEVIER

Seminars in
HEMATOLOGY

Recombinant Activated Factor VII in Severe Trauma

Bruno Riou

Trauma is the leading cause of death in young people, and the leading cause of lost years of life in industrialized countries.[1] Considerable improvement in the care of trauma patients has been accomplished by organization of pre-hospital care, development of regionalized trauma systems, and improvement in the assessment of trauma patients by modern imaging techniques. Nevertheless, hemorrhage remains the first cause of death in trauma patients. Blood transfusion is associated with late complications and has been demonstrated to be an independent risk factor for development of infections[2] and multiple organ failure (MOF).[3] Moreover, coagulopathy remains a major contributing factor to bleeding-related mortality, even after achieving surgical or radiological control of the hemorrhage in these patients. The association of coagulopathy, metabolic acidosis, and hypothermia has been described as the "lethal triad."[4]

Some promising case reports[5–8] have suggested that recombinant activated coagulation factor VII (rFVIIa; NovoSeven®, Novo Nordisk, Bagsvaerd, Denmark) could be beneficial in trauma patients. The largest series from Dutton et al[8] recently reported 81 cases of trauma patients treated with rFVIIa. These authors reported that bleeding was stopped in 61 (75%) cases. The responders required transfusion of fewer red blood cell (RBC) units post-administration than nonresponders (median, 4 *v* 23 units). It should be pointed out that the case series included not only trauma patients with massive hemorrhage (n = 46), but also those with intracranial hemorrhage (n = 20) and hemostasis abnormalities related to inherited factor deficiencies (n = 6) or anti-vitamin K treatment (n = 9). The latter group of patients may not be an ideal target for rFVIIa treatment, since other therapies exist. Comparing responders with nonresponders, Dutton et al[8] observed that, pretreatment, nonresponders required greater amounts of RBC units (27 ± 13 *v* 15 ± 15 units; $P < .002$), had lower platelet counts (86 ± 60 *v* $141 \pm 77 \times 10^9$/L; $P < .04$), and demonstrated more severe acidosis (7.02 ± 0.31 *vs* 7.29 ± 0.15; $P < .002$). This suggests that bleeding in the nonresponders was too severe and/or treated too late.

Boffard et al[9] conducted a randomized, placebo-controlled, double-blind trial of the efficacy and safety of rFVIIa (200 +100 + 100 μg/kg) as an adjunctive therapy for control of bleeding in 301 patients with severe blunt or penetrating trauma. Trauma patients were treated after they received 8 units of RBC, with additional injections of rFVIIa 1 and 3 hours later. In blunt trauma, RBC transfusion was significantly reduced following rFVIIa treatment when compared with placebo (reduction of 2.6 RBC units; $P = .02$), and the need for massive transfusion (>20 RBC units) was significantly reduced (14% *v* 33% of patients; $P = .03$). In penetrating trauma, similar analyses showed trends towards rFVIIa reducing RBC transfusion (reduction of 1.0 RBC unit; $P = .10$) and massive transfusion (7% *v* 19%; $P = .08$). A trend towards fewer predefined critical complications (MOF, acute respiratory distress syndrome [ARDS], and/or death) was noted. No significant difference in adverse events, including thromboembolic events, was noted between groups. One can conclude that rFVIIa improved bleeding control in severe trauma patients with an excellent safety profile in this high-risk population.

Nevertheless, some important issues remain to be determined. First, the precise target trauma population and the ideal timing for administration remain to be established. These important issues should probably be solved by expert guidelines. In Europe, clinicians involved in trauma care should develop national guidelines for the appropriate use of rFVIIa in these patients, and it is hoped that such guidelines will lead to the approval of rFVIIa use in trauma patients within the European community. The dose administered in the randomized trial was greater than the dose administered in previous studies (usually 100 μg/kg).[5–8] Some preliminary pharmacokinetic data indicate that there are important between-subject variations in plasma concentration in trauma patients, and that a high dose of rFVIIa is required to reach a sufficient plasma concentration in most patients. Nonetheless, the appropriate target concentration of rFVIIa is based only on in vitro studies and thus remains a matter of debate. The need to administer a second or even a third dose of rFVIIa is not obvious in every case, as suggested in previous studies.[5–8] The impact of rFVIIa administration in trauma patients, particularly from a pharmacoeconomic point of

Department of Emergency Medicine and Surgery, Hôpital Pitié Salpêtrière; Assistance Publique-Hôpitaux de Paris; Université Pierre et Marie Curie, Paris, France.

Address correspondence to Bruno Riou, MD, CHU Pitié Salpêtrière; Service d'accueil des urgences, Paris 75651, France. E-mail: bruno.riou@psl.ap-hop-paris.fr

0037-1963/06/$-see front matter Published by Elsevier Inc.
doi:10.1053/j.seminhematol.2005.11.010

view, also remains to be determined. The trend towards an improvement in the composite endpoint of the randomized trial, including death and development of ARDS and MOF (both of which consume medical resources and increase the risk of mortality), is a promising result. Finally, there is recent evidence that rFVIIa could be of interest in severe head trauma with intracranial hemorrhage.[10] Further studies in patients with severe head trauma are ongoing.

However, some caution is advised when using rFVIIa in trauma patients. Although rFVIIa seems to be effective in the trauma population, it is only an adjunctive treatment for bleeding control in such patients and should never replace or delay surgical and/or radiological (embolization) control of bleeding. Moreover, attempts to address those factors that induce coagulopathy should also be made. These factors include platelet counts, hemostatic factors, hypothermia, and acidosis, as well as hematocrit[11,12] and probably hypocalcemia, the importance of which has been underestimated in trauma patients.[13]

References

1. Capan LM, Miller SM, Turndorf H: Trauma overview, in Capan LM, Miller SM, Turndorf H (eds): Trauma: Anesthesia and Intensive Care. Philadelphia, PA, Lippincott, 1991, pp 3-28
2. Hoyt DB, Bulger EM, Knudson MM, Morris J, Ierardi R, Sugerman HJ, et al: Death in the operating room: An analysis of a multi-center experience. J Trauma 37:426-432, 1994
3. Claridge JA, Sawyer RG, Schulman AM, McLemore EC, Young JS: Blood transfusions correlate with infections in trauma patients in a dose-dependent manner. Am Surg 68:566-572, 2002
4. Moore FA, Moore EE, Sauaia A: Blood transfusion. An independent risk factor for postinjury multiple organ failure. Arch Surg 132:620-625, 1997
5. Kenet G, Walden R, Eldad A, Martinowitz U: Treatment of traumatic bleeding with recombinant factor VIIa. Lancet 354:1879, 1999
6. Martinowitz U, Kenet G, Segal E, Luboshitz J, Lubetsky A, Ingerslev J, et al: Recombinant activated factor VII for adjunctive hemorrhage control in trauma. J Trauma 51:431-439, 2001
7. O'Neill PA, Bluth M, Gloster ES, Wali D, Priovolos S, DiMaio TM, et al: Successful use of recombinant activated factor VII for trauma-associated hemorrhage in a patient without preexisting coagulopathy. J Trauma 52:400-405, 2002
8. Dutton RP, McCunn M, Hyder M, D'Angelo M, O'Connor J, Hess JR, et al: Factor VIIa for correction of traumatic coagulopathy. J Trauma 57: 709-719, 2004
9. Boffard KD, Riou B, Warren B, Choong PI, Rizoli S, et al; NovoSeven Trauma Study Group: Recombinant factor VIIa as adjunctive therapy for bleeding control in severely injured trauma patients: Two parallel randomized, placebo-controlled, double-blind clinical trials. J Trauma 59:8-18, 2005
10. Mayer SA, Brun NC, Broderick J, Davis S, Diringer MN, et al; Europe/AustralAsia NovoSeven ICH Trial Investigators: Safety and feasibility of recombinant factor VIIa for acute intracerebral hemorrhage. Stroke 36:74-79, 2005
11. Escolar G, Garrido M, Mazzara R, Castillo R, Ordinas A: Experimental basis for the use of red cell transfusion in the management of anemic-thrombocytopenic patients. Transfusion 28:406-411, 1988
12. Delaporte-Cerceau S, Samama CM, Riou B, Bonnin P, Guillosson JJ, Coriat P: Ketorolac and enoxaparin affect arterial thrombosis and bleeding in the rabbit. Anesthesiology 88:1310-1317, 1998
13. Vivien B, Langeron O, Morell E, Devilliers C, Carli PA, Coriat P, et al: Early hypocalcemia in severe trauma. Crit Care Med 33:1946-1952, 2005

Excluded Abstracts

Safety Update on rFVIIa
Stephanie Seremetis

Parvovirus B19—Culprit or Bystander?
J. Michael Soucie

ELSEVIER

Seminars in
HEMATOLOGY

XXth Congress of the International Society on Thrombosis and Haemostasis Papers

The Platelet: Form and Function

John H. Hartwig

Platelets are small subcellular fragments that are released from megakaryocytes. They are composed of a concentrate of megakaryocyte membrane, cytoplasm, granules, and organelles, and circulate throughout blood vessels and survey the integrity of the vascular system. They circulate as discs, a form specified by their internal microtubule and actin cytoskeleton. When encountering vascular damage, platelets rapidly convert into their active forms, which function to seal off the injury and prevent fluid loss. To assume the active shape, the internal cytoskeleton of each platelet is rapidly disassembled and replaced. New actin filament assembly provides the force that spreads platelets across damaged surfaces and allows the formation of filopodia, which are used to interconnect platelets in solution. In this review, we discuss the role of the cytoskeleton in defining the resting and active forms of the platelet.
Semin Hematol 43(suppl 1):S94-S100

Platelets are tiny, subcellular fragments shed by megakaryocytes, and are composed of megakaryocyte membrane, cytoplasm, granules, and organelles. Large numbers of platelets (10^{11}) are produced daily in the bone marrow; once released into the blood from bone marrow megakaryocytes, they circulate for 7 to 10 days.[1] Platelet mass is tightly controlled and, under normal conditions, maintained by feedback from thrombopoietin (TPO): circulating free TPO concentration increases as platelet counts drop, stimulating increased production and maturation of megakaryocytes. The process of making and releasing platelets from megakaryocytes is unique in cell biology. It first requires the amplification of megakaryocyte DNA to produce an extremely large polyploidy cell that can synthesize an abundance of the platelet-specific products. This is followed by the actual process of platelet assembly and release that occurs only during the final 4 to 10 hours of megakaryocyte life and during which the bulk of the megakaryocyte cytoplasm is spread out into long proplatelets. Platelets are then assembled and filled with their specific organelle/granule content at the ends of the proplatelets.[2,3]

The primary function of platelets is to maintain vascular integrity. When they encounter vascular damage, platelets rapidly convert into their active forms, which then flatten to efficiently cover the damaged surface. Conversion to the active shape is driven by the disassembly and replacement of the platelet's internal cytoskeleton, a process that involves new actin filament assembly and the extension of filopodia from the cell surface. In this review, we discuss the role of the cytoskeleton in defining the resting and active forms of the platelet.

The Resting Form of the Platelet

Once formed and filled with intracellular materials, resting platelets are released into the blood as small discs. In humans, these discs measure approximately 0.5×3.0 μm. The discoid shape is achieved solely by an internal coil formed from microtubules that sits in the cytoplasm just beneath the plasma membrane, along the thin edge of each disc (Fig 1). Microtubules are rigid, hollow polymers assembled from subunits. Each microtubule is a linear aggregate of 13 stacks of tubulin subunits, each arranged in head-to-tail alignments called protofilaments. Tubulin subunits are heterodimeric, expressed by platelets as different isoforms (β1, β2, β4, β5), as well as different isotypes.[4] With a heterodimer concentration of 70 μm, each platelet contains 3×10^5 tubulin subunits; 1.6 to 2×10^5 subunits are required to generate 100 μm of microtubule length, which supports the estimation that, at any time, 50% to 60% of the total platelet tubulin is in the polymeric state.

Division of Hematology, Karp Family Research Laboratories, Brigham and Women's Hospital, Boston, MA.

Address correspondence to John H. Hartwig, PhD, Division of Hematology, Karp Family Research Laboratories, Floor 6, Room 06-215, Brigham and Women's Hospital, Boston, MA 02115. E-mail: hartwig@rics.bwh.harvard.edu

 0037-1963/06/$-see front matter
doi:10.1053/j.seminhematol.2005.11.004

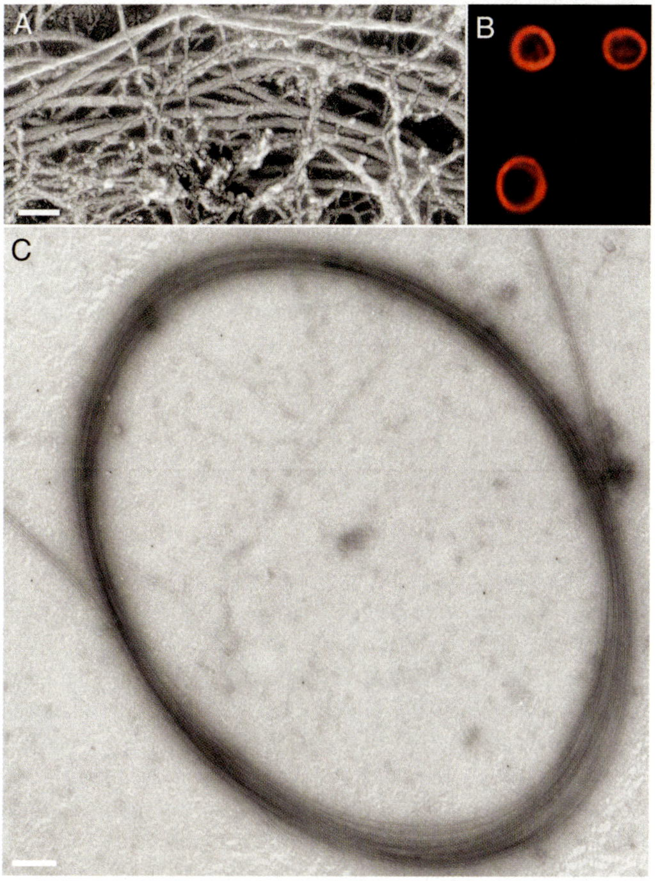

Figure 1 Microtubule ring of the resting platelet. (A) Immunofluorescent staining of tubulin in discoid platelets. (B) The microtubule can be isolated as an intact coil from lysed platelets. The free ends of the single microtubule forming the coil are observed in this negatively stained image, and the hollow structure of microtubules is revealed. (C) After coating platelet cytoskeletons with metal, the surface of the microtubule comprising the coil can be observed. Such images reveal that microtubules in resting platelets have a smooth surface and are not decorated by associated proteins. The bars in A and C are 0.1 μm.

The dominant isoform expressed in mouse and human platelets and megakaryocytes is $\beta1$. Transgenic knockout experiments in mice reveal that platelets lacking $\beta1$ can still polymerize some tubulin, but have greatly diminished amounts of tubulin polymer that organizes into an aberrant and discontinuous ring. A human polymorphism that changes Q43 to P has recently been discovered in $\beta1$-tubulin, and may be carried by up to 10% of the Caucasian population.[5] Heterozygous carriers show substantial reductions in the level of $\beta1$-tubulin expression, and a large fraction of the circulating platelets in such individuals have been reported to be spherocytic. Mouse platelets lacking $\beta1$-tubulin circulate only as spherocytes.

It remains unclear whether the microtubules, rolled into a coil in the circulating platelet, have any function in addition to conferring discoid shape, and whether there is physiological advantage gained by platelets circulating as discs. A rapid reorganization of the microtubule coil occurs once the platelet has been activated, and the cytoskeleton of the active platelet may contain multiple short microtubules that run outward from the center of the active cell into the protrusions elaborated at the edge. Alternatively, the coil may also be found in a compressed state in the center of spread cells. Microtubule dynamics per se, however, are not required for either the shape change reaction or the secretory function of the platelet, as both processes occur normally in the presence of agents that either stabilize microtubules or affect their dissolution. Although microtubule movements are essential for the assembly of platelets by megakaryocytes, as discussed below, the microtubule coil of the platelet retains all the information necessary for its assembly/disassembly, despite the fact that platelets lack defined microtubule-organizing centers. The microtubule coil disassembles when platelets are chilled, resulting in the loss of disc shape.[6] Upon rewarming, however, the microtubules reassemble and form a coil.

Microtubule dynamics and microtubule-based motors are involved in many aspects of cytoplasmic motility. Megakaryocytes and platelets express cytoplasmic dynein and kinesin, which are microtubule motor proteins that conduct adenosine triphosphate (ATP)-dependent movement along microtubules. Dynein is a minus–end-directed motor that transports cargo vesicles toward the minus end of the microtubule and, when attached to one microtubule, binds and slides a second microtubule in the plus direction. Megakaryocyte dynein is used to elongate proplatelets and form platelet bodies at the proplatelet ends.[7] Kinesins are a large family of motor molecules that bind to cargo and transport them over microtubules. Most kinesins are plus–end-directed motors, although minus–end-directed kinesins have also been described. Kinesin is used by megakaryocytes to deliver the platelet-specific granules and organelles to the nascent platelet buds at the proplatelet ends.[8] Whether microtubule-based organelle/granule movements are involved in the physiological functions of activated platelets remains to be determined.

The Actin Cytoskeleton of the Resting Platelet

Although microtubules confer the discoid shape on the resting platelet, platelet integrity is maintained by an elaborate internal actin filament cytoskeleton. This cytoskeleton has been widely studied and can be dissected into its two fundamental components: a membrane skeleton and cytoplasmic actin scaffolding (Fig 2).

Organization of the Membrane Skeleton

Platelet surfaces lack projections; instead, the surface is decorated with pits that mark the openings of enfolded plasma membrane, which forms the open canalicular system of platelets (Fig 2). A dense membrane skeleton laminates the cytoplasmic side of the plasma membrane, as well as the cytoplasmic surface of the open canalicular system. The main protein components of this network are spectrin, adducin,

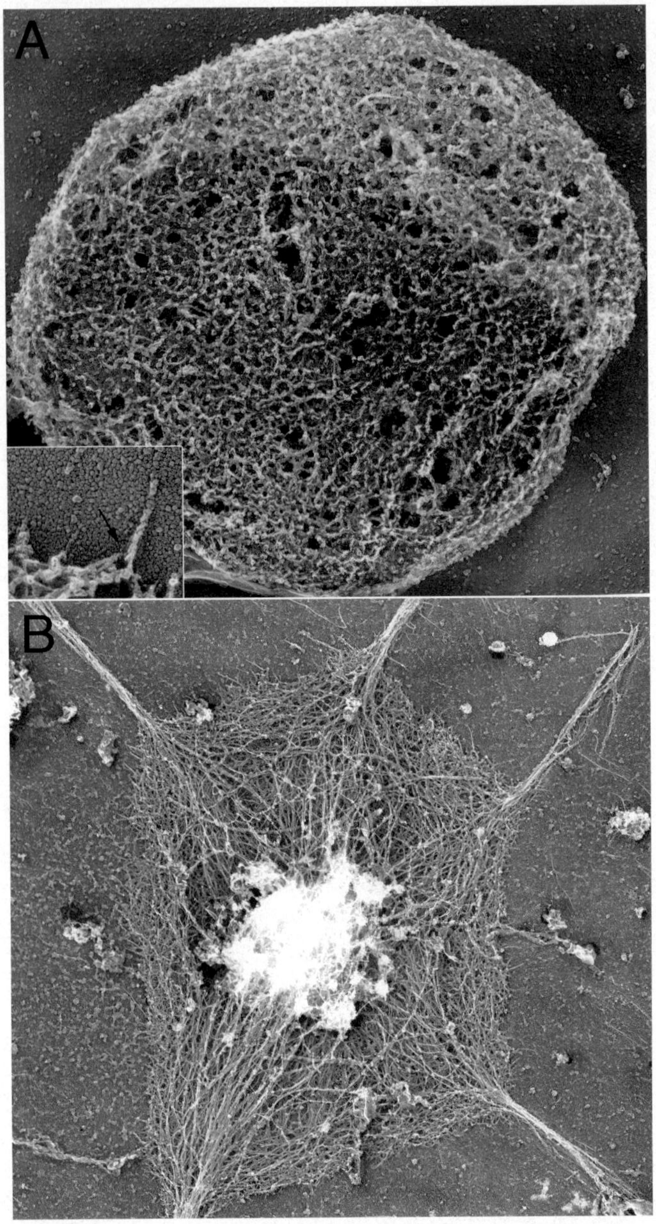

Figure 2 The cytoskeleton of the resting and active platelet. (A) Membrane skeleton of the resting platelet. The membrane skeleton is a dense fibrous coat that retains integrity after detergent extraction, rapid freezing, freeze-drying, and metal casting. The numerous small holes are the entrances to the open canalicular system. Inset. Attachment of actin filament ends to the spectrin-based membrane skeleton. Actin filaments are bound at the barbed end with respect to the binding of myosin S1 to actin (arrow). (B) Cytoskeleton of the activated platelet.

filamin (FLN), actin, and the von Willebrand factor (vWF) receptor (vWFR) (Table 1).

Platelets express 2,000 molecules of non-erythroid spectrin (also called fodrin), which self-assemble into elongated twisted strands that are 200 nm in length. Spectrin molecules are head-to-head, bipolar assemblies of two $\alpha\beta$ heterodimers, which associate lengthwise in an anti-parallel conformation. The free amino-terminus of each spectrin β-chain possesses both an actin filament and an adducin binding site, while the opposite end—the carboxyl-terminus of the β-chain and the amino-terminus of the α-chain—forms the dimer-dimer self-association site. Spectrin heterotetramers interconnect with one another using actin filaments. Of the actin contained within a resting platelet, 40% is assembled into 2,000 to 5,000 filaments. Actin forms a space-filling network within the platelet cytoplasm; filaments run from the cell center toward the plasma membrane, where they turn and run parallel with it. This configuration places the barbed ends of actin in apposition with the plasma membrane. Adducin targets the actin filament ends to membrane-associated spectrin strands. Platelet adducin molecules, which are heterodimers of α and β adducin subunits, cap the majority of actin filament barbed ends in the resting cell.[9] Adducin also has a binding site for β-spectrin subunits, and this interaction collects actin filament ends to the molecular ends of spectrin. β-spectrin also has a pleckstrin homology domain that targets it to the abundant D4-containing phosphoinositides that exist on the cytoplasmic face of the plasma membrane of the resting platelet.

An interaction between FLN A and B (FLNa/b) and the $GP1b_\alpha$ chain of the vWF receptor strengthens the adhesion of the spectrin-actin network to the plasma membrane. FLNa/b molecules self-assemble into bipolar dimers with their actin filament binding sites posited on their free ends, in a similar fashion to spectrin molecules.[10,11] FLN's amino-terminal actin binding domain is separated from its self-association site by 24 repeat units, each consisting of approximately 100 amino acids that fold into β-barrel structures. FLNa/b subunits constitutively bind to the cytoplasmic tail of $GP1b_\alpha$ using repeat 17. $GP1b_\alpha$ chains outnumber FLNa/b molecules by a ratio of 2 to 1. However, since each FLNa/b molecule has two binding sites for $GP1b_\alpha$, the stoichiometry of this interaction in platelets is theoretically near 1 to 1, and biochemical experiments have demonstrated that greater than 90% of the vWF receptor is bound to FLNa/b in the resting cell.[12] The FLN-$GP1b_\alpha$ interaction has a number of important structural consequences. First, the superimposition of this linkage over the spectrin network aids in laminating the spectrin skeleton to the cytoplasmic surface of the plasma membrane. Second, since there are six molecules of FLNa for every actin filament assembled in the resting platelet, it aligns vWF receptors into linear arrays on the cell surface that reflect the underlying organization of actin filaments. Both of these interactions are critical for platelet formation/circulation: platelets from transgenic mice engineered to lack either FLNa or $GP1b_\alpha$,[13] and platelets from human patients with Bernard-Soulier Syndrome[14] that fail to express stabile $GP1b_\alpha$ on their surfaces, are enlarged and fragile, and circulate only in small numbers. Finally, since FLNa/b is a scaffolding protein, it also brings its many partner signaling molecules to the cytoplasm-plasma membrane interface. The FLN family of proteins also functions to rigidify the underlying cytoplasm of the platelet by crosslinking actin filaments into orthogonal gel networks. Platelets also express high levels of α-actinin, which participates in the crosslinking of cytoplasmic actin filaments.

Table 1 The Major Protein Components of the Membrane Skeleton

Membrane Skeletal Protein	No. of Molecules per Platelet	Function	Regulation
$\alpha\beta$-Spectrin	2,000 tetramers	Assemble a 2D lattice on membrane	Calpain proteolysis
$\alpha\gamma$ Adducin	8,000	Barbed end capping; target barbed ends to spectrin	Negative regulation by phosphorylation: $PI_{4,5}P_2$ binding; calcium
Filamin (A, B, and C)	12,500	Attach vWFR to actin	Actin filament binding regulated by calcium-calmodulin
Actin	20,000 (2–5,000 ends)	Crosslink spectrin, provide cytoplasm with structure	At ends by nucleation/severing/depolymerization/capping
vWF receptor (GP1bab9/5)	12–25,000	Adhesion, signaling	? 14-3-3 association

Abbreviations: 2D, two dimensional; vWF, von Willebrand factor; vWFR, von Willebrand factor receptor.

The Cytoskeleton of the Active Platelet

The cytoskeletal rearrangements that occur following platelet activation have been extensively studied, and the processes involved are outlined in Fig 3A–C. Exposure of platelets to agonists results in loss of the discoid shape: platelets first become spherocytic and then rapidly extend filopodia (Fig 3C). When activation occurs on a surface, a circumferential spreading of cells is observed (Fig 3B). Reorganization of the cytoskeleton and doubling of the actin filament content of the cell drive the alterations in cell morphology. Shape change is rapid, beginning within seconds and completing within one minute after exposure to agonists.

For a platelet to change shape, the following cytoplasmic events are required: first, the membrane skeleton is disassembled; second, the cortical actin filament network is disrupted; and third, new actin filament assembly is initiated from the ends of actin filaments that abut the plasma membrane. We now understand many of the proteins that are involved in these reactions and some of the signals and signaling pathways that effect these changes.

Disassembly of the Membrane Skeleton

Upon activation, the membrane skeleton releases from actin and becomes sequestered in the center of the spread platelets. This event is mediated, at least in part, by the dissociation of adducin molecules from the barbed ends of actin filaments and from the ends of spectrin molecules. Adducin can be inactivated in vitro by a variety of different mechanisms, including protein kinase C (PKC)-mediated phosphorylation, phosphatidylinositides, or calcium-calmodulin binding.[15] When platelets are activated using soluble agonists that ligate PAR-1, GP-6 or the immunoglobulin-Fc receptor, dissociation of adducin from the cytoskeleton correlates best with its phosphorylation at serine 726 by PKC.

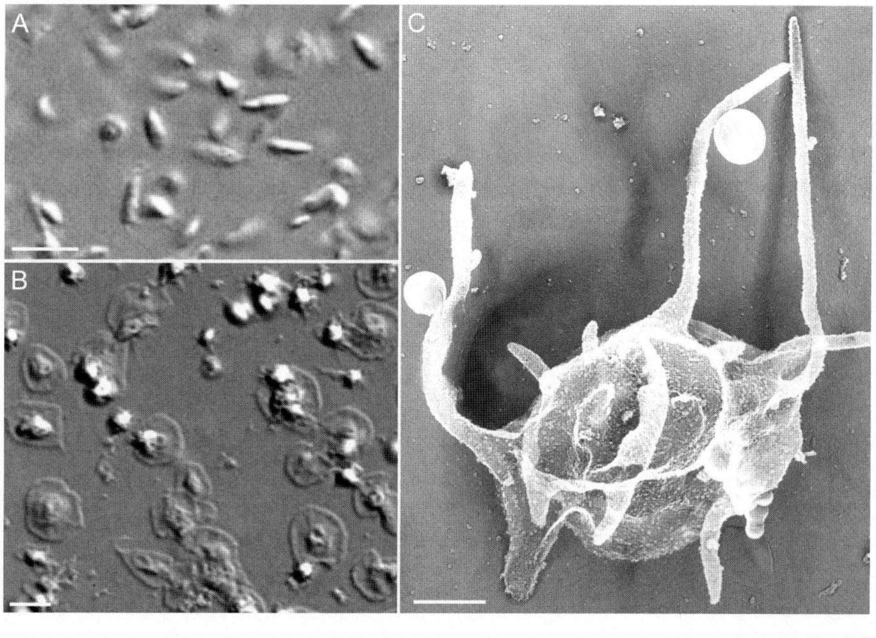

Figure 3 Shape change of the human platelet. (A) Resting platelets in a differential interference contrast photograph. (B) Platelets after spreading for 10 min on a surface coated with the tethered ligand TRAP for PAR-1. When platelets adhere, they spread and protrude filopodia. (C) Platelet activated in solution and photographed after fixation, rapid-freezing, freeze-drying, and metal casting in an electron microscope. The bars are 5 μm in A and B, and 1 μm in C.

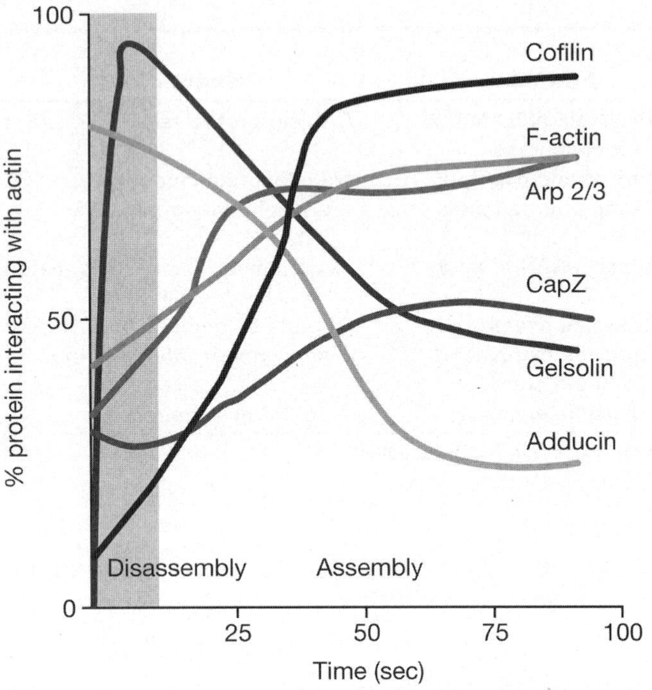

Figure 4 Regulation of platelet shape change. Platelet shape change is controlled by proteins that control the assembly/disassembly of cytoskeletal F-actin. **Disassembly.** Gelsolin and cofilin are activated while adducin is inactivated. Gelsolin and cofilin cooperate to fragment and disassemble the resting platelet actin cytoskeleton. Adducin dissociation loosens the membrane skeleton and allows it to be collected in the cell center. **Assembly.** Gelsolin inactivation provides actin fragments onto which the actin-related protein (Arp) 2/3 complex binds and nucleates a second filament. The actin assembly reaction is terminated by the binding of CapZ to the barbed filament ends.

Disruption of the Resting Actin Cytoskeleton

Before new actin assembly is used to construct filopodia and lamellae, the actin-based cytoskeleton of the resting platelet is reorganized. Reorganization is mediated by the activation of two proteins, gelsolin and cofilin, which combine to fragment actin filaments and promote net F-actin disassembly (Fig 4). Resting platelets contain copious amounts of both proteins: 5 μm gelsolin (20,000 copies per cell) and 25 μm cofilin (100,000 copies per cell). Gelsolin is a potent actin filament protein that severs and caps barbed ends. Cofilin also severs filaments and promotes the disassembly of actin subunits from the pointed end of the filaments. Gelsolin is activated when cytosolic free calcium rises into the micron range. Calcium binding mediates a conformational change in gelsolin that allows it to bind to filaments, interdigitate, and fragment them. After fragmentation, gelsolin remains tightly bound to the barbed end of the fragmented filament and can only be removed by polyphosphoinositides. Cofilin is also inactivated by polyphosphoinositide binding and by phosphorylation at serine 3. At rest, greater than 98% of gelsolin is free (not active) in platelets; however, following treatment with thrombin, gelsolin complexes to actin in seconds, an event inhibited by chelation of cytosolic calcium. In a similar fashion, cofilin, which is mostly phosphorylated in the resting platelet, is dephosphorylated in a slower reaction that requires 15 to 60 seconds to become maximal.[16] Hence, gelsolin becomes mobilized, then gelsolin-mediated filament severing is followed by cofilin activation. It is the combined activity of these two proteins, and the release of adducin from spectrin-actin, that remodels both the resting membrane and actin skeletons.

Assembly of Filopodia and Lamellipodia

Lamellae

Lamellae are broad, actin filament-rich sheets that can grow to large (many μm^2) sizes. They are used for cell spreading and locomotion. Platelets do not polarize and move directionally over a surface, as do motile cells such as leukocytes, but activated platelets spread on surfaces using circumferential lamellae. This uses large amounts of F-actin, and platelet activation doubles the content of cellular F-actin as filaments form and elongate from their barbed ends (barbed end growth).

Two convergent pathways are used in platelets to initiate actin assembly: fragmentation/uncapping of barbed filament ends, and activation of the actin-related protein (Arp) 2/3 complex, which nucleates filaments. Actin assembly is initiated when actin filament templates with exposed barbed ends are brought into contact with activated Arp 2/3 complexes. In platelets, barbed ends are provided by the severing activity of gelsolin and, to a lesser extent, of cofilin, as discussed above. After severing actin filaments, gelsolin bound to the barbed end of actin filaments dissociates. The only known mechanism to remove gelsolin from barbed filament ends is phosphoinositide binding and, as shown in Fig 4, approximately 50% of the bound gelsolin dissociates during times of maximal actin filament assembly. Experiments on platelets from transgenic mice lacking gelsolin have demonstrated the importance of gelsolin in the actin assembly reaction: gelsolin-null platelets mount only a poor actin assembly reaction, and the final actin filament content of cells responding to a variety of agonists is reduced by approximately 80% when compared with that of normal platelets. Cofilin may also participate in the production of filament ends,[17] particularly under conditions where calcium does not rise to the levels required to activate gelsolin. As with gelsolin, experiments in cultured cells have revealed that Arp 2/3 function may also be dependent on cofilin severing activity.[18,19]

Once barbed ends are exposed, actin assembly is amplified by the activity of the Arp 2/3 complex. This complex binds to the actin filament templates near their barbed ends, and nucleates a second filament from these sites. Platelets express 2 to 3 μm of the Arp 2/3 complex, of which approximately 40% is bound to the resting cytoskeleton. Upon activation, this amount increases to around 70% to 80% of total Arp 2/3 levels during the actin assembly reaction (Fig 4). Upstream proteins and phospholipids regulate the targeting of Arp 2/3 to the plasma membrane and activate its nucleation activity. Upstream proteins that bind to Arp 2/3 complex and stimulate its nucleation activity include cortactin and the Wiskott-Aldrich syndrome protein (WASp) family members, including WASp, neuronal WASp (N-WASp), and the WASp family verprolin-homologous (WAVE) proteins, although the relative role of each protein in platelet actin assembly remains to be determined. WASp-null platelets from both humans and mice have normal actin assembly reactions[20,21] but circulate poorly, accounting for the severe thrombocytopenia of patients with the human Wiskott-Aldrich Syndrome, whose myeloid cells lack WASp. Platelets express predominantly WAVE-2,[22] which has been reported to interact with Abi1, IRSp53 and rac to induce the nucleation activity of the complex. It has become widely accepted that nucleation by the Arp 2/3 complex generates the branched networks of actin that fill lamellipodia and, from many studies of platelets, it is clear that Arp 2/3 complex concentrates within lamellar actin filament networks.[23] However, in the absence of gelsolin function or without the addition of actin filament fragments in vitro, Arp 2/3 complex is a poor nucleator of actin assembly. In cells lacking gelsolin, Arp 2/3 complex no longer concentrates lamellae and is instead found in disorganized actin foci. Actin filament assembly is terminated by CapZ, a protein that constitutively caps exposed barbed filament ends in cells.

Signaling to Actin Assembly/Disassembly

A main focus in the field is to define how signals lead to actin assembly, particularly how signals can generate different actin ultrastructures such as filopodia or lamellipodia. In platelets, which circulate in blood containing relatively high levels of free calcium, calcium-initiated pathways are central in controlling actin assembly/disassembly and shape change. For example, the activation of platelets under conditions that prevent increases in cytosolic calcium results in aberrant cell shape change and poor actin filaments. Prime targets of calcium in platelets include gelsolin, myosin, and FLN. Internal calcium release results from the breakdown of phosphatidylinositol 4,5 bisphosphate ($PI_{4,5}P_2$) into diacylglycerol and inositol trisphosphate, and this pathway has been shown to increase cytosolic calcium into the micron range. Platelets can also import external calcium to drive shape change, leading to free calcium concentrations of 10 μm in the cell.

Resting platelets maintain high concentrations (approximately 200 μm) of both phosphatidylinositol 4 phosphate (PI_4P) and $PI_{4,5}P_2$. Following platelet activation by agonists, $PI_{4,5}P_2$ is hydrolyzed by phospholipase Cγ or β (depending on the agonist), causing an initial decrease in the $PI_{4,5}P_2$ concentration in the platelet. $PI_{4,5}P_2$ content is rapidly restored following platelet activation and, in fact, increases to levels 40% greater than those maintained by the resting cell (280 μm) within 15 s. Newly synthesized $PI_{4,5}P_2$ in the plasma membrane can collect actin regulatory proteins that not only interact with the membrane through their pH domains, but also inactivate capping proteins of all classes and participate in the activation of WASp family members.[24] Platelets express two pleckstrin isoforms, and the pleckstrin family of proteins is likely to be intimately involved in the regulation of phosphatidylinositol metabolism.

Small guanosine triphosphatases (GTPases) are intimately involved in the regulation of actin ultrastructure in platelets as in other motile cells. As in other cells, evidence has accumulated that rac controls lamellipodia extension while cdc42 is more involved in filopodial extension. Critical downstream targets of rac include PIP-5 kinase and WAVE. Cdc42 is known to interact with, and activate, both WASp and N-WASp.

Filopodia

Filopodia are long thin processes with actin filament bundle cores. They are protruded from the surface of all eukaryotic cells, but come in a diverse variety of shapes and sizes. Filopodia are prominent in platelets, particularly at very early times following activation when extremely long, thin filopodia are extended. They also appear later on the apical surface of adherent platelets, where they appear to be used to probe around the cell margins. In general, a coalescence of filaments appears to form the bundles that fill filopodia, and this mechanism has recently been reported to be the origin of all filopodia.[25] Despite their abundance on platelets, their mechanism of formation is poorly understood.

Nobes and Hall[26] showed that cdc42 activation causes filopodial growth in fibroblasts. Others have suggested that WASp/N-WASp is also involved,[27] and that WASp/WASP mediates signaling from cdc42 to Arp2/3 complex. GTP-Cdc42 binds to WASp/N-WASp in vitro,[28-32] and, in combination with D4 phosphoinositides, opens the WASp molecule, allowing it to bind to the Arp2/3 complex through its C-terminal VCA domain.[33,34] In turn, this activates the nucleation activity of Arp2/3 complex. However, this model for cdc42-mediated filopodia, while widely cited, fails to explain certain observations. First, cdc42-coated beads do not grow actin filament bundles in vitro, but instead assemble actin rocket tails composed of actin filament networks. Second, N-WASp–deficient fibroblasts and WASp/N-WASp–deficient platelets make abundant filopodia when stimulated, and the platelets have normal—perhaps even enhanced—actin assembly responses to ligation of PAR-1 and GP6. Third, Arp2/3 nucleation stimulated by WASp (or its Arp 2/3 activating VCA domain) is slow[35,36] unless F-actin barbed ends are added into the mix.[23] Recently, it has been reported that filopodial growth in cells can be promoted by modulating the activity of CapZ in cells.[25]. One family of proteins that appears to have this capacity is VASP/Mena,[37] originally shown to participate in the delivery of actin monomers to the barbed ends of growing filaments. Hence, critical intermediaries in the cdc42 pathway of platelets remain to be identified. Cdc42 is activated following ligation of PAR-1,[38] and addition of constitutively active cdc42 to n-octyl-β-D-glucopyranoside-permeabilized platelets leads to barbed end exposure, but quantitatively much less than the response to activated rac. The drastically different organization of filopodia versus lamellipodia in platelets is a wonderful opportunity to learn how different cell signaling pathways lead to diverse actin architectures.

References

1. Harker LA, Finch CA: Thrombokinetics in man. J Clin Invest 48:963-974, 1969
2. Italiano J Jr, Lecine P, Shivdasani RA, Hartwig JH: Blood platelets are assembled principally at the ends of proplatelet processes produced by differentiated megakaryocytes. J Cell Biol 147:1299-1312, 1999
3. Italiano J Jr, Bergmeier W, Tiwari S, Falet H, Hartwig JH, Hoffmeister KM, et al: Mechanisms and implications of platelet discoid shape. Blood 101:4789-4796, 2003
4. Lecine P, Italiano JE Jr, Kim SW, Villeval JL, Shivdasani RA: Hematopoietic-specific B1 tubulin participates in a pathway of platelet biogenesis dependent on the transcription factor NF-E2. Blood 96:1366-1373, 2000
5. Freson K, De Vos R, Wittevrongel C, Thys C, Defoor J, Vanhees L, et al: The β1-tubulin Q43P functional polymorphism reduces the risk of cardiovascular disease in men by modulating platelet function and structure. Blood 106:2356-2362, 2005
6. White J, Krivit W: An ultrastructural basis for the shape changes induced in platelets by chilling. Blood 30:625-635, 1967
7. Patel SR, Richardson JL, Schulze H, Kahle E, Galjart N, Drabek K, et al: Differential roles of microtubule assembly and sliding in proplatelet formation by megakaryocytes. Blood 106:4076-4085, 2005
8. Richardson J, et al: Mechanisms of organelle transport and capture along proplatelets during platelet production. Blood, 2005 (in press)
9. Barkalow K, Italiano JE Jr, Chou DE, Matsuoka Y, Bennett V, Hartwig JH: Alpha-adducin dissociates from F-actin filaments and spectrin during platelet activation. J Cell Biol 161:557-570, 2003
10. Gorlin J, Yamin R, Egan S, Stewart M, Stossel TP, Kwiatkowski DJ, et al: Human endothelial actin-binding protein (ABP-280, non-muscle filamin): A molecular leaf spring. J Cell Biol 111:1089-1105, 1990
11. Hartwig JH, DeSisto M: The cytoskeleton of the resting human blood platelet: Structure of the membrane skeleton and its attachment to actin filaments. J Cell Biol 112:407-425, 1991
12. Kovacsovics TJ, Hartwig JH: Thrombin-induced GPIb-IX centralization on the platelet surface requires actin assembly and myosin II activation. Blood 87:618-629, 1996
13. Ware J, Russell S, Ruggeri ZM: Generation and rescue of a murine model of platelet dysfunction: The Bernard-Soulier syndrome. Proc Natl Acad Sci USA 97:2803-2808, 2000
14. Bernard J, Soulier J: Sur une nouvelle variété de dystrophie thrombocytaire hemorragique congenitale. Sem Hop Paris 24:3217-3223, 1948
15. Matsuoka Y, Li X, Bennett V: Adducin: structure, function, and regulation. Cell Mol Life Sci 57:884-895, 2000
16. Falet H, Chang G, Brohard-Bohn B, Rendu F, Hartwig JH: Integrin αIIbβ3 signals lead to cofilin to accelerate platelet actin dynamics. Am J Physiol Cell Physiol 289:C819-C825, 2005
17. Ichetovkin I, Grant W, Condeelis J: Cofilin produces newly polymerized actin filaments that are preferred for dendritic nucleation by Arp2/3 complex. Curr Biol 12:79-84, 2002
18. Chan A, Bailly M, Zebda N, Segall JE, Condeelis JS: Role of cofilin in epidermal growth factor-stimulated actin polymerization and lamellipod protrusion. J Cell Biol 148:531-542, 2000
19. Ghosh M, Song X, Mouneimne G, Sidani M, Lawrence DS, Condeelis JS: Cofilin promotes actin polymerization and defines the direction of cell motility. Science 304:743-746, 2004
20. Gross BS, Wilde JI, Quek L, Chapel H, Nelson DL, Watson SP: Regulation and function of WASp in platelets by the collagen receptor, glycoprotein VI. Blood 94:4166-4176, 2000
21. Falet H, Hoffmeister KM, Neujahr R, Hartwig JH: Normal Arp2/3 complex activation in platelets lacking WASp. Blood 100:2113-2122, 2002
22. Oda A, Miki H, Wada I, Yamaguchi H, Yamazaki D, Suetsugu S, et al: WAVE/Scars in platelets. Blood 105:3141-3148, 2005
23. Falet H, Hoffmeister KM, Neujahr R, Italiano JE Jr, Stossel TP, Southwick FS, et al: Importance of free actin filament barbed ends for Arp2/3 complex function in platelets and fibroblasts. Proc Natl Acad Sci USA 99:16782-16788, 2002
24. Rozelle A, Machesky LM, Yamamoto M, Driessens MH, Insall RH, Roth MG, et al: Phosphatidylinositol 4,5-bisphosphate induces actin-based movement of raft-enriched vesicles through WASP-Arp2/3. Curr Biol 10:311-320, 2000
25. Mejillano MR, Kojima S, Applewhite DA, Gertler FB, Svitkina TM, Borisy GG: Lamellipodial versus filopodial mode of the actin nanomachinery: Pivotal role of the filament barbed end. Cell 118:363-373, 2004
26. Nobes CD, Hall A: Rho, rac, and cdc42 GTPases regulate the assembly of multimolecular focal complexes associated with actin stress fibers, lamellipodia, and filopodia. Cell 81:53-62, 1995
27. Miki H, Sasaki T, Takai Y, Takenawa T: Induction of filopodium formation by a WASP-related actin-depolymerizing protein N-WASP. Nature 391:93-96, 1998
28. Aspenstrom P, Lindberg U, Hall A: Two GTPases, Cdc42 and Rac, bind directly to a protein implicated in the immunodeficiency disorder Wiskott-Aldrich syndrome. Curr Biol 6:70-75, 1996
29. Kolluri R, Tolias KF, Carpenter CL, Rosen FS, Kirchhausen T: Direct interaction of the Wiskott-Aldrich syndrome protein with the GTPase Cdc42. Proc Natl Acad Sci USA 93:5615-5618, 1996
30. Symons M, Derry JM, Karlak B, Jiang S, Lemahieu V, Mccormick F, et al: Wiskott-Aldrich syndrome protein, a novel effector for the GTPase CDC42Hs, is implicated in actin polymerization. Cell 84:723-734, 1996
31. Kato M, Miki H, Imai K, Nonoyama S, Suzuki T, Sasakawa C, et al: Wiskott-Aldrich syndrome protein induces actin clustering without direct binding to Cdc42. J Biol Chem 274:27225-27230, 1999
32. Higgs HN, Pollard TD: Activation by Cdc42 and PIP2 of Wiskott-Aldrich syndrome protein (WASp) stimulates actin nucleation by Arp2/3 complex. J Cell Biol 150:1311-1320, 2000
33. Rohatgi R, Ma L, Miki H, Lopez M, Kirchhausen T, Takenawa T, et al: The interaction between N-WASP and the Arp2/3 complex links Cdc42-dependent signals to actin assembly. Cell 97:221-231, 1999
34. Le Clainche C, Didry D, Carlier MF, Pantaloni D: Activation of Arp2/3 complex by Wiskott-Aldrich syndrome protein is linked to enhanced binding of ATP to Arp2. J Biol Chem 276:46689-46692, 2001
35. Zigmond SH, Joyce M, Yang C, Brown K, Huang M, Pring M: Mechanism of Cdc42-induced actin polymerization in neutrophil extracts. J Cell Biol 142:1001-1012, 1998
36. Zigmond SH, Joyce M, Borleis J, Bokoch GM, Devreotes PN: Regulation of actin polymerization in cell-free systems by GTPgammaS and Cdc42. J Cell Biol 138:363-374, 1997
37. Gertler FB, Niebuhr K, Reinhard M, Wehland J, Soriano P: Mena, a relative of VASP and Drosophila Enabled, is implicated in the control of microfilament dynamics. Cell 87:227-239, 1996
38. Azim AC, Barkalow K, Chou J, Hartwig JH: Activation of the small GTPases, rac and cdc42, following ligation of the platelet PAR-1 receptor. Blood 95:959-964, 2000

ELSEVIER

Seminars in
HEMATOLOGY

Advances in Gene Therapy Using Factor VIIa in Hemophilia

Paris Margaritis[a] and Katherine A. High[a,b]

The development of recombinant activated factor VII (rFVIIa; NovoSeven®, Novo Nordisk, Bagsvaerd, Denmark) has provided an effective, alternative treatment strategy for hemophilia patients with inhibitors. However, its short half-life necessitates frequent infusions and results in high treatment costs. One potential solution to this problem may lie in the use of FVIIa gene transfer, which would achieve long-lasting therapeutic levels of expression from a single injection. Studies in animal models have shown that a recombinant adeno-associated viral vector can be used to insert both murine and human FVIIa into murine liver. Following FVIIa gene transfer, mice with hemophilia B demonstrated a long-term, dose-dependent increase in circulating levels of FVIIa, reduced prothrombin time, and correction of activated partial thromboplastin time into the normal range. In addition, blood loss following a modified tail-clip assay was significantly reduced. Ongoing studies in mice engineered to express a wide range of FVIIa levels aim to analyze organ histology and evaluate long-term survival, reproductive fitness, and real-time in vivo clot formation in the microvasculature. These studies are expanding our knowledge of the effects of continuously expressed rFVIIa, and it is hoped that they may eventually provide a new avenue for treatment of hemophilia.
Semin Hematol 43(suppl 1):S101-S104

Hemophilia is an X-linked bleeding disorder caused by mutations in the genes encoding factor VIII (FVIII; hemophilia A) or factor IX (FIX; hemophilia B). The disease is currently treated by repeated intravenous infusions of plasma-derived or recombinant clotting factor, given either prophylactically or in response to bleeds. The major complication of current treatment is the formation of neutralizing antibodies (inhibitors) to the infused protein in approximately 20% of patients with hemophilia A and 3% of those with hemophilia B.[1-5] Management of acute bleeding episodes in patients with inhibitors can be achieved with so-called bypassing agents. The initially available bypassing agents had variable efficacy,[6,7] although the development of recombinant activated factor VII (rFVIIa; NovoSeven®; Novo Nordisk, Bagsvaerd, Denmark) has provided a successful alternative for patients with hemophilia and inhibitors.[8,9]

In vivo, FVII is synthesized as a zymogen in the liver (Fig 1). As a component of the extrinsic coagulation pathway, FVII combines with tissue factor to form a complex that catalyzes conversion of FX to activated FX (Fig 2A). This circumvents either a deficiency of, or inhibitors to, FVIII or FIX. The rFVIIa protein product is synthesized as the zymogen form and activated by cleavage of the Arg^{152}–Ile^{153} bond during the purification process (Fig 2B). Recombinant FVIIa effects hemostasis when infused at supraphysiologic doses (90 μg/kg). However, it has a short half-life (around 2.7 hours), which necessitates frequent infusions and results in high treatment costs. Continuous infusion, with the goal of maintaining a relatively constant plasma concentration, has been proposed as an alternative to bolus infusion since it results in lower overall consumption and cost. It is worth noting however, that efficacy with rFVIIa treatment is related to the dose regimen used, especially in surgical settings,[9] as well as the delay in the onset of treatment.[10] In some cases, augmented continuous infusion using a higher bolus dose (160 to 180 μg/kg) followed by continuous infusion of 30 μg/kg/h has been more successful[11] than a regular bolus dose followed by continuous infusion of approximately 15 μg/kg/h. Lastly, high-dose regimens (>200 μg/kg) have been shown to be more effective than continuous infusion regimens[12] or lower dosing regimens.[13]

[a]The Children's Hospital of Philadelphia, Philadelphia, PA.
[b]Howard Hughes Medical Institute, Chevy Chase, MD.
Address correspondence to Katherine High, The Children's Hospital of Philadelphia, 3615 Civic Center Blvd, 302 Abramson Research Center, Philadelphia, PA 19104. E-mail: high@email.chop.edu

0037-1963/06/$-see front matter © 2006 Elsevier Inc. All rights reserved.
doi:10.1053/j.seminhematol.2005.11.015

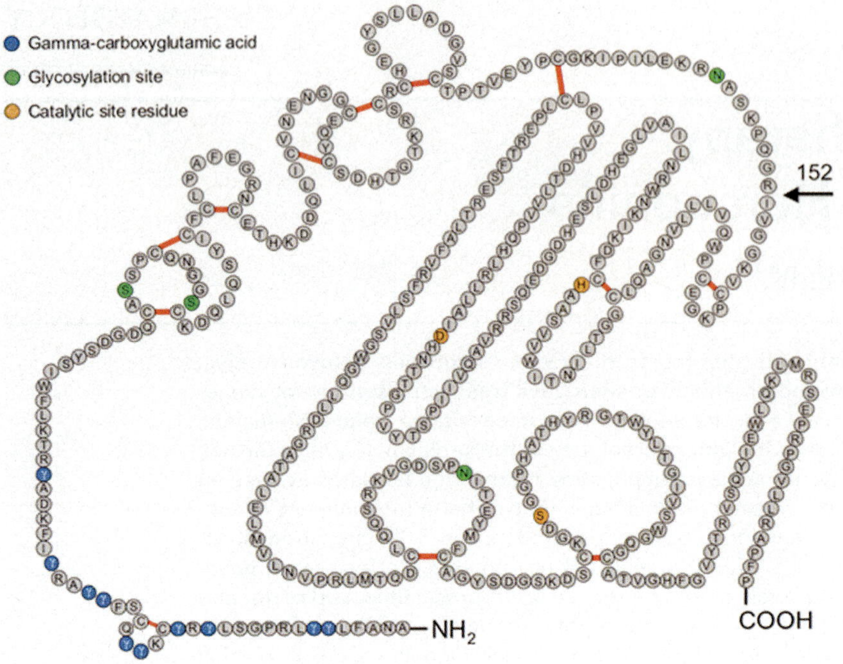

Figure 1 Amino acid sequence of mature human factor VII. The N-terminal Gla domain facilitates binding to phospholipids. This is followed by two EGF-like domains, then a catalytic domain. Activation requires cleavage of the Arg^{152}–Ile^{153} bond (marked with arrow).

Factor VIIa Gene Transfer

We have been interested in the use of gene transfer as a method of achieving hemostasis in people with hemophilia. In previous work, we have shown long-term expression of FIX in a large-animal model of hemophilia B after hepatic artery (or portal vein) infusion of a recombinant adeno-associated viral (AAV) vector (vide infra) expressing FIX.[14] The obvious advantage of this approach is that the animal can achieve therapeutic levels of expression that last for years from a single injection of vector. Such an approach would also be attractive for the expression of FVIIa, since continuous expression at appropriate levels would obviate problems arising from the short half-life of the protein. We sought to determine whether AAV-mediated expression of FVIIa could correct the hemostatic defect in animals with hemophilia.

Before discussing our experimental approach to continuous expression of FVIIa, it is appropriate to provide some background information on the use of AAV vectors in the setting of genetic disease. Adeno-associated viral vectors have been engineered from a naturally occurring parvovirus, AAV serotype 2. The wild-type virus has a 4.7-kb, single-stranded DNA genome; humans are the natural hosts, but the virus is a dependovirus and can only replicate in the presence of a helper virus such as adenovirus or herpesvirus. In fact, AAV was initially isolated as a contaminant of adenovirus (hence the name) from respiratory secretions of adenovirus-infected individuals.[15] A substantial percentage of the population carries antibodies to AAV, probably as a result of a respiratory tract infection during childhood occurring in the context of a concomitant adenoviral infection. In the mid 1990s, two groups reported that a recombinant AAV vector could direct long-term expression of a gene after introduction into skeletal muscle in mice.[16-18] This represented an important advance, at least in terms of genetic disease: in contrast to retroviral vectors, one could achieve efficient transduction even in nondividing target cells and, in contrast to adenoviral vectors, one could achieve long-term expression. The minimal cellular immune response evoked by AAV vectors also stood in stark contrast to the results achieved with adenoviral vectors.[19] Subsequent work by a number of laboratories established that AAV-2 vectors had tropism for several tissues, including liver, brain (including the retina), respiratory tract[16,17,20-22] and skeletal muscle, and that efficient transduc-

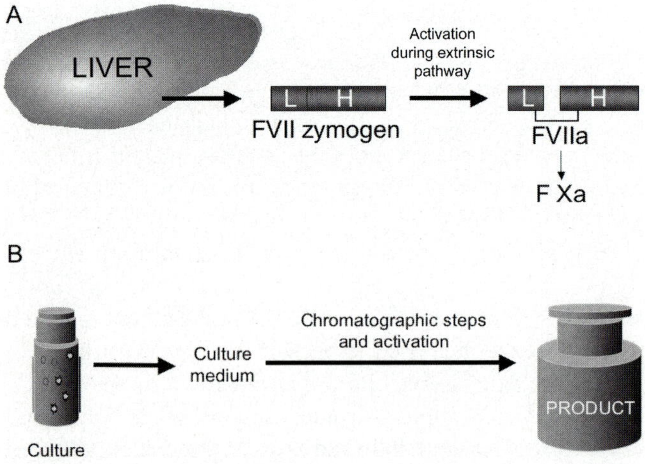

Figure 2 (A) Generation of human activated FVII (FVIIa) under physiologic conditions. FVII is synthesized as a zymogen in the liver and, through the extrinsic pathway of blood coagulation, is activated through proteolytic cleavage at position 152 to give rise to a two-chain (L, light chain; H, heavy chain) active molecule. Factor VIIa forms a complex with tissue factor to activate factor X (FX) to FXa. (B) Generation of recombinant human FVIIa (rFVIIa). Culture medium containing zymogen human FVII undergoes a series of chromatographic steps and activation to yield FVIIa.

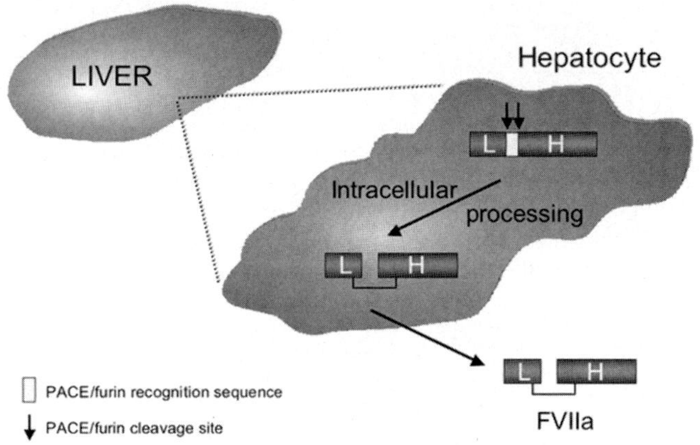

Figure 3 Gene transfer approach. A modified transgene that contains a recognition sequence (at the normal site of cleavage) for the intracellular protease, PACE/furin, is expressed in the liver. During protein expression, PACE/furin cleaves (arrows) the protein, thus generating a two-chain molecule that is secreted as FVIIa.

tion of these tissues was observed in both mice and large-animal models (including dogs and non-human primates). In particular, it was possible to achieve long-term (>3 years, with observation still ongoing) expression of FIX at therapeutic levels (5% to 10% normal) in the dog model of hemophilia B using a recombinant AAV vector infused into the liver.[14]

Given the success of long-term expression of a transgene with an AAV vector, we were interested in determining whether we could express FVIIa at therapeutically relevant levels in hemophilic animal models. It is worth noting that, if problems related to the cost and half-life of rFVIIa could be solved, the management of patients with hemophilia could be simplified; all patients, not just those with inhibitors, could be treated with AAV-FVIIa. The risk of inhibitor formation would be eliminated, since FVIIa is nonimmunogenic; all hemophilia patients are tolerant to FVIIa since it is an endogenous protein.

In order to test the feasibility of this treatment strategy, we first had to develop a transgene that could be secreted directly into the circulation as FVIIa. Factor VII is normally synthesized as a zymogen, and is activated by the cleavage of the Arg^{152}–Ile^{153} bond. The rFVIIa protein product is also synthesized as a zymogen and activated during the purification process. Our plan was to transduce liver with a vector expressing FVIIa; to achieve this, we needed a construct that could be cleaved *intracellularly* to generate FVIIa. We thus chose to introduce cleavage sites for the intracellular PACE/furin protease at the relevant site in the human FVII sequence (Fig 3). We tested three different cleavage sites in a cell culture system, and discovered that the one that underwent cleavage most efficiently (and therefore had the highest activity) was the construct containing the sequence RKRRKR. We then constructed an AAV vector expressing this construct under the control of a liver-specific promoter, and introduced the vector at a range of doses into the portal vein of mice with hemophilia B. The mice showed a dose-dependent increase in circulating levels of human FVIIa, as determined by an enzyme-linked immunosorbent assay (ELISA); those receiving a lower dose of approximately 1×10^{11} vector genomes (vg) per mouse had circulating levels in the range of 100 to 200 ng/mL FVIIa, while those receiving a 10-fold higher dose exhibited circulating levels of 700 to 1,000 ng/mL.

The FVIIa Transgene Induces Hemostasis

We had chosen to work with the human transgene initially, since antibodies for tracking human FVIIa levels are available. However, it is difficult to analyze the effects of human FVIIa on hemostasis in a mouse, since murine tissue factor does not interact well with human FVIIa. To assess the effects of the transgene on hemostasis, we constructed a second AAV vector, this one expressing mouse FVIIa (mFVIIa) under the control of a liver-specific promoter. Preliminary experiments in tissue culture established that introduction of the RKRRKR cleavage site in mFVII also resulted in efficient cleavage to mFVIIa. When the vector expressing this construct was introduced into the hepatic circulation of mice with hemophilia B, it resulted in long-term expression of mFVIIa, shortening of the prothrombin time (PT), and correction of the activated partial thromboplastin time (aPTT) into the normal range. The correction of the aPTT was remarkable, decreasing from a baseline of approximately 60 to 70 seconds to 30 to 35 seconds. In addition, a tail-clip bleeding time assay also showed correction after AAV-mFVIIa infusion into hemophilic mice. This assay, developed to monitor the adequacy of hemostasis in hemophilic mice, is usually carried out by cutting a pre-warmed (37°C in normal saline) mouse tail with a diameter of 3 mm, and measuring time to clot formation. A hemophilic mouse generally does not form a stable clot and exsanguinates within 24 hours of the tail clip. To minimize loss of vector-injected mice through exsanguination, we modified this assay to measure total blood loss over 10 minutes, at which point the tail was cauterized. Using this modified assay, we showed that expression of mFVIIa at levels of approximately 1,200 ng/mL resulted in statistically significant reduction of blood loss after tail clip compared with untreated mice with hemophilia B, although blood loss was not reduced to the minimal levels seen in hemostatically normal mice after tail clip.

Ongoing Studies

A crucial safety question raised by the gene transfer strategy for FVIIa is whether continuous expression of FVIIa could be associated with an increased risk of thrombosis. We sought to study this effect over a range of levels of expression in a transgenic mouse model. Using the same engineered mFVIIa as used for the AAV vector, we have generated mice with circulating mFVIIa levels ranging from just above physiologic levels, to as much as 7 μg/mL. Characterization of these mice in terms of long-term survival, histologic analysis of organs, reproductive fitness, and real-time in vivo clot formation in the microvasculature is underway. The goal of these studies is to define levels of FVIIa that are high enough to provide hemostasis but low enough to avoid any risk of increased thrombosis.

An intriguing area for further study is the correlation of mFVIIa effect on hemostasis assays in the microcirculation (in vivo thrombus formation in the cremaster arteriole) and in the macrocirculation (eg, $FeCl_3$ model). It is possible, for example, that increased levels of FVIIa may be adequate to provide hemostasis in the microcirculation, which is rich in tissue factor, without improving hemostatic efficacy in the macrocirculation.

In a second line of studies, we are interested in extending this work to the large-animal model of hemophilia. To this end, we have cloned the canine FVII (cFVII) gene and engineered it so that it can be processed in the liver and secreted directly in the active (cFVIIa) form (vide supra) (unpublished data). The advantage of the hemophilia dog model is that these animals experience bleeding episodes at a well-characterized rate over time; thus, it is possible to follow a clinical endpoint that is relevant to human disease. An eventual goal of these studies will be to place expression under the control of an inducible promoter, so that levels of FVIIa can be raised or lowered depending on the clinical situation.[23]

Conclusions

Preliminary work suggests that FVIIa gene transfer is feasible. However, our understanding of this process as a therapeutic strategy remains incomplete. Whether the studies outlined above can eventually provide a new avenue for the treatment of hemophilia is unclear, but they are certainly expanding our knowledge of the hemostatic effects of continuously expressed FVIIa.

References

1. Addiego J, Kasper C, Abilgaard C, Hilgartner M, Lusher J, Glader B, et al: Frequency of inhibitor development in haemophiliacs treated with low-purity factor VIII. Lancet 342:462-464, 1993
2. Bray GL, Gomperts ED, Courter S, Gruppo R, Gordon EM, Manco-Johnson M, et al: A multicenter study of recombinant factor VIII (recombinate): Safety, efficacy, and inhibitor risk in previously untreated patients with hemophilia A. The Recombinate Study Group. Blood 83:2428-2435, 1994
3. Hoyer LW: The incidence of factor VIII inhibitors in patients with severe hemophilia A. Adv Exp Med Biol 386:35-45, 1995
4. Lusher JM, Arkin S, Abildgaard CF, Schwartz RS: Recombinant factor VIII for the treatment of previously untreated patients with hemophilia A. Safety, efficacy, and development of inhibitors. Kogenate Previously Untreated Patient Study Group. N Engl J Med 328:453-459, 1993
5. Strauss HS: Acquired circulating anticoagulants in hemophilia A. N Engl J Med 281:866-873, 1969
6. Sjamsoedin LJ, Heijnen L, Mauser-Bunschoten EP, van Geijlswijk JL, van Houwelingen H, van Asten P, et al: The effect of activated prothrombin-complex concentrate (FEIBA) on joint and muscle bleeding in patients with hemophilia A and antibodies to factor VIII. A double-blind clinical trial. N Engl J Med 305:717-721, 1981
7. Lusher JM, Blatt PM, Penner JA, Aledort LM, Levine PH, White GC, et al: Autoplex versus proplex: A controlled, double-blind study of effectiveness in acute hemarthroses in hemophiliacs with inhibitors to factor VIII. Blood 62:1135-1138, 1983
8. Key NS, Aledort LM, Beardsley D, Cooper HA, Davignon G, Ewenstein BM, et al: Home treatment of mild to moderate bleeding episodes using recombinant factor VIIa (Novoseven) in haemophiliacs with inhibitors. Thromb Haemost 80:912-918, 1998
9. Shapiro AD, Gilchrist GS, Hoots WK, Cooper HA, Gastineau DA: Prospective, randomised trial of two doses of rFVIIa (NovoSeven) in haemophilia patients with inhibitors undergoing surgery. Thromb Haemost 80:773-778, 1998
10. Lusher JM: Acute hemarthroses: the benefits of early versus late treatment with recombinant activated factor VII. Blood Coagul Fibrinolysis 11:S45-S49, 2000 (suppl 1)
11. Kenet G, Lubetsky A, Gitel S, Luboshitz J, Varon D, Martinowitz U: Treatment of bleeding episodes in patients with hemophilia and an inhibitor: Comparison of two treatment protocols with recombinant activated factor VII. Blood Coagul Fibrinolysis 11:S35-S38, 2000 (suppl 1)
12. Kenet G, Lubetsky A, Luboshitz J, Martinowitz U: A new approach to treatment of bleeding episodes in young hemophilia patients: A single bolus megadose of recombinant activated factor VII (NovoSeven). J Thromb Haemost 1:450-455, 2003
13. Parameswaran R, Shapiro AD, Gill JC, Kessler CM: Dose effect and efficacy of rFVIIa in the treatment of haemophilia patients with inhibitors: Analysis from the Hemophilia and Thrombosis Research Society Registry. Haemophilia 11:100-106, 2005
14. Mount JD, Herzog RW, Tillson DM, Goodman SA, Robinson N, McCleland ML, et al: Sustained phenotypic correction of hemophilia B dogs with a factor IX null mutation by liver-directed gene therapy. Blood 99:2670-2676, 2002
15. Blacklow NR, Hoggan MD, Sereno MS, Brandt CD, Kim HW, Parrott RH, et al: A seroepidemiologic study of adenovirus-associated virus infection in infants and children. Am J Epidemiol 94:359-366, 1971
16. Kaplitt MG, Leone P, Samulski RJ, Xiao X, Pfaff DW, O'Malley KL, et al: Long-term gene expression and phenotypic correction using adeno-associated virus vectors in the mammalian brain. Nat Genet 8:148-154, 1994
17. Kessler PD, Podsakoff GM, Chen X, McQuiston SA, Colosi PC, Matelis LA, et al: Gene delivery to skeletal muscle results in sustained expression and systemic delivery of a therapeutic protein. Proc Natl Acad Sci U S A 93:14082-14087, 1996
18. Xiao X, Li J, Samulski RJ: Efficient long-term gene transfer into muscle tissue of immunocompetent mice by adeno-associated virus vector. J Virol 70:8098-8108, 1996
19. Gallo-Penn AM, Shirley PS, Andrews JL, Tinlin S, Webster S, Cameron C, et al: Systemic delivery of an adenoviral vector encoding canine factor VIII results in short-term phenotypic correction, inhibitor development, and biphasic liver toxicity in hemophilia A dogs. Blood 97: 107-113, 2001
20. Flotte TR, Afione SA, Conrad C, McGrath SA, Solow R, Oka H, et al: Stable in vivo expression of the cystic fibrosis transmembrane conductance regulator with an adeno-associated virus vector. Proc Natl Acad Sci U S A 90:10613-10617, 1993
21. Flotte TR, Carter BJ: Adeno-associated virus vectors for gene therapy. Gene Ther 2:357-362, 1995
22. Snyder RO, Xiao X: Vectors for gene therapy. Curr Prot Genet 12.01-12.1.24, 1996 (Suppl 10)
23. Rivera VM, Wang X, Wardwell S, Courage NL, Volchuk A, Keenan T, et al: Regulation of protein secretion through controlled aggregation in the endoplasmic reticulum. Science 287:826-830, 2000

ELSEVIER

Seminars in
HEMATOLOGY

Mechanism of Action of Recombinant Activated Factor VII: An Update

Ulla Hedner

Bleeding episodes in patients with hemophilia and inhibitors must be managed using agents that are hemostatically active in the absence of factor VIII or IX. Activated prothrombin complex concentrates have long been used in this context. However, the search for safer and more effective agents has led to the development of recombinant activated factor VII (rFVIIa; NovoSeven®, Novo Nordisk, Bagsvaerd, Denmark). This paper presents an update on the mechanism of action of rFVIIa, and describes how pharmacologic doses of this agent enhance thrombin production and thus contribute to the development of a stable, lysis-resistant fibrin plug at the site of vessel damage. This mechanism explains the reported efficacy of rFVIIa in a range of clinical situations characterized by impaired thrombin generation.
Semin Hematol 43(suppl 1):S105-S107

In patients with hemophilia complicated by inhibitory antibodies, hemostasis must be achieved with agents that are hemostatically active in the absence of factor VIII (FVIII) or IX (FIX). Activated prothrombin complex concentrates (aPCCs) containing both activated coagulation proteins and zymogens are still widely used for this purpose. To date, only two controlled studies have compared an aPCC with a non-activated PCC in this context, and both were published in the early 1980s.[1,2] The trials demonstrated an efficacy rate of approximately 50% to 65% for aPCCs. In addition, the reported association of these concentrates with thromboembolic events means that their efficacy and safety are far from optimal.[3]

In the search for (pharmacologic) agents with greater efficacy and more robust safety profiles, activated factor VII (FVIIa) was identified as an attractive candidate. In healthy individuals and hemophilia patients, FVII circulates in its activated form (approximately 1% of the total FVII protein mass), highlighting the fact that FVIIa is not enzymatically active by itself. It must form a complex with the tissue factor (TF) that is exposed as a result of an injury to the vessel wall before it is capable of activating factor X (FX) into activated factor X (FXa). Activated FVII is not immediately inhibited by circulating antithrombin,[4] and is therefore able to find its way to the TF at the site of injury without its activity being neutralized.

Preliminary investigations showed that purified FVIIa from human plasma could induce hemostasis in two hemophilia patients with inhibitors.[5] Based on these encouraging findings, recombinant FVIIa (rFVIIa; NovoSeven®, Novo Nordisk, Bagsvaerd, Denmark) was developed for the treatment of such patients,[6,7] and subsequent studies confirmed the utility of the agent in this indication. One report demonstrated an efficacy rate of 80% to 90% when rFVIIa was used to manage serious bleeds in hemophilic inhibitor patients[8]; furthermore, the efficacy rate during major surgery, including hip and knee arthroplasty, was found to be 90% to 100%.[9,10] Today, rFVIIa is well established as an effective hemostatic treatment for hemophilia patients who develop inhibitors to FVIII or FIX.

Mechanism of Action of rFVIIa

Normal hemostasis is initiated by the formation of a complex between TF exposed as a result of vascular injury, and activated FVII already present in the circulation. Tissue factor is expressed by a number of different cells, all of which are located in the deeper layers of the vessel wall. It is a true receptor protein, and has one intramembranous and one intracellular component. The complex formed between TF and FVIIa is tight, and enzymatically activates FX on the surface of the TF-expressing cell. As a result of these initial reactions, a limited amount of thrombin is generated, and this amount is sufficient to activate the cofactors FVIII and FV. The initial

University of Lund, Sweden, and Research and Development, Novo Nordisk A/S, Bagsvaerd, Denmark.

Address correspondence to Ulla Hedner, MD, PhD, Research and Development, Novo Nordisk A/S, Krogshøjvej 55, 2880 Bagsvaerd, Denmark. E-mail: UHE@novonordisk.com

0037-1963/06/$-see front matter
doi:10.1053/j.seminhematol.2005.11.025

thrombin generation also activates platelets, leading to the exposure of negatively charged phospholipids on their surfaces.[11] The negatively charged platelet surface forms a perfect template for the formation of the tenase and prothrombinase complexes, which in turn leads to the generation of the full thrombin burst necessary for the formation of a tight and stable hemostatic fibrin plug. The tenase complex is formed when activated FIX (FIXa), generated by the TF-FVIIa complex, binds tightly to the activated platelet surface. It then complexes with activated FVIII (FVIIIa) generated by the initially formed thrombin, leading to the activation of FX and the binding of FXa to FVa on the activated platelet surface, thus forming the prothrombinase complex.

The full thrombin burst is highly important for the fibrin structure of the hemostatic plug, as demonstrated by studies suggesting that the structure and porosity of fibrin vary according to the amount of added thrombin.[12,13] Thrombin is also required for activation of factor XIII (FXIII), the fibrin-stabilizing factor necessary for the cross-linking of fibrin monomers that makes the hemostatic plug more resistant to premature lysis. Furthermore, high thrombin concentrations are required for the full activation of thrombin-activatable fibrinolytic inhibitor (TAFI).[14] These observations suggest that a full thrombin burst is essential for the formation of a stable fibrin hemostatic plug that is resistant to premature fibrinolysis, thus providing a reliable and maintained hemostasis.

The Role of rFVIIa

The administration of pharmacologic doses of rFVIIa that reach plasma concentrations of ≥25 nmol/L induces hemostasis. This probably occurs via the enhancement of thrombin production on the surface of platelets activated by the initial thrombin generation. Ultimately, this leads to the formation of a tight, stable, hemostatic fibrin plug.

In a cell-based in vitro model, it was shown that rFVIIa binds to thrombin-activated platelet surfaces with a low affinity, requiring higher concentrations of rFVIIa than those found naturally in circulating blood.[15] In the same model, thrombin generation in the absence of FIX was substantially improved following addition of rFVIIa in concentrations of 50 to 100 nmol/L, although it never completely normalized to the levels observed with physiological concentrations of factor XI.[16]

Optimal hemostatic efficacy requires not only an effective initial hemostasis, but also a maintained hemostasis that depends on the formation of a tight, stable, hemostatic fibrin plug resistant to premature lysis. In addition to efficient thrombin generation, which is characterized by rapid onset and a high rate and sufficient peak of production, a successfully maintained hemostasis requires activation of TAFI and FXIII. Optimal thrombin generation and polymerization of fibrin play an important role in these activation processes. Indeed, in one study, a dose-dependent normalization of fibrin permeability was achieved by adding rFVIIa to hemophilia plasma containing platelets—an effect that was reflected in a tighter fibrin structure.[17]

Conclusion

The hemostatic effect of exogenous rFVIIa, when added in pharmacologic doses, seems to be mediated by an enhanced thrombin generation rate on thrombin-activated platelet surfaces. This results in further activation of platelets at the site of injury, leading to increased exposure of phospholipids on the platelet surfaces, increased platelet adhesion, and aggregation involving glycoprotein Ib.[18] Furthermore, this thrombin generation facilitates full activation of TAFI and FXIII and subsequent formation of a hemostatic plug that has a tight fibrin structure resistant to premature lysis. As a result of these processes, the fibrinolytic potential is downregulated.

To date, rFVIIa has demonstrated considerable efficacy not only in hemophilia, but also in platelet disorders such as Glanzmann's thrombasthenia (GT).[19–21] Indeed, the agent has recently been approved in Europe for use in patients with GT who have antibodies to glycoprotein IIb–IIIa and/or human leukocyte antigen, with past or present refractoriness to platelet transfusions. Recombinant FVIIa has also been successfully used in trauma- and surgery-related hemorrhages, which may trigger severe coagulopathy.[22–25] Based on the mechanism of action of rFVIIa described in this article, the hemostatic benefits provided by this agent in various situations characterized by impaired thrombin generation can be explained and understood.

References

1. Lusher JM, Blatt PM, Penner JA, Aledort LM, Levine PH, White GC, et al: Autoplex versus proplex: A controlled, double-blind study of effectiveness in acute hemarthroses in hemophiliacs with inhibitors to factor VIII. Blood 62:1135-1138, 1983
2. Sjamsoedin LJ, Heijnen L, Mauser-Bunschoten EP, van Geijlswijk JL, van Houwelingen H, van Asten P, et al: The effect of activated prothrombin-complex concentrate (FEIBA) on joint and muscle bleeding in patients with hemophilia A and antibodies to factor VIII. N Engl J Med 305:717-758, 1981
3. Lusher JM: Thrombogenicity associated with factor IX complex concentrates. Semin Hematol 28:3-5, 1991 (suppl 6)
4. Rapaport SI, Rao LV: Initiation and regulation of tissue factor-dependent blood coagulation. Arterioscler Thromb 12:1111-1121, 1992
5. Hedner U, Kisiel W: Use of human factor VIIa in the treatment of two hemophilia A patients with high-titer inhibitors. J Clin Invest 71:1836-1841, 1983
6. Thim L, Bjoern S, Christensen M, Nicolaisen EM, Lund-Hansen T, Pedersen AH, et al: Amino acid sequence and posttranslational modifications of human factor VIIa from plasma and transfected baby hamster kidney cells. Biochemistry 27:7785-7793, 1988
7. Hedner U: Factor VIIa in the treatment of haemophilia. Blood Coagul Fibrinolysis 1:307-317, 1990
8. Lusher J, Ingerslev J, Roberts H, Hedner U: Clinical experience with recombinant factor VIIa. Blood Coagul Fibrinolysis 9:119-128, 1998
9. Ingerslev J, Freidman D, Gastineau D, Gilchrist G, Johnsson H, Lucas G, et al: Major surgery in haemophilic patients with inhibitors using recombinant factor VIIa. Haemostasis 26:118-123, 1996 (suppl 1)
10. Shapiro AD, Gilchrist GS, Hoots WK, Cooper HA, Gastineau DA: Prospective, randomised trial of two doses of rFVIIa (NovoSeven) in haemophilia patients with inhibitors undergoing surgery. Thromb Haemost 80:773-778, 1998
11. Monroe DM, Hoffman M, Roberts HR: Transmission of a procoagulant signal from tissue factor-bearing cell to platelets. Blood Coagul Fibrinolysis 7:459-464, 1996
12. Blombäck B, Carlsson K, Hessel B, Liljeborg A, Procyk R, Aslund N:

Native fibrin gel networks observed by 3D microscopy, permeation and turbidity. Biochim Biophys Acta 997:96-110, 1989

13. Carr ME Jr, Alving BM: Effect of fibrin structure on plasmin-mediated dissolution of plasma clots. Blood Coagul Fibrinolysis 6:567-573, 1995
14. Bajzar L, Manuel R, Nesheim ME: Purification and characterization of TAFI, a thrombin activable fibrinolysis inhibitor. J Biol Chem 270: 14477-14484, 1995
15. Monroe DM, Hoffman M, Oliver JA, Roberts HR: Platelet activity of high-dose factor VIIa is independent of tissue factor. Br J Haematol 99:542-547, 1997
16. Allen GA, Monroe DM 3rd, Roberts HR, Hoffman M: The effect of factor X level on thrombin generation and the procoagulant effect of activated factor VII in a cell-based model of coagulation. Blood Coagul Fibrinolysis 11:S3-7, 2000 (suppl 1)
17. He S, Blombäck M, Jacobsson Ekman G, Hedner U: The role of recombinant factor VIIa (FVIIa) in fibrin structure in the absence of FVIII/FIX. J Thromb Haemost 1:1215-1219, 2003
18. Lisman T, Adelmeijer J, Cauwenberghs S, van Pampus EC, Heemskerk JW, de Groot PG: Recombinant factor VIIa enhances platelet adhesion and activation under flow conditions at normal and reduced platelet count. J Thromb Haemost 3:742-751, 2005
19. Poon MC, d'Oiron R, Hann I, Negrier C, de Lumley L, Thomas A, et al: Use of recombinant factor VIIa (NovoSeven) in patients with Glanzmann thrombasthenia. Semin Hematol 38: 21-25, 2001
20. Chuansumrit A, Suwannuraks M, Sri-Udomporn N, Pongtanakul B, Worapongpaiboon S: Recombinant activated factor VII combined with local measures in preventing bleeding from invasive dental procedures in patients with Glanzmann thrombasthenia. Blood Coagul Fibrinolysis 14: 187-190, 2003
21. Poon MC, d'Oiron R, von Depka M, Khair K, Negrier C, Karafoulidou A, et al: Prophylactic and therapeutic recombinant factor VIIa administration to patients with Glanzmann's thrombasthenia: results of an international survey. J Thromb Haemost 2:1096-1103, 2004
22. Kenet G, Walden R, Eldad A, Martinowitz U: Treatment of traumatic bleeding with recombinant factor VIIa. Lancet 354:1879, 1999
23. O'Neill PA, Bluth M, Gloster ES, Wali D, Priovolos S, DiMaio TM, et al: Successful use of recombinant activated factor VII for trauma-associated hemorrhage in a patient without preexisting coagulopathy. J Trauma 52:400-405, 2002
24. Friederich PW, Henny CP, Messelink EJ, Geerdink MG, Keller T, Kurth KH, et al: Effect of recombinant activated factor VII on perioperative blood loss in patients undergoing retropubic prostatectomy: A double-blind placebo-controlled randomised trial. Lancet 361:201-205, 2003
25. Boffard KD, Riou B, Warren B, Choong PI, Rizoli S, Rossaint R, et al: NovoSeven Trauma Study Group: Recombinant factor VIIa as adjunctive therapy for bleeding control in severely injured trauma patients: Two parallel randomized, placebo-controlled, double-blind clinical trials. J Trauma 59:8-18, 2005

Seminars in
HEMATOLOGY

High-Dose Recombinant Factor VIIa Therapy in Hemophilia Patients With Inhibitors

Gili Kenet

Recombinant activated factor VII (rFVIIa; NovoSeven®, Novo Nordisk, Bagsvaerd, Denmark) is well established as an effective hemostatic agent for the management and prophylaxis of hemorrhage in hemophilia patients with inhibitors. Treatment schedules usually involve multiple bolus doses of 90 to 120 μg/kg administered every 2 to 3 hours, but recent evidence suggests that the use of higher doses might be justified. Such high-dose regimens may overcome the rapid clearance rate observed in pediatric patients, and may be more convenient for patients with poor venous access. It has been suggested that individually tailored high-dose therapies might be beneficial in selected groups of patients, although careful monitoring of such patients is advised. Thrombelastography has demonstrated considerable success in this regard, allowing accurate assessment of both hemostatic efficacy and individual response to rFVIIa. To date, no safety issues associated with high-dose rFVIIa have been identified. However, it is hoped that further research will support these favorable observations and thus contribute towards more effective dose optimization of rFVIIa in hemophilic inhibitor patients.
Semin Hematol 43(suppl 1):S108-S110

The management and prophylaxis of bleeds in patients with hemophilia A are usually achieved using factor VIII (FVIII) concentrates to replace the missing clotting factor. However, alloantibodies to human FVIII develop in approximately 30% of patients with this disorder,[1–3] and these inhibitors render conventional factor replacement therapy ineffective.

Recombinant activated factor VII (rFVIIa; NovoSeven®, Novo Nordisk, Bagsvaerd, Denmark) is well established as an effective first-line treatment for bleeding episodes and surgical coverage in patients with congenital hemophilia A or B and inhibitors. In the European Union (EU) and several non-EU areas, the agent is also approved for use in acquired hemophilia A or B, and is considered a standard therapy for this indication in the USA.

Due to its very short half-life (approximately 2.5 hours),[4] rFVIIa treatment regimens typically involve repeated bolus injections. A dosing schedule using a bolus of 90 to 120 μg/kg, initially given every 2 hours and followed by the same dose at increasing intervals, has been shown to provide effective hemostatic prophylaxis for elective surgical procedures in hemophilia patients.[5] Similarly, a standard dosing regimen of 90 to 120 μg/kg administered every 2 to 3 hours has yielded a success rate of approximately 90% when used for the home treatment of mild or moderate bleeds in patients with hemophilia and inhibitors.[4,6,7] In this setting, an average of 2.2 injections per bleeding episode has been required for effective hemostasis using the standard dosing level.[6] Nevertheless, the agent's short half-life and rapid clearance (especially in children) require careful consideration in order to optimize the efficacy and convenience of rFVIIa administration.

The Israeli National Hemophilia Center, Sheba Medical Center, Tel-Hashomer, Israel.

Address correspondence to Gili Kenet, MD, Director, Pediatric Coagulation, The Israeli National Hemophilia Center, Sheba Medical Center, Tel-Hashomer, 52621. E-mail: Gili.Kenet@sheba.health.gov.il

Potential Rationale for the Use of Higher-Dose rFVIIa Regimens

The rate of thrombin generation is assumed to play a key role in the formation of a stable fibrin plug at the site of injury. High thrombin generation enhances platelet-surface thrombin generation, increases procoagulant microparticles, and improves the fibrin structure of the clot.[8–10]

However, the exact relationship between the bolus dose of rFVIIa administered and the patient's level of thrombin generation has yet to be defined. Substantial interindividual variation in thrombin generation has been shown following rFVIIa treatment: doses of 90 to 120 μg/kg may, in some individuals, be sufficient to produce enough throm-

 0037-1963/06/$-see front matter
doi:10.1053/j.seminhematol.2005.11.006

bin,[4–7,11,12] whereas other patients may require higher, recurrent dosing. Furthermore, the clearance rate of rFVIIa varies between individuals,[4,11–13] and a preliminary trial of children aged under 15 years indicated that the clearance rate may be 50% faster in children than in adults.[14] This finding might justify the use of higher doses of rFVIIa, especially in pediatric inhibitor patients. Administration of a higher rFVIIa dose may also avoid the current need for repeated dosing every 2 to 3 hours, and may thus be a more convenient alternative for patients with restricted venous access.

Studies and Case Series of Higher rFVIIa Dosing

Some recent studies suggest that rFVIIa doses >200 μg/kg may provide greater efficacy than conventional doses, probably by enhancing thrombin generation on activated platelets and thus promoting the formation of a more stable fibrin clot (reviewed in Abshire).[15] These findings are supported by those from a single-center, open-label trial in which a high initial dose (300 μg/kg) of rFVIIa was effective and safe when used to treat hemarthrosis in patients with hemophilia and inhibitors.[16] Several case studies also suggest that rFVIIa treatment is more effective when administered as a single, high-dose (defined as >90 μg/kg) intervention.[17–19] Analysis of data from 555 bleeding episodes in 39 hemophilic inhibitor patients reported to the Hemophilia and Thrombosis Research Society Registry suggests that single doses of >200 μg/kg rFVIIa were more effective than doses of <200 μg/kg (efficacy rates of 97% and 84%, respectively; $P < .001$).[19] Finally, in a recently completed, randomized, double-blind, cross-over trial comparing standard and high bolus doses, the efficacy, safety and patient preference were similar for both treatment arms.[20] These findings all suggest that the administration of single high doses of rFVIIa may be feasible and effective in patients with hemophilia and inhibitors.

Specific Considerations and Patient Monitoring

Some inhibitor patients may develop refractoriness not only to standard rFVIIa regimens, but also to activated prothrombin complex concentrate (aPCC) products such as FEIBA (Baxter Corp, Deerfield, IL).[21,22] For such patients, individually tailored therapy regimens should be devised. For instance, it has been suggested that therapy with sequential FEIBA and rFVIIa may be effective in these cases.[22,23] Higher rFVIIa doses may also be of potential benefit in this specific subpopulation of inhibitor patients, provided that adequate patient selection and monitoring methods are undertaken to avoid thromboembolic complications.

The ability to select the optimal rFVIIa dose for each patient, or for each bleeding episode, would be greatly enhanced if laboratory assays were capable of monitoring and evaluating the impact of therapy. However, there is currently no single laboratory test that can accurately illustrate the clinical effects of a procoagulant treatment. The prothrombin time (PT) and activated partial thromboplastin time (aPTT) cannot adequately monitor the effects of rFVIIa; factor VII activity (FVII:C) levels neither reflect thrombin generation nor measure real-time parameters; measurement of FVIIa levels is highly complex; and thrombin-antithrombin III complex (TAT) and fragment F1+2 markers are not representative of hemostatic efficacy. Furthermore, although thrombin generation tests are accurate and of potential predictive value,[24,25] they require expert technicians and cannot be performed at the bedside.

The continuous coagulation profiles provided by thrombelastography may facilitate a more accurate reflection of the in-vivo impact of rFVIIa and other procoagulant interventions, and has been used successfully for this purpose.[26] For instance, Yoshioka et al concluded that this method was more suitable than the aPTT, PT, or FVIIa level as a monitor of hemostatic effects during rFVIIa treatment in three hemophilia A patients with high-titer inhibitors.[27] More recently, Sorensen and Ingerslev showed that rotational thrombelastography (ROTEG, Pentapharm, Munich, Germany) is a valuable method for assessing both hemostatic efficacy and individual responses to rFVIIa treatment.[26,28] ROTEG has demonstrated not only that rFVIIa shortens the clot formation time (CFT) and increases maximum clot firmness (MCF) in hemophilic blood, but also that these changes correlate with the in-vivo effects of rFVIIa in a dose-dependent manner.[28]

Safety Issues

The use of standard doses of rFVIIa in patients with hemophilia and inhibitors has generated a highly favorable safety profile; post-marketing data indicate a reported incidence of just 0.09% for fatal complications. Similar results can be found in the literature. A total of 25 thrombotic events or cases of disseminated intravascular coagulation were reported among hemophilia patients after more than 700,000 rFVIIa doses, and most of these adverse events occurred in elderly patients with co-morbid risk factors for thrombosis.[29] Limited safety data currently exist for off-label use, including the use of higher doses; however, no safety issues have been identified so far in any studies of high-dose rFVIIa therapy in selected patients with hemophilia A and inhibitors.[16–20] Further study is needed to clarify and support these encouraging findings.

Conclusions

Previous studies indicate that administration of standard bolus doses of rFVIIa is generally effective for the treatment of hemarthrosis in hemophilic inhibitor patients, although multiple doses are often required. More recent evidence suggests that high-dose rFVIIa represents a safe and effective alternative to standard dosing regimens, particularly in children or in patients with poor venous access. However, caution is advised when treating high-risk patients with co-morbid conditions that predispose to thromboembolic complications. For selected patients, individually tailored therapy may provide the best outcome, but it is important to monitor these patients carefully. In such circumstances, whole blood clotting assays may offer an effective method for monitoring the hemostatic response induced by rFVIIa treatment. Future studies should aim to improve our understanding of inter-patient variation in recovery and clearance rates, and to increase our knowledge of the agent's overall efficacy and safety profile, so that more efficient dose optimization of rFVIIa can be achieved.

References

1. Santagostino E, Mancuso ME, Rocino A, Mancuso G, Mazzucconi MG, Tagliaferri A, et al: Environmental risk factors for inhibitor development in children with haemophilia A: A case-control study. Br J Haematol 130:422-427, 2005
2. White GC 2nd, Kempton CL, Grimsley A, Nielsen B, Roberts HR: Cellular immune responses in hemophilia: Why do inhibitors develop in some, but not all hemophiliacs? J Thromb Haemost 3:1676-1681, 2005
3. Lusher JM: Inhibitor antibodies to factor VIII and factor IX: Management. Semin Thromb Hemost 26: 179-188, 2000
4. Erhardtsen E: Pharmacokinetics of recombinant activated factor VII (rFVIIa). Semin Thromb Hemost 26:385-391, 2000
5. Shapiro AD, Gilchrist GS, Hoots WK, Cooper HA, Gastineau DA: Prospective, randomized trial of two doses of rFVIIa (NovoSeven) in haemophilia patients with inhibitors undergoing surgery. Thromb Haemost 80:773-778, 1998
6. Key NS, Aledort LM, Beardsley D, Cooper HA, Davignon G, Ewenstein BM: Home treatment of mild to moderate bleeding episodes using recombinant factor VIIa (Novoseven) in haemophiliacs with inhibitors. Thromb Haemost 80:912-918, 1998
7. Ingerslev J, Thykjaer H, Kudsk-Jensen O, Fredberg U: Home treatment with recombinant activated factor VII: Results from one centre. Blood Coagul Fibrinolysis 9:S107-110, 1998 (suppl 1)
8. Proulle V, Hugel B, Guillet B, Trichet C, Rafowicz A, Lambert T, et al: Injection of recombinant activated factor VII can induce transient increase in circulating procoagulant microparticles. Thromb Haemost 91:873-878, 2004
9. Carr ME Jr., Martin EJ, Kuhn JG, Seremetis SV: Effects of recombinant factor VIIa on platelet function and clot structure in blood with deficient prothrombin conversion. Thromb Haemost 89:803-811, 2003
10. He S, Ekman GJ, Hedner U: The effect of platelets on fibrin gel structure formed in the presence of recombinant factor VIIa in hemophilia plasma and in plasma from a patient with Glanzmann thrombasthenia. J Thromb Haemost 3:272-279, 2005
11. Erhardtsen E, Nony P, Dechavanne M, Ffrench P, Boissel JP, Hedner U: The effect of recombinant factor VIIa (NovoSeven) in healthy volunteers receiving acenocoumarol to an International Normalized Ratio above 2.0. Blood Coagul Fibrinolysis 9:741-748, 1998
12. Sumner WT, Monroe DM, Hoffman M: Variability in platelet procoagulant activity in healthy volunteers. Thromb Res 81:533-543, 1996
13. Schulman S, d'Oiron R, Martinowitz U, Pasi J, Briquel ME, Mauser-Bunschoten E, et al: Experiences with continuous infusion of recombinant activated factor VII. Blood Coagul Fibrinolysis 9:S97-101, 1998
14. Villar A, Aronis S, Morfini M, Santagostino E, Auerswald G, Thomsen HF, et al: Pharmacokinetics of activated recombinant coagulation factor VII (NovoSeven) in children vs. adults with haemophilia A. Haemophilia 10:352-359, 2004
15. Abshire T, Kenet G: Recombinant factor VIIa: Review of efficacy, dosing regimens and safety in patients with congenital and acquired factor VIII or IX inhibitors. J Thromb Haemost 2:899-909, 2004
16. Kenet G, Lubetsky A, Luboshitz J, Martinowitz U: A new approach to treatment of bleeding episodes in young hemophilia patients: A single bolus megadose of recombinant activated factor VII (NovoSeven). J Thromb Haemost 1:450-455, 2003
17. Cooper HA, Jones CP, Campion E, Roberts HR, Hedner U: Rationale for the use of high dose rFVIIa in a high-titre inhibitor patient with haemophilia B during major orthopaedic procedures. Haemophilia 7:517-522, 2001
18. Kenet G, Lubetsky A, Luboshitz J, Ravid B, Tamarin I, Martinowitz U: High dose recombinant activated factor VII for treatment of patients with hemophilia and inhibitors. Haemophilia 10:53-66, 2004
19. Parameswaran R, Shapiro AD, Gill JC, Kessler CM: HTRS Registry Investigators: Dose effect and efficacy of recombinant factor VIIa (rF-VIIa) in the treatment of haemophilia patients with inhibitors: Analysis from the Hemophilia and Thrombosis Research Society Registry. Haemophilia 11:100-106, 2005
20. Kavakli K, Makris M, Zulfikar B, Abrams Z, Kenet G, for the NovoSeven® Trial (F7HAEM-1510): rFVIIa (NovoSeven) for the treatment of mild/moderate joint bleeds in haemophilia patients with inhibitors: a double-blind study of a single high dose versus standard multiple doses of rFVIIa. Presented at the XXth Congress of the International Society on Thrombosis and Haemostasis, Sydney, Australia, August 6-12, 2005
21. Hayashi T, Tanaka I, Shima M, Yoshida K, Fukuda K, Sakurai Y, et al: Unresponsiveness to factor VIII inhibitor bypassing agents during haemostatic treatment for life-threatening massive bleeding in a patient with haemophilia A and a high responding inhibitor. Haemophilia 10:397-400, 2004
22. Schneiderman J, Nugent DJ, Young G: Sequential therapy with activated prothrombin complex concentrate and recombinant factor VIIa in patients with severe haemophilia and inhibitors. Haemophilia 10: 347-351, 2004
23. Martinowitz U, Livnat T, Zivelin A, Luboshitz J, Seligsohn U, Kenet G: Concomitant infusion of low doses of rFVIIa and FEIBA in severe hemophilia A patients with an inhibitor to factor VIII who are refractory to rFVIIa or FEIBA has an excellent hemostatic effect and synergistically enhances thrombin generation. Presented at the XXth Congress of the International Society on Thrombosis and Haemostasis, Sydney, Australia, August 6-12, 2005
24. Carr ME Jr, Martin EJ: Evolving techniques for monitoring clotting in plasma and whole blood samples. Clin Lab 50:539-549, 2004
25. Dargaud Y, Lienhart A, Meunier S, Hequet O, Chavanne H, Chamouard V, et al: Major surgery in a severe haemophilia A patient with high titre inhibitor: Use of the thrombin generation test in the therapeutic decision. Haemophilia 11:552-558, 2005
26. Sorensen B, Ingerslev J: Tailoring haemostatic treatment to patient requirements—An update on monitoring haemostatic response using thrombelastography. Haemophilia 11:1-6, 2005 (suppl 1)
27. Yoshioka A, Nishio K, Shima M: Thrombelastgram as a hemostatic monitor during recombinant factor VIIa treatment in hemophilia A patients with inhibitor to factor VIII. Haemostasis 26:139-142, 1996 (suppl 1)
28. Sorensen B, Ingerslev J: Whole blood clot formation phenotypes in hemophilia A and rare coagulation disorders. Patterns of response to recombinant factor VIIa. J Thromb Haemost 2:102-110, 2004
29. Abshire TC: Dose optimization of recombinant factor VIIa for control of mild to moderate bleeds in inhibitor patients: Improved efficacy with higher dosing. Semin Hematol 41:3-7, 2004 (suppl 1)

ELSEVIER

Seminars in
HEMATOLOGY

Haemostasis Award Winner

Protein S Multimers Are Generated In Vitro and Affect Protein S Structure-Function Analyses

Kristin M. Seré, George M. Willems, Jan Rosing, and Tilman M. Hackeng

Purified human protein S preparations contain small amounts of multimeric protein S. Protein S multimers are absent in plasma, suggesting that multimerization results from purification. Protein S multimers effectively inhibit phospholipid-dependent reactions at low phospholipid concentrations, and may therefore interfere during functional analysis of protein S. We have demonstrated that anion-exchange chromatography, as well as high ionic strength or low pH elution conditions used in immunoaffinity purification of protein S, induce protein S multimer formation. When protein S multimers were removed from protein S preparations by size-exclusion chromatography, multimers spontaneously reappeared in the protein S monomer fraction. In model systems, high phospholipid concentrations (>50 μmol/L) completely abrogate the inhibitory effect of protein S multimers on prothrombinase complex activity. In addition, C4BP does not bind to protein S multimers. Thus, at low phospholipid concentrations, addition of C4BP to purified protein S will not affect the inhibitory activity of protein S multimers. In conclusion, to avoid misinterpretations during protein S structure-function analysis due to multimers present in purified protein S preparations, we recommend studying the anticoagulant activities of protein S either in plasma, where protein S is in its unmodified natural form, or at high phospholipid concentrations in model systems with purified proteins.
Semin Hematol 43(suppl 1):S111-S120

Protein S is a vitamin K-dependent protein that is present in human plasma at a concentration of 25 mg/L.[1,2] Protein S is an important natural anticoagulant, since deficiencies in protein S are associated with thrombotic complications.[3-5] Approximately 60% of plasma protein S is present in a high affinity 1:1 stoichiometric complex with C4b-binding protein (C4BP), a regulator of the classic complement pathway.[6] The C-terminal domain of protein S consists of a sex hormone-binding globulin (SHBG) homology region that is involved in C4BP binding.[7] Amino acid residues in the second (C-terminal) laminin G module domain of SHBG have been shown to be essential for the interaction between protein S and C4BP.[8] The free protein S present in plasma is a cofactor of activated protein C (APC)[9,10] in the inactivation of coagulation factors Va and VIIIa.[11,12] In addition, protein S has been reported to inhibit prothrombin activation in the absence of APC[13] via direct interactions with the components of the prothrombinase complex.[14-17] Identification of binding sites for FVa and activated factor X (FXa) on protein S support this theory.[18,19] Complexation of protein S by C4BP has been shown to abolish its APC-cofactor activity but not its APC-independent anticoagulant activity.[14,20,21]

Binding of the N-terminal γ-carboxyglutamic acid-rich (Gla) domain of protein S to phospholipid surfaces is essential for the expression of both the APC-cofactor and the APC-independent anticoagulant activities of protein S.[17,22,23] Compared with other vitamin K-dependent proteins, the affinity of protein S for lipid surfaces is high,[24] and reported K_d values for purified protein S preparations vary from 7 to 74 nmol/L.[17] However, purified protein S preparations are a heterogeneous mixture of protein S monomers and multimers.[25] A small percentage of the protein S molecules (<5%) exist in multimeric forms that bind with a much higher affinity (K_d <1 nmol/L) to anionic phospholipids than do the protein S monomers (K_d ~250 nmol/L). Therefore, the reported K_d values likely represent an average phospholipid

Department of Biochemistry, Cardiovascular Research Institute Maastricht, University Maastricht, Maastricht, The Netherlands
Supported in part by a fellowship of the Netherlands Organization for Scientific Research (NWO-VIDI 917.36.372 to T.M.H.).
Address correspondence to Tilman M. Hackeng, PhD, Department of Biochemistry, Cardiovascular Research Institute Maastricht, University Maastricht, PO Box 616, 6200 MD Maastricht, The Netherlands. E-mail: t.hackeng@bioch.unimaas.nl

0037-1963/06/$-see front matter
doi:10.1053/j.seminhematol.2005.11.027

binding affinity of multimeric and monomeric protein S forms in the preparations used.

It has been proposed that protein S inhibits prothrombin activation in the absence of APC by competing with prothrombin, FXa and FVa for binding to phospholipid membranes.[17,26] Because of their high affinity for phospholipids, multimeric forms of protein S are potent competitors and therefore efficiently inhibit prothrombin activation at low phospholipid concentrations.[25] However, the fact that multimers could not be detected in plasma suggests that, in plasma, a different mechanism must underlie the observed APC-independent activity of protein S.[27] This is underscored by the observations that, in the absence of APC, protein S is an effective inhibitor of tissue factor-induced thrombin generation, and that the APC-independent anticoagulant activity of protein S in plasma is not affected by variation of the phospholipid concentration between 0.1 and 100 μmol/L.[27] Considering the above, protein S multimers are not physiologically relevant and their presence in purified protein S preparations should be avoided.

The presence of multimeric forms in purified protein S preparations has been observed previously in lipid-binding and activity experiments[17,26,28] and appears to be characteristic for purified protein S preparations. The present study describes the steps during protein S purification at which multimers are generated, and provides information on how to adjust experimental conditions to circumvent unwanted influences of protein S multimers on structure-function analyses of protein S.

Experimental Procedures

Materials

HEPES (*N*-2-hydroxyethylpiperazine-*N'*-2-ethanesulfonic acid), MES (2-[*N*-morpholino]ethanesulfonic acid) and Tris buffer, EDTA (ethylenedinitrilotetra acetic acid), benzamidine-HCl, BSA (bovine serum albumin), ovalbumin, and DAB (diaminobenzidine) were purchased from Sigma-Aldrich (St Louis, MO). NaCl, $CaCl_2$, NaN_3, and ammonium sulfate were obtained from Merck (Darmstadt, Germany). 3-[(3-cholamidopropyl)dimethylammonio]-1-propane-sulfonate (CHAPS) was from ICN Biomedicals (Aurora, OH) and D-phenylalanyl-L-phenylalanyl-L-arginine-chloromethylketone (PPACK) was supplied by Behring Diagnostics (La Jolla, CA). 1,2-dioleoyl-*sn*-glycero-3-phosphocholine (DOPC), 1,2-dioleoyl-*sn*-glycero-3-phosphoserine (DOPS) and 1,2-dioleoyl-*sn*-glycero-3-phosphoethanolamine (DOPE) were obtained from Avanti Polar Lipids (Alabaster, AL). The chromogenic substrate D-Phe-(pipecolyl)-Arg-pNA (S2238) was supplied by Chromogenix (Mölndal, Sweden). Column materials were obtained from Amersham Biosciences (Uppsala, Sweden). CNBr-activated Sepharose 4B was from Pharmacia Biotech. Gradient polyacrylamide gels (4% to 15%) and sodium dodecyl sulphate (SDS) were from Biorad (Hercules, CA). Immobilon polyvinylidene fluoride (PVDF) membranes were from Millipore (Bedford, MA). Factor Xa was obtained from Enzyme Research Laboratories (South Bend, IN). Prothrombin,[29] factor Va,[30] and beta-chain containing C4BP[31] were purified as described previously.

Protein S Purification

Purification of protein S was performed as reported by Koedam et al[29] with some modifications. Seven units (~2000 mL) of freshly frozen human plasma were thawed and pooled, enzyme inhibitors were added (2 μmol/L PPACK, 25 mmol/L benzamidine-HCl) and 240 mL 1 mol/L $BaCl_2$ was added drop-wise while stirring. The barium citrate precipitate was washed twice with 0.1 mol/L $BaCl_2$ and 25 mmol/L benzamidine-HCl and was suspended in 25 mmol/L benzamidine-HCl. Following 30% ammonium sulfate precipitation, the supernatant, which contained protein S, was dialyzed against MES-buffered saline (MBS: 10 mmol/L MES, 150 mmol/L NaCl, pH 6.0) containing 2 μmol/L PPACK, 10 mmol/L EDTA, 0.02% NaN_3, 1 mmol/L benzamidine, and subsequently applied to a QAE Sephadex column (5 × 40 cm) for anion exchange chromatography. Proteins were eluted with a linear gradient of 150 to 500 mmol/L NaCl in MBS. The fractions containing protein S were pooled, concentrated (70% ammonium sulfate vol/vol) and dialyzed in Tris-buffered saline (TBS: 50 mmol/L Tris, 150 mmol/L NaCl, pH 7.4) containing 2 mmol/L EDTA and 0.02% NaN_3. Subsequent affinity chromatography on a Blue Sepharose column separated protein S from protein C. In the final purification step, protein S-containing fractions were subjected to anion exchange chromatography on Q Sepharose fast flow. Protein S was eluted with calcium-containing TBS (25 mmol/L Tris, 110 mmol/L NaCl, 20 mmol/L $CaCl_2$, pH 7.4), dialyzed against HEPES-buffered saline (HBS: 25 mmol/L HEPES, 175 mmol/L NaCl, pH 7.7), and stored at −80°C. All steps were performed at 4°C except for Blue Sepharose and Q Sepharose fast flow chromatography, which were performed at RT (RT). Protein S concentrations were determined with an enzyme-linked immunosorbent assay (ELISA) using protein S from Enzyme Research Laboratories (#1540), the concentration of which was determined from the absorbance at 280 nm (A_{280}) using $\epsilon^{1\%}_{1cm,280nm} = 9.6$,[1] as a standard. Samples were taken throughout the purification procedure and analyzed on SDS-polyacrylamide gel electrophoresis (PAGE) or native PAGE immunoblot as described previously.[25]

In addition, protein S was purified from plasma-derived protein S-C4BP complex essentially as described by Koenen et al.[31] Reversed phase high-performance liquid chromatography (HPLC) of the purified complex resulted in a complete separation of C4BP and protein S in a linear gradient of acetonitrile in water/0.1% trifluoroacetic acid (TFA).[31] Neutralization of pH of the protein S-containing fractions caused precipitation of the protein. After centrifugation, the precipitate was resolved in 0.1 mol/L Tris-HCl, pH 8.0, containing 6 mol/L guanidine-HCl and the solution was dialyzed against HBS.

Stability and C4BP Binding of Protein S Monomers and Multimers

Protein S monomers and multimers, present in a purified protein S preparation, were separated by centrifugation of a mixture of protein S and liposomes in HBS containing 5 mg/mL BSA as described previously.[25] Subsequently, the formation and/or stability of protein S multimers and monomers were tested by incubating (1) protein S multimers (75 μL of 40 nmol/L) with 10 mmol/L CHAPS for 1 hour at 37°C (total volume of 100 μL) and subsequent dialysis against HBS; (2) protein S monomers (20 μL of 800 nmol/L) with 50 μL potassium thiocyanate (4 mol/L KSCN, pH 7.4) for 15 minutes at RT, and dialysis (twice) against 1 L HBS containing 10 mmol/L EDTA for 1 hour at RT; (3) protein S monomers (15 μL of 800 nmol/L) with 30 μL 0.1 mol/L glycine pH 2.7 for 20 minutes at RT and subsequent neutralization of the pH to ~7.5 by addition of 3 μL 1 mol/L Tris-HCl pH 8.8; and (4) protein S monomers (15 μL of 800 nmol/L) with 33 μL glycine/Tris-HCl pH ~7.5 for 20 minutes at RT (control). Complex formation of C4BP with protein S was achieved by incubating 220 nmol/L protein S with an excess of C4BP (290 nmol/L) in HBS containing 5 mg/mL BSA and 0.5 mmol/L $CaCl_2$ for 30 minutes at RT.

Removal of Protein S Multimers Using Size-Exclusion Chromatography

Small unilamellar 20/80 DOPC/DOPE vesicles were prepared as described previously.[30] A 4-mL aliquot of a 10-mmol/L vesicle solution in HBS containing 3 mmol/L $CaCl_2$ was applied to a HiLoad 26/60 Superdex 200 column and eluted with HBS containing 3 mmol/L $CaCl_2$ at a flow rate of 1 mL/min. Four fractions of ~2 mmol/L from the void volume were collected and incubated with purified protein S for 3 hours at RT and the solution was gently mixed occasionally. Final concentrations were 19 μmol/L protein S and ~0.9 mmol/L phospholipid vesicles in HBS with 3 mmol/L $CaCl_2$. Subsequently, 8.75 mL of the protein S/phospholipid mixture was loaded on the Superdex size-exclusion chromatography column and eluted with HBS containing 3 mmol/L $CaCl_2$ at a flow rate of 1 mL/min. Fractions of 1 mL were collected and protein S concentration was determined by measuring A_{280}. Then, 0.02% NaN_3 was added to all fractions. Immediately after size-exclusion chromatography, the fraction with the highest concentration of protein S was analyzed for the presence of multimers. Protein adsorption on a phospholipid bilayer was quantified by ellipsometry as described in a previous report.[25] This fraction was stored for several weeks at 4°C and occasionally tested in the ellipsometer. The remaining fractions of the size-exclusion column which contained high protein S concentrations were pooled. Aliquots (1 mL) of the pooled fractions (600 μg/mL protein S) were incubated with BSA (5 mg/mL) and/or ammonium sulfate (70%) and stored at 4°C. Diluted aliquots of the protein S pool (75 μg/mL protein S) were incubated in the same way. After 48 hours, the ammonium sulfate pellet was resuspended, and all preparations were analyzed for the presence of multimers by ellipsometry.

Ellipsometric Determination of Protein S Adsorption to Lipid Bilayers

Protein adsorption to planar bilayers was measured by ellipsometry.[32] Briefly, planar bilayers deposited on silicon slides were prepared as described previously[33] by immersion of the hydrophilic silicon slide for 5 minutes in a stirred suspension of small unilamellar lipid vesicles (30 μmol/L) in binding buffer (50 mmol/L Tris, 120 mmol/L NaCl, 3 mmol/L $CaCl_2$, pH 7.5). The instrument and data analysis have been described earlier.[34] Measurements were performed using silicon slides at an angle of incidence to the light beam (HeNe Laser) of 68 degrees.[21] Experiments were performed in binding buffer containing 0.5 mg/mL BSA at RT (20 to 22°C) with continuous stirring in a trapezoidal cuvette.

Influence of Phospholipid Concentration on Anticoagulant Activity of Protein S

The inhibition of prothrombin activation by protein S was measured in a prothrombinase assay. Factor Va, factor Xa, phospholipid vesicles (20/60/20 DOPS/DOPC/DOPE) and protein S were incubated for 15 minutes at 37°C in HBS containing 3 mmol/L $CaCl_2$ and 5 mg/mL BSA. Prothrombin was added and, after various time intervals, aliquots from the activation mixture were diluted in ice-cold TBS-buffered saline (25 mmol/L Tris-HCl, 175 mmol/L NaCl, pH 7.9) containing 20 mmol/L EDTA and 0.5 mg/mL ovalbumin. Thrombin concentrations were determined with chromogenic substrate S2238. Final concentrations in the prothrombin activation mixture were 10 pmol/L FVa, 10 pmol/L FXa, 0.1 to 50 μmol/L phospholipid vesicles, 1,500 nmol/L prothrombin, and 0 or 100 nmol/L protein S.

Results

Standard Protein S Purification

In a previous study, we observed that purified human protein S preparations contain a small fraction (<5%) of multimeric protein S forms.[25] However, no multimers could be identified in plasma, suggesting that multimerization occurs during purification of protein S from plasma or plasma concentrates. This hypothesis was tested by following the protein S multimerization process on native PAGE and Western blot through the full purification procedure of protein S from plasma. The starting material—pooled freshly frozen plasma from healthy donors—did not contain any detectable multimeric form of protein S (Fig 1, lane a). Two protein S bands were visible, a band with a low mobility at the top of the gel representing protein S in complex with C4BP, and a higher mobility band representing monomeric, free protein S. The presence of abundant plasma proteins (eg, albumin) likely hindered the electrophoretic migration of the free protein S monomers. Subsequently, vitamin K-dependent plasma proteins were isolated from plasma by barium citrate precipitation, and further fractionated by ammonium sulfate precipitation. No protein S multimerization was observed after these purification steps as shown on native PAGE and Western blot (Fig 1, lane b). The protein concentrate was subjected to anion-exchange chromatography (QAE Sephadex) and protein S was eluted with 250 to 300 mmol/L NaCl in a linear NaCl gradient. During the anion-exchange purification step protein S multimers were generated (Fig 1, lane c). Fractions

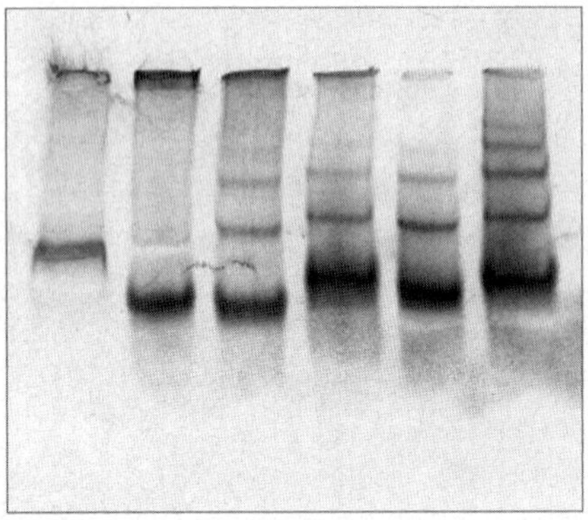

a b c d e f

Figure 1 Protein S multimerization during purification. Protein S (250 ng) obtained at different stages of purification was subjected to native PAGE and transferred to a PVDF membrane and visualized with peroxidase-conjugated polyclonal antibodies against protein S. Freshly frozen pooled human plasma (lane a); protein S after barium citrate precipitation and ammonium sulfate fractionation (lane b); pool of protein S-containing fractions from the QAE Sephadex column (lane c); protein S-containing fractions from the QAE Sephadex column after ammonium sulfate fractionation (lane d); pool of protein S-containing fractions from the Blue Sepharose column (lane e); pool of protein S-containing fractions after Q Sepharose fast flow chromatography (lane f). For further details see Experimental Procedures.

containing protein S were pooled and subsequent precipitation (70% ammonium sulfate) followed by dialysis did not alter the relative amount of multimers in the protein S concentrate (Fig 1, lane d). Blue Sepharose chromatography was used to further purify protein S and, under the conditions used, protein S was not retained by the column and was eluted in the void volume. No increase in the amount of protein S multimers was observed after Blue Sepharose chromatography (Fig 1, lane e). The final purification step was anion-exchange chromatography on Q Sepharose and elution of protein S was based on Ca^{2+}-dependent conformational change of vitamin K-dependent proteins. Protein S-containing fractions were pooled and dialyzed against HBS and the protein S preparation was analyzed on native PAGE and Western blot (Fig 1, lane f). An increase in protein S multimerization was observed after this final anion-exchange purification step. Based on a concentration determination by ELISA, all lanes of the native PAGE/Western blot shown in Fig 1 contained equal amounts of protein S. The staining intensities of the various protein bands on the blot indicate that multimer formation occurred during the first anion-exchange QAE Sephadex step and increased after the second Q Sepharose Fast Flow anion-exchange step. Barium citrate precipitation, ammonium sulfate precipitation, and Blue Sepharose chromatography did not induce multimerization of protein S.

Immunoaffinity Purification of Protein S

As an alternative to ion-exchange chromatography, protein S can be purified by immunoaffinity chromatography using Sepharose-bound polyclonal antibodies against protein S. Elution of protein S from the antibody column requires stringent conditions such as 3 mol/L KSCN at pH 7.4 or 0.1 mol/L glycine at pH 2.7. To study the effect of high concentrations of chaotropic reagents or low pH on the multimerization of protein S, purified protein S monomers (Fig 2, lane a) were subjected to the following treatments: (1) protein S was incubated with 3 mol/L KSCN at pH 7.4 for 20 minutes at RT and dialyzed against HBS (Fig 2, lane b); (2) protein S was brought to low pH by the addition of 0.1 mol/L glycine, pH 2.7, and after incubation at RT for 20 minutes the mixture was brought to neutral pH with 1 mol/L Tris buffer pH 8.8 (Fig 2, lane c); (3) protein S was treated with 0.1 mol/L glycine at neutral pH 7.5 (control, Fig 2, lane d). When protein S was treated with the chaotropic agent KSCN or with glycine at low pH, multimers were readily generated (Fig 2). The presence of glycine at neutral pH does not induce multimerization of protein S. Considering the above, it would be virtually impossible to purify protein S from plasma by classic ion-exchange chromatography or by affinity chromatography without generation of protein S multimers.

Reversing Protein S Multimerization by Detergent Treatment

As purification of monomeric protein S from plasma was unsuccessful, an attempt was made to dissociate the protein S multimers present in a purified protein S preparation by the addition of detergent. Protein S multimers are not SDS resistant and when isolated protein S multimers (Fig 3, lane a) were applied to SDS-PAGE and Western blot analysis, a single protein S band was observed (Fig 3, lane c), indicating

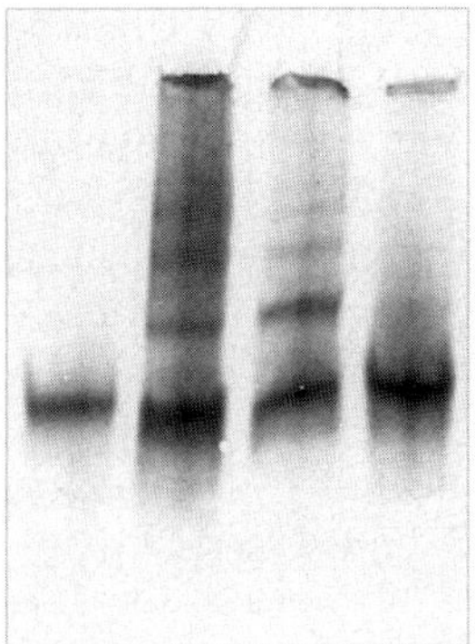

a b c d

Figure 2 Protein S multimerization by affinity chromatography elution conditions. Isolated protein S monomers were treated (a) with HBS for 20 minutes at RT; (b) with 4 mol/L KSCN, pH 7.4, for 15 minutes at RT, then dialyzed against HBS containing 10 mmol/L EDTA; (c) with 0.1 mol/L glycine, pH 2.7, for 20 minutes at RT, then pH was restored to ~7.5 with 1 mol/L Tris-HCl, pH 8.8; (d) with 0.1 mol/L glycine, pH ~7.5, for 20 minutes at RT. After incubation, free $CaCl_2$ was complexed by the addition of HBS containing 10 mmol/L EDTA (a, c, d). Protein S (300 ng) was subjected to native PAGE immunoblot and protein S was visualized with peroxidase-conjugated polyclonal antibodies against protein S. For further details see Experimental Procedures.

that the interaction between protein S molecules that leads to multimer formation is noncovalent. Because detergent removal would be necessary for subsequent functional studies with purified protein S, zwitterionic CHAPS was used instead of anionic SDS because of the difficulties of removing SDS by dialysis. Isolated protein S multimers were incubated with CHAPS for 1 hour and then dialyzed against HBS. Native PAGE and Western blot analysis showed that only some of the protein S multimers could be reverted to monomers and the majority of multimers remained (Fig 3, lane b).

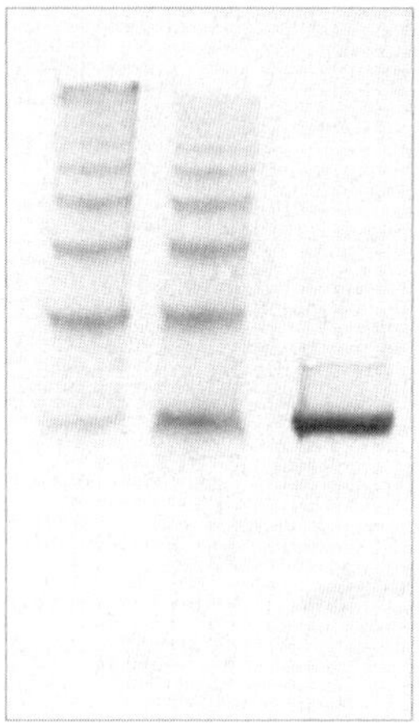

Figure 3 Dissociation of protein S multimers. Isolated protein S multimers were incubated without (a) or with (b) 10 mmol/L CHAPS for 1 hour at 37°C and then dialyzed against HBS. Protein S (30 ng) was subjected to native PAGE and transferred to a PVDF membrane by Western blotting. Lane c represents Western blotting of 30 ng protein S multimers (untreated) subjected to SDS-PAGE. Protein S was visualized using peroxidase-conjugated polyclonal antibodies against protein S. * For reasons of clarity, protein S monomer bands were aligned, as mobility in native- and SDS-PAGE can not be compared.

Separation of Protein S Multimers and Monomers by Size-Exclusion Chromatography

As conversion of protein S multimers into monomers by detergent treatment was unsuccessful, an attempt was made to remove protein S multimers from a protein S preparation by size-exclusion chromatography on Superose 6. Protein S multimers elute slightly earlier from the Superose 6 column than protein S monomers. Although protein S multimers were enriched in the early eluting fractions, no clear separation from monomers could be achieved.[25]

In the next step, the high affinity of protein S multimers for anionic phospholipids was used to separate protein S monomers and multimers. A purified protein S preparation containing monomers and multimers was incubated for 3 hours with small unilamellar phospholipid vesicles (20/80 DOPS/DOPC) in $CaCl_2$-containing buffer under conditions where protein S multimers, but not monomers, quantitatively bind to the vesicles. Subsequently, the protein S/phospholipid mixture was loaded onto a size-exclusion chromatography column (HiLoad 26/60 Superdex 200). Absorbance measurements at 280 nm showed that 2 separate peaks eluted from the column (Fig 4A). The phospholipid vesicles eluted in the void volume peak 1 (~110 mL) and caused a high absorbance at 280 nm likely due to light scattering by the vesicles (Fig 4A). The protein S concentration in the column fractions was determined by ELISA. Less than 10% of the total protein S applied to the column was bound to the vesicles as multimers. The majority of protein S was retarded on the column and eluted in a symmetrical peak at ~180 mL. This peak only contained protein S monomers and 1 hour after size-exclusion chromatography, the protein S peak 2 fraction (0.6 mg/mL) was tested for phospholipid binding in an ellipsometer and compared with the starting material.

Time-dependent protein S adsorption ($\mu g/cm^2$) to a planar phospholipid bilayer (20/80 DOPS/DOPC) was followed over time at a final concentration of 25 nmol/L protein S (Fig 4B) using ellipsometry essentially as described.[25] The starting material, which was a mixture of protein S monomers and multimers, showed the characteristic biphasic adsorption as observed before[25] (Fig 4B, curve a). The abundant protein S monomers in the preparation (~95%) with a low affinity for phospholipids resulted in a fast, initial adsorption phase, which was completed within 50 seconds after addition of protein S to the ellipsometer cuvette. Following the initial adsorption of the protein S monomers, the fraction of protein S multimers (~5%) with a high affinity for phospholipids resulted in a second slow continuing adsorption of protein S to the phospholipid bilayer. During this second phase, the protein S multimers with a high affinity for phospholipids (K_d <1 nmol/L) quantitatively replaced the low-affinity protein S monomers (K_d = ~250 nmol/L).[25] This was illustrated by the observation that almost no protein S multimers dissociated from the lipid bilayer when the nonbound protein S was removed by flushing the cuvette with buffer containing $CaCl_2$ (at ~3,500 seconds). Binding of protein S multimers was Ca^{2+}-dependent as addition of EDTA resulted in complete desorption (at ~3,700 seconds).

Adsorption of protein S from the second peak of the Superdex chromatography run only showed the fast, initial adsorption phase that was reversible upon flushing with buffer containing $CaCl_2$ at ~1,800 seconds (Fig 4B). This confirmed that the second protein S peak from the Superdex column was essentially protein S multimer-free and only contained protein S monomers. When, after 1 week, the monomeric protein S was analyzed on native PAGE and Western blot, traces of multimers were observed (not shown), which raised the question of whether multimer formation occurred spontaneously within purified (monomeric) protein S preparations.

In an additional Superdex chromatography experiment, the fraction containing monomeric protein S (peak 2) was kept at 4°C and tested in the ellipsometer after 1, 2, and 5 weeks of storage (Fig 4C). New formation of multimeric protein S forms was clearly observed. The phospholipid-binding rate of protein S on the phospholipid bilayer during the second slow adsorption phase increased with storage time, indicating that there was a time-dependent increase in the formation of protein S multimers (Fig 4C). In addition, the amount of bound protein S that was removed upon washing with $CaCl_2$-containing buffer decreased with storage time, confirming the time-dependent formation of protein S multimers. Calculation of the initial adsorption slope of the second slow phase of binding showed that, after 1, 2, and 5 weeks of storage, the protein S preparation contained 9%, 17%, and 25%, respectively, of the amount of protein S multimers present in the starting protein S preparation (Fig 4B).

In an attempt to prevent generation of protein S multimers in the purified protein S monomer preparation, freshly isolated monomeric protein S (600 μg/mL) was stored in a buffer containing BSA (0.5%), precipitated with ammonium sulfate (70%), or both. Under all conditions, protein S multimers were formed (not shown). In addition, dilution of monomeric protein S fractions to 75 μg/mL prior to addition of BSA and/or ammonium sulfate still resulted in multimer formation. Therefore, we were not able to obtain a purified protein S preparation devoid of multimeric forms that could be used for structure-function analysis, unless used immediately (<1 day) after size-exclusion chromatography in the presence of small unilamellar phospholipid vesicles as described above.

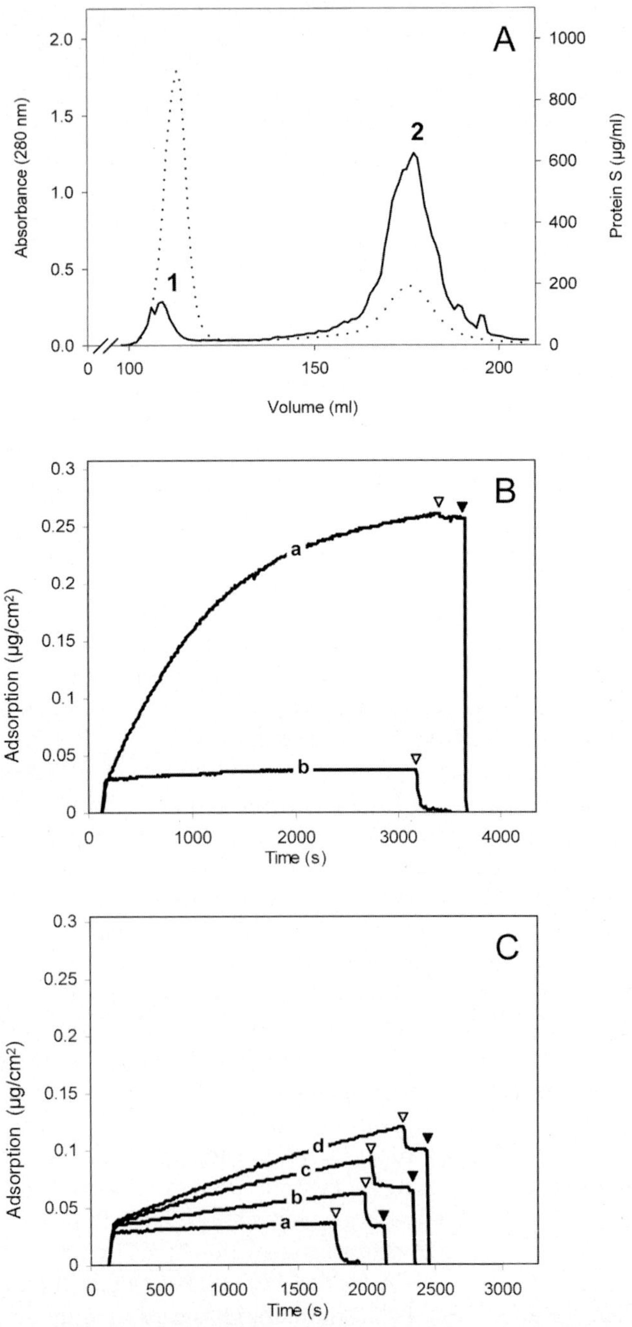

Inhibition of Prothrombin Activation by Protein S at Various Concentrations of Phospholipid

Protein S multimers bind with high affinity to anionic phospholipids (K_d <1 nmol/L) and effectively inhibit phospholipid-dependent enzyme processes at low phospholipid concentrations. Purified protein S has been reported to inhibit prothrombin activation at phospholipid concentrations less than 1 μmol/L[17,26] and differences in the extent of inhibition between protein S preparations could be attributed to differences in the multimer content of the protein S preparations.[25] In order to find experimental conditions under which protein S multimers cannot exert their inhibitory activity, two protein S preparations were tested for their ability to inhibit prothrombin activation as a function of phospholipid concentration. Protein S_1 was purified from plasma as described in the Experimental Procedures section, and contained multimeric protein S forms (Fig 1, lane f). Protein S_2 was derived from plasma-purified protein S-C4BP complex and separated from C4BP by reverse phase HPLC as described in the Experimental Procedures section. Factor Xa, FVa and phospholipids were pre-incubated in Ca^{2+}-containing buffer for 15 minutes in the absence or presence of 100 nmol/L protein S (final

←

Figure 4 Separation of protein S multimers and monomers by size-exclusion chromatography. Purified protein S (19 μmol/L) was incubated with 0.9 mmol/L small unilamellar phospholipid vesicles (20/80 DOPS/DOPC) in HBS containing 3 mmol/L $CaCl_2$ for 3 h at RT. After incubation, the mixture was applied to a HiLoad 26/60 Superdex 200 column, which was equilibrated with HBS containing 3 mmol/L $CaCl_2$. (A) The absorption profile at 280 nm (dashed line) and the protein S concentrations in the column fractions determined by ELISA (solid line). (B) Adsorption of protein S on a DOPS/DOPC phospholipid bilayer (20 mol% DOPS) was quantified using ellipsometry. Protein S (25 nmol/L) was added to the ellipsometer cuvette at ~200 seconds and the mass of protein adsorbed to the lipid bilayer (Γ) was followed in time. The protein S starting preparation (a) and the Superdex fraction 2 (b) are shown. After binding, the cuvette was flushed with HBS containing $CaCl_2$ (open triangles) and HBS containing EDTA (filled triangles) (C) Fraction 2 was stored at 4°C and analyzed by ellipsometry at 1 hour (a), 1 week (b), 2 weeks (c), and 5 weeks (d) after size-exclusion chromatography. Ellipsometry experiments were performed at RT in a buffer (50 mmol/L Tris-HCl, 100 mmol/L NaCl, 3 mmol/L $CaCl_2$, pH 7.5) containing 5 mg/mL BSA.

concentration). Thrombin formation was initiated by addition of prothrombin to the reaction mixture. At 0.2 μmol/L phospholipid, thrombin generation was nearly completely inhibited by 100 nmol/L protein S_1 (Fig 5). Increasing the phospholipid concentration resulted in a gradual loss of the inhibitory activity of protein S_1. The protein S_2 preparation contained a higher amount of multimeric forms than protein S_1 due to the exposure of protein S to low pH during HPLC purification procedures (data not shown), and was a more effective inhibitor of thrombin formation than protein S_1 (Fig 5). Half-maximal inhibition of prothrombin activation was reached at 3.2 μmol/L phospholipid for protein S_2 and 0.7 μmol/L phospholipid for protein S_1, suggesting an approximately fourfold higher multimer-concentration in protein S_2. At high phospholipid concentrations (>50 μmol/L), both protein S preparations only slightly inhibited prothrombin activation (<10%).

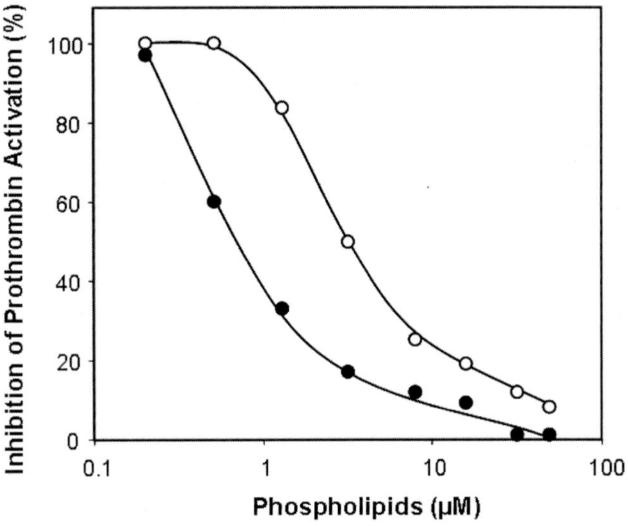

Figure 5 Inhibition of prothrombin activation by protein S multimers at varying phospholipid concentrations. Factor Va, FXa and phospholipid vesicles (20/80 DOPS/DOPC) were incubated with or without protein S in HBS containing 3 mmol/L $CaCl_2$ and 5 mg/mL BSA for 15 minutes at 37°C. Prothrombin was added and thrombin formation was followed in time as described in the Experimental Procedures section. Final concentrations were 10 pmol/L FVa, 10 pmol/L FXa, 1.5 μmol/L prothrombin, 0 or 100 nmol/L protein S and 0.2-50 μmol/L phospholipid vesicles. Inhibition of prothrombin activation by protein S_1 (●) and protein S_2 (○) is presented as a function of the phospholipid concentration.

C4BP-Protein S Complex Formation

C4BP has a profound influence on protein S function[14,20,21] and is often used to modulate protein S activity in model systems. Because of the actual risk of misinterpretation of protein S activity at low phospholipid concentrations due to the presence of protein S multimers, it is important to test whether C4BP is able to bind to protein S multimers. A protein S preparation that contained multimers (Fig 6, lane a) was incubated with excess β chain-containing C4BP in a buffer with $CaCl_2$. Subsequent analysis on Western blot showed a shift of the major protein S monomer band to a low mobility protein S-C4BP band on top of the gel (Fig 6, lane b). No change in intensity or mobility was observed for bands corresponding to protein S multimers. When isolated protein S monomers (Fig 6, lane c) were incubated with C4BP, a shift of the protein S monomer band was again observed as a result of complex formation between protein S and C4BP (Fig 6, lane d), but protein S-C4BP complex formation was not accompanied by protein S multimerization.

Discussion

Purified human protein S preparations contain 2 forms of protein S: a major fraction consisting of protein S monomers and a minor fraction (<5%) of protein S multimers.[25] In plasma these multimers are absent, implying that multimerization occurs during the purification of protein S. We have shown that protein S multimers were generated during standard anion-exchange chromatography that is used for isolation of protein S from plasma. In addition, high ionic strength as well as denaturing conditions like low pH and treatment with chaotropic reagents, used in immunoaffinity purification of protein S, induce multimer formation.

When multimers were quantitatively removed from a protein S preparation by applying a pre-incubated mixture of purified protein S and phospholipid vesicles to size-exclusion chromatography, spontaneous generation of multimers occurred in the isolated fraction of protein S monomers. This observation contradicts our earlier report, where it was suggested that a multimer-free protein S preparation was stable for several weeks.[25] In that study, liposome centrifugation was used to separate protein S multimers bound to the liposomes from the monomers in the supernatant. We now believe that this procedure likely introduces phospholipid remnant structures into the monomeric protein S fraction, which tightly bind traces of protein S multimers. These multimers can subsequently be missed in phospholipid binding analyses using ellipsometry and functional protein S studies.

The question remains as to what initiates multimer formation. In vitro purification conditions clearly induced protein S multimerization. When protein S multimers were removed from a purified protein S preparation, they spontaneously reappeared. The presence of either BSA or ammonium sulfate did not prevent multimer formation. As no contaminants could be detected in the purified monomeric protein S preparation, the origin of multimer formation seems to lie in the monomeric protein S molecule itself. This might imply a limited proportion of protein S molecules acting as nuclei to propagate multimerization.

Partly denatured intermediates of proteins that are relatively stable may reflect the so-called "molten-globule" state.[35] Such intermediates have the same secondary structure as the native counterpart but their amino acid sidechains are more disordered. The latter results in (partial) loss of tertiary structure and in increased hydrophobicity. Exposure of hydrophobic residues to the solvent will likely result in aggregation of proteins. Such partial unfolding can be induced in denaturing conditions like low pH or increased

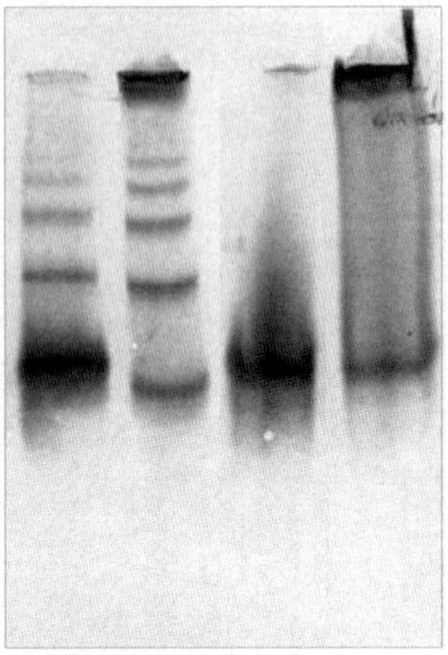

Figure 6 Protein S-C4BP complex formation. Purified protein S preparations (220 nmol/L) were incubated with or without β chain-containing C4BP (290 nmol/L) in HEPES-buffered saline (25 mmol/L HEPES, 175 mmol/L NaCl, pH 7.7) containing 5 mg/mL BSA and 0.5 mmol/L $CaCl_2$ for 30 minutes at RT and subsequently subjected to native PAGE (4-15% acrylamide), transferred to a PVDF membrane by Western blotting and visualized with peroxidase-conjugated polyclonal antibodies against protein S. Lane a: total purified protein S; lane b: total purified protein S with C4BP; lane c: isolated protein S monomers; lane d: isolated protein S monomers with C4BP.

temperature.[36] Loss of tertiary structure can also occur under physiologic conditions when the stabilizing environment of a protein is absent. Thus, the lack of the plasma (protein) environment may induce minor modifications in the protein S molecule resulting in (partial) aggregation of purified protein S. Interestingly, the aggregation of recombinant human factor VIII was described as originating from "a small transition in the tertiary structure of the protein which produced a nucleating species that led to the formation of inactive soluble aggregates."[37] The observations for factor VIII and protein S seem to be similar and emphasize the need for prudence with the use of purified proteins in structure-function analysis.

Prevention of protein S multimerization during purification from plasma appears virtually impossible, and it is therefore likely that the presence of protein S multimers is a general characteristic of purified protein S preparations. Protein S multimers have also been observed in previous reports. In 1990, Schwalbe et al[28] reported that the binding of purified human protein S to phospholipids had a biphasic nature and that multiple protein layers were formed on the phospholipid surface. van 't Veer et al[26] reported that the APC-independent activity of protein S increased with prolonged incubation times, which is likely a result of the time-dependent increase in adsorption of the high-affinity, low-abundance protein S multimers to the phospholipid surface. Since the first report on the anticoagulant effect of protein S in the absence of APC, up to 10-fold differences in APC-independent activity of protein S have been reported,[15,17] and the activity of a protein S preparation has been correlated with its affinity for anionic phospholipids.[17] Today we know that these observations can be ascribed to variable amounts of protein S multimers present in different protein S preparations.[25] In addition, the influence of the protein S purification procedure on the activity of a preparation has been recognized[15,38] and it has been suggested that modifications in the protein S molecule occur during purification.[15,16]

At low phospholipid concentrations, the multimeric protein S present in purified protein S preparations will likely inhibit all lipid-dependent coagulation processes, not only in model systems of factor X or prothrombin activation,[17,25,26] but also in plasma reconstitution experiments.[17] Moreover, it is possible that other processes occurring on a negatively charged phospholipid surface will be influenced by multimers as well. For example, we have observed that protein S multimers introduce cross-linking of liposomes (unpublished observations). The possibility that this also occurs with cells expressing phosphatidylserine on their surface cannot be excluded, which might be interesting in view of the stimulatory effect of purified protein S on phagocytosis of apoptotic cells.[39]

Multimerization not only influences the interaction of protein S with a phospholipid surface; protein S multimers no longer form a complex with C4BP. Apparently, the binding site for C4BP on the protein S molecule is altered or obstructed in protein S multimers. Moreover, multimerization of protein S is not a result of C4BP-protein S interactions. The loss of the C4BP binding site on protein S might be due to steric hindrance or a specific alteration in the protein S molecule. In the absence of APC, the presence of C4BP did not affect the ability of purified protein S to inhibit prothrombin activation.[14] This observation can now be explained by the fact that protein S multimers present in the protein S preparations were responsible for the inhibition of prothrombin activation, and that addition of C4BP, which does not form a complex with protein S multimers, therefore does not affect their inhibitory activity.

Protein S multimers bind tightly to phospholipids (K_d <1 nmol/L)[25] and therefore can effectively compete for phospholipid binding sites with prothrombin, the substrate of the prothrombinase complex, and/or interfere with the assembly of the prothrombinase complex. Consequently, the inhibitory activity of protein S multimers on prothrombin activation can easily reach 100% at concentrations of phospholipids less than 1 μmol/L (Fig 5). The use of high phospholipid concentrations is therefore a prerequisite for studying the anticoagulant activity of purified protein S in model systems. The fact that protein S monomers have a low affinity for phospholipids suggests that monomeric protein S inhibits thrombin formation via a mechanism other than competition for binding sites on the phospholipid surface. Direct interactions of protein S with FXa and FVa may cause inhibition of prothrombin activation, and it has been hypothesized that such interactions could explain the APC-independent anticoagulant activity of protein S in plasma.[27] However, in our model system using purified components, 100 nmol/L protein S hardly inhibited prothrombin activation at phospholipid concentrations greater than 50 μmol/L, whereas in plasma experiments protein S considerably inhibited thrombin formation independent of the phospholipid concentration.[27]

The results of the present study indicate that protein S structure-function analysis in model systems using purified proteins should be performed at phospholipid concentrations ≥50 μmol/L to ensure that unwanted activities of protein S multimers are avoided. Furthermore, the inhibition of prothrombin activation by protein S in the absence of APC in model systems using purified proteins at low phospholipid concentrations is nonphysiologic and a result of in vitro purification procedures: that mechanism is different from the mechanism by which protein S inhibits thrombin generation in plasma in the absence of APC.

Acknowledgment

The authors thank Dr Guido Tans for stimulating discussions.

References

1. DiScipio RG, Davie EW: Characterization of protein S, a gamma-carboxyglutamic acid containing protein from bovine and human plasma. Biochemistry US 18:899-904, 1979
2. Griffin JH, Gruber A, Fernandez JA: Reevaluation of total, free, and bound protein S and C4b-binding protein levels in plasma anticoagulated with citrate or hirudin. Blood 79:3203-3211, 1992
3. Comp PC, Esmon CT: Recurrent venous thromboembolism in patients with a partial deficiency of protein S. N Engl J Med 311:1525-1528, 1984
4. Makris M, Leach M, Beauchamp NJ, Daly ME, Cooper PC, Hampton KK, et al: Genetic analysis, phenotypic diagnosis, and risk of venous thrombosis in families with inherited deficiencies of protein S. Blood 95:1935-1941, 2000
5. Schwarz HP, Fischer M, Hopmeier P, Batard MA, Griffin JH: Plasma protein S deficiency in familial thrombotic disease. Blood 64:1297-1300, 1984
6. Dahlback B, Frohm B, Nelsestuen G: High affinity interaction between C4b-binding protein and vitamin K-dependent protein S in the presence of calcium. Suggestion of a third component in blood regulating the interaction. J Biol Chem 265:16082-16087, 1990
7. Evenas P, Garcia De Frutos P, Linse S, Dahlback B: Both G-type domains of protein S are required for the high-affinity interaction with C4b-binding protein. Eur J Biochem 266: 935-942, 1999
8. Fernandez JA, Griffin JH, Chang GT, Stam J, Reitsma PH, Bertina RM, et al: Involvement of amino acid residues 423-429 of human protein S in binding to C4b-binding protein. Blood Cells Mol Dis 24:101-112; discussion 113, 1998
9. Walker FJ: Regulation of activated protein C by a new protein. A possible function for bovine protein S. J Biol Chem 255:5521-5524, 1980
10. Walker FJ, Fay PJ: Regulation of blood coagulation by the protein C system. FASEB J 6:2561-2567, 1992
11. O'Brien LM, Mastri M, Fay PJ: Regulation of factor VIIIa by human activated protein C and protein S: Inactivation of cofactor in the intrinsic factor Xase. Blood 95:1714-1720, 2000
12. Rosing J, Hoekema L, Nicolaes GA, Thomassen MC, Hemker HC, Varadi K, et al: Effects of protein S and factor Xa on peptide bond cleavages during inactivation of factor Va and factor VaR506Q by activated protein C. J Biol Chem 270:27852-27858, 1995
13. van't Veer C, Hackeng TM, Biesbroeck D, Sixma JJ, Bouma BN: Increased prothrombin activation in protein S-deficient plasma under flow conditions on endothelial cell matrix: An independent anticoagulant function of protein S in plasma. Blood 85:1815-1821, 1995
14. Hackeng TM, van 't Veer C, Meijers JC, Bouma BN: Human protein S inhibits prothrombinase complex activity on endothelial cells and platelets via direct interactions with factors Va and Xa. J Biol Chem 269:21051-21058, 1994
15. Heeb MJ, Mesters RM, Tans G, Rosing J, Griffin JH: Binding of protein S to factor Va associated with inhibition of prothrombinase that is independent of activated protein C. J Biol Chem 268:2872-2877, 1993
16. Heeb MJ, Rosing J, Bakker HM, Fernandez JA, Tans G, Griffin JH: Protein S binds to and inhibits factor Xa. Proc Natl Acad Sci U S A 91:2728-2732, 1994
17. van Wijnen M, Stam JG, van't Veer C, Meijers JC, Reitsma PH, Bertina RM, et al: The interaction of protein S with the phospholipid surface is essential for the activated protein C-independent activity of protein S. Thromb Haemost 76:397-403, 1996
18. Heeb MJ, Kojima Y, Rosing J, Tans G, Griffin JH: C-terminal residues 621-635 of protein S are essential for binding to factor Va. J Biol Chem 274:36187-36192, 1999
19. Stenberg Y, Muranyi A, Steen C, Thulin E, Drakenberg T, Stenflo J: EGF-like module pair 3-4 in vitamin K-dependent protein S: Modulation of calcium affinity of module 4 by module 3, and interaction with factor X. J Mol Biol 293: 653-665, 1999
20. Dahlback B: Inhibition of protein Ca cofactor function of human and bovine protein S by C4b-binding protein. J Biol Chem 261:12022-12027, 1986
21. Nishioka J, Suzuki K: Inhibition of cofactor activity of protein S by a complex of protein S and C4b-binding protein. Evidence for inactive ternary complex formation between protein S, C4b-binding protein, and activated protein C. J Biol Chem 265:9072-9076, 1990
22. Dahlback B, Hildebrand B, Malm J: Characterization of functionally important domains in human vitamin K-dependent protein S using monoclonal antibodies. J Biol Chem 265:8127-8135, 1990
23. Hackeng TM, Hessing M, van 't Veer C, Meijer-Huizinga F, Meijers JC, de Groot PG, et al: Protein S binding to human endothelial cells is required for expression of cofactor activity for activated protein C. J Biol Chem 268:3993-4000, 1993
24. McDonald JF, Shah AM, Schwalbe RA, Kisiel W, Dahlback B, Nelsestuen GL: Comparison of naturally occurring vitamin K-dependent proteins: Correlation of amino acid sequences and membrane binding properties suggests a membrane contact site. Biochemistry US 36: 5120-5127, 1997
25. Sere KM, Janssen MP, Willems GM, Tans G, Rosing J, Hackeng TM: Purified protein S contains multimeric forms with increased APC-independent anticoagulant activity. Biochemistry US 40:8852-8860, 2001
26. van 't Veer C, Butenas S, Golden NJ, Mann KG: Regulation of prothrombinase activity by protein S. Thromb Haemost 82:80-87, 1999
27. Sere KM, Rosing J, Hackeng TM: Inhibition of thrombin generation by protein S at low procoagulant stimuli: Implications for maintenance of the hemostatic balance. Blood 104:3624-3630, 2004
28. Schwalbe R, Dahlback B, Hillarp A, Nelsestuen G: Assembly of protein S and C4b-binding protein on membranes. J Biol Chem 265: 16074-16081, 1990
29. Koedam JA, Meijers JC, Sixma JJ, Bouma BN: Inactivation of human factor VIII by activated protein C. Cofactor activity of protein S and protective effect of von Willebrand factor. J Clin Invest 82:1236-1243, 1988
30. Rosing J, Bakker HM, Thomassen MC, Hemker HC, Tans G: Characterization of two forms of human factor Va with different cofactor activities. J Biol Chem 268:21130-21136, 1993
31. Koenen RR, Gomes L, Tans G, Rosing J, Hackeng TM: The Ser460Pro mutation in recombinant protein S Heerlen does not affect its APC-cofactor and APC-independent anticoagulant activities. Thromb Haemost 91:1105-1114, 2004
32. Willems GM, Janssen MP, Pelsers MAL, Comfurius P, Galli M, Zwaal RFA, et al: Role of divalency in the high-affinity binding of anticardiolipin antibody-beta(2)-glycoprotein I complexes to lipid membranes. Biochemistry US 35:13833-13842, 1996
33. Giesen PLA, Willems GM, Hermens WT: Production of thrombin by the prothrombinase complex is regulated by membrane-mediated transport of prothrombin. J Biol Chem 266:1379-1382, 1991
34. Cuypers PA, Corsel JW, Janssen MP, Kop JM, Hermens WT, Hemker HC: The adsorption of prothrombin to phosphatidylserine multilayers quantitated by ellipsometry. J Biol Chem 258:2426-2431, 1983
35. Ptitsyn OB: How the molten globule became. Trends Biochem Sci 20: 376-379, 1995

36. Dobson CM: Protein misfolding, evolution and disease. Trends Biochem Sci 24:329-332, 1999
37. Grillo AO, Edwards KL, Kashi RS, Shipley KM, Hu L, Besman MJ, et al: Conformational origin of the aggregation of recombinant human factor VIII. Biochemistry US 40:586-595, 2001
38. Mitchell CA, Kelemen SM, Salem HH: The anticoagulant properties of a modified form of protein S. Thromb Haemost 60:298-304, 1988
39. Anderson HA, Maylock CA, Williams JA, Paweletz CP, Shu H, Shacter E: Serum-derived protein S binds to phosphatidylserine and stimulates the phagocytosis of apoptotic cells. Nat Immunol 4:87-91, 2003

Seminars in
HEMATOLOGY

Abstracts

Dynamics of Thrombus Formation

Bruce Furie

Hemostasis and thrombosis are, respectively, complex physiologic and pathologic processes that involve the vessel wall, circulating blood cells with their receptors and ligands, soluble blood coagulation and regulatory proteins, and blood cell-derived microparticles. Although we and others have worked with purified systems to examine this complexity and subsequently to develop models of the processes involved, it has become increasingly important to analyze hemostasis and thrombosis in a living animal where all of the components are present simultaneously. Furthermore, the availability of genetically altered mice that lack the ability to synthesize a specific protein offers the opportunity to study these processes in a mouse model of thrombosis. The confluence of the development of knockout technology in the mouse, improved microscopic imaging instrumentation, and high-speed computers has supported the development of a novel system for high-speed, intravital, digital videomicroscopy in the microcirculation of a living mouse. The goal has been to visualize thrombus formation following vessel wall injury in this model using an intravital, confocal, and wide-field microscopy imaging system (Fig 1). Using this system, we have studied, or are studying, P-selectin/P-selectin glycoprotein ligand-1 (PSGL-1)-mediated tissue factor-bearing microparticle accumulation in the developing thrombus; calcium mobilization during platelet activation; the role of protease-activated receptor and glycoprotein VI in platelet activation; factor XI participation in thrombin generation; and the relevant membrane surfaces that support thrombin generation in vivo. Furthermore, this system has been useful for evaluating the efficacy of platelet antagonists during experimental thrombosis in vivo. By revisiting and testing the models and hypotheses that have been developed from in vitro studies, we have been able to determine that many of these models and hypotheses are correct, whereas others may need some significant modification. The study of biochemistry and cell biology in a living animal offers opportunities to understand physiology and pathology in complex biological systems.

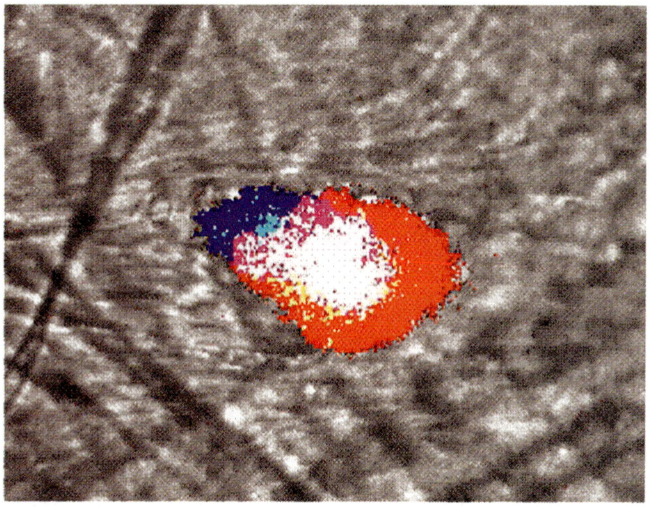

Figure 1 Intravital imaging of platelet, tissue factor, and fibrin deposition in the developing thrombus of a living wild-type mouse following laser-induced vessel wall injury. Blood flow is from left to right. Alexa 660-conjugated CD41 Fab fragments, Alexa 488-conjugated rabbit anti-mouse tissue factor antibodies, and Alexa 350-conjugated mouse anti-human fibrin antibodies were infused into the systemic circulation. Thrombus components in four separate channels were identified in pseudocolors as well as a black and white brightfield image, and a composite image generated. Platelets (red); tissue factor (green); fibrin (blue); platelets + tissue factor (yellow); tissue factor + fibrin (turquoise); platelets + fibrin (magenta); platelets + fibrin + tissue factor (white). This image was acquired 100 seconds following injury.

Center for Hemostasis and Thrombosis Research, Beth Israel Deaconess Medical Center, Harvard Medical School, Boston, MA.

Address correspondence to Bruce Furie, Chief, Division of Hemostasis-Thrombosis, Beth Israel Deaconess Medical Center, Harvard Medical School, 330 Brookline Ave, Boston MA 02215. E-mail: bfurie@bidmc.harvard.edu

doi:10.1053/j.seminhematol.2005.11.014

ELSEVIER

Seminars in
HEMATOLOGY

Recombinant Factor VIIa and COAT Platelets

Marianne Kjalke and Rasmus Rojkjaer

Activation of platelets with a combination of collagen and thrombin generates a subpopulation of highly procoagulant platelets, the so-called COAT (collagen- and thrombin-activated) platelets, characterized by a high surface expression of fibrinogen and other coagulation proteins. We found greatly enhanced binding of recombinant factor VIIa (rFVIIa; NovoSeven®, Novo Nordisk, Bagsvaerd, Denmark) to COAT platelets compared with single-agonist-activated platelets. The rFVIIa–COAT platelet interaction was dependent on the rFVIIa Gla-domain and platelet activation-mediated exposure of negatively charged phospholipids, as rFVIIa lacking the Gla-domain did not bind COAT platelets and the addition of annexin V inhibited binding. In a tissue factor-initiated cell-based model system, addition of an agonist to the platelet collagen receptor, glycoprotein VI, dramatically enhanced thrombin generation. Upon induction of hemophilia A-like conditions, reduced thrombin generation and reduced COAT platelet fibrinogen expression were observed. Addition of rFVIIa (30 to 300 nmol/L) dose-dependently enhanced thrombin generation but did not restore platelet surface fibrinogen expression. Our data suggest that rFVIIa is retained preferentially on platelets activated with dual agonists, thereby ensuring that enhanced thrombin generation is localized at the site of injury where both collagen and tissue factor are exposed.

Novo Nordisk A/S, Måløv, Denmark.

Address correspondence to Marianne Kjalke, PhD, Novo Nordisk A/S, Novo Nordisk Park C9.1.31, DK-2760 Måløv, Denmark. E-mail: mkja@novonordisk.com

 0037-1963/06/$-see front matter Published by Elsevier Inc.
doi:10.1053/j.seminhematol.2005.11.007

Excluded Abstracts

Contribution of rFVIIa to Clot Stability In Vivo
Emrys Kirkman, Wayne Sapsford, and Graham Cooper

Seminars in HEMATOLOGY

Neal S. Young · Photis Beris

Editors

Peter A. Miescher, *Founding Editor* Ernst R. Jaffé, *Co-Editor Emeritus*

Seminars in Hematology (ISSN 0037-1963) is published quarterly by Elsevier, 1600 John F. Kennedy Blvd, Ste 1800, Philadelphia, PA 19103-2899. (For Post Office use only: Volume 42 issue 2 of 4.) Months of issue are January, April, July, and October. Corporate and Editorial Offices: 6277 Sea Harbor Dr, Orlando, FL 32887-4800. Periodicals postage paid at Orlando, FL 32887-4800, and at additional mailing officies.

POSTMASTER: Send change of address to *Seminars in Hematology,* Elsevier, Periodicals Department, 6277 Sea Harbor Dr, Orlando, FL 32887-4800.

Editorial correspondence should be addressed to Photis Beris, MD, Division d'Hématologie, Hôpital Cantonal Universitaire, 25 rue Micheli-du-Crest, 1211 Geneve 14, Switzerland, or Neal S. Young, MD, 4400 17th Street, NW, Washington, DC 20011.

Business correspondence (subscriptions, change of address) should be addressed to the Publisher, Elsevier, 6277 Sea Harbor Dr, Orlando, FL 32887-4800; Email elspcs@elsevier.com.

Change of address notices, including both the old and new addresses of the subscriber, should be sent at least one month in advance.

Customer Service: 1-800-654-2452; outside the United States and Canada, (407) 345-4000.

Yearly subscription rates: United States and possessions: individual, $169.00; institution, $267.00; single issues, $81.00. All other countries: individual, $239.00; institution, $339.00; single issues, $81.00. Student and resident: United States and possessions, and Canada: $85.00; all other countries: $122.00. To receive student/resident rate, orders must be accompanied by name of affiliated institution, date of term, and the *signature* of program/residency coordinator on institution letterhead. Orders will be billed at individual rate until proof of status is received. Current prices are in effect for back volumes and back issues. Single issues, both current and back, exist in limited quantities and are offered for sale subject to availability. Back issues sold in conjunction with a subscription are on a prorated basis. Prices are subject to change without notice. *Checks* should be made payable to Elsevier and sent to *Seminars in Hematology,* Elsevier, Periodicals Department, PO Box 628239, Orlando, FL 32862-8239.

Other correspondence (copyediting, production) should be addressed to Elsevier, 1600 John F. Kennedy Blvd, Ste 1800, Philadelphia, PA 19103-2899.

The contents of *Seminars in Hematology* are indexed in *Index Medicus* and *MEDLINE, Current Contents/Clinical Medicine, Current Contents/Life Sciences,* Science Citation Index, and *EMBASE/* Excerpta Medica.

The *Seminars in Hematology* home page is located at *www.seminhematol.org.*

W.B. Saunders **Philadelphia, PA**

Seminars in HEMATOLOGY

Vol 43, No 2, April 2006

Acute Leukemia in the Elderly

Elihu H. Estey
Guest Editor

Introduction: Acute Leukemia in the Elderly 81
Elihu H. Estey

Etiology of Acute Myeloid Leukemia in the Elderly 82
David T. Bowen

General Approach to, and Perspectives on Clinical Research in, Older Patients With Newly Diagnosed Acute Myeloid Leukemia 89
Elihu H. Estey

Treatment of Older Patients With Acute Myeloid Leukemia—New Agents 96
Alan K. Burnett and Unmesh Mohite

Allogeneic Transplantation for the Elderly Patient With Acute Myelogenous Leukemia or Myelodysplastic Syndrome 107
Marcos de Lima and Sergio Giralt

Immunologic Approaches to Acute Leukemia in the Elderly 118
Sherif S. Farag and Michael A. Caligiuri

Management of Acute Lymphoblastic Leukemia in Older Patients 126
Richard A. Larson

Approach to the Complications of Treatment for Acute Leukemia in the Elderly 134
Joel Gingerich and Eric J. Bow

Cover Illustration: The past three decades have seen little improvement in life expectancy for older patients with acute myeloid leukemia. This issue of *Seminars* deals with the etiology of, and new therapeutic approaches to, acute leukemia in the older patient. (Figure from Burnett and Mohite, pages 96-106.)

Seminars in HEMATOLOGY

Previous Issues

2005

Vol 42, No 1, January	**von Willebrand Factor in Hemostasis and Thrombosis** *Pier M. Mannucci, Guest Editor*
Vol 42, No 2, April	**Immune Hemolytic Anemia** *George Garratty, Guest Editor*
Vol 42, No 3, July	**Transplant Immunobiology** *Effie W. Petersdorf, Guest Editor*
Vol 42, No 4, October	**Chronic Myeloproliferative Disorders** *Radek Skoda and Josef T. Prchal, Guest Editors*

2004

Vol 41, No 1, January	**Thrombotic Thrombocytopenic Purpura: Advances in Pathophysiology, Diagnosis, and Treatment** *Bernhard Lämmle and James N. George, Guest Editors*
Vol 41, No 2, April	**Erythrocyte Membrane Proteins and Their Diseases** *Narla Mohandas, Guest Editor*
Vol 41, No 3, July	**Chronic Lymphocytic Leukemia** *Kanti R. Rai and Jacques Louis Binet, Guest Editors*
Vol 41, No 4, October	**Gene Therapy in Hematology** *Cynthia E. Dunbar, Guest Editor*

2003

Vol 40, No 1, January	**Management of Chronic Myeloid Leukemia** *John M. Goldman, Guest Editor*
Vol 40, No 2, April	**Herpesvirus in Hematology** *Giovanna Tosato, Guest Editor*
Vol 40, No 3, July	**Hematologic Malignancies of Cytotoxic Cells** *Thomas P. Loughran Jr, Guest Editor*
Vol 40, No 4, October	**Genomics in Hematology** *Louis M. Staudt, Guest Editor*

Seminars in
HEMATOLOGY

Future Topics

Vol 43, No 3, July	**Constitutional Marrow Failure** *Grover C. Bagby, Guest Editor*
Vol 43, No 4, October	**Aggressive Treatment of Aggressive Lymphomas** *Richard Fisher, Guest Editor*
Vol 44, No 1, January	**Transfusion Medicine in the Early 21st Century** *Harvey Klein, Guest Editor*
Vol 44, No 2, April	**Inherited Thrombophilias** *Michael Greaves, Guest Editor*

Seminars in
HEMATOLOGY

Forthcoming Issue
July 2006

Constitutional Marrow Failure
Grover C. Bagby, *Guest Editor*

Fanconi Anemia — *Grover C. Bagby and Blanche P. Alter*

Dyskeratosis Congenita — *Tom Vulliamy and Inderjeet Dokal*

Diamond Blackfan Anemia: New Paradigms for a "Not So Pure" Inherited Red Cell Aplasia — *Jeffrey M. Lipton*

Shwachman-Diamond Syndrome — *Akiko Shimamura*

Inherited Thrombocytopenia: Congenital Amegakaryocytic Thrombocytopenia and Thrombocytopenia With Absent Radii — *Amy E. Geddis*

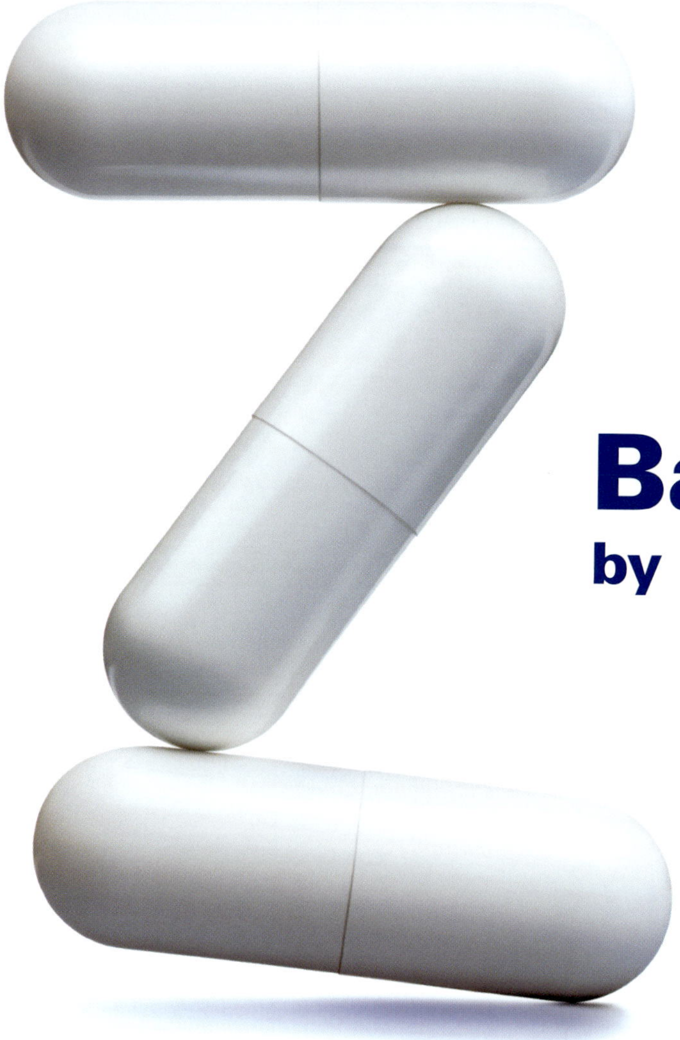

For adults with mild-to-moderate ***type 1 Gaucher disease*** *for whom enzyme replacement therapy is not an option*

Balance
by Substrate Reduction

Substrate Reduction Therapy (SRT) With Zavesca Provides Important Benefits

- Liver and spleen volume reductions seen as early as month 6—continued reductions over 24 months
- Hemoglobin concentration and platelet count improvements seen as early as month 6—significant improvements seen at 24 months

Zavesca Maintained Benefits of Long-Term Enzyme Replacement Therapy (ERT)

- In patients on ERT for a mean of 5.6 years, liver and spleen volume, as well as hemoglobin concentration and platelet count, were maintained after 6 months of Zavesca monotherapy

Important Safety Information

- Peripheral neuropathy has been reported in patients receiving Zavesca
- Zavesca may cause fetal harm if administered to a pregnant woman
- There is a risk of impaired fertility in men

Convenient Oral Dosing

- Recommended at 100 mg tid
- May be taken with or without food

Zavesca may be prescribed only by physicians knowledgeable in the management of Gaucher disease

- **Visit www.ZAVESCA.com or call 1.866.228.3546**

ZAVESCA® 100mg
(miglustat) capsules

Please see brief summary of full prescribing information on following page.

ACTELION

ELSEVIER

Seminars in
HEMATOLOGY

Volume 43, Number 2 **April 2006**

Introduction: Acute Leukemia in the Elderly

It is readily accepted that the prognosis of older patients with acute leukemia is extraordinarily poor. To a large extent this reflects our lack of knowledge about the differences between the blasts seen in acute leukemia and their normal counterparts. Exploration of the etiology and epidemiology of acute myeloid leukemia (AML) in the elderly may help us understand these distinctions. Accordingly, the first chapter in this issue of *Seminars*, by David Bowen, discusses the etiology of AML in the elderly. The chapter emphasizes the interplay between environmental factors and polymorphic variants in several genes responsible for maintaining the integrity of the genome. In the second chapter, Dr Estey focuses on the general management of AML in the elderly and in particular on which patients are candidates for clinical trials of new drugs, for standard therapy, or for palliative care. The topic of new drugs is pursued in much more depth by Burnett and Mohite. Both this chapter and Estey's propose new designs for clinical trials in older patients; these designs are intended to allow more rapid screening of the large number of therapies that will become available in the future. Novel therapies are further discussed by De Lima and Giralt and by Farag and Caligiuri. In the former, the authors describe the applicability of reduced intensity allogeneic transplantation in older patients. It is clear that such "mini-transplants" have extended the age limit beyond which transplantation can be performed. The latter chapter notes recent advances in understanding the importance of natural killer (NK) cell receptors in recognizing and lysing AML cells, emphasizing strategies to harness NK cells. Although AML is considerably more frequent, older patients can also develop acute lymphoblastic leukemia (ALL). Thus, Richard Larson discusses management of ALL in older patients, stressing the frequency of Philadelphia chromosome (*BCR/ABL*)-positive ALL in older patients and the resultant potential for use of tyrosine kinase inhibitors. Older patients with acute leukemia are obviously more prone than younger patients to develop complications of these diseases and their treatment. Thus, in the final chapter Gingerich and Bow describe methods to predict risk of these complications in various types of older patients and discuss methods for managing common sequelae of treatment, such as mucositis and infection.

We hope the readers find this issue of *Seminars* both informative and thought-provoking.

Elihu H. Estey
M.D. Anderson Cancer Center
Houston, TX
Guest Editor

0037-1963/06/$-see front matter
doi:10.1053/j.seminhematol.2006.03.001

ELSEVIER

Seminars in HEMATOLOGY

Etiology of Acute Myeloid Leukemia in the Elderly

David T. Bowen

The biologic and epidemiologic study of acute myeloid leukaemia (AML) in the elderly is in its infancy. Most epidemiologic data attempting to ascertain the etiology of AML have been obtained from younger cohorts or patients with therapy-related AML. The increasing prevalence of deletional and complex karyotypes in elderly AML patients implies a cumulative genotoxicity over time for this subgroup, given the similar spectrum of abnormalities following exposure to known genotoxic agents such as alkylating chemotherapeutic drugs. Exposure to benzene, radiation, and tobacco smoke are clear but weak risk factors for AML. Polymorphic variants in several genes responsible for genomic protection and integrity are now also weak risk factors for AML. Future epidemiologic studies should correlate exposure data with well-defined biologic subtypes of AML.
Semin Hematol 43:82-88

Most patients with acute myeloid leukemia (AML) could be considered "elderly," with a median age at presentation in unselected series of approximately 67 years.[1] The biology of AML represents a continuum of change from predominantly translocational genomic abnormalities in younger adults to an increasing prevalence of adverse and complex karyotypic abnormalities with increasing age.[1–3] The number of cases with a normal karyotype also increases with age. Inevitably, the etiology of AML in the elderly will differ from that in younger patients, reflecting the biologic differences.

While the scientific study of genomic variants (single-nucleotide polymorphisms [SNPs]) as risk factors for disease moves rapidly forward, the epidemiologic study of exposure to environmental toxins remains difficult. Indeed, the magnitude of the contribution of the environment to the etiology of AML remains uncertain and the potential for intrinsic damage associated with hematopoietic stem cell "aging" to play a major role is very real.

Detailed descriptive demographic and molecular epidemiology of AML in the elderly is required in order to generate hypotheses to direct the study of the etiology of biologically defined subtypes of AML.

Demographics

Large-scale, population-based demographic study of AML has been a surprisingly neglected area, largely due to the lack of comprehensive registration programs in most healthcare systems. The incidence of AML increases with age. However, the incidence of AML with balanced translocations is influenced less by age than is that of AML with both normal karyotype and complex aberrant karyotypes.[3] The most common translocational abnormality, t(15;17), changes little with age.[4] Thus in the decades beyond aged 70 years, translocational abnormalities account for less than 5% of AML cases, with the majority either a normal karyotype, deletions (structural and numerical), or trisomies.[1]

Most studies indicate a male predominance for AML[1,5] but when corrected for population-based age and sex distribution, the male predominance becomes less striking.[6] When age- and sex-corrected, female predominance cannot be identified in any karyotypic subgroup.[6]

Biology

Advances in molecular technology are beginning to separate distinct biologic subtypes of AML characterized by combinations of known abnormalities. Most reported cohorts are trial-based and selected for patients fit for intensive chemotherapy. A steady evolution from the study of trial-based patient cohorts to population-based cohorts will be more informative for the biology of AML in the elderly, whose entry into clinical trials remains relatively low.

Molecular signatures can be defined at several levels: *chromosomal* by G-banding karyotype or molecular cytogenetics (fluorescence-in-situ hybridization [FISH] or comparative genomic hybridization [CGH]), *genomic* (DNA) by gene mutation studies, *transcriptional* (RNA) by gene expression profiling, or *protein* profiling by proteomics. For elderly AML, there is a moderate dataset for G-banding karyotyping, less

Department of Haematology, Leeds Gerneral Infirmary, Leeds, UK.
Address correspondence to David T. Bowen, MD, Consultant Haematologist, Leeds General Infirmary, Great George Street, Leeds LS1 3EX, UK. E-mail: david.bowen@leedsth.nhs.uk

 0037-1963/06/$-see front matter
doi:10.1053/j.seminhematol.2006.01.005

for gene mutation studies, and little for the remainder of techniques. The predominant karyotypic abnormalities in elderly AML in order of frequency are normal, deletional, and trisomic, with normal karyotype in approximately 50% cases. Molecularly defined subgroups of patients with normal karyotype are now emerging from the study of younger, predominantly trial-based AML patient cohorts. Genetic pathways to the subtypes of therapy-related AML[7] may also apply to de novo cases, and the genetics of t-AML more closely resemble that of older patients with AML than younger. Thus several biologically defined subgroups of potential relevance to older AML patients are emerging, including the following:

- A relatively good prognosis group with normal karyotype, mutation in the Nucleophosmin (*NPM*) gene, but lacking internal tandem duplication (ITD) or activation loop mutation of *FLT3*[8]
- A poorer prognosis group with normal karyotype and *FLT3* ITD/mutation
- A very poor prognosis group with complex karyotype and p53 dysfunction, usually lacking *NPM* or *FLT3* abnormalities[9]
- Subgroups with distinct differences in overall survival defined by gene expression profile patterns only[10]

These scientific studies use the bulk AML tumor, in which many of the molecularly defined abnormalities are unstable, often differing between diagnosis and relapse.[8,11] These abnormalities may be predominantly post-initiation events and are more likely to provide clues to the pathogenesis of AML tumor promotion as opposed to initiation. Thus the study of AML stem cell biology is likely to be more fruitful in unraveling the etiologic events that lead to the initiation of AML.

Environmental and Occupational Exposures

Thus far, there have been no published large scale questionnaire-based epidemiologic studies that have correlated data with detailed molecular/cytogenetic studies in AML. Thus, conclusions drawn from epidemiologic studies alone will very likely be applicable only to some molecularly defined AML subtypes and not to others.

Case-Control Studies

Several small- to medium-sized case control studies of occupational and environmental exposures have been reported,[12-15] but none has been of sufficient size to meaningfully separate different AML subtypes, and different methodologies have been employed. Although no consistent exposures are identified across all studies, two trials have highlighted pesticide exposure as a risk factor,[12,13] another implicated solvent exposure,[14] and another tobacco smoke exposure.[15] Pesticide and solvent exposure have also been suggested as risk factors for myelodysplastic syndromes (MDS),[16,17] but given the relatively low odds ratios in all studies, if this risk is real then it is of low magnitude. Tobacco smoke exposure is a consistent but weak risk factor for the development of MDS[18] and AML (vide infra).

Case-control studies addressing specific exposures such as benzene or rubber are discussed below.

Exposure to Specific Toxins

Benzene

The data for occupational exposure to high concentrations of benzene indicate a cause and effect for the development of AML, following seminal studies of Turkish shoe workers[19] and employees in Pliofilm manufacture.[20] These exposures are now historical, with strict exposure limits now imposed on modern Western industry. The data for the relationship between exposure to low doses of benzene and the development of AML are contentious, and usually rely on models of linear extrapolation from high-dose exposure studies.[21,22] Environmental exposure to benzene is predominantly in tobacco smoke and unleaded petrol. Although tobacco smoke exposure is a weak risk factor for AML (vide infra), there are hundreds of alternative carcinogens contained within. No consistent increased risk of developing AML has been identified for automobile users, gas station employees, vehicle mechanics,[23] or anyone with exposure to diesel exhaust.[24]

In vitro incubation of either $CD34^+$ cells or lymphocytes with benzene metabolites induces predominantly aneuploid cytogenetic abnormalities (Fig 1), also described in AML.[25-27]

Radiation

There is clear evidence from atomic bomb survivors that relatively high-dose exposure to ionizing radiation can cause AML, with an increased risk that peaked at 10 years after exposure and persisted for approximately 15 years after exposure.[28] The data for incidence of AML after nuclear testing in the Pacific are inconsistent.[29,30] Occupational exposure to high doses of radiation also increases the risk of AML, but these are historical cohorts (usually before 1940) and such a risk no longer appears to be identifiable.[31,32] Radiotherapy for nonmalignant conditions can also increase the risk of subsequent AML[33-37] but is no longer offered. Local radiotherapy for cancer is probably not a significant risk factor for AML development when used as the only treatment, but this remains uncertain.[38,39] Radiotherapy in combination with chemotherapy,[40] particularly when radiotherapy is more generalized such as in autologous stem cell transplantation, may be a weak risk factor for the subsequent development of AML.[41] There is no consistent evidence for an association between AML and ultraviolet or electromagnetic radiation exposure but this has not been systematically studied. Studies of exposure to cosmic radiation have similarly produced contradictory data.[42-44] While direct genotoxic effects of ionizing radiation are well described[45] (Fig 1), a significant contribution may arise from bystander damage to cells adjacent to the hematopoietic stem cell.[46]

Others

The risk of cancer including leukemias has been studied across a number of occupations. For many of these studies, the different types of leukemia have not been separated, and for none of the studies have sufficient cases of AML been identified to further differentiate the biologic subtypes. Thus data exist for an excess of leukemias in painters,[47] seamen on tankers,[48] and synthetic rubber workers.[49] Other occupations with a reported excess of myeloid leukemia or AML are workers in the meat industry[50] and embalmers/funeral directors.[51] The excess risk in all of these studies is always small (less than threefold).

Lifestyle Factors

Diet

Although not extensively studied, there is no evidence to implicate diet in the etiology of AML. The diet is nevertheless a source of phenol and quinone exposure, and hypotheses have been proposed to link dietary exposure mechanistically to that of benzene.[52] However, limited study of diet within large prospective cohorts has failed to reveal an excess of AML or other leukemias associated with specific variation in dietary intake.[53,54] This area requires more extensive study.

Tobacco Smoking

Exposure to tobacco smoke is a consistent but weak risk factor for the development of AML. The largest reported studies are from a relatively younger cohort of patients, aged 16 to 69 years,[55] and the median age is 62 years.[56] The risk appears strongest in current smokers and probably declines to baseline at more than 10 years since cessation. The only carcinogen implicated in the etiology of AML and present in tobacco smoke is benzene. However, the estimated exposure levels to benzene in smokers are considerably lower than those observed in subjects with occupational benzene poisoning. Nevertheless, the leukemogenic effects of low-level benzene exposure remain unclear, and some investigators believe that benzene exposure explains up to three fifths of smoking-related AML mortality.[57]

Others

There are limited and inconclusive data for exposure to other lifestyle factors, including alcohol consumption[58] and hair dye usage.[59,60]

Inflammatory/ Infectious Disorders

Many paradigms exist linking cancer to inflammatory or infectious disease. Although no such strong associations can be identified for AML, there are weak associations reported with inflammatory bowel disease.[61,62] However, it is difficult to separate the risk associated with the inflammatory bowel disease from that associated with disease-modifying therapy, which now includes biologic response modifiers with immunosuppressive properties, in addition to potentially mutagenic cytotoxic immunosuppressant drugs.

Similarly there appears to be no clear link between infectious disease and AML, but again this has not been systematically studied. No significant association between AML and hepatitis virus antibody positivity could be found in a case-control study,[63] and a weak association (odds ratio = 1.89) was identified between AML and a history of chicken pox or measles.[64]

Molecular Epidemiology

As the mechanisms of mutagenesis are better understood, and the molecular lesions within the bulk AML tumor are better defined, so mechanistic causative hypotheses centered on intracellular biochemical pathways can begin to be proposed. AML is characterized by large-scale genomic abnormalities (aneuploidy, predominantly deletional), chromosomal translocations, and a spectrum of more localized genomic damage, namely, point mutations, tandem duplications, and small deletions, among many others. The mechanisms underlying aneuploidy and indeed chromosomal translocation remain poorly understood.

Mechanisms inducing point mutation in vitro include oxidative DNA damage and spontaneous cytosine deamination.[65] Oxidative and nitrosative free radical damage results from cellular exposure to many xenobiotic toxins—environmental, endogenous, and iatrogenic. This toxic stress is defended by a combination of detoxifying enzymes (including cytochrome P450s and glutathione *S*-transferases), and antioxidant processes (enzymatic and nonenzymatic). Any genotoxic damage is in turn efficiently repaired by a battery of DNA repair enzymes.[66]

The study of genetic predisposition to AML is gathering momentum. It is clear that inherited syndromes predispose to AML, including Fanconi anemia,[67] Bloom's syndrome,[68] and familial thrombocytopenia.[69] Murine models also indicate an inherited component for predisposition to both benzene-[70] and radiation-induced[71] genomic instability. This creates a paradigm for lower penetrance genetic predisposition, which in turn may produce a weak propensity to leukemogenesis. Theoretically, this predisposition could evolve from functional genetic polymorphisms in key defense genes within detoxification, antioxidant, DNA repair, and genome stabilization pathways. Many such polymorphic variants are described and large-scale genotyping of DNA from AML patients and controls are beginning to be reported. The larger cohorts reported thus far are from patients entered into clinical trials,[72] those with therapy-related AML,[72-75] or a relatively young nonselected population (Table 1).[76-78] Some studies have correlated polymorphic variant frequency with biologic (cytogenetic) subgroups, and include associations between inv(16) and *NQO1* C609T variant,[78] and *CYP 1A1*2B* variant and *NRAS* gene mutation.[79] These subgroup analyses require verification within larger cohorts. Extrapolation of these data to the etiology of AML in the elderly may or may not be appropriate.

No large cohorts correlating environmental/occupational exposure with biologic subtypes of AML (and/or polymorphic variant frequency) have been published. Such studies in a small cohort of MDS patients suggest an association between an abnormal karyotype and a history of exposure to solvents/pesticides,[17] but this has not been consistently demonstrated in AML.[80]

Therapy-Related MDS/AML

Prior exposure to cytotoxic chemotherapy is the most consistent and strongest risk factor for the development of

Table 1 Pathways and Genes Implicated as Predisposing to AML Through Functional Genomic Polymorphic Variation

Pathway	Enzyme Gene Variant	AML Type	Odds Ratio (95% confidence interval)
Phase 1 detoxification	*CYP 1A1 *2B*	AML (<69 yr) with mutated *NRAS* gene	2.36 (1.01–5.53)
	CYP2C19 poor metabolizer	AML < 60 yr	1.68 (0.97–2.92)
	CYP2D6 poor metabolizer	AML < 69 yr	1.69 (1.17–2.43)
Phase 2 detoxification	*NQO1 C609T*	AML < 69 yr	1.47 (1.13–1.90)
	GST P1 Val105	t-AML	1.81 (1.11–2.94)
DNA repair	*XPD Gln/Gln codon 751*	t-AML >60 yr	2.22 (1.04–4.74)
	XRCC1 399Gln	AML all ages	0.44 (0.20–0.93)*
Immunomodulation	*FAS G1377A*	AML < 69 yr	1.69 (1.32–2.16)

Abbreviations: CYP, cytochrome P450; GST, glutathione *S*-transferase; NQO1, NADP(H) quinone oxidoreductase 1; XPD, xeroderma pigmentosa; XRCC, x-ray repair cross-complementing; t-AML, therapy-related AML.
*Protective effect.

AML and MDS. These cases account for approximately 13% of AML patients.[81] This topic has been extensively reviewed elsewhere.[7] The similarities between the more common karyotypic abnormalities in therapy-related MDS/AML (t-MDS/AML) and poor risk de novo AML have prompted the hypothesis that exposure to environmental genotoxic agents may be implicated in this de novo AML subtype (Fig 1). Separate genetic pathways to t-MDS/AML can now be defined, and these are also observed in de novo AML.[6,9] Among the poor-risk karyotypic group, the more prevalent subgroups are those involving chromosome 5 abnormalities, often with chromosome 17 deletion and mutation within the *p53* gene, and chromosome 7 abnormalities associated with *RAS* gene mutation.[7] These subgroups have distinct gene expression profiles, confirming their karyotypic classification.[82] t-MDS/AML following exposure to alkylating agents and anthracyclines is characterized by abnormalities of chromosomes 5 and 7 and perhaps most closely mirrors the poor-risk de novo AML in the elderly. The latency of onset from start of previous therapy to the development of t-MDS/AML following exposure to alkylating agent chemotherapy was 63 months (range, 7 to 173 months) in a recent large series.[81]

Rare t-MDS/AML subgroups involving translocational ab-

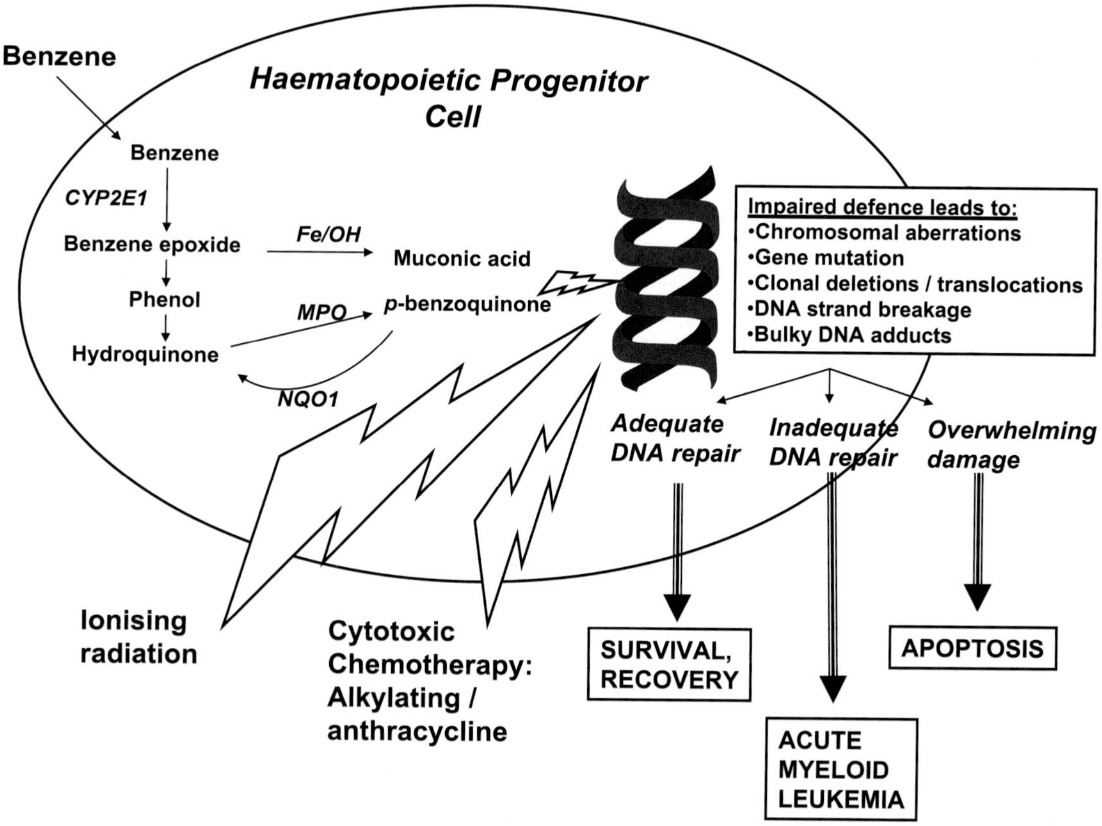

Figure 1 Potential genotoxic mechanisms and consequences in the etiology of AML.

normalities are less likely to be relevant to the etiology of de novo AML in the elderly.

Conclusion

AML is a heterogeneous disease. Clear predisposing factors have been identified, but given the low relative risks associated with these it is likely that they account for only a small component of disease etiology. Furthermore, it is certain that different biologic subtypes of AML will have different etiologies, and efforts to refine the biologic classification of these subtypes will provide the starting point for revisiting epidemiologic research in the future.

References

1. Preiss BS, Kerndrup GB, Schmidt KG, Sorensen AG, Clausen NA, Gadeberg OV, et al: Cytogenetic findings in adult de novo acute myeloid leukaemia. A population-based study of 303/337 patients. Br J Haematol 123:219-234, 2003
2. Moorman AV, Roman E, Willett EV, Dovey GJ, Cartwright RA, Morgan GJ: Karyotype and age in acute myeloid leukemia. Are they linked? Cancer Genet Cytogenet 126:155-161, 2001
3. Schoch C, Kern W, Krawitz P, Dugas M, Schnittger S, Haferlach T, et al: Dependence of age-specific incidence of acute myeloid leukemia on karyotype. Blood 98:3500, 2001 (letter)
4. Vickers M, Jackson G, Taylor P: The incidence of acute promyelocytic leukemia appears constant over most of a human lifespan, implying only one rate limiting mutation. Leukemia 14:722-726, 2000
5. Cartwright RA, Gurney KA, Moorman AV: Sex ratios and the risks of haematological malignancies. Br J Haematol 118:1071-1077, 2002
6. Sanderson RN, Johnson PRE, Moorman AV, Roman E, Willett E, Proctor SJ, et al: Population-based demographic study of karyotypes in 1709 patients with adult acute myeloid leukemia. Leukemia 2006 Jan 19 [Epub ahead of print]
7. Pedersen-Bjergaard J, Andersen MK, Christiansen DH, Nerlov C: Genetic pathways in therapy-related myelodysplasia and acute myeloid leukemia. Blood 99:1909-1912, 2002
8. Suzuki T, Kiyoi H, Ozeki K, Tomita A, Yamaji S, Suzuki R, et al: Clinical characteristics and prognostic implications of NPM1 mutations in acute myeloid leukemia. Blood 101:2770-2794, 2005
9. Schoch C, Kern W, Kohlmann A, Hiddemann W, Schnittger S, Haferlach T: Acute myeloid leukemia with a complex aberrant karyotype is a distinct biological entity characterized by genomic imbalances and a specific gene expression profile. Genes Chromosomes Cancer 43: 227-238, 2005
10. Valk PJ, Verhaak RG, Beijen MA, Erpelinck CA, Barjesteh van Waalwijk van Doorn-Khosrovani S, Boer JM, et al: Prognostically useful gene-expression profiles in acute myeloid leukemia. N Engl J Med 350:1617-1628 2004
11. Kottaridis PD, Gale RE, Langabeer SE, Frew ME, Bowen DT, Linch DC: Studies of FLT3 mutations in paired presentation and relapse samples from patients with acute myeloid leukemia: Implications for the role of FLT3 mutations in leukemogenesis, minimal residual disease detection, and possible therapy with FLT3 inhibitors. Blood 100:2393-2398, 2002
12. Richardson S, Zittoun R, Bastuji Garin S, Lasserre V, Guihenneuc C, Cadiou M, et al: Occupational risk factors for acute leukaemia: A case-control study. Int J Epidemiol 21:1063-1073, 1992
13. Ciccone G, Mirabelli D, Levis A, Gavarotti P, Rege-Cambrin G, Davico L, et al: Myeloid leukemias and myelodysplastic syndromes: Chemical exposure, histologic subtype and cytogenetics in a case-control study. Cancer Genet Cytogenet 68:135-139, 1993
14. Lazarov D, Waldron HA, Pejin D: Acute myeloid leukaemia and exposure to organic solvents—A case-control study. Eur J Epidemiol 16: 295-301, 2000
15. Speer SA, Semenza JC, Kurosaki T, Anton-Culver H: Risk factors for acute myeloid leukemia and multiple myeloma: A combination of GIS and case-control studies. J Environ Health 64:9-16, 2002
16. Nisse C, Haguenoer JM, Grandbastien B, Preudhomme C, Fontaine B, Brillet JM, et al: Occupational and environmental risk factors of the myelodysplastic syndromes in the North of France. Br J Haematol 112: 927-935, 2001
17. Rigolin GM, Cuneo A, Roberti MG, Bardi A, Bigoni R, Piva N, et al: Exposure to myelotoxic agents and myelodysplasia: Case-control study and correlation with clinicobiological findings. Br J Haematol 103:189-197, 1998
18. Bjork J, Albin M, Mauritzson N, Stromberg U, Johansson B, Hagmar L: Smoking and myelodysplastic syndromes. Epidemiology 11:285-291, 2000
19. Aksoy M, Erdem S: Followup study on the mortality and the development of leukemia in 44 pancytopenic patients with chronic exposure to benzene. Blood 52:285-292, 1978
20. Paustenbach DJ, Bass RD, Price P: Benzene toxicity and risk assessment, 1972-1992: Implications for future regulation. Environ Health Perspect 101:177-200, 1993 (suppl 6)
21. Smith MT: Mechanistic studies of benzene toxicity—Implications for risk assessment. Adv Exp Med Biol 387:259-266, 1996
22. Zeise L, McDonald TA: California perspective on the assessment of benzene toxicological risks. J Toxicol Environ Health A 61:479-483, 2000
23. Hotz P, Lauwerys RR: Hematopoietic and lymphatic malignancies in vehicle mechanics. Crit Rev Toxicol 27:443-494, 1997
24. Boffetta P: Risk of acute myeloid leukemia after exposure to diesel exhaust: A review of the epidemiologic evidence. J Occup Environ Med 46:1076-1083, 2004
25. Smith MT, Zhang LP, Wang YX, Hayes RB, Li GL, Wiemels J, et al: Increased translocations and aneusomy in chromosomes 8 and 21 among workers exposed to benzene. Cancer Res 58:2176-2181, 1998
26. Zhang L, Wang Y, Shang N, Smith MT: Benzene metabolites induce the loss and long arm deletion of chromosomes 5 and 7 in human lymphocytes. Leuk Res 22:105-113, 1998
27. Smith MT, Zhang L, Jeng M, Wang Y, Guo W, Duramad P, et al: Hydroquinone, a benzene metabolite, increases the level of aneusomy of chromosomes 7 and 8 in human CD34-positive blood progenitor cells. Carcinogenesis 21:1485-1490, 2000
28. Shimizu Y, Schull WJ, Kato H: Cancer risk among atomic bomb survivors. The RERF Life Span Study. Radiation Effects Research Foundation. JAMA 264:601-604, 1990
29. Pearce N, Prior I, Methven D, Culling C, Marshall S, Auld J, et al: Follow up of New Zealand participants in British atmospheric nuclear weapons tests in the Pacific. BMJ 300:1161-1166, 1990
30. Darby SC, Kendall GM, Fell TP, Doll R, Goodill AA, Conquest AJ, et al: Further follow up of mortality and incidence of cancer in men from the United Kingdom who participated in the United Kingdom's atmospheric nuclear weapon tests and experimental programmes. BMJ 307: 1530-1535, 1993
31. Doody MM, Mandel JS, Lubin JH, Boice JD Jr: Mortality among United States radiologic technologists, 1926-90. Cancer Causes Control 9:67-75, 1998
32. Cardis E, Gilbert ES, Carpenter L, Howe G, Kato I, Armstrong BK, et al: Effects of low doses and low dose rates of external ionizing radiation: Cancer mortality among nuclear industry workers in three countries. Radiat Res 142:117-132, 1995
33. Weiss HA, Darby SC, Fearn T, Doll R: Leukemia mortality after x-ray treatment for ankylosing spondylitis. Radiat Res 142:1-11, 1995
34. Inskip PD, Monson RR, Wagoner JK, Stovall M, Davis FG, Kleinerman RA, et al: Leukemia following radiotherapy for uterine bleeding. Radiat Res 122:107-119, 1990
35. Urowitz MB, Rider WD: Myeloproliferative disorders in patients with rheumatoid arthritis treated with total body irradiation. Am J Med 78:60-64, 1985
36. Inskip PD, Kleinerman RA, Stovall M, Cookfair DL, Hadjimichael O, Moloney WC, et al: Leukemia, lymphoma, and multiple myeloma after pelvic radiotherapy for benign disease. Radiat Res 135:108-124, 1993
37. Griem ML, Kleinerman RA, Boice JD Jr, Stovall M, Shefner D, Lubin JH:

Cancer following radiotherapy for peptic ulcer. J Natl Cancer Inst 86:842-849, 1994
38. Travis LB, Curtis RE, Storm H, Hall P, Holowaty E, Vanleeuwen FE, et al: Risk of second malignant neoplasms among long-term survivors of testicular cancer. J Natl Cancer Inst 89:1429-1439, 1997
39. Curtis RE, Boice JD Jr, Stovall M, Bernstein L, Greenberg RS, Flannery JT, et al: Risk of leukemia after chemotherapy and radiation treatment for breast cancer. N Engl J Med 326:1745-1751, 1992
40. Curtis RE, Boice JD Jr, Stovall M, Bernstein L, Greenberg RS, Flannery JT, et al: Risk of leukemia after chemotherapy and radiation treatment for breast cancer. N Engl J Med 326:1745-1751, 1992
41. Armitage JO, Carbone PP, Connors JM, Levine A, Bennett JM, Kroll S: Treatment-related myelodysplasia and acute leukemia in non-Hodgkin's lymphoma patients. J Clin Oncol 21:897-906, 2003
42. Gundestrup M, Storm HH: Radiation-induced acute myeloid leukaemia and other cancers in commercial jet cockpit crew: A population-based cohort study. Lancet 354:2029-2031, 1999
43. Ballard T, Lagorio S, De Angelis G, Verdecchia A: Cancer incidence and mortality among flight personnel: A meta-analysis. Aviat Space Environ Med 71:216-224, 2000
44. Pukkala E, Aspholm R, Auvinen A, Eliasch H, Gundestrup M, Haldorsen T, et al: Cancer incidence among 10,211 airline pilots: A Nordic study. Aviat Space Environ Med 74:699-706, 2003
45. Reynolds TY, Rockwell S, Glazer PM: Genetic instability induced by the tumor microenvironment. Cancer Res 56:5754-5757, 1996
46. Lorimore SA, Coates PJ, Scobie GE, Milne G, Wright EG: Inflammatory-type responses after exposure to ionizing radiation in vivo: A mechanism for radiation-induced bystander effects? Oncogene 20:7085-7095, 2001
47. Chen R, Seaton A: A meta-analysis of painting exposure and cancer mortality. Cancer Detect Prev 22:533-539, 1998
48. Nilsson RI, Nordlinder R, Horte LG, Jarvholm B: Leukaemia, lymphoma, and multiple myeloma in seamen on tankers. Occup Environ Med 55:517-521, 1998
49. Sathiakumar N, Delzell E, Hovinga M, Macaluso M, Julian JA, Larson R, et al: Mortality from cancer and other causes of death among synthetic rubber workers. Occup Environ Med 55:230-235, 1998
50. Metayer C, Johnson ES, Rice JC: Nested case-control study of tumors of the hemopoietic and lymphatic systems among workers in the meat industry. Am J Epidemiol 147:727-738, 1998
51. Hayes RB, Blair A, Stewart PA, Herrick RF, Mahar H: Mortality of U.S. embalmers and funeral directors. Am J Ind Med 18:641-652, 1990
52. McDonald TA, Holland NT, Skibola C, Duramad P, Smith MT: Hypothesis: Phenol and hydroquinone derived mainly from diet and gastrointestinal flora are causal factors in leukemia. Leukemia 15:10-20, 2001
53. Ross JA, Kasum CM, Davies SM, Jacobs DR, Folsom AR, Potter JD: Diet and risk of leukemia in the Iowa Women's Health Study. Cancer Epidemiol Biomarkers Prev 11:777-781, 2002
54. Hursting SD, Margolin BH, Switzer BR: Diet and human leukemia—An analysis of international data. Prevent Med 22:409-422, 1993
55. Kane EV, Roman E, Cartwright R, Parker J, Morgan G: Tobacco and the risk of acute leukaemia in adults. Br J Cancer 81:1228-1233, 1999
56. Bjork J, Albin M, Mauritzson N, Stromberg U, Johansson B, Hagmar L: Smoking and acute myeloid leukemia: Associations with morphology and karyotypic patterns and evaluation of dose-response relations. Leuk Res 25:865-872, 2001
57. Korte JE, Hertz-Picciotto I, Schulz MR, Ball LM, Duell EJ: The contribution of benzene to smoking-induced leukemia. Environ Health Perspect 108:333-339, 2000
58. Brown LM, Gibson R, Burmeister LF, Schuman LM, Everett GD, Blair A: Alcohol consumption and risk of leukemia, non-Hodgkin's lymphoma, and multiple myeloma. Leuk Res 16:979-984, 1992
59. Mele A, Szklo M, Visani G, Stazi MA, Castelli G, Pasquini P, et al: Hair dye use and other risk factors for leukemia and pre-leukemia: A case-control study. Italian Leukemia Study Group. Am J Epidemiol 139: 609-619, 1994
60. Correa A, Mohan A, Jackson L, Perry H, Helzlsouer K: Use of hair dyes, hematopoietic neoplasms, and lymphomas: A literature review. I. Leukemias and myelodysplastic syndromes. Cancer Invest 18:366-380, 2000
61. Caspi O, Polliack A, Klar R, Ben Yehuda D: The association of inflammatory bowel disease and leukemia—Coincidence or not? Leuk Lymphoma 17:255-262, 1995
62. Askling J, Brandt L, Lapidus A, Karlen P, Bjorkholm M, Lofberg R, et al: Risk of haematopoietic cancer in patients with inflammatory bowel disease. Gut 54:617-622, 2005
63. Gentile G, Mele A, Monarco B, Vitale A, Pulsoni A, Visani G, et al: Hepatitis B and C viruses, human T-cell lymphotropic virus types I and II, and leukemias: A case-control study. The Italian Leukemia Study Group. Cancer Epidemiol Biomarkers Prev 5:227-230, 1996
64. Cooper GS, Kamel F, Sandler DP, Davey FR, Bloomfield CD: Risk of adult acute leukemia in relation to prior immune-related conditions. Cancer Epidemiol Biomarkers Prev 5:867-872, 1996
65. Parry TE: The non-random distribution of point mutations in leukaemia and myelodysplasia—A possible pointer to their aetiology. Leuk Res 21:559-574, 1997
66. Wood RD, Mitchell M, Sgouros J, Lindahl T: Human DNA repair genes. Science 291:1284-1289, 2001
67. Kutler DI, Singh B, Satagopan J, Batish SD, Berwick M, Giampietro PF, et al: A 20-year perspective on the International Fanconi Anemia Registry (IFAR). Blood 101:1249-1256, 2003
68. Poppe B, Van Limbergen H, Van Roy N, Vandecruys E, De Paepe A, Benoit Y, et al: Chromosomal aberrations in Bloom syndrome patients with myeloid malignancies. Cancer Genet Cytogenet 128:39-42, 2001
69. Song WJ, Sullivan MG, Legare RD, Hutchings S, Tan X, Kufrin D, et al: Haploinsufficiency of CBFA2 causes familial thrombocytopenia with propensity to develop acute myelogenous leukaemia. Nat Genet 23: 166-175, 1999
70. Gowans ID, Lorimore SA, McIlrath JM, Wright EG: Genotype-dependent induction of transmissible chromosomal instability by gamma-radiation and the benzene metabolite hydroquinone. Cancer Res 65: 3527-3530, 2005
71. Boulton E, Cole C, Knight A, Cleary H, Snowden R, Plumb M: Low-penetrance genetic susceptibility and resistance loci implicated in the relative risk for radiation-induced acute myeloid leukemia in mice. Blood 101:2349-2354, 2003
72. Seedhouse C, Faulkner R, Ashraf N, Das-Gupta E, Russell N: Polymorphisms in genes involved in homologous recombination repair interact to increase the risk of developing acute myeloid leukemia. Clin Cancer Res 10:2675-2680, 2004
73. Larson RA, Wang Y, Banerjee M, Wiemels J, Hartford C, Le Beau MM, et al: Prevalence of the inactivating 609C→T polymorphism in the NAD(P)H:quinone oxidoreductase (NQO1) gene in patients with primary and therapy-related myeloid leukemia. Blood 94:803-807, 1999
74. Allan JM, Wild CP, Rollinson S, Willett EV, Moorman AV, Dovey GJ, et al: Polymorphism in glutathione S-transferase P1 is associated with susceptibility to chemotherapy-induced leukemia. Proc Natl Acad Sci U S A 98:11592-11597, 2001
75. Worrillow LJ, Travis LB, Smith AG, Rollinson S, Smith AJ, Wild CP, et al: An intron splice acceptor polymorphism in hMSH2 and risk of leukemia after treatment with chemotherapeutic alkylating agents. Clin Cancer Res 9:3012-3020, 2003
76. Sibley K, Rollinson S, Allan JM, Smith AG, Law GR, Roddam PL, et al: Functional FAS promoter polymorphisms are associated with increased risk of acute myeloid leukemia. Cancer Res 63:4327-4330, 2003
77. Bowen DT, Frew ME, Rollinson S, Roddam PL, Dring A, Smith MT, et al: Cytochrome P450 1A1 *2B (Val) allele is over-represented in a sub-group of acute myeloid leukemia patients with poor-risk karyotype associated with NRAS mutation, but not associated with FLT3 internal tandem duplication. Blood 2002–01, 2002
78. Smith MT, Wang Y, Kane E, Rollinson S, Wiemels JL, Roman E, et al: Low NAD(P)H:quinone oxidoreductase 1 activity is associated with increased risk of acute leukemia in adults. Blood 97:1422-1426, 2001
79. Bowen DT, Frew ME, Rollinson S, Roddam PL, Dring A, Smith MT, et al: CYP1A1*2B (Val) allele is overrepresented in a subgroup of acute myeloid leukemia patients with poor-risk karyotype associated with

NRAS mutation, but not associated with FLT3 internal tandem duplication. Blood 101:2770-2774, 2003
80. Crane MM, Strom SS, Halabi S, Berman EL, Fueger JJ, Spitz MR, et al: Correlation between selected environmental exposures and karyotype in acute myelocytic leukemia. Cancer Epidemiol Biomarkers Prev 5:639-644, 1996
81. Mauritzson N, Albin M, Rylander L, Billstrom R, Ahlgren T, Mikoczy Z, et al: Pooled analysis of clinical and cytogenetic features in treatment-related and de novo adult acute myeloid leukemia and myelodysplastic syndromes based on a consecutive series of 761 patients analyzed 1976-1993 and on 5098 unselected cases reported in the literature 1974-2001. Leukemia 16:2366-2378, 2002
82. Qian Z, Fernald AA, Godley LA, Larson RA, Le Beau MM: Expression profiling of CD34+ hematopoietic stem/progenitor cells reveals distinct subtypes of therapy-related acute myeloid leukemia. Proc Natl Acad Sci U S A 99:14925-14930, 2002

ELSEVIER

Seminars in
HEMATOLOGY

General Approach to, and Perspectives on Clinical Research in, Older Patients With Newly Diagnosed Acute Myeloid Leukemia

Elihu H. Estey

Most patients aged ≥55 to 60 years who are treated for newly diagnosed acute myeloid leukemia (AML) receive a combination of an anthracycline plus cytarabine (ara-C). A principal thesis of this chapter is that such therapy is unsatisfactory for the great majority of such patients. In particular, the ≥15% risk of death in the month following the start of treatment is difficult to justify given median survivals of less than 1 year in the patients who do not die early. Thus, investigational therapy should be recommended for most, if not all, older patients. In patients for whom such therapy is not feasible, low-dose ara-C is a reasonable alternative except for patients with de novo disease and a normal karyotype, who might benefit more from an anthracycline + ara-C combination, and patients with either a poor performance status, abnormal organ function, or age ≥80, for whom supportive/palliative care only is recommended. Distinctions are made between investigational therapies likely associated with lower and higher risks of treatment-related mortality (TRM). The former are preferable initial treatment in patients aged 70 and above, or with abnormal cytogenetics. Three topics are discussed that are likely to be relevant to future clinical research in older patients: the possibility of delaying therapy to gain information about prognosis with initial induction therapy, the clinical value of responses less than conventional complete remission (CR), and the possibility of looking for larger differences between treatments in randomized clinical trials
Semin Hematol 43:89-95

Multivariate analyses indicate that several covariates, described below, other than age, affect outcome of patients with newly diagnosed acute myeloid leukemia (AML). Because associations between age and these covariates are quite imperfect, the concept of "older AML" is per se oversimplified, and any dichotomization of patients into "older" and "younger" is arbitrary. Nonetheless, the former term is typically applied to patients over age 55 to 60 years, and this chapter will proceed accordingly. If treated, the majority of older patients receive an anthracycline (daunorubicin or idarubicin) plus cytarabine (ara-C), a combination hereafter called AA. Emphasizing survival as the crucial outcome, the chapter will contend that, in the vast majority of older patients, the potential benefits of AA are not commensurate with the risks. Accordingly, the first option for such patients should be investigational therapies. The chapter will somewhat arbitrarily distinguish between two types of investigational therapies according to their associated risk of therapy-related mortality and point out patients in whom one type therapy, or the other, might be preferable. Finally, there will be a general discussion focusing on (1) the benefits and risks of delaying treatment to allow integration of prognostic information into therapeutic decision-making, (2) the recently noted entity "complete remission with incomplete platelet recovery" (CRp), and (3) perceived problems with clinical trial methodology as applied to randomized clinical trials, which remain the principal method for assessing the benefit of new therapies.

Inadequacy of AA: The Rationale for General Use of Investigational Therapy

Table 1 lists series reporting outcome with AA in older patients.[1–5] Despite variations in post-remission therapy in these studies (for example, one course of high-dose ara-C in

Department of Leukemia, M.D. Anderson Cancer Center, Houston, TX.
Address correspondence to Elihu H. Estey, MD, Department of Leukemia, M.D. Anderson Cancer Center, 15151 Holcombe Blvd, Box 428, Houston, TX 77030. E-mail: ehestey@mdanderson.org

0037-1963/06/$-see front matter
doi:10.1053/j.seminhematol.2006.01.002

Table 1 Outcomes With Anthracycline + ara-C

Study	Patients*	Median Survival	Probability Survival at 2 Years	CR Rate	Induction Death Rate	Comment
ECOG[1]	234 Age ≥ 56 yr	7–8 mo	~20%	41%	19%	Results same with daunorubicin, idarubicin, or mitoxantrone and ± GM-CSF priming
MRC (AML 11)[2]	328 Age ≥ 56 yr	~12 mo	~25%	62%	16%	Results same with 1 or 4 courses post-CR and ± G-CSF starting 8 days after end induction
SWOG[3]	161 Age ≥ 56 yr	9 mo	19%	43%	15%	Survival worse with mitoxantrone + etoposide
HOVON[4]	211 Age ≥ 60 yr	~10 mo	~25%	48%	15%	Results same ± PSC-833
M.D. Anderson[5]	31 Age ≥ 65 yr	~12 mo	~20%	48%	Not given	ara-C at 1.5 g/m² daily × 3; survival worse with single-agent gemtuzumab

*The listed patients received only AA; for example, the patients given mitoxantrone + ara-C in the ECOG study are excluded, as are the patients given AA + PSC-833 in the Hovon study.

the Eastern Cooperative Oncology Group [ECOG] study, one or four courses of lower ara-C doses + anthracyclines in the Medical Research Council [MRC] trial, two such courses in the Southwest Oncology Group [SWOG] study), and possible differences in therapy after relapse, Table 1 indicates that the average older patient with untreated AML can expect to live 8 to 12 months if given AA as the initial therapy designed to produce complete remission (CR). The argument that the risk/benefit ratio of AA is unfavorable follows from observations in 186 patients patients aged 60 and above, but with Zubrod performance status 0 to 2 and pretreatment serum bilirubin and creatinine values each less than 2.0 mg/dL, given AA from 1995 through present at M.D. Anderson Cancer Center. Although these patients received doses of ara-C higher than usually given (1.5 g/m² daily × 3, rather than 100 to 200 mg/m² daily × 7), their 8-month median survival was typical of that shown in Table 1. Fifteen percent of the 186 patients were dead within 4 weeks, quantifying the risk associated with AA, while the 9- to 10-month median survival of the remaining 85% quantifies the benefit. While similar outcomes might have been observed without treatment, the point is that the risk/benefit ratio of AA is high. Attempts to improve this ratio by reducing the doses/duration of AA from those used in the studies noted in Table 1 have decreased both early mortality and the anti-AML efficacy of treatment, resulting in no improvement in survival.[6] Interventions such as addition of granulocyte colony-stimulating factor (G-CSF) or granulocyte-macrophage colony-stimulating factor (GM-CSF) to AA or substitution of mitoxantrone for an anthracycline have also failed to lengthen survival (Table 1).

It is well known that the outcome of patients with AML is so variable that to speak, as in the previous paragraph, of an "average" outcome is potentially misleading. Perhaps 30% of this variability can be explained by currently known prognostic factors (covariates).[7] Those most readily assessable are leukemia cell cytogenetics,[8] presence of an antecedent hematologic disorder (AHD; such as an abnormal blood count suggesting a previously undocumented diagnosis of myelodysplastic syndrome),[9] a history of cytotoxic chemotherapy for another illness (secondary, as opposed to de novo AML),[10] performance status, organ function, and age, with younger patients (ages 55 to 69) having a better prognosis. The reports in Table 1 describe such covariates' effects singly (for example, the effect of age >69, the effect of abnormal cytogenetics, etc). For clinical purposes however, examining the effect of several covariates simultaneously (such as the effect of age >69 when combined with abnormal cytogenetics) is more useful. In particular, it is instructive to examine outcome following administration of AA to the most prognostically favorable older patients. These are those age less than 70 with Zubrod performance status 0 to 2, pretreatment bilirubin and creatinine less than 2.0 mg/dL, normal cytogenetics, and with de novo AML without an AHD. Only 26 of the above-noted 186 M.D. Anderson patients (14%) met these criteria. Although just two died in the first 4 weeks after beginning treatment and although the CR rate was 73%, median survival was only 1.1 years, with only a 20% probability of living 2 years after beginning treatment (Fig 1).

The outcomes described above probably overestimate the true situation. Specifically, therapeutic trials in older patients with AML most likely enroll a disproportionate number of patients with relatively favorable prognoses. First, the trials' eligibility criteria generally bar the entry of patients who are not ambulatory or who have abnormal hepatic, renal, or cardiac function; such patients constitute 25% of older patients with untreated AML (M.D. Anderson data). Second and more difficult to quantify, eligible patients are sometimes not enrolled because they may be thought too "sick." Evidence of such selection bias is provided by the rarity with which reports such as those in Table 1 note that *consecutive* eligible patients were entered. There is also no doubt that treatment for AML interferes with patients' lives. Although the extent of

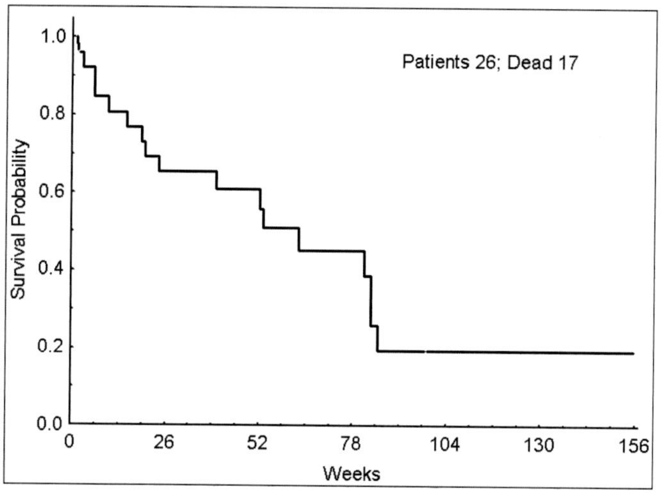

Figure 1 Survival in the 14% best prognosis older patients.

such interference is difficult to quantify, its existence further calls into question the benefit/risk ratio of AA.

Given the data in Table 1 and the considerations discussed in the preceding paragraphs, it is appropriate to recommend investigational therapy for all older patients with untreated AML. This view is supported by analogy to practice in patients with lung or pancreatic cancer in whom new drugs are often administered as initial treatment; life expectancy in these patients is not much worse than in the "favorable" AML patients referred to above. Furthermore, the National Comprehensive Cancer Network, a consortium of prominent American cancer centers, explicitly cites "clinical trial" as the preferred option in patients with untreated AML age 60 and above.[11] There is, of course, no assurance that results with an investigational therapy will not be worse than those obtainable with AA. For example, a Cancer and Leukemia Group B (CALGB) study in older patients was stopped before accrual was completed because patients randomized to the investigational arm (daunorubicin+ ara-C + etoposide + PSC-833) had a higher death rate than patients randomized to the same three drugs without PSC-833.[12] However, it seems fair to ask: "how much worse than AA can an investigational therapy be?" Some patients in the most favorable group of older patients might value the results with AA more than other patients. The former would reply "a lot" to the above question and would choose AA over investigational therapy. Other patients would offer the opposite reply and choose investigational therapy. Obviously, the weight given to the recommendation for investigational therapy should increase as the number of unfavorable prognostic factors (age >69, abnormal cytogenetics, an AHD or secondary AML, poor performance status, or abnormal organ function) increases.

The exception to the generalization that abnormal cytogenetics confer a poor prognosis are cases with t(8; 21) and inv(16).[8] These abnormalities were found in only 2% of 962 patients age ≥60 with AML seen at M.D. Anderson from 1995 to present. Since such patients had a median survival of 21 months following ara-C–containing therapy, such therapy should be the first option in such patients.

Role of Allogeneic Stem Cell Transplant

As discussed further in the chapter by de Lima and Giralt, allogeneic stem cell transplant (SCT) in older patients generally employs nonmyeloablative chemotherapy intended primarily to facilitate engraftment.[13] Such "minitransplants" are usually done in first CR or at initial relapse. Alyea et al have suggested that survival after minitransplantation is at least as good as that after myeloablative allogeneic SCT in patients age ≥50.[14] However, the median age of their 30 patients receiving a minitransplant was only 58 years, and only 7% had AML in first CR. Furthermore, it seems likely that myeloablative allogeneic SCT itself is without benefit, or with only marginal benefit, in patients under age 60 with AML in first CR, assuming that given the somewhat arbitrary distinction between such patients and older patients, results in the former are relevant to the latter; in particular, groups that do poorly with AA also do poorly with myeloablative transplantation.[15–17] Thus, there is reason to question the effectiveness of minitransplant. Consequently, the procedure should be recommended only if done in an investigational context. Data suggesting the questionable relevance, and the likely effect of selection bias on interpretation of the results of minitransplant, were provided by Tibes et al. They described a systematic attempt to perform the procedure in first CR in all M.D. Anderson patients age ≥50 with an abnormal karyotype and a sibling or matched unrelated donor.[18] Ninety-nine patients entered CR, a donor search was not performed in 37, donors were found in 25 of the remaining 62, and transplants were performed in 11 of the 25. Although these 11 had the best outcomes, they also were the youngest, leaving aside the likely operation of other, less quantifiable, selection biases

Cases Where Investigational Therapy Is Not an Option

Here the options are AA, low-dose ara-C (LDAC), or "supportive care." A frequently referenced randomized study compared, in patients age 65 and above, immediate AA to observation/supportive care with use of hydroxyurea or LDAC only if progression occurred, that is, a rise in white blood cell (WBC) count above 50,000/μL, fall in platelet count below 15,000/μL, or development of symptoms.[19] Median survival was 21 weeks in the AA arm and 10 weeks in the observation arm, and the number of days spent in hospital was essentially identical. However, 80% of the 60 patients enrolled had a performance status less than 3, and all patients had relatively normal organ function. Furthermore, 50% of the patients randomized to observation had to begin therapy within 1 month, suggesting that they were on the verge of progression when randomized. Thus, data from this trial can be used to support immediate AA only in patients who are relatively fit and relatively likely to progress. In its AML14 trial in patients age 60 and above not considered fit for AA by community physicians, the MRC terminated randomization between LDAC and hydroxyurea because of longer survival (medians of approximately 6 v 4 months) with LDAC; number of days in hospital were similar.[20] Although the authors suggest that the results support the adoption of LDAC as standard treatment in older patients thought unfit for AA, only 12% of their patients had a performance status of 3 to 4, with another 18% having a performance status of 2; furthermore, it is unclear, although likely, that hydroxyurea and supportive care are exchangeable. Finally, Tilly et al found equivalent survival in older patients randomized between LDAC and AA, but with less time spent in hospital in the LDAC group[21]; patients with abnormal organ function or poor performance status were excluded.

Although the differences in survival between LDAC, or AA, and supportive care are thus relatively modest, it appears reasonable to administer LDAC (for example, 20 mg twice daily for 10 days every 4 to 6 weeks, as in AML14) to older patients who are unable to receive investigational therapy but have a performance status of Zubrod 0 to 2, and relatively preserved organ function. Because higher doses of ara-C produce better outcomes in patients with a normal karyotype, use of AA rather than LDAC should be strongly considered in such patients; however, it must be noted that the comparisons were between high-dose ara-C and AA in younger patients, rather than between AA and LDAC in older patients.[22] In patients with very poor performance status (Zubrod 3 to 4), severely abnormal organ function, or perhaps who are age ≥80, supportive care should be the first option given the strong association between these covariates and treatment-related mortality (TRM) and the absence of data suggesting that such patients, unlike those with a better performance status, benefit from LDAC or AA. Similarly, a low and stable WBC would add support to a choice of supportive care, since experience suggests that at least some such older patients can survive for 1 to 2 years without undue morbidity.

Any discussion of choice of therapy, particularly between AA and supportive care, in older patients would be incomplete without reference to the findings of Sekeres et al.[23] They noted that 74% of older patients estimated that their chances of cure with AA were at least 50%; in contrast, 85% of their physicians estimated this chance to be less than 10%. While the most plausible cause of this discrepancy is patients' natural tendency to believe what they want to believe, there may also be gaps in communication between physicians and patients.

Two Types of Investigational Therapy

Recent years have seen use of "targeted" therapy, rather than more conventional chemotherapy, in untreated older patients (see, for example, Lancet et al[24] and Stone et al[25]); this trend is likely to continue. Much of the appeal of such therapy stems from its presumed specific toxicity for hematopoietic cells and, in particular, AML blasts. What constitutes targeted therapy is a question of semantics. For example, remissions produced by AA would not occur if AA were not at least somewhat specific for (targeted to) AML blasts; thus AA, as well as therapies such as tipifarnib, and others described in Dr Burnett's chapter in this issue, might be considered "targeted." Here distinction between therapies will be based, somewhat arbitrarily, on their associated risk of TRM. "Noncytotoxic therapies," for example, tipifarnib but also LDAC, plausibly produce relatively low rates (<5%). "Cytotoxic therapies," for example, AA but also new chemotherapeutic agents such as clofarabine or cloretazine, as well as minitransplantation, produce greater damage to normal organs (gastrointestinal mucosa, lung). They are thus associated with TRM rates of 15% to 20% (and higher in patients over age 69 and, particularly in patients with a poor performance status). A combination of tipifarnib + LDAC is considered noncytotoxic therapy, while a combination of tipifarnib + AA is considered cytotoxic therapy.

Assuming investigational therapy will be administered, which patients should receive cytotoxic therapy and which noncytotoxic therapy as initial treatment? The advantage of beginning with noncytotoxic treatment is a reduced risk of TRM. The advantage of beginning with noncytotoxic treatment is that it may produce more anti-AML effect, with such effect (for example, CR) necessary to reverse bone marrow failure, which is the usual cause of death in AML. Although patients often prefer to receive cytotoxic therapy only after noncytotoxic therapy has failed, this approach risks increasing the duration of bone marrow failure, with consequent development of infections, etc, that may reduce the success rate with subsequent cytotoxic therapy. Because equally compelling arguments can be made for either a noncytotoxic or a cytotoxic first approach, a randomized trial comparing the effect of each approach on survival would be of great interest. Of course, findings might be therapy-specific. However, given the above-noted increase in the number of trials of noncytotoxic treatment as initial therapy, it appears worthwhile to demonstrate, in at least one case, that a noncytotoxic first approach does not shorten survival; optimally, such a trial would include quality-of-life assessments.

Given the strong opinions of physicians and patients, it may be unrealistic to expect that such a trial will be undertaken. Under these circumstances the following recommendations might be made. Patients who are age ≥70 or who have a poor performance status (Zubrod 2 to 4) or abnormal organ function receive noncytotoxic therapy (such as tipifarnib + LDAC) in deference to the risk of TRM with cytotoxic therapy. Patients age 55/60–69 with a good performance status and normal organ function receive cytotoxic therapy (such as clofarabine + ara-C) if they have a normal karyotype and noncytotoxic therapy if they do not. This recommendation follows from (1) a presumed greater importance of dose in the former patients, and (2) recognition of the effect of age on TRM even in older patients with good performance status and normal organ function; in particular, benefit/risk considerations do not favor cytotoxic therapy in those of such patients who have abnormal karyotypes. Table 2 summarizes the recommendations for therapy made in this chapter.

Table 2 Treatment Recommendations

Relative Risk of TRM	Relative Risk of Resistance to AA in Absence of TRM	Therapeutic Options (in order of preference)
Low (age 55/60–69, good performance status, normal organ function)	Low (normal cytogenetics and de novo AML without AHD)	1. Investigational cytotoxic 2. AA
Low	High (abnormal cytogenetics,* secondary AML or AHD)	1. Investigational noncytotoxic 2. LDAC
High (either Zubrod performance status 2, mildly–moderately abnormal organ function, or age 70–79)	High or low	1. Investigational noncytotoxic 2. LDAC
Very high (either Zubrod performance status 3–4, severely abnormal organ function, or age ≥ 80)	High or low	1. Investigational noncytotoxic 2. Supportive care only

Abbreviations: TRM, treatment-related mortality; AA, anthracycline + ara-C (cytarabine); AHD, antecedent hematologic disorder; LDAC, low-dose ara-C.
*Except inv(16) or t(8;21); patients with these abnormalities should receive AA.

Delaying the Start of Therapy to Permit Use of Prognostic Information

The future will undoubtedly see the development of molecularly based tests that will either, like cytogenetics, refine our ability to know which patients will/won't benefit from a general therapy (such as AA) or will allow prognostication of response to specific therapies, for example, bcl-2 antisense combined with AA. Application of this knowledge to assign initial induction therapy is clearly desirable given such therapy's generally high risk/benefit ratio and the ability of such therapy to significantly affect remission duration (see, for example, Bishop et al[26]). However, it may require several weeks to obtain the results of these tests; such is often the case with cytogenetics. Whether the desirability of obtaining results outweighs the risks associated with delaying therapy is thus likely to become an important question. Clearly, therapy must begin immediately in patients with rapidly rising WBC counts, WBC counts greater than 100,000/μL, or lung or brain failure due to leukostasis or infiltration. However, older patients usually do not present with these features. Among AA-treated patients age ≥ 55 , the ECOG reported a CR rate of 38% in 235 patients in whom there was a delay of 3 to 5 days in initiating therapy versus 50% in 113 patients in whom there was no delay (P = .03).[1] The delay reflected logistical factors inherent in a blinded randomization to priming with GM-CSF versus placebo in the 235 patients; in contrast, priming, which ultimately had no effect on CR rate, was not studied in the initial group of 113 patients. While the report noted that risk factors in patients in the delay and the no delay groups were similar, it is unclear whether a multivariate analysis was done or whether risk factors other than cytogenetics, WBC count, and age were analyzed. In contrast, among 197 patients given idarubicin (12 mg/m^2 daily × 3 days + ara-C 1.5 g/m^2 daily × 3 to 4 days by continuous infusion) at M.D. Anderson, multivariate analysis indicated that age and unfavorable cytogenetics were independent predictors of CR, but that days from M.D. Anderson diagnosis to treatment, performance status (only 8% of patients with Zubrod performance status >2), WBC count, and serum levels of albumin, bilirubin, creatinine were not; findings were similar in older and younger patients.[27] A median of only 4 days elapsed between M.D. Anderson diagnosis and start of treatment and a delay of greater than 9 days occurred in only 25% of patients. However, since 2000, survival is equivalent in the 49 patients age ≥60 beginning treatment more than 1 month from M.D. Anderson diagnosis and in the 560 similarly aged patients beginning treatment sooner. Although selection bias may influence these findings, they suggest that the risk of waiting to ascertain results of tests that might influence choice of therapy is less than the risk of giving therapy that is unlikely to be successful and may, as with AA, be associated with significant rates of TRM. Furthermore, both the ECOG and M.D. Anderson data undoubtedly overestimate the interval from diagnosis to treatment since neither includes the interval from diagnosis by referring physicians to confirmation of diagnosis at the tertiary center.

New Criteria for Response

For many years response to induction therapy for AML was classified as CR or no CR. Recently, initially with respect to gemtuzumab ozogamicin, responses less than CR, such as CR with incomplete platelet recovery (CRp), have also been recognized.[28] Attaining CRp suggests that a treatment is more "active" than if neither CR nor CRp had occurred ("resistant"). However, the question of whether CRp conveys clinical benefit has received relatively little attention; in particular, what is the effect of CRp on subsequent survival probability relative to CR or resistant?

There seems to be little doubt that potential cure, defined as being in CR for at least 3 years,[29] requires attainment of CR. Thus, 90% of 84 such patients age ≥60 seen at M.D. Anderson from 1980 to 2005 achieved CR with initial therapy, with the remainder doing so with subsequent therapy. However, responses less than CR may still be associated with a survival benefit, if not cure. We addressed this question by comparing survival in three groups of patients age ≥60 treated at M.D. Anderson since 2000: (1) patients achieving CR, (2) patients

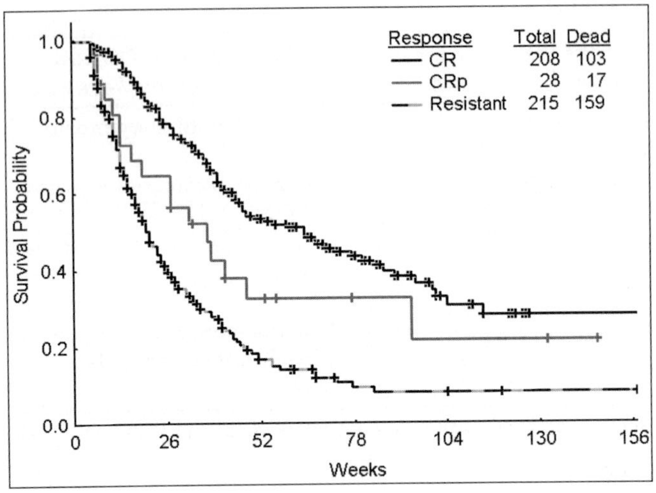

Figure 2 Survival according to whether CR, CRp, or neither ("resistant") occurred. All patients had to live a minimum of 40 days from start of treatment; 40 days was the median time to CRp. Results were the same if 30 or 60 days was used rather than 40 days.

achieving CRp, and (3) patients with resistant disease. Patients in each group had to live ≥40 days, which was the median time needed to achieve CRp (*v* 32 days for patients achieving CR). Figure 2 indicates that while CR conferred longer survival than CRp, CRp was superior to resistant. The finding that the relative advantage of CRp to resistant was approximately the same as that of CR to CRp applied regardless of whether patients were required to live a minimum of 30, 40, or 60 days (by which time 85% of the CRps had been observed). The number of CRps relative to the number of CRs was greater in patients with abnormal cytogenetics. This suggests that some of the negative effect of CRp relative to CR might be due to the former's association with prognostically unfavorable cytogenetics.

Perspectives on Clinical Trial Methodology

Randomized trials in older patients with AML typically enroll 100 to 200 patients per treatment arm. Such numbers are needed to have 80% power (type 2 error 20%) to detect often small absolute differences, for example 20% in CR rate, with a false positive rate (type 1 error) less than 5%. Assuming that most CRs will be brief, such differences are likely to translate into relatively small differences, usually a few months, in survival. Under these circumstances, it seems fair to inquire whether trials should be concerned with detection of larger, more medically significant, differences, thus requiring fewer patients per treatment arm. Compounding the problem is the nearly universal use of type 1 and type 2 error rates of 5% and 20%, respectively. These rates are sensible when studying a new drug in a disease where standard treatment is reasonably good, and thus where the principal concern is to prevent use of a falsely promising drug that might usurp standard therapy. In contrast, AML in the elderly is a disease for which there is no satisfactory treatment. Thus, there may be more reason to protect against a false negative result than a false positive result. Thus, it might be reasonable to specify type 1 and type 2 errors of 20 % each. The point is that type 1 and type 2 error rates should not be taken as constants.

Enrolling fewer patients per treatment arm allows more treatments to be studied. This will become particularly desirable as understanding of the differences between normal and AML blasts increases, spawning a large number of new treatments, whose relative usefulness can only be established with the aid of clinical data. It is true that such trials will be nominally "underpowered." However, this argument ignores the false negative rate inherent in the selection of which investigational regimen to study. For example, if there are three potential regimens that could be investigated and if preclinical rationale is an imperfect predictor of clinical results, limiting investigation to one regimen in effect potentially entails a false negative rate of 67%. In particular, the most egregious false negative results when a treatment is not studied at all.[30]

References

1. Rowe JM, Neuberg D, Friedenberg W, Bennett JM, Paietta E, Makary AZ, et al: A phase 3 study of three induction regimens and of priming with GM-CSF in older adults with AML: A trial by the Eastern Cooperative Oncology Group. Blood 103:479-485, 2004
2. Goldstone AH, Burnett AK, Wheatley K, Smith AG, Hutchinson RM, Clark RE: Attempts to improve treatment outcomes in AML in older patients: The results of the United Kingdom Medical Research Council AML11 trial. Blood 98:1302-1311, 2001
3. Anderson JE, Kopecky KJ, Willman CL, Head D, O'Donnell MR, Luthardt FW, et al: Outcome after induction chemotherapy for older patients with AML is not improved with mitoxantrone and etoposide compared to daunorubicin and cytarabine: A Southwest Oncology Group Study. Blood 100:3869-3876, 2002
4. Van der Holt B, Loewenberg B, Burnett AK, Knauff WU, Sheperd J, Paolo P, et al: The value of the MDR1 reversal agent PSC-833 in addition to daunorubicin and cytarabine in the treatment of elderly patients with previously untreated AML in relation to MDR1 status at diagnosis. Blood 106:2646-2654, 2005
5. Estey EH, Thall PF, Giles FG, Wang X-M, Cortes JE, Beran M, et al: Gemtuzumab ozogamycin with or without interleukin 11 in patients 65 years of age or older with untreated AML or high-risk MDS: Comparison with idarubicin plus high-dose continuous infusion cytosine arabinoside. Blood 99:4343-4349, 2002
6. Kahn SB, Begg CB, Mazza JJ, Bennett JM, Bonner H, Glick JH: Full dose vs. attenuated dose daunorubicin, cytosine arabinoside and 6-thioguanine in the treatment of acute non-lymphocytic leukemia in the elderly. J Clin Oncol 2:865-870, 1984
7. Simon R: Importance of prognostic factors in cancer clinical trials. Cancer Treat Rep 68:185-192, 1984
8. Grimwade D, Walker H, Harrison G, Oliver F, Chatters S, Harrison CJ, et al: The predictive value of hierarchical cytogenetic classification in older adults with AML:analysis of 1,065 patients entered into the MRC AML 11 trial. Blood 98:1312-1320, 2001
9. Estey E, Thall P, Beran M, Kantarjian H, Pierce S, Keating M: Effect of diagnosis (refractory anemia with excess blasts, refractory anemia with excess blasts in transformation, or AML) on outcome of AML-type chemotherapy. Blood 90:2969-2977, 1997
10. Goldstone AH, Burnett AK, Avivi I, Hills R, Wheatley K: Secondary AML has a worse outcome than de novo AML even taking into account cytogenetics and age. AML 10,11,12 MRC trials. Blood 100:88a, 2002 (abstr)
11. National Comprehensive Cancer Network (NCCN) AML Panel: AML clinical practice guidelines. J Natl Compr Cancer Network 1:520-539, 2003
12. Baer MR, George SL, Dodge RK, O'Laughlin KL, Minderman H, Cali-

giuri M, et al: Phase 3 study of the multidrug resistance modulator PSC-833 in previously untreated patients 60 years of age and older with acute myeloid leukemia: Cancer and Leukemia Group B study 9720. Blood 100:1224-1232, 2002

13. Giralt S, Estey E, Albitar M, van Besien K, Rhondon G, Anderlini P, et al: Engraftment of allogeneic hematopoietic progenitor cells with purine analog-containing chemotherapy: Harnessing graft- versus-leukemia without myeloablative therapy. Blood 89:4531-4536, 1997
14. Alyea EP, Kim HT, Ho V, Cutler C, Gribben J, DeAngelo DJ, et al: Comparative outcome of nonmyeloablative and myeloablative allogeneic hematopoietic cell transplantation for patients older than 50 years of age. Blood 105:1810-1814, 2005
15. Burnett AK, Wheatley K, Stevens R, Goldstone AH, Hann I, Prentice AG, et al: Further data to question the use of allo bone marrow transplant in AML 1st remission in addition to intensive chemotherapy: The MRC experience in 715 patients under age 44 years with donors available. Blood 100;74a, 2002 (abstr)
16. Burnett AK, Goldstone AH, Stevens R, Hann IM, Rees JK, Wheatley K: Biologic characteristics determine the outcome of allogeneic or autologous BMT in AML CR1. Blood 86:614a, 1995 (abstr)
17. Kottaridis PD, Gale RE, Holt MP, Wheatley K, Goldstone AH, Burnett AK, et al: Consolidation of AML therapy with autograft and allograft procedures does not negate the poor prognostic impact of flt3 internal tandem duplications-results from the UK MRC 10 and 12 trials. Blood 100:75a, 2002 (abstr)
18. Tibes R, de Lima M, Estey E, Shahjahan R, Champlin R: Non-myeloablative HSCT in elderly AML/MDS patients in 1st CR. Proc Am Soc Clin Oncol 2005 (abstr 6655)
19. Lowenberg B, Zittoun R, Kerkhofs H, Jehn U, Abels J, Debusscher L, et al: On the value of intensive remission induction therapy in elderly patients of 65+ years with AML: A randomized phase III study of the European Organization for Research and Treatment of Cancer Group. J Clin Oncol 7:1268-1274, 1989
20. Burnett AK, Milligan D, Prentice AG, Goldstone AW, McMullin MF, Wheatley K, et al: Low dose ara-C versus hydroxyurea with or without retinoid in older patients not considered fit for intensive chemotherapy: The UK NCRI AML14 trial. Blood 104:872, 2002 (abstr)
21. Tilly H, Castaigne S, Bordessoule D, Casassus P, LePrise PY, Tertain G, et al: Low dose cytarabine vs. intensive chemotherapy in the treatment of acute nonlymphocytic leukemia in the elderly. J Clin Oncol 8:272-279, 1990
22. Bloomfield CD, Lawrence D, Byrd JC, Carroll A, Pettenati MJ, Tantravahi R, et al: Frequency of prolonged remission after high-dose cytarabine intensification in AML varies by cytogenetic subtype. Cancer Res 58:4173-4179, 1998
23. Sekeres MA, Stone RM, Zahrieh D, Morrison V, DeAngelo DJ, Galinsky I, et al: Decision-making and quality of life in older adults with AML or advanced MDS. Leukemia 18:809-816, 2004
24. Lancet JE, Gojo I, Gotlib J, Greer J, Kaufmann SH, Liesveld JL, et al: Tipifarnib in previously untreated poor-risk AML and MDS: Interim results of a phase II trial. Blood 102:176a, 2003 (abstr)
25. Stone RM, DeAngelo DJ, Klimek V, Galinsky I, Estey E, Nimer SD, et al: Patients with AML and an activating mutation in FLT3 respond to a small-molecule FLT3 tyrosine kinase inhibitor, PKC412. Blood 105: 54-60, 2005
26. Bishop JF, Matthews JP, Young GA, Bradstock K, Lowenthal RM: Intensified induction chemotherapy with high dose cytarabine and etoposide for acute myeloid leukemia: A review and updated results of the Australian Leukemia Study Group. Leuk Lymphoma 28:315-327, 1998
27. Estey E, Wang X-M, Thall P, Pierce S, Koller C, Faderl S, et al: Plausibility of delaying induction therapy in untreated AML. Blood 104: 879, 2004 (abstr)
28. Sievers EL, Larson RA, Stadtmauer EA, Estey E, Loweneberg B, Dombret H, et al: Efficacy and safety of gemtuzumab ozogamicin in patients with CD33-positive AML in first relapse. J Clin Oncol 19:3244-3254, 2001
29. de Lima M, Strom S, Keating M, Kantarjian H, Pierce S, O'Brien S, et al: Implications of potential cure in AML: Development of subsequent cancer and return to work. Blood 90:4719-4724, 1997
30. Estey E: Clinical trials in AML of the elderly: Should we change our methodology? Leukemia 18:1772-1774, 2004

ELSEVIER

Seminars in
HEMATOLOGY

Treatment of Older Patients With Acute Myeloid Leukemia—New Agents

Alan K. Burnett and Unmesh Mohite

The experience of most collaborative study groups is that the outcome for older patients has, unlike in younger patients, failed to improve over the last two decades. In addition there are a substantial number of older patients who do not enter collaborative group trials because they are not considered suitable for an intensive chemotherapy approach. During this era many combinations of chemotherapeutic agents at different dose levels have been tried. It is clear that novel agents and new approaches must be used to improve the situation, and should include options for patients who are not fit for intensive treatment. Fortunately, the increased understanding of the molecular basis and heterogeneity of the disease has fostered the development of novel agents. Chemo-resistance is a key characteristic of acute myeloid leukaemia (AML) in older patients and a number of randomized trials have now been completed to assess this approach. New possibilities of selectively killing leukemic cells and/or modifying toxicity are in prospect with the development of antibody directed chemotherapy in the form of gemtuzumab ozogamicin (Mylotarg; Wyeth, Philadelphia, PA). New drugs such as clofarabine or cloretazine are being evaluated. Molecular mechanisms, whether recognized or not, have been targeted by the use of *FLT-3* and farnesyl transferase (FT) inhibitors. With several new agents to evaluate, novel approaches to trial design aimed at detecting options likely to make a useful impact are needed.
Semin Hematol 43:96-106

One of the features of trials on acute myeloid leukaemia (AML) conducted by all collaborative groups over the last 30 years is how little improvement in overall survival has been observed. While remission rates may have improved, probably due to improved supportive care, this has not converted into a survival improvement (Fig 1). In addition, most large phase III trials have failed to reveal a difference between the arms, or, if a difference is shown, the benefits are marginal. For example the UK Medical Research Council (MRC) has undertaken 5,155 randomizations to nine questions in 2,790 patients over 60 years of age in the last 10 years. In none of the questions relating to conventional intensive treatment was a difference between the treatments seen. Only one question—low-dose cytarabine (Ara-C) versus hydroxyurea—for patients not considered fit for an intensive approach showed a difference. The conclusion is that new agents and new strategies need to be developed. Fortunately, an increased understanding of the biology of the disease is resulting in new approaches to treatment becoming available.

Department of Haematology, University Hospital of Wales, Cardiff, UK.
Address correspondence to Alan K. Burnett, MD, Department of Haematology, University Hospital of Wales, Heath Park, Cardiff CF14 4XW, UK. E-mail: burnettak@cardiff.ac.uk

Consideration must also be given to the fact that median age of patients with AML is in the mid 60s, and recruitment to trials in this age range is acknowledged to be selective so it is not easy to extrapolate the results from trials to the older AML population as a whole. There is also a large, and potentially increasing, group of older patients who are not fit for an intensive treatment approach. There have been very few trials designed for these patients. A relatively small European Organization for Research and Treatment of Cancer (EORTC) study established that in patients who were considered fit to be randomized to receive conventional chemotherapy or a non-intensive approach, intensive treatment was superior.[1] However, the best approach for patients for whom intensive treatment is not an option is unclear. The availability of new drugs that may have an improved side effect profile and in some cases bioavailability may offer future improvement for this neglected group. Some of the more promising new agents (Table 1) will be discussed.

Low-Dose Ara-C

Administration of low-dose Ara-C subcutaneously is a practical and well tolerated treatment for older patients. It

0037-1963/06/$-see front matter
doi:10.1053/j.seminhematol.2006.01.003

Improvements in CR rate over time 1970s to 2005

	Pre 1980	1980-84	1985-89	1990-94	1995-99	2000-05
Age 60-69	25%	52%	47%	58%	60%	65%
Age 70+	18%	36%	40%	48%	47%	62%
Overall	34%	66%	70%	74%	77%	79%

Improvements in survival over time 1970 to 2005.

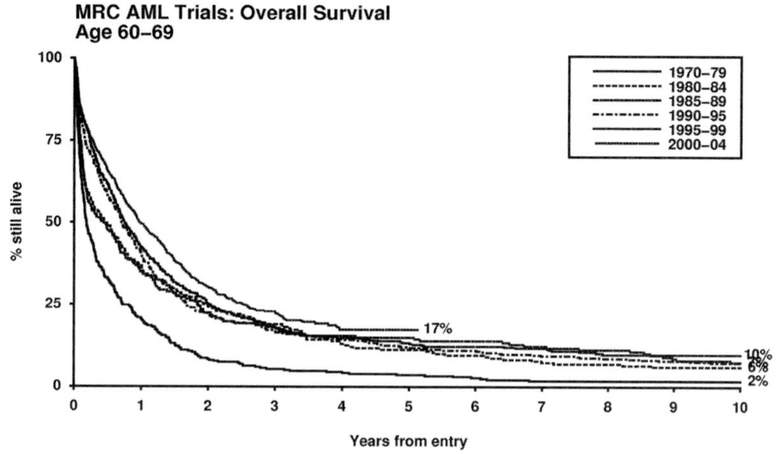

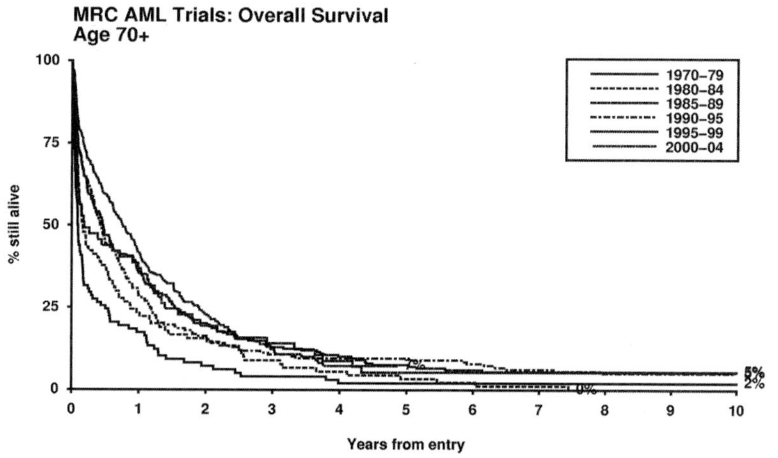

Figure 1 Changes in outcome in older patients over three decades.

is not new. Several years ago a number of unrandomized studies in AML and myelodysplastic syndrome showed that useful responses, including complete remissions (CRs), were achievable.[2–6] Various dose schedules were used and it has been debated as to whether the activity is mediated by cytotoxicity or differentiation induction.[7,8] The UK MRC group recently completed a comparison of low dose Ara-C given in a schedule of 20 mg twice daily subcutaneously for 10 days every 4 to 6 weeks versus hydroxyurea for patients who were not considered fit for standard chemotherapy. Each arm was also randomized to receive All-*trans* retinoic acid (ATRA) based on preclinical data that ATRA can sensitize AML blasts to Ara-C. This study recruited 217 patients. The independent Data and Ethics Monitoring Committee recommended premature closure of the trial because the remission rate and survival on the low-dose Ara-C arm was significantly superior. Eighteen percent of low-dose Ara-C patients achieved CR and the median duration of remission was 82 weeks.[9] The overall benefit was entirely attributable to patients who entered CR, which reinforces the point that for survival benefit—even in the older patients—the main target for success is the achievement of CR. No clearly beneficial effect of the addition of ATRA was seen. While the overall survival in patients receiving low-dose Ara-C is poor, this trial does provide a simple treatment schedule that is well

Table 1 New Agents for Older Patients

• Low-dose Ara-C
• Resistance modulators
• Antibody-directed treatment
• Novel nucleoside analogs—clofarabine
• Cloretazine
• *FLT-3* inhibitors
• Farnesyl transferase inhibitors

tolerated and could be the comparator for future studies of newer agents, either alone or in combination, in this group of patients.

Circumventing Drug Resistance

Several studies have been able to correlate a resistance phenotype with clinical outcome in AML; the most convincing relationship is with high expression of the gene product of the *MDR1* gene, P-glycoprotein (Pgp). Notwithstanding early differences in the technique of measurement, it has become clear that phenotypic and functional overexpression of Pgp correlates with increased age, adverse karyotype, a lower remission rate, and in some studies a higher relapse rate.[10–12] Other proteins are also associated with drug export and cell resistance such as MRP (multi-resistance protein), LRP (lung resistance protein), BCRP, and BCL_2.[13–15] As a therapeutic target, Pgp has been the main priority partly because anthracyclines, which are Pgp substrates, are such an important component of AML treatment.

Considerable preclinical data demonstrate that substrate drug retention is much less in Pgp-expressing cells and that the efflux pumping function can be blocked by a number of agents, including quinine, cyclosporine, and the cyclosporine derivative PSC-833. In the major study of quinine, the Groupe Ouest Est Leucémies Aiguës Myéloblastiques (GOELAMS) randomized 425 patients under 60 years of age to have, or not, a continuous infusion of quinine with standard therapy.[16] Overall there was no difference in response or overall survival between the arms. In a subset of patients who were Pgp phenotypically and functionally positive, quinine improved the remission rate from 48% to 83% but did not change overall survival.

Cyclosporine is effective at blocking efflux in vitro. Two randomized trials in relapsed or high-risk disease have been reported. The Southwest Oncology Group (SWOG trial 9126) showed a significant improvement in survival by combining cyclosporine 16 mg/kg with daunorubicin and Ara-C.[17] The schedule gave a 72-hour continuous infusion of daunorubicin covered with a continuous infusion of cyclosporine. Patients who entered remission had the treatment repeated. In the 226 patients evaluable for induction, resistance to treatment was considerably reduced (33% *v* 40%) and 2-year survival was significantly improved (22% *v* 12%). In a second study on relapsed disease, the UK MRC group randomized patients to cyclosporine at a lower dose (5 to 10 mg/kg/d), but saw no benefit. Indeed the study in older patients was closed prematurely due to an excess of deaths in patients over age 60 years that could not be attributed to any single cause such as immunosuppression or renal failure.[18] No clinical benefit on CR rate, relapse risk, or overall survival was found. The difference between these two trials may have been the higher cyclosporine dose given in the SWOG trial, or possibly a benefit of administering daunorubicin as a continuous infusion.

One of the consequences of Pgp blockage is the effect on the pharmacodynamics of the substrate drugs (daunorubicin or etoposide in the case of AML trials). A possible explanation for the benefits in the Pgp-positive subset could be the persistence of higher blood levels of drug, thus providing some of the rationale for testing higher doses of anthracycline as a separate strategy.

PSC-833 (Valspodar; Novartis, Basle, Switzerland) is a cyclosporine analog that is less myelosuppressive and less nephrotoxic.[19] It has become a standard reversal agent in vitro to measure Pgp function. Phase I and II studies suggested that considerable Pgp inhibition can be induced in vivo at feasible doses of PSC-833, although to avoid toxicity the daunorubicin or etoposide dose was reduced.[20–22] Four major randomized trials have been initiated. Two are completed and reported, one was stopped prematurely, and one study remains open. In what was intended to be a registration study, a joint trial organized by the Dutch Haemato-Oncologie voor Volwaasener Nederland (HOVON) and the UK MRC collaborative groups randomized 428 patients to receive daunorubicin 35 mg/m^2 with PSC-833 plus Ara-C or daunorubicin 45 mg/m^2 with Ara-C.[23] This was repeated in patients who achieved remission. The remission rates were not different. No effect on relapse and overall survival was observed with a median follow-up of 56 months. The second completed trial was conducted by the MRC in patients over age 60 years. Here, 601 patients were randomized to one of two doses of daunorubicin (50 mg/m^2 or 35 mg/m^2) and one of two dose levels of Ara-C (200 mg/m^2 or 400 mg/m^2 per day).[24] Patients allocated to daunorubicin 35 mg were randomized to receive PSC-833 or not. No benefit was found in the PSC-833 arm; in fact, the remission rate was lower (56% *v* 65%) due to a significant increase in induction deaths, again in older patients. The overall survival at 5 years was significantly inferior (16% *v* 21%) in the PSC-833 arm. The rationale of comparing two doses of daunorubicin in this trial was based on the possibility that if PSC + daunorubicin 35 mg turned out to be the same as daunorubicin (50 mg), this could have been interpreted as PSC-833 compensating for a reduced anthracycline dose. However, in a comparison of 890 patients, no difference was seen. The Cancer and Leukemia Group B (CALGB) performed extensive studies to establish the doses of daunorubicin and etoposide in an ADE (Ara-C, daunorubicin, etoposide) schedule that could be combined with PSC-833.[25–27] In these nonrandomized studies, there was a suggestion of an improved outcome in patients who received PSC-833. This led to a randomized phase III trial in patients over 60 years of age (CALGB 9720); however, the trial was closed after 120 patients due to excess toxicity.[28] A similar trial (CALGB 19808) in younger patients comparing ADE and ADE + PSC-833 is now reaching completion of recruitment.

So far the overall strategy of modulation of drug resistance has been disappointing, particularly in older patients.[29] The preclinical in vitro data were seductive. It is likely that subsets of patients could be identified where modulation can be shown to be beneficial. For example, there appears to be a benefit in patients with Pgp overexpression. Newer generation agents may be more effective.[30–32]

Antibody-Directed Treatment

Antibody-directed therapy has finally emerged as a possibility in AM.[33] The first convincing evidence was with an unconjugated monoclonal antibody directed against the CD33 epitope used in patients with acute promyelocytic leukemia (APL). Half of 22 cases that were molecularly positive were rendered negative by unconjugated antibody.[34] However, the data in other AML subtypes were less convincing.[35] Combining this antibody with standard chemotherapy was feasible, but the randomized comparison did not demonstrate any benefit.[36] CD33 has emerged as the favored target, and although not leukemia-specific, it was expressed on the blast cells of 85% to 90% of cases.[33] However, it is expressed on normal hemopoietic tissues but not on stem cells—at least at the level normally considered to give a designation of "positive."[37] As far as is known, no expression is found on nonhemopoietic tissue. Since naked human antibody reliant on antibody-dependent cellular cytotoxicity (ADCC) was disappointing, the next development was to exploit this epitope for antibody-targeted chemotherapy. This has several theoretic advantages: it may represent a useful antileukemic modality in frail patients by minimizing collateral toxicity; it may add to the antileukemic effects of standard chemotherapy; it may be useful for incorporation into transplant preparative protocols; and it may be used as maintenance. Combination with standard chemotherapy, which may be defined as simultaneous or sequential scheduling, is feasible in the induction phase or consolidation phase or both.[38]

These possibilities have become available with development of the first example of antibody-directed chemotherapy originally designated CMA-676 and now known as gemtuzumab ozogamicin (Mylotarg; Wyeth, Philadelphia, PA). This comprises a humanized anti-CD33 monoclonal antibody of the IgG_4 subclass to which is chemically linked the powerful antitumor antibiotic calicheamicin.[39] As free drug, calicheamicin is several logs more potent against leukemic cell lines than some clinically established drugs. It induces cytotoxicity by intercalation into DNA, and its potency excludes its use as a free drug. The key features of gemtuzumab ozogamicin are that the chemical linker to the antibody is only severed in the acidic intercellular environment of the lysosyme. Very little or no free drug is found in the product or patient's circulation. The second advantage is that when the antibody complexes with the CD33 epitope, the complex is rapidly internalized. This represents a theoretically advantageous drug delivery mechanism. However, there is concern that calicheamicin might be a substrate for biochemical resistance mechanisms, such as Pgp-mediated efflux. In vitro models suggest this is the case, but the clinical evidence is so far scant and early clinical trials indicated that Pgp-positive cases were less likely to respond.[40] Although the number of patents on which this observation was based was small, it nevertheless creates a rationale for combining Pgp modulation with this immunoconjugate.

Developmental phase I and II studies were conducted in relapsed AML. The phase I study examined several dose levels from 1 to 9 mg/m^2. Saturation of CD33 receptors was maintained over several hours at doses from 4 mg/m^2, being maximal at 9 mg/m^2. CRs were observed at dose levels as low as 4 mg/m^2.[40] The 9-mg/m^2 dose level was taken into phase II evaluation to be given as two single doses 14 days apart. Two unrandomized phase II studies were conducted in first relapse.[41,42] The study in the United States included patients who had relapsed after a minimal length of first remission of at least 3 months. A European trial included patients with a minimum length of 6 months but also patients who had received transplants. The overall marrow remission rate was 32%, but this included almost 16% of patients who failed to achieve full platelet recovery, although most were transfusion-independent, designated as CRp. The impact of new agents in relapsed patients in unrandomized trials is difficult to assess because of the heterogeneity of relapse risk, being as it is the length of first remission, patient age, and cytogenetics at diagnosis that determine treatment response.[43] While gemtuzumab ozogamicin is clearly active, and the ability to induce a CR with a single infusion is impressive, it is not clear that it represents a better way to treat relapse than currently available alternative approaches. Nevertheless it received approval in the United States and Japan in older patients.

Apart from the infusion reactions and myelosuppression that are expected because of the CD33 positivity of normal precursors, the treatment was well tolerated. Of potential importance with respect to intercurrent infections, gut toxicity usually does not occur. There has been some concern about liver toxicity. This is usually transient, but about 1% of patients develop liver sinusoidal injury manifest as features similar to veno-occlusive disease of the liver. However, expert opinion regards this not as a thrombotic manifestation but as a sinusoidal obstructive syndrome, which can be fatal.

Several prospective trials are underway to determine the correct niche for this agent. In younger patients, preliminary unrandomized phase I/II studies confirmed that it was possible to give Mylotarg and standard chemotherapy simultaneously, although the dose has to be modified.[38] Even at the modified doses, the observed remission rates were encouraging enough to justify major phase III trials. The UK MRC AML15 trial randomizes Mylotarg in a single dose of 3 mg/m^2 with the first course of induction therapy and/or with course 3 in consolidation. After approximately 600 courses administered, there has been no excessive toxicity. The SWOG 0106 trial compared daunorubicin/Ara-C induction with or without Mylotarg (6 mg/m^2), followed by Mylotarg given monthly (5 mg/m^2 $\times$ 3) as maintenance. Although these trials primarily recruit younger patients, the AML15 trial has recruited 88 patients over the age of 60 years. In these randomized patients the overall remission rate is 81%, which has encouraged the development of a trial using the same approach to induction in older patients.

The Dutch HOVON–Swiss Group for Clinical Cancer (SAKK) 43 trial is recruiting patients over 60 years and randomizing them to receive maintenance Mylotarg (6 mg/m^2 monthly × 3) or no maintenance. These major trials are at an advanced stage. The European/Italian EORTC/Gruppo Italiana Malathie Ematologiche Maligre dell Adulto (GIMEMA) group has focused exclusively on older patient groups. Following feasibility studies, the AML17 trial will randomize patients to receive or not two doses (6 mg/m^2) of Mylotarg before commencing standard chemotherapy. In consolidation, patients will also be randomly allocated to receive Mylotarg (3 mg/m^2) for two courses simultaneously with chemotherapy. For older patients who are not fit for an intensive approach, induction will be either 3 or 6 mg/m^2 alone for two doses followed by maintenance at 2 mg/m^2 monthly for 8 months, that is, Mylotarg as monotherapy. Based on the low-dose Ara-C experience, the UK MRC has recently concluded a randomized phase II comparison of low-dose Ara-C with or without a single dose (5 mg) of Mylotarg with each course in older patients not fit for an intensive approach. The Eastern Cooperative Oncology Group (ECOG) E1900 study will test whether the administration of Mylotarg (6 mg/m^2) added to the myeloablative schedule reduces the relapse rate after autologous stem cell transplantation. Apart from these important major trials, and including similar approaches in children, several unrandomized studies continue to evaluate the use of this agent, but so far there are no phase III data to define a role for Mylotarg.[44]

Based on anecdotal experience of obtaining polymerase chain reaction (PCR)-negative CRs in relapsed APL,[45] the group in Italy is evaluating the use of Mylotarg alone to treat relapse, while Estey and colleagues have shown that sustained molecular negativity can be achieved as first-line treatment in combination with ATRA with no or very little additional chemotherapy,[46] an approach that has been tested in older patients with APL.

Novel Nucleoside Analogs

Clofarabine

Nucleoside analogs (Ara-C, fludarabine, and cladrabine) have found key roles in the treatment of hematologic malignancies and Ara-C in various dose schedules remains the mainstay of AML treatment. To be active and effective, these agents need to be phosphorylated intracellularly to the triphosphate form, which depends on deoxycytidine kinase availability. They are all susceptible to deamination by adenosine deaminase. Ara-C is the only one of this generation of nucleoside analogs that, with respect to AML, has stood the test of time. At doses required to be effective in AML, fludarabine is associated with prohibitive neurotoxicity,[47,48] although it is more resistant to deamination. Clofarabine has been designed to combine the beneficial properties of fludarabine and cladrabine for inhibiting DNA synthesis by terminal incorporation into DNA (like fludarabine), and inhibition of ribonucleotide reductase (like cladrabine).[49] Cleavage of the glycosidic bond by purine nucleoside phosphorylase results in the presence of 2-F-adenosine, which has no cytotoxic merit but contributes to toxicity. Chemical substitution at the 2′ carbon position by a fluorine made the compound resistant to phosphorolysis and resulted in less neurotoxicity.

These specific modifications have resulted in clofarabine (Cl-F-ara-A; 2 chloro-2′-fluoro-deoxy-9-β-D-arabinofuranosyladenine), which is aimed at combining the advantages of fludarabine and cladrabine as well as being stable in acidic environment, giving it the potential to be available as an oral agent.[50] Clinical experience to date in acute leukemia has used a 5-day schedule of daily 1- to 2-hour intravenous infusions. These are well tolerated and not associated with alopecia.[51]

In a subsequent phase II study including relapsed or refractory AML, 31 patients received 40 mg/m^2 for 5 days.[52] The median age was 54 years (range, 19 to 82). Eleven patients (35%) entered CR and a further four achieved marrow remission with incomplete platelet recovery, giving an overall response rate of 48%. Eighteen of 19 (42%) AML cases achieved CR: on treatment of first relapse, six of eight patients (75%) with a first remission longer than 12 months, and five of 12 patients (42%) in second or subsequent relapse. Approximately 25% of patients developed reversible grade 3 or 4 liver toxicity. Hematologic recovery of patients achieving CR was 31 days for platelets to 100 × 10^9/L and 28 days for neutrophils to 1.0 × 10^9/L. The choice of a 40-mg/m^2 dose was supported by in vitro data suggesting that sustained blood levels of triphosphate were required for efficacy and a daily dose at this level was required to do that. Because of the tolerability and efficacy of clofarabine in AML demonstrated by the M.D. Anderson Cancer Center investigators, the UK MRC group initiated a trial using single-agent clofarabine as first-line treatment for patients not considered fit for an intensive treatment approach.[53] Such treatment must have an acceptable side effect profile and have the potential to be given on an outpatient basis with reasonable efficacy. The potential for oral administration is in the future. However, a dose level of 30 mg/m^2 was chosen to try to avoid liver toxicity and possibly shorten the duration of cytopenia.

Twenty-nine patients were recruited with a median age of 72 years (range, 61 to 82). Nine had high-risk cytogenetics. Little significant liver toxicity was seen, and that which occurred was transient. Sixteen patients (53%) achieved CR after one course and a further two had marrow remissions without count recovery. The median duration of survival of patients who entered CR was approximately 26 weeks. The aspirations of the trial were largely met; however, myelosuppression remained an issue. Neutrophil recovery to 1.0 × 10^9/L took 28 days (range, 19 to 39) and platelet recovery to 100 × 10^9/L required 28 days (range, 19 to 180). This was associated with neutropenic sepsis in virtually all patients. Thus, even at the reduced dose, efficacy was encouraging but myelosuppression remained problematic. Studies at lower doses, irrespective of the in vitro triphosphate data, are still justified.

Clofarabine in Combination

Since preclinical data suggested a direct relationship between Ara-C triphosphate (Ara-CTP) and clinical response,[52] various maneuvers have been introduced to increase the accumulation of Ara-CTP in leukemic cells. This was the intention in combining Ara-C with fludarabine or cladrabine. Since clofarabine has been designed to incorporate the cytotoxic mechanisms of both drugs, there is a logic to testing combinations of clofarabine and Ara-C given in a sequential manner.

In a phase I/II trial involving 25 relapsed AML patients, clofarabine was given in the usual schedule (40 mg/m^2/d for 5 days), on each day of which Ara-C 1 g/m^2 was given 4 hours later.[54] Seven of 25 patients (28%) achieved a CR, and a further three had marrow remission with incomplete peripheral blood recovery for an overall response rate of 40%. In a subsequent phase II study using the same scheduling in older untreated patients (>50 years), 31 of 60 patients (52%) achieved CR and a further five achieved CR with incomplete platelet recovery, giving an overall response rate of 60%.[55] This combination is feasible, but in the absence of a randomized comparison it is difficult to judge whether it is likely to be more efficacious than standard anthracycline/Ara-C or even Ara-C alone. Several studies are underway or are planned to evaluate further this interesting new drug in combination therapy.[56]

Cloretazine

Cloretazine is a novel sulfonylhydrazine alkylating agent that showed a degree of activity in a phase I trial in advanced myeloid malignancy.[57] A dose-finding study that included 28 AML cases concluded that, since no significant extramedullary toxicity was seen at 600 mg/m^2, this level as a single dose would be taken forward. One patient in second relapse achieved CR. A subsequent phase I trial was undertaken to find out what dose of cloretazine could be combined with high-dose Ara-C in relapsed or refractory patients or in untreated patients with poor prognostic factors. With a constant Ara-C dose schedule (1.5 g/m^2/d continuous infusion over 4 days), the dose of cloretazine was escalated from 200 to 600 mg/m^2. Significant gut toxicity and prolonged myelosuppression were seen but could be avoided by limiting the Ara-C schedule to 3 days combined with 600 mg/m^2 of cloretazine. Among 31 patients, eight achieved complete marrow remission. Since several of the patients in these studies were over 60 years, it is conceivable that further development could benefit older patients, but further schedules may be more efficacious. At present, a multicenter randomised phase III trial is being undertaken to compare the combination of cloretazine/Ara-C versus placebo/Ara-C in patients in first relapse.

FLT-3 Inhibition

FLT-3 is a member of the class III receptor tyrosine kinase family, which includes *FLT1*, *FMS*, *PDGFRβ*, and *KIT*. It is normally expressed on hematopoietic precursors and is overexpressed in unmutated form in AML cells.[58] It appears to be the most common single mutation in AML, occurring as an internal tandem duplication (ITD) in the juxtamembrane domain of the receptor, in about 30% of patients so far reported.[59–61] This is a consistent finding in several reports, although the frequency appears to be less (approximately 15%) in older patients, possibly reflecting the lower frequency in patients with myelodysplasia. A further 7% have a single point mutation at various positions in the activation loop of the receptor, usually at position 835. The effect of the mutations or ITDs is the removal of an autoinhibitory function that would normally keep the kinase in inactive form. This results in constitutive activation of *FLT-3* kinase and downstream activation of the *STAT5*, *RAS/MAPK*, and *P13K* pathways. The biologic consequence of this, seen in cell lines transfected with *FLT-3* ITDs, is factor-independent growth.[62–64] In the clinic, the interest has been the consistent observation that these mutations confer a poor prognosis, being particularly associated with a higher risk of relapse in several series. On multivariate analysis the predictive power is at least as strong as cytogenetics and indeed can further stratify the major cytogenetic risk groups. The mutations are not evenly distributed across the French-American-British (FAB) or cytogenetic groups. Paradoxically, the highest frequencies are seen in the M3-APL subgroup, where the frequency can be as high as 40%, and correlated with high white blood cell counts, where the frequency is 70%.[65] However, there is no major impact on survival. It is in the intermediate-risk group—particularly in association with normal karyotype and trisomy 8—that the adverse impact is more obvious. Here the relapse rate of 48% can be increased by 50%.[61]

Mutated *FLT-3* is clearly a candidate for therapeutic intervention. So far there is insufficient evidence from retrospective analysis to confirm that transplantation should be recommended.[66] Preclinical in vitro and in vivo models are persuasive that a number of agents are capable of targeting the molecular consequences of the mutations with the desired effect on the cell phenotype.

Early clinical trials have explored the tolerability and efficacy of these agents. An attraction for older patients is that the agents are orally bioavailable with an acceptable side effect profile. Although the frequency of mutation appears to be lower in older patients, the utility of these agents in unmutated cases with a high level of expression is worthy of explo-

Table 2 *FLT-3* Inhibitors in Phase II Trials

Company	Compound	Chemical Group	Trial Status
Sugen	SU5416	Indolin-2-one	Phase II
	SU11248		Phase I
Cephalon	CEP701	Indoloearbazole alkaloid	Phase II
Novartis	PKC416	Indolinone derivative	Phase II
Millennium	MLN518	Piperazinyl quinaxoline	Phase II

ration. At least five agents have had preliminary clinical evaluation (Table 2).

SU5416

SU5416 has had extensive clinical exposure, alone and in combination with chemotherapy in a variety of cancers, because it is potentially anti-angiogenic with anti-*VEGF* receptor *FLT-3* receptor properties. In the first study in AML comprising 43 refractory or elderly patients, one patient had a greater than 50% reduction in marrow blasts and seven had at least a 50% reduction in either bone marrow or peripheral blood blasts.[67] When responses occurred, they lasted 1 to 5 months. The associated biologic studies were limited so it is not clear whether the treatment resulted in dephosphorylation of *FLT-3*. None of the patients who responded had a mutation, so the mechanism of response is not clear. In a subsequent study, however, inhibition of phosphorylation after the infusion was demonstrated, but the effect was not sustained, which will limit the potential use of this compound.[68]

SU11248

SU11248, another indolinone derivative, is an orally available agent with several receptor inhibition properties. In a phase I study, inhibition of phosphorylation of various targets was seen, but the dose level required was associated with unacceptable toxicity.[69]

PKC412

Also an indolinone derivative, PKC412 is not a new compound, having originally attracted interest as a protein kinase C inhibitor. In vitro studies in *FLT3* mutation models encouraged examination of its *FLT-3* inhibitory potential.[70]

An unrandomized phase II study was conducted on 20 patients with relapsed or refractory AML who had a *FLT-3* mutation.[71] Ten patients were over 60 years of age. Overall, 14 showed a clinical response, mostly as a reduction in marrow blasts, and three cleared blasts to less than 5%. In vitro studies showed that responses were correlated with inhibition of *FLT-3*, with a plasma half-life of 6 to 9 hours. In the first unrandomized phase II study, 17 patients with relapsed or refractory AML with *FLT-3* mutations were treated.[72] Eleven patients were 60 years or older. The dose schedule was 60 mg orally twice a day for 56 days, which was thought sufficient to achieve the plasma levels required to inhibit *FLT-3* phosphorylation. The correlative in vitro studies confirmed this. Some patients received an 80-mg dose. The study permitted coincident treatment with hydroxyurea to control the white blood cell count. Five of the 14 patients showed clinical activity with a significant reduction of peripheral blood or bone marrow blasts. There were no CRs.

A second study exclusively in older patients who were not considered fit for intensive chemotherapy has been reported.[73] Here CEP-701 was given as first-line treatment in 29 patients who had a median age of 72 years (range, 67 to 80). Because of the possibility of efficacy in patients who do not have an *FLT-3* mutation, the presence of a mutation was not a trial entry requirement. The dose schedule was the same as that in refractory/relapsed patients with the provision to increase to 80 mg daily. Inhibition of the *FLT-3* receptor was demonstrated. Of the 29 patients, five had an activating mutation. As in other studies, the treatment was usually well tolerated and in 19 patients the dose was increased to 80 mg with two experiencing grade 3/4 nausea. Twenty-seven patients were evaluable for response. Clinical responses were seen in three of the five mutated cases, and six of the 22 wild-type patients. No patients achieved a CR. Five (all wild-type) patients had a marrow blast cell reduction, defined as a reduction in blasts to less than 15% or a 50% reduction, and four patients had a reduction in peripheral blasts. Two cases showed normalization of peripheral blood counts 2 or 3 months after completion of the 56-day treatment course, but marrow confirmation of CR was not obtained.

MLN518

A more recent phase II trial has evaluated MLN 518, a piperazinyl quinaxoline compound, in 20 patients so far.[74] Clinical responses, defined as a greater than 90% reduction in peripheral blasts and a mean reduction of marrow blasts of 62%, were seen in six or 15 evaluable patients. No complete or partial remissions have been observed so far.

It seems likely that the currently available *FLT-3* inhibitors, although fulfilling some of the requirements for older patients, namely, good tolerability and oral bioavailability, have limited potential as monotherapy. However, preclinical studies suggest that there may be synergism when combined with chemotherapy, which is the rationale of studies that are currently underway.[75] Second-generation agents may soon be available.

Farnesyl Transferase Inhibition

Farnesyl transferase (FT) is the enzyme responsible for the transfer of farnesyl to the cysteine residue of the C-terminal CAAX motif of *RAS* and other proteins—so-called prenylation. This is a crucial step in intracellular signaling and involves *RAS*, *RhoB*, *Ras* and *TGFβ*. This allows *RAS* to anchor to the inner aspect of the cell membrane, facilitating binding with guanine nucleotides. Since *RAS* is widely expressed in various cancers, including AML, this process is of potential interest as a therapeutic target. Four classes of FT inhibition have been developed. However, the limitations of the early generation of inhibitors led to the development of nonpeptidomimetric compounds, which, although structurally different, compete with the −CAAX peptides for FT binding, thereby inhibiting prenylation. The most developed in AML is R115777 or tipifarnib (Zarnestra; Johnson & Johnson). Cell lines show sensitivity in vitro, which is not *RAS*-dependent.[76–78] It is a selective nonpeptidomimetric inhibitor of FT, and thus acts by preventing attachment of candidate proteins to the inner aspect of the membrane, which is a requirement for activity. It is a methyl-quinoline with potent competitive inhibition action on FT, and it is active in cell lines in concentrations of 5 nmol/L to 100 nmol/L. Such levels are clinically achievable. Peak plasma levels can be achieved within a few hours after oral administration. The oral bioavailability is 34%, which is increased if taken with food. Overall, in several clinical settings, it has been well tolerated, with the most frequent side effects being myelosuppression, rash, and gastrointestinal effects. In an unrandomized phase II trial of 252 patients, there was no suggestion of increased side effects with higher patient age.

Experience in AML

In a dose-finding trial in poor-risk AML (patients with refractory or relapsed disease), two complete (8%) and eight partial (32%) responses were seen across all dose levels, which ranged from 100 to 1,200 mg twice daily. Responses usually occurred after several treatment cycles.[78]

In a phase II trial of relapsed or refractory disease using a dose schedule of 600 mg twice daily for 21 days out of a 28-day cycle, only three of 252 patients achieved a CR or CR with incomplete platelet recovery.[79] However, the mean response (12 months) was durable. A subsequent phase II trial in previously untreated older patients, using the same dosing schedule, was more encouraging. One hundred seventy patients were enrolled in the multicenter nonrandomized phase II trial (Cancer Therapy Evaluation Program [CTEP]-20).[80] Of these, 148 patients were evaluable for response; 160 had AML, and the median age was 73 years (range, 34 to 85). Half were over 75 years,with almost all having poor-risk features like antecedent myelodysplasia or unfavorable cytogenetics. Eighteen percent achieved CR and a further 16% had a partial remission. Twenty percent of patients over 75 achieved CR. The overall survival of patients was 5.6 months, which is a little better than the median seen in the MRC trial (3.3 months) with low-dose Ara-C, and the survival of remitters was 14.4 months, similar to that seen with patients receiving low-dose Ara-C who achieved a CR. The side effects were mainly gastrointestinal toxicity or infections, which occurred in about half of the patients, with a median number of days in hospital per patient of 12 days. The final analysis of the data may change slightly, but it can be concluded that inhibition of farnesylation is an effective therapeutic strategy with the convenience of oral administration, acceptable side effects, and useful duration of responses in those who responded.

None of these studies was randomized, but an international study is now underway aimed at untreated older patients (>70 years) who are not considered fit for intensive treatment. They will receive tipifarnib (Zarnestra) or best supportive care, which may include hydroxyurea. It is possible that this agent may be useful when augmenting conventional chemotherapy. Such studies are in the advanced stages of planning. Other agents capable of farnesyl inhibition are in the early stages of development.[81,82]

New Approaches to Trial Design

The last 15 to 20 years have been characterized by substantial effort by Collaborative Groups to improve treatment by the traditional phase III trials that have recruited sufficient patients to ensure the reliability of the conclusions. However, the conclusion has usually been, first, that no differences between treatment options are apparent and that relatively large numbers of patients have been required to be sure of that conclusion. The second conclusion is that, as illustrated earlier, there is little sign that treatment is getting better. In younger patients, phase III trials have also usually not shown a difference in the study arms, but at least improvement has taken place over the years. There is also a large proportion of patients who are not considered fit for intensive treatment, and few trials have been developed for these patients over the years. Meanwhile, several new agents are emerging that require testing alone or in combination.

These three issues should lead trialists to take stock of the conventional ways of seeking improvement. Given the lack of progress and the emerging new treatment options, it is relevant to consider more rapid ways of accumulating evidence. New drugs are likely to be expensive, and it is reasonable to approach the problem by looking for new treatments that may produce a larger benefit rather than concentrating on large trials, which consume a lot of patients, designed to detect or disprove small differences.

For example, in older unfit patients it would be reasonable to improve the remission rate from 18% (low-dose Ara-C) to say 30%. By using a "pick a winner" approach, several agents could be randomized against a standard arm (such as low-dose Ara-C). After a certain number of events, an interim analysis could be made as to whether the desired improvement was likely to be achieved. In light of the probability that this sort of benefit was likely, the "winner" would be carried forward to a conventional phase III design and power. By including the patients in the initial randomized phase II component, more optimal use is made of the recruitment. Because of the small numbers, there is a possibility of missing a beneficial effect. Possible scenarios might be, for example, if after 50 patients the observed remission rate was 15%, this would mean that the probability of the actual CR rate being the aspirational 30% would be 6%, in which case the comparison would be abandoned. Under these circumstances it would be considered unlikely to achieve the benefit that is being looked for if more patients were to be recruited. If the observed remission rate was 20%, then the probability of the actual CR being 30% will be 15%. This might be considered too uncertain to make a decision, and therefore the cohort could be expanded to 100 patients before a decision is made to continue or discontinue. If a CR rate of 25% was seen, it might be reasonable to commit to a phase III comparison. It is recognized that with small numbers, and a potentially heterogeneous group of patients, there is a chance of missing a positive effect, and on the other hand of pursuing a "loser" into phase III. Whatever the risks, the urgency for improvement requires a new strategic approach, particularly with the novel agents that will be available as single agents or in combination.

References

1. Lowenberg B, Zittoun R, Kerkhofs H, Jehn U, Abels J, Debusscher L , et al: On the value of intensive remission-induction chemotherapy in

elderly patients of 65+ years with acute myeloid leukemia: A randomized phase III study of the European Organization for Research and Treatment of Cancer Leukemia Group. J Clin Oncol 7:1268-1274, 1989
2. Wisch JS, Griffin JD, Kufe DW: Response of preleukemia syndromes to continuous infusion of low-dose H cytarabine. N Eng J Med 309:1599-1602, 1983
3. Tilly H, Castaigne S, Bordessoule D, Sigaux F, Daniel MT, Monconduit M, et al: Low-dose cytosine arabinoside treatment for acute non-lymphocytic leukemia in elderly patients. Cancer 55:1633-1636, 1985
4. Roberts JD, Ershler WB, Tindle BH, Stewart JA: Low-dose cytosine arabinoside in the myelodysplastic syndromes and acute myelogenous leukemia. Cancer 56:1001-1005, 1985
5. Degos L, Castaigne S, Tilly H, Sigaux F, Daniel MT: Treatment of leukemia with low-dose ara-C: A study of 160 cases. Semin Oncol 12:196-199, 1985
6. Cheson BD, Japerse DM, Simon R, Friedman MA: A critical appraisal of low-dose cytosine arabinoside in patients with acute non-lymphocytic leukemia and myelodysplastic syndromes. J Clin Oncol 4:1857-1864, 1986
7. Pinkerton PH, London B, Cowan DH: Low-dose cytosine arabinoside in acute myeloid leukemia: Remission is not due to induction of differentiation. Am J Hematol 19:415-417, 1985
8. Leyden M, Manoharan A, Boyd A, Cheng ZM, Sullivan J: Low dose cytosine arabinoside: Partial remission of acute myeloid leukaemia without evidence of differentiation. Br J Haematol 57:301-307, 1984
9. Burnett AK, Milligan D, Prentice AG, Goldstone A, McMullin MF, Wheatley K: Low dose Ara-C with or without retinoid in older patients not considered fit for intensive chemotherapy: The UK NCRI AML14 trial. Blood 104:249a, 2004 (abstr)
10. Leith CP, Chen IM, Kopecky KJ, Appelbaum FR, Head DR, Godwin JE, et al: Correlation of multidrug resistance (MDR1) protein expression with functional dye/drug efflux in acute myeloid leukemia by multiparameter flow cytometry: Identification of discordant MDR-/efflux+ and MDR1+/efflux- cases. Blood 86:2329-2342, 1995
11. Leith CP, Kopecky K, Godwin JE, McConnell TS, Slovak M, Chen IM, et al: Acute myeloid leukemia in the elderly: Assessment of multidrug resistance (MDR1) and cytogenetics distinguishes biologic subgroups with remarkably distinct responses to standard chemotherapy. A Southwest Oncology Group study. Blood 89:3323-3329, 1997
12. Leith CP, Kopecky KJ, Chen IM, Eijdems L, Slovak ML, McConnell TS, et al: Frequency and clinical significance of the expression of the multidrug resistance proteins MDR1/P-glycoprotein, MRP1 and LRP in acute myeloid leukemia: A Southwest Oncology Group study. Blood 94:1086-1099, 1999
13. Hart SM, Ganeshaguru K, Hoffbrand AV, Prentice HG, Mehta AB: Expression of the multidrug resistance-associated protein (MRP) in acute leukaemia. Leukemia 8:2163-2168, 1994
14. Hart SM, Ganeshaguru K, Scheper RJ, Prentice HG, Hoffbrand AV, Mehta AB: Expression of the human major vault protein (LRP) in acute myeloid leukemia. Exp Hematol 25:1227-1232, 1997
15. Pirker R, Pohl G, Stranzl T, Suchomel RW, Scheper RJ, Jager U, et al: The lung resistance protein (LRP) predicts poor outcome in acute myeloid leukemia. Adv Exp Med Bio 457:133-139, 1999
16. Solary E, Drenou B, Campos L, de Cremoux P, Mugneret F, Moreau P, et al: Quinine as a multidrug resistance inhibitor: A phase 3 multicentric randomized study in adult de novo acute myelogenous leukemia. Blood 102:1202-1210, 2003
17. List AF, Kopecky KJ, Willman CL, Spier R, Dorr R, Flaherty L, et al: Benefit of cyclosporin (CsA) modulation of anthracycline resistance in high-risk AML: A Southwest Oncology Group (SWOG) study. Blood 92:312, 1998 (abstr)
18. Yin JAL, Wheatley K, Rees JK, Burnett AK: Comparison of 'sequential' versus 'standard' chemotherapy as re-induction treatment, with or without cyclosporin, in refractory/relapsed acute myeloid leukaemia (AML): Results of the UK Medical Research Council AML-R trial. Br J Haematol 113:713-726, 2001
19. Boesch D, Gaveriaux C, Jachez B, Pourtier-Manzanedo A, Bollinger P, Loor F: In vivo circumvention of P-glycoprotein-mediated multidrug resistance of tumor cells with SDZ PSC833. Cancer Res 51:4226-4233, 1991
20. Visani G, Milligan D, Leoni F, Chang J, Kelsey S, Marcus R, et al: Combined action of PSC833 (Valspodar), a novel MDR reversing agent, with mitoxantrone, etoposide and cytarabine in poor-prognosis acute myeloid leukemia. Leukemia 15:764-771, 2001
21. Advani R, Saba HI, Tallman MS, Rowe JM, Wiernick PH, Ramek J, et al: Treatment of refractory and relapsed acute myelogenous leukemia with combination chemotherapy plus the multidrug resistance modulator PSC 833 (Valspodar). Blood 93:787-795, 1999
22. Sonneveld P, Lowenberg B, Vossebeld P, Malkhandi J, Covelli A, Dekker AW: Dose-finding study of PSC833, a novel MDR reversing agent, with daunorubicin and ara-C in untreated elderly patients with acute myeloid leukemia. Blood 90:566a, 1997 (abstr)
23. van der Holt B, Lowenberg B, Burnett AK, Knauf WU, Shepherd J, Piccaluga PP, et al: The value of the MDR1 reversal agent PSC-833 in addition to daunorubicin and cytarabine in the treatment of elderly patients with previously untreated acute myeloid leukemia (AML), in relation to MDR1 status at diagnosis. Blood 106:2646-2654, 2005
24. Burnett AK, Hills RK, Goldstone AH, Prentice AG, Milligan D, Pallis M: Attempts to modulate chemoresistance in older patients with AML using PSC-833 - Results of LRF AML14 Trial. Blood 102:614a, 2003 (abstr)
25. Greenberg PL, Advani R, Tallman M, Letendre H, Saba K, Dugan K: Treatment of refractory/relapsed AML with PBSC833 plus mitroxantrone, etoposide, cytarabine (PBS-MEC) vs MEC: Randomised phase III trial (E2995). Blood 94:383a, 1999 (abstr)
26. Kolitz JE, George SL, Dodge RK, Hoke E, Hurd DD, Powell BL: Dose escalation studies of Ara-C (A), daunorubicin (D) and etoposide (E) with and without multidrug resistance (MDR) modulation with PSC-833 (P) in untreated adults with acute myeloid leukemia (AML) <60 years: Final induction results of CALGB 9621. Blood 98:461a, 2001 (abstr)
27. Baer MR, George SL, Dodge RK, O'Loughlin KL, Minderman H, Caligiuri MA: Phase 3 study of the multidrug resistance modulator PSC-833 in previously untreated patients 60 years of age and older with acute myeloid leukemia: Cancer and Leukemia Group B study 9720. Blood 100:1224-1232, 2002
28. Lee EJ, George SL, Caligiuri M, Szatrowski TP, Powell BL, Lemke S, et al: Parallel phase I studies of daunorubicin given with cytarabine and etoposide with or without the multidrug-resistance modulator PSC-833 in previously untreated patients 60 years of age or older with acute myeloid leukemia: Results of Cancer and Leukemia Group B study 9420. J Clin Oncol 17:2831-2839, 1999
29. Larson RA: Is modulation of multidrug resistance a viable strategy for acute myeloid leukemia? Leukemia 17:488-491, 2003
30. Oza AM: Clinical development of P glycoprotein modulations in oncology. Novartis Found Symp 243:103-115, 2002
31. Peck RA, Hewett J, Harding MW, Wang YM, Chaturvedi PR, Bhatnagar A, et al: Phase I and pharmacokinetic study of the novel MDR1 and MRP1 inhibitor biricodar administered alone and in combination with doxorubicin. J Clin Oncol 19:3130-3141, 2001
32. Slapak CA, Dahlheimer J, Piwnica-Worms D: Reversal of multi-drug resistance with LY335979: Functional analysis of p-glycoprotein-mediated transport activity and its modulation in vivo. J Clin Pharmacol 29S-38S, 2001 (suppl)
33. Scheinberg DA, Tanimoto M, McKenzie S, Strife A, Old LJ, Clarkson BD: Monoclonal antibody M195: A diagnostic marker for acute myelogenous leukemia. Leukemia 3:440-445, 1989
34. Jurcic JG, DeBlasio T, Dumont L, Yao T-J, Scheinberg DA: Molecular remission induction with retinoic acid and anti-CD33 monoclonal antibody HuM195 in acute promyelocytic leukemia. Clin Cancer Res 6:372-380, 2000
35. Caron PC, Jurcic JG, Scott AM, Finn RD, Divgi CR, Graham MC: A phase 1B trial of humanized monoclonal antibody M195 (anti-CD33) in myeloid leukemia: Specific targeting without immonogenicity. Blood 83:1760-1768, 1994
36. Feldman EJ, Brandwein J, Stone R, Kalaycio M, Moore J, O'Connor J, et al: Phase III randomized multicenter study of a humanized anti-

CD33 monoclonal antibody, lintuzumab, in combination with chemotherapy, versus chemotherapy alone in patients with refractory or first-relapsed acute myeloid leukemia. J Clin Oncol 23:4110-4116, 2005
37. Tanimoto M, Scheinberg DA, Cordon-Cardo C, Huie D, Clarkson BD, Old LJ, et al: Restricted expression of an early myeloid and monocytic cell surface antigen defined by monoclonal antibody M195. Leukemia 5:339-348, 1989
38. Kell WJ, Burnett AK, Chopra R, Yin JA, Clark RE, Rohatiner A, et al: A feasibility study of simultaneous administration of gemtuzumab ozogamicin with intensive chemotherapy in induction and consolidation in younger patients with acute myeloid leukemia. Blood 102:4277-4283, 2003
39. Zein N, Sinha AM, McGahren WJ, Ellestad GA: Calicheamicin gamma 1I: An antitumor antibiotic that cleaves double-stranded DNA site specifically. Science 240:1198-1201, 1988
40. Sievers EL, Appelbaum FR, Spielberger RT, Forman SJ, Flowers D, Smith FO, et al: Selective ablation of acute myeloid leukemia using antibody-targeted chemotherapy: A phase I study of an anti-CD33 calicheamicin immunoconjugate. Blood 93:3678-3684, 1999 (abstr)
41. Sievers E, Larson R, Estey E, et al: Final report of prolonged disease-free survival in patients with acute myeloid leukemia in first relapse treated with gemtuzumab ozogamicin followed by haematopoietic stem cell transplant. Blood 100:11, 2002 (abstr 89a)
42. Larson RA, Boogaerts MA, Estey E, Karanes C, Stadtmauer EA, Sievers EL, et al: Antibody-targeted chemotherapy of older patients with acute myeloid leukemia in first relapse using Mylotarg (gemtuzumab ozogamicin). Leukemia 16:1627-1636, 2002
43. Breems DA, van Putten WL, Huijgens PC, Ossenkoppele GJ, Verhoef GE, Verdonck LF, Vellenga E,et al: Prognostic index for adult patients with acute myeloid leukemia in first relapse. J Clin Oncol 23:1969-1978, 2005
44. Nabhan C, Rundhaugen LM, Riley MB, Boehlke L, Jatoi M, Tallman MS: Phase II trial of gemtuzumab ozogamicin (GO) as first line therpy in acute myeloid leukemia patients age 65 or older. Blood 102:618a, 2003 (abstr)
45. Petti MC, Pinazzi MB, Diverio D, Romano A, Petrucci MT, De Santis S, et al: Prolonged molecular remission in advanced acute promyelocytic leukaemia after treatment with gemtuzumab ozogamicin (Mylotarg CMA-676). Br J Haematol 115:63-65, 2001
46. Estey E, Giles F, Beran M, O'Brien S, Pierce S, Faderl S, et al: Experience with gemtuzumab ozogamicin ("mylotarg") + all-trans retinoic acid in untreated acute promyelocytic leukemia. Blood 99:4222-4224, 2002
47. Warrell RP, Berman E: Phase I and II study of fludarabine phosphate in leukemia: Therapeutic efficacy with delayed central nervous system toxicity. J Clin Oncol 4:74-79, 1986
48. Spriggs DR, Stopa E, Mayer RJ, Schoene W, Kufe DW: Fludarabine phosphate (NSC 312878) infusions for the treatment of acute leukemia: Phase I and neuropathological study. Cancer Res 46:5953-5958, 1986
49. Vahdat L, Wong ET, Wile MJ, Rosenblum M, Foley KM Jr, Warrell RP: Therapeutic and neurotoxic effects of 2-chlorodeoxyadenosine in adults with acute myeloid leukemia. Blood 84:3429-3434, 1994
50. Montgomery JA, Shortnacy-Fowler AT, Clayton SD, Riordan JM, Secrist JA 3rd: Synthesis and biological activity of 2′-fluoro-2-halo derivatives of 9-β-D-arabinofurano-syladenine. J Med Chem 35:397-401, 1992
51. Kantarjian HM, Gandhi V, Kozuch P, Faderl S, Giles F, Cortes J, et al: Phase I clinical and pharmacology study of clofarabine in patients with solid and hematological cancers. J Clin Oncol 21:1167-1173, 2003
52. Kantarjian H, Gandhi V, Cortes J, Verstovsek S, Du M, Garcia-Manero G, et al: Phase 2 clinical and pharmacologic study of clofarabine in patients with refractory or relapsed acute leukemia. Blood 102):2379-2386, 2003
53. Burnett AK, Russell N, Kell W J, Milligan D, Culligan D: A phase 2 evaluation of single agent clofarabine as first line treatment for older patients with AML who are not considered fit for intensive chemotherapy. Blood 104:248a, 2004 (abstr)
54. Faderl S, Gandhi V, O'Brien S, Bonate P, Cortes J, Estey E, et al: Results of a phase 1-2 study of clofarabine in combination with cytarabine (ara-C) in relapsed and refractory acute leukemias. Blood 105:940-947, 2005
55. Faderl S, Gandhi V, Verstovsek S, et al: Clofarabine plus cytarabine (ara-C) combination is active in newly diagnosed patients (pts) ≥age 50 with acute myeloid leukemia (AML) and myelodysplastic syndrome (MDS). Blood 104:250a, 2004 (abstr)
56. Faderl S, Ferrajoli A, Wierda W, et al: Phase I study of clofarabine plus idarubicin and clofarabine plus idarubicin plus cytarabine (ara-C) in patients (pts) with relapsed and primary refractory acute myeloid leukemia (AML), myelodysplastic syndrome (MDS), and myeloid blast phase of chronic myeloid leukemia (CML). Blood 104:501a, 2004 (abstr 1809)
57. Giles F, Thomas D, Garcia-Manero G, Faderl S, Cortes J, Verstovsek S, et al: A phase I and pharmacokinetic study of VNP40101M, a novel sulfonylhydrazine alkylating agent, in patients with refractory leukemia. Clin Cancer Res 10:2908-2917, 2004
58. Birg F, Courcoul M, Rosnet O, Bardin F, Pebusque MJ, Marchetto S, et al: Expression of the FMS/KIT-like gene FLT3 in human acute leukemias of the myeloid and lymphoid lineages. Blood 80:2584-2593, 1992
59. Kiyoi H, Towatari M, Yokota S, Hamaguchi M, Ohno R, Saito H, et al: Internal tandem duplication of the FLT3 gene is a novel modality of elongation mutation which causes constitutive activation of the product. Leukemia 12:1333-1337, 1998
60. Nakao M, Yokota S, Iwai T, Kaneko H, Horiike S, Kashima K: Internal tandem duplication of the flt3 gene found in acute myeloid leukemia. Leukemia 10:1911-1918, 1996
61. Kottaridis PD, Gale RE, Frew ME, Harrison G, Langabeer S, Belton AA, et al: The presence of a FLT3 internal tandem duplication in patients with acute myeloid leukemia (AML) adds important prognostic information to cytogenetic risk group and response to the first cycle of chemotherapy: analysis of 854 patients from the United Kingdom Medical Research Council AML 10 and 12 Trials. Blood 98:1752-1759, 2001
62. Gilliland DG, Griffin JD: The roles of FLT3 in hematopoiesis and leukemia. Blood 100:1532-1542, 2002
63. Griffith J, Black J, Faerman C, Swenson L, Wynn M, Lu F, et al: The structural basis for autoinhibition of FLT3 by the juxtamembrane domain. Mol Cell 13:169-178, 2004
64. Levis M, Small D: FLT3: IT does matter in leukemia. Leukemia 17: 1738-1752, 2003
65. Gale RE, Hills RK, Pizzey AR, Kottaridis PD, Swirsky D, Gilkes AF, Nugent E, Mills KI, Wheatley K, Solomon E, Burnett AK, Linch DC, Grimwade D: The relationship between FLT3 mutation status, biological characteristics and response to targeted therapy in acute promyelocytic leukemia. Blood 106:3768-3776, 2005
66. Gale RE, Hills RK, Kottaridis PD, Srirangan S, Wheatley K, Burnett AK, Linch DC: No evidence that FLT3 status should be considered as an indicator for transplantation in acute myeloid leukemia (AML): An analysis of 1135 patients excluding acute promyelocytic leukemia from the UK MRC AML10 and 12 trials. Blood 106:3658-3665, 2005
67. Fiedler W, Mesters R, Tinnefeld H, Loges S, Staib P, Duhrsen U, et al: A phase II clinical study of SU5416 in patients with refractory acute myeloid leukemia. Blood 102:2763-2767, 2003
68. Giles FJ, Cooper MA, Silverman L, Karp JE, Lancet JE, Zangari M, et al: Phase II study of SU5416-a small-molecule, vascular endothelial growth factor tyrosine-kinase receptor inhibitor-in patients with refractory myeloproliferative diseases. Cancer 97:1920-1928, 2003
69. O'Farrell A-M, Foran JM, Fiedler W, Serve H, Paquette RL, Cooper MA, et al: An innovative phase I clinical study demonstrates inhibition of FLT3 phosphorylation by SU11248 in acute myeloid leukemia patients. Clin Cancer Res 9:5465-5476, 2003
70. Weisberg E, Boulton C, Kelly LM: Inhibition of mutant FLT3 receptors in leukemia cells by the small molecule tyrosine kinase inhibitor PKC412. Cancer Cell 1:433-443, 2002
71. Stone RM, Deangelo DJ, Klimek V, Galinsky I, Estey E, Nimer SD: Patients with acute myeloid leukemia and an activating mutation in FLT3 respond to a small-molecule FLT3 tyrosine kinase inhibitor, PKC412. Blood 105:54-60, 2005

72. Smith BD, Levis M, Beran M, Giles F, Kantarjian H, Berg K, et al: Single-agent CEP-701, a novel FLT3 inhibitor, shows biologic and clinical activity in patients with relapsed or refractory acute myeloid leukemia. Blood 103:3669-3676, 2004
73. Knapper S, Burnett AK, Kell WJ, Clark R, Craig J, Chopra R, et al: A Phase II trial of the FLT3 inhibitor CEP701 as first line treatment for older patients with acute myeloid leukaemia not considered fit for intensive chemotherapy. Proc Am Soc Hematol (abstr, submitted)
74. De Angelo DJ, Stone RM, Heaney ML, Nimer SD, Paquette R, Bruner-Klisovic R, et al: Phase II evaluation of the tyrosine kinase inhibitor MLN518 in patients with acute myeloid leukemia (AML) bearing a FLT3 internal tandem duplication (ITD) mutation. Blood 104:496a-497a, 2004
75. Levis M, Pham R, Smith BD, Small D: In vitro studies of a FLT3 inhibitor combined with chemotherapy: Sequence of administration is important to achieve synergistic cytotoxic effects. Blood 104:1145-1150, 2004
76. End DW, Smets G, Todd AV, Applegate TL, Fuery CJ, Angibaud P, et al: Characterization of the antitumor effects of the selective farnesyl protein transfease inhibitor R115777 in vivo and in vitro. Cancer Res 61:131-137, 2001
77. Kelland LR, Smith V, Valenti M, et al: Preclinical antitumor activity and pharmacodynamic studies with the farnesyl protein transferase inhibitor R115777 in human breast cancer. Clin Cancer Res 7:3544-3550, 2001
78. Karp JE, Lancet JE, Kaufmann SH, End DW, Wright JJ, Bol K, et al: Clinical and biologic activity of the farnesyltransferase inhibitor R115777 in adults with refractory and relapsed acute leukemias: A phase 1 clinical-laboratory correlative trial. Blood 97:3361-3369, 2001
79. Harousseau JL, Reiffers J, Lowenberg B, Thomas X, Huguet F, Fenaux P, et al. Zarnestra (R115777) in patients with relapsed and refractory acute myelogenous leukemia (AML): Results of a multicenter phase 2 study. Blood 102:614, 2003 (abstr)
80. Lancet JE, Gotlib J, Gojo I, Feldman EJ, Morris L, Thibault A, et al: Tipifarnib (ZARNESTRA) in previously untreated poor risk AML of the elderly: Updated results of a multicenter phase 2 trial. Blood 104:249a, 2004 (abstr)
81. Kurzrock R, Cortes J, Kantarjian H: Clinical development of farnesyltransferase inhibitors in leukemias and myelodysplastic syndrome. Semin Hematol 39:20-24, 2002 (suppl 3)
82. Feldman EJ, Cortes J, Holyoake TL, et al: Continuous oral lonafarnib (Sarasar) for the treatment of patients with myelodysplastic syndrome. Blood 102:421a, 2003 (abstr)

ELSEVIER

Seminars in
HEMATOLOGY

Allogeneic Transplantation for the Elderly Patient With Acute Myelogenous Leukemia or Myelodysplastic Syndrome

Marcos de Lima and Sergio Giralt

Acute myelogenous leukemia (AML) and myelodysplastic syndrome (MDS) are diseases of the elderly. Allogeneic hematopoietic stem cell transplantation (HSCT) offers the possibility of cure for these malignancies, but until recently its use was restricted to younger patients due to prohibitive treatment-related mortality. Improvements in supportive care and development of reduced-intensity preparative regimens have allowed patients in the sixth, seventh, and to a lesser extent, eighth decade of life to be treated with allogeneic transplantation. Major obstacles to extending this form of treatment to older patients are lack of promptly available donors, graft-versus-host disease (GVHD), delayed immune recovery, and the high prevalence of refractory and relapsed disease intrinsic to the natural history of these myeloid malignancies. Here we review current results of allogeneic blood and marrow transplantation for AML and MDS in the elderly.
Semin Hematol 43:107-117

Aging has been defined by Bortz as "the result of entropic decay inherent in metabolic processes, which is partially but incompletely offset by countering mechanisms. Aging is wear and tear minus repair."[1] The end result of this irreversible sequence of events is progressive deterioration of performance that leads ultimately to death. Frailty very often precedes death, in a scenario of weakness, low exercise tolerance, biochemical abnormalities such as hypoalbuminemia, and intellectual disarray. Furthermore, aging is frequently associated with other morbid conditions that likely leave the host with decreased reserve in terms of organ function. Therefore, many of the physiologic changes and disease processes associated with older age impair the general ability to tolerate aggressive treatment such as standard dose induction chemotherapy for acute myelogenous leukemia (AML) and allogeneic hematopoietic stem cell transplantation (HSCT).

Department of Blood and Marrow Transplantation, M.D. Anderson Cancer Center, Houston, TX.

Address correspondence to Marcos de Lima, MD, Associate Professor of Medicine, Department of Blood and Marrow Transplantation, M.D. Anderson Cancer Center, 1515 Holcombe Blvd, Unit 423, Houston, TX 77033. E-mail: mdelima@mdanderson.org

The Impact of Aging on the Incidence and Biology of AML and Myelodysplastic Syndrome

A review of Surveillance, Epidemiology and End Results (SEER)[2] data for the years 1998 to 2002 shows that AML is primarily a disease of the seventh to eighth decades of life. The median age of patients with AML at diagnosis is 68 years, while it is 77 years for the SEER category "aleukemic, and subleukemic." The age-adjusted incidence of AML is 1.8 per 100,000 for subjects less than 65 years old, increasing to 16.3 for those older than 64 years. The incidence per 100,000 increases from 3.5 in the population age 50 to 54 years to 21.3 among those older than 80 years. For the general population, the incidence per 100,000 is 3.6 (1999 data). The risk of developing AML doubles during the first 45 years of life but increases 10-fold in the subsequent 40 years.

The AML phenotype is characterized by impaired cellular differentiation capabilities and a proliferative advantage for the malignant clone, developing in a multi-step series of events.[3,4] Myeloid leukemias in the elderly are associated with higher frequencies of chromosomal abnormalities and/or *MDR1* expression, which are associated with worse prognosis, as is the tendency for AML in the elderly to evolve from a myelodysplastic syndrome (MDS).

In mice, changes at the stem cell level may explain the increase in the incidence of myeloid leukemias with aging.

0037-1963/06/$-see front matter
doi:10.1053/j.seminhematol.2006.01.004

Increased stem cell self-renewal, diminished potential to generate committed lymphoid progenitors with downregulation of "lymphoid" genes, and upregulation of "myeloid" genes have been described, as well as a high level of expression of genes associated with leukemic transformation.[5]

Results of Therapy for AML in the Elderly

The different biology of AML in the elderly is reflected in the poorer outcomes of therapy. SEER data illustrate the contrast in the likelihood of successful treatment of AML as a function of age.[2] The 5-year relative survival rates (years 1992 to 1998) for patients under and above age 65 years was 30.7% versus 4.1%, respectively. Most patients with AML will die of their disease, as indicated by Eastern Cooperative Oncology Group (ECOG) and M.D. Anderson Cancer Center data.[6,7] ECOG data points to a lack of improvement in the survival of patients aged 55 years or older treated in multiple trials conducted from 1973 to 1997, with a median survival time of 3 to 8 months and a 5-year survival rate of 6% to 12%. Complete remission rate and duration of remission are significantly reduced in the elderly.[8] Furthermore, in the ECOG experience, induction death rates increased from 10% for patients younger than age 60 years to 20% to 35% for those older than 60 years.[6] It is reasonable to speculate from these results that treatment of AML and MDS in the elderly is further complicated by our inability to effectively deliver therapies considered "standard" for younger subjects.

The issue of selection bias in the literature adds to the complexity of the problem, limiting somewhat the interpretation of current results of various therapies for this disease. Given that AML and MDS are diseases of the elderly, it is clear that patients in the higher incidence age range are underrepresented in clinical trials and are less likely to be referred for treatment. Selection bias has to be taken into account in the interpretation of results of allogeneic HSCT in this context, as discussed in a subsequent section of this review.

Allogeneic Transplantation

Allogeneic transplantation is associated with a graft-versus-leukemia (GVL) effect, mediated by donor lymphocytes and thought to be in great part responsible for the cure of leukemia after transplantation. Although occasional reports indicate the possibility of the GVL effect occurring in the absence of long-term engraftment of donor cells, sustained donor-derived hematopoiesis is generally considered a required step for this phenomenon to occur. Engraftment is achieved by inducing host immunosuppression, usually in conjunction with myelosuppression. The preparative regimen given prior to HSCT should provide both myelosuppression and immunosuppression. Traditional "ablative" transplants (such as those employing 12 Gy of total body irradiation [TBI]-based regimens) induce complete donor chimerism and intense myelosuppression, and are associated with higher toxicity rates and poor tolerance by older patients. The concept of reduced-intensity or "mini" transplants evolved from the realization of the importance of the GVL effect in several hematologic malignancies, such as chronic myelogenous leukemia (CML), where infusion of donor lymphocytes can induce remission of relapsed disease after allogeneic transplantation. The basic hypothesis is that if the intensity of the regimen can be decreased while retaining the ability to immunosuppress the recipient, one can induce chimerism at the expense of less toxicity, thus allowing older and frailer patients to be treated. The assumption is that the donor cells will have a greater role in keeping the malignancy in check.[9–11]

Nonmyeloablative and Reduced-Intensity Regimens for Allogeneic Transplantation

The intensity of the preparative regimen is an important contributor to treatment success after allogeneic transplantation, and to some extent also correlates with the incidence of graft-versus-host disease (GVHD) and decreased quality of life. Thus traditional ablative allogeneic stem cell transplantation has been restricted to younger patients with good performance status, excluding many candidates due to advanced age or comorbid conditions. Given the peak age incidence of the majority of the hematologic malignancies for which allogeneic transplantation is used, ablative regimens appear to preclude access to transplantation for the majority of the patients in need.

The existence of the graft-versus-malignancy effect in humans may be inferred by indirect evidence, such as the lower relapse rate in subjects developing GVHD or the higher relapse rates after syngeneic transplants or among recipients of T-cell–depleted allografts. More direct evidence is derived from the observation that infusions of donor lymphocytes can induce remission in patients relapsing after allogeneic transplant.[10] A less intensive preparative regimen that is sufficiently immunosuppressive to prevent graft rejection may be used to explore the graft-versus-malignancy effect. In addition, achievement of stable mixed or complete hematopoietic donor chimerism may be curative for several nonmalignant genetic diseases, a scenario where complete marrow ablation may be unnecessary.

Diseases that can be considered highly sensitive to the graft-versus-malignancy effect include CML, low-grade lymphoma, mantle cell lymphoma, and chronic lymphocytic leukemia. AML, MDS, intermediate-grade lymphoma, multiple myeloma, and Hodgkin's disease are usually considered to be of intermediate sensitivity, while acute lymphocytic leukemia and the high-grade lymphomas are relatively insensitive. Accordingly, the likelihood of success after nonmyeloablative or reduced-intensity transplants is highly influenced by the diagnosis and disease stage. Given the low intensity of the conditioning and the relatively delayed time for the graft immune effect to be effective, rapidly progressing malignancies are less likely to benefit from this approach. Post-transplantation immune interventions are frequently employed to maximize the GVL effect, such as early immunosuppression withdrawal or donor lymphocyte infusions.[11,12]

Truly nonmyeloablative conditioning regimens include fludarabine + cyclophosphamide, fludarabine + idarubicin + cytarabine, and 2 Gy TBI-based regimens, while "reduced-intensity" ablative regimens include combinations of fludarabine with intermediate doses of melphalan or busulfan. The less ablative regimens are generally associated with a higher proportion of recipient-derived hematopoiesis after transplantation and decreased duration of myelosuppression. Nonablative regimens are supposed to not require stem cell support and allow autologous hematopoietic recovery given the low dose of cytotoxic agents employed. However, these definitions are somewhat arbitrary and a wide variety of new regimens are now used by different groups, making the distinction between nonmyeloablative and reduced-intensity regimens very difficult.[12–14]

A major complication of allogeneic HSCT is graft-versus-host disease (GVHD), a product of alloreacting donor lymphocytes. Although GVL may occur without GVHD, it is frequently documented in the context of this complication. A key component of the pathophysiology of GVHD is inflammation and tissue damage induced by the preparative regimen. Reducing the intensity of the conditioning, conversely, may be associated with decreased rates of acute GVHD.[15–17] Development of grade III to IV acute GVHD (more severe grades of this complication) is usually associated with worse prognosis, even in the context of reduced-intensity transplantation.[18,19]

Immunologic Senescence

Aging is associated with a multiplicity of immunologic changes, most of which are likely to influence allogeneic transplantation outcomes. A proinflammatory milieu is frequently identified in older individuals, although it is unclear if this is a product of the aging process or the underlying diseases. This is exemplified by elevated levels of interleukin-6, tumor necrosis factor-α, prostaglandin E2, and other mediators of inflammation. Furthermore, macrophage function may decrease with aging, and the innate immune system function as a whole may be impaired by the imbalance in proinflammatory and anti-inflammatory mediators, with inappropriate responses to stress.[20] Host antigen-presenting cells are important in the generation of acute GVHD, and interestingly, antigen-presenting cells from older mice have enhanced allostimulatory activity.[21,22] This may provide an additional explanation for the reported increased incidence of GVHD in elderly individuals.

T lymphocytes from aged mice have defects in the activation process, and overall have slower responses than younger mice. B-lymphocyte function is also affected, and collectively these changes result in increased susceptibility to infections, which very often precede the transplant and complicate the treatment of the underlining malignancy. In addition, thymic function is severely impaired, especially from the fifth decade of life onwards, leading to an inability to build a diverse T-cell repertoire. Around the seventh decade of life, the repertoire diversity of naive $CD4^+$ T lymphocytes starts a rapid decline, which is no longer (or to a lesser extent) compensated by proliferation of post-thymic T cells. Individuals in the seventh to eighth decades of life commonly show a significant decrease in memory and naive T-lymphocyte compartments.[23,24] Collectively, these changes may provide an environment that favors the development of GVHD, and decrease the ability of the recipient to tolerate even minor degrees of this complication, as well as infectious problems. Current evidence would indicate that the aging immune system provides a less than ideal scenario for an allogeneic HSCT to be performed. However, the transplant itself may ameliorate some of these defects, given time and absence of major complications, especially GVHD.

It is unclear if the use of older donors' hematopoietic stem cells will recapitulate these immunologic problems in the recipient. Interestingly, in an analysis of National Marrow Donor Program (NMDP) data it was shown that the use of older donors was associated with higher incidence of GVHD in recipients of unrelated donor bone marrow transplants.[25] Conversely, it is not known if the use of younger donors provides advantages in terms of immune recovery.

Impact of Comorbidities

The prevalence of co-morbid conditions increases with aging. The development of AML or MDS is likely to exacerbate or trigger clinical problems that may contribute to morbidity and mortality during the transplantation process.[26] Several indices have been created to measure the influence of comorbidities on the outcome of treatment of a given primary disease, and some have been applied to allogeneic transplantation. Reduced-intensity regimens now allow patients with other diseases besides the primary indication for transplantation to receive allogeneic HSCT. Comorbidity indices have been proposed as a counseling and selection tool.[27] The Charlson Comorbidity Index (CCI) is commonly used in several clinical contexts. It assigns weights to chronic conditions in relation to their association with mortality, and adds points to each decade of life after age 50 years.[28] The Seattle group used the CCI to analyze outcomes after allogeneic related and unrelated HSCT. In the related-donor study, patients with a variety of hematologic malignancies were prepared with an ablative regimen (busulfan and cyclophosphamide or 12 Gy TBI and cyclophosphamide) or a nonablative regimen (2 Gy TBI with or without fludarabine). Assignment to each type of regimen was not randomized, and the low-dose TBI approach was used for older patients with more comorbidities. Other potential confounding factors included the retrospective nature of the study and the use of a different GVHD prophylaxis combination for ablative (cyclosporine and methotrexate) and nonablative patients (cyclosporine and mycophenolate). Nonrelapse mortality at 1 year in the ablative group was 56% for patients with a CCI score of 1 or greater, compared to 22% in the nonablative cohort (P = .002). There was no statistically significant difference in nonrelapse mortality in the subgroup of patients with a score of 0 (22% *v* 12%, respectively).[29] Interestingly, the incidence of acute grade III to IV GVHD was similar in both groups, a finding that may be explained in part by the early cyclosporine withdrawal used in the nonmyeloablative regimen.

The unrelated-donor publication followed a comparable design. Similarly, recipients of ablative regimens were younger and had less comorbidities. The incidence of acute GVHD was lower after nonmyeloablative conditioning (77% *v* 91%, $P = .01$), while the incidence of chronic GVHD was equivalent. Ablative transplants induced significantly higher rates of grade IV toxicity, while differences in day 100 and 1-year nonrelapse mortality were not statistically significant (18% *v* 12% and 32% *v* 20%, respectively). Higher CCI scores correlated with higher risks of nonrelapse mortality and severe toxicity in both groups. Nonrelapse mortality at 1 year was 28% for ablative patients with a score of 0, versus 67% for those with a score of 1 or 2.[17] Both studies did not analyze overall survival and relapse rates in depth, and were limited by the intrinsic fact that patients with high CCI scores are not generally treated with ablative regimens. Other CCI-related limitations include the use of morbid conditions unusually seen in transplantation, leading to a high prevalence of low scores. A new score has been proposed by the Seattle group, in an attempt to correct these limitations.[27] However, all of these indices have not been prospectively evaluated as tools for regimen intensity assignment or for patient selection in clinical trials.

Preparative Regimen Intensity

AML and MDS are considered to be of intermediate sensitivity to the GVL effect. Given this relative insensitivity, they may need the maximum conditioning strength that can be safely delivered, keeping in mind that nonrelapse mortality may increase with higher dose intensity, negating the decrease in relapse rates.[30,31] This is illustrated in the following study conducted at the M.D. Anderson Cancer Center. We compared outcomes of AML/MDS patients treated with the reduced intensity regimen of fludarabine and melphalan (FM) or the nonablative combination of fludarabine, cytarabine (ara-c) and idarubicin (FAI regimen). The former group had most patients with refractory and relapsed disease at HSCT, while the latter was composed of older patients (median age of 61 *v* 54 years), with a higher proportion of subjects in complete remission at the time of transplantation. Unrelated donors were used only in the FM group, while the majority of patients received human leukocyte antigen (HLA)-identical related bone marrow or peripheral blood stem cell transplants. The more intense regimen was associated with higher rates of nonrelapse mortality and morbidity, while the nonablative FAI regimen produced significantly poorer disease control and higher relapse rates, despite the higher prevalence of lower risk disease at transplant.[30]

Long-term follow-up (median, 29 months) of 112 patients with AML or MDS treated with FM in our institution with HLA-identical sibling or matched unrelated donor transplants indicates that durable disease control can be achieved. This cohort was comprised mostly of high-risk patients (80% with active disease at transplantation) with a median age of 55 years. The majority of the patients with relapsed or refractory disease at HSCT achieved a complete remission (remission rate was 75%). Relapse-free and overall survival are illustrated in Fig 1. The impact of disease status on the mortality rate is exemplified by the fact that 100-day mortality of patients treated in complete remission was zero, as opposed to 32% for heavily pretreated, relapsed disease subjects. The Seattle experience treating AML in first complete remission with a nonmyeloablative low-dose TBI-based regimen resulted in low treatment-related mortality, but a significant relapse rate. The 1-year progression-free survival rate was 42% in a group of patients with a median age of 59 years treated with HLA-identical sibling peripheral blood stem cell transplants.[32]

The most commonly used reduced-intensity regimens reported to the International Bone Marrow Transplant Registry (IBMTR) are combinations of fludarabine with low-dose TBI, as investigated by the Seattle group[19] (31%); with cyclophosphamide, as investigated by the group at the National Institutes of Health (17%)[33]; with busulfan, as developed by the group in Israel (27%)[34]; with melphalan, as investigated by the group at the M.D. Anderson Cancer Center (15%)[35]; or with other drugs (10%). In 45% of the cases reported to the IBMTR, antithymocyte globulin (ATG) or alemtuzumab was added to the regimen, as an in vivo recipient or graft T-cell depletion procedure, most often employed for mismatched related or unrelated donor transplants. There is extensive controversy surrounding the use of these T-cell–depleting agents, with the proponents of their use highlighting decreases in GVHD and rejection rates and the opponents indicating poor immune recovery and increased relapse rates as major drawbacks of the drugs.

The European Group for Blood and Marrow Transplantation (EBMT) compared outcomes of patients with AML older than age 50 years treated with HLA-identical sibling HSCT after regimens of reduced intensity or of myeloablative intensity. The former consisted mainly of fludarabine with busulfan or low-dose TBI, while the latter incorporated 10 Gy or greater TBI-based regimens or busulfan-based combinations with more than 8 mg/kg of the drug. Study groups had comparable disease status at transplantation (approximately 70% of patients in remission) and proportion of poor prognosis cytogenetics (16% and 12%, respectively). Recipients of reduced-intensity transplants were older (57 *v* 54 years) but had significantly less grade II to IV acute GVHD and transplant-related mortality, with a statistically significant higher rate of relapse. Interestingly, incidence of grade III to IV acute GVHD was similar. However, leukemia-free survival was not statistically different in the two groups. Relapse incidence (using death as a competing event) for patients in first or second remission or with advanced disease was as follows (myeloablative *v* reduced-intensity groups): 16 ± 3 versus 33 ± 4, 18 ± 6 versus 28 ± 6, and 45 ± 5 versus 64 ± 5. The 2-year cumulative incidence of treatment-related mortality (myeloablative *v* reduced-intensity groups) was: 30 ± 3 versus 22 ± 3, 34 ± 8 versus 16 ± 6, and 34 ± 4 versus 14 ± 3, respectively, for patients in first or second remission, or with advanced disease.[36]

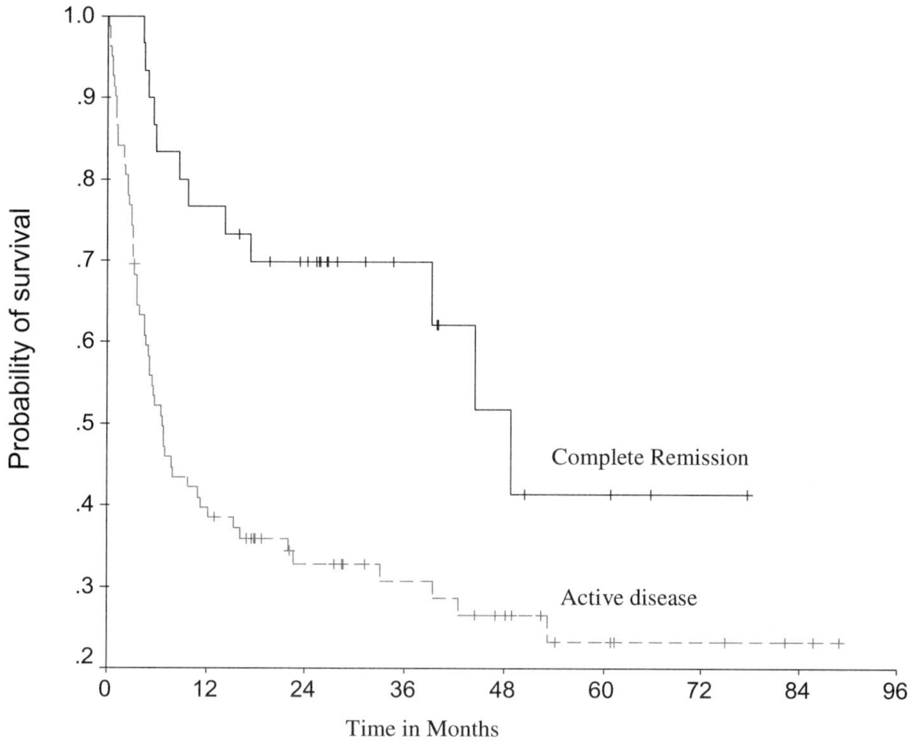

Figure 1 Overall survival of patients treated with fludarabine and melphalan, and allogeneic HLA-identical sibling or matched unrelated-donor transplants at the M.D. Anderson Cancer Center. Log-rank $P = .001$ for the comparison of patients in remission versus those not in remission at transplantation.

A common denominator in most series comparing different regimen intensities is the high early mortality associated with high-dose oral busulfan- or 12 Gy TBI-based combinations. As discussed above, several retrospective comparisons indicated higher rates of morbidity and infection after ablative regimens.[17,36,37] The Dana Farber experience with cyclophosphamide and 12 Gy TBI for patients with hematologic malignancies older than 50 years of age indicated worse nonrelapse mortality when compared to patients treated with fludarabine and busulfan (0.8 mg/kg for four doses, equivalent to 4 mg of the oral formulation). Early (100 days) treatment-related mortality was 6% versus 30%, while the cumulative incidence of transplant-related deaths was 32% versus 50%, respectively for nonablative and ablative transplants. The study cohort included 152 patients, of which 66 (43%) had AML or MDS. Nonablative patients received more unrelated donor transplants and were more heavily pretreated than recipients of ablative regimens. The tradeoff between dose intensity, toxicity, and disease control was again present: relapse rate was higher after nonablative transplants (46% *v* 30%, $P = .052$). However, a subset analysis of AML/ MDS patients beyond first remission (31 in the nonablative group and 29 in the ablative cohort) showed similar progression-free survival, and overall survival of 28% versus 16% in favor of the nonablative treatment ($P = .08$).[37]

The controversy surrounding preparative regimens is magnified by the fact that there is growing evidence indicating that the safety of myeloablative regimens can be improved. Lowering nonrelapse mortality while keeping a higher degree of myeloablation will potentially allow older patients to be treated and optimize disease control and survival. The Seattle group reported on their historic experience with 52 patients older than 60 years of age treated from 1979 to 2002. Preparative regimens employed high-dose oral busulfan in combination with cyclophosphamide or fludarabine, cyclophosphamide and high-dose TBI, and cyclophosphamide alone. The median age was 62.8 years. Nonrelapse mortality rates at 100 days and at 3 years post transplantation were estimated at 27% and 43%, respectively.[38] The success rate was higher for transplants performed after 1993. Our experience at the M.D. Anderson Cancer Center indicates that use of intravenous busulfan-based preparative regimens has significantly reduced morbidity and mortality in the treatment of patients with AML and MDS.[39] We have treated 56 patients older than age 55 years (median age, 58 years) with MDS (n = 13), AML (n = 33), or CML/myeloproliferative disorder (n = 10) from 1997 to 2004 on two consecutive protocols. Conditioning used fludarabine 40 mg/m^2 and once-daily busulfan 130 mg/m^2 for 4 days (n = 36), or busulfan 0.8 mg/kg for 16 doses combined with cyclophosphamide 120 mg/kg (n = 20). GVHD prophylaxis was based on tacrolimus and minimethotrexate. Donors were unrelated in 40% of the transplants, and most patients were not in complete remission. At a median follow-up of 15 months, 100-day and 1-year treatment-related mortality rates were 11% and 29%, respectively. Major causes of treatment failure were relapse and GVHD. Patients up to age 65 years are now eligible for our protocol using fludarabine and high-dose busulfan.[40,41]

The group at Chaim Sheba Medical Center in Israel has reported improved results in the context of unrelated donor transplantation for patients older than age 55 years with the use of an intravenous busulfan-based regimen. Furthermore, in their experience, the use of fludarabine in association to myeloablative doses of intravenous busulfan (0.8 mg/kg for 16 doses) provided better disease control for patients with AML/MDS than the same combination given with reduced doses of busulfan (eight doses), without increased treatment-related mortality.[42,43]

However, controversy remains as to whether there is a better regimen for reduced intensity or nonablative transplants. It is unclear if alkylating agent–containing regimens are better than TBI-based conditioning, as it is not known if a given alkylator produces better results than others. It is likely that the answer to this type of question will only come from large randomized trials that may be conducted by large cooperative groups. Meanwhile, it is recommended that older patients with AML and MDS should be treated within clinical trials whenever possible and available, given the multiplicity of questions surrounding the treatment of these conditions with allogeneic HSCT. The Cancer and Leukemia Group B (CALGB) and Bone Marrow Transplant–Clinical Trials Network are now implementing a single-arm clinical protocol investigating the role of allogeneic transplantation as consolidation for patients with AML older than age 60 years in first remission. Results of published series of AML/MDS patients in the sixth and seventh decades of life treated with allogeneic HSCT are summarized in Table 1.

Timing of Transplantation for MDS and the Confounding Effect of Selection Bias on Results of Transplantation

MDS is a heterogeneous disease, with dissimilar survival among the various subtypes. Accordingly, it is difficult to generalize when making treatment recommendations, and even more difficult to put into context results of any therapy for this disease, given the confounding effect of patient selection. Furthermore, the treatment of MDS is undergoing major changes as new medications are investigated, such as farnesyltransferase inhibitors, hypomethylating agents, FLT3 kinase inhibitors, and lenalidomide, to cite a limited list. The incorporation of immunologic approaches such as vaccines is also likely to be effective at least for a subset of patients with this condition. This revolution is logically welcome, but it certainly adds to the complicated issue of timing of allogeneic transplantation for MDS, especially taking into account the traditionally very high morbidity and mortality rates associated with transplantation.

An IBMTR study investigated retrospectively three transplantation strategies for newly diagnosed MDS: transplantation at diagnosis or at leukemic progression, or transplantation at a later time point from diagnosis but prior to leukemic transformation. A transplant and a nontransplant data set were used. Low and intermediate-1 International Prognostic Scoring System (IPSS) groups benefited from delayed transplantation, with maximum effect if the transplant was performed prior to leukemic transformation. Delaying HSCT had a stronger positive impact on survival for a subset of patients younger than age 40 years. For patients in the IPSS categories intermediate-2 and high, early HSCT was the best approach. This study did not include recipients of unrelated or mismatched-related donor transplants. All patients received ablative regimens, and had a median age of 40.4 years and median bone marrow blasts of 8.2% prior to transplantation. Median survival of the transplantation cohort by IPSS category was as follows: 40.2 , 20.5, 14.8, and 6.1 months, respectively, for the IPSS categories low, intermediate-1, intermediate-2, and high.[44] The major limitation of this study is its retrospective nature and the lack of randomization, making it impossible to determine the criteria that guided patient assignment, and to what extent selection per se determined the results.

The experience of the Department of Leukemia at the M.D. Anderson Cancer Center would indicate that AML-type chemotherapy can also produce long-term survival for younger patients with diploid cytogenetics. Between 1991 and 2000, 156 patients younger than age 60 years with high-risk MDS (IPSS categories high or intermediate-2) were so treated.[45] Chemotherapy consisted of high-dose ara-c–based regimens. The median age was 50 years, 43% were scored as IPSS intermediate-2, and 57% as IPSS high. Probability of event-free survival at 3 years was 0.12 $\pm$ 03 for all patients, while it was 0.23 $\pm$ 07 for 38 patients with diploid cytogenetics. Patients with cytogenetics other than diploid, inversion 16, or t(8;21), however, had a very poor probability of 3-year event-free survival of 0.04 $\pm$ 02. Our results in the same institution transplanting AML/MDS patients in complete remission at the time of transplantation indicate a 3-year survival of 70% (Fig 1). Considering that the Department of Leukemia is our major referral basis, the question of patient selection begs to be answered.

From 2000 to 2003, a study was implemented in our institution by which all subjects older than 50 years were to be referred for a transplantation consult during induction. The treatment plan was to proceed to a reduced-intensity transplant after achievement of first remission, should a donor be identified. The complete remission rate in the cohort of 259 patients was 39% (n = 99). Median age of those achieving remission was 65 years; 63 had AML and 36 high-risk MDS. The median number of siblings was one. A transplant consultation was done in 63% of the remission cases, and a donor identified in 40% of the consulted patients (26% of all patients in remission). Ultimately, 14 patients were transplanted in first remission at a median of 11 weeks from remission (15% of all patients who achieved a remission, or 56% of those with an identified donor). The proportion of patients with deletions of chromosome 5 or 7 was 14% in the transplanted group, while it was 36% in the group in remission with a donor that did not receive a transplant in first remission, 57% in the group without a donor, and 46% in the group that was never consulted. Disease relapse was the major reason for patients not being transplanted in first remis-

Table 1 Results of Allogeneic HSCT for Patients With AML/MDS With Median Age in the Sixth or Seventh Decade of Life

Authors	Disease (no. of patients)	Median Age, yr (range)	Disease Status at Transplant	Preparative Regimen	Donor	GVHD Prophylaxis	Median Follow-up	aGVHD and cGVHD Rates	TRM	PFS/Relapse Rate	Survival
Martino et al[54]	MDS = 20 AML = 31 CML = 9 Other = 2	56 (35–66) targeted busulfan; 59 (22–69) nontargeted	Early = 51% Late stage = 49%	Reduced-intensity: fludarabine and busulfan (targeted busulfan *v* nontargeted)	HLA-identical sibling (100%)	CsA and methotrexate	45 mo	Targeted *v* nontargeted busulfan Gd II–IV 20% *v* 22%; cGVHD 65% *v* 61%	Targeted *v* nontargeted busulfan (differences not significant) 100-d 5% *v* 3%; 2-yr = 12% *v* 19%	Targeted v nontargeted busulfan 2-yr 21% *v* 29%; 2-yr PFS 61% *v* 51% (*P* = .4)	Targeted *v* nontargeted 2-yr overall survival 65% *v* 53% (*P* = .4)
Maris et al[55]	MDS = 21 Ac leuk = 17 Other = 51	53 (5–69)	90% high-risk (several diagnoses)	Nonmyeloablative: 2 Gy TBI ± fludarabine	MUD 100%	CsA and MMF	42 pts alive at a median of 13 mo	Gd II–IV 52%; Gd III–IV 10%; cGVHD extensive 37%	100-d 11%; 1-year 16% (all patients)	1-year PFS: 38% (all patients)	1-yr overall survival: 52% (all patients)
Sorror et al[17*]	MDS = 13 Ac leuk = 12 Other = 35	54 (5–69)	78% high-risk (several diagnoses)	Nonmyeloablative: fludarabine, 2 Gy TBI	MUD 100%	CsA and MMF	Not given	Gd III–IV 17%; cGVHD extensive 53%	100-d 12%; 1-yr 20% (all patients)	Not given	1-yr = 60% (patients with low comorbidity scores) 25% (high morbidity scores)
de Lima et al[30]	MDS = 26 AML = 68	FAI: 61 (27–74) FM: 54 (22–75)	Remission = 24 (26%) Not in remission = 70 (74%) Remission: FAI: 44% vs FM: 16%	Reduced-intensity (FM): fludarabine and melphalan (n = 62) Nonmyeloablative (FAI): fludarabine, ara-C, and idarubicin (n = 32)	HLA-identical sibling 54%; MUD or mismatched related 46%	Tacrolimus and mini-methotrexate	40 mo	Gd II–IV 34%; Gd III–IV 16%; cGVHD 34%	100-d 21%; 3-yr cumulative incidence: FAI = 15.6%; FM = 39.2%	3-yr cumulative incidence of relapse: FAI = 53.4%; FM = 26%	Actuarial 3-yr survival: 33%
Bertz et al[56]	MDS = 3 AML = 15 Other = 1	64 (60–70)	Untreated = 6 Rel1 = 5 CR1 = 1 - CR2 = 2 PIF = 5	Reduced intensity: fludarabine, carmustine, and melphalan	HLA-identical sibling = 7 MUD = 12	CsA-based	825 d (595–1,028)	GdII–IV 59%; Gd III–IV 29%; cGVHD 65%	1-yr 22%	1-yr 61%	1-yr 68%
Wallen et al[57]	MDS = 35 AML = 6 CML = 8 Other = 3	62.8 (60.1–67.8)	AML rel1 = 5 CR1 = 1 MDS RA = 13 RAEB = 17 RAEBt = 4 CMML = 1	Ablative: BuCy (67%), CyTBI (21%), BuFlu (10%), Cy (2%)	All related-HLA identical (n = 48)/ mismatch (n = 4)	CsA-based (n = 48) Other: 4	4.6 yr (0.8–9.1)	Gd III–IV 20%; extensive cGVHD 53%	100-day 27%; 3-yr 43%	Relapse rate: MDS 20%; AML 50%	MDS 40% at median of 2.8 yrs; AML no survivors
Spyridonidis et al[58]	AML = 28 MDS = 6	All patients > 59 yr	Active disease: 91%	Reduced-intensity: fludarabine, BCNU, melphalan, and ATG	MUD 100%	CsA and MMF	913 d (55–1,591)		2-yr 19.6%	2-yr cumulative risk of relapse 27.3%	2-yr overall survival 62.7%; 2-yr PFS 53.1%
Wong et al[59]	AML = 13 MDS = 7 CML = 9	59 (55–69), all patients > 54 yr	AML/MDS: Remission = 4 pts (20%) CML: 1st chronic phase = 1 patient (11%) All others in advanced phase of disease	Reduced-intensity: fludarabine and melphalan (n = 24); fludarabine and busulfan (n = 5)	MUD 10%	Tacrolimus and mini-methotrexate	27 mo	Gd II–IV 41%; cGVHD 63%	1-yr 55%	1-yr EFS 37%	1-yr 44%

Table 1 Continued

Authors	Disease (no. of patients)	Median Age, yr (range)	Disease Status at Transplant	Preparative Regimen	Donor	GVHD Prophylaxis	Median Follow-up	aGVHD and cGVHD Rates	TRM	PFS/Relapse Rate	Survival
Schmid et al[60]	MDS = 10 AML = 65	52.3 (18.5–65.8)	CR1 = 8 CR2 = 8 REL1–2 = 28 PIF = 21 Unt = 10	Chemotherapy with Flu, amsacrine, and ara-C, followed in 3 days by 4 Gy TBI, ATG, Cy; prophylactic DLI in 12 patients	HLA identical sibling (n = 31)/ MUD or mismatch related (n = 44)	CsA and MMF	35.1 mo (13.6–47.6)	Gd II–IV 49%; cGVHD 45%	HLA-identical sibling donor: 22.6% MUD or mismatched related: 50%	2-yr leukemia-free survival 40%	2-yr overall survival 42%
van Besien et al[52]	MDS = 11 AML = 11	52 (17–71)	CR1 = 9 CR2 = 4 AML active disease = 28 MDS = 11	Fludarabine, melphalan, and alemtuzumab	HLA identical sibling (n = 23)/ MUD or mismatch related (n = 29)	Tacrolimus	18 mo (2–34)	Gd II–IV 33%; Gd III–IV 10%; Ext cGVHD 18%	1-yr 33%	Relapse rate 27%; 1-yr PFS 38%	1-yr survival 48%

Abbreviations: PFS, progression-free survival; aGVHD, acute graft-versus-host disease; cGVHD, chronic graft-versus-host disease; MDS, myelodysplastic syndrome; RA, refractory anemia; RAEB, refractory anemia with excess blasts; RAEBt, refractory anemia with excess blasts in transformation; CMML, chronic myelomonocytic leukemia; AML, acute myelogenous leukemia; CML, chronic myelogenous leukemia; CsA, cyclosporine; MMF, mycophenolate mophetyl; rel1, first relapse; CR1, first complete remission; Unt, untreated; Rel1–2, first or second relapse; PIF, primary induction failure; BuCy, busulfan and cyclophosphamide; CyTBI, cyclophosphamide and total-body irradiation; BuFlu, busulfan and cyclophosphamide; MUD, matched unrelated donor; Ac leuk, acute leukemia;
*Results of ablative transplants (median age below 50) are not summarized here.

sion, with patient frailty as the secondary reason. Relapse-free survival of the transplanted patients has not been reached, which is presumed to be a consequence of the GVL effect. However, assessment of transplant efficacy is confounded by the younger age, better cytogenetics, less comorbidities, lead-time bias, or unknown selection factors. We were able to perform the HSCT in 15% of patients achieving a remission, or 5% of the whole cohort of patients older than age 50 years. This study determined that the major obstacle to extending HSCT to more patients is the disease per se, since most patients never achieved a remission in the first place. It also highlights the fact that novel approaches will be necessary in order to extend allografting to a larger proportion of older patients.[46]

It is unclear if chemotherapy prior to HSCT influences the outcome of the transplant. The Seattle group found no effect of prior systemic chemotherapy on the outcome of a group of patients with MDS and AML with multilineage dysplasia undergoing allografts.[47] It is also largely unclear if the newer approaches to MDS will impact positively on the outcomes of subsequent transplants. Current results of MDS therapy are sub optimal, with or without transplantation. This should serve as incentive for a larger number of patients to participate in clinical trials and to receive investigational treatments.

Other Unsolved Controversies in Transplantation

Older patients are less likely to have healthy, HLA-compatible donors in the family, given aging and increasing prevalence of clinical problems. If one is to extend allogeneic HSCT to patients in the sixth and seventh decades of life, unrelated donors will have to be increasingly used. Younger donors are the preferred choice for bone marrow or peripheral blood stem cell donation, whenever possible.[25] There are a number of theoretical and practical issues associated with this choice. Aging may affect homing and engraftment of hematopoietic stem cells.[48] Older stem cells have an increased frequency of DNA repair defects, which may affect longevity and increase the likelihood of malignant transformation.[49] It is unclear, however, if using stem cells from older donors has a negative impact on outcome of older or younger recipients of HSCT. Donor issues are also to be taken into consideration. The donation process is usually better tolerated by younger individuals, although successful donations of hematopoietic stem cells have been reported in the eighth decade of life.

The issue of unrelated stem cell source (peripheral blood versus bone marrow) is under investigation in a multicenter Bone Marrow Transplant–Clinical Trials Network. As in many other questions surrounding transplantation, there are strong opinions in favor of one source or the other, a controversy that will hopefully be addressed with the ongoing clinical study.

The incidence of GVHD increases with age, but the variation in reported GVHD rates reflects confounding variables such as regimen intensity, donor type and level of HLA typing. The ability to tolerate the effects of GVHD and its treatment are usually decreased in the elderly. It is reasonable to expect that, for older subjects, allele level HLA typing will have the effect of decreasing GVHD rates for HLA-A, -B, -C, -DRB1, and -DQB1 matched unrelated donor-recipient pairs, similarly to what has been documented in younger recipients. Our experience treating 66 patients with myeloid leukemias in complete remission (AML, MDS, and CML) with unrelated donor transplantation using high-resolution typing can be summarized as follows. Median age was 45 years. Survival after transplantation where the donor-recipient pairs were matched at HLA-A, -B, -C, -DRB1, and -DQB1 was significantly better than in situations where one or two mismatches were present. Unfortunately, age greater than 59 years negatively influenced event-free, overall, and acute grade II–IV GVHD-free survival.[50]

Alemtuzumab is a humanized immunoglobulin monoclonal antibody that recognizes the CD52 antigen. It induces profound T-cell depletion in the recipient. Given its half-life, it may also cause graft T-cell depletion, reducing the incidence of acute and chronic GVHD.[51] The experience of the group at the University of Chicago (Table 1) and at the King's College Hospital in London treating AML and MDS patients showed a very low rate of acute and chronic GVHD.[52] In the British series, 62 patients with AML or MDS, median age 56 and 52 years for recipients of related or unrelated donor transplants, respectively, were treated with fludarabine, oral busulfan (8 mg/kg), and alemtuzumab (20 mg daily) for five doses. Donor lymphocyte infusions were required by 67% of the recipients of sibling transplants and 26% of the recipients of unrelated donor HSCT, in order to reverse donor chimerism loss or to treat relapse. Cumulative incidence of cytomegalovirus reactivation was 59% for high-risk patients. Disease-free survival rates at 1 year were 61% and 59%, respectively, for recipients of sibling and unrelated donor transplants.[53] However, it is unclear if longer follow-up will show increased relapse rates with this promising approach. Similar questions surround the use of ATG in this context. We recommend its use for unrelated donor transplants but not for HLA-identical sibling HSCT, as proposed by other groups.[34]

Conclusion

Selected older patients are now routinely offered the possibility of an allogeneic HSCT, and a significant fraction of those treated will achieve long-term disease control. The complete remission rate is usually higher than that achieved with any form of salvage chemotherapy, likely the result of the immune GVL effect. Relapse, however, is the major cause of treatment failure for patients treated with active disease at transplantation, while GVHD remains a problem, especially among recipients of unrelated donor transplants. Unfortunately, most patients in the sixth, seventh or eighth decades of life will have refractory or relapsed disease. Furthermore, the number of available family donors decreases with aging. If the use of HSCT is to be extended to more patients in need, one will have to use donors other than HLA-identical siblings, and develop strategies designed to decrease the relapse and GVHD rates after transplantation.

References

1. Bortz W: Biological basis of determinants of health. Am J Public Health 95:389-392, 2005
2. SEER: Surveillance, Epidemiology and End Results (SEER). SEER CANCER GOV (accessed on August, 2005)
3. Godwin J, Smith T: Acute myeloid leukemia in the older patient. Crit Rev Oncol Hematol 48S:17-26, 2003
4. Kelly L, Gilliland DG: Genetics of myeloid leukemias. Annu Rev Genomics Hum Genet 3:179-198, 2002
5. Rossi D, Bryder D, Zahn J, Ahlenius H, Sonu R, Wagers A: Cell intrinsic alterations underlie hematopoietic stem cell aging. Proc Natl Acad Sci U S A 102:9194-9199, 2005
6. Appelbaum FR, Rowe JM, Radich J, Dick JE: Acute myeloid leukemia. Hematology (Am Soc Hematol Educ Program) 62-86, 2001
7. de Lima M, Strom SS, Keating M, Kantarjian H, Pierce S, O'Brien S, et al: Implications of potential cure in acute myelogenous leukemia: Development of subsequent cancer and return to work. Blood 90:4719-4724, 1997
8. de Lima M, Ghaddar H, Pierce S, Estey E: Treatment of newly diagnosed acute myelogenous leukemia in-patients age 80 years and above. Br J Haematol 93:89-95, 1996
9. Giralt S, Anagnostopoulos A, Shahjahan M, Champlin R: Nonablative stem cell transplantation for older patients with acute leukemias and myelodysplastic syndromes. Semin Hematol 39:57-62, 2002
10. Kolb HJ, Schattenberg A, Goldman JM, Hertenstein B, Jacobsen N, Arcese W, et al: Graft-versus-leukemia effect of donor lymphocyte transfusions in marrow grafted patients. Blood 86:2041-2050, 1995
11. Champlin R, Khouri I, Anderlini P, de Lima M, Hosing C, McMannis J, et al: Nonmyeloablative preparative regimens for allogeneic hematopoietic transplantation. Biology and current indications. Oncology (Williston Park) 17:94-100, 2003
12. Khouri IF, Lee MS, Saliba RM, Jun G, Fayad L, Younes A, et al: Nonablative allogeneic stem-cell transplantation for advanced/recurrent mantle-cell lymphoma. J Clin Oncol 21:4407-4412, 2003
13. Maris M, Storb R: The transplantation of hematopoietic stem cells after non-myeloablative conditioning: A cellular therapeutic approach to hematologic and genetic diseases. Immunol Res 28:13-24, 2003
14. van Besien K, Artz A, Stock W: Unrelated donor transplantation over the age of 55. Are we merely getting (b)older? Leukemia 19:31-33, 2005
15. Couriel DR, Saliba RM, Giralt S, Khouri I, Andersson B, de Lima M, et al: Acute and chronic graft-versus-host disease after ablative and nonmyeloablative conditioning for allogeneic hematopoietic transplantation. Biol Blood Marrow Transplant 10:178-185, 2004
16. Sorror M, Maris M, Diaconescu R, Storb R: Lessened severe graft-versus-host after "minitransplantations." Blood 105:2614, 2005
17. Sorror ML, Maris MB, Storer B, Sandmaier BM, Diaconescu R, Flowers C, et al: Comparing morbidity and mortality of HLA-matched unrelated donor hematopoietic cell transplantation after nonmyeloablative and myeloablative conditioning: Influence of pretransplantation comorbidities. Blood 104:961-968, 2004
18. Corradini P, Zallio F, Mariotti J, Farina L, Bregni M, Valagussa P, et al: Effect of age and previous autologous transplantation on nonrelapse mortality and survival in patients treated with reduced-intensity conditioning and allografting for advance hematologic malignancies. J Clin Oncol 23:6690-6698, 2005
19. Baron F, Maris MB, Sandmaier BM, Storer BE, Sorror M, Diaconescu R, et al: Graft-versus-tumor effects after allogeneic hematopoietic cell transplantation with nonmyeloablative conditioning. J Clin Oncol 23: 1993-2003, 2005
20. Gomez CR, Boehmer ED, Kovacs EJ: The aging innate immune system. Curr Opin Immunol 17:1-6, 2005
21. Shlomchik WD, Couzens MS, Tang CB, McNiff J, Robert ME, Liu J, et al: Prevention of graft versus host disease by inactivation of host antigen-presenting cells. Science 285:412-415, 1999

22. Ordemann R, Hutchinson R, Friedman J, Burakoff SJ, Reddy P, Duffner U, et al: Enhanced allostimulatory activity of host antigen-presenting cells in old mice intensifies acute graft-versus-host disease. J Clin Invest 109:1249-1256, 2002
23. Akha A, Miller R: Signal transduction in the aging immune system. Curr Opin Immunol 17:1-6, 2005
24. Goronzy J, Weyand CM: T cell development and receptor diversity during aging. Curr Opin Immunol 17:1-8, 2005
25. Kollman C, Howe CW, Anasetti C, Antin JH, Davies SM, Filipovich AH, et al: Donor characteristics as risk factors in recipients after transplantation of bone marrow from unrelated donors: The effect of donor age. Blood 98:2043-2051, 2001
26. Alamo J, Shahjahan M, Lazarus HM, de Lima M, Giralt SA: Comorbidity indices in hematopoietic stem cell transplantation: A new report card. Bone Marrow Transplant 36:475-479, 2005
27. Sorror ML, Maris MB, Storb R, Baron F, Sandmaier BM, Maloney DG, et al: Hematopoietic cell transplantation-specific comorbidity index: A new tool for risk assessment before allogeneic HCT. Blood 2005
28. Charlson ME, Pompei P, Ales KL, MacKenzie CR: A new method of classifying prognostic comorbidity in longitudinal studies: Development and validation. J Chronic Dis 40:373-383, 1987
29. Diaconescu R, Flowers CR, Storer B, Sorror ML, Maris MB, Maloney DG, et al: Morbidity and mortality with nonmyeloablative compared with myeloablative conditioning before hematopoietic cell transplantation from HLA-matched related donors. Blood 104:1550-1558, 2004
30. de Lima M, Anagnostopoulos A, Munsell M, Shahjahan M, Ueno N, Ippoliti C, et al: Nonablative versus reduced-intensity conditioning regimens in the treatment of acute myeloid leukemia and high-risk myelodysplastic syndrome: Dose is relevant for long-term disease control after allogeneic hematopoietic stem cell transplantation. Blood 104: 865-872, 2004
31. Clift RA, Buckner CD, Appelbaum FR, Sullivan KM, Storb R, Thomas ED: Long-term follow-up of a randomized trial of two irradiation regimens for patients receiving allogeneic marrow transplants during first remission of acute myeloid leukemia. Blood 92:1455-1456, 1998
32. Feinstein LC, Sandmaier BM, Hegenbart U, McSweeney PA, Maloney DG, Gooley TA, et al: Non-myeloablative allografting from human leucocyte antigen-identical sibling donors for treatment of acute myeloid leukaemia in first complete remission. Br J Haematol 120:281-288, 2003
33. Childs R, Clave E, Contentin N, et al: Engraftment kinetics after non-myeloablative allogeneic peripheral blood stem cell transplantation: Full donor T-cell chimerism precedes alloimmune responses. Blood 94:3234-3241, 1999
34. Slavin S, Nagler A, Naparstek E, Kapelushnik Y, Aker M, Cividalli G, et al: Nonmyeloablative stem cell transplantation and cell therapy as an alternative to conventional bone marrow transplantation with lethal cytoreduction for the treatment of malignant and nonmalignant hematologic diseases. Blood 91:756-763, 1998
35. Giralt S, Estey E, Albitar M, van Besien K, Rondon G, Anderlini P, et al: Engraftment of allogeneic hematopoietic progenitor cells with purine analog-containing chemotherapy: harnessing graft-versus-leukemia without myeloablative therapy. Blood 89:4531-4536, 1997
36. Aoudjane M, Labopin M, Gorin N, Shimoni A, Ruutu M, Kolb H, et al: Comparative outcome of reduced intensity and myeloablative conditioning regimen in HLA identical sibling allogeneic hematopoietic stem cell transplantation for patients older than 50 years of age with acute myeloblastic leukaemia: A retrospective survey from the acute leukemia party (ALWP) of the European group for Blood and Marrow Transplantation (EBMT). Leukemia [Epub ahead of print:1-9, 2005]
37. Alyea E, Kim H, Ho VT, Cutler C, Gribben J, DeAngelo D, et al: Comparative outcome of nonmyeloablative and myeloablative allogeneic hematopoietic stem cell transplantation for patients older than 50 years of age. Blood 105:1810-1814, 2005
38. Wallen H, Gooley T, Deeg HJ, Pagel JM, Press OW, Appelbaum FR, et al: Ablative allogeneic hematopoietic cell transplantation in adults 60 years of age and older. J Clin Oncol 23:3439-3446, 2005
39. de Lima M, Couriel D, Thall PF, Wang X, Madden T, Jones R, et al: Once-daily intravenous busulfan and fludarabine: Clinical and pharmacokinetic results of a myeloablative, reduced-toxicity conditioning regimen for allogeneic stem cell transplantation in AML and MDS. Blood 104:857-864, 2004
40. de Lima M, Champlin R, Andersson B: Treatment of AML/MDS with allogeneic hematopoietic stem cell transplantation after intravenous busulfan-based conditioning therapy. Biol Blood Marrow Transplant Rev 15:10-11, 2005
41. de Lima M, Couriel D, Ghosh S, Jones R, Shpall EJ, Giralt S, et al: Outcomes of older patients with myeloid leukemias treated with myeloablative intravenous busulfan-based conditioning regimens and allogeneic blood or marrow transplantation. Blood 106:660a, 2005 (abstr)
42. Shimoni A, Kroger N, Zabelina T, Ayuk F, Hardan I, Yeshurun M, et al: Hematopoietic stem-cell transplantation from unrelated donors in elderly patients (age >55 years) with hematologic malignancies: Older age is no longer a contraindication when using reduced intensity conditioning. Leukemia 19:7-12, 2005
43. Nagler A: Myeloablative conditioning using IV busulfan reduces toxicity to the level observed in low-intensity conditioning regimens: dose does matter. Biol Blood Marrow Transplant 15:8-9, 2005
44. Cutler CS, Lee SJ, Greenberg P, Deeg HJ, Perez WS, Anasetti C, et al: A decision analysis of allogeneic bone marrow transplantation for the myelodysplastic syndromes: Delayed transplantation for low-risk myelodysplasia is associated with improved outcome. Blood 104:579-585, 2004
45. Estey E: The Thompson/Luger article reviewed. Oncology 19:542-543, 2005
46. Tibes R, de Lima M, Estey E, Pierce S, Champlin R, Giralt S: Prospective feasibility analysis of reduced intensity conditioning regimens (RIC) for hematopoietic stem cell transplantation (HSCT) in elderly patients with AML and MDS. Blood 106:2892a, 2005 (abstr)
47. Scott BL, Storer B, Loken MR, Storb R, Appelbaum FR, Deeg HJ: Pretransplantation induction chemotherapy and posttransplantation relapse in patients with advanced myelodysplastic syndrome. Biol Blood Marrow Transplant 11:65-73, 2005
48. Liang Y, Van Zant G, Szilvassy SJ: Effects of aging on the homing and engraftment of murine hematopoietic stem and progenitor cells. Blood 106:1479-1487, 2005
49. Park Y, Gerson S: DNA repair defects in stem cell function and aging. Annu Rev Med 56:508, 2005
50. Parmar S, Fernandez-Vina M, Liu P, Cano P, Andersson B, Munsell M, et al: Influence of allele level HLA typing on unrelated donor (UD) transplantation for high-risk myeloid leukemias. Blood 106:2916a, 2005 (abstr)
51. Chakraverty R, Peggs K, Chopra R, Milligan D, Kottaridis PD, Verfuerth S, et al: Limiting transplantation-related mortality following unrelated donor stem cell transplantation by using a nonmyeloablative conditioning regimen. Blood 99:1071-1078, 2002
52. van Besien K, Artz A, Smith D, Cao D, Rich L, Gooley D, et al: Fludarabine, melphalan, and alemtuzumab conditioning in adults with standard-risk advanced acute myeloid leukemia and myelodysplastic syndrome. J Clin Oncol 23:5728-5738, 2005
53. Ho AY, Pagliuca A, Kenyon M, Parker JE, Mijovic A, Devereux S, Mufti GJ: Reduced-intensity allogeneic hematopoietic stem cell transplantion for myelodysplastic syndrome and acute myeloid leukemia with multilineage dysplasia using fludarabine, busulfan and alemtuzumab (FBC) conditioning. Blood 104:1616-1623, 2004
54. Martino R, Perez-Simon J, Moreno E, Queralto J, Caballero D, Mateos M, et al: Reduced-intensity conditioning allogeneic blood stem cell transplantation with fludarabine and oral busulfan with or without pharmacokinetically targeted busulfan dosing in patients with myeloid leukemia ineligible for conventional conditioning. Biol Blood Marrow Transplant 11:437-447, 2005
55. Maris MB, Niederwieser D, Sandmaier BM, Storer B, Stuart M, Maloney D, et al: HLA-matched unrelated donor hematopoietic cell transplantation after nonmyeloablative conditioning for patients with hematologic malignancies. Blood 102:2021-2030, 2003
56. Bertz H, Patthoff K, Finke J: Allogeneic stem-cell transplantation from

related and unrelated donors in older patients with myeloid leukemia. J Clin Oncol 21:1480-1484, 2003
57. Wallen H, Gooley TA, Deeg HJ, Pagel JM, Press OW, Appelbaum FR, et al: Ablative allogeneic hematopoietic cell transplantation in adults 60 years of age and older. J Clin Oncol 23:3439-3446, 2005
58. Spyridonidis A, Bertz H, Ihorst G, Grullich C, Finke J: Hematopoietic cell transplantation from unrelated donors as an effective therapy for older patients (>= 60 years) with active myeloid malignancies (letter). Blood 105:4147-4148, 2005
59. Wong R, Giralt SA, Martin T, Couriel DR, Anagnostopoulos A, Hosing C, et al: Reduced-intensity conditioning for unrelated donor hematopoietic stem cell transplantation as treatment for myeloid malignancies in patients older than 55 years. Blood 102:3052-3059, 2003
60. Schmid C, Schleuning M, Ledderose G, Tischer J, Kolb H: Sequential regimen of chemotherapy, reduced-intensity conditioning for allogeneic stem-cell transplantation, and prophylactic donor-lymphocyte transfusion in high-risk acute myeloid leukemia and myelodysplastic syndrome. J Clin Oncol 23:5675-5687, 2005

Seminars in
HEMATOLOGY

Immunologic Approaches to Acute Leukemia in the Elderly

Sherif S. Farag and Michael A. Caligiuri

The outcome of older patients with acute leukemia remains poor with few long-term survivors, indicating the need for treatment approaches that target pro-apoptotic pathways not influenced by chemotherapy resistance. For a long time, natural killer (NK) cells have held promise for cancer immunotherapy because, unlike T lymphocytes, they can kill tumor cells without the need for tumor-specific antigen recognition. In the treatment of acute leukemia, NK cell-based therapies have focused on in vivo expansion and activation with cytokines with only modest success. However, recent understanding of the importance of NK receptors for the recognition and lysis of leukemia cells suggests novel therapeutic strategies. The balance of inhibitory and activating signals through surface receptors, recognizing major histocompatibility complex (MHC) class I and class I–like molecules on target cells, determines whether NK cells activate killing. In this review, we discuss the biologic rationale for therapeutic strategies harnessing NK cells and focus on novel directions for their future use in elderly patients with acute leukemia.
Semin Hematol 43:118-125

While the incidence of acute leukemia generally increases with age in adults, proportionally acute myeloid leukemia (AML) is significantly more common than acute lymphoblastic leukemia (ALL) in older patients. In those aged 60 years or older, the prevalence of ALL is reported to be between 16% to 31% of all adult cases,[1] while more than 50% of AML cases occur in this population. Significantly, however, the vast majority of older patients with acute leukemia die of their disease. Despite advances in supportive care, the long-term outcome has not significantly improved over the past 20 years, with less than 10% to 20% of AML patients 60 years or older alive beyond 5 years[2,3] and the outcome for ALL patients significantly worse.[4] Resistance to cytotoxic chemotherapy remains the main cause of treatment failure, suggesting the need to explore alternative strategies that target pro-apoptotic pathways not influenced by chemotherapy resistance. Immune-based approaches that exploit effectors of the innate and adaptive arms of immune system represent such strategies that may hold promise for the treatment of acute leukemia.

Division of Hematology and Oncology, Department of Internal Medicine and The Comprehensive Cancer Center, The Ohio State University, Columbus, OH.

Address correspondence to Sherif S. Farag, MD, PhD, The Ohio State University, B312 Starling Loving Hall, 320 W 10th Ave, Columbus, OH 43210. E-mail: sherif.farag@osumc.edu

Immunologic approaches to acute leukemia have to date largely focused on harnessing the graft-versus-leukemia (GvL) effect, mediated by cytotoxic T lymphocytes, following allogeneic hematopoietic stem cell transplantation. The development of reduced-intensity or nonmyeloablative preparative regimens has allowed older patients with acute leukemia to undergo allogeneic stem cell transplantation with significantly less morbidity and mortality,[5,6] and is discussed elsewhere in this issue. On the other hand, while cytotoxic T lymphocytes directed against leukemic blasts have been described in patients with acute leukemia, their role in immune responses against autologous leukemia cells remains uncertain. Furthermore, the requirement for tumor-specific antigens, which are poorly defined for the majority of patients, limits this strategy. Effector cells of the innate immune system, however, do not require the recognition of tumor-specific antigens for killing target cells. As critical effectors of the innate immune response, natural killer (NK) cells have been shown to lyse leukemia, as well as other tumor cells, without prior exposure to antigen.[7,8] Furthermore, their anti-tumor activity can be enhanced by clinically available cytokines, such as interleukin (IL)-2 and IL-12. As such, NK cells may have wider potential applicability in the treatment of leukemia. This review will discuss the biologic rationale for therapeutic strategies harnessing NK cells and focus on novel directions for their future use in elderly patients with acute leukemia.

 0037-1963/06/$-see front matter
doi:10.1053/j.seminhematol.2006.01.006

Biology of Natural Killer Cells

NK cells are large granular lymphocytes that comprise approximately 10% to 15% of peripheral blood lymphocytes, and are defined by the surface expression of CD56, a neural cell adhesion molecule of uncertain function, and absence of the T-cell–specific antigen called CD3.[9] Functionally, NK cells have the capacity for direct cytolytic activity against target cells (such as virus-infected cells or tumor cells) and are an important source of immunoregulatory cytokines (for example, interferon-gamma [IFN-γ], tumor necrosis factor-α [TNF-α], TNF-β, IL-10, granulocyte-macrophage colony-stimulating factor [GM-CSF]).[9] In addition, NK cells can also mediate antibody-dependent cellular cytotoxicity (ADCC) via FcγRIII receptors (CD16) that bind to the Fc portion of IgG expressed on the majority of the cells.[9]

Two functionally distinct subsets of human NK cells have been defined based on the surface expression of CD56.[10] Approximately 90% of circulating NK cells express low levels of CD56 ($CD56^{dim}$) but high levels of CD16, while the remaining NK cells are $CD56^{bright}$ but $CD16^{neg/dim}$. The $CD56^{bright}$ subset is the primary population of NK cells that produces immunoregulatory cytokines following monokine stimulation, but has less potential for direct cytotoxicity and ADCC compared to $CD56^{dim}$ cells.[10] In addition, relative to $CD56^{bright}$ NK cells, $CD56^{dim}$ NK cells express high levels of receptors important in mediating killing of target cells, which might also account for the observed differences in cytotoxic capacity.[10] Finally, while all NK cells express the intermediate-affinity heterodimeric IL-2 receptor (IL-2R$\beta\gamma$), only $CD56^{bright}$ NK cells constitutively express the high-affinity heterotrimeric IL-2 receptor (IL-2R$\alpha\beta\gamma$) and expand in vitro and in vivo in response to low (picomolar) concentrations of IL-2 with little cytotoxic activity.[11–13] In contrast, $CD56^{dim}$ cells express only the intermediate-affinity IL-2 receptor and proliferate weakly in response to high (nanomolar) concentrations of IL-2, even after induction of the high-affinity IL-2 receptor. Although resting $CD56^{bright}$ NK cells exhibit less cytotoxicity than $CD56^{dim}$ cells, the former can exhibit similar or enhanced cytotoxicity against NK targets compared to $CD56^{dim}$ cells after IL-2 activation.[14,15] As discussed below, the differences in response to IL-2 have important implications for the design of therapeutic approaches that expand and activate NK cells in vivo using cytokines.

Human NK cells develop from hematopoietic progenitor cells that reside in the $CD34^+$ cell compartment under the influence of cooperating cytokines produced by bone marrow stromal cells. The early-acting cytokines, flt-3 ligand and c-kit ligand (stem cell factor), stimulate $CD34^+$ NK cell progenitors to develop into intermediate precursors that are capable of responding to IL-15, which is able to induce terminal NK cell differentiation.[16] The IL-15 receptor shares common receptor signaling subunits (β and γ chains) with that of IL-2, which together form the intermediate heterodimeric receptor complex, IL-2/IL-15R$\beta\gamma$, that is upregulated by flt-3 ligand and c-kit ligand.[17] However, IL-15 and IL-2 each utilize specific α subunits (IL-2/IL-15Rα) that confer high-affinity specific binding to their specific high-affinity receptors. Recent evidence suggests that differentiation of $CD56^{bright}$ NK cells occurs primarily in lymph nodes from a rare and unique population of precursor cells that has low expression of CD34 but constitutively expresses CD45RA and has a high surface density of L-selectin, β_7-integrin, and the high-affinity receptor IL-2R$\alpha\beta\gamma$ ($CD34^{dim}$ $CD45RA^+\beta_7^{high}$).[18] Among $CD34^+$ hematopoietic precursor cells, the $CD34^{dim}CD45RA^+\beta_7^{high}$ subpopulation is uniquely enriched within lymph nodes in the parafollicular T-cell–rich regions, and comprising almost all of the $CD34^+$ cell population found in this site, compared to approximately 6% of $CD34^+$ cells in peripheral blood and less than 1% in bone marrow.[18] It is likely, therefore, that the earliest stage of NK cell development occurs in the bone marrow with the generation of $CD34^{dim}CD45RA^+\beta_7^{high}$ NK cell precursors. These precursors then traffic to lymph nodes where, under the influence of IL-2 produced from activated T cells during infection or other antigen challenge, and/or IL-15 from antigen-presenting cells, they differentiate into $CD56^{bright}$ NK cells. The site of development of $CD56^{dim}$ NK cells, as well as the developmental relationship between $CD56^{bright}$ and $CD56^{dim}$ NK cell subsets, however, remains unknown. It remains uncertain if $CD56^{bright}$ and $CD56^{dim}$ NK cells represent two functionally distinct subsets possibly emerging from a common precursor or are different stages of NK cell maturation with different adaptive functions.

Unlike T and B lymphocytes, NK cells do not rearrange genes encoding receptors for antigen recognition in the context of human leukocyte antigen (HLA) class I or II molecules. However, HLA class I molecules are important in modulating NK cell recognition and activation. Early studies indicated that self-HLA class I molecules inhibit the lysis of normal autologous cells by NK cells.[19] Inhibition is mediated by a number of inhibitory receptors that specifically recognize groups of classical (HLA-A, -B, or -C) or nonclassical (HLA-E and -G) HLA class I molecules.[20–22] Autologous cells that have altered or lost self-HLA class I expression may be selectively lysed by NK cells.[23] It is important to note that major histocompatability complex (MHC) class I expression is not always necessary for protection from lysis by NK cells,[24] and that inhibition by MHC class I is not always sufficient to prevent NK cytotoxicity,[25,26] suggesting the presence of other modulating receptors. It is now known that each NK cell expresses its own repertoire of activating and inhibitory receptors, and cytotoxicity is ultimately regulated by a balance of intracellular signals resulting from these receptors interacting with their cognate ligands expressed on target cells.

The receptors on NK cells include two families of paired inhibitory and activating receptors: the killer immunoglobulin (Ig)-like receptor (KIR) family, which primarily recognize HLA-A, -B, and -C; and the heterodimeric CD94/NKG2 C-type lectin receptor family, which recognizes HLA-E.[20,21,27] In addition, unpaired receptors important in mediating activating signals include the natural cytotoxicity receptors (NCR),[28–30] whose ligands are poorly defined, and the C-type lectin receptor NKG2D, which recognizes a number of MHC class I–like ligands, including the polymorphic MHC class I chain-related (MIC) peptides, MICA and MICB, and the human cytomegalovirus UL16 binding proteins (ULBP-1, −2, and −3).[31–33] Although the ligands for the NCR remain poorly defined, the NCR have been implicated in the recognition and lysis of a variety of tumor (including leukemia) cells by NK cells.[28–30,34] Differences in susceptibility to NK cell-mediated killing, however, suggest that tumor cells are likely to vary significantly in their expression of NCR ligands.[34] The ligands of NKG2D are either absent or expressed only in low density on normal tissues but are induced or upregulated on target cells following stress and neoplastic transformation. Variable expression of NKG2D ligands has been demonstrated in a number of malignant cell lines, including leukemia cells,[34,35] and more recently in primary AML blasts.[36] A number of other receptors, including FcγRIII, function primarily as coreceptors and in some cases their ligands remain unknown. The reader is referred to excellent reviews on NK receptor biology that have recently been published.[20,37,38] Table 1 lists the human NK cell activating and inhibitory receptors and their ligands.

Table 1 Major Human NK Cell Receptors and Known Ligands

Receptor		Ligand
Paired Activating and Inhibitory Receptors		
a) Killer Ig-like receptors (KIR)		
Inhibitory	Activating*	
KIR2DL1	KIR2DS1	Group 2 HLA-C Asn77Lys80 alleles
KIR2DL2	KIR2DS2	Group 1 HLA-C Ser77Asn80 alleles
KIR2DL3		
	KIR2DL4†	HLA-G
	KIR2DS4	Unknown
KIR2DL5	KIR2DS5	Unknown
	KIR3DS1	Unknown
KIR3DL1		HLA-Bw4
KIR3DL2		HLA-A3, -A11
KIR3DL7		Unknown
b) Heterodimeric C-type lectin receptors		
Inhibitory	Activating	
CD94/NKG2A/B‡	CD94/NKG2C	HLA-E
	CD94/NKG2E/H‡	Unknown
Unpaired Activating Receptors		
a) NKG2D		MICA, MICB, ULBP-1, -2, -3
b) Natural cytotoxicity receptors (NCR)		
NKp30		Unknown
NKp46		Unknown
NKp44		Unknown
Activating Coreceptors		
FcγRIII (CD16)		Fc of IgG
CD2		CD58 (LFA-3)
LFA-1		ICAM-1
2B4		CD48
NKp80		Unknown
CD69		Unknown
CD40 ligand		CD40

*Although activating KIR have similar extracellular domains to their inhibitory counterparts, their ligands are uncertain in many cases.

†Although KIR2DL4 has ITIM motifs in its long cytoplasmic tail, it is functionally an activating KIR that indicates NK cell secretion of IFN-γ without inducing cytotoxicity.

‡NKG2A and NKG2B, and NKG2E and NKG2H are splice variants, respectively.

Cytokine Therapy of Acute Leukemia

The improved understanding of the cytokines involved in modulating effector cells of the innate immune system, together with recent understanding of the NK cell recognition and killing of target cells, has provided a basis for the rational investigation of immunoregulatory cytokine combinations in the treatment of leukemia.

Recombinant human IL-2 (rhuIL-2) is the first immunoregulatory cytokine approved by the US Food and Drug Administration for the treatment of human cancer. IL-2 is a growth factor for T lymphocytes that is produced primarily by activated T-helper cells, but also has activity on B cells, NK cells, and monocytes. Although rhuIL-2 differs slightly from native IL-2 in not being glycosylated and in one amino acid substitution (serine substituted for cysteine at position 125), the two have similar immunomodulatory activities. rhuIL-2 has no direct antileukemic activity, and its therapeutic effect is entirely mediated by its ability to modulate immune reactions. In spite of its wide spectrum of activity on different immune effector cells, however, investigations of rhuIL-2 for the treatment of leukemia has largely focused on its ability to in vivo modulate NK cells.

Numerous clinical trials using rhuIL-2 have been conducted in patients with acute leukemia, predominantly AML, using a variety of doses and schedules. The majority of these studies have been small pilot trials, which have only tested tolerability and feasibility of treatment, making it difficult to properly assess efficacy. As high doses are required to activate NK cells in vivo, early clinical trials used high-dose IL-2, alone or in combination with IL-2–activated blood lymphocytes, for the treatment of patients with relapsed and refractory acute leukemia with modest success.[39–43] In a pilot trial of 24 patients with relapsed or refractory AML with ≤30% marrow blasts, treated with high-dose (8 to 18 × 10^6 IU/m^2) rhuIL-2 by continuous intravenous infusion, 13 achieved a complete response (CR), suggesting promising activity.[44] In contrast, a multicenter phase II trial of 39 AML and 19 ALL patients with relapsed or refractory disease treated with high-dose intravenous bolus infusions (8 × 10^6 IU/m^2 every 8 to 12 hours) of rhuIL-2 showed only modest responses.[39] Only two AML patients achieved CR, while no patient with ALL responded. Although significant biologic effects, in terms of an increase in cells with lymphokine-activated killer (LAK) activity, were demonstrated, treatment was associated with severe hematologic, hemodynamic, and metabolic toxicity. Based on the demonstrated activity in patients with lower disease burden and the toxicity associated with the high-dose schedules, lower doses of rhuIL-2 have been used to prevent disease relapse in AML patients already in complete remission,[45–47] or following autologous hematopoietic progenitor cell transplantation.[48–53]

We previously demonstrated that low-doses of IL-2 can induce in vivo selective expansion of $CD56^{bright}$ NK cells due to the binding of IL-2 to its high-affinity receptor.[11,13,54] Initial phase I/II trials in patients with human immunodeficiency virus (HIV) infection and malignancy demonstrated that low-dose rhuIL-2 (1×10^6 IU/m^2/d) is well tolerated and consistently resulted in expansion of NK cells in vivo.[55,56] Interestingly, the expanded $CD56^{bright}$ NK cell population demonstrated significant cytotoxicity against NK-resistant cells only when incubated in higher concentrations of IL-2 that saturate the intermediate-affinity receptors.[11,13,54] Based on these observations, a regimen of extended low-dose rhuIL-2 with interval intermediate-dose rhuIL-2 pulsing was developed and found to be well tolerated following intensive chemotherapy in AML patients.[36] Of relevance to therapy, the expansion of NK cells following low-dose IL-2 results from enhanced NK cell differentiation from bone marrow progenitors, combined with an IL-2–dependent delay in NK cell death, rather than proliferation of mature NK cells in the periphery.[57] This suggests that use of rhuIL-2 with recombinant human stem cell factor (rhuSCF) may be a more therapeutically effective combination for in vivo expansion of NK cells because it enhances the generation of NK cells from CD34(+) hematopoietic progenitors.[16] Exogenous SCF would result in NK progenitor differentiation into NK precursors that are in turn responsive to exogenous IL-2. We are currently investigating the safety and efficacy of low-dose rhuIL-2 with rhuSCF in patients with HIV-related malignancy.

While the lower doses of rhuIL-2 appear to be better tolerated,[58,59] the efficacy of in vivo expansion and activation of NK cells using IL-2 in acute leukemia patients remains uncertain. The reported in vivo antitumor activity of IL-2 therapy has generally been modest or difficult to convincingly demonstrate. A multicenter randomized trial comparing low-dose to high-dose rhuIL-2 in 110 patients with refractory anemia with excess blasts in transformation and secondary AML, who were in first remission after induction and consolidation, showed no significant difference in relapse-free or overall survival.[60] The results of randomized trials specifically testing the efficacy of rhuIL-2 compared to observation in AML patients after remission induction and consolidation are awaited. An interim analysis of a Cancer and Leukemia Group B (CALGB) study of AML patients ≥60 years of age randomized to receive low-dose IL-2 with intermediate-dose pulse IL-2 as maintenance therapy, in first remission or observation following intensive induction and consolidation, has shown no benefit to the group under treatment with IL-2 compared to those patients not receiving IL-2 (Richard Larson, personal communication, 2002). An additional large randomized trial in younger AML patients treated with low-dose rhuIL-2 and intermediate-dose pulse therapy following autologous stem cell transplantation is currently ongoing through the CALGB and the results are awaited. It is of interest that a randomized trial of intermediate-dose rhuIL-2 (12×10^6 IU/m^2/d) in 130 acute leukemia patients in remission following autologous bone marrow transplantation has shown no benefit.[61]

Novel Approaches to Improve IL-2 Immunotherapy

In spite of the ability of IL-2 to in vivo expand and activate NK cells, the results have generally been disappointing regardless of the dose and schedule used. Furthermore, while the addition of other cytokines such as rhuSCF may improve the ability to in vivo expand NK cells, it is also likely that the efficacy of this approach will remain modest. Improved understanding of NK cell receptors and signaling mechanisms is likely to lead to novel approaches to optimize the in vivo activity of IL-2.

One approach has been to use histamine hydrochloride in combination with rhuIL-2. Early studies demonstrated that NK cells (and T cells) within tumors had impaired cytotoxic activity related to downmodulation of the CD3ζ signaling pathway.[62,63] While NK cells do not express CD3, they express the activating NCR, including NKp30 and NKp46, and NKp44 following IL-2 stimulation, which mediate their activating signal through coupling with immunotyrosine activating motif (ITAM)-containing CD3ζ chains. This signal is inhibited by monocyte/macrophage-derived reactive oxygen species (ROS).[63] In addition to inhibiting anti-tumor cytotoxicity, ROS have also been shown to inhibit cell cycle proliferation and IL-2–induced gene transcription with eventual apoptosis of NK cells.[63,64] Histamine, acting via H2 receptors on monocytes/macrophages, has been shown to protect NK cells from functional inhibition and apoptosis.[64,65] Preclinical and clinical data have indicated positive activity with the combination of histamine hydrochloride and rhuIL-2 compared to IL-2 alone.[66–68] Recently, a randomized phase III study involving 320 patients with AML in complete remission reported that the combination of histamine hydrochloride and rhuIL-2 improved leukemia-free survival compared to no such treatment largely due to a reduction in relapses in patients treated in first remission.[69]

Despite the improvement in the anti-leukemic activity of rhuIL-2 when combined with histamine hydrochloride, it is likely that any major improvement in outcome will need to take into account the interactions of NK cell receptors with their ligands on leukemic cells. For example, the interaction of HLA class I molecules expressed on tumor cells with inhibitory KIR on autologous NK cells is likely to mediate an important inhibitory signal to rhuIL-2 (with or without any other cytokine) expanded NK cells, and limit successful killing and efficacy of cytokine treatment. Indeed, in vitro studies using fresh leukemic blasts have shown a strong inverse correlation between the numbers of HLA class I molecules expressed on blasts and NK cell-mediated lysis.[70] While the range of expression of HLA class I molecules on leukemic cells is not well studied, limited studies suggest that HLA class I expression is normal in the majority of cases of primary

AML cells.[71] However, significant differences in NK cell receptor ligand expression by leukemia cells appear to exist,[36] which may in turn affect the susceptibility to NK cell lysis and therefore cytokine immunomodulation. It may be hypothesized that patients whose leukemic cells express high levels of NKG2D ligands (and potentially NCR ligands as well) and/or low levels of HLA class I may be most susceptible to NK cell lysis. To test this hypothesis, correlation of NKG2D ligand expression on leukemic blasts with relapse-free survival in patients treated with rhuIL-2 may allow identification of potential subsets of patients who may or may not benefit from rhuIL-2. If this is confirmed, future studies should prospectively target such patients whose leukemic cells are most susceptible to autologous NK cell lysis.

Antibody-Dependent Cellular Cytotoxicity

The increasing availability of monoclonal antibodies has permitted the investigation of ADCC as a therapeutic approach. Although multiple mechanisms have been proposed for the activity of monoclonal antibodies, recent work has demonstrated that ADCC is an important mechanism in vivo.[72] However, while NK cells are important effectors of ADCC, their ability to function in ADCC may be reduced in advanced malignancy,[73] possibly due to defective expression of NK cell-triggering receptors.[74] The reduced ADCC activity can be enhanced in vitro by cytokines, including IL-12, IFN-α, GM-CSF, IL-15, and IL-2,[75–77] which among other effects also upregulate expression of the activating receptors, including NKp44 on NK cells.

While the combination of rhuIL-2 and monoclonal antibody in lymphoid disorders has been investigated, few studies have investigated ADCC in acute leukemia. Lintuzumab (HuM195) is an unconjugated humanized murine monoclonal antibody directed against CD33 that has been investigated in patients with relapsed or refractory AML.[78] In contrast to gemtuzumab ozagomycin, an anti-CD33 antibody conjugated to the cytotoxic calicheamicin,[79] lintuzumab has been shown to induce cell death by ADCC,[78] as well as by complement-mediated lysis and a direct pro-apoptotic effect. Although a recent randomized study involving 191 patients with active AML has shown no improvement in complete remission rate when lintuzumab was combined with induction chemotherapy,[80] few studies have investigated its potential for mediating ADCC in vivo. A single phase I study of lintuzumab in combination with rhuIL-2 has been conducted in patients with relapsed or refractory AML, with only modest activity observed.[81] However, studies have so far been conducted in a setting that does not optimally favor ADCC. The success of harnessing the ADCC potential of monoclonal antibodies depends critically on the presence of adequate numbers of functional immune effector cells, which are not likely to be present in sufficient numbers in patients with active leukemia. Therefore, lintuzumab with rhuIL-2 should be investigated in AML patients in remission where NK cell numbers are likely to be satisfactory.

In Vivo Blockade of Inhibitory Interactions Between NK Cells and Leukemia Cells

Another potential strategy under investigation is the therapeutic use of monoclonal antibodies to block the inhibitory interactions of HLA class I molecules on leukemic cells with KIR on NK cells. Such blocking antibodies may target either KIR or HLA class I molecules. In-vitro studies have demonstrated that blocking HLA class I molecules by anti-HLA antibodies renders NK cell-resistant leukemic blasts susceptible to lysis.[70] The feasibility of such an approach in vivo was recently demonstrated in a mouse model, whereby treatment with $F(ab')_2$ anti-Ly49C (mouse counterpart of human KIR) enhanced in vivo NK cell-mediated tumor activity and protected mice from leukemic death.[82] Significantly, treatment with $F(ab')_2$ anti-Ly49C did not result in significant pancytopenia that would be expected from killing of normal hematopoietic cells. Currently, anti-human KIR antibodies are being developed for therapeutic use and should provide an opportunity to clinically test this approach (Fig 1). Although not yet tested, it is possible that simultaneous blockade of CD94/NKG2A/B interactions with HLA-E might further increase anti-tumor activity. As NK cells recover rapidly following induction and consolidation chemotherapy in patients with acute leukemia, anti-KIR or anti-HLA blocking antibodies will be best suited as postremission therapy to delay or prevent relapse. The combination of KIR-HLA class I interaction blocking antibodies with cytokines that in vivo expand and activate NK cells will also be an important approach to investigate.

KIR Ligand Mismatched Allogeneic NK Cells

Although the use of antibodies to block the inhibitory interactions between HLA class I molecules and KIR on NK cells is necessary to overcome the limitation of immunologic approaches depending on autologous NK cells, the problem may be completely obviated by the use of allogeneic NK cells which provide a readily available means of overcoming inhibitory interactions by the appropriate choice of donor and recipient pairs who are mismatched for KIR ligands. In younger patients, the efficacy of this approach has been demonstrated in the setting of haplotype-mismatched hematopoietic stem cell transplantation. With KIR ligand mismatching between donor and recipient in the graft-versus-host (GVH) direction, engrafting NK cells have been shown to exert an important anti-leukemia effect following T-cell–depleted, haplotype-mismatched stem cell transplants.[83] Following transplant, NK cells with KIR repertoire identical to that of the donor rapidly reconstitute with a high-frequency of donor-versus-recipient alloreactive NK clones.[83] As reconstituting donor NK cells do not recognize mismatched HLA class I ligands expressed on the recipient's leukemic cells, an important inhibitory effect on NK cells is not operative and the balance of signals favors activation and killing of leukemic cells. In a recent update of the clinical experience in AML patients, the 5-year risk of relapse was 79% in the absence of

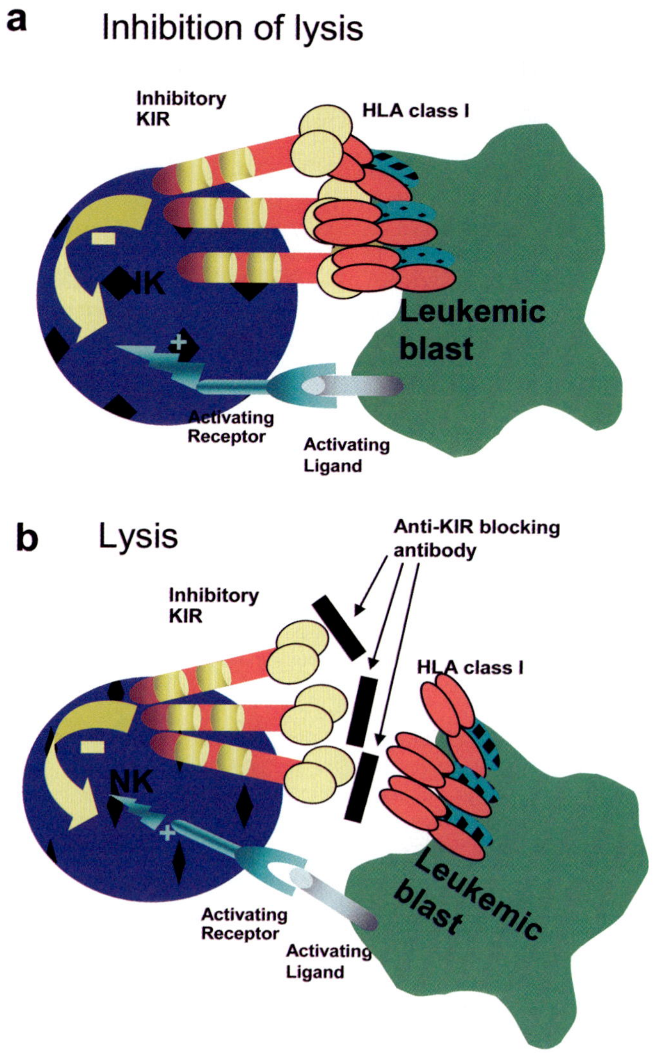

Figure 1 Potential therapeutic use of anti-KIR blocking antibody to break tolerance to autologous leukemic cells. (a) Inhibitory interactions mediated by inhibitory KIR on NK cells and self-HLA class I molecules on autologous leukemic cells predominate over activating receptor-ligand interactions resulting in a net negative signal that prevents NK cell lysis of the leukemic blast. This mechanism of tolerance to autologous cells may limit the efficacy of NK cell-based immunotherapy approaches in the autologous setting. (b) The use of anti-KIR antibodies (or anti-HLA antibodies not shown) can block HLA class I–KIR interactions and break tolerance with resultant killing of autologous leukemic blasts.

KIR ligand-mismatching compared to 17% where KIR ligand mismatch in the GVH direction existed ($P < .005$). The 5-year survival for the KIR-mismatched group was 59% compared to 7% in KIR-matched patients ($P < .005$). Of note, however, an anti-leukemic effect of engrafted NK cells was not observed in patients with ALL where the tumor cells did not express the adhesion molecule lymphocyte function antigen-1 (LFA-1),[83] indicating that other molecules, in addition to KIR and their ligands, are also important. However, the possibility that the difference between ALL and AML blasts with regard to their susceptibility to alloreactive NK cell-mediated killing might also be related to differences in expression of activating ligands has not been examined. At present, the application of KIR ligand-mismatched, haplotype-mismatched stem cell transplantation to a significant proportion of older leukemia patients is unlikely given the potential toxicity of the preparative regimen in this population. In this respect, development of better tolerated immunoablative regimens that may facilitate engraftment without significant organ toxicity in older patients will be important.

A recent report has also indicated that infusion of T-depleted, purified alloreactive NK cells may also be effective without the need for stem cell transplantation. Infusion of purified alloreactive NK cells and IL-2 following immunosuppression with fludarabine and high-dose cyclophosphamide resulted in transient remissions in five of 19 patients with AML.[84] In this study, which included patients older than 60 years, responses correlated with engraftment of NK cells. While proving the principle, better application of this approach in older patients will depend on the development of more immunosuppressive regimens to prevent rejection and the use of repeated infusions of NK cells.

Conclusions

Harnessing the anti-leukemic activity of NK cells is a potentially powerful immunologic approach in the treatment of acute leukemias, including those in older patients. The optimal use of NK cells in the treatment, however, will depend on careful consideration of NK cell receptor mechanisms in leukemia cell recognition. Novel directions exploiting the cytotoxic potential of autologous NK cells using combinations of cytokines to efficiently expand NK cells in vivo for use with tumor-specific monoclonal antibodies should be further investigated. A particularly exciting approach will be the use of antibodies to block inhibitory interactions of autologous NK cells with tumor cells. Such antibodies are currently under development for clinical use, and the next few years should allow a better appreciation of the feasibility and efficacy of this approach. The use of alloreactive NK cells, with or without infusion of stem cells, holds promise but will depend on overcoming rejection of donor cells using better tolerated immunosuppressive regimens. While most investigations have focused on KIR receptors on NK cells, it is likely that better appreciation of activating ligand expression on leukemia cells will lead to better patient and disease selection for NK cell-based immunotherapy.

References

1. Taylor PR, Reid MM, Proctor SJ: Acute lymphoblastic leukaemia in the elderly. Leuk Lymphoma 13:373-380, 1994
2. Mayer RJ, Davis RB, Schiffer CA, Berg DT, Powell BL, Schulman P, et al: Intensive postremission chemotherapy in adults with acute myeloid leukemia. Cancer and Leukemia Group B. N Engl J Med 331:896-903, 1994
3. Stone RM, Berg DT, George SL, Dodge RK, Paciucci PA, Schulman PP, et al: Postremission therapy in older patients with de novo acute myeloid leukemia: A randomized trial comparing mitoxantrone and intermediate-dose cytarabine with standard-dose cytarabine. Blood 98:548-553, 2001
4. Pagano L, Mele L, Casorelli I, Fianchi L, Di Febo A, Leone G: Acute lymphoblastic leukemia in the elderly. A twelve-year retrospective, single center study. Haematologica 85:1327-1329, 2000
5. Bertz H, Potthoff K, Finke J: Allogeneic stem-cell transplantation from

related and unrelated donors in older patients with myeloid leukemia. J Clin Oncol 21:1480-1484, 2003
6. Alyea EP, Kim HT, Ho V, Cutler C, Gribben J, DeAngelo DJ, et al: Comparative outcome of nonmyeloablative and myeloablative allogeneic hematopoietic cell transplantation for patients older than 50 years of age. Blood 105:1810-1814, 2005
7. Landay AL, Zarcone D, Grossi CE, Bauer K: Relationship between target cell cycle and susceptibility to natural killer lysis. Cancer Res 47:2767-2770, 1987
8. Allavena P, Damia G, Colombo T, Maggioni D, D'Incalci M, Mantovani A: Lymphokine-activated killer (LAK) and monocyte-mediated cytotoxicity on tumor cell lines resistant to antitumor agents. Cell Immunol 120:250-258, 1989
9. Trinchieri G: Biology of natural killer cells. Adv Immunol 47:187-376, 1989
10. Cooper MA, Fehniger TA, Turner SC, Chen KS, Ghaheri BA, Ghayur T, et al: Human natural killer cells: A unique innate immunoregulatory role for the CD56(bright) subset. Blood 97:3146-3151, 2001
11. Caligiuri MA, Zmuidzinas A, Manley TJ, Levine H, Smith KA, Ritz J: Functional consequences of interleukin 2 receptor expression on resting human lymphocytes. Identification of a novel natural killer cell subset with high affinity receptors. J Exp Med 171:1509-1526, 1990
12. Baume DM, Robertson MJ, Levine H, Manley TJ, Schow PW, Ritz J: Differential responses to interleukin 2 define functionally distinct subsets of human natural killer cells. Eur J Immunol 22:1-6, 1992
13. Caligiuri MA, Murray C, Robertson MJ, Wang E, Cochran K, Cameron C, et al: Selective modulation of human natural killer cells in vivo after prolonged infusion of low dose recombinant interleukin 2. J Clin. Invest 91:123-132, 1993
14. Nagler A, Lanier LL, Phillips JH: Constitutive expression of high affinity interleukin 2 receptors on human CD16-natural killer cells in vivo. J Exp Med 171:1527-1533, 1990
15. Robertson MJ, Soiffer RJ, Wolf SF, Manley TJ, Donahue C, Young D, et al: Response of human natural killer (NK) cells to NK cell stimulatory factor (NKSF): Cytolytic activity and proliferation of NK cells are differentially regulated by NKSF. J Exp Med 175:779-788, 1992
16. Mrozek E, Anderson P, Caligiuri MA: Role of interleukin-15 in the development of human $CD56^+$ natural killer cells from $CD34^+$ hematopoietic progenitor cells. Blood 87:2632-2640, 1996
17. Fehniger TA, Caligiuri MA: Interleukin 15: Biology and relevance to human disease. Blood 97:14-32, 2001
18. Freud AG, Becknell B, Roychowdhury S, Mao HC, Ferketich AK, Nuovo GJ, et al: A human CD34(+) subset resides in lymph nodes and differentiates into CD56bright natural killer cells. Immunity 22:295-304, 2005
19. Shimizu Y, DeMars R: Demonstration by class I gene transfer that reduced susceptibility of human cells to natural killer cell-mediated lysis is inversely correlated with HLA class I antigen expression. Eur J Immunol 19:447-451, 1989
20. Lanier LL: Activating and inhibitory NK cell receptors. Adv Exp Med Biol 452:13-18, 1998
21. Lopez-Botet M, Bellon T, Llano M, Navarro F, Garcia P, de Miguel M: Paired inhibitory and triggering NK cell receptors for HLA class I molecules. Hum Immunol 61:7-17, 2000
22. Lopez-Botet M, Llano M, Navarro F, Bellon T: NK cell recognition of non-classical HLA class I molecules. Semin Immunol 12:109-119, 2000
23. Ljunggren HG, Karre K: In search of the 'missing self': MHC molecules and NK cell recognition. Immunol Today 11:237-244, 1990
24. Zijlstra M, Auchincloss H Jr, Loring JM, Chase CM, Russell PS, Jaenisch R: Skin graft rejection by beta 2-microglobulin-deficient mice. J Exp Med 175:885-893, 1992
25. Moretta A, Bottino C, Pende D, Tripodi G, Tambussi G, Viale O, et al: Identification of four subsets of human $CD3^-CD16^+$ natural killer (NK) cells by the expression of clonally distributed functional surface molecules: Correlation between subset assignment of NK clones and ability to mediate specific alloantigen recognition. J Exp Med 172:1589-1598, 1990
26. Malnati MS, Lusso P, Ciccone E, Moretta A, Moretta L, Long EO: Recognition of virus-infected cells by natural killer cell clones is controlled by polymorphic target cell elements. J Exp Med 178:961-969, 1993
27. Braud VM, Allan DS, O'Callaghan CA, Soderstrom K, D'Andrea A, Ogg GS, et al: HLA-E binds to natural killer cell receptors CD94/NKG2A, B and C. Nature 391:795-799, 1998
28. Pende D, Parolini S, Pessino A, Sivori S, Augugliaro R, Morelli L, et al: Identification and molecular characterization of NKp30, a novel triggering receptor involved in natural cytotoxicity mediated by human natural killer cells. J Exp Med 190:1505-1516, 1999
29. Cantoni C, Bottino C, Vitale M, Pessino A, Augugliaro R, Malaspina A, et al: NKp44, a triggering receptor involved in tumor cell lysis by activated human natural killer cells, is a novel member of the immunoglobulin superfamily. J Exp Med 189:787-796, 1999
30. Pessino A, Sivori S, Bottino C, Malaspina A, Morelli L, Moretta L, et al: Molecular cloning of NKp46: A novel member of the immunoglobulin superfamily involved in triggering of natural cytotoxicity. J Exp Med 188:953-960, 1998
31. Bauer S, Groh V, Wu J, Steinle A, Phillips JH, Lanier LL, et al: Activation of NK cells and T cells by NKG2D, a receptor for stress-inducible MICA. Science 285:727-729, 1999
32. Bahram S: MIC genes: From genetics to biology. Adv Immunol 76:1-60, 2000
33. Sutherland CL, Chalupny NJ, Schooley K, VandenBos T, Kubin M, Cosman D: UL16-binding proteins, novel MHC class I-related proteins, bind to NKG2D and activate multiple signaling pathways in primary NK cells. J Immunol 168:671-679, 2002
34. Pende D, Cantoni C, Rivera P, Vitale M, Castriconi R, Marcenaro S, et al: Role of NKG2D in tumor cell lysis mediated by human NK cells: Cooperation with natural cytotoxicity receptors and capability of recognizing tumors of nonepithelial origin. Eur J Immunol 31:1076-1086, 2001
35. Groh V, Rhinehart R, Randolph-Habecker J, Topp MS, Riddell SR, Spies T: Costimulation of CD8alphabeta T cells by NKG2D via engagement by MIC induced on virus-infected cells. Nat Immunol 2:255-260, 2001
36. Farag SS, George SL, Lee EJ, Baer M, Dodge RK, Becknell B, et al: Postremission therapy with low-dose interleukin 2 with or without intermediate pulse dose interleukin 2 therapy is well tolerated in elderly patients with acute myeloid leukemia: Cancer and Leukemia Group B study 9420. Clin Cancer Res 8:2812-2819, 2002
37. Middleton D, Curran M, Maxwell L: Natural killer cells and their receptors. Transplant Immunol 10:147-164, 2002
38. Farag SS, Fehniger TA, Ruggeri L, Velardi A, Caligiuri MA: Natural killer cell receptors: New biology and insights into the graft-versus-leukemia effect. Blood 100:1935-1947, 2002
39. Maraninchi D, Vey N, Viens P, Stoppa AM, Archimbaud E, Attal M, et al: A phase II study of interleukin-2 in 49 patients with relapsed or refractory acute leukemia. Leuk Lymphoma 31:343-349, 1998
40. Meloni G, Foa R, Vignetti M, Guarini A, Fenu S, Tosti S, et al: Interleukin-2 may induce prolonged remissions in advanced acute myelogenous leukemia. Blood 84:2158-2163, 1994
41. Meloni G, Vignetti M, Andrizzi C, Capria S, Foa R, Mandelli F: Interleukin-2 for the treatment of advanced acute myelogenous leukemia patients with limited disease: updated experience with 20 cases. Leuk Lymphoma 21:429-435, 1996
42. Olive D, Chambost H, Sainty D, Stoppa AM, Blaise D, el Marsafy S, et al: Modifications of leukemic blast cells induced by in vivo high-dose recombinant interleukin-2. Leukemia 8:1230-1235, 1994
43. Lim SH, Newland AC, Kelsey S, Bell A, Offerman E, Rist C, et al: Continuous intravenous infusion of high-dose recombinant interleukin-2 for acute myeloid leukaemia—A phase II study. Cancer Immunol Immunother 34:337-342, 1992
44. Meloni G, Vignetti M, Pogliani E, Ivernizzi R, Allione B, Mirto S, et al: Interleukin-2 therapy in relapsed acute myelogenous leukemia. Cancer J Sci Am 3:S43-S47, 1997
45. Bergmann L, Heil G, Kolbe K, Lengfelder E, Puzicha E, Martin H, et al: Interleukin-2 bolus infusion as late consolidation therapy in 2nd remission of acute myeloblastic leukemia. Leuk Lymphoma 16:271-279, 1995
46. Wiernik PH, Dutcher JP, Todd M, Caliendo G, Benson L: Polyethylene glycolated interleukin-2 as maintenance therapy for acute myelogenous leukemia in second remission. Am J Hematol 47:41-44, 1994
47. Sievers EL, Lange BJ, Sondel PM, Krailo MD, Gan J, Liu-Mares W, et al: Feasibility, toxicity, and biologic response of interleukin-2 after consolidation chemotherapy for acute myelogenous leukemia: A report from the Children's Cancer Group. J Clin Oncol 16:914-919, 1998

48. Fefer A, Benyunes M, Higuchi C, York A, Massumoto C, Lindgren C, et al: Interleukin-2 +/- lymphocytes as consolidative immunotherapy after autologous bone marrow transplantation for hematologic malignancies. Acta Haematol 89:2-7, 1993
49. Benyunes MC, Massumoto C, York A, Higuchi CM, Buckner CD, Thompson JA, et al: Interleukin-2 with or without lymphokine-activated killer cells as consolidative immunotherapy after autologous bone marrow transplantation for acute myelogenous leukemia. Bone Marrow Transplant 12:159-163, 1993
50. Massumoto C, Benyunes MC, Sale G, Beauchamp M, York A, Thompson JA, et al: Close simulation of acute graft-versus-host disease by interleukin-2 administered after autologous bone marrow transplantation for hematologic malignancy. Bone Marrow Transplant 17:351-356, 1996
51. Robinson N, Benyunes MC, Thompson JA, York A, Petersdorf S, Press O, et al: Interleukin-2 after autologous stem cell transplantation for hematologic malignancy: A phase I/II study. Bone Marrow Transplant 19:435-442, 1997
52. Meehan KR, Badros A, Frankel SR, Cahill R, Areman E, Jenson M, et al: A pilot study evaluating interleukin-2-activated hematopoietic stem cell transplantation for hematologic malignancies. J Hematother 6:457-464, 1997
53. Benyunes MC, Higuchi C, York A, Lindgren C, Thompson JA, Buckner CD, et al: Immunotherapy with interleukin 2 with or without lymphokine-activated killer cells after autologous bone marrow transplantation for malignant lymphoma: A feasibility trial. Bone Marrow Transplant 16:283-288, 1995
54. Caligiuri MA, Murray C, Soiffer RJ, Klumpp TR, Seiden M, Cochran K, et al: Extended continuous infusion low-dose recombinant interleukin-2 in advanced cancer: Prolonged immunomodulation without significant toxicity. J Clin Oncol 9:2110-2119, 1991
55. Bernstein ZP, Porter MM, Gould M, Lipman B, Bluman EM, Stewart CC, et al: Prolonged administration of low-dose interleukin-2 in human immunodeficiency virus-associated malignancy results in selective expansion of innate immune effectors without significant clinical toxicity. Blood 86:3287-3294, 1995
56. Bernstein ZP, Khatri V, Poiesz B: Phase I/II study of daily subcutaneous (sc) low dose interleukin-2 (IL-2) in AIDS-associated lymphomas (AIDS-NHL). Blood 92:625a, 1998 (abstr)
57. Fehniger TA, Bluman EM, Porter MM, et al: Potential mechanisms of human natural killer cell expansion in vivo during low-dose IL-2 therapy. J Clin Invest 106:117-124, 2000
58. Farag SS, George SL, Lee EJ, Mrozek E, Cooper MA, VanDeusen JB, et al: Postremission therapy with low-dose interleukin 2 with or without intermediate pulse dose interleukin 2 therapy is well tolerated in elderly patients with acute myeloid leukemia: Cancer and Leukemia Group B study 9420. Clin Cancer Res 8:2812-2819, 2002
59. Cortes JE, Kantarjian HM, O'Brien S, Giles F, Keating MJ, Freireich EJ, et al: A pilot study of interleukin-2 for adult patients with acute myelogenous leukemia in first complete remission. Cancer 85:1506-1513, 1999
60. Ganser A, Heil G, Seipelt G, Hofmann W, Fischer JT, Langer W, et al: Intensive chemotherapy with idarubicin, ara-C, etoposide, and m-AMSA followed by immunotherapy with interleukin-2 for myelodysplastic syndromes and high-risk Acute Myeloid Leukemia (AML). Ann Hematol 79:30-35, 2000
61. Blaise D, Attal M, Reiffers J, Michallet M, Bellanger C, Pico JL, et al: Randomized study of recombinant interleukin-2 after autologous bone marrow transplantation for acute leukemia in first complete remission. Eur Cytokine Network 11:91-98, 2000
62. Mizoguchi H, O'Shea JJ, Longo DL, Loeffler CM, McVicar DW, Ochoa AC: Alterations in signal transduction molecules in T lymphocytes from tumor-bearing mice. Science 258:1795-1798, 1992
63. Kono K, Salazar-Onfray F, Petersson M, Hansson J, Masucci G, Wasserman K, et al: Hydrogen peroxide secreted by tumor-derived macrophages down-modulates signal-transducing zeta molecules and inhibits tumor-specific T cell-and natural killer cell-mediated cytotoxicity. Eur J Immunol 26:1308-1313, 1996
64. Hansson M, Asea A, Ersson U, Hermodsson S, Hellstrand K: Induction of apoptosis in NK cells by monocyte-derived reactive oxygen metabolites. J Immunol 156:42-47, 1996
65. Hansson M, Hermodsson S, Brune M, Mellqvist UH, Naredi P, Betten A, et al: Histamine protects T cells and natural killer cells against oxidative stress. J Interferon Cytokine Res 19:1135-1144, 1999
66. Johansson S, Landstrom M, Hellstrand K, Henriksson R: The response of Dunning R3327 prostatic adenocarcinoma to IL-2, histamine and radiation. Br J Cancer 77:1213-1219, 1998
67. Hellstrand K, Naredi P, Lindner P, Lundholm K, Rudenstam CM, Hermodsson S, et al: Histamine in immunotherapy of advanced melanoma: A pilot study. Cancer Immunol Immunother 39:416-419, 1994
68. Agarwala SS, Glaspy J, O'Day SJ, Mitchell M, Gutheil J, Whitman E, et al: Results from a randomized phase III study comparing combined treatment with histamine dihydrochloride plus interleukin-2 versus interleukin-2 alone in patients with metastatic melanoma. J Clin Oncol 20:125-133, 2002
69. Brune M, Castaigne S, Catalano J, Kurt Gehlsen, Wolf-Karsten Hofmann, Anthony Ho, et al: Improved leukemia-free survival after post-consolidation treatment with histamine hydrochloride and interleukin-1 in AML: A randomized phase III trial. Blood 104:261, 2004 (abstr)
70. Handgretinger R, Lang P, Schumm M, Pfeiffer M, Gottschling S, Demirdelen B, et al: Immunological aspects of haploidentical stem cell transplantation in children. Ann N Y Acad Sci 938:340-357, 2001
71. Wetzler M, Baer MR, Stewart SJ, Donohue K, Ford L, Stewart CC, et al: HLA class I antigen cell surface expression is preserved on acute myeloid leukemia blasts at diagnosis and at relapse. Leukemia 15:128-133, 2001
72. Clynes RA, Towers TL, Presta LG, Ravetch JV: Inhibitory Fc receptors modulate in vivo cytoxicity against tumor targets. Nat Med 6:443-446, 2000
73. Kono K, Takahashi A, Ichihara F, Sugai H, Fujii H, Matsumoto Y: Impaired antibody-dependent cellular cytotoxicity mediated by herceptin in patients with gastric cancer. Cancer Res 62:5813-5817, 2002
74. Costello RT, Sivori S, Marcenaro E, Lafage-Pochitaloff M, Mozziconacci MJ, Reviron D, et al: Defective expression and function of natural killer cell-triggering receptors in patients with acute myeloid leukemia. Blood 99:3661-3667, 2002
75. Dabholkar M, Tatake R, Amin K, Advani S, Gangal S: Modulation of natural killer and antibody-dependent cellular cytotoxicity by interferon and interleukin-2 in chronic myeloid leukemia patients in remission. Oncology 46:123-127, 1989
76. Carson WE, Parihar R, Lindemann MJ, Personeni N, Dierksheide J, Meropol NJ, et al: Interleukin-2 enhances the natural killer cell response to Herceptin-coated Her2/neu-positive breast cancer cells. Eur J Immunol 31:3016-3025, 2001
77. Friedberg JW, Neuberg D, Gribben JG, Fisher DC, Canning C, Koval M, et al: Combination immunotherapy with rituximab and interleukin 2 in patients with relapsed or refractory follicular non-Hodgkin's lymphoma. Br J Haematol 117:828-834, 2002
78. Caron PC, Co MS, Bull MK, Avdalovic NM, Queen C, Scheinberg DA: Biological and immunological features of humanized M195 (anti-CD33) monoclonal antibodies. Cancer Res 52:6761-6767, 1992
79. Linenberger ML: CD33-directed therapy with gemtuzumab ozogamicin in acute myeloid leukemia: Progress in understanding cytotoxicity and potential mechanisms of drug resistance. Leukemia 19:176-182, 2005
80. Feldman EJ, Brandwein J, Stone R, Kalaycio M, Moore J, O'Connor J, et al: Phase III randomized multicenter study of a humanized anti-CD33 monoclonal antibody, lintuzumab, in combination with chemotherapy, versus chemotherapy alone in patients with refractory or first-relapsed acute myeloid leukemia. J Clin Oncol 23:4110-4116, 2005
81. Kossman SE, Scheinberg DA, Jurcic JG, Jimenez J, Caron PC: A phase I trial of humanized monoclonal antibody HuM195 (anti-CD33) with low-dose interleukin 2 in acute myelogenous leukemia. Clin Cancer Res 5:2748-2755, 1999
82. Koh CY, Blazar BR, George T, Welniak LA, Capitini CM, Raziuddin A, et al: Augmentation of antitumor effects by NK cell inhibitory receptor blockade in vitro and in vivo. Blood 97:3132-3137, 2001
83. Ruggeri L, Capanni M, Casucci M, Volpi I, Tosti A, Perruccio K, et al: Role of natural killer cell alloreactivity in HLA-mismatched hematopoietic stem cell transplantation. Blood 94:333-339, 1999
84. Miller JS, Soignier Y, Panoskaltsis-Mortari A, McNearney SA, Yun GH, Fautsch SK, et al: Successful adoptive transfer and in vivo expansion of human haploidentical NK cells in patients with cancer. Blood 105: 3051-3057, 2005

ELSEVIER

Seminars in
HEMATOLOGY

Management of Acute Lymphoblastic Leukemia in Older Patients

Richard A. Larson

Although the median age for adults with acute lymphoblastic leukemia (ALL) is older than 60 years, relatively few of these patients have been enrolled on prospective clinical trials. The presence of coexisting medical disorders and unfavorable cytogenetic and biologic disease characteristics within this population presents considerable challenges for successful treatment using conventional chemotherapy programs. Selected patients have achieved remission and long-term survival following intensive chemotherapy. Philadelphia (Ph) chromosome (*BCR/ABL*)-positive ALL is particularly common among older patients. The availability of specific tyrosine kinase inhibitors is changing the prognosis for this challenging subset.
Semin Hematol 43:126-133

The success that has been achieved treating children and younger adults with acute lymphoblastic leukemia (ALL) has not been paralleled in older adults. Likely reasons include the presence of coexisting medical disorders leading to decreased tolerance for chemotherapy as well as fundamental biologic differences in the spectrum of ALL seen in this population. In this review, as in most of the available literature, the older adult age group is generally 60 years and older, although some series start at 55 years and others at 65 years old.

Age-Related Clinical and Biologic Differences

Available data on ALL in older patients are relatively scarce. One population-based registry reported that 31% of all cases occurred in patients 60 years or older. Although the most common malignant disease in childhood, ALL is rare in adults.[1] The age-specific annual incidence in the United States is only 0.4 to 0.6 cases per 100,000 individuals between 25 and 50 years of age (Fig 1). However, the incidence rises steadily during the older decades and is two- to threefold higher above the age of 60 years (0.9 to 1.6 cases per 100,000). According to the US Census Bureau, one fifth of the population in 2050 will be older than 65 years; the fastest growing segment of the elderly population is 85 years and older.

There is considerable evidence that the clinical and biologic characteristics of the disease change dramatically between childhood, the middle adult years, and older age groups. For example, the ratio of males to females declines from 1.75 in younger adults to 0.97 in older adults (Table 1). Comparative data on clinical characteristics are available from large treatment centers, although these are not free of referral bias. Sixty-nine patients between 60 and 89 years of age (median, 68 years) were evaluated at the Edouard Herriot Hospital in Lyon, France between 1980 and 1998, and were compared with 309 younger adults 15 to 59 years (median, 29 years).[2] Of note, 14% of the older adults had previously had a malignant disease compared with 3% of the younger patients. The older adults were less likely to have peripheral lymphadenopathy (21% *v* 51%) or a mediastinal mass (1% *v* 14%) or splenomegaly (26% *v* 45%), but there were no differences in hepatomegaly or central nervous system (CNS) involvement. Weight loss was slightly more common among older patients, but fever, infection, and bleeding were less common.

Modest differences were noted in presenting blood counts. The median white blood cell (WBC) count was 8,400/μL (range, 500 to 520,000/μL) among the older patients compared with 13,200/μL (range, 500 to 1,440,000/μL) among the younger adults (P = .05). There were no differences in the initial median hemoglobin levels (9.7 g/dL *v* 10.1 g/dL) or platelet counts (47,000/μL *v* 55,000/μL). Pretreatment data from 909 adults enrolled on multicenter clinical trials by the

Department of Medicine and the Cancer Research Center, University of Chicago, Chicago, IL.
Supported in part by grants from the National Institutes of Health CA-14599, CA-31946, CA-41287, and CA-33601.
Address correspondence to Richard A. Larson, MD, University of Chicago, MC-2115, 5841 S Maryland Ave, Chicago, IL 60637. E-mail: rlarson@medicine.bsd.uchicago.edu

 0037-1963/06/$-see front matter
doi:10.1053/j.seminhematol.2006.01.007

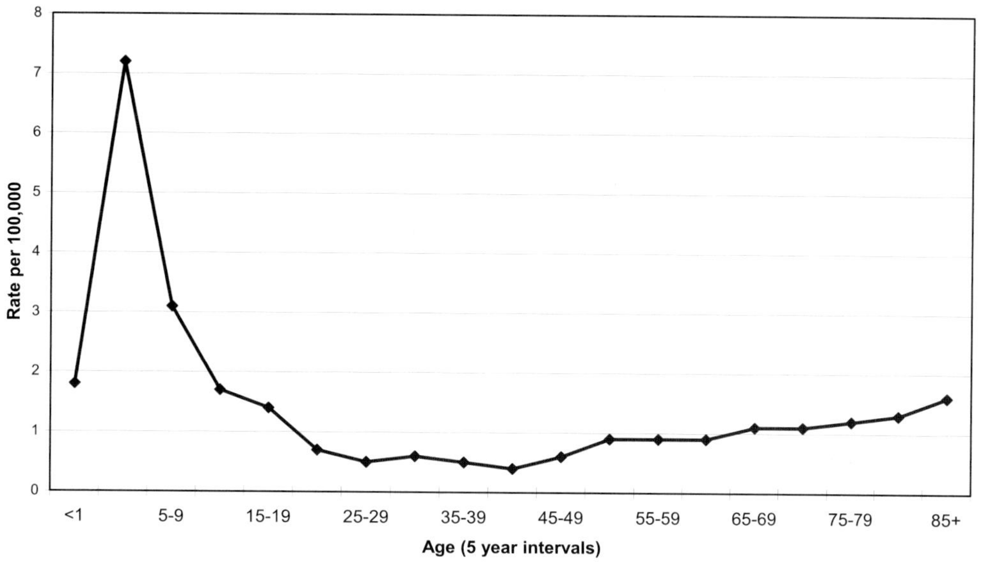

Figure 1 Age-sepcific annual incidence of ALL (US SEER data, 1998 to 2002).

Cancer and Leukemia Group B (CALGB) between 1988 and 2005 show similar trends (Table 1).

The most significant age-related differences in the Lyon series were noted in the immunophenotype and karyotype results. Lymphoblasts were of B-cell lineage in 89% of the older patients compared with 66% of the younger adults (P = .0004). Conversely, T-cell ALL was present in only 8% of older patients compared with 29% of the younger patients (P = .0007). Myeloid antigens were coexpressed by 19% of the older adult cases compared with 11% of the younger cases; lymphoblasts from 69% of older ALL patients also expressed CD34.

Table 1 Pretreatment Characteristics by Age Cohort for 909 Adults With Newly Diagnosed ALL Enrolled on CALGB Studies Between 1988 and 2005

Feature	Age Group at Diagnosis (yr)		
	16–29	30–59	≥60
No. of patients	318	425	166
Median age (yr)	22	43	66
Gender			
Male (%)	69	55	51
Race/ethnic group			
White (%)	73	83	88
Black (%)	10	8	8
Hispanic (%)	13	6	2
History of other cancer (%)	0	3	13
Infection			
Fever (%)	50	44	34
Pneumonia (%)	9	11	20
Septicemia (%)	6	2	7
Skin/mucosa (%)	12	10	13
Lymphadenopathy (%)	41	28	17
Splenomegaly (%)	32	23	12
Hepatomegaly (%)	18	17	11
Mediastinal mass (%)	12	9	1
CNS leukemia (%)	1	2	1
Median blood counts			
Hemoglobin (g/dL)	9.6	9.5	9.8
Platelets (/μL)	56,000	53,000	45,000
Leukocytes (/μL)	13,800	12,500	7,600
Blasts (%)	57	42	36
Neutrophils (%)	8	13	12
Median marrow cellularity (%)	100	95	95
Median marrow blasts (%)	90	88	90

A similar analysis has been reported by the German Multicenter ALL Study Group (GMALL), although the older age group was truncated at 65 years old.[3] Between 1984 and 1999, 342 patients (12%) aged 55 to 65 years were enrolled on one of four prospective clinical trials and were compared with 2,463 patients (88%) aged 15 to 54 years. The older patients less frequently had peripheral lymph node involvement, mediastinal tumor, and splenomegaly. A common or pre-B immunophenotype was more frequent among older patients (75% *v* 59%; $P = .001$), whereas T-cell ALL was less frequent (3% *v* 14%), and the frequencies of null plus pro-B ALL were similar (13% *v* 12%). Among T-ALL cases, mature T-ALL (2% *v* 7%) and thymic T-ALL (3% *v* 14%) occurred less commonly in older patients. In a recent multicenter series of older ALL patients from Poland, no remarkable differences in pretreatment characteristics were reported between 64 patients aged 60 to 69 years and 23 patients 70 years and older.[4]

Age-Related Cytogenetic Differences

Cytogenetic abnormalities characterize the biologic heterogeneity of ALL and provide a strong and independent prognostic factor for treatment outcome.[5] The incidence of Philadelphia (Ph) chromosome–positive ALL, a subset that is resistant to conventional chemotherapy, clearly increases with age.[6] Clonal chromosomal abnormalities were found at diagnosis in 378 of 443 adults (85%) by the Groupe Francais de Cytogenetique Hematologique; 60 (13%) were older than 60 years (range, 60 to 84 years).[7] In this series, 18% of those less than 40 years old and 46% of those 40 to 60 years old were Ph^+ compared with 35% of those older than 60 years. Among 276 patients (ages 16 to 83 years) with centrally reviewed karyotypes enrolled on a prospective study by the CALGB, 76% had a clonal abnormality; 28% overall and 33% of those older than 60 years had a t(9;22).[8] In a recent report from the Southwest Oncology Group, the frequency of Ph^+ ALL increased from 6% in those less than 25 years old to 14% for those aged 25 to 35 years, 33% for those aged 36 to 55 years, and 53% for patients older than 56 years.[9] In the large GMALL series described above, among those with common or pre–B-ALL, the incidence of Ph^+ or *BCR/ABL*$^+$ ALL was significantly higher among adults older than 55 years than younger adults (54% *v* 37%; $P = .001$).[3] In the French series from Lyon, the Ph chromosome or *BCR/ABL* fusion gene was detected in 24% of older patients and 19% of young patients.[2] In contrast, a rearrangement of chromosome 11q23 was observed in only 2% of older and 5% of younger patients (χ^2 statistic, $P = .001$). An analysis of the age distribution of chromosomal abnormalities in 1,500 British cases of ALL has been reported.[10]

Prospective Clinical Trials in Older Adults

With a few exceptions, older patients with ALL have often been excluded from clinical trials by eligibility criteria. Regimens developed for younger adults have been truncated at 60 or 65 years old. For the past two decades, the CALGB has not had an upper age limit for enrollment into its frontline ALL treatment studies. Approximately 18% of clinical trial subjects have been 60 years or older (median, 66 years; range, 60 to 83 years). Similarly, investigators at the M.D Anderson Cancer Center in Houston, TX have actively enrolled older patients into their frontline ALL studies.[11] The fraction older than 60 years has been 22%. In both this multicenter example and a single-center experience, the proportion of older patients enrolled appears less than the proportion in the community.

In general, older cancer patients have been underrepresented in prospective clinical trials, and this can have serious consequences on the development of better therapies for these patients.[12] This is particularly notable for patients greater than 75 years old. Although it is estimated that 54% of patients with leukemia in the United States are greater than 65 years of age, only 24% of subjects enrolled in new drug trials for leukemia filed with the Food and Drug Administration (FDA) are older than 65 years.[13] In the United Kingdom, where on average 68 patients 60 years or older develop ALL every year, only three to eight patients (4% to 15%) were enrolled each year in the national Medical Research Council (MRC) UKALL X and XA studies.[14] Criteria for decision-making regarding which older patients should be recommended for treatment have not been adequately addressed.

Very few clinical trials have focused on therapies designed specifically for older patients with ALL, and fewer still have sufficient numbers to deal with the clinical and biologic heterogeneity within this age group. Even when treated on the same trial as younger adults, older patients often receive attenuated doses of myelosuppressive drugs.[15,16] Figure 2 demonstrates the effect of increasing age on the outcomes of 759 adults with newly diagnosed ALL treated on five sequential CALGB studies between 1988 and 2002. The complete remission (CR) rate declined from 90% for those under age 30, to 81% between 30 and 59 years old, and to 57% for those 60 years and older. The overall survival at 3 years was estimated to be 58% (95% confidence limits, 52% to 64%) for those less than 30 years old, 38% (33% to 43%) for those 30 to 59 years old, and only 12% (7% to 19%) for the 129 patients older than 60 years. Similar results have been reported by other cooperative groups and large leukemia centers (Table 2).

The GMALL Study Group reported on a pilot study designed for patients older than 65 years.[17] Favorable factors for achievement of CR were pro–B-ALL or T-ALL (69% compared with 36% for pre–B-ALL), no Ph chromosome (64% *v* 19% for Ph^+), and WBC count less than 30,000/μL (60% compared with 25%). The CR rate was 74% for patients without any of these risk factors. In contrast, 52% of patients had one or more of these risk factors, and they had a CR rate of only 19% ($P = .001$). Survival was also significantly better for the group with no risk factors (median, 17 months *v* 6 months, $P = .002$). Recently updated to include 94 patients,

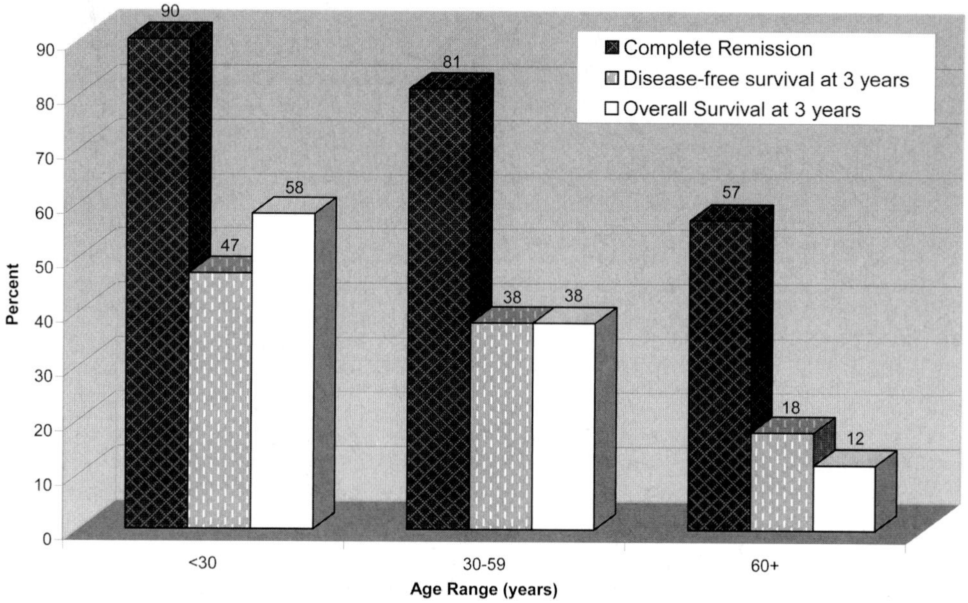

Figure 2 Treatment outcome by age cohort (CALGB studies with 759 ALL patients, 1988 to 2002).

the CR rate overall was 48%, but survival was less than 10%.[18] In recent reviews of the literature describing the outcomes of older ALL patients reported between 1990 and 2004,[19,20] the weighted mean CR rate was 56% for the 519 patients older than 60 years who received intensive chemotherapy on a prospective trial; 23% of patients had early deaths, and 30% had chemotherapy-resistant disease. The median remission duration was 9 months, and the median survival overall was 7 months.

Palliative chemotherapy approaches are sometimes recommended to older patients because of poor performance status or the presence of comorbid disorders such as diabetes, cardiac disease, or renal insufficiency. In a report from the Instituto di Demeitotica Medica in Rome, 37 (31%) of 119 patients, newly diagnosed with ALL between 1986 and 1998, were older than 65 years; 25 received intensive chemotherapy and 12 received only vincristine and corticosteroids.[21] A CR was achieved in 80% of the intensively treated older patients and their median survival duration was 14 months (range, 2 to 82 months). Among the patients managed with palliative treatment, 42% had a CR; the median survival for all 12 patients was only 2.6 months (range, 0.3 to 19 months).

Similar results were reported when practice patterns in the northern region of England were surveyed.[22] Among 62 consecutive, newly diagnosed ALL patients older than 60 years, 28 (median age, 67 years; range, 60 to 80) received "curative" therapy, 25 (median age, 74 years) received palliative therapy, and nine (median age, 83 years) received no treatment. A CR was achieved in 10 (36%) of the intensively treated group and four (16%) of the palliative therapy group. The median survival for each treatment group was only 3 months, although several patients survived longer than 3 years after intensive therapy.

Management of Older Patients With ALL

Pharmacologic changes associated with aging do not necessarily apply to all persons above a specific age.[23,24] Comorbid conditions, interactions with multiple other medications, nutritional status, and adherence to complex treatment regimens all influence the pharmacokinetic profile in older adults. There is little evidence that drug absorption is affected by the chronologic age of the patient. However, the volume of distribution of a drug may be less than in younger adults due to different proportions of body fat to lean body mass, hydration status, and plasma protein levels. Hepatic blood flow and renal clearance may be diminished in older patients. However, older adults with normal calculated renal function appear to tolerate chemotherapy drugs and have similar toxicity profiles to younger adults.

Nevertheless, the pharmacodynamic effects of particular drugs may be greater in older individuals. The number of hematopoietic stem cells declines with age; thus, the neutrophil nadir may be lower and recovery from myelotoxic chemotherapy more prolonged in older adults.[25] Mucositis appears more frequent and more severe in older patients, and the consequences with regard to pain, diminished nutrition, and infection may be more grave. Pain may respond to considerably lower doses of analgesics in older patients. Delirium during treatment is under-recognized and misdiagnosed. It must be treated promptly by removing the causative factors or with psychotropic medications such as haloperidol. Interestingly, nausea and vomiting after chemotherapy have been reported to be less common in older adults.

Specific leukemia drugs have well known toxicities that require special attention in older patients. Vincristine may cause severe constipation, and thus laxatives should be used prophylactically. Corticosteroids can exacerbate diabetes, and hyperglycemia may lead to infection and fluid and electrolyte abnormalities. L-asparaginase causes cognitive impairment leading to encephalopathy more often in older adults than in children. The appearance of somnolence and confusion in such cases can be mistakenly attributed to depression or viral encephalitis. Discontinuation of the enzyme and prompt refeeding or infusion of amino acid solutions containing glutamine can yield a dramatic improvement in mental status. Discontinuation of extraneous medications that many older adults take for chronic but mild disorders can prevent serious drug interactions during chemotherapy.

Among randomized clinical trials testing the use of hematopoietic growth factors during chemotherapy for ALL, older patients have enjoyed the greatest benefits. In a CALGB study of 185 ALL patients who were randomly assigned to receive either granulocyte colony-stimulating factor (G-CSF) or placebo during induction and consolidation therapy, 36 were 60 years or older.[15] The time to recovery of greater than 1,000 neutrophils/μL during remission induction was shortened from 29 days in the placebo group to 16 days in the G-CSF group ($P <.001$). For these older patients the corresponding CR rates were 69% in the placebo group and 85% in the G-CSF group, and the induction death rate fell from 31% to 5% with G-CSF support. Older patients who received placebo had a median time to platelet recovery greater than 50,000/μL of 26 days, whereas the older patients who received G-CSF had a median of 17 days. It has become routine practice within the CALGB to use G-CSF during treatment of ALL in older adults.

The Challenge of Ph$^+$ ALL

The diagnosis of Ph$^+$ ALL should be considered in all patients with precursor B-ALL, particularly in older patients and those with biphenotypic morphology or coexpressing myeloid markers.[26] The t(9;22) is found most often in CD10$^+$ ALL, both common and pre–B-ALL.[27] The disease is characterized by a variable but somewhat higher WBC count, surface expression of CD19 and often CD10 and CD34 antigens, and frequent coexpression of CD13.[28] Although Ph$^+$ ALL patients have an increased risk of developing meningeal leukemia during their clinical course, CNS leukemia is not significantly more frequent at diagnosis.[29] At least one third to perhaps as many as one half of patients older than 60 years with precursor-B–ALL are *BCR/ABL*$^+$.[5–10,27] About 70% of these adults have the p190 protein in contrast to about 90% of children with Ph$^+$ ALL, and the remainder have the p210 protein characteristic of chronic myelogenous leukemia.[27] Cytogenetic or molecular analyses are required to confirm the diagnosis and can generally be obtained within a few days.

The prognosis of adult patients with Ph$^+$ ALL treated only with chemotherapy has been poor, with rare long-term survivors. Although CR rates ranged from 60% to 80%, the median remission duration was short, ranging from 9 to 16 months.[6–8,11,15,16,27] Allogeneic stem cell transplantation (SCT) in first CR is the treatment of choice, with a 27% to 65% long-term survival rate.[30]

The development of selective ABL tyrosine kinase inhibitors has improved the prognosis for Ph$^+$ ALL patients, and especially for those unable to undergo SCT. In early studies in patients with relapsed or refractory Ph$^+$ ALL, oral imatinib mesylate in doses of 400 to 800 mg per day led to remission or clearance of peripheral blood blasts in about 60% of patients, including a few with CRs.[31–33] However, these responses were short even though patients continued to receive imatinib therapy. The estimated median times to progression and overall survival were only 2.2 and 4.9 months, respectively.[32]

More recently, imatinib has been added to initial induction and consolidation chemotherapy for newly diagnosed Ph$^+$ patients. A group from the M.D. Anderson Cancer Center has reported updated results of a phase II study combining imatinib with the first 14 days of hyperCVAD chemotherapy.[34] Twenty-five of 26 patients (96%) achieved a CR, suggesting synergy between imatinib and concurrent chemotherapy. Approximately one-half of patients had a molecular response, defined as a negative bone marrow reverse transcriptase–polymerase chain reaction (RT-PCR) assay for *BCR/ABL*. There were no unexpected toxicities related to the addition of imatinib. Similar results were reported by the Japan Adult Leukemia Study Group, when imatinib was started after 1 week of induction therapy and then continued concurrently with chemotherapy during the remainder of the induction.[35] During consolidation, imatinib was alternated with courses of high-dose methotrexate/cytarabine. The CR rate was 95%, and the molecular response rate reached 73%. The event-free and overall survival rates at 1 year were estimated at 78% and 88%. Subsequent SCT did not appear to be adversely affected by preceding imatinib therapy in these studies.

The optimal schedule for combining imatinib with chemotherapy has not been established. Alternating and concurrent imatinib plus chemotherapy combinations were compared in two sequential patient cohorts treated within a recent GMALL trial.[36] Efficacy analyses based on *BCR/ABL* transcript levels showed an advantage of the concurrent over the alternating schedule, with approximately 50% of patients achieving PCR negativity. Both schedules enabled a high percentage of patients to undergo SCT. Patients with Ph$^+$ ALL have an increased risk of developing CNS leukemia. Imatinib does not cross the blood:brain barrier so that cerebrospinal fluid concentrations are only 1% to 2% of serum levels.[37] Therefore, conventional CNS prophylaxis must be given.

In view of the favorable toxicity profile of imatinib, several studies have explored single-agent imatinib induction therapy in older patients with newly diagnosed Ph$^+$ ALL. In a GIMEMA study, patients greater than 61 years of age received imatinib at 800 mg/d in combination with prednisone for 30 days, followed by imatinib alone as postremission treatment; 92% of patients achieved a CR.[38] The GMALL evaluated imatinib monotherapy in older Ph$^+$ ALL patients in a prospective, randomized trial.[39] Patients with a median age of 67 years were randomly assigned to receive a 4-week course of Imatinib at 600 mg/d or standard induction chemotherapy. After achieving a CR or partial remission (PR), all patients then received imatinib concurrently with consolidation chemotherapy. Imatinib induction was significantly superior to chemotherapy alone, with 93% achieving a CR and 7% a PR. In contrast, 46% of evaluable patients allocated to the chemotherapy arm failed to enter remission. Severe infections were less frequent in patients allocated to imatinib induction, and there was no induction mortality.[39]

Newer Drugs for ALL

It is not likely that escalating the doses of currently available chemotherapy agents or altering their sequence of administration will markedly improve the outcome of treatment for ALL in adults. New drugs are needed. Because a large fraction of older patients have Ph$^+$ ALL, major advances in the treatment of *BCR/ABL*$^+$ leukemia offer hope for considerable improvement. There is considerable evidence that the tyrosine kinase inhibitor imatinib mesylate should be incorporated into induction and postremission therapy for these patients. Second generation ABL kinase inhibitors such as AMN107 (Novartis, East Hanover, NJ) and dasatinib (BMS354825; Bristol Myers Squibb, Princeton, NJ) are now completing phase II trials in patients with imatinib-resistant Ph$^+$ ALL. If successful, these agents should be evaluated next in frontline therapy and in combination with chemotherapy.

Other targeted therapies currently being evaluated in ALL include monoclonal antibodies. Rituximab binds to CD20 which is expressed on more than 20% of lymphoblasts in about half of common or pre-B ALL cases. Investigators at the M.D. Anderson Cancer Center have incorporated rituximab into frontline hyperCVAD therapy for CD20$^+$ ALL.[40] In a pilot study by the GMALL, when rituximab was given before each cycle of chemotherapy, the CR rate was 63% and survival after 1 year was 54% for 19 CD20$^+$ patients older than 55 years (median, 66 years).[18]

The antigen CD52 is expressed on normal and malignant lymphocytes and is the target for alemtuzumab. Approved for the treatment of B-cell chronic lymphocytic leukemia, this antibody has also shown single agent activity in a small number of patients with refractory ALL. It is currently being tested by the CALGB in both young and older adults with CD52$^+$ ALL in first remission.[41] Approximately 69% of ALL cases have been shown to express CD52 on more than 10% of the blasts. A dose-escalation pilot study has demonstrated the safety of administering 30 mg subcutaneously three times per week for 4 weeks between courses of intensive consolidation chemotherapy at a time when minimal residual disease is likely to be present.

The newest drug to be approved by the FDA for the treatment of ALL in children is clofarabine.[42] This purine analog has also shown single-agent activity in adults with relapsed ALL or acute myeloid leukemia (AML) and has been combined with cytarabine for initial treatment of older patients with AML or myelodysplastic syndrome. Clofarabine acts by inhibiting ribonucleotide reductase and DNA polymerase, depleting the amount of intracellular dNTPs available for DNA replication, and also resulting in premature DNA chain termination. Dose-limiting toxicities have been reversible hepatotoxicity and rash.

Nelarabine (compound 506U78; Glaxo Smith Kline, Philadelphia, PA) has completed phase II trials in both children and adults with relapsed or refractory T-ALL.[43] Although neurotoxicity has been dose-limiting, the drug can be given safely at 900 mg/m^2/d by continuous intravenous infusion for 5 days in children, or at 1.5 g/m^2/d on days 1, 3, and 5 in adults.[44,45] Nelarabine has considerably less activity against B-lineage ALL. Forodesine (BCX-1777; BioCryst, Birmingham, AL), a novel inhibitor of purine nucleotide phosphorylase, has shown activity in cutaneous T-cell lymphoma and is now being investigated in phase I and II trials in relapsed T-ALL.[46] However, because of the low incidence of T-ALL in

Table 2 Treatment Outcomes for Young, Middle-Age, and Older Adults With ALL

Research Group	Age Group (yr)	No. of Patients	Complete Remission (%)	Leukemia-Free Survival Median (mo)	Leukemia-Free Survival 3-Year (%)	Overall Survival Median (mo)	Overall Survival 3-Year (%)
Cancer and Leukemia Group B (CALGB)							
	<30	280	90%	30	47	56	58
	30–59	350	81	21	38	22	38
	≥60	129	57	10	18	8	12
Hopital Edouard Herriot, Lyon[2]							
	<35	192	84	16	35	24	39
	35–60	118	85	15	31	18	34
	>60	66	58	8	11	6	11
M.D. Anderson Cancer Center, Houston[10]							
	<30	65	98	NR	52	NR	54 (5 yr)
	30–50	64	89	NR	55	NR	42 (5 yr)
	50–59	31	93	NR	34	NR	29 (5 yr)
	≥60	44	79	NR	36	NR	17 (5 yr)
German Multicenter Study Group for Adult ALL (GMALL)[16]							
	>65	63	46	NR	NR	11	24 (2 yr)

Abbreviation: NR, not reported.

Table 3 New Drugs Under Development for ALL

New Agent	Mechanism	Notes
Tyrosine kinase inhibitors		
Imatinib	Inhibits BCR/ABL	Approved for Ph+ ALL
Dasatinib (BMS354825)	Inhibits SRC and ABL kinases	Effective against imatinib-resistant Ph+ ALL
AMN107	Inhibits BCR/ABL	Effective against imatinib-resistant Ph+ ALL
Monoclonal antibodies		
Rituximab	Anti-CD20	May potentiate chemotherapy in B-cell malignancies
Alemtuzumab	Anti-CD52	Can be given intravenously or subcutaneously
Antimetabolites		
Clofarabine	Nucleoside analog; inhibits ribonucleotide reductase and DNA polymerase	Approved for relapsed childhood ALL
Nelarabine	Pro-drug of ara-G inhibits purine nucleoside phosphorylase (PNP)	Effective in T-ALL
Forodesine	Inhibits PNP	Under evaluation in T-ALL
Trimetrexate	Competitive inhibitor of dihydrofolate reductase	Not dependent on facilitated transport into cells
Aminopterin	Anti-folate	Excellent oral bioavailability
Liposomal encapsulated drugs		
Liposomal vincristine		Diminished neurotoxicity
Liposomal daunorubicin		Diminished cardiotoxicity
Pegylated asparaginase		Long half-life (6 days)

patients older than 60 years, these latter two drugs are unlikely to impact on the outcomes of many older patients.

Drugs with proven efficacy against ALL, such as vincristine and daunorubicin, have been modified as liposomal sphingomyelin/cholesterol preparations, and are in clinical trials.[47] The liposomal preparations offer the ability to infuse higher total doses of the native drug, yielding greater tumor cell uptake with no increase in neurotoxicity or cardiac toxicity.[48] Liposomal encapsulation provides pharmacokinetic advantages such as a prolonged half-life compared with the free drug and possibly preferential uptake into tumor cells. Italian investigators have reported on a small trial using liposomal daunorubicin with vincristine and dexamethasone in 15 newly diagnosed older ALL patients (median age, 69 years).[49] The CR rate was 73%, the median disease-free survival (DFS) was 21 months, and the 2-year DFS was 36%.

Many new drugs await further testing and incorporation into frontline regimens (Table 3).[50] It is possible that some combination of these agents will overcome the innate resistance present in older patients with ALL and at the same time improve the overall tolerance to treatment.

Acknowledgment

The author thanks Ben L. Sanford, MS, and Daohai Yu, PhD in the Cancer and Leukemia Group B Statistical Center at Duke University for their analysis of the CALGB data.

References

1. National Cancer Institute, Surveillance, Epidemiology, and End Results Program. www.seer.cancer.gov
2. Thomas X, Olteanu N, Charrin C, Lheritier V, Magaud JP, Fiere D: Acute lymphoblastic leukemia in the elderly: The Edouard Herriot Hospital experience. Am J Hematol 67:73-83, 2001
3. Göbuget N, Hoelzer D, Arnold R, Bohme A, Bartram CR, Freund M, et al: Subtypes and treatment outcome in adult acute lymphoblastic leukemia less than or greater than 55 years. Hematol J 1:186, 2001 (suppl 1)
4. Robak T, Szmigielska-Kaplon A, Wrzesien-Kus A, Wierzbowska A, Skotnicki AB, Piatkowska-Jakubas B, et al: Acute lymphoblastic leukemia in elderly: The Polish Adult Leukemia Group experience. Ann Hematol 83:225-231, 2004
5. Mrozek K, Heerema NA, Bloomfield CD: Cytogenetics in acute leukemia. Blood Rev 18:115-136, 2004
6. Secker-Walker LM, Prentice HG, Durrant J, Richards S, Hall E, Harrison G, MRC Adult Leukaemia Working Party: Cytogenetics adds independent prognostic information in adults with acute lymphoblastic leukaemia on MRC trial UKALL XA. Br J Haematol 96:601-610, 1997
7. Groupe Francais de Cytogenetique Hematologique: Cytogenetic abnormalities in adult acute lymphoblastic leukemia: Correlations with hematologic findings and outcome. Blood 87:3135-3142, 1996
8. Wetzler M, Dodge RK, Mrozek K, Carroll AJ, Tantravahi R, Block AW, et al: Prospective karyotype analysis in adult acute lymphoblastic Leukemia. The Cancer and Leukemia Group B experience. Blood 93:3983-3993, 1999
9. Appelbaum FR: Impact of age on the biology of acute leukemia, in Perry MC (ed): American Society of Clinical Oncology Educational Book. 2005, pp 528-532
10. Secker-Walker LM, Clark R, Hawkins JM, Maritineau M, Moorman AV: Age distribution of good and poor risk chromosomal subgroups among the first 1500 cases in the LRF UKCCG karyotype database in acute lymphoblastic leukemia. Br J Haematol 97:45, 1997 (suppl 1, abstr)
11. Kantarjian HM, O'Brien S, Smith TL, Cortes J, Giles FJ, Beran M, et al: Results of treatment with hyper-CVAD, a dose-intensive regimen, for adult acute lymphoblastic leukemia. J Clin Oncol 18:547-561, 2000
12. Lewis JH, Kilgore ML, Goldman DP, Trimble EL, Kaplan R, Montello MJ, et al: Participation of patients 65 years of age or older in cancer clinical trials. J Clin Oncol 21:1383-1389, 2003
13. Talarico L, Chen G, Pazdur R: Enrollment of elderly patients in clinical

trials for cancer drug registration: A 7-year experience by the US Food and Drug Administration. J Clin Oncol 22:4626-4631, 2004
14. Chessels JM, Hall E, Prentice HG, Durrant J, Bailey CC, Richards SM: The impact of age on outcome in lymphoblastic leukaemia; MRC UKALL X and XA compared: A report from the MRC Paediatric and Adult Working Parties. Leukemia 112:463-473, 1998
15. Larson RA, Dodge RK, Burns CP, Lee EJ, Stone RM, Schulman P, et al: A five-drug remission induction regimen with intensive consolidation for adults with acute lymphoblastic leukemia: Cancer and Leukemia Group B study 8811. Blood 85:2025-2037, 1995
16. Larson RA, Dodge RK, Linker CA, Stone RM, Powell BL, Lee EJ, et al: A randomized controlled trial of filgrastim during remission induction and consolidation chemotherapy for adults with acute lymphoblastic leukemia: CALGB study 9111. Blood 92:1556-1564, 1998
17. Gökbuget N, de Wit M, Gerhardt A, Lipp T, Rieder H, Schwartz S, et al: Results of a shortened, dose reduced treatment protocol in elderly patients with acute lymphoblastic leukemia. Blood 96:718a, 2000 (suppl 1, abstr 3104)
18. Hoelzer D, Gökbuget N, Beck J, Burmeister T, Giagounidis A, Glasmacher A, et al: Subtype adjusted therapy improves outcome of elderly patients with acute lymphoblastic leukemia. Blood 104: 2004 (suppl 1, abstr 2732)
19. Hoelzer D, Gökbuget N: Treatment of elderly patients with acute lymphoblastic leukemia, in Perry MC (ed): American Society of Clinical Oncology Educational Book. 2005, pp 533-539
20. Pagano L, Mele L, Trape G, Leone G: The treatment of acute lymphoblastic leukaemia in the elderly. Leuk Lymph 45:117-123, 2004
21. Pagano L, Mele L, Casorelli I, Fianchi L, Di Febo A, Leone G: Acute lymphoblastic leukemia in the elderly. A twelve-year retrospective, single center study. Haematologica 85:1327-1329, 2000
22. Taylor PRA, Reid MM, Proctor SJ: Acute lymphoblastic leukaemia in the elderly. Leuk Lymph 13:373-380, 1994
23. Crome P: What's different about older people? Toxicology 192:49-54, 2003
24. Bressler R, Bahl J: Principles of drug therapy for the elderly patient. Mayo Clin Proc 78:1564-1577, 2003
25. Lipschitz DA: Age related decline in hematopoietic reserve capacity. Semin Oncol 22:3-5, 1995
26. Ottmann OG, Wassmann B: Treatment of Philadelphia chromosome positive acute lymphoblastic leukemia, in Berliner N (ed): Hematology 2005. Washington, DC, American Society of Hematology, 2005, pp 118-122
27. Gleissner B, Gokbughet N, Bartram CR, et al: Leading prognostic relevance of the BCR-ABL translocation in adult acute B-lineage lymphoblastic leukemia: A prospective study of the German Multicenter Trial Group. Blood 99:1536-1543, 2002
28. Czuczman MS, Dodge RK, Stewart CC, Frankel SR, Davey FR, Powell BL, et al: Value of immunophenotyping in intensively treated adult acute lymphoblastic leukemia: Cancer and Leukemia Group B study 8364. Blood 93:3931-3939, 1999
29. Radich JP: Philadelphia chromosome-positive acute lymphocytic leukemia. Hematol Oncol Clin North Am 15:21-36, 2001
30. Avivi I, Goldstone AH: Bone marrow transplant in Ph+ ALL patients. Bone Marrow Transplant 31:623-632, 2003
31. Druker BJ, Sawyers CL, Kantarjian H, Resta DJ, Reese SF, Ford JM, et al: Activity of a specific inhibitor of the BCR-ABL tyrosine kinase in the blast crisis of chronic myeloid leukemia and acute lymphoblastic leukemia with the Philadelphia chromosome. N Engl J Med 344:1038-1042, 2001
32. Ottmann OG, Druker BJ, Sawyers CL, Goldman JM, Reiffers J, Silver RT, et al: A phase 2 study of imatinib in patients with relapsed or refractory Philadelphia chromosome-positive acute lymphoid leukemias. Blood 100:1965-1971, 2002
33. Wassmann B, Pfeifer H, Scheuring UJ, Binckebanck A, Gökbuget N et al: Early prediction of response in patients with relapsed or refractory Philadelphia-chromosome positive acute lymphoblastic leukemia (Ph^+ ALL) treated with imatinib mesylate (Glivec). Blood 103:1495-1498, 2004
34. Thomas D, Faderl S, Cortes J, O'Brien S, Giles F et al: Update of the hyper-CVAD and imatinib mesylate regimen in Philadelphia (Ph) positive acute lymphocytic leukemia. Blood 104: 2004, (abstr 2738)
35. Towatari M, Yanada M, Usui N, Takeuchi J, Sugiura I, Takeuchi M, Yagasaki F, et al: Combination of intensive chemotherapy and imatinib can rapidly induce high-quality complete remission for a majority of patients with newly diagnosed BCR-ABL-positive acute lymphoblastic. Blood 104:3507-35, 2004
36. Ottmann OG, Wassmann B, Pfeifer H, Gökbuget N, Bug G et al: Imatinib given concurrently with induction chemotherapy is superior to imatinib subsequent to induction and consolidation in newly diagnosed Philadelphia-positive acute lymphoblastic leukemia. Blood 104: 2004 (abstr 685)
37. Pfeifer H, Wassmann B, Hoffmann WK, Komor M, Scheuring U, et al: Risk and prognosis of central nervous system leukemia in patients with Philadelphia chromosome positive acute leukemias treated with imatinib mesylate (Glivec). Clin Cancer Res 9:4674-4681, 2003
38. Vignetti M, Fazi P, Meloni G, Chiarenza A, Malagola M, et al: Dramatic improvement in CR rate and CR duration with imatinib in adult and elderly Ph+ ALL patients: Results of the GIMEMA prospective study LAL0201. Blood 104: 2004 (abstr 2739)
39. Ottmann OG, Wassmann B, Gökbuget N, Binckebanck A, Pfeifer H, Bruck R, et al: A randomized phase II study comparing imatinib with chemotherapy as induction therapy in elderly patients with newly diagnosed Philadelphia-positive acute lymphoid leukemias. Hematology J 5:S112, 2004 (suppl, abstr)
40. Thomas DA, Cortes J, Giles FJ, et al: The modified hyper-CVAD regimen in newly diagnosed adult acute lymphoblastic leukemia. Blood 98:590a, 2001 (suppl 1, abstr 2474)
41. Stock W, Yu D, Sanford B, Lozanski G, Cataland S, Vik R, et al: Incorporation of alemtuzumab into front-line therapy of adult acute lymphoblastic leukemia is feasible: A phase I/II study from the Cancer and leukemia Group B (CALGB 10102). Blood 106:46a, 2005 (suppl 1, abstr 145)
42. Faderl S, Gandhi V, Keating MJ, Jeha S, Plunkett W, Kantarjian HM. The role of clofarabine in hematologic and solid malignancies—Development of a next-generation nucleoside analog. Cancer 103:1985-1995, 2005
43. Kurtzberg J, Ernst TJ, Keating MJ, et al: Phase I study of 506U78 administered on a consecutive 5-day schedule in children and adults with refractory hematologic malignancies. J Clin Oncol 23:3396-3403, 2005
44. Berg SL, Blaney SM, Devidas M, et al: Phase II study of nelarabine (compound 506U78) in children and young adults with refractory T-cell malignancies: A report from the Children's Oncology Group. J Clin Oncol 23:3376-3382, 2005
45. DeAngelo DJ, Yu D, Dodge RK, et al: A phase II study of 2-amino-9-beta-D-arabinosyl-6-methoxy-9H-purine (506U78) in patients with relapsed or refractory T-lineage acute lymphoblastic leukemia or lymphoblastic lymphoma: CALGB study 19801. Blood 100:198a, 2003 (suppl 1, abstr 743)
46. Isola L, Furman RR, Gandhi V, Thomas DA, Bennett JC, Banita S, et al: Antileukemic activity and pharmacodynamics of intravenous forodesine (BCX-1777), a novel purine nucleoside phosphorylase (PNP) inhibitor, in phase I/II trials in patients with advanced T-cell malignancies. Blood 104: 2004 (abstr 4501)
47. Gelmon KA, Tolcher A, Diab AR, et al: Phase I study of liposomal vincristine. J Clin Oncol 17:697-705, 1999
48. Thomas DA, Sarris A, O'Brien S, et al: Phase II study of liposomal vincristine in relapsed or refractory adult acute lymphoblastic leukemia. Blood 94:238b, 1999 (suppl 1, abstr 4269)
49. Offidani M, Corvatta L, Centurioni R, Leoni F, Malerba L, Mele A, et al: High-dose daunorubicin as liposomal compound (Daunoxome) in elderly patients with acute lymphoblastic leukemia. Hematol J 4:47-53, 2003
50. Thomas DA, Cortes J, Kantarjian HM. New agents in the treatment of acute lymphoblastic leukemia. Best Pract Res Clin Haematol 15:771-790, 2003

Seminars in
HEMATOLOGY

Approach to the Complications of Treatment for Acute Leukemia in the Elderly

Joel Gingerich[a] and Eric J. Bow[b]

Acute leukemia is common in the elderly and, due to the aging population and poorer prognosis, represents a major challenge. Elderly acute leukemia patients have been arbitrarily defined as ≥55 to 65 years of age and are underrepresented in clinical trials. There are physiologic differences between elderly and non-elderly patients. A comprehensive understanding of these differences allows the development of a systematic approach to assessing the risks for treatment-related complications. Use of a comprehensive geriatric assessment (CGA), initially developed and validated in the general geriatric population, may allow more accurate assessment of the likelihood of chemotherapy-induced complications and allow for proactive risk minimization. Once complications to therapy develop, aggressive treatment is essential. Treatment related to common complications that arise from therapy will be reviewed. Further research directed at this population is required.
Semin Hematol 43:134-143

The elderly population is growing. In 2001, people over the age of 60 years represented 16.9% of the total population of Canada. This group is expected to nearly double by the year 2026 and will represent 28.4% of the Canadian population.[1] These findings are similar to other industrialized nations.

Cancer affects the elderly disproportionately. It is estimated that in 2005, 68% of new cancer diagnoses will be in patients 60 years and older and that the percentage of deaths in patients over the age of 60 will represent 81% of all cancer deaths in Canada.[2] Acute myeloid leukemia (AML) is an example of a malignancy that disproportionately affects elderly patients. The median age of AML diagnosis in the United States is 65 years.[3] The probability of developing AML doubles by the age of 45 but increases almost 10-fold during the remainder of a person's life.[4] Unlike AML, acute lymphoblastic leukemia (ALL) is rare in elderly patients but may become an increasing problem in the future because of the aging population.[5] Elderly patients with acute leukemia have a poorer prognosis when compared to their younger counterparts. For example, the rates of complete remission and 5-year survival in AML, after induction chemotherapy with cytarabine and an anthracycline, are lower in older patients when compared to younger patients (45% *v* 75%, and 12% *v* 37%, respectively).[6–8] Similar findings have been found in elderly ALL patients as well.[5] Because elderly patients are a growing segment of the population, because they develop AML more commonly than younger patients, and because elderly patients with acute leukemia do poorly, acute leukemia in this subset of patients will become an increasingly important issue. This review will focus on considerations for an approach to the management of complications of acute leukemia therapy in the elderly by (1) defining the elderly population, (2) identifying physiologic differences that exist between elderly and non-elderly acute leukemia patients, (3) highlighting ways to identify elderly acute leukemia patients at risk of complications, and (4) discussing treatment strategies for complications that arise in acute leukemia patients.

Defining the Elderly Acute Leukemia Patient Population

Geriatric oncology is a relatively new field. Clinical trials dealing with acute leukemia have arbitrarily defined the lower age boundary of the elderly population as between 55

[a]Section of Haematology/Oncology, Department of Internal Medicine, the University of Manitoba, and the Department of Medical Oncology and Haematology, Cancer Care Manitoba, Winnipeg, Manitoba, Canada.
[b]Sections of Infectious Diseases and Haematology/Oncology, Department of Internal Medicine, the University of Manitoba, and Department of Medical Oncology and Haematology, CancerCare Manitoba, Winnipeg, Manitoba, Canada.
E.J.B. is a Consultant and Investigator for Pfizer Global Pharmaceuticals, Astellas Pharma Canada, Inc, Merck Frosst Canada Ltd, AMGEN Canada Inc, Enzon Pharmaceuticals, Schering-Plough Pharmaceuticals, and Wyeth Pharmaceuticals.
Address correspondence to E.J. Bow, MD, GD600, Health Sciences Centre, 820 Sherbrook St, Winnipeg, Manitoba, Canada R3A 1R9. E-mail: ebow@hsc.mb.ca

 0037-1963/06/$-see front matter © 2006 Elsevier Inc. All rights reserved.
doi:10.1053/j.seminhematol.2006.01.001

and 65 years.[9,10] The Surveillance, Epidemiology, and End Results (SEER) Program for all cancer sites has defined elderly as the age group ≥65 years.[11] Moreover, consensus has further divided elderly patients into three groups: the "young old," age 65 to 74 years; the "older old," age 75 to 84 years; and the "oldest old," age ≥85 years.[11] These age cut-offs seem fitting in acute leukemia since the pathophysiology and natural history of AML appears to change in patients after 60 years of age.[12,13] Along with an increased incidence of AML during and after the sixth decade of life, this group of patients also has a poorer prognosis, an increased proportion of cytogenetic abnormalities, and an increased risk of expressing a multidrug resistance gene (*MDR1*) phenotype and they are less likely to benefit from transplantation.[14–17] The pathophysiology of ALL seems to change with age as well since the presence of Philadelphia chromosomes, pre–B-cell ALL, and common ALL are all more common in the elderly while the prevalence of T-cell ALL is rarer in this population.[18]

Elderly acute leukemia patients are underrepresented in clinical trials.[19,20] A comparison of the 1992 accrual to National Cancer Institute–sponsored Cooperative Group Cancer Treatment trials with the 1990 SEER incidence data showed a significant discordance between the proportion of male patients ≥65 years accrued into leukemia trials (9.6%) compared to the proportion of males with leukemia that were ≥65 years (55.6%).[11,19] The Southwestern Oncology Group (SWOG) also noted that the proportion of patients with acute leukemia who were older than 65 years of age and were enrolled in clinical trials (27%) was much less than what was expected based on the percentage of patients greater than 65 years of age with acute leukemia in the general population.[20] Large cooperative leukemia trials tend to accrue selected cohorts of patients based on strict inclusion and exclusion criteria. Less than half of consecutive elderly AML patients receiving medical attention may be sufficiently fit to permit intensive remission-induction therapy.[21] This bias may lead to overestimation of response and survival outcomes.[22]

Despite earlier systematic observations suggesting similar toxicities among younger and older patients undergoing cytotoxic therapy,[23] the elderly are perceived to be less able than younger patients to tolerate standard chemotherapy regimens because of their decreased hematopoietic reserves, high prevalence of comorbidities, and greater risk of toxicity.[24] This belief may lead to dose reductions and delays that may compromise outcomes. Thus, it is difficult to accurately articulate from the medical literature the incidence of treatment-related toxicities in elderly leukemia patients.

Identifying Important Age-Related Physiologic Differences

An understanding of the physiologic differences between the young and old is important in developing a systematic approach to assess the risks for treatment-related complications. Elderly patients have more comorbidities[25] and there is evidence, at least in solid tumors, that these comorbidities limit clinical trial enrollment, adversely affect prognosis and survival, and increase the risk of chemotherapy-induced toxicity.[26–28]

However, not all comorbid conditions exert the same degree of health risk to an individual, and the variance in severity of a specific comorbidity among enrollees may be considerable. Two comorbidity scales that objectively characterize the impact of comorbidities on survival are the Charlson Comorbidity scale[29] and the Cumulative Illness Rating Scale-Geriatric (CIRS-G).[30] While not specific to elderly acute leukemia patients, these scales are widely accepted in the geriatric oncology literature and may be used to identify the impact of comorbidities on treatment decisions.[9] The impact on treatment outcome seen in patients with increased comorbid conditions appears to be independent of functional status.[31]

Nutritional deficiencies occur often in elderly patients and are thought to be common in acute leukemia patients.[9,32] There are many reasons for malnutrition in elderly leukemia patients, including poor dentition, depression, and poor socioeconomic status.[9] Anorexia may develop due to tumor-induced cytokine production and its affect on the hypothalamus or because of drug-induced taste modification.[32] Gastrointestinal changes may interfere with nutritional absorption. Tumor necrosis factor-alpha and cachectin promote glucose intolerance, increased gluconeogenesis, and increased lactate production and have been implicated in the pathogenesis of malnutrition.[32] Malnutrition is associated with impairment of B- and T-cell function, which may increase the risk of infection in cancer patients.[33] Deficiencies in vitamin C, vitamin E, the beta-carotenes, vitamin B_6, and vitamin B_{12} have been linked to an increased risk for pressure ulcers, poor wound healing, and cognitive defects in the elderly.[34,35]

The relationship of increased myelotoxicity with older age remains controversial.[36] The progressive age-related decline in functional end-organ reserve may also apply to myelopoiesis,[37] although supporting empirical evidence is inconsistent.[38] Other factors such as cytokines may interfere and blunt the normal stem cell response to stress.[37] Elevated levels of interleukin-6 have been associated with anemia, functional impairment, frailty, depression, and mortality in elderly patients.[39,40]

Cognitive changes, including learning and recall ability, information processing, reaction times, and nonverbal intelligence, occur with age and are linked to increased mortality.[41,42] Therefore, elderly acute leukemia patients may have more difficulty than their younger counterparts absorbing the complexities of acute leukemia decision making, understanding the realistic prognosis, and processing the treatment-related side effects. Patients with significant cognitive impairment may not benefit from aggressive therapy.[43] Various validated tools, such as the Mini-Mental State Examination, have been produced that assess the cognitive function of elderly patients.[44] Other potentially reversible medical conditions that can cause symptoms of dementia in elderly patients, including uncontrolled hypertension, vitamin B_{12} deficiencies, folate deficiencies, uncontrolled diabetes, chronic obstructive pulmonary disease, sleep apnea, thyroid dysfunction, psychotropic medications, and depression, should be explored.[41]

Drug-related toxicity in elderly patients is common.[45] An understanding of age-related changes in the volume of distribution, renal clearance, gastrointestinal absorption, hepatic metabolism, and tendency to polypharmacy can help prevent excess drug toxicity. The volume in which a particular drug diffuses, the volume of distribution, provides a reference for the plasma concentration of that particular drug. With age, particularly in cancer patients, intracellular water, serum albumin concentration, and red blood cell mass all decrease and the proportion of fat content to body weight increases[9,46,47]; the result is a decrease and increase in the volumes of distribution for charged and uncharged compounds, respectively. These changes may have important clinical ramifications; for example, the plasma concentrations of the anthracycline antibiotics, which bind to erythrocytes and serum albumin, are inversely proportional to the concentrations of these blood components.[9] Accordingly, anthracycline-related toxicity may be enhanced in the setting of severe anemia and hypoalbuminemia.[9,48]

Kidney function changes with age. The measured glomerular filtration rate (GFR) and the renal plasma flow both decrease by 10% per year beginning between the fourth and fifth decade of life for most but not all populations.[49] These changes are important since chemotherapeutic agents or their metabolites typically used in acute leukemia treatment (cytarabine, daunorubicin, or methotrexate, for example) are excreted through the kidneys. Formulae created to calculate the GFR include the Cockcroft-Gault equation[50] (Creatinine clearance, CrCl, in milliliters per minute = ([140 − age] × [weight, in kilograms] × [1 − (0.15 × sex, where male = 0 and female = 1)])/(0.814 × serum Cr)), the Jellife equation[51] (CrCL in milliliters per minute = [((98 − 0.8) × (age − 20) × (1 − (0.01 × sex)) × (Body surface area, BSA/1.73))/(Serum creatinine, SCr, × 0.0113)]), and the Wright equation[52] (GFR, in milliliters per minute, = [(6,580 − (38.8 × age)) × (BSA × (1 − (0.168 × sex))/SCr]). Since the Cockcroft and Gault and the Jelliffe formulas may be less accurate in older individuals because of the unpredictable rate of decline in the GFR and muscle mass with age, a more recent review suggests that the Wright formula may be preferable.[52]

The ability to administer drugs by mouth to elderly leukemia patients is important for effective supportive care strategies. However, with age, changes in gastrointestinal mobility, gastrointestinal secretion, and gastrointestinal blood flow affect drug absorption.[47] In addition, chemotherapy-induced gastrointestinal injury is more common in elderly patients.[48,53] Cytotoxic agents interfere with intestinal epithelial cell metabolism, repair, and division, resulting in loss of mucosal integrity and function.[54–56] These changes may affect the therapeutic effectiveness of oral anti-nauseants, antiemetics, antimicrobials, anti-pyretics, analgesics and other oral medications used to treat pre-existing comorbid conditions, particularly at the time halfway through the treatment course when these agents are most needed.

Hepatic metabolism may be affected in the elderly leukemia patients. With age, splanchnic blood flow and the total number of hepatocytes decrease.[57] In parallel, elderly patients seem to be at increased risk of P-450 cytochrome–related drug interactions. The proteins of the P-450 cytochrome pathway, which are important in the metabolism of many drugs, may themselves be up- or downregulated through interactions with different pharmaceutical agents.[58] For example, cytarabine and the anthracycline, idarubicin, used in the management of AML, are both metabolized in part through the cytochrome P450 pathway.[59] Itraconazole, a commonly used anti-fungal triazole, may inhibit components of this pathway, thereby reducing the metabolism of cytarabine and increasing the risk of hematopoietic and intestinal epithelial toxicities. Similar concerns have been expressed with regard to triazole-related perturbations of cyclophosphamide metabolism.[60] Age-related physiologic effects together with pharmaceutical agent–related interactions with hepatic metabolic pathways may enhance the overall adverse clinical drug reactions in elderly leukemic patients.

Elderly patients often require multiple medications to manage cumulative health problems and, accordingly, are at risk of poly-pharmacy.[61] The elderly are the biggest users of pharmaceutical drugs.[36] Elderly patients have about a 5% risk of one or more adverse drug events per year and an approximately 20% risk of using one or more inappropriate medications.[45] Furthermore, the acute leukemia patient is exposed not only to his/her regular medication but also to cytotoxic, immunosuppressive, and symptom control medications. Poly-pharmacy may well be an independent risk factor for chemotherapy-induced toxicity.[62]

Elderly patients are at increased risk of chemotherapy-induced cardiotoxicity. Anthracyclines, commonly used in the treatment of both AML and ALL, are known to be cardiotoxic.[63] Known risk factors include older age, increased drug exposure, mediastinal radiotherapy, female sex, pre-existing heart disease, and hypertension.[63] Drug-induced cardiotoxicity is more likely in the presence of underlying cardiac disease or cardiac risk factors, which are more common in elderly patients.[9,25] The underlying mechanism of myocyte injury leading to myofibrillar loss is likely multifactorial; however, it is believed that oxygen-free-radical formation created by the semiquinone moiety of the anthracycline molecule may cause lipid peroxidation leading to cellular injury.[63] The exact incidence of anthracycline-related cardiotoxicity in the elderly is difficult to ascertain.

Performance status measurements are important predictors of survival in acute leukemia patients, although they are not specific to the elderly.[64] Two markers of functional status have been developed for use in the general elderly population, including the Katz Activities of Daily Living (ADL) scale[65] and the Lawton Instrumental Activities of Daily Living (IADL) scale.[66] The ADL scale measures functional ability in the basic tasks of dressing, eating, ambulating, toileting, and personal hygiene. The IADL scale measures the ability to perform more complex tasks such as shopping, housekeeping, accounting, food preparation, and transferring. Dependence in either ADL or IADL are predictors of increased mortality in the general elderly population.[67] The ADL and IADL scale measurements add useful information to the assessment of performance status in elderly cancer patients and it has been argued that dependence by these measurements may predict a risk for a poor outcome sufficient to preclude aggressive chemotherapy.[25,43]

Defining Which Patients Should be Treated

The second step in the management of complications of acute leukemia therapy in the elderly should be the proactive identification of patients at high risk for regimen-related toxicity for whom high-dose induction chemotherapy would have limited benefit. There is growing advocacy in the geriatric oncology literature for a standardized method for assessment in this regard. Tools such as the Functional Assessment of Cancer Therapy Scale[68] and the Canadian Study of Health and Aging Clinical Frailty Scale have been developed to supplement clinicians' assessments of performance status.[69] Outcomes have been superior among older patients undergoing a Comprehensive Geriatric Assessment (CGA).[70,71] While the CGA has not been validated in the elderly acute leukemia setting, this tool systematically examines variables pertinent to prognosis and outcome expectations.[43,48] The main components of the CGA include the identification of comorbidities, mental status deficiencies, depression, level of social support, nutritional status, evidence for poly-pharmacy, home environmental barriers, and deficiencies in the activities of daily living.[43] Many of these categories are themselves markers for survival in elderly cancer patients. For example, a retrospective review noted European ethnicity with intact social support structures in place to be an independent predictor of prolonged overall and event-free survival in AML patients.[72] The CGA identifies domains of deficiency often underappreciated on routine history taking.[73–75] For example, in 200 consecutive cancer patients ≥70 years of age, the prevalence of dependence in a variety of CGA domains was high: ADL and IADL (18% and 72%, respectively), serious comorbidity (36%), memory impairment (22%), poor nutrition (19%) and poly-pharmacy (41%).[48]

Three categories of elderly acute leukemia patients can be recognized from the CGA: (1) low-risk fit patients able to tolerate regular therapy, (2) intermediate-risk patients at risk of increased toxicity and who require close monitoring during treatment or treatment dose-reduction, and (3) high-risk frail patients unable to tolerate intense therapy and for whom symptom control and palliation may be most appropriate.[25,43] Intermediate-risk patients may display dependence in IADL, mild memory impairment, mild depression, or non-severe comorbidities. Frail high-risk patients are defined by dependence in ≥1 ADL, presence of ≥1 geriatric syndromes, or ≥3 severe comorbidities. The timed "Up & Go" test has been used to identify frail patients based on the timed ability to emerge from an armchair, walk 3 meters, turn, return to the chair, and sit down.[76] Extreme caution should be used before deciding to administer aggressive induction chemotherapy to patients over the age of 85.[25,43]

An integration of the results of assessment tools like the CGA with other known disease-specific prognostic factors in acute leukemia including the cytogenetics profile, prior myelodysplastic disorders and *MDR1* phenotype, together with a review of life tables of elderly patients without cancer, can provide the clinician with a balanced assessment about the relative benefits of remission-induction therapy versus a symptom-control palliative approach.[14,15,77,78]

Treating the Complications of Therapy

Aggressive proactive minimization and treatment of toxic side effects such as myelosuppression, infection, mucositis, diarrhea, nausea, vomiting, and pain is particularly important in older individuals. Age-related physiologic changes decrease capacity to tolerate many of the side effects produced by aggressive therapy.

The Role of Myeloid Growth Factors

The role of myeloid growth factors after induction chemotherapy in elderly AML patients remains controversial.[79] The products that have been studied include glycosylated yeast-derived granulocyte-macrophage colony-stimulating factor (GM-CSF),[80,81] glycosylated Chinese hamster ovary-derived granulocyte colony-stimulating factor (G-CSF),[82–85] nonglycosylated *Escherichia coli*–derived G-CSF,[86–90] and nonglycosylated *E coli*–derived GM-CSF.[91–94] Eight trials have examined the efficacy of myeloid growth factors in elderly leukemia patients.[80,82,84,85,89,91,92,94] These trials are hard to systematically compare given the heterogeneity of study design, product studied, timing of administration, and state of the marrow at the time of initiation of therapy.[79] Taken together, the results of these trials have been unable to demonstrate treatment effects on outcomes such as complete remission rates, overall survival, or disease-free survival.[13,95,96] However, beneficial treatment effects have included shortened times to neutrophil recovery by a mean of 4.3 days (range, 2 to 8 days),[80,82,84,85,89–94,97] shortened duration of hospitalization from 2.5 to 6 days,[85,90] and reduced duration of antibiotic therapy by a mean of 3.4 days (range, 2.8 to 4 days).[89,90,98] The 2000 updated American Society of Clinical Oncology guidelines, based on nine randomized controlled trials encompassing 2,295 randomized subjects,[80,82,84,89–94] suggest that the use of growth factors in elderly AML patients has significant cost implications and should be at the discretion of the treating physician or based on local practice guidelines.[99] Cost savings from the prophylactic use of hematopoietic growth factors in elderly leukemia patients have been reported in some studies of GM-CSF[100,101] but not in others of G-CSF.[102] Since there are no large randomized controlled comparative studies, the relative values of G-CSF and GM-CSF cannot be detemined.

Oral and Gastrointestinal Mucositis

Guidelines for the management of oral and gastrointestinal mucositis[103] and associated diarrhea[104] in cancer patients have been published. These guidelines do not differentiate patients by age or underlying malignancy. The pathogenesis and epidemiology have been recently reviewed.[55] Up to 100% of patients receiving high-dose cytotoxic myeloablative therapy will develop mucositis. Cytotoxic therapy mucositis score increments of a single point have been associated with measurable increases in days of fever, risk of infection, days of parenteral nutrition, intravenous narcotic analgesia, hospital charges, and mortality.[105] The magnitude of the functional impairment of the gastrointestinal barrier induced by cytotoxic therapy is discontinuous over time, reaching a zenith at approximately day 14 from the first day of the cytotoxic therapy course.[53,106–108] At this time the risks for fever and invasive infection are highest. Interventions such as keratinocyte growth factors that promote restoration of the functional integrity of the gastrointestinal mucosal surface analogous to the effect of hematopoietic growth factors on committed hematopoietic progenitors can significantly reduce the severity, duration, and incidence of these outcomes.[109]

The etiology of drug-induced diarrhea is similar to that of mucositis and has already been discussed. Treatment begins by assessing the severity of the diarrhea. Grade 3 toxicity consists of ≥7 stools per day, incontinence, or the need for parenteral support because of dehydration. Grade 4 toxicity includes the requirement of intensive care or the development of hemodynamic collapse.[104] Prompt replacement of fluids and electrolytes as well as treatment with loperamide are important. For patients with grade 3 or 4 diarrhea or in patients who develop diarrhea while neutropenic, the administration of octreotide should be considered and a work-up should be instituted to evaluate for other potentially cofounding diagnoses.[104] Of note, in patients with abdominal pain, neutropenia, and fever, evaluation for neutropenic enterocolitis is warranted and has been found in 5.3% of acute leukemia patients undergoing induction therapy.[110]

Management of Pain

Pain requiring analgesia has been estimated to occur in 60% to 70% of elderly patients receiving chemotherapy.[111] The pathophysiology of age-associated pain remains controversial.[112] Untreated pain in elderly patients affects mood and cognition.[113] Identifying the source of pain, if possible, and minimizing potential confounding variables are essential.[113] When possible, acetaminophen should be used first as it has a favorable toxicity profile. Nonsteroidal anti-inflammatory drugs should be avoided, especially if administration over prolonged periods is planned given the associated risks for promoting bleeding diatheses and renal insufficiency, particularly in the elderly.[111,112] Opioids are frequently required and as a class have similar analgesic properties. Although morphine remains the most commonly used opioid, other opioids may have advantages in particular situations. For example, when compared to morphine, hydromorphone is associated with decreased purities and sedation, oxycodone is associated with decreased hallucinations and nausea, and fentanyl is associated with decreased constipation, daytime drowsiness, and improved safety profile in acute renal insufficiency. Once an opioid is initiated, its effects should be monitored for an optimal balance between pain control and adverse consequences such as delirium, increased likelihood of drug-drug interactions, respiratory depression, or sedation.[111] Therefore, frequent reassessment and drug dose adjustment may be required. Patient education and exercise may enhance the analgesic effects achieved by medication.[112]

Fever, Neutropenia, and Infection

More than 80% of adult patients are expected to develop at least one febrile neutropenic episode during remission-induction therapy for acute leukemia.[114] This incidence is independent of age.[115] A febrile neutropenic episode can add approximately 20% to the daily cost of inpatient management for elderly patients with AML.[102] Cost containment can be achieved by a systematic protocol-specific approach to the prevention and management of infection in the neutropenic leukemia patient.[116]

Strategies for prevention of bacterial infections have focused on chemoprophylaxis using orally absorbable antibacterial agents,[117] particularly the oral fluoroquinolones. Several systematic reviews based on the published clinical trials in this field have examined the efficacy and safety of this approach.[118–122] The advantages[123] and disadvantages[124] of fluoroquinolone-based antibacterial chemoprophylaxis have been recently reviewed. In summary, in an environment wherein the prevalence of fluoroquinolone-resistant aerobic gram-negative bacilli is low, prophylactic administration can significantly reduce and even eliminate the risk of invasive gram-negative bacillary infection-related morbidity and mortality. Overuse of fluoroquinolones in the community is associated with increased risk of infection by fluoroquinolone-resistance gram-negative bacilli.[125–127].The practice increases the risk of infection due to micro-aerophilic gram-positive cocci such as the coagulase-negative Staphylococci and viridans group Streptococci, particularly in a setting where cytarabine and proton pump inhibitors are being used.[128–131]

The role of anti-fungal chemoprophylaxis in high-risk patients has been studied in multiple randomized controlled clinical trials. These trials have been the subject of a number of systematic reviews.[132–136] While most of the focus has been on patients at highest risk for invasive fungal infection during allogeneic hematopoietic stem cell transplantation, meta-regression analysis has been able to identify nontransplant subgroups for which efficacy can be demonstrated,[134] in particular patients such as those with AML undergoing intensive cytotoxic therapy with the expectation of severe neutropenia (absolute neutrophil count $<0.5 \times 10^9/L$) lasting longer than 14 days. Fluconazole-based chemoprophylaxis is effective for reducing invasive yeast infections, particularly those due to susceptible species of *Candida*,[134] where the event rate among untreated subjects is greater than 15%,[133] and if daily doses of greater than 200 mg are administered.[134] Moreover, treatment effects for fungal infection-related mortality and overall mortality have been observed, particularly among the highest risk patients.[134,135] Itraconazole has been effective for reducing the risk of invasive mould infection such as that due to

Aspergillus spp, as well as infections due to opportunistic yeasts,[135] provided patients comply with the regimen.[137] The optimal duration for chemoprophylaxis strategies remains to be determined; however, it seems prudent to apply the strategy over the period of risk, defined for elderly acute leukemia patients as the period beginning with induction therapy until recovery from severe neutropenia. Of note, for leukemia patients treatment effects have only been observed during remission-induction or reinduction therapy but not during postremission consolidation.[138] Accordingly, fluconazole chemoprophylaxis during postremission consolidation therapy is not recommended.

Management guidelines for low-risk and high-risk patients have recently been published from the Infectious Diseases Society of America,[139] the Infectious Diseases Working Party of the German Society of Hematology and Oncology,[140] the National Comprehensive Cancer Network,[141] Japan,[142–144] and the Sociedad Espanola de Quimioterapia (SEQ) in Spain.[145] Elderly acute leukemia patients who develop febrile neutropenic episodes during induction therapy are considered at high risk for medical complications.[140,146] A number of empirical antibacterial regimens are recommended; however, the weight of evidence favors initial monotherapy with a third-generation cephalosporin such as ceftazidime or cefepime, a carbapenem such as imipenem/cilastatin or meropenem, or a broad-spectrum anti-pseudomonal penicillin combined with a β-lactamase inhibitor such as piperacillin plus tazobactam. Aminoglycoside-based combination therapy has no advantages over monotherapy regimens and has the disadvantage of additional nephrotoxicity that may be a greater threat to the elderly patient.[147,148] Initial empirical therapy with glycopeptide-based combinations has not been shown to be beneficial[149] and is not recommended.[139] Furthermore, the empirical addition of glycopeptide antibiotics for persistent neutropenic fever has also not been shown to be effective[150] and is not recommended. The median expected time to defervescence for responders to empirical antibacterial therapy is 5 days.[114,151] Accordingly, regimen modification for persistent fever in patients who are otherwise stable is unnecessary.[114,150]

Empirical administration of anti-fungal therapy for persistent or recrudescent fever despite broad-spectrum antibacterial therapy in severely neutropenic patients has become a standard practice[139,141] despite the lack of compelling evidence for efficacy in systematic review.[152]. The agent of choice, amphotericin B desoxycholate, has been largely supplanted by less toxic agents including lipid formulations of amphotericin B,[153,154] itraconazole,[155] voriconazole,[156] and caspofungin.[157] While the optimal agent for use in the elderly has not yet been defined, it seems prudent given the availability of other choices to avoid the predictable metabolic and renal toxicities associated with the polyene anti-fungal agents.

The expectations of outcomes of treatment for invasive fungal infection have been made more realistic by the introduction of standardized definitions for these infections.[158] The mortality in one series of patients with invasive fungal infection varied with the robustness of the diagnosis when defined by the European Organization for Research and Treatment of cancer (EORTC) and Mycoses Study Group criteria as possible (20%), probable (57%), and proven (80%).[159]

The differential diagnosis of persistent and recrudescent neutropenic fever includes both infectious and non-infectious processes. Examples of the former include invasive fungal infection, central venous catheter-related infection,[160] myeloid reconstitution syndrome,[161] skin and soft tissue infections,[162] nosocomial pneumonia syndromes,[163] and neutropenic enterocolitis.[110,164] Clinicians should be mindful that blood product transfusion still represents one of the most common non-infectious causes of recrudescent fever in leukemia patients undergoing intensive cytotoxic therapy.

Conclusions

The prevalence of older patients at risk for developing acute leukemia is rising. The spectrum of complications associated with anti-leukemia treatment in elderly patients is influenced by the underlying pathophysiologic mechanisms giving rise to the leukemia that influence response to treatment, the number and severity of existing comorbidities, and the physiologic changes that normally characterize the aging process. Standardized functional assessments can be used to predict the likelihood of tolerance to treatment and thereby estimate the balance of potential benefit of anti-leukemic therapy and risk for treatment-related complications. Our understanding of the optimal supportive care strategies for elderly acute leukemia patients is still incomplete and further research specifically directed at this population is needed.

References

1. Statistics Canada: Canadian statistics: Population and demography: Population characteristics: Population projections for 2110, 2006, 2011, 2016, 2021, and 2026, update. http://www.statcan.ca, accessed July 1, 2005
2. Mclaughlin JR, Dryer D, Mao Y, Marrett L, Mills C, Morrison H, et al. Canadian cancer statistics. Canadian Cancer Society/National Cancer Institute of Canada, http://www.cancer.ca, accessed July 1, 2005
3. Heath CH: Epidemiology and hereditary aspects of acute leukemia, in Wiernik PH, Canellos GP, Dutcher JP, Kyle RA (eds): Neoplastic Disease of the Blood (ed 3). New York, NY, Churchill-Livingston, 1996, p 177
4. Lichtman MA, Rowe JM: The relationship of patient age to the pathobiology of the clonal myeloid diseases. Semin Oncol 31:185-197, 2004
5. Pagano L, Mele L, Trape G, Leone G: The treatment of acute lymphoblastic leukaemia in the elderly. Leuk Lymphoma 45:117-123, 2004
6. Mayer RJ, Davis RB, Schiffer CA, Berg DT, Powell BL, Schulman P, et al: Intensive postremission chemotherapy in adults with acute myeloid leukemia. Cancer and Leukemia Group B. N Engl J Med 331: 896-903, 1994
7. Rees JK, Gray RG, Swirsky D, Hayhoe FG: Principal results of the Medical Research Council's 8th acute myeloid leukaemia trial. Lancet 2:1236-1241, 1986
8. Appelbaum FR, Rowe JM, Radich J, Dick JE: Acute myeloid leukemia. Hematology (Am Soc Hematol Educ Program) 2001:62-86
9. Balducci L: The geriatric cancer patient: Equal benefit from equal treatment. Cancer Control 8:1-25, 2001
10. Zagonel V, Monfardini S, Tirelli U, Carbone A, Pinto A: Management of hematologic malignancies in the elderly: 15-year experience at the

Aviano Cancer Center, Italy. Crit Rev Oncol Hematol 39:289-305, 2001
11. Yancik R: Cancer burden in the aged: An epidemiologic and demographic overview. Cancer 80:1273-1283, 1997
12. Jemal A, Thomas A, Murray T, Thun M: Cancer statistics, 2002. CA Cancer J Clin 52:23-47, 2002
13. Godwin JE, Smith SE: Acute myeloid leukemia in the older patient. Crit Rev Oncol Hematol 48:S17-S26, 2003
14. Grimwade D, Walker H, Harrison G, Oliver F, Chatters S, Harrison CJ, et al: The predictive value of hierarchical cytogenetic classification in older adults with acute myeloid leukemia (AML): Analysis of 1065 patients entered into the United Kingdom Medical Research Council AML11 trial. Blood 98:1312-1320, 2001
15. Leith CP, Kopecky KJ, Godwin J, McConnell T, Slovak ML, Chen IM, et al: Acute myeloid leukemia in the elderly: Assessment of multidrug resistance (MDR1) and cytogenetics distinguishes biologic subgroups with remarkably distinct responses to standard chemotherapy. A Southwest Oncology Group study. Blood 89:3323-3329, 1997
16. Wahlin A, Markevarn B, Golovleva I, Nilsson M: Improved outcome in adult acute myeloid leukemia is almost entirely restricted to young patients and associated with stem cell transplantation. Eur J Haematol 68:54-63, 2002
17. Wahlin A, Markevarn B, Golovleva I, Nilsson M: Prognostic significance of risk group stratification in elderly patients with acute myeloid leukaemia. Br J Haematol 115:25-33, 2001
18. Robak T: Acute lymphoblastic leukaemia in elderly patients: Biological characteristics and therapeutic approaches. Drugs Aging 21:779-791, 2004
19. Trimble EL, Carter CL, Cain D, Freidlin B, Ungerleider RS, Friedman MA: Representation of older patients in cancer treatment trials. Cancer 74:2208-2214, 1994
20. Hutchins LF, Unger JM, Crowley JJ, Coltman CA Jr, Albain KS: Underrepresentation of patients 65 years of age or older in cancer-treatment trials. N Engl J Med 341:2061-2067, 1999
21. Taylor PR, Reid MM, Stark AN, Bown N, Hamilton PJ, Proctor SJ: De novo acute myeloid leukaemia in patients over 55-years-old: A population-based study of incidence, treatment and outcome. Northern Region Haematology Group. Leukemia 9:231-237, 1995
22. Rathnasabapathy R, Lancet JE: Management of acute myelogenous leukemia in the elderly. Cancer Control 10:469-477, 2003
23. Begg CB, Carbone PP: Clinical trials and drug toxicity in the elderly. The experience of the Eastern Cooperative Oncology Group. Cancer 52:1986-1992, 1983
24. Dale DC: Poor prognosis in elderly patients with cancer: The role of bias and undertreatment. J Support Oncol 1:11-17, 2003
25. Basso U, Monfardini S: Multidimensional geriatric evaluation in elderly cancer patients: A practical approach. Eur J Cancer Care (Engl) 13:424-433, 2004
26. Satariano WA, Silliman RA: Comorbidity: Implications for research and practice in geriatric oncology. Crit Rev Oncol Hematol 48:239-248, 2003
27. Yancik R, Wesley MN, Ries LA, Havlik RJ, Edwards BK, Yates JW: Effect of age and comorbidity in postmenopausal breast cancer patients aged 55 years and older. JAMA 285:885-892, 2001
28. Mandelblatt JS, Edge SB, Meropol NJ, Senie R, Tsangaris T, Grey L, et al: Predictors of long-term outcomes in older breast cancer survivors: Perceptions versus patterns of care. J Clin Oncol 21:855-863, 2003
29. Charlson ME, Pompei P, Ales KL, MacKenzie CR: A new method of classifying prognostic comorbidity in longitudinal studies: Development and validation. J Chronic Dis 40:373-383, 1987
30. Miller MD, Paradis CF, Houck PR, Mazumdar S, Stack JA, Rifai AH, et al: Rating chronic medical illness burden in geropsychiatric practice and research: Application of the Cumulative Illness Rating Scale. Psychiatry Res 41:237-248, 1992
31. Extermann M, Overcash J, Lyman GH, Parr J, Balducci L: Comorbidity and functional status are independent in older cancer patients. J Clin Oncol 16:1582-1587, 1998
32. De Cicco M, Bortolussi R, Fantin D, Matovic M, Fracasso A, Fabiani F, et al: Supportive therapy of elderly cancer patients. Crit Rev Oncol Hematol 42:189-211, 2002
33. Dewys WD, Begg C, Lavin PT, Band PR, Bennett JM, Bertino JR, et al: Prognostic effect of weight loss prior to chemotherapy in cancer patients. Eastern Cooperative Oncology Group. Am J Med 69:491-497, 1980
34. Harris CL, Fraser C: Malnutrition in the institutionalized elderly: The effects on wound healing. Ostomy Wound Manage 50:54-63, 2004
35. Gonzalez-Gross M, Marcos A, Pietrzik K: Nutrition and cognitive impairment in the elderly. Br J Nutr 86:313-321, 2001
36. Lichtman SM: Guidelines for the treatment of elderly cancer patients. Cancer Control 10:445-453, 2003
37. Balducci L: Anemia, cancer, and aging. Cancer Control 10:478-486, 2003
38. Christman K, Muss HB, Case LD, Stanley V: Chemotherapy of metastatic breast cancer in the elderly. The Piedmont Oncology Association experience. JAMA 268:57-62, 1992
39. Ershler WB: Biological interactions of aging and anemia: A focus on cytokines. J Am Geriatr Soc 51:S18-S21, 2003
40. Hamerman D, Berman JW, Albers GW, Brown DL, Silver D: Emerging evidence for inflammation in conditions frequently affecting older adults: Report of a symposium. J Am Geriatr Soc 47:1016-1025, 1999
41. Craft S, Cholerton B, Reger M: Aging and cognition. What is normal?, in Hazzard WR, Blass JP, Halter JB, Ouslander JG, Tinetti ME (eds): Principles of Geriatric Medicine and Gerontology (ed 5). York, PA, McGraw-Hill, 2003, pp 1355-1372
42. Noale M, Maggi S, Minicuci N, Marzari C, Destro C, Farchi G, et al: Dementia and disability: Impact on mortality. The Italian Longitudinal Study on Aging. Dement Geriatr Cogn Disord 16:7-14, 2003
43. Balducci L, Yates J: General guidelines for the management of older patients with cancer. Oncology (Williston Park) 14:221-227, 2000
44. Folstein MF, Folstein SE, McHugh PR: "Mini-Mental State." A practical method for grading the cognitive state of patients for the clinician. J Psychiatr Res 12:189-198, 1975
45. Hanlon JT, Lindblad CI, Hajjar ER, McCarthy TC: Update on drug-related problems in the elderly. Am J Geriatr Pharmacother 1:38-43, 2003
46. Baker SD, Grochow LB: Pharmacology of cancer chemotherapy in the older person. Clin Geriatr Med 13:169-183, 1997
47. Yuen GJ: Altered pharmacokinetics in the elderly. Clin Geriatr Med 6:257-267, 1990
48. Balducci L, Extermann M: Management of cancer in the older person: A practical approach. Oncologist 5:224-237, 2000
49. Wiggins J: Changes in renal function, in Hazzard WR, Blass JP, Halter JB, Ouslander JG, Tinetti ME (eds): Principles of Geriatric Medicine and Gerontology (ed 5). York, PA, McGraw-Hill, 2003, pp 543-581
50. Cockcroft DW, Gault MH: Prediction of creatinine clearance from serum creatinine. Nephron 16:31-41, 1976
51. Jelliffe RW: Estimation of creatinine clearance when urine cannot be collected. Lancet 1:975-976, 1971
52. Marx GM, Blake GM, Galani E, Steer CB, Harper SE, Adamson KL, et al: Evaluation of the Cockroft-Gault, Jelliffe and Wright formulae in estimating renal function in elderly cancer patients. Ann Oncol 15: 291-295, 2004
53. Bow EJ, Sutherland JA, Kilpatrick MG, Williams GJ, Clinch JJ, Shore TB, et al: Therapy of untreated acute myeloid leukemia in the elderly: remission-induction using a non-cytarabine-containing regimen of mitoxantrone plus etoposide. J Clin Oncol 14:1345-1352, 1996
54. Duncan M, Grant G: Oral and intestinal mucositis—Causes and possible treatments. Aliment Pharmacol Ther 18:853-874, 2003
55. Sonis ST, Elting LS, Keefe D, Peterson DE, Schubert M, Hauer-Jensen M, et al: Perspectives on cancer therapy-induced mucosal injury: Pathogenesis, measurement, epidemiology, and consequences for patients. Cancer 100:1995-2025, 2004
56. Sonis ST: Pathobiology of mucositis. Semin Oncol Nurs 20:11-15, 2004
57. Balducci L, Corcoran MB: Antineoplastic chemotherapy of the older cancer patient. Hematol Oncol Clin North Am 14:193-212, 2000

58. Nebert DW, Russell DW: Clinical importance of the cytochromes P450. Lancet 360:1155-1162, 2002
59. Colburn DE, Giles FJ, Oladovich D, Smith JA: In vitro evaluation of cytochrome P450-mediated drug interactions between cytarabine, idarubicin, itraconazole and caspofungin. Hematology 9:217-221, 2004
60. Marr KA, Leisenring W, Crippa F, Slattery JT, Corey L, Boeckh M, et al: Cyclophosphamide metabolism is affected by azole antifungals. Blood 103:1557-1559, 2004
61. Rollason V, Vogt N: Reduction of polypharmacy in the elderly: A systematic review of the role of the pharmacist. Drugs Aging 20:817-832, 2003
62. Extermann M, Chen H, Cantor AB, Corcoran MB, Meyer J, Grendys E, et al: Predictors of tolerance to chemotherapy in older cancer patients: A prospective pilot study. Eur J Cancer 38:1466-73, 2002
63. Shan K, Lincoff AM, Young JB: Anthracycline-induced cardiotoxicity. Ann Intern Med 125:47-58, 1996
64. Kansal V, Omura GA, Soong SJ: Prognosis in adult acute myelogenous leukemia related to performance status and other factors. Cancer 38: 329-334, 1976
65. Katz S, Ford AB, Moskowitz RW, Jackson BA, Jaffe MW: Studies of illness in the aged. The index of ADL: A standardized measure of biological and psychological function. JAMA 185:914-919, 1963
66. Lawton MP, Brody EM: Assessment of older people: Self-maintaining and instrumental activities of daily living. Gerontologist 9:179-186, 1969
67. Reuben DB, Rubenstein LV, Hirsch SH, Hays RD: Value of functional status as a predictor of mortality: Results of a prospective study. Am J Med 93:663-669, 1992
68. Cella DF, Tulsky DS, Gray G, Sarafian B, Linn E, Bonomi A, et al: The Functional Assessment of Cancer Therapy scale: Development and validation of the general measure. J Clin Oncol 11:570-579, 1993
69. Rockwood K, Song X, MacKnight C, Bergman H, Hogan DB, McDowell I, et al: A global clinical measure of fitness and frailty in elderly people. CMAJ 173:489-495, 2005
70. Stuck AE, Siu AL, Wieland GD, Adams J, Rubenstein LZ: Comprehensive geriatric assessment: a meta-analysis of controlled trials. Lancet 342:1032-1036, 1993
71. Balducci L: New paradigms for treating elderly patients with cancer: The comprehensive geriatric assessment and guidelines for supportive care. J Support Oncol 1:30-37, 2003
72. Alcalai R, Ben-Yehuda D, Ronen I, Paltiel O: Ethnicity and prognosis in acute myeloid leukemia. Am J Hematol 72:127-134, 2003
73. Lachs MS, Feinstein AR, Cooney LM Jr, Drickamer MA, Marottoli RA, Pannill FC, et al: A simple procedure for general screening for functional disability in elderly patients. Ann Intern Med 112:699-706, 1990
74. Extermann M, Meyer J, McGinnis M, Crocker TT, Corcoran MB, Yoder J, et al: A comprehensive geriatric intervention detects multiple problems in older breast cancer patients. Crit Rev Oncol Hematol 49:69-75, 2004
75. McCorkle R, Strumpf NE, Nuamah IF, Adler DC, Cooley ME, Jepson C, et al: A specialized home care intervention improves survival among older post-surgical cancer patients. J Am Geriatr Soc 48:1707-1713, 2000
76. Podsiadlo D, Richardson S: The timed "Up & Go": A test of basic functional mobility for frail elderly persons. J Am Geriatr Soc 39:142-148, 1991
77. Walter LC, Brand RJ, Counsell SR, Palmer RM, Landefeld CS, Fortinsky RH, et al: Development and validation of a prognostic index for 1-year mortality in older adults after hospitalization. JAMA 285:2987-2994, 2001
78. Walter LC, Covinsky KE: Cancer screening in elderly patients: A framework for individualized decision making. JAMA 285:2750-2756, 2001
79. Rowe JM: Treatment of acute myeloid leukemia with cytokines: Effect on duration of neutropenia and response to infection. Clin Infect Dis 26:1290-1294, 1998
80. Rowe JM, Andersen JW, Mazza JJ, Bennett JM, Paietta E, Hayes FA, et al: A randomized placebo-controlled phase III study of granulocyte-macrophage colony-stimulating factor in adult patients (> 55 to 70 years of age) with acute myelogenous leukemia: A study of the Eastern Cooperative Oncology Group (E1490). Blood 86:457-462, 1995
81. Buchner T, Hiddemann W, Koenigsmann M, Zuhlsdorf M, Wormann B, Boeckmann A, et al: Recombinant human granulocyte-macrophage colony-stimulating factor after chemotherapy in patients with acute myeloid leukemia at higher age or after relapse. Blood 78:1190-1197, 1991
82. Dombret H, Chastang C, Fenaux P, Reiffers J, Bordessoule D, Bouabdallah R, et al: A controlled study of recombinant human granulocyte colony-stimulating factor in elderly patients after treatment for acute myelogenous leukemia. AML Cooperative Study Group. N Engl J Med 332:1678-1683, 1995
83. Link H, Wandt H, Schonrock-Nabulsi R, Ehninger G, Franke A, Gackle R, et al: G-CSF (lenograstim) after chemotherapy for acute myeloid leukemia: A placebo controlled trial. Blood 88:2654a, 1996 (suppl 1, abstr)
84. Goldstone AH, Burnett AK, Wheatley K, Smith AG, Hutchinson RM, Clark RE: Attempts to improve treatment outcomes in acute myeloid leukemia (AML) in older patients: The results of the United Kingdom Medical Research Council AML11 trial. Blood 98:1302-1311, 2001
85. Amadori S, Suciu S, Jehn U, Stasi R, Thomas X, Marie JP, et al: Use of glycosylated recombinant human G-CSF (lenograstim) during and/or after induction chemotherapy in patients 61 years of age and older with acute myeloid leukemia: Final results of AML-13, a randomized phase-3 study. Blood 106:27-34, 2005
86. Ohno R, Tomonaga M, Koboyashi T, Kanamaru A, Shirakawa S, Masaoka T, et al: Effect of granulocyte colony stimulating factor after intensive induction therapy in relapsed or refractory acute leukemia. N Engl J Med 323:871-877, 1990
87. Ohno R, Naoe T, Kanamaru A, Yoshida M, Hiraoka A, Kobayashi T, et al: A double-blind controlled study of granulocyte colony-stimulating factor stared two days before induction chemotherapy in refractory acute myeloid leukemia. Blood 83:2086-2092, 1994
88. Estey E, Thall P, Andreef M, Beran M, Kantarjian H, O'Brien S, et al: Use of granulocyte colony-stimulating factor before, during, and after fludarbine plus cytarabine induction therapy of newly diagnosed acute myelogenous leukemia or myelodysplastic syndromes: Comparison with fludarabine plus cytarabine without granulocyte colony-stimulating factor. J Clin Oncol 12:671-678, 1994
89. Godwin JE, Kopecky KJ, Head DR, Willman CL, Leith CP, Hynes HE, et al: A double-blind placebo-controlled trial of granulocyte colony-stimulating factor in elderly patients with previously untreated acute myeloid leukemia: A Southwest Oncology Group study (9031). Blood 91:3607-3615, 1998
90. Heil G, Hoelzer D, Sanz MA, Lechner K, Liu Yin JA, Papa G, et al: A randomized, double-blind, placebo-controlled, phase III study of filgrastim in remission induction and consolidation therapy for adults with de novo acute myeloid leukemia. The International Acute Myeloid Leukemia Study Group. Blood 90:4710-4718, 1997
91. Stone RM, Berg DT, George SL, Dodge RK, Paciucci PA, Schulman P, et al: Granulocyte-macrophage colony-stimulating factor after initial chemotherapy for elderly patients with primary acute myelogenous leukemia. Cancer and Leukemia Group B. N Engl J Med 332:1671-1677, 1995
92. Lowenberg B, Suciu S, Archimbaud E, Ossenkoppele G, Verhoef GE, Vellenga E, et al: Use of recombinant GM-CSF during and after remission induction chemotherapy in patients aged 61 years and older with acute myeloid leukemia: Final report of AML-11, a phase III randomized study of the Leukemia Cooperative Group of European Organisation for the Research and Treatment of Cancer and the Dutch Belgian Hemato-Oncology Cooperative Group. Blood 90:2952-2961, 1997
93. Zittoun R, Suciu S, Mandelli F, De Witte T, Thaler J, Stryckmans P, et al: Granulocyte-macrophage colony-stimulating factor associated with induction treatment of acute myelogenous leukemia: A randomized trial by the European Organization for Research and Treatment of

Cancer Leukemia Cooperative Group. J Clin Oncol 14:2150-2159, 1996

94. Witz F, Sadoun A, Perrin MC, Berthou C, Briere J, Cahn JY, et al: A placebo-controlled study of recombinant human granulocyte-macrophage colony-stimulating factor administered during and after induction treatment for de novo acute myelogenous leukemia in elderly patients. Groupe Ouest Est Leucemies Aigues Myeloblastiques (GOELAM). Blood 91:2722-2730, 1998
95. Schiffer CA : Hematopoietic growth factors as adjuncts to the treatment of acute myeloid leukemia. Blood 88:3675-3685, 1996
96. Geller RB: Use of cytokines in the treatment of acute myelocytic leukemia: A critical review. J Clin Oncol 14:1371-1382, 1996
97. Lofgren C, Paul C, Astrom M, Hast R, Hedenius M, Lerner R, et al: Granulocyte-macrophage colony-stimulating factor to increase efficacy of mitoxantrone, etoposide and cytarabine in previously untreated elderly patients with acute myeloid leukaemia: A Swedish multicentre randomized trial. Br J Haematol 124:474-480, 2004
98. Amadori S, Suciu S, Willemze R, Mandelli F, Selleslag D, Stauder R, et al: Sequential administration of gemtuzumab ozogamicin and conventional chemotherapy as first line therapy in elderly patients with acute myeloid leukemia: A phase II study (AML-15) of the EORTC and GIMEMA leukemia groups. Haematologica 89:950-956, 2004
99. Ozer H, Armitage JO, Bennett CL, Crawford J, Demetri GD, Pizzo PA, et al: 2000 update of recommendations for the use of hematopoietic colony-stimulating factors: Evidence-based, clinical practice guidelines. J Clin Oncol 18:3558-3585, 2000
100. Bennett CL, Stinson TJ, Tallman MS, Stadtmauer EA, Marsh RW, Friedenberg W, et al: Economic analysis of a randomized placebo-controlled phase III study of granulocyte macrophage colony stimulating factor in adult patients (>55 to 70 years of age) with acute myelogenous leukemia. Eastern Cooperative Oncology Group (E1490). Ann Oncol 10:177-182, 1999
101. Woronoff-Lemsi MC, Witz F, Arveux P, Cahn JY, Harousseau JL: Cost effectiveness of GM-CSF in the treatment of acute myeloblastic leukemia in aged patients: protocol of GOELAM Sa3. Therapie 56:131-133, 2001
102. Bennett CL, Hynes D, Godwin J, Stinson TJ, Golub RM, Appelbaum FR: Economic analysis of granulocyte colony stimulating factor as adjunct therapy for older patients with acute myelogenous leukemia (AML): Estimates from a Southwest Oncology Group clinical trial. Cancer Invest 19:603-610, 2001
103. Rubenstein EB, Peterson DE, Schubert M, Keefe D, McGuire D, Epstein J, et al: Clinical practice guidelines for the prevention and treatment of cancer therapy-induced oral and gastrointestinal mucositis. Cancer 100:2026-2046, 2004
104. Benson AB III, Ajani JA, Catalano RB, Engelking C, Kornblau SM, Martenson JA Jr, et al: Recommended guidelines for the treatment of cancer treatment-induced diarrhea. J Clin Oncol 22:2918-2926, 2004
105. Sonis ST, Oster G, Fuchs H, Bellm L, Bradford WZ, Edelsberg J, et al: Oral mucositis and the clinical and economic outcomes of hematopoietic stem-cell transplantation. J Clin Oncol 19:2201-2205, 2001
106. Bow EJ, Loewen R, Cheang MS, Shore TB, Rubinger M, Schacter B: Cytotoxic therapy-induced D-xylose malabsorption and invasive infection during remission-induction therapy for acute myeloid leukemia in adults. J Clin Oncol 15:2254-2261, 1997
107. Blijlevens NM, Donnelly JP, De Pauw BE: Prospective evaluation of gut mucosal barrier injury following various myeloablative regimens for haematopoietic stem cell transplant. Bone Marrow Transplant 35: 707-711, 2005
108. Blijlevens NM, van't Land B, Donnelly JP, M'Rabet L, De Pauw BE: Measuring mucosal damage induced by cytotoxic therapy. Support Care Cancer 12:227-233, 2004
109. Spielberger R, Stiff P, Bensinger W, Gentile T, Weisdorf D, Kewalramani T, et al: Palifermin for oral mucositis after intensive therapy for hematologic cancers. N Engl J Med 351:2590-2598, 2004
110. Gorschluter M, Mey U, Strehl J, Ziske C, Schepke M, Schmidt-Wolf IG, et al: Neutropenic enterocolitis in adults: Systematic analysis of evidence quality. Eur J Haematol 75:1-13, 2005
111. Rao A, Cohen HJ: Symptom management in the elderly cancer patient: Fatigue, pain, and depression. J Natl Cancer Inst Monogr 32:150-157, 2004
112. Ferrell BA, Chodosh J: Pain management, in Hazzard WR, Blass JP, Halter JB, Ouslander JG, Tinetti ME (eds): Principles of Geriatric Medicine and Gerontology (ed 5). York, PA, McGraw-Hill, 2003, pp 303-321
113. Agostini JV, Inouye SK: Delirium, in Hazzard WR, Blass JP, Halter JB, Ouslander JG, Tinetti ME (eds): Principles of Geriatric Medicine and Gerontology (ed 5). York, PA, McGraw-Hill, 2003, pp 1503-1516
114. Bow EJ: Infectious complications in patients receiving cytotoxic therapy for acute leukemia: History, background and approaches to management, in Wingard JR, Bowden RA (eds): Management of Infection in Oncology Patients. London, UK, Martin Dunitz, 2003, pp 71-104
115. Garcia-Suarez J, Krsnik I, Reyes E, De MD, Hernanz N, Barr-Ali M, et al: Elderly haematological patients with chemotherapy-induced febrile neutropenia have similar rates of infection and outcome to younger adults: A prospective study of risk-adapted therapy. Br J Haematol 120:209-216, 2003
116. Masaoka T: Economic issues: Toward a cost-effective approach to the management of febrile neutropenia in Japan. Clin Infect Dis 39:S68-S69, 2004 (suppl 1)
117. Yoshida M, Ohno R: Antimicrobial prophylaxis in febrile neutropenia. Clin Infect Dis 39:S65-S67, 2004 (suppl 1)
118. Cruciani M, Rampazzo R, Malena M, Lazzarini L, Todeschini G, Messori A, et al: Prophylaxis with fluoroquinolones for bacterial infections in neutropenic patients: A meta-analysis. Clin Infect Dis 23:795-805, 1996
119. Cruciani M, Malena M, Bosco O, Nardi S, Serpelloni G, Mengoli C: Reappraisal with meta-analysis of the addition of gram-positive prophylaxis to fluoroquinolone in neutropenic patients. J Clin Oncol 21:4127-4137, 2003
120. Rotstein C, Mandell L, Goldberg N: Fluoroquinolone prophylaxis for profoundly neutropenic cancer patients: A meta-analysis. Curr Oncol 4:S2-S7, 1997 (suppl 2)
121. Engels EA, Lau J, Barza M: Efficacy of quinolone prophylaxis in neutropenic cancer patients: A meta-analysis. J Clin Oncol 16:1179-1187, 1998
122. Gafter-Gvili A, Fraser A, Paul M, Leibovici L: Meta-analysis: Antibiotic prophylaxis reduces mortality in neutropenic patients. Ann Intern Med 142:979-995, 2005
123. Bow EJ: Point: Fluoroquinolone-based antibacterial chemoprophylaxis in neutropenic cancer patients works for defined populations, but must be used wisely. J Natl Compr Cancer Network 2:433-444, 2004
124. Kleinberg M. Counterpoint: Routine anti-bacterial prophylaxis is not indicated in neutropenic patients with hematological maligancies. J Natl Compr Cancer Network 2:445-451, 2004
125. Pena C, Albareda JM, Pallares R, Pujol M, Tubau F, Ariza J: Relationship between quinolone use and emergence of ciprofloxacin-resistant *Escherichia coli* in bloodstream infections. Antimicrob Agents Chemother 39:520-524, 1995
126. Perea S, Hidalgo M, Arcediano A, Ramos MJ, Gomez C, Hornedo J, et al: Incidence and clinical impact of fluoroquinolone-resistant *Escherichia coli* in the faecal flora of cancer patients treated with high dose chemotherapy and ciprofloxacin prophylaxis. J Antimicrob Chemother 44:117-120, 1999
127. Gomez L, Garau J, Estrada C, Marquez M, Dalmau D, Xercavins M, et al: Ciprofloxacin prophylaxis in patients with acute leukemia and granulocytopenia in an area with a high prevalence of ciprofloxacin-resistant *Escherichia coli*. Cancer 97:419-424, 2003
128. Bochud P-Y, Eggiman P, Calandra T, Van Melle G, Saghafi L, Francioli P: Bacteremia due to viridans streptococcus in neutropenic patients with cancer: Clinical spectrum and risk factors. Clin Infect Dis 18:25-31, 1994
129. Viscoli C, Bruzzi P, Castagnola E, Boni L, Calandra T, Gaya H, et al: Factors associated with bacteremia in febrile, granulocytopenic cancer patients. Eur J Cancer 30A:430-437, 1994
130. Elting LS, Rubenstein EB, Rolston KV, Bodey GP: Outcomes of bacteremia in patients with cancer and neutropenia: Observations from

two decades of epidemiological and clinical trials. Clin Infect Dis 25:247-259, 1997
131. Elting LS, Bodey GP, Keefe BH: Septicemia and shock syndrome due to viridans streptococci: A case-control study of predisposing factors. Clin Infect Dis 14:1201-1207, 1992
132. Gotzsche PC, Johansen HK: Meta-analysis of prophylactic or empirical antifungal treatment versus placebo or no treatment in patients with cancer complicated by neutropenia. BMJ 314:1238-1244, 1997
133. Kanda Y, Yamamoto R, Chizuka A, Hamaki T, Suguro M, Arai C, et al: Prophylactic action of oral fluconazole against infection in neutropenic patients—A meta-analysis of 16 randomized, controlled trials. Cancer 89:1611-1625, 2000
134. Bow EJ, Laverdiere M, Lussier N, Rotstein C, Cheang MS, Ioannou S: Antifungal prophylaxis for severely neutropenic chemotherapy recipients: A meta analysis of randomized-controlled clinical trials. Cancer 94:3230-3246, 2002
135. Glasmacher A, Prentice A, Gorschluter M, Engelhart S, Hahn C, Djulbegovic B, et al: Itraconazole prevents invasive fungal infections in neutropenic patients treated for hematologic malignancies: Evidence from a meta-analysis of 3,597 patients. J Clin Oncol 21:4615-4626, 2003
136. Cornely OA, Ullmann AJ, Karthaus M: Evidence-based assessment of primary antifungal prophylaxis in patients with hematologic malignancies. Blood 101:3365-3372, 2003
137. Marr KA, Crippa F, Leisenring W, Hoyle M, Boeckh M, Balajee SA, et al: Itraconazole versus fluconazole for prevention of fungal infections in patients receiving allogeneic stem cell transplants. Blood 103:1527-1533, 2004
138. Rotstein C, Bow EJ, Laverdiere M, Ioannou S, Carr D, Moghaddam N: Randomized placebo-controlled trial of fluconazole prophylaxis for neutropenic cancer patients: Benefit based on purpose and intensity of cytotoxic therapy. The Canadian Fluconazole Prophylaxis Study Group. Clin Infect Dis 28:331-340, 1999
139. Hughes WT, Armstrong D, Bodey GP, Bow EJ, Brown AE, Calandra T, et al: 2002 guidelines for the use of antimicrobial agents in neutropenic patients with cancer. Clin Infect Dis 34:730-751, 2002
140. Link H, Bohme A, Cornely OA, Hoffken K, Kellner O, Kern WV, et al: Antimicrobial therapy of unexplained fever in neutropenic patients—Guidelines of the Infectious Diseases Working Party (AGIHO) of the German Society of Hematology and Oncology (DGHO), Study Group Interventional Therapy of Unexplained Fever, Arbeitsgemeinschaft Supportivmassnahmen in der Onkologie (ASO) of the Deutsche Krebsgesellschaft (DKG-German Cancer Society). Ann Hematol 82:S105-S117, 2003 (suppl 2)
141. Freifeld AG, Baden LR, Brown AE, Elting L, Gelfand M, Greene JN, et al: Fever and neutropenia. J Natl Comp Cancer Network 2:390-432, 2004
142. Masaoka T: Febrile neutropenia—Guideline in Japan. Gan To Kagaku Ryoho 27:161-165, 2000
143. Crivellari D, Lombardi D, Spazzapan S, Veronesi A, Toffoli G: New oral drugs in older patients: A review of idarubicin in elderly patients. Crit Rev Oncol Hematol 49:153-163, 2004
144. Masaoka T: Evidence-based recommendations for antimicrobial use in febrile neutropenia in Japan: Executive summary. Clin Infect Dis 39:S49-S52, 2004 (suppl 1)
145. Garcia-Rodriguez JA, Gobernado M, Gomis M, Mensa J, Picazo J, Prieto J, et al: Clinical guide for the evaluation and treatment of patients with neutropenia and fever. Rev Esp Quimioter 14:75-83, 2001
146. Klastersky J, Paesmans M, Rubenstein EB, Boyer M, Elting L, Feld R, et al: The Multinational Association for Supportive Care in Cancer risk index: A multinational scoring system for identifying low-risk febrile neutropenic cancer patients. J Clin Oncol 18:3038-3051, 2000
147. Paul M, Soares-Weiser K, Leibovici L: Beta lactam monotherapy versus beta lactam-aminoglycoside combination therapy for fever with neutropenia: Systematic review and meta-analysis. BMJ 326:1111-1120, 2003
148. Furno P, Bucaneve G, Del Favero A: Monotherapy or aminoglycoside-containing combinations for empirical antibiotic treatment of febrile neutropenic patients: a meta-analysis. Lancet Infect Dis 2:231-242, 2002
149. Viscoli C: Management of infection in cancer patients. studies of the EORTC International Antimicrobial Therapy Group (IATG). Eur J Cancer 38:S82-S87, 2002 (suppl 4)
150. Wade JC, Glasmacher A: Vancomycin does not benefit persistently febrile neutropenic people with cancer. Cancer Treat Rev 30:119-126, 2004
151. Bow EJ, Noskin GA, Schwarer AP, Laverdiere M, Vesole DH: Efficacy of piperacillin/tazobactam as initial empiric therapy for febrile neutropenia in patients with hematological malignancy. Blood 102:281a, 2003 (abstr 1000)
152. Bow EJ, Laverdière M, Rotstein C: A systematic review of the efficacy of azoles and lipid-based formulations of amphotericin B as empirical anti-fungal therapy in persistently febrile neutropenic patients despite broad-spectrum anti-bacterial therapy. 40th Interscience Conference on Antimicrobial Agents and Chemotherapy, Toronto, Canada, September 17-20, 2000, p 364 (abstr 702)
153. Walsh TJ, Finberg RW, Arndt C, Hiemenz J, Schwartz C, Bodensteiner D, et al: Liposomal amphotericin B for empirical therapy in patients with persistent fever and neutropenia. National Institute of Allergy and Infectious Diseases Mycoses Study Group. N Engl J Med 340:764-771, 1999
154. Barrett JP, Vardulaki KA, Conlon C, Cooke J, Daza-Ramirez P, Evans EG, et al: A systematic review of the antifungal effectiveness and tolerability of amphotericin B formulations. Clin Ther 25:1295-1320, 2003
155. Boogaerts M, Winston DJ, Bow EJ, Garber G, Reboli AC, Schwarer AP, et al: Intravenous and oral itraconazole versus intravenous amphotericin B deoxycholate as empirical antifungal therapy for persistent fever in neutropenic patients with cancer who are receiving broad-spectrum antibacterial therapy. A randomized, controlled trial. Ann Intern Med 135:412-422, 2001
156. Walsh TJ, Pappas P, Winston DJ, Lazarus HM, Petersen F, Raffalli J, et al: Voriconazole compared with liposomal amphotericin B for empirical antifungal therapy in patients with neutropenia and persistent fever. N Engl J Med 346:225-234, 2002
157. Walsh TJ, Teppler H, Donowitz GR, Maertens JA, Baden LR, Dmoszynska A, et al: Caspofungin versus liposomal amphotericin B for empirical antifungal therapy in patients with persistent fever and neutropenia. N Engl J Med 351:1391-1402, 2004
158. Ascioglu S, Rex JH, de Pauw B, Bennett JE, Bille J, Crokaert F, et al: Defining opportunistic invasive fungal infections in immunocompromised patients with cancer and hematopoietic stem cell transplants: An international consensus. Clin Infect Dis 34:7-14, 2002
159. Martino R, Subira M, Rovira M, Solano C, Vazquez L, Sanz GF, et al: Invasive fungal infections after allogeneic peripheral blood stem cell transplantation: Incidence and risk factors in 395 patients. Br J Haematol 116:475-482, 2002
160. Mermel LA, Farr BM, Sherertz RJ, Raad II, O'Grady N, Harris JS, et al: Guidelines for the management of intravascular catheter-related infections. Clin Infect Dis 32:1249-1272, 2001
161. Azoulay E, Darmon M, Delclaux C, Fieux F, Bornstain C, Moreau D, et al: Deterioration of previous acute lung injury during neutropenia recovery. Crit Care Med 30:781-786, 2002
162. Barnes SG, Sattler FR, Ballard JO: Perirectal infections in acute leukemia—Improved survival after incision and debridement. Ann Intern Med 100:515-518, 1984
163. Maschmeyer G, Link H, Hiddemann W, Meyer P, Helmerking M, Eisenmann E, et al: Pulmonary infiltrates in febrile patients with neutropenia. Risk factors and outcome under empirical antimicrobial therapy in a randomized multicenter study. Cancer 73:2296-2304, 1994
164. Gomez L, Martino R, Rolston KV: Neutropenic enterocolitis: Spectrum of the disease and comparison of definite and possible cases. Clin Infect Dis 27:695-699, 1998

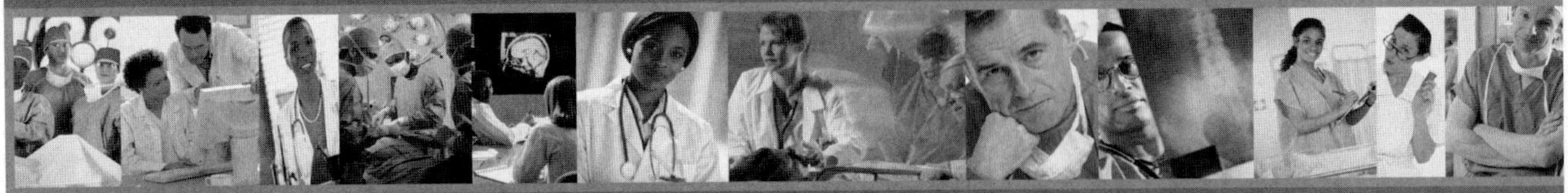

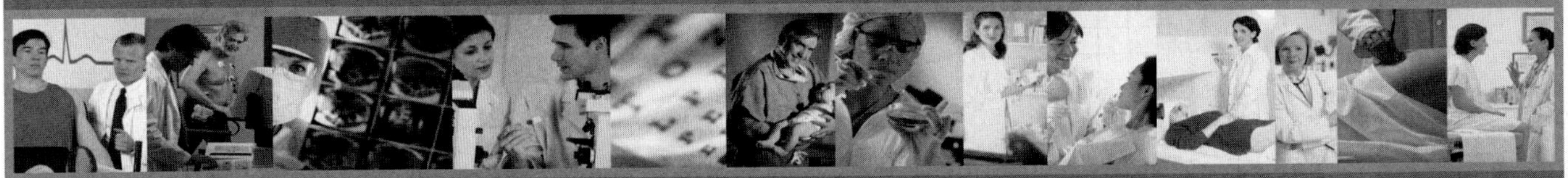

Hematology from Elsevier

Manual of Pediatric Hematology and Oncology FOURTH EDITION

Philip Lanzkowsky

Schneider Children's Hospital, New Hyde Park, NY, U.S.A.

Entirely updated to reflect modern thinking and protocols, the **Manual of Pediatric Hematology and Oncology** provides concise information needed for the day-to-day management of children with pediatric hematologic and oncologic diseases. The clear style allows readers to make an accurate diagnosis and permits him/her to treat patients even if they have not had extensive previous hematologic or oncologic experience. Pertinent advances in molecular genetics, cytogenetics, immunology, transplantation and biochemistry are the result of 40 years of practical experience by the author in the management of patients and incorporates various contributors who have had extensive clinical experience.

KEY FEATURES:

- Features numerous tables, flow diagrams, protocols, and algorithms for quick access of essential clinical information necessary for the diagnosis and management of these diseases in children
- Designed as a concise, easy-to-use guide for medical students, residents, fellows, pediatric hematologists/oncologists, pediatric nurses and nurse practitioners
- Much of the practical information contained in this manual is not found in standard textbooks

June 2005, Hardback, 856 pp.,
ISBN: 0120885247
$149.95 / £95.00 / €135.00

Encyclopedia of Heart Diseases

M. Gabriel Khan

Cardiologist at the Ottawa General Hospital and Associate Professor of Medicine at the University of Ottawa, Canada

The Encyclopedia of Heart Diseases is a sizeable source of in-depth information on the diseases that kill more than 12 million individuals worldwide each year. In fact, cardiovascular diseases are more prevalent than the combined incidence of all forms of cancer, diabetes, asthma and leukemia. In one volume, this Encylopedia thoroughly covers these ailments and also includes in-depth analysis of less common and rare heart conditions. Researchers, clinicians, and students alike will find this resource an invaluable tool for quick reference before approaching the primary literature.

July 2005, Hardback, 584 pp.,
ISBN: 0124060617
$129.95 / £80.00 / €115.00

Blood Substitutes

Robert M. Winslow

Sangart Inc., San Diego, CA, U.S.A.

Blood substitutes are solutions designed for use in patients who need blood transfusions, but for whom whole blood is not available, or is not safe. This interest has intensified in the wake of the AIDS and hepatitis C epidemics. **Blood Substitutes** describes the rationale, current approaches, clinical efficacy, and design issues for all blood substitutes now in clinical trials. The many summary diagrams and tables help make the book accessible to readers such as surgeons and blood bankers, who have less technical expertise than the biochemists and hematologists who are designing and testing blood substitutes.

September 2005, Hardback, 576 pp.,
ISBN: 0127597603
$199.95 / £125.00 / €180.00

ALSO AVAILABLE FROM ELSEVIER

Handbook of Pediatric Transfusion Medicine

Editor-in-Chief

Christopher Hillyer

Emory University, School of Medicine, Atlanta, GA, U.S.A.

Structured to be a companion to the **Handbook of Transfusion Medicine**, the **Handbook of Pediatric Transfusion Medicine** is dedicated to pediatric hematology-oncology and transfusion medicine, a field which remains ambiguous and which has generated few comprehensive texts. This book stands alone as one of the few texts that addresses transfusion issues specific to pediatric medicine. Written in an eminently readable style, this authoritative handbook is a requirement for any pediatric physician or caregiver.

February 2004, Hardback, 394 pp.,
ISBN: 0123487765
$129.95 / £80.00 / €115.00

The Blood Group Antigen FactsBook SECOND EDITION

Marion E. Reid
Christine Lomas-Francis

New York Blood Center, NY, U.S.A.

The second edition of **The Blood Group Antigen FactsBook** provides key information relating to human red blood cell membrane components carrying blood group antigens, the molecular basis of the antigens, their serological characteristics, and the clinical significance of blood group antibodies.

September 2003, Paperback, 584 pp.,
ISBN: 0125865856
$65.00 / £39.99 / €57.95

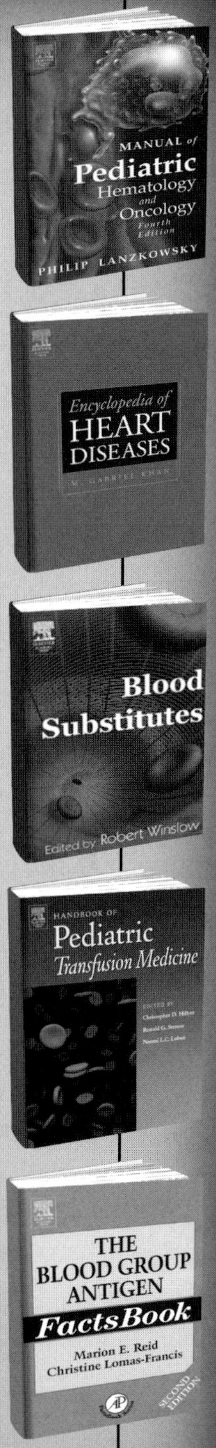

ELSEVIER
ACADEMIC PRESS

Visit books.elsevier.com/microbio for more information on these titles. Secure online ordering available.

Vol 43, No 2, Suppl 2 April 2006

Supplement to

Seminars in HEMATOLOGY

Neal S. Young · Photis Beris
Editors

Purine Analogues in the Treatment of Lymphoid Malignancies

Francine Foss and Julie M. Vose
Guest Editors

W.B. Saunders

Seminars in
HEMATOLOGY

Neal S. Young · Photis Beris
Editors

Peter A. Miescher, *Founding Editor* Ernst R. Jaffé, *Co-Editor Emeritus*

Editorial correspondence should be addressed to Photis Beris, MD, Division d'Hématologie, Hôpital Cantonal Universitaire, 25 rue Micheli-du-Crest, 1211 Geneve 14, Switzerland, or Neal S. Young, MD, 4400 17th Street, NW, Washington, DC 20011.

Business correspondence (subscriptions, change of address) should be addressed to the Publisher, Elsevier, 6277 Sea Harbor Dr, Orlando, FL 32887-4800; Email elspcs@elsevier.com.

Change of address notices, including both the old and new addresses of the subscriber, should be sent at least one month in advance.

Customer Service: 1-800-654-2452; outside the United States and Canada, (407) 345-4000.

Yearly subscription rates: United States and possessions: individual, $169.00; institution, $267.00; single issues, $81.00. All other countries: individual, $239.00; institution, $339.00; single issues, $81.00. Student and resident: United States and possessions, and Canada: $85.00; all other countries: $122.00. To receive student/resident rate, orders must be accompanied by name of affiliated institution, date of term, and the *signature* of program/residency coordinator on institution letterhead. Orders will be billed at individual rate until proof of status is received. Current prices are in effect for back volumes and back issues. Single issues, both current and back, exist in limited quantities and are offered for sale subject to availability. Back issues sold in conjunction with a subscription are on a prorated basis. Prices are subject to change without notice. *Checks* should be made payable to Elsevier and sent to *Seminars in Hematology*, Elsevier, Periodicals Department, PO Box 628239, Orlando, FL 32862-8239.

Other correspondence (copyediting, production) should be addressed to Elsevier, 1600 John F. Kennedy Blvd, Ste 1800, Philadelphia, PA 19103-2899.

The contents of *Seminars in Hematology* are indexed in *Index Medicus* and *MEDLINE, Current Contents/Clinical Medicine, Current Contents/Life Sciences,* Science Citation Index, and *EMBASE/* Excerpta Medica.

The *Seminars in Hematology* home page is located at *www.seminhematol.org*.

W.B. Saunders **Philadelphia, PA**

Seminars in HEMATOLOGY

Vol 43, No 2, Supplement 2, April 2006

Purine Analogues in the Treatment of Lymphoid Malignancies

Francine Foss and Julie M. Vose
Guest Editors

Purine Analogues in the Treatment of Lymphoid Malignancies S1
Francine Foss and Julie M. Vose

Pentostatin for the Treatment of Indolent Lymphoproliferative Disorders S2
Anthony D. Ho and Manfred Hensel

Purine Analogue Combinations for Indolent Lymphomas S11
Nicholas Di Bella and Farhad Ravandi

Role of Single-Agent Purine Analogues in Therapy of Peripheral T-Cell Lymphomas S22
Claire E. Dearden

Purine Analogues in Advanced T-Cell Lymphoid Malignancies S27
Razelle Kurzrock and Farhad Ravandi

The Role of Purine Analogues in Low-Intensity Regimens With Allogeneic Hematopoietic Stem Cell Transplantation S35
Francine M. Foss

Purine Analogue-Based Chemotherapy Regimens for Second-Line Therapy in Patients With Chronic Lymphocytic Leukemia S44
Nicole Lamanna and Mark A. Weiss

Purine Analogue-Based Chemotherapy Regimens for Patients With Previously Untreated B-Chronic Lymphocytic Leukemia S50
Neil E. Kay

Seminars in
HEMATOLOGY

Purine Analogues in the Treatment of Lymphoid Malignancies

Francine Foss and Julie M. Vose
Guest Editors

The articles in this supplement are based on presentations made during educational symposia held in 2005 during the Lymphoma Meeting in Lugano, Switzerland and the Pan Pacific Meeting in Hawaii.

This sole-sponsored supplement is being supported by an unrestricted educational grant from SuperGen. The opinions or views expressed in this supplement are those of the authors. It should not be assumed that they are expressing the opinions of their institutions, SuperGen, The Med Ed Group, Inc. or the publisher.

ELSEVIER

Seminars in
HEMATOLOGY

Volume 43, Number 2, Supplement 2 **April 2006**

Purine Analogues in the Treatment of Lymphoid Malignancies

Although some patients with lymphoid malignancies can be cured with standard chemotherapy, a large percentage of patients require alternative chemotherapy or stem cell transplantation for recurrent or resistant disease. T-cell non-Hodgkin's lymphomas (NHL) in particular have a worse outcome with standard chemotherapy and require novel agents for therapy. The purine analogues such as fludarabine, cladrabine, and pentostatin have now demonstrated activity in many cases of lymphoid malignancies and have been incorporated into several different combination chemotherapy regimens as well as in reduced intensity transplantation regimens.

Due to the wide range of uses for purine analogues, the current information on purine analogue treatment for NHL and chronic lymphocytic leukemia is reviewed in this series of articles. In this supplement, the use of purine analogues as well as alkylating agents and antibody therapy for lymphoplasmocytic lymphoma is reviewed by Dr Anthony Ho. In the next chapter, Drs Nicholas Di Bella and Farhad Ravandi review the use of purine analogue combinations for indolent NHL. Due to the difficulty in treating T-cell NHL, the current use of purine analogues and combinations for peripheral T-cell lymphoma and cutaneous T-cell lymphomas is reviewed by Drs Dearden, Kurzrock, and Ravandi. The use of purine analogues for the treatment of chronic lymphocytic leukemia either as first-line or second-line therapy is reviewed in two articles by Drs Lamanna and Weiss as well as Dr Kay. Finally, the use of purine analogues as part of a reduced intensity conditioning regimen for hematologic malignancies is reviewed by Dr Francine Foss.

These chapters all have a common theme outlining the usefulness of purine analogues in various clinical setting for indolent lymphoid malignancies. New combinations and the use of purine analogues in alternative clinical situations such as stem cell transplantation offer new modalities of treatments for these resistant lymphomas which need to be further explored in clinical trials.

Francine Foss, MD
Director of Immunology
Professor of Medicine
Yale Cancer Center
New Haven, CT

Julie M. Vose, MD
Neumann M. and Mildred E. Harris, Professor
Chief, Section of Hematology/Oncology
Department of Internal Medicine
University of Nebraska Medical Center
Omaha, NE
Guest Editors

Address correspondence to Francine Foss, MD, Director of Immunology, Professor of Medicine, Yale Cancer Center, Medical Oncology, 333 Cedar St, PO Box 208032, New Haven, CT 06520-8032. E-mail: Francine.foss@yale.edu

doi:10.1053/j.seminhematol.2005.12.014

ELSEVIER

Seminars in
HEMATOLOGY

Pentostatin for the Treatment of Indolent Lymphoproliferative Disorders

Anthony D. Ho and Manfred Hensel

Purine analogues have been shown to be active in a variety of B- and T-cell malignancies. Among them, pentostatin is also a tight binding inhibitor of adenosine deaminase (ADA), a key enzyme of purine metabolism. ADA is present in all human tissues, with the highest levels in the lymphoid system. Early clinical trials with pentostatin used high doses for acute lymphoblastic leukemias, which were characterized by high levels of ADA. Through the efforts of a few investigators, low-dose regimens that are active and well tolerated for indolent lymphoid malignancies have been developed. Myelosuppressive adverse effects have been shown to be minimal using these schedules. Lymphoplasmacytic lymphoma (LL) is an indolent chronic B-cell lymphoproliferative disorder moderately responsive to alkylating agents. All of the purine analogues have shown activity in LL. However, the advantage of pentostatin over the other agents is the relatively specific toxicity to lymphoid cells and the paucity of myelosuppression as a single agent. No direct comparisons of the agents have been investigated, although pentostatin may be considered to be preferred since it has not been associated with toxicity to myeloid progenitors in colony assays. This is of significance for patients who might benefit from high-dose chemotherapy with autologous stem cell transplantation.
Semin Hematol 43(suppl 2):S2-S10

Adenosine deaminase (ADA) is a key enzyme of purine metabolism and catalyzes the irreversible conversion of adenosine to inosine and deoxyadenosine to deoxyinosine.[1] Interest in the purine degradative enzymes was stimulated by the discovery that inherited deficiency was associated with immunodeficiency diseases.[2,3] Congenital deficiency of ADA, for example, is associated with a specific defect in lymphocyte maturation and function. Children born with this congenital error of metabolism present with lymphopenia and severe combined immunodeficiency disease (SCID) but without deleterious effects on the other hematopoietic elements and organ systems.[2] Deficiency of purine nucleoside phosphorylase (PNP), another purine degradative enzyme, is associated with severely defective T-cell immunity but normal B-cell immunity.[3,4]

ADA is present in virtually all human tissues, but the highest levels are found in the lymphoid system, such as lymph nodes, spleen, and thymus.[5,6] Among these, activity in T cells is higher than in B cells,[7] a relationship that remains true for neoplastic T and B cells.[8,9]

Two mechanisms have been proposed to account for the toxicity of congenital ADA deficiency to lymphocyte precursors. Accumulation of dATP may inhibit the enzyme ribonucleotide reductase and thus cause starvation of the other deoxyribonucleotides, dCTP and dGTP.[10] Alternatively, accumulation of adenosine may lead to a build-up of S-adenosyl homocysteine (SAH) and inhibition of SAH-hydrolase.[10-12] This in turn causes a fall in cellular S-adenosyl methionine (SAM) concentration and thus an Inhibition of methylation reactions in DNA, RNA, and protein synthesis.[11-14]

The observation that congenital deficiency of ADA is associated with a specific defect in lymphocyte function and SCID but normal development of other organ systems has suggested that inhibition of this enzyme may provide an avenue for selective chemotherapy.[1,9,15]

2′-Deoxycoformycin (pentostatin)

Pentostatin (2′-deoxycoformycin) (Nipent®, Supergen, Dublin, CA) was isolated from culture broths of *Streptomyces antibioticus*[16] and has been shown to be a tight-binding inhibitor of ADA.[17] Early clinical trials performed in the 1970s and 1980s have suggested that T-cell neoplasms characterized by

Department of Medicine V, University of Heidelberg, Heidelberg, Germany.
Address correspondence to Anthony D. Ho, MD, Department of Medicine V, University of Heidelberg, Im Neuenheimer Feld 410, 69120 Heidelberg, Germany. E-mail: Anthony_dick.ho@urz.uni-heidelberg.de

 0037-1963/06/$-see front matter
doi:10.1053/j.seminhematol.2005.12.005

high levels of ADA were responsive to pentostatin.[18-20] Thus, t-cell acute lymphoblastic leukemia (tALL) blasts, which have extremely high ADA levels, responded readily whereas common acute lymphoblastic leukemia (cALL) cells with comparatively lower ADA levels were not responsive.[19,20] However, in the dose levels and schedules used at that time, significant renal, pulmonary, and central nervous system toxicities were noted.[18,20,21] Of major concern also was the fact that toxicity was unpredictable: some patients tolerated up to 30 mg/m²/d for 5 days with minimal adverse effects, while others succumbed to toxicity at lower doses.

Through the efforts of a few investigators, well-tolerated and effective regimens have emerged. With low-dose regimens (4-5 mg/m²/d once every week or once every other week or 2 to 3 consecutive days every 2 to 3 weeks) encouraging results have been obtained in hairy cell leukemia (HCL), refractory non-Hodgkin's lymphomas (NHLs), and in B-cell chronic lymphocytic leukemia (CLL).[22-25]

The assumption that pentostatin would be more effective in T-cell neoplasms has been proven incorrect. This drug is active in cells of both T- and B-cell origin. The activity of pentostatin might, to a certain extent, depend on the enzyme profile of the malignant lymphoid cells to be treated. A lower dose of the drug is active in indolent lymphoid neoplasms with low intracellular concentrations of ADA, which can be inhibited by small amounts of the drug.[22-25]

Another remarkable feature of pentostatin is that it is cytotoxic to nondividing cells. The exact mechanism in nonproliferative cells is still unknown, but it may be caused by DNA strand breaks,[24,26] NAD depletion,[26] inhibition of S-adenosyl homocysteine hydrolase,[11-13] or incorporation of the drug into DNA.[27]

Clinical Applications of Pentostatin

Although clinical trials in the 1980s have demonstrated remarkable activity of pentostatin in HCL and B-cell chronic lymphocytic leukemia (B-CLL), its role for treatment of other lymphoproliferative diseases has not been adequately exploited until recent years. During this period, it was shown that indolent lymphoid malignancies with the lowest concentrations of ADA are extremely responsive to pentostatin.

Hairy Cell Leukemia

HCL is a relatively rare B-cell lymphoproliferative disorder. The incidence is estimated to be 2% of leukemias in adults, with 3.5 new cases per 1 million people per year.[28] The disease is characterized by infiltration of bone marrow and spleen by mononuclear cells of B-lymphocyte origin. The most remarkable features are massive splenomegaly and pancytopenia. Symptoms include fatigue, bleeding, and especially infection as a result of neutropenia and monocytopenia. Before 1980, the standard treatment for HCL was splenectomy, while chemotherapy was shown to induce further cytopenia without any benefits. In the early 1980s, treatment with interferon-alfa was found to improve hematologic parameters in symptomatic patients but complete remissions (CRs) were rare.[29-31] The activity of pentostatin in HCL was first reported in 1984.[24] Phase II studies in pretreated as well as in untreated patients demonstrated that pentostatin was highly active as a single agent, with CR rates of 60% to 90%.[32-36] A large phase III study directly compared pentostatin with interferon in 313 untreated patients. Patients who received pentostatin (4 mg/m² intravenously every 2 weeks) had a significantly higher clinical remission rate with remarkably durable responses.[37] This pivotal trial was the basis for the Food and Drug Administration (FDA) to approve pentostatin as first-line treatment with HCL.

Long-term follow-up of this trial also showed that only 18% of patients who achieved a CR upon treatment with pentostatin have relapsed and 83% of patients are still alive.[38] The median observation period was 9 years. In contrast, long-term follow-up on patients treated with cladribine showed that 36% of patients with an initial CR relapsed after a median follow-up of 9 years.[39] Based on two single-arm trials with a total of 124 patients, cladribine (Leustatin, Ortho Biotech Bridgewater, NJ) was approved by the FDA for the first- and second-line treatment of active HCL.

Toxicity spectrum associated with pentostatin compared favorably with cladribine.[37-40] Hematologic toxicities of grade 3/4 neutropenia occurred only in 19% of patients, with no significant thrombocytopenia or anemia. This confirms the relative specific activity of pentostatin towards lymphoid cells. Neutropenic fever was reported in 27% of patients treated with pentostatin, whereas neutropenic fever associated with cladribine was observed in 40% of patients.

B-Cell Chronic Lymphocytic Leukemia

B-CLL represents the most common adult leukemia and is characterized by monoclonal proliferation of abnormal B lymphocytes in blood, bone marrow, and lymph nodes, infiltrating the liver and the spleen. Chlorambucil has been the standard first-line treatment option for decades, inducing hematologic improvements in 60% to 70% of patients. Combination chemotherapy regimens such as CVP (cyclophosphamide, vincristine, and prednisone) and CHOP (cyclophosphamide, doxorubicin, vincristine, and prednisone) have been applied, but response and survival rates were not found to be superior to chlorambucil.[41] Fludarabine (Fludara, Berlex Laboratories, Richmond, CA) is approved for relapsed or refractory B-CLL following treatment with alkylating agents, and has been investigated extensively in first-line use.

The efficacy of fludarabine was compared to chlorambucil in the primary treatment of CLL in a randomized trial of 509 patients.[42] The overall response rate in the fludarabine arm was 63%, compared with 37% in the chlorambucil arm. Responses in the combination arm were similar to single-agent fludarabine. Median time to progression was significantly prolonged among patients who received fludarabine (20 months *v* 14 months in the chlorambucil arm); however, overall survival was the same in both treatment arms.

Pentostatin was shown in phase I/II clinical trials to be active in heavily pretreated patients. In a study of 28 patients

Table 1 Comparison of Purine Analogue-Induced Hematologic Toxicities

	Neutropenia		Thrombocytopenia		Anemia	
	Grade 3	Grade 4	Grade 3	Grade 4	Grade 3	Grade 4
HCL						
Pentostatin						
Grever et al[37] (n = 158)	5%	14%	3%	0	1%	0
Cladribine						
Saven et al[40] (n = 135)	16%	71%	10%	10%	20%	2%
CLL (relapsed/refractory)						
Pentostatin						
Dillman et al[43] (n = 39)	0		26%		23%	
Ho et al[25] (n = 26)	15%		12%		0%	
Johnson et al[44] (n = 29)	17%		10%		3%	
Fludarabine						
Keating et al[84]	56%		25%		NR	
Pentostatin + cyclophosphamide (600–900 mg/m^2)	31%*		30%		0	
Weiss et al[46] (n = 23)						
Cladribine + cyclophosphamide (350 mg/m^2)	41%*		24%		24%	
Montillo et al[85] (n = 29)						
Fludarabine + cyclophosphamide (300–350 mg/m^2)	88%		40%		NA	
O'Brien et al[86] (n = 128)						
Low-grade NHL						
Pentostatin + rituximab	10%		NR		2%	
Drapkin et al[87] (n = 60)						
Fludarabine + rituximab	73%		10%		8%	
Czuczman et al[88] (n = 40)						

Abbreviations: CLL, chronic lymphocytic leukemia; HCL, hairy cell leukemia; IFN, interferon alpha; NHL, non-Hodgkin's lymphoma; NR, not reported.
*Prophylactic growth factors

with pretreated B-CLL, Grever et al[23] reported that one CR, four partial responses (PRs), and four hematologic improvements were achieved with pentostatin. Dillmann et al[43] showed that an overall response rate of 26% could be attained in 39 patients with B-CLL pretreated with one prior regimen or without pretreatment. In a group of 26 patients who have been heavily pretreated, Ho et al reported seven PRs (27%) and five clinical improvements in patients treated with with pentostatin.[25] Whereas comparable activity could be observed using fludarabine or cladribine as a single agent, pentostatin was unique as responses could be achieved with only slight and transient myelosuppression (Table 1). Remissions could be achieved even in patients who did not respond to fludarabine, suggesting a lack of cross-resistance.[44,45] Lacking comparative trials, the relative merits of pentostatin, fludarabine, and cladribine are not definitively known. However, as pentostatin has been shown to be less myelotoxic than all other agents, the combination of pentostatin with chlorambucil, cyclophosphamide or antibodies might be beneficial as front line therapy.

In a phase II study, the combination of pentostatin and cyclophosphamide has been evaluated in 23 patients with previously treated CLL.[46] These patients received a median of three prior regimens and 87% of the patients had exposure to fludarabine and 78% to alkylating agents. Pentostatin was administered at a dose of 4 mg/m^2, in combination with 600 mg/m^2 or with 900 mg/m^{2}of cyclophosphamide. There were 17 responses (74%; 95% confidence interval, 63% to 85%), including four CRs (17%) and 13 PRs (57%). In the 13 patients treated with fludarabine, there were 10 responses (77%), including one CR.

A phase I/II study in untreated CLL evaluated the combination of pentostatin, chlorambucil, and prednisone.[47] In the phase I portion of the study, 2 mg/m^2 was established as the preferred dose for pentostatin in this combination. Subsequently, patients received pentostatin 2 mg/m^2, chlorambucil 30 mg/m^2, and prednisone 80 mg/d, on days 1 to 5 of each 14-day cycle. The overall response rate was 87%, including CRs in 45% of patients. The CR rate for patients with stage I/II disease was 55%, compared with 30% in patients who entered the study with grade III/IV disease. The median response duration was 33 months. Severe neutropenia was reported in 41% of patients. Three patients died of treatment-related infections and a total of 29 patients (74%) had at least one episode of documented infection.

Indolent Non-Hodgkin's Lymphoma

Indolent NHL refers to a group of B-cell neoplastic diseases that include follicular lymphoma, small lymphocytic lymphoma (SLL), lymphoma of mucosa-associated lymphoid tissue (MALT), and lymphoplasmacytic lymphoma (LL or Waldenström macroglobulinemia [WM]). Although these disease entities have a relatively benign course and respond favorably to radiation or chemotherapy treatment strategies, they have a propensity to recur and are currently considered to be incurable, with a median survival of 6 to 8 years. Once the disease is disseminated and advanced, the management has been considered to be palliative. Initially, watchful waiting seems to be the appropriate therapeutic approach. Indications for treatment include symptoms related to cytopenias, tumor-related compression, and recurrent infections.

The combination of pentostatin plus rituximab was evaluated in a phase II study of 60 patients with indolent NHL.[48] Rituximab 375 mg/m^2 and pentostatin 4 mg/m^2 were administered once weekly for 4 weeks, followed by a 1-week rest. The overall response rate was 77%. Twenty-three percent of patients had a CR, 35% a PR, and 10.5% an unconfirmed PR. Median duration of response was 11 months (range, 2.3 to 22 months); median time to progression was 15 months (range, <1 to 25 months). Severe neutropenia was the most common adverse event and was limited to six patients (10%). Based on the results from this trial of pentostatin plus rituximab, a pilot study was initiated that also added mitoxantrone to this combination regimen. The overall confirmed response rate was 71% (CR, 38%; PR, 33%); with the inclusion of unconfirmed CR, the overall response rate was 83%. The median time to disease progression was 14 months (range, 2.8 to 17.5 months). Severe neutropenia occurred in 67% of patients; febrile neutropenia was reported in 17% of patients. The addition of mitoxantrone moderately increased response rates but was also associated with an increased rate of myelosuppression.

Lymphoplasmacytic Lymphoma (Waldenström macroglobulinemia)

LL or WM is a rare chronic B-cell lymphoproliferative disorder associated with monoclonal immunoglobulin M (IgM).[49] Waldenström originally described it in 1944.[50] According to the Revised European-American Lymphoma (REAL) classification and World Health Organization (WHO) criteria, it is characterized by bone marrow infiltration through small lymphocytes showing plasmacytoid or plasma cell differentiation, and IgM monoclonal protein of any concentration.[51] At diagnosis, most of the patients show symptoms that are related to tumor infiltration or monoclonal IgM. LL always involves the bone marrow and most prominent manifestations related to tumor infiltration are cytopenias. Other symptoms include fever, night sweats, and weight loss, and about one third of the patients presents with lymphadenopathy, splenomegaly, or hepatomegaly. Manifestations related to circulating IgM include hyperviscosity, cryoglobulinemia, cold agglutinin disease, neuropathy, and amyloidosis.

However, some patients fulfill the criteria for the diagnosis without any symptoms or signs, organomegaly or lymphadenopathy, and are classified as asymptomatic WM.[49] As such patients might remain stable for years, they should not receive specific treatment. Initiation of specific therapy is appropriate for patients who develop symptoms and signs related to IgM and /or tumor infiltration as mentioned above.[52] Thus, patients who develop a hemoglobin level of less than 100 g/L, or platelet count of less than 100×10^9/L, bulky adenopathy, or organomegaly should be considered for treatment. Hemoglobin and β_2-microglobulin levels of less than 100 g/L and less than 3.0 mg/dL, respectively, could be considered as major poor prognostic factors.[49,52]

Response criteria for WM/LL have thus far been heterogeneous. The Second International Workshop on WM delineated common response criteria.[53] CR is defined as complete disappearance of serum and urine monoclonal protein by immunofixation, resolution of lymphadenopathy and organomegaly, and absence of malignant cells by bone marrow histologic evaluation. PR is defined as a greater than 50% reduction of serum monoclonal protein and a greater than 50% reduction of lymphadenopathy or organomegaly. Symptoms due to LL must have resolved.

Treatment of Waldenström Macroglobulinemia

Plasmapheresis

For patients whose predominant symptoms are associated with elevated serum viscosity, plasmapheresis is an effective means of rapidly reducing circulation IgM.[49,52] Plasmapheresis could be repeated daily or every other day until symptoms have resolved. However, systemic chemotherapy must be initiated to achieve long-term effects. Longer-term plasma exchange might be justified in patients who suffer predominantly from hyperviscosity and who are refractory to systemic treatment.

Chemotherapy

The standard primary therapy for WM has been the administration of oral alkylating agents such as chlorambucil, melphalan, or cyclophosphamide.[49,52] Chlorambucil has been most commonly used. Approximately 50% of the patients achieve a PR, and CRs are rare. Chlorambucil has been administered either on a daily basis at low doses or intermittently at higher doses, with similar outcomes. Addition of corticosteroids has been beneficial for patients with autoimmune hemolytic anemia, mixed cryoglobulinemia, or cold agglutinin disease but has not been shown to increase response rates or survival.

Fludarabine

Fludarabine has been reported in the treatment of WM since 1990.[54] An initial attempt with fludarabine as a single agent in 10 pretreated patients and one untreated patient showed that this agent is active, with five objective responses. The median time to 50% reduction of IgM was 5.2 months and the median response duration was 1 year.

A more recent study in 182 patients (35% of them pretreated) showed an overall response rate of 36% with 3% achieving a CR.[55] Fludarabine was administered at a dose of 30 mg/m^2 daily for 5 days and repeated monthly. Four to eight cycles were given. Median event-free survival was 28 months and overall survival was 84 months. There was no difference in response rate between the 118 patients who

Table 2 Response to Pentostatin and Cyclophosphamide (PC) (n = 4) or Pentostatin, Cyclophosphamide, and Rituximab (R-PC) (n = 13) in Patients With Waldenström Macroglobulinemia[77]

	Pretreated (n = 8)	Primary (n = 9)	All (n = 17)
Median no. of cycles			4 (1–6)
Complete response	2	0	2 (11.7%)
Partial response	3	6	9 (58.8%)
Overall response	5 (62.5%)	6 (66.6%)	11 (64.7%)
Stable disease	3	3	6 (35.2%)
Median follow-up			13 mo (2–48)

were untreated and the 64 who were pretreated with systemic therapy.

The activity of fludarabine in WM has been shown by a randomized trial that compared salvage treatment with either fludarabine alone, or cyclophosphamide, doxorubicin, and prednisone.[56] Twenty-eight percent of fludarabine-treated patients responded, versus 11% of patients who received combination chemotherapy. The median time of disease-free survival was also significantly longer in patients who received fludarabine, whereas the survival was similar in both arms.

Fludarabine has led to severe suppression of $CD4^+$ cells, resulting in impaired cell-mediated immunity. Frequent opportunistic infections have been observed. Severe myelosuppression could also be seen if more than six cycles of fludarabine have been administered.[57-59]

Cladribine

Cladribine has been shown to be active in patients with WM. In one of the first studies, 29 patients, nine of them without previous treatment, received cladribine as a continuous infusion at a dosage of 0.1 mg/kg body weight daily for 7 days for two courses. Fifty-nine percent of the patients responded. One treatment-related death was reported.[60] These results have been confirmed using cladribine by continuous infusion as a 2-hour daily infusion, or subcutaneous injection with response rates of 38 to 54%.[61-63]

Although the immediate toxicity of cladribine is mild, the principle dose-limiting toxicity of cladribine is bone marrow suppression.[64,65,66] Fever is often observed after cladribine administration as well as immunosuppression and subsequent fatal infections. Renal and neurologic side effects and local skin reactions have also been reported. Immune-mediated hemolysis has developed after cladribine therapy, and two of the four patients died as a consequence.[67]

Rituximab

As the monoclonal antibody rituximab targeting CD20 has been used successfully for the treatment of various B-cell malignancies and as CD20 is always present on the malignant WM cells, it becomes a rational treatment for this disease. Since 1999, the results of at least six clinical trials using rituximab as single agent for WM have been reported.[68-73] Response rates in pretreated patients varied between 20% to 75% and in untreated patients, 35%. In the early studies, rituximab was administered at a dose of 375 mg/m²/ wk for 4 weeks. The median time to treatment failure was about 8 months. Subsequent studies applied an extended schedule of two sets of four infusions at weeks 1 to 4 and 12 to 16. Forty-eight percent of the patients (14 of 26 evaluable patients) achieved a PR and 17% (five patients), a minor response. Time to maximum response was slow and exceeded 3 months.

As rituximab is an active and nonmyelosuppressive drug, its combination with chemotherapy became a logical rationale. It has been combined with cladribine and cyclophosphamide and a PR was reported in 94% of 17 patients.[53] Treon et al[74] have combined rituximab with fludarabine and an objective response was accomplished in 80% of patients .

Our group has combined rituximab with pentostatin for patients with low-grade NHL, ie, LL, and small lymphocytic, well-differentiated lymphoma (B-CLL). The results for WM or LL are described below.

Pentostatin

Although the activity of pentostatin for treatment of WM was already demonstrated in 1980s,[75] no further reports on the efficacy of pentostatin have been published until recently.

Based on our experience in achieving a dramatic and durable response in a 43-year-old woman with refractory WM and severe hemolytic anemia (Ho et al, unpublished results), our group has initiated a clinical trial using the combination pentostatin (4 mg/m²) and cyclophosphamide (600 mg/m²), repeated once every 21 days. The patient we observed developed refractory disease to chlorambucil, and subsequently to the combination chemotherapy CVP in 1998. She achieved a CR after six cycles of pentostatin and cyclophosphamide. Thereafter, progenitor cells could be harvested from the peripheral blood after one leukapheresis procedure for eventual autologous transplantation. However, she has remained in a remission since then and high-dose therapy was never performed.

Encouraged by the data reported by Lamanna et al,[76] we have subsequently added rituximab to the combination.[77] The result of the induction therapy is shown in Table 2. The responders subsequently received rituximab maintenance treatment in the following schedule: 375 mg/m², every 3 months, for 24 months. In the pilot phase we observed no disease progression in nine responders receiving maintenance rituximab. In three patients who achieved PR, the remission status improved upon maintenance therapy. In two patients, the IgM levels have normalized whereas the criteria for a CR could be accomplished in one patient. Toxicities are

Table 3 Toxicity of Rituximab, Pentostatin, and Cyclophosphamide (R-PC) Compared to Other Combinations of Purine Analogues in Patients With CLL and Waldenström's Macroglobulinemia

					Toxicity WHO Grade 3/4			
					Neutrophils (% of courses)		Platelets (% of courses)	
Trial	Therapy	n	ORR (%)	CR (%)	3°	4°	3°	4°
Wierda et al[89] (treated)	FC-R	177	73	25	21	41	10	7
Keating et al[90] (untreated)	FC-R	224	95	70	24	28	4	1
Robak et al[91] (untreated)	2-CDA/C	152	82	28	28		16	
Hensel et al[92] (CLL/WM, treated/untreated)	PC-R	23	74	6.6	3.3		5.5	2.2

Abbreviations: F, fludarabine; C, cyclophosphamide; R, rituximab; P, pentostatin; CDA, cladribine; ORR, overall response rate; CR, complete response; °, grade; WHO, World Health Organization; CLL, chronic lymphocytic leukemia; WM, Waldenström's macroglobulinemia.

mild to moderate in the dose schedule administered. Hematologic toxicity is favourable as compared to other combinations of purine analogues in patients with CLL (Table 3). The definitive role of pentostatin in combination with rituximab is being explored in ongoing studies.

Hematopoietic Progenitor Cell Transplantation

As high-dose chemotherapy followed by autologous progenitor cell transplantation (APCT) has been shown to be beneficial for several B-cell chronic malignancies such as B-CLL and multiple myeloma, several studies have explored the efficacy of this strategy in WM.[78-82] The number of patients in each of these analyses was limited. Nevertheless, Dreger et al[81] reported a median progression-free survival of 70 months and a 4-year estimate of overall survival of 93% in 14 patients treated with high-dose cyclophosphamide and total body irradiation. Despite all the limitations, APCT seems to be feasible, safe and might induce durable remissions. It was also shown that prior therapy with the purine analogues fludarabine or cladribine might induce protracted myelosuppression and collection of an adequate amount of progenitor cells thereafter might not be feasible. This is most probably not the case with pentostatin.

Experience with allogeneic transplantation for patients with WM has been even more limited. Conventional conditioning regimens are associated with severe and life-threatening toxicities but allogeneic transplantation after nonmyeloablative conditioning might be a novel treatment option for young patients with advanced and refractory disease.[81]

Future Perspectives

Although clinical trials in the 1980s have demonstrated a remarkable activity of pentostatin in HCL and B-CLL with minimal myelosuppression, its role for treatment of other lymphoproliferative diseases has not been adequately exploited until recent years. During the 1980s, investigations on the correlations between enzyme make-up of the disease entities and response, as well as between biochemical sequels of pentostatin treatment on the malignant cells and clinical response, were reported extensively. It could be shown that indolent lymphoid malignancies with the lowest concentrations of ADA are extremely responsive to pentostatin. Diseases such as Sézary syndrome and T-CLL, characterized by higher cellular ADA levels, are moderately responsive to the low-dose schedule. Probably a "titration" of the drug, ie, higher dose levels adjusted to the enzyme profile of the disease might be necessary.[1,9,13]

In dose levels and schedules that are active in HCL, B-CLL, the myelosuppressive side effect has been confirmed to be minimal and such dose levels have been shown to be active also in other indolent NHL such as LL/WM. The combination with cyclophosphamide and subsequently with rituximab has demonstrated significant activity for treatment of both pretreated and untreated WM. The advantage of pentostatin containing regimens instead of other purine analogues is its low rate of severe myelosuppression. The latter side effect might render collection of hematopoietic progenitor cells impossible after pretreatment with fludarabine[83] or with cladribine.

Although there are no data from prospective randomized studies to recommend the use of one purine analogue over another, the relative specificity of pentostatin might render it the preferable agent in disease entities that are similarly responsive to the three agents. This is especially so for patients who might benefit from autologous stem cell transplantation. Exposure to pentostatin is unlikely to influence stem cell collection, but future trials have to address this question. Pending further confirmation, pentostatin might be the preferred agent for most of the rare and indolent lymphoproliferative diseases.

References

1. Ho AD, Knauf W, Ganeshaguru K, Hunstein W, Hoffbrand AV: Purine degradative enzymes in circulating malignant cells of patients with chronic B cell neoplasia. Hematol Oncol 5:9-17, 1987
2. Giblett ER, Anderson JE, Cohen F, Pollara B, Meuwissen HJ: Adenosine-deaminase deficiency in two patients with severely impaired cellular immunity. Lancet 2:1067-1069, 1972
3. Giblett ER, Ammann AJ, Wara DW, Sandman R, Diamond LK: Nucleoside-phosphorylase deficiency in a child with severely defective T-cell immunity and normal B-cell immunity. Lancet 1:1010-1013, 1975

4. Biggar WD, Giblett ER, Ozere RL, Grover BD: A new form of nucleoside phosphorylase deficiency in two brothers with defective T-cell function. J Pediatr 92:354-357, 1978
5. Barton R, Martiniuk F, Hirschhorn R, Goldschneider I: The distribution of adenosine deaminase among lymphocyte populations in the rat. J Immunol 122:216-220, 1979
6. Chechik BE, Schrader WP, Minowada J: An immunomorphologic study of adenosine deaminase distribution in human thymus tissue, normal lymphocytes, and hematopoietic cell lines. J Immunol 126: 1003-1007, 1981
7. Tung R, Silber R, Quagliata F, Conklyn M, Gottesman J, Hirschhorn R: Adenosine deaminase activity in chronic lymphocytic leukemia. Relationship to B- and T-cell subpopulations. J Clin Invest 57:756-761, 1976
8. Ganeshaguru K, Lee N, Llewellin P, Prentice HG, Hoffbrand AV, Catovsky D, et al: Adenosine deaminase concentrations in leukaemia and lymphoma: Relation to cell phenotypes. Leuk Res 5:215-222, 1981
9. Ho AD, Ganeshaguru K: Enzymes of purine metabolism in lymphoid neoplasms, clinical relevance for treatment with enzyme inhibitors. Klin Wochenschr 66:467-474, 1988
10. Cohen A, Hirschhorn R, Horowitz SD, Rubinstein A, Polmar SH, Hong R, et al: Deoxyadenosine triphosphate as a potentially toxic metabolite in adenosine deaminase deficiency. Proc Natl Acad Sci U S A 75:472-476, 1978
11. Hershfield MS, Kredich NM: Resistance of an adenosine kinase-deficient human lymphoblastoid cell line to effects of deoxyadenosine on growth, S-adenosylhomocysteine hydrolase inactivation, and dATP accumulation. Proc Natl Acad Sci U S A 77:4292-4296, 1980
12. Hershfield MS, Kredich NM, Koller CA, Mitchell BS, Kurtzberg J, Kinney TR, et al: S-adenosylhomocysteine catabolism and basis for acquired resistance during treatment of T-cell acute lymphoblastic leukemia with 2′-deoxycoformycin alone and in combination with 9-beta-D-arabinofuranosyladenine. Cancer Res 43:3451-3458, 1983
13. Ho AD, Ganeshaguru K, Knauf WU, Dietz G, Trede I, Hunstein W, et al: Clinical response to deoxycoformycin in chronic lymphoid neoplasms and biochemical changes in circulating malignant cells in vivo. Blood 72:1884-1890, 1988
14. Ganeshaguru K, Ho AD, Piga A, Catovsky D, Hoffbrand AV: Biochemical mechanisms of deoxycoformycin toxicity in chronic leukemias. Leuk Res 11:941-945, 1987
15. Gelfand EW, Lee JJ, Dosch HM: Selective toxicity of purine deoxynucleosides for human lymphocyte growth and function. Proc Natl Acad Sci U S A 76:1998-2002, 1979
16. Woo PWK, Dion HW, Lange SM, Dahl LF, Durham LJ: A novel adenosine and araA deaminase inhibitor, (R)-3-(2-deoxy-β-D-Erythropento-furanosyl)-3,6,7,8-tetra-hydroimidazo (4,5-d) (1,3) diazepin-8-ol. J Heterocyclic Chem 11:641-643, 1974
17. Agarwal RP, Spector T, Parks REJ: Inhibition of adenosine deaminase by various inhibitors. Biochem Pharmacol 26:359-367, 1977
18. Poplack DG, Sallan SE, Rivera G, Holcenberg J, Murphy SB, Blatt J, et al: Phase I study of 2′-deoxycoformycin in acute lymphoblastic leukemia. Cancer Res 41:3343-3346, 1981
19. Prentice HG, Smyth JF, Ganeshaguru K, Wonke B, Bradstock KF, Janossy G, et al: Remission induction with adenosine-deaminase inhibitor 2′-deoxycoformycin in Thy-lymphoblastic leukaemia. Lancet 2:170-172, 1980
20. Prentice HG, Russell NH, Lee N, Ganeshaguru K, Blacklock H, Piga A, et al: Therapeutic selectivity of and predication of response to 2′-deoxycoformycin in acute leukaemia. Lancet 2:1250-1254, 1981
21. Smyth JF, Paine RM, Jackman AL, Harrap KR, Chassin MM, Adamson RH, et al: The clinical pharmacology of the adenosine deaminase inhibitor 2′-deoxycoformycin. Cancer Chemother Pharmacol 5:93-101, 1980
22. Grever MR, Siaw MF, Jacob WF, Neidhart JA, Miser JS, Coleman MS, et al: The biochemical and clinical consequences of 2′-deoxycoformycin in refractory lymphoproliferative malignancy. Blood 57:406-417, 1981
23. Grever MR, Leiby JM, Kraut EH, Wilson HE, Neidhart JA, Wall RL, et al: Low-dose deoxycoformycin in lymphoid malignancy. J Clin Oncol 3:1196-1201, 1985
24. Spiers AS, Ruckdeschel JC, Horton J: Effectiveness of pentostatin (2′-deoxycoformycin) in refractory lymphoid neoplasms. Scand J Haematol 32:130-134, 1984
25. Ho AD, Thaler J, Stryckmans P, Coiffier B, Luciani M, Sonneveld P, et al: Pentostatin in refractory chronic lymphocytic leukemia: A phase II trial of the European Organization for Research and Treatment of Cancer. J Natl Cancer Inst 82:1416-1420, 1990
26. Seto S, Carrera CJ, Kubota M, Wasson DB, Carson DA: Mechanism of deoxyadenosine and 2-chlorodeoxyadenosine toxicity to nondividing human lymphocytes. J Clin Invest 75:377-383, 1985
27. Siaw MF, Coleman MS: In vitro metabolism of deoxycoformycin in human T lymphoblastoid cells. Phosphorylation of deoxycoformycin and incorporation into cellular DNA. J Biol Chem 259:9426-9433, 1984
28. Polliack A: Hairy cell leukemia: Biology, clinical diagnosis, unusual manifestations and associated disorders. Rev Clin Exp Hematol 6:366-388, 2002
29. Quesada JR, Reuben J, Manning JT, Hersh EM, Gutterman JU: Alpha interferon for induction of remission in hairy-cell leukemia. N Engl J Med 310:15-18, 1984
30. Ratain MJ, Golomb HM, Vardiman JW, Vokes EE, Jacobs RH, Daly K: Treatment of hairy cell leukemia with recombinant alpha 2 interferon. Blood 65:644-648, 1985
31. Golomb HM, Jacobs A, Fefer A, Ozer H, Thompson J, Portlock C, et al: Alpha-2 interferon therapy of hairy-cell leukemia: A multicenter study of 64 patients. J Clin Oncol 4:900-905, 1986
32. Ho AD, Thaler J, Mandelli F, Lauria F, Zittoun R, Willemze R, et al: Response to pentostatin in hairy-cell leukemia refractory to interferon-alpha. The European Organization for Research and Treatment of Cancer Leukemia Cooperative Group. J Clin Oncol 7:1533-1538, 1989
33. Kraut EH, Bouroncle BA, Grever MR: Pentostatin in the treatment of advanced hairy cell leukemia. J Clin Oncol 7:168-172, 1989
34. Cassileth PA, Cheuvart B, Spiers AS, Harrington DP, Cummings FJ, Neiman RS, et al: Pentostatin induces durable remissions in hairy cell leukemia. J Clin Oncol 9:243-246, 1991
35. Johnston JB, Eisenhauer E, Corbett WE, Scott JG, Zaentz SD: Efficacy of 2′-deoxycoformycin in hairy-cell leukemia: A study of the National Cancer Institute of Canada Clinical Trials Group. J Natl Cancer Inst 80:765-769, 1988
36. Golomb HM, Dodge R, Mick R, Budman D, Hutchison R, Horning SJ, et al: Pentostatin treatment for hairy cell leukemia patients who failed initial therapy with recombinant alpha-interferon: A report of CALGB study 8515. Leukemia 8:2037-2040, 1994
37. Grever M, Kopecky K, Foucar MK, Head D, Bennett JM, Hutchison RE, et al: Randomized comparison of pentostatin versus interferon alfa-2a in previously untreated patients with hairy cell leukemia: An intergroup study. J Clin Oncol 13:974-982, 1995
38. Flinn IW, Kopecky KJ, Foucar MK, Head D, Bennett JM, Hutchison R, et al: Long-term follow-up of remission duration, mortality, and second malignancies in hairy cell leukemia patients treated with pentostatin. Blood 96:2981-2986, 2000
39. Goodman GR, Burian C, Koziol JA, Saven A: Extended follow-up of patients with hairy cell leukemia after treatment with cladribine. J Clin Oncol 21:891-896, 2003
40. Saven A, Burian C, Koziol JA, Piro LD: Long-term follow-up of patients with hairy cell leukemia after cladribine treatment. Blood 92:1918-1926, 1998
41. Flinn IW, Grever MR: Chronic lymphocytic leukemia. Cancer Treat Rev 22:1-13, 1996
42. Rai KR, Peterson BL, Appelbaum FR, Kolitz J, Elias L, Shepherd L, et al: Fludarabine compared with chlorambucil as primary therapy for chronic lymphocytic leukemia. N Engl J Med 343:1750-1757, 2000
43. Dillman RO, Mick R, McIntyre OR: Pentostatin in chronic lymphocytic leukemia: A phase II trial of Cancer and Leukemia Group B. J Clin Oncol 7:433-438, 1989
44. Johnson SA, Catovsky D, Child JA, Newland AC, Milligan DW, Janmohamed R: Phase I/II evaluation of pentostatin (2′-deoxycoformycin) in a five day schedule for the treatment of relapsed/refractory B-cell chronic lymphocytic leukaemia. Invest New Drugs 16:155-160, 1998

45. Dearden CE, Matutes E, Catovsky D: Clinical overview of pentostatin (Nipent) use in lymphoid malignancies. Semin Oncol 27:22-26, 2000
46. Weiss MA, Maslak PG, Jurcic JG, Scheinberg DA, Aliff TB, Lamanna N, et al: Pentostatin and cyclophosphamide: An effective new regimen in previously treated patients with chronic lymphocytic leukemia. J Clin Oncol 21:1278-1284, 2003
47. Oken MM, Lee S, Kay NE, Knospe W, Cassileth PA: Pentostatin, chlorambucil and prednisone therapy for B-chronic lymphocytic leukemia: A phase I/II study by the Eastern Cooperative Oncology Group study E1488. Leuk Lymphoma 45:79-84, 2004
48. Di Bella N, Reynolds C, Faragher D, Muscato J, Boehm KA, Asmar L: An open-label pilot study of pentostatin, mitoxantrone, and rituximab in patients with previously untreated, stage III or IV, low-grade non-Hodgkin lymphoma. Cancer 103:978-984, 2005
49. Dimopoulos MA, Kyle RA, Anagnostopoulos A, Treon SP: Diagnosis and management of Waldenstrom's macroglobulinemia. J Clin Oncol 23:1564-1577, 2005
50. Waldenstrom J: Incipient myelomatosis of "essential" hyperglobulinemia with fibrinogenopenia: A new syndrome. Acta Med Scand 117: 216-222, 1944
51. Lin P, Medeiros LJ: Lymphoplasmacytic lymphoma/Waldenstrom macroglobulinemia: An evolving concept. Adv Anat Pathol 12:246-255, 2005
52. Gertz MA: Waldenstrom macroglobulinemia: A review of therapy. Am J Hematol 79:147-157, 2005
53. Weber DM, Dimopoulos MA, Delasalle K, Rankin K, Gavino M, Alexanian R: 2-Chlorodeoxyadenosine alone and in combination for previously untreated Waldenstrom's macroglobulinemia. Semin Oncol 30: 243-247, 2003
54. Kantarjian HM, Alexanian R, Koller CA, Kurzrock R, Keating MJ: Fludarabine therapy in macroglobulinemic lymphoma. Blood 75:1928-1931, 1990
55. Dhodapkar MV, Jacobson JL, Gertz MA, Rivkin SE, Roodman GD, Tuscano JM, et al: Prognostic factors and response to fludarabine therapy in patients with Waldenstrom macroglobulinemia: Results of United States intergroup trial (Southwest Oncology Group S9003). Blood 98:41-48, 2001
56. Leblond V, Levy V, Maloisel F, Cazin B, Fermand JP, Harousseau JL, et al: Multicenter, randomized comparative trial of fludarabine and the combination of cyclophosphamide-doxorubicin-prednisone in 92 patients with Waldenstrom macroglobulinemia in first relapse or with primary refractory disease. Blood 98:2640-2644, 2001
57. Fenchel K, Wijermans P, Mitrou PS, Hoelzer D, Bergmann L: Fludarabine is an effective agent in immunocytic lymphoma. Onkologie 17: 508-513, 1994
58. Bjorkholm M, Celsing F, Runarsson G, Waldenstrom J: Successful intravenous immunoglobulin therapy for severe and persistent astrovirus gastroenteritis after fludarabine treatment in a patient with Waldenstrom's macroglobulinemia. Int J Hematol 62:117-120, 1995
59. Costa P, Luzzati R, Nicolato A, Perboni G, Scalzini A, Lazzarini L, et al: Cryptococcal meningitis and intracranial tuberculoma in a patient with Waldenstrom's macroglobulinemia treated with fludarabine. Leuk Lymphoma 28:617-620, 1998
60. Dimopoulos MA, O'Brien S, Kantarjian H, Estey EE, Keating MJ, Alexanian R: Treatment of Waldenstrom's macroglobulinemia with nucleoside analogues. Leuk Lymphoma 11:105-108, 1993 (suppl 2)
61. Liu ES, Burian C, Miller WE, Saven A: Bolus administration of cladribine in the treatment of Waldenstrom macroglobulinaemia. Br J Haematol 103:690-695, 1998
62. Hellmann A, Lewandowski K, Zaucha JM, Bieniaszewska M, Halaburda K, Robak T: Effect of a 2-hour infusion of 2-chlorodeoxyadenosine in the treatment of refractory or previously untreated Waldenstrom's macroglobulinemia. Eur J Haematol 63:35-41, 1999
63. Betticher DC, Hsu Schmitz SF, Ratschiller D, von Rohr A, Egger T, Pugin P, et al: Cladribine (2-CDA) given as subcutaneous bolus injections is active in pretreated Waldenstrom's macroglobulinaemia. Swiss Group for Clinical Cancer Research (SAKK). Br J Haematol 99:358-363, 1997
64. Bryson HM, Sorkin EM: Cladribine. A review of its pharmacodynamic and pharmacokinetic properties and therapeutic potential in haematological malignancies. Drugs 46:872-894, 1993
65. Van Den Neste E, Louviaux I, Michaux JL, Delannoy A, Michaux L, Hagemeijer A, et al: Myelodysplastic syndrome with monosomy 5 and/or 7 following therapy with 2-chloro-2′-deoxyadenosine. Br J Haematol 105:268-270, 1999
66. Van Den Neste E, Delannoy A, Feremans W, Ferrant A, Michaux L: Second primary tumors and immune phenomena after fludarabine or 2-chloro-2′-deoxyadenosine treatment. Leuk Lymphoma 40:541-550, 2001
67. Tetreault SA, Saven A: Delayed onset of autoimmune hemolytic anemia complicating cladribine therapy for Waldenstrom macroglobulinemia. Leuk Lymphoma 37:125-130, 2000
68. Weber DM, Gavino M, Huh Y: Phenotypic and clinical evidence supports rituximab for Waldenstrom's macroglobulinemia. Blood 94:125a, 1999 (abstr 551)
69. Foran JM, Rohatiner AZ, Cunningham D, Popescu RA, Solal-Celigny P, Ghielmini M, et al: European phase II study of rituximab (chimeric anti-CD20 monoclonal antibody) for patients with newly diagnosed mantle-cell lymphoma and previously treated mantle-cell lymphoma, immunocytoma, and small B-cell lymphocytic lymphoma. J Clin Oncol 18:317-324, 2000
70. Treon SP, Agus TB, Link B, Rodrigues G, Molina A, Lacy MQ, et al: CD20-directed antibody-mediated immunotherapy induces responses and facilitates hematologic recovery in patients with Waldenstrom's macroglobulinemia. J Immunother 24:272-279, 2001
71. Dimopoulos MA, Zervas C, Zomas A, Kiamouris C, Viniou NA, Grigoraki V, et al: Treatment of Waldenstrom's macroglobulinemia with rituximab. J Clin Oncol 20:2327-2333, 2002
72. Treon SP, Emmanouilides C, Kimby E, Kelliher A, Preffer F, Branagan AR, et al: Extended rituximab therapy in Waldenstrom's macroglobulinemia. Ann Oncol 16:132-138, 2005
73. Gertz MA, Rue M, Blood E, Kaminer LS, Vesole DH, Greipp PR: Multicenter phase 2 trial of rituximab for Waldenstrom macroglobulinemia (WM): An Eastern Cooperative Oncology Group Study (E3A98). Leuk Lymphoma 45:2047-2055, 2004
74. Treon SP, Branagan AR, Wasi P: Combination therapy with rituximab and fludarabine in Waldenstrom's macroglobulinemia. 3rd International Workshop on Waldenstrom's Macroglobulinemia. Paris, France, October 7-10, 2004, p 57
75. Riddell S, Johnston JB, Rayner HL, Israels LG: Response of Waldenstrom's macroglobulinemia to pentostatin (2′-deoxycoformycin). Cancer Treat Rep 70:546-548, 1986
76. Lamanna N, Kalaycio M, Maslak PG, Jurcic JG, Scheinberg DA, Gencarelli AN, et al: Pentostatin and cyclophosphamide with or without rituximab has significant activity in patients with previously treated chronic lymphocytic leukemia and other low grade lymphoid neoplasms. Blood 104:950a, 2004 (abstr)
77. Hensel M, Krasniqi F, Villabos M, Kornacker M, Ho AD: Pentostatin and cylcophosphamide followed by maintenance therapy with rituximab for previously treated patients with B-cell chronic lymphocytic leukaemia, and Walendstroem's macroglobulinemia. Blood 102:404a, 2003 (abstr)
78. Desikan R, Dhodapkar M, Siegel D, Fassas A, Singh J, Singhal S, et al: High-dose therapy with autologous haemopoietic stem cell support for Waldenstrom's macroglobulinaemia. Br J Haematol 105:993-996, 1999
79. Anagnostopoulos A, Dimopoulos MA, Aleman A, Weber D, Alexanian R, Champlin R, et al: High-dose chemotherapy followed by stem cell transplantation in patients with resistant Waldenstrom's macroglobulinemia. Bone Marrow Transplant 27:1027-1029, 2001
80. Tournilhac O, Leblond V, Tabrizi R, Gressin R, Senecal D, Milpied N, et al: Transplantation in Waldenstrom's macroglobulinemia—The French experience. Semin Oncol 30:291-296, 2003
81. Dreger P, Stilgenbauer S, Seyfarth B: Autologous and allogeneic stem cell transplantation for treatment of Waldenstrom's macroglobulinemia. 3rd International Workshop on Waldenstrom's Macroglobulinemia. Paris, France, October 7-10, 2004, p 70
82. Fassas A, Dhodapkar M, McCoy J: Management of Waldenstrom's mac-

roglobulinemia in the pre-rituximab era: Update on US Intergroup Trial S9003 and the Arkansas autotransplant experience. 3rd International Workshop on Waldenstrom's Macroglobulinemia. Paris, France, October 7-10, 2004, p 59
83. Leo E, Scheuer L, Schmidt-Wolf IG, Kerowgan M, Schmitt C, Leo A, et al: Significant thrombocytopenia associated with the addition of rituximab to a combination of fludarabine and cyclophosphamide in the treatment of relapsed follicular lymphoma. Eur J Haematol 73:251-257, 2004
84. Keating MJ, Kantarjian H, Talpaz M, Redman J, Koller C, Barlogie B, et al: Fludarabine: A new agent with major activity against chronic lymphocytic leukemia. Blood 74:19-25, 1989
85. Montillo M, Tedeschi A, O'Brien S, Di Raimondo F, Lerner S, Ferrajoli A, et al: Phase II study of cladribine and cyclophosphamide in patients with chronic lymphocytic leukemia and prolymphocytic leukemia. Cancer 97:114-120, 2003
86. O'Brien SM, Kantarjian HM, Cortes J, Beran M, Koller CA, Giles FJ, et al: Results of the fludarabine and cyclophosphamide combination regimen in chronic lymphocytic leukemia. J Clin Oncol 19:1414-1420, 2001
87. Drapkin R, Di Bella NJ, Faragher DC, Harden E, Matei C, Hyman W, et al: Results of a phase II multicenter trial of pentostatin and rituximab in patients with low grade B-cell non-Hodgkin's lymphoma: An effective and minimally toxic regimen. Clin Lymphoma 4:169-175, 2003
88. Czuczman MS, Koryzna A, Mohr A, Stewart C, Donohue K, Blumenson L, et al: Rituximab in combination with fludarabine chemotherapy in low-grade or follicular lymphoma. J Clin Oncol 23:694-704, 2005
89. Wierda W, O'Brien S, Wen S, Faderl S, Garcia-Manero G, Thomas D, et al: Chemoimmunotherapy with fludarabine, cyclophosphamide, and rituximab for relapsed and refractory chronic lymphocytic leukemia. J Clin Oncol 23:4070-4078, 2005
90. Keating MJ, O'Brien S, Albitar M, Lerner S, Plunkett W, Giles F, et al: Early results of a chemoimmunotherapy regimen of fludarabine, cyclophosphamide, and rituximab as initial therapy for chronic lymphocytic leukemia. J Clin Oncol 23:4079-4088, 2005
91. Robak T, Blonski JZ, Gora-Tybor J, Kasznicki M, Dwilewicz-Trojaczek J, Tomaszewska A, et al: Cladribine alone or in combination with cyclophosphamide or cyclophosphamide and mitoxantrone as first line treatment in chronic lymphocytic leukemia: An early report of prospective randomized study. Blood 104:337a, 2004 (abstr)
92. Hensel M, Villalobos M, Kornacker M, Krasniqi F, Ho AD: Pentostatin/cyclophosphamide with or without rituximab: An effective regimen for patients with Waldenstrom's macroglobulinemia/lymphoplasmacytic lymphoma. Clin Lymphoma Myeloma 6:131-135, 2005

ELSEVIER

Seminars in
HEMATOLOGY

Purine Analogue Combinations for Indolent Lymphomas

Nicholas Di Bella[a] and Farhad Ravandi[b]

Indolent lymphomas are a group of lymphoid malignancies with differing patterns of behavior and responses to treatment. The progress in treating patients with hairy cell leukemia (HCL) using nucleoside analogues can be used as a model for other indolent B-lymphoproliferative disorders, such as follicular lymphoma. Recent advancements in therapeutic options available for these patients include combination therapy with agents that have differing mechanisms of action and non-overlapping toxicity. It has been shown that patients who are candidates for aggressive therapy might receive benefit, including disease-free survival and overall survival, from combination purine analogue therapy. Using these more aggressive therapeutic approaches earlier in the disease course and as maintenance therapy may further enhance outcomes. With the advent of these new therapies along with the molecular evaluation of these regimens, we may be nearing the time where the goal for more advanced indolent lymphoma will be to achieve a cure.
Semin Hematol 43(suppl 2):S11-S21

Indolent lymphomas are a group of lymphoid malignancies with differing patterns of behavior and responses to treatment. They generally have a long course, with a history of responses and relapses. Therapy of these diseases has been mainly palliative; however, with recent data showing significant activity of newer therapies, including the purine analogues, the goals are becoming aggressive in hopes of achieving long-term remissions and cure. This report will provide an overview of available data of purine analogues in the most common indolent lymphoma, follicular lymphoma.

Overview of Indolent Lymphoma

Lymphomas are a heterogenous group of malignancies that are caused by malignant transformation of immune cells in lymphoid tissues. Based on histopathology, these malignancies are classified into two distinct types: Hodgkin's and non-Hodgkin's lymphoma (B- or T-cell lymphocyte markers). Of these, non-Hodgkin's lymphoma (NHL) is more common with an expected 56,390 new cases and 19,200 deaths in 2005.[1] NHL is the fifth most common cause of newly diagnosed cancer in the United States and accounts for about 4% of all cancers. The incidence of NHL is more common among Caucasians, and men are more likely to develop the disease than women. The average age at the time of diagnosis is 65 years.[1] Lymphoma is one of two cancers where the incidence has increased over the past three decades. The exact cause for this increase is unknown.

The cause of NHL is currently unknown, although there have been several factors implicated in its etiology, including environmental, infectious, genetic, and occupational factors.[2] The role of immune dysregulation in the etiology is strongly supported by the increased incidence of NHL in congenital and acquired immunodeficiency states. In fact, immunodeficiency is one of the strongest risk factors known to increase NHL risk.[2] The risk of NHL is increased 100- to 300-fold in patients with HIV infection and this has played a role in the increasing incidence of NHL over the past few years. Epidemiologic studies suggest that environmental toxins such as phenoxyacetic acid herbicides, organophosphate insecticides, triazine herbicide, and fertilizers are associated with an increased risk of NHL. This may help explain why certain occupations like farmers and agricultural workers have a higher risk of NHL. These occupational and environment risk factors may be responsible for the increased incidence of NHL over the years.[2] Chromosomal translocations are hallmarks of lymphoid malignancies, specifically t(1;14), t(11;18), and t(14;18).[3] The translocation t(14;18), which results in mutation of the *bcl-2* oncogene, is found in most patients with follicular lymphoma and can be used clinically

[a]Rocky Mountain Cancer Centers, Aurora, CO.
[b]Department of Leukemia, University of Texas–M.D. Anderson Cancer Center, Houston, TX.
Address correspondence to Nicholas Di Bella, MD, FACP, Chairman Hematology Research Committee, US Oncology, Medical Director, Rocky Mountain Cancer Centers. 1700 Potomac. Aurora, CO 80012. E-mail: nick.dibella@usoncology.com

0037-1963/06/$-see front matter
doi:10.1053/j.seminhemato1.2005.12.006

Table 1 WHO Classification of Lymphoid Neoplasms[5]

B-Cell Neoplasms	T-Cell and NK Cell Neoplasms
Precursor B-cell neoplasm	Precursor T-cell neoplasm
Precursor B-lymphoblastic leukemia/lymphoma	Precurosr T-lymphoblastic lymphoma/leukemia
Mature (peripheral) B-cell neoplasms	Mature (peripheral) T-cell neoplasms
B-cell CLL/small lymphocytic lymphoma	T-cell prolymphocytic leukemia
B-cell prolymphocytic leukemia	T-cell granular lymphocytic leukemia
Lymphoplasmacytic lymphoma	Aggressive NK cell leukemia
Splenic marginal zone B-cell lymphoma	Adult T-cell lymphoma/leukemia
Hairy cell leukemia*	Extranodal NK/T-cell lymphoma (nasal)
Plasma cell myeloma/plasmacytoma	Enteropathy-type T-cell lymphoma
Extranodal marginal zone B-cell (MALT) type	Anaplastic large-cell lymphoma, T/null cell, primary cutaneous type
Nodal marginal zone B-cell lymphoma	Subcutaneou panniculitis-like T-cell
Follicular lymphoma*	Mycosis fungoides/Sézary syndrome
Mantle-cell lymphoma	Peripheral T-cell not characterized
Diffuse large B-cell lymphoma	Angioimmunoblstic T-cell
Primary effusion lymphoma	Anaplastic large cell, T/null cell, primary systemic
Burkitt's lymphoma/Burkitt cell leukemia	
Hodgkin's Lymphoma	
Nodular lymphocyte-predominant Hodgkin's lymphoma	
Classical Hodgkin's lymphoma	
Nodular sclerosis Hodgkin's lymphoma (grades 1 and 2)	
Lymphocytes-rich classical Hodgkin's lymphoma	
Mixed cellularity Hodgkin's lymphoma	
Lymphocyte depletion Hodgkin's lymphoma	

*Entities discussed further in this review.
Abbreviations: NK, natural killer; CLL, chronic lymphocytic leukemia.

to monitor for minimal residual disease (MRD).[3] Newer techniques such as cytogenetic and molecular analyses along with gene expression arrays may assist in further recognizing the etiology of NHL.

Classification of Lymphoid Malignancies

The classification of NHL has undergone numerous revisions since the first description in 1982, which was based primarily on morphologic appearance. In 1994 the Revised European-American Lymphoma (REAL) classification distinguished lymphomas by histology in addition to immunophenotypic, genetic, and clinical characteristics.[4] This system was then further modified to the universally accepted World Health Organization (WHO) classification[5] (Table 1). The REAL-WHO classification categorizes lymphoma into three categories: B-cell lymphomas, T-cell lymphomas, and Hodgkin's lymphomas. In 1995 the usage of terms "indolent," "aggressive," and "very aggressive" lymphoma was proposed to reflect the natural history of the disease irrespective of it response to therapy. Although these terms are not included in the REAL-WHO classification, they are commonly used in clinical practice. The term "indolent" lymphoma applies to lymphoid tumors with a survival measurable in years. These lymphoproliferative disorders have variable clinical courses and are thus subcategorized into three categories: disseminated leukemias/lymphomas, extranodal forms, and nodal forms. The Ann Arbor staging system is used to describe the degree of spread of the disease. Stage I is early disease, while stage IV is widespread disease.[6]

Follicular lymphoma comprises 19% of NHLs in the United States and is the most common indolent lymphoma.[7] The WHO classification includes criteria for grading follicular lymphoma based on the number of centroblasts per high-power field (hpf): grade 1 (0–5 centroblasts/hpf), grade 2 (6–15 centeroblasts/hpf), and grade 3 (>15 centeroblasts/hpf).[5] Indolent lymphoma is usually referred to as grade 1 or 2, while grade 3 is usually treated as an aggressive lymphoma. Most patients have advanced disease by the time of diagnosis but approximately 30% will have either stage I or II disease.[8] The course of the disease is characterized by an initial response to treatment followed by remissions and relapses with occasional transformation to a more aggressive NHL. Median survival approximates 8 to 10 years.[9] An international cooperative study retrospectively reviewed 5,000 patients worldwide over an 8-year period to develop what is now known as the Follicular Lymphoma International Prognostic Index (FLIPI).[10] Five factors that are collected clinically in all patients are used (age, Ann Arbor stage, number of nodal sites, serum lactate dehydrogenase level, and hemoglobin level) to build a three-category prognostic index (Table 2). This index, together with new biologic markers such as gene profiling and proteomics, can help in improving treatment choices, comparing clinical trials, and designing studies to evaluate new therapies. A disadvantage of this index is the lack of inclusion of computed tomography (CT) findings. The FLIPI changed our understanding of the biology of the disease and future studies evaluating therapy for indolent lymphoma should incorporate the FLIPI.

Table 2 Follicular Lymphoma International Prognostic Index[10]

Risk Groups	No. of Adverse Factors	% of Patients	5-Year OS % (SE)	10-Year OS 5 (SE)
Low-risk	0–1	36	90.6 (1.2)	70.7 (2.7)
Intermediate risk	2	37	77.6 (1.6)	50.9 (2.7)
Poor risk	≥3	27	52.5 (2.3)	35.5 (2.8)
Adverse prognostic factors				
Age >60 years				
Disseminated disease with Ann Arbor stage III/IV*				
Hemoglobin level <12 g/dL				
>4 nodal areas				
Serum LDH above normal				
Ann Arbor staging system*[6]				
I A single nodal region or single extranodal site				
II Two or more nodal regions or an extranodal site and regional nodal involvement on the same side of the diaphragm				
III Lymphatic involvement on both sides of the diaphragm				
IV Live or bone marrow or extensive involvement of another extralymphatic organ				

NOTE. N = 1,795.

Abbreviations: LDH, lactate dehydrogenase; OS, overall survival. SE, standard error.

From: Solal-Celigny et al. Follicular lymphoma international prognostic index. *Blood* 2004;104:1258-65. Copyright American Society of Hematology, used with permission.

Treatment Principles of Indolent Lymphoma

Follicular Lymphoma

The treatment choices for patients with indolent lymphoma have been controversial. In years past, the treatment choices consisted of "watch and wait," single-agent chemotherapy (eg, chlorambucil), combination chemotherapy (eg, cyclophosphamide, vincristine, prednisone or CHOP), radiation therapy either alone or in combination with chemotherapy, chemotherapy with maintenance biologic therapy, or high-dose chemotherapy with autologous bone marrow transplantation. Various treatment options have been evaluated and no consensus has been developed as to optimal initial therapy. The decision-making process has become complex with the availability of multiple new therapeutic options. First, the clinician must decide whether the goal of therapy is palliative versus attempted remission ("curative"). The patient with poor performance status and multiple comorbidities may be best managed conservatively with either watchful waiting or single-agent therapy at the time of progression, while the patient who is in better clinical condition can be considered for more aggressive therapy with the aim of a complete remission (CR) of disease. The FLIPI may be useful in helping make the decision as to which patient might benefit from aggressive therapy.

Radiation therapy has been the treatment standard for patients with early-stage follicular lymphoma with disease-free survival rates of 40% to 50% and overall survival rates of 60% and 70% at 10 years.[11] The combination of radiotherapy with chemotherapy appears to be more effective than radiotherapy alone, with 82% overall survival rates.[12] Therefore, the goal in managing these patients is cure. The management of advanced disease is where the controversy has developed since none of the standard therapeutic approaches have been shown to be curative despite the initial response to therapy. CR can be achieved in 50% to 80% of patients with chemotherapy or biologic therapy; however, the median time to relapse is 18 to 36 months.[13] Therefore, two different initial treatment approaches have been adopted for these patients, described as either conservative or aggressive. Patients treated with the conservative approach receive no initial therapy followed by single-agent chemotherapy or radiation therapy when treatment is needed. Patients who are usually considered for this approach are those who are older, asymptomatic, and have minimal tumor burden. Patients must be followed closely as stable disease can rapidly change to aggressive disease. All other patients should be considered for more aggressive approaches. There are no convincing data that either approach is superior to the other.[13] Therefore, the goal of therapy in these patients is to attain a good response since this stage of the disease is currently considered to be incurable. However, long-term follow-up data in patients with other indolent lymphoid malignancies such as hairy cell leukemia (HCL) who were treated with nucleoside analogues suggest that achievement of a CR is important for duration of relapse-free survival.[14,15] This confirms that the goal of initial therapy in patients with a good performance status should be to achieve a CR.

Oral alkylating agents were the mainstay chemotherapy for follicular lymphoma, especially as palliative therapy. More intensive regimens have not been shone to improve overall outcome. However, neither an alkylating agent alone or in combination with vincristine and prednisone (CVP) nor CVP with doxorubicin has shown a significant impact on survival.[11] Rituximab represented a significant treatment advancement for patients with indolent lymphoma and has made the watch and wait approach less of an option. Based on the activity of rituximab in relapsed or refractory patients, it is increasingly being used as first-line therapy. Initial response rates to single-agent are in the region of 60% to 70%.[16] When continued as maintenance therapy, the overall response rate improved to 73% at 24 months with a 37% CR rate (with the courses repeated every 6 months).[17] The role of maintenance rituximab is being further investigated alone and in combination with other agents.

Purine Analogues for Indolent Lymphoma

There is a great need for new treatment options to increase response rates and reduce relapses for patients with indolent NHL. A number of treatment approaches are being investigated including the use of purine analogues, such as pentostatin (Nipent®, Supergen, Dublin, CA). There is rationale for the use of these agents in patients with NHL. These drugs have been shown to be cytotoxic to all lymphocytes both in vitro and in vivo and they have the ability to induce apoptosis of lymphocytes.[18]

The purine analogues, pentostatin and cladribine (Leustatin, Ortho Biotech, Bridgewater, NJ), have emerged as the treatment of choice for patients with HCL. Fludarabine does not appear to be as active against HCL as the other agents.[19] The rationale for the use of these agents was described over 30 years ago by Giblett et al[20] who reported that children with severe combined immunodeficiency syndrome lacked the enzyme adenosine deaminase (ADA). The absence of lymphocytes was attributed to the accumulation of the triphosphorylated form of deoxyadenosine. Thus inhibition of ADA pharmacologically emerged as a potential antilymphocyte strategy. A significant treatment milestone for HCL was the discovery that hairy cells are sensitive to purine analogues (cladribine and pentostatin) with a 70% to 85% CR rate and 7- to 8-year disease-free survival rates of 60% to 75%.[14,21-26] The progress in treating patients with HCL using nucleoside analogues can be used as a model for other indolent B-lymphoproliferative disorders where perhaps combination therapy can lead to similar results.

Differences Between Purine Analogues

The purine analogues are structurally similar analogues of adenosine but they differ in their interaction with ADA. This enzyme participates in the purine metabolism of adenosine to inosine and deoxyadenosine to deoxyinosine resulting in accumulation of deoxyadenosine triphoasphate (dATP). These metabolites block DNA synthesis through inhibition of ribonucleotide reductase.[27] 2′-Deoxycoformycin (pentostatin) is an irreversible inhibitor ADA, which results in accumulation of deoxyadenosine and subsequent toxicity to lymphocytes. In comparison, 2-chlorodeoxyadenosine (cladribine) and 2-fluro-ara-AMP (fludarabine; Fludara,, Berlex Laboratories, Richmond, CA) are purine analogues that do not inhibit ADA but instead are resistant to the deaminating enzyme. Fludarabine and cladribine must be phosphorylated to be active. These agents accumulate in the lymphoid cells since they are rich in deoxycytidine kinase. This enzyme phosphorylates cladribine and fludarabine creating a deoxynucleotide that cannot readily exit the cell.[28] These agents are incorporated into DNA, producing chain termination. Cladribine is not as potent a chain terminator as fludarabine.[29] Purine analogues affect both dividing and nondividing cells, unlike conventional chemotherapy.[30] Pentostatin has several theoretical advantages over the other agents in patients with NHL, including the following: (1) pentostatin is not incorporated into DNA like the other agents; (2) pentostatin is the least myelosuppressive so there is less need to reduce the doses of drugs when used in combination; and (3) in vitro data suggest that pentostatin has less effect on stem cells and thus does not eliminate the utility of stem cell transplantation as a treatment option.[31,32]

The purine analogues have a similar spectrum of toxicities, including moderate myelosuppression, profound immunosuppression, and neurotoxicity. A concern with the use of purine analogues is the development of infections. Profound immunosuppression is associated with a decrease in lymphocytes, primarily $CD4^+$ cells. $CD4^+$ counts may decrease to levels similar to those observed in patients with AIDS and may remain depressed for a year or longer following administration.[33-35] However, the use of lower dosing schedules has reduced the risk of infections in these patients.

Review of Single-Agent Therapy Response Rates

Fludarabine first entered clinical trials 20 years ago and focused primarily on chronic lymphocytic leukemia (CLL) where it has shown significant activity. Fludarabine was the first of the purine analogues to also show significant activity in indolent lymphoma. Single-agent fludarabine for indolent lymphoma has an overall response rate of 50% with a CR rate of 10% to 15%.[36-41] CR (40%) is more common in patients who receive fludarabine as initial treatment.[42] Cladribine has also shown activity as single-agent therapy in indolent lymphoma, with overall response rates between 32% and 88%.[41-44] Responses were seen in previously untreated patients, with response rates upwards of 89%,[43] and in those with refractory disease. Pentostatin was explored as single-agent therapy in four different studies in patients with NHL.[45-48] The overall response rate was 16% to 23%, and patients with indolent lymphoma responded better than those with aggressive lymphoma. These data evaluating purine analogues as single-agent therapy are very old and may not be reliable since we are unsure of the histology of the patients reported.

Purine Analogue Combination Therapy

No single agent is likely to have a substantial impact on survival of patients with indolent lymphoma; therefore, recent studies have focused on combining purine analogues with other agents that have shown activity in this disease. Since purine analogues have a low incidence of nonhematologic adverse effects, it makes them a reasonable option to use with other regimens.

Table 3 Fludarabine Combination Therapy Summary for Indolent Lymphoma

Reference	N	Regimen	CR(%)	Survival Measure	Toxicity
64	64	F: 25 mg/m^2 d 1–3 C: 250 mg/m^2 d 1–3	29	5-yr OS 55%	G3-4 neutropenia 35%
53	73	F: 25 mg/m^2 d 1–3 N: 10 mg/m^2 d 1 D: 20 mg d 1–5 Or	67	5-yr FFS 41%	G3-4 neutropenia 81%
	69	ATT	59	5-yr FFS 50%	G3-4 neutropenia 94%
55	17	F: 25 mg/m^2 d 1–3 M: 10 mg/m^2 d 1	76	92% 2-yr survival	G3-4 hematologic 17%
71	40	R: 375 mg/m^2 × 2 F: 25 mg/m^2/d × 5 d	80	Median TTP not reached at 44 mo	G3-4 neutropenia 80%*
66	60	F: 25 mg/m^2 d 1–3 C: 300 mg/m^2 d 1–3 M: 10 mg/m^2 d 1	77	83% survival 31 mo	G3-4 granulocytopenia 60%
72	62 FL = 30	F: 25 mg/m^2 d 1–3 C: 200 mg/m^2 d 1–3 M: 8 mg/m^2 d 1 Or	23	PFS 10 mo	G3-4 lymphocytopenia 39% G3-4 granulocytopenia 41%
	66 FL = 35	R: 375 mg/m^2 prior to FCM FCM regimen as above	40	PFS 16 mo	G3-4 lymphocytopenia 51% G3-4 granulocytopenia 40%

Abbreviations: CR, complete remission; F, fludarabine; C, cyclophosphamide; OS, overall survival; N or M, mitoxantrone; D, dexamethasone; FFS, failure-free survival; R, rituximab; PFS, progression free survival; FL, follicular lymphoma; G3-4, grade 3–4; ATT, alternating triple therapy (CHOD-Bleo, ESHAP, NOPP).
*Toxicity reported in first 10 patients prior to alteration in dosing schedule.

Fludarabine Combinations

The initial positive results of fludarabine as single-agent therapy led to its investigation in combination with other agents such as mitoxantrone (Table 3). Fludarabine (25 mg/m^2 × 3 days) combined with dexamethasone (20 mg/d × 5 days) and mitoxantrone (10 mg/m^2 on day 1) (FND) was evaluated in 51 previously treated patients with indolent NHL.[49] Prior to this trial, a phase I study determined the optimal dosing strategy for this combination.[50] There was a 47% CR rate, with an overall response rate of 94%. The incidence of immunosuppression observed led the investigators to add cotrimoxazole as prophylaxis against *Pneumocystis carinii* (PCP) pneumonia. In a similar patient group where the same combination was evaluated except that prednisone was substituted for dexamethasone, an overall response rate of 83% and a 35% CR rate were reported.[51] The major adverse effects reported were infections and neutropenia. The FND combination has also shown similar response rate profiles when administered to first-line therapy.[52]

There are also reports of comparative combination regimens using fludarabine in patients with indolent lymphoma. The FND combination was compared to alternating triple therapy (CHOD-Bleo, ESHAP, and NOPP) (ATT) in 142 patients with stage IV disease.[53] Maintenance interferon alfa-2a/dexamethasone was given for 1-year in both treatment groups. Responses in this study included both clinical and molecular evaluations. The overall clinical response rate for both regimens was 97% with 5-year failure free survival rates of 41% in the FND group and 50% in the ATT group (P = .02). ATT was associated with a greater incidence of grade 3/4 toxicities than FND. Molecular responses were reported at least once in 81% of patient in the FND arm and 67% in the ATT arm (P = .17), but there were only nonsignificant trends for better outcomes in these molecular responders.[53] The study population that received FND was monitored long-term for evaluation of immunosuppression and infectious complications.[54] This combination resulted in a decline in CD4 counts and immunoglobulin levels with a return to normal levels by 3 years. Based on these data, the investigators suggested that prophylaxis against opportunistic infections, particularly PCP, be administered to patients receiving this combination.

Because of the concern of profound immunosuppression when corticosteroids are combined with purine analogues, the combination of fludarabine and mitoxantrone (FM) was evaluated omitting the steroid component. The combination of FM was evaluated in 27 previously treated indolent lymphoma patients with the majority of patients having follicular lymphoma (n = 17).[55] A 67% CR rate with an overall response rate of 89% was reported after six treatment cycles. Interestingly, the patients with follicular lymphoma had the highest response rates (76% CR, 94% overall response rate) and 2-year survival (92%). The regimen was well tolerated with only five patients developing 3/4 hematologic toxicity.[55] Other investigators have also confirmed similar response rates with the FM combination with reduced risk of infections and in previously untreated patients.[56-59]

Synergistic cytotoxicity between purine analogues and alkylating agents has been reported in vitro.[29] Cyclophosphamide enhances DNA damage, allowing for increased opportunities for incorporation of purine analogues into DNA. Initial reports of fludarabine (25 mg/m^2) and cyclophosphamide (300 to 350 mg/m^2) given in combination as salvage therapy to small groups of indolent NHL patients showed overall response rates of 70% to 80%.[60,61] However, significant toxicity has been reported for this regimen, including infections, myelosuppression, and nausea/vomiting. In fact, toxicity was unacceptable in an Eastern Cooperative Oncology Group phase III study comparing fludarabine with cyclophosphamide (FC) to CVP (cyclophosphamide, vincristine, prednisone), leading to an early closure of the fludarabine arm of the trial.[9] A pivotal study evaluating FC in 128 patients using a similar dosing regimen reported severe neutropenia in 33% to 50% of the population and infections in 25%.[62] Not all regimens evaluating FC have shown this same degree of toxicity; however, some of these trials evaluated patients who had not received previous therapy[63] and used alternative dosing schedules.[64,65] Tam et al[64] used an attenuated dosing schedule of FC (F: 25 mg/m^2 and C: 250 mg/m^2 on days 1 to 3) and reported an overall response rate of 86% with 29% CRs and a more acceptable toxicity profile.

Mitoxantrone has been added to the FC combination (FCM) for treating previously untreated patients[66] and those with refractory disease.[67] The regimen for those who were previously untreated included fludarabine 25 mg/m^2 on days 1 to 3, cyclophosphamide 300 mg/m^2 on days 1 to 3, and mitoxantrone 10 mg/m^2 on day 1,[66] while the regimen in patients who were previously treated used 250 mg/m^2 of cyclophosphamide and 5 mg/m^2 of mitoxantrone.[67] Patients in both of these studies received cotrimoxazole prophylaxis and growth factors when clinically indicated. In the previously untreated patients, there was an 87% overall response rate with FCM (77% CR) with 83% survival rate at 31 months.[66] Similarly, the refractory patients had an overall response rate of 78.5% with 32% CRs and a median survival of 19 months.[67] Toxicity was less in patients who had not received previous therapy. Molecular evaluation of response was conducted in the study of untreated patients. The majority of patients (76%) treated with FCM converted to polymerase chain reaction (PCR) *bcl*-2 negativity.[66] A comparison study was also conducted between FC and FCM in refractory patients.[68] The overall responses were similar between the two groups (CRs with FC = 54% *v* FCM = 61%) along with the reported toxicity. The administration of prophylactic oral antibiotics along with growth factors when indicated lessened the degree of infectious side effects reported.[68]

The combination of rituximab and fludarabine in vitro has been shown to be more active than either agent alone.[69] The combination of these agents seems rational since they do not have overlapping mechanisms of action or toxicities. A phase I/II study evaluated fludarabine 30 mg/m^2 on days 1 to 4 and rituximab 125, 250, or 375 mg/m^2 on day 5 at intervals of 28 days for eight cycles in a population that consisted of 64% indolent lymphoma patients.[70] The overall response rate was 82.8% with a 34.5% CR rate; however, four patients were removed from the study due to prolonged hematopoietic toxicity. In a recent report, Czuczman et al[71] evaluated the fludarabine/rituximab combination in a phase II study that enrolled 40 patients. Patients received two infusions of rituximab 375 mg/m^2 given 4 days apart and then 72 hours later fludarabine 25 mg/m^2/d for 5 days was administered. An overall response rate of 90% (80% CRs) was achieved, with responses being similar between previously treated and treatment-naive patients. Among patients who were positive for the t14;18 translocation, molecular remission was achieved in 88% of the cases with patients remaining negative for up to 4 years. The investigators did report a 15% incidence of herpes simplex/zoster infections; otherwise toxicity was manageable.[71]

Rituximab has been shown to improve remission rates and overall survival when added to the FCM regimen (R-FCM) for patients with relapsed or refractory follicular and mantle cell lymphomas.[72] A total of 147 patients were randomized to receive four courses of therapy with fludarabine 25 mg/m^2 on days 1 to 3, 200 mg/m^2 cyclophosphamide on days 1 to 3, and 8 mg/m^2 mitoxantrone on day 1 (FCM, n = 62) alone or in combination with rituximab 375 mg/m^2 (R-FCM, n = 66). R-FCM had an overall response rate of 79% compared to 58% with FCM. In addition, patients in the R-FCM group had significantly better progression-free survival and overall survival. The CR rates in patients with follicular lymphoma for R-FCM compared to FCM were 40% and 30%, respectively. Toxicity was similar in the two groups.[72] These encouraging results may lead to a new second-line treatment standard if similar results are confirmed in other randomized trials.

Cladribine Combinations

Saven et al[73] were the first to show that cladribine may be combined with mitoxantrone in a study of 23 patients with indolent NHL who had received previous treatment. Cladribine was given by continuous infusion 0.1 mg/kg/d for 7 days and mitoxantrone was delivered on day 1 at doses escalating by 2.5-mg/m^2 increments from 5 mg/m^2. The investigators reported an overall response rate of 70% with CRs in 22% of the patients and a median response duration of 15 months. The dose-limiting toxicities were myelosuppression and infection, and at the median follow-up of 14 months 11 of the 23 patients had died.[73] Other investigators have proposed using a lower dosing schedule of cladribine to reduce the incidence of late toxicity.[44,74] The schedule used was 5 mg/m^2/d over 3 consecutive days by a 2-hour infusion along with mitoxantrone at 8 mg/m^2 on days 1 and 2 for untreated patients or 12 mg/m^2 for relapsed patients. The reported overall response rate for the reduced dose regimen was 90% with a 44% CR rate and a median duration of remission of 25 months. Myelosuppression was the major toxicity observed with the combination (grade 4 = 48%) resulting in more hematologic toxicity than previously reported for cladribine monotherapy (grade 4 = 3%). However, the incidence of infection was low, with 3% of patients experiencing pneumonia.[44,74]

Corticosteroids have also been used in combination with cladribine and mitoxantrone in two studies. Saven et al[73] originally used prednisone in the study that was previously discussed, but it was later omitted from the regimen because of the increased risk of infection without an improvement in response rates. Dexamethasone (20 mg/d on days 1 to 5) has

Table 4 Cladribine Combination Therapy Summary for Indolent Lymphoma

Reference	N	Regimen	CR (%)	Survival Measure	Toxicity
76	7	Cd: 0.1 mg/kg/d d 1–3 C: 500 mg/m² d 1 P: 40 mg d 1–5	22	68% at 3 yrs	G3-4 hematologic 26%
74	32	Cd: 5 mg/m² × 3 d M: 8 mg/m² d 1–2 (12 mg/m² for relapsed patients)	47	RFS 25 mo	G3 granulocytopenia 23% G4 granulocytopenia 50%
75	14	Cd: 0.12 mg/kg/d × 5 d M: 10 mg/m² × d 1 D: 20 mg d 1–5	7.1	NR	G3-4 myelosuppression 36%
77	14	Cd: 0.12 mg/kg/d × 3–5 d M: 10 mg/m² D1 C: 650 mg/m² D1	12	NR	G3-4 neutropenia 29%
78	11	R: 375 mg/m² D1 Cd: 0.12 mg/kg/d D2–6	27.3	FFS 6.5 mo	G3-4 infections 15.4% G3-4 neutropenia 11.5%

Abbreviations: CR, complete remission; Cd, cladribine; C, cyclophosphamide; P, prednisone; M, mitoxantrone; D, dexamethasone; NR, not reported; FFS, failure-free survival; R, rituximab; RFS, relapse-free survival; G3-4, grade 3–4.

also been combined with this regimen (cladribine 0.12 mg/kg/d × 5 days + mitoxantrone 10 mg/m² on day 1) in 14 patients with recurrent indolent lymphoma.[75] An overall response rate of 29% (7% CRs) was reported; however, 35% of patients developed infection.[75] This study suggested that this combination was inferior to single-agent cladribine therapy, although it was conducted in a small number of patients.

Cladribine has been evaluated in combination with standard chemotherapy regimens, including cyclophosphamide and prednisone.[76,77] Laurencet et al[76] were the first to evaluate this combination in a phase II study in 19 patients (seven with NHL). Cladribine was administered at 0.2 mg/kg subcutaneously on days 1 to 3 along with intravenous cyclophosphamide 500 mg/m² on day 1 with oral prednisone 40 mg/m² on days 1 to 5 at 4-weekly intervals up to six courses. The overall response rate was 88% with a 22% CR rate. The combination was associated with a moderate degree of myelosuppression and very few infections. This may have been related to selection bias where the majority of patients were previously untreated or to the fact that cladribine was only given for 3 days.[76] Robak et al[77] then evaluated the combination of cladribine (0.12 mg/kg/d × 3 or 5 days), mitoxantrone (10 mg/m² on day 1), and cyclophosphamide (650 mg/m² on day 1) in 33 patients, 14 with indolent NHL. The overall response rate was 49% with 12% CRs. Myelosuppression was more pronounced in the patients who received the 5-day infusion.[77]

Recently, a combination of cladribine with rituximab was investigated in 26 CD20 antigen-positive patients, including 11 patients with refractory indolent NHL.[78] The regimen consisted of rituximab 375 mg/m² over 6 hours on day 1 followed by cladribine 0.12 mg/kg/d on days 2 through 6 with the courses repeated at 4-week intervals. This sequence of administration was based on data showing that rituximab sensitizes lymphoma cells to subsequent chemotherapy.[79] The overall response rate of the study population was 69%, and 73% in patients with indolent NHL. CR was achieved in 15% of the patients, the majority of whom had indolent lymphoma. Grade 3 neutropenia was only observed in 11.5% of patient and infections were reported in only four patients.[78] This combination appears to be better tolerated than previously investigated regimens. This study shows that the combination of these two agents induces higher response and CR rates than when the agents are given as monotherapy. Further study is necessary for evaluation of this regimen in a larger number of patients. Table 4 summarizes cladribine combination therapy regimens.

Pentostatin Combinations

The US Oncology group performed two sequential studies of pentostatin combinations (Table 5). The first combination included a two-drug regimen of pentostatin (4 mg/m²) and rituximab (375 mg/m²) weekly for 4 weeks with the fifth week off in 60 patients with previously treated and untreated indolent NHL (PR regimen).[80] In order to be considered evaluable, a patient had to receive two 5-week cycles. Patients with partial responses or stable disease received two additional cycles. Most of the patients had follicular lymphoma (68%) and 50% had stage III or IV disease. Expression of CD20 was not a requirement for inclusion in the study and only one third of the population was CD20-positive. Among 57 evaluable patients, 73% responded (22.3% CR rate). The response rate was 73% in patients who were treatment-naive (29% CR rate) compared with 69% in previously treated patients (19% CR rate). The median duration of response was 11 months and median time to progression was 15 months. Grade 3–4 neutropenia, which occurred in 10%, was the most common toxicity reported and overall the combination was well tolerated.[80]

The second study was a phase II trial, which included only chemotherapy-naive patients, used mitoxantrone (10 mg/m² and day 1) in addition to pentostatin 4 mg/m² on days 1 and 8 and rituximab 375 mg/m² on days 1 and 8 (only given on day 8 in the first course) every 28 days in 24 patients with stage III-IV indolent NHL (PMR regimen).[81] Lymphomas in this study had to be CD20-positive. Among the 24 evaluable

Table 5 Pentostatin Combination Therapy Summary for Indolent Lymphoma

Reference	N	Regimen	CR (%)	Duration of Response	Toxicity
80	60	P (4 mg/m²) + R (375 mg/m²) Weekly × 4 wk with 1 wk off × 4	22.3	11 mo	G3-4 neutropenia 10%
81	24	P (4 mg/m²) + R (375 mg/m² d 1 & 8) M (10 mg/m² d1) Repeat every 28 d	50	10 mo	G3-4 neutropenia 67%, leukopenia 17%, febrile neutropenia 17%, sepsis 8%
83	32	P (5 mg/m² d 1 & 8) + Pred (100 mg d 1 & 8) M (10 mg/m² d 1) B (8 mg/m² d 8) Repeat every 3 wk × 6	30	38 mo 3-yr OS 71% 3-yr FFS 23%	G3-4 leukopenia 37%, G3 thrombocytopenia 7%

Abbreviations: P, pentostatin; R, rituximab; G, grade; Pred, prednisone; B, bleomycin; OS, overall survival; FFS, failure-free survival.

patients, the overall response rate was 84% with 50% CRs. The median duration of response was 10 months, likely due to the dosage reductions that were necessary. Eighteen (75%) patients required dose reduction or delay due to toxicity, mainly neutropenia. This is most likely attributable to the intensity of the regimen and the fact that growth factors were not permitted. Grade 3–4 neutropenia was observed in 67% of patients, although there were only four occurrences of febrile neutropenia and two documented infections.[81] We believe that this pilot study demonstrated the safety and increased response rate of the PMR regiment compared to the PR combination but feel that the use of growth factors would lessen the myelotoxicity and likely improve the duration of remission. In a follow-up study we propose to administer the same PMR regimen but with pegilfastrim on day 9 and four cycles will be administered. Prophylaxis with cotrimoxazole, acyclovir, and allopurinol will be given to all patients.

Another avenue of therapy will be the investigation into maintenance therapy with pentostatin. Based on data from Ghielmini et al,[82] who demonstrated the rituximab maintenance following rituximab induction in patients with indolent lymphoma resulted in prolonged progression-free survival, we propose to use a maintenance program following induction with PMR. All patients except those with progression of NHL will be randomized to rituximab alone (357 mg/m² every 2 months) or rituximab plus pentostatin 4 mg/m² every 2 months for four courses. Randomization will occur at the time of entry into the study, prior to receiving induction therapy. End points will include duration of progression-free survival, overall survival, and percentage increase in response in the two arms. Toxicity will also be compared and molecular assessment of response will be evaluated.

A four-drug combination including pentostatin 5 mg/m² on days 1 and 8, mitoxantrone 10 mg/m² on day 1, bleomycin 8 mg/m² on day 8, and prednisone 100 mg on days 1 and 8 for 3-week intervals for up to six cycles was evaluated in 32 patients with refractory and relapsed indolent NHL. The overall response rate was 60% with 33% CRs. The median duration of remission was 38 months with a 3-year survival of 71%. Toxicity consisted of frequent leukopenia but was not associated with infection and a few cases of thrombocytopenia.[83] This regimen appears to be suitable for patients in need of salvage therapy and may not be candidates for high-dose chemotherapy approaches.

Assessment of Combination Therapy With Molecular Diagnostics

Treatments for indolent lymphoma that produce a higher frequency of CR do not necessarily result in better survival outcomes than treatments that produce lower CR rates. In order to appropriately determine the success of a given treatment other modalities beside the clinical assessment of CR are essential. Recent improvements in technology have enabled the quantitative assessment of response at the molecular level including polymerase chain reaction (PCR) and flow cytometry. These methods have become more sensitive and quantitative over the last few years. One method that is being investigated is the achievement of a molecular complete response defined by evaluating the eradication of MRD from either peripheral blood or bone marrow to the point where it is undetectable. MRD describes the presence of cancer cells below the level of detection by standard light microscopy. The *bcl*-2 gene is rearranged in 80% to 90% of patients with follicular lymphomas.[84] The significance of this molecular response is unknown; however, molecular response is probably necessary to achieve total irradication of lymphoma.

Molecular remission, defined by eradication of detectable *bcl*-2–rearranged cells, has been associated with prolonged failure-free survival following both stem cell transplantation and chemotherapy.[85-88] Patients who have rearranged *bcl*-2 cells have been reported to have a better prognosis than those with *bcl*-2 germ line cells.[89] Rambaldi et al[90] monitored for MRD in follicular lymphoma patients who received CHOP and rituximab. Results of this study supported the concept that failure free survival is associated with achievement of PCR negativity. They also suggest that patients who remain PCR-positive may need to receive additional therapy. However, the predictave value of molecular remission may not be perfect. Some studies have reported that long-term remissions are achieved in patients who are persistently PCR-positive.[91,92] Clearly, standardization of criteria of molecular response will be necessary in the future in order to evaluate the utility of this surrogate marker.

Conclusions/Future Directions

Indolent lymphomas primarily affect elderly patients who commonly have significant comorbidities and poor performance status thus limiting their ability to tolerate combined therapeutic modalities. Therefore, it is essential to identify new options for these patients in order to affect the natural history of the disease. Over the past few decades the treatment of another indolent lymphoid malignancy, HCL, has been highly successful with several new therapeutic options. Purine analogues appear to have changed the natural history of HCL with the high CR rates that have been reported and serve as the basis for investigating these agents for indolent lymphomas. Several lessons can be learnt from the HCL story that may be applicable to the treatment of follicular lymphomas. First, achievement of an initial CR is desirable and associated with longer duration of response. Second, despite the high efficacy of nucleoside analogues in this disease, single-agent therapy does not appear to be curative in all patients and the progression-fre survival curve after therapy with pentostatin or cladribine does not appear to have a plateau. As such, combination regimens, perhaps with monoclonal antibodies, are desirable. Finally, achievement of CR can not be considered to be equivalent to a "cure" and relapse is likely to be a function of MRD. Recent advancements in therapeutic options available for patients with follicular lymphoma include combination therapy with agents that have differing mechanisms of action and non-overlapping toxicity. It has been shown that patients who are candidates for aggressive therapy might receive benefit, including disease-free survival and overall survival, from combination purine analogue therapy. Using these more aggressive therapeutic approaches earlier in the disease and as maintenance therapy may further enhance outcomes. With the advent of these new therapies along with the molecular evaluation of these regimens, we may be nearing the time where the goal for more advanced indolent lymphoma will be to achieve a cure. In fact, the survival of patients with follicular lymphoma has improved over the last 25 years, which may be a result of the availability of new treatment options and improved supportive care.[93] Further randomized clinical trials with longer term follow-up will be necessary to establish the most effective and safe regimen that will have an impact on the course of the disease.

References

1. Jemal A, Murray T, Ward E, Samuels A, Tiwari RC, Ghafoor A, et al: Cancer statistics, 2005. CA Cancer J Clin 55:10-30, 2005
2. Vose JM, Chiu BC, Cheson BD, Dancey J, Wright J: Update on epidemiology and therapeutics for non-Hodgkin's lymphoma. Hematology (Am Soc Hematol Educ Program):241-262, 2002
3. Pileri SA, Zinzani PL, Went P, Pileri A Jr, Bendandi M: Indolent lymphoma: The pathologist's viewpoint. Ann Oncol 15:12-18, 2004
4. Harris NL, Jaffe ES, Stein H, Banks PM, Chan JK, Cleary ML, et al: A revised European-American classification of lymphoid neoplasms: A proposal from the International Lymphoma Study Group. Blood 84: 1361-1392, 1994
5. Harris NL, Jaffe ES, Diebold J, Flandrin G, Muller-Hermelink HK, Vardiman J, et al: World Health Organization classification of neoplastic diseases of the hematopoietic and lymphoid tissues: Report of the Clinical Advisory Committee meeting—Airlie House, Virginia, November 1997. J Clin Oncol 17:3835-3849, 1999
6. Armitage JO: Treatment of non-Hodgkin's lymphoma. N Engl J Med 328:1023-1030, 1993
7. Groves FD, Linet MS, Travis LB, Devesa SS: Cancer surveillance series: Non-Hodgkin's lymphoma incidence by histologic subtype in the United States from 1978 through 1995. J Natl Cancer Inst 92:1240-1251, 2000
8. A clinical evaluation of the International Lymphoma Study Group classification of non-Hodgkin's lymphoma. The Non-Hodgkin's Lymphoma Classification Project. Blood 89:3909-3918, 1997
9. Winter JN, Gascoyne RD, Van Besien K: Low-grade lymphoma. Hematology (Am Soc Hematol Educ Program):203-220, 2004
10. Solal-Celigny P, Roy P, Colombat P, White J, Armitage JO, Arranz-Saez R, et al: Follicular lymphoma international prognostic index. Blood 104:1258-1265, 2004
11. Horning SJ: Natural history of and therapy for the indolent non-Hodgkin's lymphomas. Semin Oncol 20:75-88, 1993
12. Miller TP, Dahlberg S, Cassady JR, Adelstein DJ, Spier CM, Grogan TM, et al: Chemotherapy alone compared with chemotherapy plus radiotherapy for localized intermediate- and high-grade non-Hodgkin's lymphoma. N Engl J Med 339:21-26, 1998
13. Cheson BD: New chemotherapeutics strategies for the treatment of indolent lymphoid malignancies. Semin Hematol 36:26-33, 1999
14. Dearden CE, Matutes E, Hilditch BL, Swansbury GJ, Catovsky D: Long-term follow-up of patients with hairy cell leukaemia after treatment with pentostatin or cladribine. Br J Haematol 106:515-519, 1999
15. Flinn IW, Kopecky KJ, Foucar MK, Head D, Bennett JM, Hutchison R, et al: Long-term follow-up of remission duration, mortality, and second malignancies in hairy cell leukemia patients treated with pentostatin. Blood 96:2981-2986, 2000
16. Cohen Y, Solal-Celigny P, Polliack A: Rituximab therapy for follicular lymphoma: A comprehensive review of its efficacy as primary treatment, treatment for relapsed disease, re-treatment and maintenance. Haematologica 88:811-823, 2003
17. Hainsworth JD, Litchy S, Burris HA 3rd, Scullin DC Jr, Corso SW, Yardley DA, et al: Rituximab as first-line and maintenance therapy for patients with indolent non-Hodgkin's lymphoma. J Clin Oncol 20: 4261-4267, 2002
18. Robertson LE, Chubb S, Meyn RE, Story M, Ford R, Hittelman WN, et al: Induction of apoptotic cell death in chronic lymphocytic leukemia by 2-chloro-2′-deoxyadenosine and 9-beta-D-arabinosyl-2-fluoroadenine. Blood 81:143-150, 1993
19. Kantarjian HM, Schachner J, Keating MJ: Fludarabine therapy in hairy cell leukemia. Cancer 67:1291-1293, 1991
20. Giblett ER, Anderson JE, Cohen F, Pollara B, Meuwissen HJ: Adenosine-deaminase deficiency in two patients with severely impaired cellular immunity. Lancet 2:1067-1069, 1972
21. Grever M, Kopecky K, Foucar MK, Head D, Bennett JM, Hutchison RE, et al: Randomized comparison of pentostatin versus interferon alfa-2a in previously untreated patients with hairy cell leukemia: an intergroup study. J Clin Oncol 13:974-982, 1995
22. Catovsky D, Matutes E, Talavera JG, O'Connor NT, Johnson SA, Emmett E, et al: Long term results with 2'deoxycoformycin in hairy cell leukemia. Leuk Lymphoma 14:109-113, 1994 (suppl 1)
23. Saven A, Burian C, Koziol JA, Piro LD: Long-term follow-up of patients

with hairy cell leukemia after cladribine treatment. Blood 92:1918-1926, 1998
24. Goodman GR, Beutler E, Saven A: Cladribine in the treatment of hairy-cell leukaemia. Best Pract Res Clin Haematol 16:101-116, 2003
25. Grever MR, Doan CA, Kraut EH: Pentostatin in the treatment of hairy-cell leukemia. Best Pract Res Clin Haematol 16:91-99, 2003
26. Spiers AS, Parekh SJ, Bishop MB: Hairy-cell leukemia: Induction of complete remission with pentostatin (2′-deoxycoformycin). J Clin Oncol 2:1336-1342, 1984
27. Brogden RN, Sorkin EM: Pentostatin. A review of its pharmacodynamic and pharmacokinetic properties, and therapeutic potential in lymphoproliferative disorders. Drugs 46:652-677, 1993
28. Cohen A, Hirschhorn R, Horowitz SD, Rubinstein A, Polmar SH, Hong R, et al: Deoxyadenosine triphosphate as a potentially toxic metabolite in adenosine deaminase deficiency. Proc Natl Acad Sci U S A 75:472-476, 1978
29. Zinzani PL: Non-Hodgkin's lymphoma: The evolving role of purine analogues. Best Pract Res Clin Haematol 15:505-516, 2002
30. Seto S, Carrera CJ, Kubota M, Wasson DB, Carson DA: Mechanism of deoxyadenosine and 2-chlorodeoxyadenosine toxicity to nondividing human lymphocytes. J Clin Invest 75:377-383, 1985
31. Sheridan W, Gordon DS, Fullen AJ, Olson A, Vogler WR, Winton E: Preclinical studies on deoxycoformycin and deoxyadenosine as pharmacologic T cell purging tools. Bone Marrow Transplant 4:511-517, 1989
32. Aye MT, Dunne JV: Effect of 2′-deoxycoformycin on erythroid, granulocytic, and T-lymphocyte colony growth. Blood 58:1043-1046, 1981
33. Seymour JF, Kurzrock R, Freireich EJ, Estey EH: 2-Chlorodeoxyadenosine induces durable remissions and prolonged suppression of $CD4^+$ lymphocyte counts in patients with hairy cell leukemia. Blood 83:2906-2911, 1994
34. O'Brien S, Kantarjian H, Beran M, Smith T, Koller C, Estey E, et al: Results of fludarabine and prednisone therapy in 264 patients with chronic lymphocytic leukemia with multivariate analysis-derived prognostic model for response to treatment. Blood 82:1695-1700, 1993
35. Steis RG, Urba WJ, Kopp WC, Alvord WG, Smith JW 2nd, Longo DL: Kinetics of recovery of $CD4^+$ T cells in peripheral blood of deoxycoformycin-treated patients. J Natl Cancer Inst 83:1678-1679, 1991
36. Hochster HS, Kim KM, Green MD, Mann RB, Neiman RS, Oken MM, et al: Activity of fludarabine in previously treated non-Hodgkin's low-grade lymphoma: Results of an Eastern Cooperative Oncology Group study. J Clin Oncol 10:28-32, 1992
37. Redman JR, Cabanillas F, Velasquez WS, McLaughlin P, Hagemeister FB, Swan F Jr, et al: Phase II trial of fludarabine phosphate in lymphoma: an effective new agent in low-grade lymphoma. J Clin Oncol 10:790-794, 1992
38. Hiddemann W, Unterhalt M, Pott C, Wormann B, Sandford D, Freund M, et al: Fludarabine single-agent therapy for relapsed low-grade non-Hodgkin's lymphomas: A phase II study of the German Low-Grade Non-Hodgkin's Lymphoma Study Group. Semin Oncol 20:28-31, 1993
39. Falkson CI: Fludarabine: A phase II trial in patients with previously treated low-grade lymphoma. Am J Clin Oncol 19:268-270, 1996
40. Whelan JS, Davis CL, Rule S, Ranson M, Smith OP, Mehta AB, et al: Fludarabine phosphate for the treatment of low grade lymphoid malignancy. Br J Cancer 64:120-123, 1991
41. Tondini C, Balzarotti M, Rampinelli I, Valagussa P, Luoni M, De Paoli A, et al: Fludarabine and cladribine in relapsed/refractory low-grade non-Hodgkin's lymphoma: A phase II randomized study. Ann Oncol 11: 231-233, 2000
42. Zinzani PL, Lauria F, Rondelli D, Benfenati D, Raspadori D, Bocchia M, et al: Fludarabine: an active agent in the treatment of previously-treated and untreated low-grade non-Hodgkin's lymphoma. Ann Oncol 4:575-578, 1993
43. Saven A, Emanuele S, Kosty M, Koziol J, Ellison D, Piro L: 2-Chlorodeoxyadenosine activity in patients with untreated, indolent non-Hodgkin's lymphoma. Blood 86:1710-1716, 1995
44. Betticher DC, von Rohr A, Ratschiller D, Schmitz SF, Egger T, Sonderegger T, et al: Fewer infections, but maintained antitumor activity with lower-dose versus standard-dose cladribine in pretreated low-grade non-Hodgkin's lymphoma. J Clin Oncol 16:850-858, 1998
45. Mercieca J, Matutes E, Dearden C, MacLennan K, Catovsky D: The role of pentostatin in the treatment of T-cell malignancies: Analysis of response rate in 145 patients according to disease subtype. J Clin Oncol 12:2588-2593, 1994
46. Cummings FJ, Kim K, Neiman RS, Comis RL, Oken MM, Weitzman SA, et al: Phase II trial of pentostatin in refractory lymphomas and cutaneous T-cell disease. J Clin Oncol 9:565-571, 1991
47. Duggan DB, Anderson JR, Dillman R, Case D, Gottlieb AJ: 2′ Deoxycoformycin (pentostatin) for refractory non-Hodgkin's lymphoma: A CALGB phase II study. Med Pediatr Oncol 18:203-206, 1990
48. Monfardini S, Sorio R, Cavalli F, Cerny TH, Van Glabbeke M, Kaye S, et al: Pentostatin (2′-deoxycoformycin, dCF) in patients with low-grade (B-T-cell) and intermediate- and high-grade (T-cell) malignant lymphomas: Phase II study of the EORTC Early Clinical Trials Group. Oncology 53:163-168, 1996
49. McLaughlin P, Hagemeister FB, Romaguera JE, Sarris AH, Pate O, Younes A, et al: Fludarabine, mitoxantrone, and dexamethasone: An effective new regimen for indolent lymphoma. J Clin Oncol 14:1262-1268, 1996
50. McLaughlin P, Hagemeister FB, Swan F Jr, Cabanillas F, Pate O, Romaguera JE, et al: Phase I study of the combination of fludarabine, mitoxantrone, and dexamethasone in low-grade lymphoma. J Clin Oncol 12:575-579, 1994
51. Zinzani PL, Bendandi M, Magagnoli M, Gherlinzoni F, Merla E, Tura S: Fludarabine-mitoxantrone combination-containing regimen in recurrent low-grade non-Hodgkin's lymphoma. Ann Oncol 8:379-383, 1997
52. Bordonaro R, Petralia G, Restuccia N, Todaro AM, Serraino D, Giuffrida D, et al: Fludarabine, mitoxantrone and dexamethasone as front-line therapy in elderly patients affected by newly-diagnosed, low-grade non-Hodgkin's lymphomas with unfavorable prognostic factors: Results of a phase II study. Leuk Lymphoma 45:93-100, 2004
53. Tsimberidou AM, McLaughlin P, Younes A, Rodriguez MA, Hagemeister FB, Sarris A, et al: Fludarabine, mitoxantrone, dexamethasone (FND) compared with an alternating triple therapy (ATT) regimen in patients with stage IV indolent lymphoma. Blood 100:4351-4357, 2002
54. Tsimberidou AM, Younes A, Romaguera J, Hagemeister FB, Rodriguez MA, Feng L, et al: Immunosuppression and infectious complications in patients with stage IV indolent lymphoma treated with a fludarabine, mitoxantrone, and dexamethasone regimen. Cancer 104:345-353, 2005
55. Zinzani PL, Magagnoli M, Bendandi M, Gherlinzoni F, Orcioni GF, Cellini C, et al: Efficacy of fludarabine and mitoxantrone (FN) combination regimen in untreated indolent non-Hodgkin's lymphomas. Ann Oncol 11:363-365, 2000
56. Seymour JF, Grigg AP, Szer J, Fox RM: Fludarabine and mitoxantrone: Effective and well-tolerated salvage therapy in relapsed indolent lymphoproliferative disorders. Ann Oncol 12:1455-1460, 2001
57. Emmanouilides C, Rosen P, Rasti S, Territo M, Kunkel L: Treatment of indolent lymphoma with fludarabine/mitoxantrone combination: A phase II trial. Hematol Oncol 16:107-116, 1998
58. Velasquez WS, Lew D, Grogan TM, Spiridonidis CH, Balcerzak SP, Dakhil SR, et al: Combination of fludarabine and mitoxantrone in untreated stages III and IV low-grade lymphoma: S9501. J Clin Oncol 21:1996-2003, 2003
59. Dimopoulos MA, Fountzilas G, Papageorgiou E, Kiamouris C, Mantzios G, Anagnostopoulos A, et al: Primary treatment of low-grade non-Hodgkin's lymphoma with the combination of fludarabine and mitoxantrone: A phase II study of the Hellenic Cooperative Oncology Group. Leuk Lymphoma 43:111-114, 2002
60. Lossos IS, Paltiel O, Polliack A: Salvage chemotherapy using a combination of fludarabine and cyclophosphamide for refractory or relapsing indolent and aggressive non-Hodgkin's lymphomas. Leuk Lymphoma 33:155-160, 1999
61. Lazzarino M, Orlandi E, Montillo M, Tedeschi A, Pagnucco G, Astori C, et al: Fludarabine, cyclophosphamide, and dexamethasone (FluCyD)

combination is effective in pretreated low-grade non-Hodgkin's lymphoma. Ann Oncol 10:59-64, 1999
62. O'Brien SM, Kantarjian HM, Cortes J, Beran M, Koller CA, Giles FJ, et al: Results of the fludarabine and cyclophosphamide combination regimen in chronic lymphocytic leukemia. J Clin Oncol 19:1414-1420, 2001
63. Eucker J, Schille C, Schmid P, Jakob C, Schetelig J, Kingreen D, et al: The combination of fludarabine and cyclophosphamide results in a high remission rate with moderate toxicity in low-grade non-Hodgkin's lymphomas. Anticancer Drugs 13:907-913, 2002
64. Tam CS, Wolf MM, Januszewicz EH, Prince HM, Westerman D, Seymour JF: Fludarabine and cyclophosphamide using an attenuated dose schedule is a highly effective regimen for patients with indolent lymphoid malignancies. Cancer 100:2181-2189, 2004
65. Rohatgi N, LaRocca RV, Bard V, Sethuraman G, Foon KA: Phase II trial of sequential therapy with fludarabine followed by cyclophosphamide, mitoxantrone, vincristine, and prednisone for low-grade follicular lymphomas. Am J Hematol 70:181-185, 2002
66. Santini G, Chisesi T, Nati S, Porcellini A, Zoli V, Rizzoli V, et al: Fludarabine, cyclophosphamide and mitoxantrone for untreated follicular lymphoma: A report from the non-Hodgkin's lymphoma co-operative study group. Leuk Lymphoma 45:1141-1147, 2004
67. Hendry L, Bowen A, Matutes E, Swansbury J, Catovsky D: Fludarabine, cyclophosphamide and mitoxantrone in relapsed or refractory chronic lymphocytic leukemia and low grade non-Hodgkin's lymphoma. Leuk Lymphoma 45:945-950, 2004
68. Santini G, Nati S, Spriano M, Gallamini A, Pierluigi D, Congiu AM, et al: Fludarabine in combination with cyclophosphamide or with cyclophosphamide plus mitoxantrone for relapsed or refractory low-grade non-Hodgkin's lymphoma. Haematologica 86:282-286, 2001
69. Di Gaetano N, Xiao Y, Erba E, Bassan R, Rambaldi A, Golay J, et al: Synergism between fludarabine and rituximab revealed in a follicular lymphoma cell line resistant to the cytotoxic activity of either drug alone. Br J Haematol 114:800-809, 2001
70. Savage DG, Cohen NS, Hesdorffer CS, Heitjan D, Oster MW, Garrett TJ, et al: Combined fludarabine and rituximab for low grade lymphoma and chronic lymphocytic leukemia. Leuk Lymphoma 44:477-481, 2003
71. Czuczman MS, Koryzna A, Mohr A, Stewart C, Donohue K, Blumenson L, et al: Rituximab in combination with fludarabine chemotherapy in low-grade or follicular lymphoma. J Clin Oncol 23:694-704, 2005
72. Forstpointner R, Dreyling M, Repp R, Hermann S, Hanel A, Metzner B, et al: The addition of rituximab to a combination of fludarabine, cyclophosphamide, mitoxantrone (FCM) significantly increases the response rate and prolongs survival as compared with FCM alone in patients with relapsed and refractory follicular and mantle cell lymphomas: Results of a prospective randomized study of the German Low-Grade Lymphoma Study Group. Blood 104:3064-3071, 2004
73. Saven A, Lee T, Kosty M, Piro L: Cladribine and mitoxantrone dose escalation in indolent non-Hodgkin's lymphoma. J Clin Oncol 14: 2139-2144, 1996
74. Rummel MJ, Chow KU, Karakas T, Jager E, Mezger J, von Grunhagen U, et al: Reduced-dose cladribine (2-CdA) plus mitoxantrone is effective in the treatment of mantle-cell and low-grade non-Hodgkin's lymphoma. Eur J Cancer 38:1739-1746, 2002
75. Robak T, Gora-Tybor J, Urbanska-Rys H, Krykowski E: Combination regimen of 2-chlorodeoxyadenosine (cladribine), mitoxantrone and dexamethasone (CMD) in the treatment of refractory and recurrent low grade non-Hodgkin's lymphoma. Leuk Lymphoma 32:359-363, 1999
76. Laurencet FM, Zulian GB, Guetty-Alberto M, Iten PA, Betticher DC, Alberto P: Cladribine with cyclophosphamide and prednisone in the management of low-grade lymphoproliferative malignancies. Br J Cancer 79:1215-1219, 1999
77. Robak T, Gora-Tybor J, Lech-Maranda E, Blonski JZ, Kasznicki M: Cladribine in combination with mitoxantrone and cyclophosphamide(CMC) in the treatment of heavily pre-treated patients with advanced indolent lymphoid malignancies. Eur J Haematol 66:188-194, 2001
78. Robak T, Smolewski P, Urbanska-Rys H, Gora-Tybor J, Blonski JZ, Kasznicki M: Rituximab followed by cladribine in the treatment of heavily pretreated patients with indolent lymphoid malignancies. Leuk Lymphoma 45:937-944, 2004
79. Wilson WH: Chemotherapy sensitization by rituximab: Experimental and clinical evidence. Semin Oncol 27:30-36, 2000
80. Drapkin R, Di Bella NJ, Faragher DC, Harden E, Matei C, Hyman W, et al: Results of a phase II multicenter trial of pentostatin and rituximab in patients with low grade B-cell non-Hodgkin's lymphoma: an effective and minimally toxic regimen. Clin Lymphoma 4:169-175, 2003
81. Di Bella N, Reynolds C, Faragher D, Muscato J, Boehm KA, Asmar L: An open-label pilot study of pentostatin, mitoxantrone, and rituximab in patients with previously untreated, stage III or IV, low-grade non-Hodgkin lymphoma. Cancer 103:978-984, 2005
82. Ghielmini M, Schmitz SF, Cogliatti SB, Pichert G, Hummerjohann J, Waltzer U, et al: Prolonged treatment with rituximab in patients with follicular lymphoma significantly increases event-free survival and response duration compared with the standard weekly × 4 schedule. Blood 103:4416-4423, 2004
83. Federico M, Callea V, Danesi R, Montanini A, Di Renzo N, Petrini M, et al: Mitoxantrone, prednisone, pentostatin and bleomycin for patients with indolent non-Hodgkin's lymphoma relapsed or unresponsive to previous treatments. Results of a phase II study conducted by the Gruppo Italiano per lo Studio dei Linfomi (GISL). Cancer Ther 1:63-70, 2003
84. Buckstein R, Pennell N, Berinstein NL: What is remission in follicular lymphoma and what is its relevance? Best Pract Res Clin Haematol 18:27-56, 2005
85. Gribben JG, Neuberg D, Freedman AS, Gimmi CD, Pesek KW, Barber M, et al: Detection by polymerase chain reaction of residual cells with the bcl-2 translocation is associated with increased risk of relapse after autologous bone marrow transplantation for B-cell lymphoma. Blood 81:3449-3457, 1993
86. McLaughlin P, Hagemeister FB, Swan F, Cabanillas F, Romaguera J, Rodriguez MA, et al: Intensive conventional-dose chemotherapy for stage IV low-grade lymphoma: High remission rates and reversion to negative of peripheral blood bcl-2 rearrangement. Ann Oncol 5:73-7, 1994 (suppl 2)
87. Lopez-Guillermo A, Cabanillas F, McLaughlin P, Smith T, Hagemeister F, Rodriguez MA, et al: The clinical significance of molecular response in indolent follicular lymphomas. Blood 91:2955-2960, 1998
88. Lopez-Guillermo A, Cabanillas F, McLaughlin P, Smith T, Hagemeister F, Rodriguez MA, et al: Molecular response assessed by PCR is the most important factor predicting failure-free survival in indolent follicular lymphoma: Update of the MDACC series. Ann Oncol 11:137-140, 2000 (suppl 1)
89. Lopez-Guillermo A, Cabanillas F, McDonnell TI, McLaughlin P, Smith T, Pugh W, et al: Correlation of bcl-2 rearrangement with clinical characteristics and outcome in indolent follicular lymphoma. Blood 93:3081-3087, 1999
90. Rambaldi A, Lazzari M, Manzoni C, Carlotti E, Arcaini L, Baccarani M, et al: Monitoring of minimal residual disease after CHOP and rituximab in previously untreated patients with follicular lymphoma. Blood 99: 856-862, 2002
91. Price CG, Meerabux J, Murtagh S, Cotter FE, Rohatiner AZ, Young BD, et al: The significance of circulating cells carrying t(14;18) in long remission from follicular lymphoma. J Clin Oncol 9:1527-1532, 1991
92. Lambrechts AC, Hupkes PE, Dorssers LC, van't Veer MB: Clinical significance of t(14; 18)-positive cells in the circulation of patients with stage III or IV follicular non-Hodgkin's lymphoma during first remission. J Clin Oncol 12:1541-1546, 1994
93. Swenson WT, Wooldridge JE, Lynch CF, Forman-Hoffman VL, Chrischilles E, Link BK: Improved survival of follicular lymphoma patients in the United States. J Clin Oncol 23:5019-5026, 2005

Seminars in
HEMATOLOGY

Role of Single-Agent Purine Analogues in Therapy of Peripheral T-Cell Lymphomas

Claire E. Dearden

Peripheral T-cell lymphomas (PTCLs) comprise a heterogeneous group of lymphomas with different clinical presentation and morphologic, immunophenotypic, and cytogenetic markers. Many of these malignancies follow an aggressive course and current therapeutic strategies are limited. The prognosis for these patients is usually very poor. The purine analogues are a class of drugs that have been shown to be active in patients who have T-cell lymphoma. T cells have a very high concentration of adenosine deaminase (ADA), a key enzyme in the purine degradation pathway, which is blocked by this class of agent. Pentostatin has been the most extensively studied of these drugs in PTCL and has shown variable response rates. However, many of the reports are limited to small single-center studies. Larger prospective randomized trials will be necessary to examine this therapy and to further explore combination regimens, which may result in increased responses.
Semin Hematol 43(suppl 2):S22-S26

T-cell lymphoproliferative disorders are a heterogenous group of rare disorders that result from clonal proliferation of mature postthymic lymphocytes. The World Health Organization classification of T-cell lymphoma (Table 1) includes nodal and extranodal peripheral T-cell lymphomas (PTCLs), anaplastic large cell lymphoma (ALCL), T-cell prolymphocytic leukemia (T-PLL), T-large granular lymphocyte leukaemia (T-LGL), and cutaneous T-cell lymphoma (CTCL). PTCLs account for 10% to 12% of all lymphoid neoplasms. There is considerable geographic and racial variation in the incidence of the different subtypes of T-cell lymphoma. Based on cases from the Non-Hodgkin's Lymphoma Classification Project, the lowest frequency of PTCL was in North America (3%) and the highest frequency was in the Far East (18%).[1] This difference is largely due to the increased number of natural killer (NK) lymphomas seen in the Far East.

PTCL usually affects adults and most entities are more commonly reported in men. The median reported age for patients with PTCL is 61 years (range, 17 to 90 years).[1] The more aggressive leukaemic subtypes, T-cell prolymphocytic leukemia (T-PLL), Sézary syndrome (SS), and adult T-cell leukemia lymphoma (ATLL), usually present with involvement of multiple sites. T-PLL is characterized by high white blood cell count (WBC) and usually follows a very aggressive course with a median survival of 7.5 months in historic series.[2,3] Some centers have reported cases that present initially with an indolent course but progression is inevitable.[4] T-LGL usually follows an indolent course and is characterized by marked neutropenia with recurrent infections. T-LGL is also associated with rheumatoid arthritis.[5] ATLL is associated with the retrovirus human T-lymphotropic virus type 1 (HTLV-1) and positive serology for HTLV-1 is mandatory for the diagnosis. The prevalence of the disease parallels the endemic distribution of the virus, which includes Japan, the Caribbean, Africa, and parts of the southeastern United States.[6] The acute form of ATLL is characterized by a rapid clinical progression in the setting of a high WBC, lymphadenopathy, hepatosplenomegaly, and hypercalcemia. There are also chronic clinical subtypes.[7]

The overall prognosis for patients with PTCL, excluding anaplastic large-cell lymphoma (ALCL), is poor. The overall survival (OS) has been reported to be 25% at 3 years with failure-free survival rates of 20%.[1] The similarity in progression-free survival (PFS) and OS is an indication of the poor response to second-line therapies. Most PTCL patients present with unfavorable international prognostic index (IPI) scores (>3) and poor performance status. Average blast counts may also be an important prognostic indicator for PTCL unspecified. Based on the Non-Hodgkin's Lymphoma Classification Project, all patients could be stratified into four prognostic groups. The first group contains subgroups that have overall 5-year survival rates greater than 70% and includes only ALCL. The second group has 5-year OS rates between 50% and 70% and includes marginal zone B-cell lymphomas, lymphoplasmacytoid, and small cell B-cell non-Hodgkin's lymphoma. The third group with OS rates between 30% and 50% includes Burkitt's lymphomas, dif-

The Royal Marsden Hospital and Institute of Cancer Research, London, UK.
Address correspondence to Claire E. Dearden, MD, FRCP, MRCPath, The Royal Marsden Hospital and Institute of Cancer Research, London SM2 5PT, UK. E-mail: claire.dearden@rmh.nhs.uk

 0037-1963/06/$-see front matter © 2006 Elsevier Inc. All rights reserved.
doi:10.1053/j.seminhematol.2005.12.008

Table 1 The WHO Classification of Mature T- and NK Cell Neoplasma

Leukemic/disseminated
T-cell prolymphocytic leukemia
T-large granular lymphocyte leukemia
Aggressive NK cell leukemia
Adult T-cell leukemia/lymphoma
Nodal lymphomas
Angioimmunoblastic T-cell lymphoma
Peripheral T-cell lymphoma unspecified
Anaplastic large cell lymphoma
Cutaneous and extranodal lymphomas
Cutaneous T-cell lymphoma
Mycosis fungoides/Sézary syndrome
Extranodal NK/T-cell lymphoma
Intestinal T-cell lymphoma
Hepatosplenic (gamma-delta) T-cell lymphoma
Subcutaneous panniculitis-like T-cell lymphoma

fuse large B-cell lymphomas, and B-cell lymphoblastic lymphomas. Finally, the fourth group with an overall 5-year survival rate of less than 10% includes T-cell lymphoblastic lymphomas, PTCL, and mantle cell lymphomas.[1]

Mature T-cell neoplasms are distinguished by their clinical, morphologic, cytogenetic, and immunophenotypic characteristics. Unlike B-cell neoplasms, there is no clonal immunophenotypic marker and molecular genetic techniques are required to confirm monoclonality. The morphology of circulating lymphoid cells in mature T-cell leukemias helps to distinguish between the different subtypes. The prolymphocytes in T-PLL have irregular basophilic cytoplasm and a prominent single nucleolus. In comparison, the lymphocytes in T-LGL are larger with pale cytoplasm containing azurophilic granules. The lymphocytes in ATLL and SS have an irregular outline, while ALCL and PTCL unspecified may present with small and large pleomorphic lymphocytes. There are several immunophenotypic markers that are present in all mature T-cell leukemias: TdT^-, $CD2^+$, $CD5^+$, and $CD52^+$. Table 2 shows other specific markers that are present for the different disease subtypes. Cytogenetic abnormalities that have been reported in PTCL include chromosomal rearrangements and deletions in chromosomes 6, 7, 8, 13, and 14.[8] There are various cytogenetic abnormalities that have been associated with specific subtypes. In T-PLL abnormalities of chromosome 14 are common, with the most frequent being inv(14)(q11;q32,1), seen in 75% of cases, along with chromosome 8 abnormalities, which are present in 50% of cases (iso (8q), trisomy 8, t(8;8)).[2] ALCL is associated with t(2,5) and expression of nucleophosmin-anaplastic large cell lymphoma kinase (NPM-ALK) protein.[8]

Overview of Purine Analogues

The purine analogues are one of the most active classes of drugs in patients with T-cell lymphoma. T-cells have high levels of adenosine deaminase (ADA), a key enzyme in the purine degradation pathway. The potential role of purine analogues was first identified based on the observation that children with congenital deficiency of ADA had impaired lymphoid development.[9] This initiated the search for agents that might interfere with ADA activity. The purine analogues, including pentostatin, fludarabine, and cladribine, are a group of structurally similar agents that were developed to target ADA. Although they differ in their action, ultimately they all result in impairment of DNA repair. Thus they have synergy with cytotoxic agents (eg, alkylating agents) that cause DNA damage. Pentostatin is a tight binding inhibitor of ADA, while fludarabine and cladribine have active metabolites that exert pharmacologic actions. The active metabolite of fludarabine, 2-fluro-ara-ATP, inhibits ribonucleotide reductase, DNA polymerase α, and DNA primase. The active metabolite of cladribine, ara-CTP, is incorporated into DNA, causing chain termination. In the earliest clinical trials pentostatin was used in high doses to treat patients with T-ALL. This was associated with treatment-limiting toxicities. Since that time purine analogues in lower, well-tolerated, doses have shown remarkable activity in patients with hairy-cell leukemia, CLL, and low-grade B-cell malignancies, as well as in T-cell lymphomas/leukemias.

Purine Analogue Therapy in PTCL

The majority of data evaluating purine analogues in T-cell lymphomas are based on trials in cutaneous T-cell lymphoma (CTCL), which is discussed in another section of this supplement. There are also reports that support the activity of these agents in other mature T-cell malignancies. Of the purine analogues, pentostatin has been the most extensively studied for these disorders.

Pentostatin

In the early 1980s, there were small reports describing the effectiveness of pentostatin in patients with T-cell leukemias, including patients refractory to other therapy.[10-12] The European Organization for Research and Treatment for Cancer Leukemia Cooperative Study Group (EORTC) conducted a phase II trial in 76 patients with advanced T-cell malignancies, including 25 patients with what was then termed "T-CLL"[13] (see Table 3). The response rate with pentostatin was 8%, with a median disease-free survival of 22 weeks. T-CLL has been reclassified by the World Helath Organization (WHO) as T-PLL, which has been shown in other studies to be responsive to pentostatin. The first

Table 2 Immunophenotype Markers of Mature T-Cell Leukemias

Marker	T-PLL	SS	ATLL	T-LGLL
CD3	+/−	+	+	+
CD7	++	−	−	+/−
CD4	+/−	+	+	−
CD8	+/−	−	−	+
CD25	+/−	+/−	++	−

Abbreviations: T-PLL, T-cell prolymphocytic leukemia; SS, Sézary syndrome; ATLL, adult T-cell leukemia lymphoma; T-LGLL, T-cell large granular leukemia. + = marker expressed; ++ = marker strongly expressed; +/− = variable expression; − = marker not expressed.

Table 3 Summary of Pentostatin Studies in Peripheral T-Cell Lymphomas

Reference	Dosing	N	Patient Subset	ORR(%)	CR(%)	Median Survival
Matutes[2]	4 mg/m² every wk	31	T-PLL	48 58*	9	16 mo (responders) 10 mo (non-rspd) 7 mo (not tx pento)
Dearden[17]	4 mg/m² every wk × 4 wks then every 2 wk until response	69	T-PLL = 31 ATLL = 20 LGL = 4	48 (58)* 15 (18)* 25 (50)*	9 10 25	T-PLL = 16 mo ATLL = NR LGL = NR
Dohner[15]	4 mg/m² every wk × 6 wks then every 2 wk × 5 doses	20	T-PLL = 6	33	0	NR
Ho[13]	4 mg/m² every wk × 3 wks then every 2 wks × 6 wk then every mo × 6 mo	76	T-PLL = 24	8	0	DFS = 22 wk
Mercieca[18]	4 mg/m² every wk × 4 wk then every 2 wk until response	145	T-PLL = 55 LGL = 5 ATLL = 25	45 40 12	9 40 8	NR
Tsimberidou[19]	3.75-5 mg/m²/d × 3 days then every 3 wk	42	PTCL = 4 ATLL = 3 ALCL = 1	100 33 0	50 0 0	18 mo†

Abbreviations: ORR, overall response rate; CR, complete response; not tx pento, patients not treated with pentostatin; T-PLL, T-cell prolymphocytic leukemia; ATLL, adult T-cell leukemia lymphoma; LGL, NK-large granular lymphocytic leukemia; PTCL, peripheral T-cell; NR, not reported; ALCL, anaplastic large cell lymphoma; DFS, disease-free survival

*Response rates for subset of patients with $CD4^+$ $CD8^-$.

†Overall response duration is 18 months; however, the majority of patients enrolled in the trial had Sézary syndrome/mycosis fungoides.

case study was published in 1986, showing that two patients achieved remission following pentostatin.[14] In the early 1990s, Matutes et al[2] published a report of 78 patients with T-PLL describing the clinical and laboratory features of the disease. Of the 78 patients, 31 were treated with pentostatin. There were 15 responses (48%), including three complete responses (CRs) and 12 partial responses (PRs). Patients with a T-helper-cell phenotype, $CD4^+CD8^-$, had a slightly better outcome (response rate, 58%). Overall there were no lengthy remissions.[2] Another phase II study conducted by the EORTC treated 20 patients with T- or B-prolymphocytic leukemia with weekly pentostatin.[15] Of the 20 patients, six had T-PLL. There were nine overall responders in the entire study population (45%), including two (33%) of the patients with T-PLL. All of the responders had PRs and the median duration of response was 9 months (range, 2 to 30 months).[15] The majority of patients (85%) enrolled in this study had received prior chemotherapy.

By far the largest experience with pentostatin in mature T-cell malignancies has been at the Royal Marsden Hospital in London[16-18] (see Table 3). A total of 165 patients who had a range of relapsed/refractory postthymic T-cell malignancies received pentostatin at a dose of 4 mg/m² weekly for 4 weeks and then every 2 weeks to maximize response. Responses were seen in 34% of patients, with a median response duration of 6 months (range, 3 months to 15 years). Some patients had durable remissions, with disease subtypes the main predictor of response; T-PLL and SS had the best response rates of 45% and 62%, respectively. Only a minority of these responses were complete. Although some of the remissions have been prolonged, most patients relapsed within 1 year.[18] Activity in ATLL was disappointing and this has been confirmed by a number of studies in Japan.

Tsimberidou et al[19] published the most recent report of pentostatin in PTCL (see Table 3). Forty-two patients, including 32 (76%) with mycosis fungoides/SS and 10 patients (24%) with other T-cell leukemias or lymphomas, were enrolled. The overall response rate was 54.8% (CR = 14.3% and PR = 40.5%). Durable responses were observed mainly in patients with SS or PTCL. The median duration of response was 4.3 months (range, 1 to 61 months).[19] The use of pentostatin alone and in combination with other agents deserves further investigation in these malignancies.

Other Agents

Most of the studies evaluating the other purine analogues have been in relapsed refractory CTCL patients and have recruited small patient numbers (Tables 4 and 5). There is some published experience in the form of single-center case reports for other T-cell malignancies, including T-LGL,

Table 4 Cladribine Monotherapy in Previously Treated CTCL

Study	N	CR (%)	OR (%)
Saven[40]	16	29	47
O'Brien[20]	22	18	41
Kuzel[41]	21	14	28
Kong[42]	25	12	24
Betticher[43]*	31	13	29
Total	115	15	32

Abbreviations: CTCL, cutaneous T-cell lymphoma; CR, complete response; OR, overall response.

*Subcutaneous cladribine.

Table 5 Fludarabine Monotherapy in Previously Treated CTCL

Study	N	CR (%)	OR (%)
Von Hoff[44]	31	3	19
Redman[45]	5	0	40
Total	36	3	22

Abbreviations: CTCL, cutaneous T-cell lymphoma; CR, complete response; OR, overall response.

ATLL, T-PLL, angioimmunoblastic T-cell lymphoma, and $\gamma\delta$ T-cell lymphoma.[20-28]

Cladribine

O'Brien et al[20] treated 22 patients with cladribine (4 mg/m² over 7 days), including 11 patients with T-cell leukemia, and three patients with T-cell lymphoma. The overall response rate was 41% with four of the patients achieving a CR and three of the these patients remaining in remission at 23 months.[20] A phase II study was recently published describing the activity of cladribine in ATLL.[23] The study planned to administer cladribine 0.09 mg/kg/d for 7 days every 4 weeks for up to three courses in 30 patients. After enrollment of 15 patients, only one patient showed an objective response and 11 patients showed progressive disease. The independent monitoring committee advised discontinuation of patient enrollment and thus it was concluded that cladribine is not worthy for further investigation for the treatment of ATLL.[23]

Fludarabine

Kantarjian et al[27] reported the results of fludarabine (30 mg/m² for 5 days every 4 weeks) therapy in 17 patients with prolymphocytic leukemia. The overall response rate was 35% with an 18% CR rate. The responses were found to be durable and the investigators concluded that fludarabine showed encouraging results and deserves further investigation.[27] A study group formed in Frankfurt is currently investigating the role of combination therapy with fludarabine (30 mg/m² days 1 to 3), cyclophosphamide (1,000 mg/m² day 1), and doxorubicin (25 mg/m² days 2 and 3) for patients with T-cell malginancies.[29]

Future Directions

There are several other purine analogues, which are being investigated for PTCL. Gemcitabine is a novel analog of cytarabine with clinical activity in both solid tumors and hematologic malignancies. This agent inhibits DNA synthesis through chain termination and ribonucleotide reductase inhibition. Gemcitabine has been administered as salvage therapy in relapsed/refractory T-cell malignancies and has response rates between 60% and 70%.[30-34] In addition, it has been administered to 20 previously untreated patients and produced an overall response rate of 70%.[35] Nelarabine is a novel nucleoside analog, which is a pro-drug of Ara-G. Goy et al[36] used nelarabine (1.5 g/m² on days 1, 3, and 5 every 4 weeks for 6 weeks) in 13 pretreated patients with PTCL. They reported that the agent was well tolerated and had a 50% overall response rate.

Monoclonal antibody therapy is also emerging as a promising approach to treating PTCL. Campath-1H is an effective and well-tolerated therapy and has produced durable responses in two thirds of heavily pretreated patients with T-PLL.[37] The overall response rate was 76% (60% CRs and 16% PRs), including patients who were resistant to other therapies. The median disease-free interval was 10 months (up to 45 months) and survival was significantly prolonged in patients who achieved a CR (median, 2 years) compared with partial responders (9 months) and nonresponders (3 months). There was no evidence that Campath-1H alone is curative; however, it is associated with significantly higher response rates than that reported with previous conventional therapies.[37] Acute, infusion-related effects are almost always associated with the initial dose but can be well controlled by premedication. The most significant adverse effect of this agent is prolonged lymphopenia that is associated with reactivation of viruses such as cytomegalovirus, herpes virus, and other opportunistic infections. The combination of Campth-1H and purine analogues deserves further exploration. However, the increased risk of infection must be considered.

Other agents have also been explored in small numbers of patients with PTCL. Unmodified anti-CD5 and anti-CD4 monoclonal antibodies have shown some success.[38,39] In addition, denileukin diftitox (ONTAK) and histone deacetylase (HDAC) inhibitors have been reported to demonstrate activity in PTCL. Further study will be necessary to delineate the role of any of these agents.

Conclusions

The PTCLs are a diverse group of diseases with varying clinical manifestations and courses. Response to traditional chemotherapy is poor. The data evaluating purine analogues in patients with PTCL are limited to small, nonrandomized, single-center studies. The response rates in patients with relapsed/refractory disease have varied with monotherapy between 25% and 60%. The majority of data in T-cell disease are in CTCL, with very limited data available for the other disease subtypes. The best results among the purine analogues have been reported with pentostatin and gemcitabine. Combination therapy with purine analogues and other agents, particularly monoclonal antibodies or small molecule inhibitors, will need to be explored in the future in order to see increased response rates, although this must be balanced with the potential increased toxicities. The role of purine analogues in previously untreated patients with PTCL has yet to be established.

References

1. Rudiger T, Weisenburger DD, Anderson JR, Armitage JO, Diebold J, MacLennan KA, et al: Peripheral T-cell lymphoma (excluding anaplastic large-cell lymphoma): Results from the Non-Hodgkin's Lymphoma Classification Project. Ann Oncol 13:140-149, 2002
2. Matutes E, Brito-Babapulle V, Swansbury J, Ellis J, Morilla R, Dearden C, et al: Clinical and laboratory features of 78 cases of T-prolymphocytic leukemia. Blood 78:3269-3274, 1991
3. Matutes E, Taylor GP, Cavenagh J, Pagliuca A, Bareford D, Domingo A, et al: Interferon alpha and zidovudine therapy in adult T-cell leukaemia lymphoma: Response and outcome in 15 patients. Br J Haematol 113: 779-784, 2001
4. Garand R, Goasguen J, Brizard A, Buisine J, Charpentier A, Claisse JF, et al: Indolent course as a relatively frequent presentation in T-prolym-

phocytic leukaemia. Groupe Francais d'Hematologie Cellulaire. Br J Haematol 103:488-494, 1998
5. Liu JH, Wei S, Lamy T, Epling-Burnette PK, Starkebaum G, Djeu JY, et al: Chronic neutropenia mediated by fas ligand. Blood 95:3219-3222, 2000
6. Manns A, Hisada M, La Grenade L: Human T-lymphotropic virus type I infection. Lancet 353:1951-1958, 1999
7. Broder S, Bunn PA Jr, Jaffe ES, Blattner W, Gallo RC, Wong-Staal F, et al: NIH conference. T-cell lymphoproliferative syndrome associated with human T-cell leukemia/lymphoma virus. Ann Intern Med 100: 543-557, 1984
8. Lepretre S, Buchonnet G, Stamatoullas A, Lenain P, Duval C, d'Anjou J, et al: Chromosome abnormalities in peripheral T-cell lymphoma. Cancer Genet Cytogenet 117:71-79, 2000
9. Giblett ER, Anderson JE, Cohen F, Pollara B, Meuwissen HJ: Adenosine-deaminase deficiency in two patients with severely impaired cellular immunity. Lancet 2:1067-1069, 1972
10. Yu AL, Mendelsohn J, Matsumoto SS: Induction of complete remission in T-cell acute lymphoblastic leukemia with deoxycoformycin (dcf) and 9-beta-D-arabinofuranosyladenine (ara-A). Adv Exp Med Biol 195: 491-496, 1986
11. Spiers AS, Ruckdeschel JC, Horton J: Effectiveness of pentostatin (2'-deoxycoformycin) in refractory lymphoid neoplasms. Scand J Haematol 32:130-134, 1984
12. Spiers AS, Davis MP, Levine M, Li CY, Mangan KF, Mazza JJ, et al: T-cell chronic lymphocytic leukaemia: Anomalous cell markers, variable morphology, and marked responsiveness to pentostatin (2'-deoxycoformycin). Scand J Haematol 34:57-67, 1985
13. Ho AD, Suciu S, Stryckmans P, De Cataldo F, Willemze R, Thaler J, et al: Pentostatin in T-cell malignancies—A phase II trial of the EORTC. Leukemia Cooperative Group. Ann Oncol 10:1493-1498, 1999
14. el'Agnaf MR, Ennis KE, Morris TC, Robertson JH, Markey G, Alexander HD: Successful remission induction with deoxycoformycin in elderly patients with T-helper prolymphocytic leukaemia. Br J Haematol 63: 93-104, 1986
15. Dohner H, Ho AD, Thaler J, Stryckmans P, Sonneveld P, de Witte T, et al: Pentostatin in prolymphocytic leukemia: Phase II trial of the European Organization for Research and Treatment of Cancer Leukemia Cooperative Study Group. J Natl Cancer Inst 85:658-662, 1993
16. Dearden C, Matutes E, Catovsky D: Pentostatin treatment of cutaneous T-cell lymphoma. Oncology (Williston Park) 14:37-40, 2000
17. Dearden C, Matutes E, Catovsky D: Deoxycoformycin in the treatment of mature T-cell leukaemias. Br J Cancer 64:903-906, 1991
18. Mercieca J, Matutes E, Dearden C, MacLennan K, Catovsky D: The role of pentostatin in the treatment of T-cell malignancies: Analysis of response rate in 145 patients according to disease subtype. J Clin Oncol 12:2588-2593, 1994
19. Tsimberidou AM, Giles F, Duvic M, Fayad L, Kurzrock R: Phase II study of pentostatin in advanced T-cell lymphoid malignancies: Update of an M.D. Anderson Cancer Center series. Cancer 100:342-349, 2004
20. O'Brien S, Kurzrock R, Duvic M, Kantarjian H, Stass S, Robertson LE, et al: 2-Chlorodeoxyadenosine therapy in patients with T-cell lymphoproliferative disorders. Blood 84:733-738, 1994
21. Lorand-Metze I, Oliveira GB, Aranha FJ: Treatment of prolymphocytic leukemia with cladribine. Ann Hematol 76:85-86, 1998
22. Rondelli D, Lauria F, Zinzani PL, Raspadori D, Ventura MA, Galieni P, et al: 2-Chlorodeoxyadenosine in the treatment of relapsed/refractory chronic lymphoproliferative disorders. Eur J Haematol 58:46-50, 1997
23. Tobinai K, Uike N, Saburi Y, Chou T, Etoh T, Masuda M, et al: Phase II study of cladribine (2-chlorodeoxyadenosine) in relapsed or refractory adult T-cell leukemia-lymphoma. Int J Hematol 77:512-517, 2003
24. Uike N, Choi I, Tokoro A, Goto T, Yufu Y, Kozuru M, et al: Adult T-cell leukemia-lymphoma successfully treated with 2-chlorodeoxyadenosine. Intern Med 37:411-413, 1998
25. Sallah AS, Bernard S: Treatment of angioimmunoblastic lymphadenopathy with dysproteinemia using 2-chlorodeoxyadenosine. Ann Hematol 73:295-296, 1996
26. Witzig TE, Weitz JJ, Lundberg JH, Tefferi A: Treatment of refractory T-cell chronic lymphocytic leukemia with purine nucleoside analogues. Leuk Lymphoma 14:137-139, 1994
27. Kantarjian HM, Childs C, O'Brien S, Huh Y, Beran M, Schachner J, et al: Efficacy of fludarabine, a new adenine nucleoside analogue, in patients with prolymphocytic leukemia and the prolymphocytoid variant of chronic lymphocytic leukemia. Am J Med 90:223-228, 1991
28. Whelan JS, Davis CL, Rule S, Ranson M, Smith OP, Mehta AB, et al: Fludarabine phosphate for the treatment of low grade lymphoid malignancy. Br J Cancer 64:120-123, 1991
29. Weidmann E, Boehrer S, Chow KU, Engels K, Harder L, Hinz T, et al: Treatment of aggressive, or progressing indolent peripheral T- and NK-cell neoplasias by combination of fludarabine, cyclophosphamide and doxorubicine. Onkologie 24:162-164, 2001
30. Dumontet C, Morschhauser F, Solal-Celigny P, Bouafia F, Bourgeois E, Thieblemont C, et al: Gemcitabine as a single agent in the treatment of relapsed or refractory low-grade non-Hodgkin's lymphoma. Br J Haematol 113:772-778, 2001
31. Sallah S, Wan JY, Nguyen NP: Treatment of refractory T-cell malignancies using gemcitabine. Br J Haematol 113:185-187, 2001
32. Zinzani PL, Baliva G, Magagnoli M, Bendandi M, Modugno G, Gherlinzoni F, et al: Gemcitabine treatment in pretreated cutaneous T-cell lymphoma: Experience in 44 patients. J Clin Oncol 18:2603-2606, 2000
33. Zinzani PL, Magagnoli M, Bendandi M, Orcioni GF, Gherlinzoni F, Albertini P, et al: Therapy with gemcitabine in pretreated peripheral T-cell lymphoma patients. Ann Oncol 9:1351-1353, 1998
34. Marchi E, Alinari L, Tani M, Stefoni V, Pimpinelli N, Berti E, et al: Gemcitabine as frontline treatment for cutaneous T-cell lymphoma: Phase II study of 32 patients. Cancer 104:2437-2441, 2005
35. Talpur R, Apisarnthanaraz N, Ward S, Kerne H, Chiao N, Kurzrock R, et al: Phase II Evaluation of gemcitabine as a single agent for cutaneous T-cell lymphoma. Blood 102:404a, 2003 (abstr)
36. Goy A, Bleyer A, Hagemeister F, Fayad PB, Romaguera J, Samaniego F, et al: Phase II study of compound GW506U78 (AraG) for patients with indolent B-cell or peripheral T-cell lymphoma previously treatment with chemotherapy. Blood 102:639a, 2003 (abstr)
37. Dearden CE, Matutes E, Cazin B, Tjonnfjord GE, Parreira A, Nomdedeu B, et al: High remission rate in T-cell prolymphocytic leukemia with CAMPATH-1H. Blood 98:1721-1726, 2001
38. Dillman RO, Beauregard J, Shawler DL, Halpern SE, Markman M, Ryan KP, et al: Continuous infusion of T101 monoclonal antibody in chronic lymphocytic leukemia and cutaneous T-cell lymphoma. J Biol Response Mod 5:394-410, 1986
39. Knox S, Hoppe RT, Maloney D, Gibbs I, Fowler S, Marquez C, et al: Treatment of cutaneous T-cell lymphoma with chimeric anti-CD4 monoclonal antibody. Blood 87:893-899, 1996
40. Saven A, Carrera CJ, Carson DA, Beutler E, Piro LD: 2-Chlorodeoxyadenosine: An active agent in the treatment of cutaneous T-cell lymphoma. Blood 80:587-592, 1992
41. Kuzel TM, Hurria A, Samuelson E, Tallman MS, Roenigk HH Jr, Rademaker AW, et al: Phase II trial of 2-chlorodeoxyadenosine for the treatment of cutaneous T-cell lymphoma. Blood 87:906-911, 1996
42. Kong LR, Samuelson E, Rosen ST, Roenigk HH, Jr., Tallman MS, Rademaker AW, et al: 2-Chlorodeoxyadenosine in cutaneous T-cell lymphoproliferative disorders. Leuk Lymphoma 26:89-97, 1997
43. Betticher DC, Ratschiller D, Hsu Schmitz SF, von Rohr A, Hess U, Zulian G, et al: Reduced dose of subcutaneous cladribine induces identical response rates but decreased toxicity in pretreated chronic lymphocytic leukaemia. Swiss Group for Clinical Cancer Research (SAKK). Ann Oncol 9:721-726, 1998
44. Von Hoff DD, Dahlberg S, Hartstock RJ, Eyre HJ: Activity of fludarabine monophosphate in patients with advanced mycosis fungoides: A Southwest Oncology Group study. J Natl Cancer Inst 82:1353-1355, 1990
45. Redman JR, Cabanillas F, Velasquez WS, McLaughlin P, Hagemeister FB, Swan F Jr, et al: Phase II trial of fludarabine phosphate in lymphoma: An effective new agent in low-grade lymphoma. J Clin Oncol 10:790-794, 1992

ELSEVIER

Seminars in
HEMATOLOGY

Purine Analogues in Advanced T-Cell Lymphoid Malignancies

Razelle Kurzrock[a] and Farhad Ravandi[b]

T-cell lymphomas account for 10% to 15% of all lymphoid malignancies. In advanced stages of T-cell lymphoma, single or multiagent chemotherapy and bioimmunotherapeutic agents have been used. Purine analogues have demonstrated activity in both refractory cutaneous T-cell lymphoma and peripheral T-cell lymphoma with response rates ranging from 20% to 70%. Response rates have been higher with pentostatin (60%) than with the other compounds in this class. The potential limitation to this therapy is the prolonged immunosuppression, which increases the risk of opportunistic injections in patients who are already at heightened risk for infections. Patients should be monitored closely with CD4 counts and surveillance for opportunistic infections. Future studies of purine analogues should evaluate patients who are less heavily pretreated and combination therapy with other agents such as alemtuzumab should be investigated in order to prolong the duration of disease remission.
Semin Hematol 43(suppl 2):S27-S34

T-cell lymphomas account for 10% to 15% of all lymphoid malignancies. Primary cutaneous T-cell lymphomas (CTCL) are heterogeneous lymphoproliferative disorders derived from clonal neoplastic T-cell lymphocytes that infiltrate the skin or other organs. The most common types of CTCL are mycosis fungoides (MF) and Sézary syndrome (SS). Although multiple therapies are available, patients are rarely cured and therefore most will experience relapse of their disease and eventually die. In advanced stages of T-cell lymphoma, single or multiagent chemotherapy and bioimmunotherapeutic agents have been used. Currently there is an emerging role for the use of purine analogues. Here, we review the literature on purine analogues in patients with advanced T-cell lymphoma, specifically focusing on CTCL.

Overview of T-Cell Lymphoid Malignancies

Non-Hodgkin's lymphomas (NHLs) are neoplasms derived from the monoclonal proliferation of malignant B or T lymphocytes and their precursors. T-cell NHLs are a heterogeneous group of diseases that differ in their clinical behavior and prognosis. Only about 15% of NHLs in the United States is T cell in origin with peripheral (T-cell) lymphoma (PTCL) representing the largest majority (7%).[1] Patients with T-cell NHL are often treated similarly to patients with intermediate grade B-cell NHL, although patients with T-cell NHL have been reported to have lower overall survival rates than patients with B-cell NHL.[2]

The Revised European American Lymphoma (REAL) and new World Health Organization (WHO) classification categorizes lymphoid malignancies into three major categories: B-cell lymphomas, T-cell lymphomas, and Hodgkin's lymphoma. The classification of T-cell lymphoproliferative disorders is contained in Table 1. Within T-cell neoplasm categories, there are two major categories based on their composition: precursor (thymic or lymphoblastic) or peripheral (mature or post thymic) lymphocytes.[3] The indolent or low-risk disorders include entities such as MF; aggressive intermediate risk disorders include PTCL; while very aggressive, high-risk disorders include T-cell lymphoblastic lymphoma, T-cell prolymphocytic leukemia, and human T-lymphotropic virus type 1 (HTLV-1) associated T-cell leukemia/lymphoma as well as others.[4]

CTCL is a term coined in 1979 to describe a group of lymphoproliferative disorders characterized by localization of neoplastic T lymphocytes to the skin at presentation. Of all primary cutaneous lymphomas, 65% are of the T-cell type. The most common types of CTCL are MF and SS. Although

[a]Department of Bioimmunotherapy, University of Texas–M.D. Anderson Cancer Center, Houston, TX.

[b]Department of Leukemia, University of Texas–M.D. Anderson Cancer Center, Houston, TX.

Address correspondence to Razelle Kurzrock, MD, Department of Bioimmunotherapy, Unit 422, University of Texas-M.D. Anderson Cancer Center, 1515 Holcombe Blvd, Houston, TX 77030. E-mail: rkurzroc@mdanderson.org

0037-1963/06/$-see front matter
doi:10.1053/j.seminhematol.2005.12.010

Table 1 WHO Classification of T-Cell and NK Cell Neoplasms[3]

Precursor T-cell neoplasm
Precursor T-lymphoblastic lymphoma/leukemia
Mature (peripheral) T-cell neoplasms
T-cell prolymphocytic leukemia
T-cell granular lymphocytic leukemia
Aggressive NK cell leukemia
Adult T-cell lymphoma/leukemia (HTLV-1)
Extranodal NK/T-cell lymphoma, nasal type
Enteropathy-type T-cell lymphoma
Hepatosplenic gamma-delta T-cell lymphoma
Subcutaneous panniculitis-like T-cell lymphoma
Mycosis fungoides/Sézary syndrome
Anaplastic large-cell lymphoma, T/null cell, primary cutaneous type
Peripheral T-cell lymphoma, not otherwise characterized
Angioimmunoblastic T-cell lymphoma
Anaplastic large cell lymphoma, T/null cell, primary systemic type

Abbreviations: WHO, World Health Organization; NK, natural killer; HTLV-1, human T-lymphotropic virus type 1.

MF/SS are called CTCL they should be differentiated from other NHLs that involve the skin such as PTCL and adult T-cell leukemia/lymphoma. The severity of cutaneous manifestations has been described based on the degree of skin involvement. The diagnosis rests on the clinical presentation along with histopathologic findings of an epidermotropic lymphoma with light microscopy showing a dermal infiltrate of lymphocytes with hyperconvoluted cerebriform nuclei and Pautrier's microabscesses.[5] At diagnosis, MF may present as patches or plaques involving 10% or less total body surface area (42%), extensive plaques involving greater than 10% total body surface area (30%), cutaneous tumors (16%), or erythroderma (12%). SS is considered the erythrodermic leukemic variant of MF, with circulating Sézary cells in peripheral blood. Clinical manifestations include scaling of the palms and soles, pruritus, and frequent infections related to the skin.[6] Extracutaneous visceral involvement is more evident as the stage of CTCL increases. The most common sites of visceral involvement are spleen, lung, and liver.[4] The malignant cells usually have a $CD4^+$ T-helper cell phenotype.

There have been several staging systems that have been developed starting in 1978 to establish the prognosis for patients with CTCL. Each of these systems take into account extent of skin, nodal, and visceral involvement along with histopathologic information from both lymph node and bone marrow biopsies.[6] The most recent staging system, described by Sausville et al,[7] simplified the system proposed by the Committee on Staging and Classification of Cutaneous T-Cell Lymphoma in 1979 (Table 2). This staging system distinguishes patients with low (Ia, Ib, IIa), intermediate (IIb, III), and high (IV) risk disease.[7]

MF/SS is typically a disease of middle-age adults with the average age being 50 years. There have been rare reports in children and it is not uncommon to diagnosis the disease in adults younger than 50 years of age. Over the last several years there has been an increase in incidence, with approximately 1,000 new cases per year. The etiology of CTCL is unknown, although many theories have implicated infectious agents, oncogenes, cytokines, or occupational/environment exposures as causative factors.[5] Patients with MF/SS have an extremely long natural history of disease where the condition may be confined to the skin for many years. The median duration of disease onset to diagnosis is 6 years. The 5-year survival rates for patients with early, intermediate, and advanced disease are 90%, 50%, and 5%, respectively.[7] Cases that undergo transformation to $CD30^+$ large cell lymphoma (8% to 23% of patients) have a worse prognosis, with a mean survival ranging from 2 to 19 months. The 5-year survival for patients with SS is 33.5%.[8] The major cause of death is infection due to the immune abnormalities noted in these patients.[5] Some of the abnormalities include decreased cell-mediated cytotoxicity, eosinophilia, increased levels of immunoglobulin E and A, decreased natural killer cell and lymphokine-activated killer cell activity, and decreased cutaneous hypersensitivity.[6]

Current Treatment Principles

Treatment strategies for CTCL depend on the extent of clinical manifestations and the patient's overall quality of life. Current treatment can be divided into two categories: skin-directed therapy and systemic therapy. Skin-directed therapy includes psoralens plus ultraviolet light (PUVA), radiation therapy, and topical chemotherapy (ie, carmustine, corticosteroids, mechlorethamine, bexarotene). Systemic therapy includes chemotherapy with cytotoxic agents, retinoids, photopheresis, interferon-α (IFN), and other biological response-modifying agents.[9] Oral methotrexate, retinoids, or IFN can be added to topical therapy to increase the response rate. Aggressive cytotoxic therapy has shown a trend towards higher response rates compared to conservative systemic therapy; however, there has not been any difference in disease-free survival or overall survival but an increased incidence of adverse effects associated with cytotoxic therapy.[10] Some of these results may be dependent on the type of chemotherapy used, with doxorubicin-containing regimens being studied frequently. However, these regimens may be less effec-

Table 2 Staging and Classification of Cutaneous T-Cell Lymphoma[7]

Stage	Clinical Features	Risk Group
Ia	Limited patch/plaque (<10% BSA)	Low
Ib–IIa	Extensive patch/plaque (>10% BSA)	Low
IIb	Tumors	Intermediate
III	Erythroderma with or without Sézary cells	Intermediate
IV	Lymph node or visceral involvement	High

Abbreviation: BSA, body surface area.

tive than other polychemotherapy, such as that containing methotrexate, or newer drugs such as Doxil (OrthoBiotech, Bridgewater, NJ) or gemcitabine. Single agent therapy appears to be just as effective as combination chemotherapy.[11]

The current goal of therapy is to provide symptom relief and cosmetic improvement since it was generally accepted that a cure was unattainable with the currently available therapies. For patients with early-stage disease (low-risk group), treatment with palliative topical therapies often results in excellent and durable responses.[12] However, patients with more advanced or intermediate- to high-risk disease are often placed on palliative systemic therapies either alone or in combination even though there are no convincing data that show a favorable effect on survival. The advent of newer therapeutic approaches, such as purine analogues, has generated hope for a possible cure in the future.

Purine Analogues for Advanced T-Cell Lymphoid Malignancies

Adenosine deaminase (ADA) is detectable in all mammalian tissues; however, its activity is the greatest in the lymphoid system. There are high levels of ADA in T cells. ADA deficiency is known to be toxic to lymphoid cells.[13] Therefore, pharmacologic intervention with purine analogues, which inhibit ADA, make a rational treatment approach. Purine analogues have shown significant activity in the management of relapsed low-grade lymphoproliferative disorders.[14]

Pentostatin (Nipent; Supergen, Dublin, CA) blocks the deamination of adenosine to inosine and deoxyadenosine to deoxyinosine, resulting in an accumulation of deoxyadenosine and deoxyadenosine triphosphate. These metabolites block DNA synthesis through the inhibition of ribonucleotide reductase. Fludarabine (Fludara; Berlex Laboratories, Inc, Richmond, CA) is a fluorinated purine analog, which acts on nonreplicating cells by inhibiting DNA repair mechanisms to induce apoptosis.[15] Cladribine (Leustatin; Ortho Biotech, Bridgewater, NJ) is a chlorinated purine analog that accumulated in lymphocytes with high deoxycytidine kinase activity, resulting in DNA strand breaks and cell death. In vitro studies have shown the sensitivity of T-lymphoblastoid cell lines to cladribine.[16]

Fludarabine

The initial evaluation of fludarabine in patients with MF/SS was reported in 1990[17] (Table 3). A total of 31 patients were treated with 25 mg/m^2/d for 5 days of fludarabine. Only five patients (19%) responded, which included one complete response (CR) and four partial responses (PRs).[17] Other studies and case reports have suggested the possible role of fludarabine monotherapy in CTCL; however, the duration of responses was not long.[18,19] Subsequent studies have addressed combination therapy with fludarabine.

Foss et al[20] were the first to evaluate combination therapy including fludarabine in patients with advanced or refractory CTCL. Thirty-five patients were treated with fludarabine (25 mg/m^2) on days 1 to 5 every 28 days along with interferon-α2a (IFN) 5 million units (MU)/m^2 subcutaneously three times per week for up to eight cycles. The dose of IFN was increased to 7.5 MU/m^2 at day 29 if no grade 3 or 4 toxicity was noted. The overall response rate was 51% (four CRs and 14 PRs). The median progression-free-survival in patients who responded was 5.9 months with an overall survival duration of 19.6 months. As expected hematologic toxicity was the most frequently reported adverse effect. Approximately 62% of the patients developed grade 3 or 4 neutropenia and 18 patients developed infections. The opportunistic infections observed were herpes zoster (n = 5), *Pneumocystis carinii* (n = 1), extrapulmonary tuberculosis (n = 1), and disseminated toxoplasmosis (n = 2).[20] This combination appears to be active in MF/SS patients who have been heavily pretreated.

A pilot study was conducted evaluating the combination of fludarabine and cyclophosphamide in 12 patients with advanced, refractory CTCL.[21] Synergistic activity between fludarabine and cyclophosphamide has been shown in vitro.[22] Patients received intravenous fludarabine (18 mg/m^2) and cyclophosphamide (250 mg/m^2) for 3 days monthly for 3 to 6 months. Of the patients enrolled, eight met the criteria for SS and the rest had tumor-stage MF. The response data from this combination study were better than those reported for fludarabine as single-agent therapy. Five patients with SS had a response (one CR and four PRs) and one patient with MF had stable disease. The mean duration of response was 10 months. However, the major problem was toxicity of the combination. Six patients had to be withdrawn from treatment due to bone marrow suppression (n = 5) and progressive disease (n = 1). Only one patient completed two full courses of therapy. The investigators concluded that this combination should only be used with caution as palliative therapy.

Quaglino et al[23] evaluated the clinical safety and efficacy of fludarabine as monotherapy in 44 patients with advanced CTCL. They also sought to evaluate if the sequential use of extracorporeal photochemotherapy (ECP) in selected patients would improve the response rate and lengthen the remission duration. Flow cytometry was utilized to evaluate the modifications of helper/inducer and cytotoxic/suppressor T cells during the treatment period. The overall response rate was 29.5%, with a higher response rate in patients with SS (35.3%) than in those with MF (25.9%). The response rate in the combined fludarabine ECP group was higher (63.2%) than with fludarabine monotherapy. However, there was no significant difference between combination and monotherapy in the time to progression (13 months *v* 7 months). The treatment was relatively well tolerated with only three patients experiencing grade 3 toxicity (liver and granulocytes). There were four cases of infections in SS patients. A decrease in the $CD4^+CD26^-$ subset was reported among responders, which paralleled a reduction in circulating Sézary cells. The investigators concluded that fludarabine monotherapy did not compare favorably with other therapeutic approaches for advanced stage MF patients.[23] Future studies may be necessary to confirm the positive response rate observed between fludarabine and ECP.

Pentostatin

Initial studies with pentostatin demonstrated responses in two patients with CTCL; however, higher dose pentostatin was administered and was associated with considerable toxicity.[24] All of the early phase I/II trials enrolled patients who had received previous therapy and failed to respond. A phase I study using much lower doses was initiated in four patients with advanced, refractory MF.[25] One patient received 4 mg/m^2 daily for three doses, two patients received 8 mg/m^2, and one received 10 mg/m^2 for a 28-day cycle. Two of the patients (4 mg/m^2 and 10 mg/m^2) achieved a CR, which lasted for 7 and 9 months, respectively. The remaining two patients achieved a PR, which lasted for 4 and 9 months. Three of the patients achieved 100% inhibition of ADA.[25]

The Eastern Cooperative Oncology Group evaluated pentostatin 5 mg/m^2 for 3 days every 21 days.[26] This study enrolled a total of 25 patients, eight of whom had CTCL. Four of these eight patients had a PR. One of these patients had a response that lasted 1.6 years; the overall median survival for the study was 25.4 months. While pentostatin showed significant activity, this dosing schedule was associated with significant toxicity. Three of the patients with CTCL developed life-threatening infections.[26]

A phase II European Organization for Research in Treatment of Cancer (EORTC) trial included 19 patients with MF or SS.[27] At the time, this was the largest trial evaluating pentostatin in CTCL. Patients received 4 mg/m^2 weekly for 3 weeks followed by every other week. One patient achieved a CR (5%) and four achieved a PR (21%).[27] In a more recent EORTC trial, a similar response rate was reported in patients with MF and SS.[28] The overall response rate was 33% (one CR and six PRs) in the SS group and 23% (five PRs) in the MF group.[27]

Higher response rates were reported in two other studies that focused on enrolling patients with CTCL. Greiner et al[29] enrolled 18 patients with stage I to IV refractory CTCL to differing dosing schedules of pentostatin. One patient received 4 mg/m^2 weekly and three patients received 5 mg/m^2 for 3 days every 28 days, while all other patients received 4 mg/m^2 every other week. The overall response rate was 39%. Two patients (11%) achieved CRs that lasted for 4 months and 6 years; both had advanced disease (stage III and IV). Five patients (28%) had PRs that lasted from 1.5 to 6 months. There was a significant association between disease duration and response ($P = .018$).[29] Similarly, Grever et al[30] evaluated patients with advanced CTCL who received a lower dose of pentostatin (4 mg/m^2 for 3 days repeated every 21 days). The overall response rate was 33%, with two patients achieving CRs that lasted for 7 to 10 months and four patients achieving PRs lasting 1 to 3 months.

Mercieca et al[31] evaluated 145 patients with PTCL and other T-cell malignancies, including 16 patients with SS, four with Sézary cell leukemia, and 13 with other CTCLs. The best responses occurred in patients with SS, three of whom had a CR and seven a PR, with a median duration of response of 9 months. Of the four patients with Sézary cell leukemia, two achieved a PR. There were no responders in patients with other CTCLs.[31] Dearden et al[32] reported a 100% response rate (14 % CR and 86% PR) in patents with SS.

The promise shown from the previously discussed phase I/II trials led to further investigation of pentostatin as single-agent therapy and in combination with other agents. Kurzrock et al[33] began to expand the experience of maximum tolerated doses of pentostatin in advanced, refractory MF/SS or PTCL. The starting dose was between 3.75 and 5.0 mg/m^2/d for 3 days every 3 weeks. Doses were increased to 6.25 mg/m^2/d or decreased to 2.8 mg/m^2/d based on the toxicity experienced. Patients with SS had an overall response rate of 71% (four CRs and six PRs), while the response rate in MF was 57% (one CR and three PRs). Median response duration was shorter in patients with tumor-stage MF, while two of the patients with SS had prolonged responses. The most common adverse effects were granulocytopenia, nausea, and non-neutropenic fever. Most patients developed significant lowering of their CD4 counts. Herpes zoster was seen within 1 year following pentostatin therapy in 19% of the patients.[33]

The most recent report of pentostatin in 42 patients with refractory T-cell lymphomas was in 2003 from Tsimberidou et al.[34] This study reported response rates at the higher end of the spectrum compared to the other studies. Of the 42 patients enrolled, 32 patients with MF or SS were included. Patients were given the same dose escalating/reduction described above. The overall response rate was 54.8% in all patients enrolled and 56% in patients with MF or SS. Response rates were more durable in patients with SS than with MF. The median overall survival was 18 months with a median failure-free survival of 2.1 months. The adverse effects were mainly hematologic. Infections, mainly bacterial, occurred in 48% of patients. Grade 3–4 neutropenia and thrombocytopenia occurred in 21% and 10% of patients, respectively. Long-term toxicity was related to lowered CD4 counts. CD4 counts increased slowly approximately 1 year after treatment was stopped. There were five cases of fungal infections and five cases of herpes zoster, which occurred within 1 year after therapy in the first 19 patients enrolled. Starting with patient no. 20, prophylaxis with valacyclovir was initiated after the second course. Of special interest, long-term responses were noted in a small number of chemotherapy-refractory patients with PTCL. In addition, a dramatic response to pentostatin has been described in a patient with end-stage Hodgkin's disease, after having failed numerous chemotherapies, autologous transplant, and phase I agents.[35]

A combination study of pentostatin with intermittent, high-dose IFN was conducted in 41 patient with advanced or refractory CTCL.[36] The dose of pentostatin used was 4 mg/m^2/d for 3 days every 42 days, alternating with IFN at a dose of 10 MU on day 22 and 50 MU on days 23 to 26. The overall response rate was 41%, with two CRs and 15 PRs. Both of the CRs occurred in patients with SS. In general, patients with erythroderma had higher response rates that those with other skin stages, although no significant correlation was reported.

The overall survival duration was 15.8 months with a median progression-free survival of 13.1 months. Even though the overall response rate of this combination is not different from single-agent pentostatin, the response duration appears to be prolonged following combination therapy. The most common adverse effect was grade 3–4 granulocytopenia, with 13 patients developing infections.[36]

Cladribine

Cladribine has also been investigated in CTCL. Saven et al[36] conducted a pilot study in 16 patients with refractory disease. Cladribine was administered as a continuous infusion (0.05 to 0.15 mg/kg/d) for 7 days. Overall 47% of patients responded for a median duration of 5 months. Three (20%) of the patients were classified as CR. Myelosuppression was the principle toxicity reported, which occurred in 53% of patients. Three of the patients (20%) had infectious complications.[37]

O'Brien et al[38] treated 22 patients with T-cell lymphoproliferative disorders. Of these patients, 11 were classified as CTCL. Cladribine was administered as a continuous infusion (4 mg/m²/d) for 7 days. The overall response rate was 41% with only one of the patients with CTCL showing a response, which was a CR. The most significant toxicity was fever and infection, occurring in 38% of the courses. Two patients died during the first course of cladribine due to disseminated *Candida* infection. There also appeared to be evidence of cumulative myelotoxicity and immunosuppression associated with cladribine.[38]

Cladribine activity in CTCL has also been reported by Kuzel et al.[39] A total of 21 patients with relapsed of refractory MF/SS received a continuous infusion of cladribine of 0.1 mg/kg/d for 7 days initially (n = 13), but the treatment was reduced to 5 days (n = 9) due to hematologic toxicity, for a 28-day cycle. An overall response rate of 28% was observed with a 14% CR rate. The median duration of CR was 4.5 months. The overall median survival was 11 months. The most significant adverse effects reported were bone marrow suppression (62%) and infectious complications (62%). The development of myelosuppression appeared to be related to multiple cycles of therapy and was prolonged.[39] Coadministration of growth factors may limit this toxicity.

Adverse Effects of Purine Analogs in Advanced T-Cell Lymphoid Malignancies

Purine analogues are immunosuppressants and would be expected to increase the risk of opportunistic infections, particularly in patients with T-cell lymphoma. The exact mechanisms responsible for their immunosuppressive effects are unclear. In addition to their desired effects on malignant lymphoid cells, these agents also have deleterious effects on normal lymphocytes. This may result in prolonged lymphopenia, especially in the CD4 subset of T cells. The most consistent adverse effect reported in clinical trials with these compounds is a decrease in CD4 counts, which places the patient at increased risk for opportunistic infections.[40] This immunosuppression is prolonged with the counts recovering very slowly. Our experience has

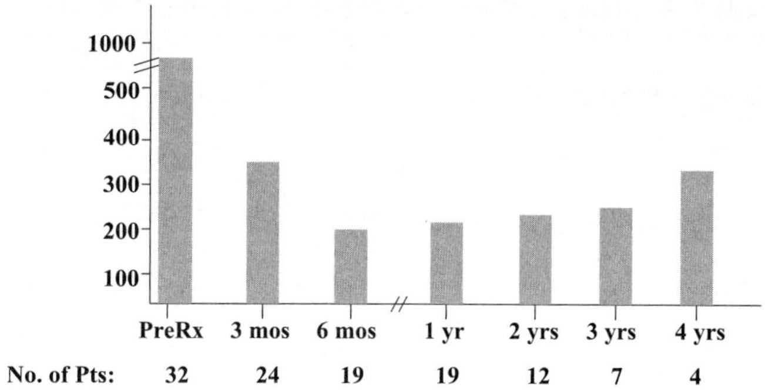

Figure 1 Peripheral blood CD4 counts before and after pentostatin therapy. CD4 counts increased slowly starting 1 year after treatment was stopped. Reprinted with permission.[34]

shown that CD4 counts recover following pentostatin at 4 years (Fig 1). This may be even more prolonged following fludarabine and cladribine. The immunosuppressant effects appear to be dose-related, which may explain why patients with T-cell malignancies who receive higher doses experience a higher rate of infection compared to hairy cell leukemia. Many of the CTCL patients in the purine analog trials, particularly with cladribine, were unable to complete multiple courses of therapy due to this toxicity.

Tam et al[41] developed a model for predicting infectious complications with fludarabine-based combination chemotherapy in patients with indolent lymphomas. Six risk factors were identified from this study: age greater than 60 years, ≥3 previous therapies, previous fludarabine exposure, time from diagnosis to current treatment of longer than 3 years, performance status ≥2, and baseline absolute neutrophil count less than 2×10^9/L. Patients who had ≥3 risk facts had significantly higher infection rates, more grade 4 neutropenia, and more neutropenic sepsis. The use of predictive models such of this may be valuable in assessing patients who should receive prophylactic therapy.

Future Directions

Alemtuzumab

Monoclonal antibodies have become and established therapy for a variety of malignancies. Alemtuzumab is a humanized monoclonal antibody against CD52, a small glycosylphosphatidylinositol-anchored glycoprotein expressed on normal T and B lymphocytes, and on a large number of malignant lymphoid cells but not on hematopoietic progenitor cells.[42] Alemtuzumab has been approved by the Food and Drug Administration for the treatment of fludarabine-refractory chronic lymphocytic leukemia.

There is a growing body of evidence suggesting the role of alemtuzumab in patients with T-cell lymphoma, including CTCL.[43-46] Malignant T cells express high numbers of CD52 cell-surface markers and the intensity of this expression is related to the clinical effects.[47] A very high CR rate (60%) was previously reported in patients with T-cell prolymphocytic leukemia following treatment with alemtuzumab. The median dis-

Table 3 Summary of Purine Analogue Activity for Cutaneous T-Cell Lymphoma

Drug/Reference	N	Regimen	CTCL Patients	RR (%)	CR (n)	Overall Survival (mo)
Fludarabine						
17	31	25 mg/m² × 5	31	19	1	NR
20	35	25 mg/m² days 1–5 every 28 d IFN 5 MU/m² 3 ×/wk	35	51	4	19.6
21	12	18 mg/m² × 3 every 4 wks	8 SS	63	1	11 (overall)
		C: 250 mg/m² × 3 every 4 wks	4 MF	25	0	
23	44	25 mg/m² × 5 d monthly	17 SS	35.3	3	19.3 (overall)
			26 MF	25.9	1	
Cladribine						
36	15	0.05–0.15 mg/kg/d × 7 d	15	47	3	NR
38	21	0.1 mg/kg/d × 7 d or 5 d	21	28	3	11
37	22	4 mg/m²/d × 7 d	11	13	1	12 (overall)
Pentostatin						
27	97	4 mg/m² weekly × 3 wks then QOW	19	26	1	10.2
29	18	4 mg/m² weekly × 3 5 mg/m² QD × 3 every 28 d 4 mg/m² QOW	18	39	2	4
25	4	4 mg/m² QD × 3 every 28 d 8 mg/m² QD × 3 every 28 d 10 mg/m² QD × 3 every 28 d	4	100	2	7–9
30	18	4 mg/m² QD × 3 every 21 d	18	33	2	3.1
28	76	4 mg/m²/wk × 3 wks then every 2 wks × 6 wks then every mo × 6 mos	21 SS	33	1	7.5
			22 MF	23	0	13.4
26	37	5 mg/m² × 3 d every 21 d	6	67	0	25.3
31	145	4 mg/m²/wk × 4 wks	16 SS	63	3	9
			4 SL	50	0	9–12
			13 other CTCL	0	0	0
32	68	4 mg/m²/wk × 4 wks (increased to 5 mg/m²/wk if suboptimal response)	7 SS	100	1	NR
			6 MF	0	0	
33	24	3.75–5 mg/m² × 3	14 SS	71	4	3.5
		every 3 wks (starting dose)	7 MF	57	1	2
36	41	4 mg/m² × 3 every 42 days alternating with IFN	41	42	2	15.8
		10 MU day 22, 50 MU days	23–26			
34	42	3.75–5 mg/m² × 3 every 3 wks (starting dose)	32	56	4	18 (overall)

Abbreviations: RR, response rate; CR, complete response; SS, Sézary syndrome; SL, Sézary cell leukemia; MF, mycosis fungoides; QD, every day; QOW, every other week; IFN, interferon-α2a; MU, million units; C, cyclophosphamide; NR, not reported.

ease-free interval was 7 months in this study. The most significant toxicity associated with this therapy is prolonged lymphopenia and associated reactivation of viruses and other opportunistic infections.[43] Lundin et al[46] evaluated the response of alemtuzumab in 22 patients with advanced MF/SS. The overall response rate was 55%, with 32% achieving CR. Sézary cells were cleared from the blood in 86% of patients. The median time to treatment failure was 12 months. Cytomegalovirus reactivation occurred in 18% of the patients.[46] Based on these initial reports, alemtuzumab appears to also show promise in the treatment of T-cell lymphoma.

Combination therapy with alemtuzumab and purine analogues is another avenue of therapy that deserves investigation as a means of providing more durable responses in patients with CTCL. Ravandi and Faderl[48] reported a case of combination alemtuzumab and pentostatin therapy in a patient with adult T-cell leukemia. This patient experienced a CR.[48] A clinical trial evaluating the combination in patients with T-cell lymphoproliferative disorders including CTCL has been initiated. Patients received pentostatin 4 mg/m² weekly, then 4 mg/m² every other week until CR, best response, or for 10 more doses in combination with alemtuzumab 30 mg three times weekly for a maximum of 3 months. All patients in the trial received prophylaxis with allopurinol, cotrimoxazole, fluconazole, and valacyclovir. A total of nine patients have received this combination to date, with six patients experiencing a response (five CRs). Six of the patients had infectious complications, but two had a previous history of the infection. Interim results indicate that this combination is safe and effective especially in younger patients. The concern with the use of this combination is the increased risk of infection; however, the incidence may be minimized with appropriate use of prophylactic regimens.

Other Novel Agents

Some of the other novel agents that have been evaluated in CTCL include ^{90}Y-T101, FD228 (depsipeptide), intermediate-dose interleukin-2 (IL-2), temozolomide, IL-12 in combination with low-dose IL-2, anti-CD4 monoclonal antibody, and anti-Tac pseudomonas exotoxin immunoconjugate.[6] The peripheral blood mononuclear cells from patients with MF/SS are deficient in the production of interferon gamma (IFNγ) and IL-12. IL-12 is also a stimulus for IFNγ production, which may be important in these patients since IFNγ production may reverse many of the immunologic abnormalities. IL-12 may also be important in the therapeutic benefit of retinoids.[49] Response rates as high as 67% has been reported in a small number of patients treated with IL-2.[50] About 50% of patients with MF/SS express significant levels of IL-2 receptors on their malignant cells. Patients with Sézary T cells have shown an increased histone acetylation and a patient with PTCL has shown a CR following treatment with the histone deacetylase inhibitor, depsipeptide.[51] Seven of eight patients with MF treated with chimeric anti-CD4 monoclonal antibody had a least a minor response, with an average freedom from progression of 25 weeks.[52]

Conclusions

The treatment of CTCL presents a challenge to the clinician. The use of immunosuppressive agents in these patients may increase the already increased risk of infection. Cytotoxic agents have been shown to induce clinical response but the duration of the response was short and offered no benefit in terms of survival. Recent attention has focused on purine analogues. Purine analogues have demonstrated activity in both refractory CTCL and PTCL with response rates ranging from 20% to 70%. Response rates have been higher with pentostatin (60%) than with the other compounds in this class. Durable responses have been described in SS and in chemotherapy-refractory PTCL with the use of pentostatin.[34] Recently, we reported a striking response in a patient with refractory end-stage Hodgkin's disease. The potential limitation to this therapy is the prolonged immunosuppression, which increases the risk of opportunistic injections in patients who are already at heightened risk for infections. Patients should be monitored closely with CD4 counts and surveillance for opportunistic infections. Because of a high incidence of herpes zoster infection after repeated courses of pentostatin, we use prophylactic valacyclovir in this setting. Future studies of purine analogues should evaluate patients who are less heavily pretreated and combination therapy with other agents such as alemtuzumab should be investigated in order to prolong the duration of disease remission. In addition, larger cohorts of patients with PTCL and Hodgkin's disease should be evaluated after pentostatin treatment, since impressive responses have been achieved in small numbers of patients treated on an exploratory basis.

References

1. A clinical evaluation of the International Lymphoma Study Group classification of non-Hodgkin's lymphoma. The Non-Hodgkin's Lymphoma Classification Project. Blood 89:3909-3918, 1997
2. Greer JP, Kinney MC, Loughran TP Jr: T cell and NK cell lymphoproliferative disorders. Hematology (Am Soc Hematol Educ Program):259-281, 2001
3. Jaffe ES, Harris NL, Diebold J, Muller-Hermelink HK: World Health Organization Classification of lymphomas: A work in progress. Ann Oncol 9:S25-S30, 1998 (suppl 5)
4. Foss F: Overview of cutaneous T-cell lymphoma: Prognostic factors and novel therapeutic approaches. Leuk Lymphoma 44:S55-S61, 2003 (suppl 3)
5. Diamandidou E, Cohen PR, Kurzrock R: Mycosis fungoides and Sezary syndrome. Blood 88:2385-2409, 1996
6. Connors JM, Hsi ED, Foss FM: Lymphoma of the skin. Hematology (Am Soc Hematol Educ Program):263-282, 2002
7. Sausville EA, Eddy JL, Makuch RW, Fischmann AB, Schechter GP, Matthews M, et al: Histopathologic staging at initial diagnosis of mycosis fungoides and the Sezary syndrome. Definition of three distinctive prognostic groups. Ann Intern Med 109:372-382, 1988
8. Bernengo MG, Quaglino P, Novelli M, Cappello N, Doveil GC, Lisa F, et al: Prognostic factors in Sezary syndrome: A multivariate analysis of clinical, haematological and immunological features. Ann Oncol 9:857-863, 1998
9. Siegel RS, Pandolfino T, Guitart J, Rosen S, Kuzel TM: Primary cutaneous T-cell lymphoma: Review and current concepts. J Clin Oncol 18: 2908-2925, 2000
10. Kaye FJ, Bunn PA Jr, Steinberg SM, Stocker JL, Ihde DC, Fischmann AB, et al: A randomized trial comparing combination electron-beam radiation and chemotherapy with topical therapy in the initial treatment of mycosis fungoides. N Engl J Med 321:1784-1790, 1989
11. Rosen ST, Foss FM: Chemotherapy for mycosis fungoides and the Sezary syndrome. Hematol Oncol Clin North Am 9:1109-1116, 1995
12. Zackheim HS, Kashani-Sabet M, Amin S: Topical corticosteroids for mycosis fungoides. Experience in 79 patients. Arch Dermatol 134:949-954, 1998
13. Dissing J, Knudsen B: Adenosine-deaminase deficiency and combined immunodeficiency syndrome. Lancet 2:1316, 1972
14. Cabanillas F: Purine nucleoside analogs in indolent non-Hodgkin's lymphoma. Oncology (Williston Park) 14:13-15, 2000
15. Sandoval A, Consoli U, Plunkett W: Fludarabine-mediated inhibition of nucleotide excision repair induces apoptosis in quiescent human lymphocytes. Clin Cancer Res 2:1731-1741, 1996
16. Seto S, Carrera CJ, Kubota M, Wasson DB, Carson DA: Mechanism of deoxyadenosine and 2-chlorodeoxyadenosine toxicity to nondividing human lymphocytes. J Clin Invest 75:377-383, 1985
17. Von Hoff DD, Dahlberg S, Hartstock RJ, Eyre HJ: Activity of fludarabine monophosphate in patients with advanced mycosis fungoides: A Southwest Oncology Group study. J Natl Cancer Inst 82:1353-1355, 1990
18. Nikko AP, RutherFord CJ, Pandya AG: Successful treatment of Sezary syndrome with lymphomatous transformation to large cell lymphoma with fludarabine phosphate. Arch Dermatol 132:978-979, 1996
19. Kantarjian HM, Redman JR, Keating MJ: Fludarabine phosphate therapy in other lymphoid malignancies. Semin Oncol 17:66-70, 1990
20. Foss FM, Ihde DC, Linnoila IR, Fischmann AB, Schechter GP, Cotelingam JD, et al: Phase II trial of fludarabine phosphate and interferon alfa-2a in advanced mycosis fungoides/Sezary syndrome. J Clin Oncol 12:2051-2059, 1994
21. Scarisbrick JJ, Child FJ, Clift A, Sabroe R, Whittaker SJ, Spittle M, et al: A trial of fludarabine and cyclophosphamide combination chemotherapy in the treatment of advanced refractory primary cutaneous T-cell lymphoma. Br J Dermatol 144:1010-1015, 2001
22. Bellosillo B, Villamor N, Colomer D, Pons G, Montserrat E, Gil J: In vitro evaluation of fludarabine in combination with cyclophosphamide and/or mitoxantrone in B-cell chronic lymphocytic leukemia. Blood 94:2836-2843, 1999
23. Quaglino P, Fierro MT, Rossotto GL, Savoia P, Bernengo MG: Treatment of advanced mycosis fungoides/Sezary syndrome with fludarabine and potential adjunctive benefit to subsequent extracorporeal photochemotherapy. Br J Dermatol 150:327-336, 2004
24. Grever MR, Siaw MF, Jacob WF, Neidhart JA, Miser JS, Coleman MS, et

al: The biochemical and clinical consequences of 2′-deoxycoformycin in refractory lymphoproliferative malignancy. Blood 57:406-417, 1981

25. Grever MR, Bisaccia E, Scarborough DA, Metz EN, Neidhart JA: An investigation of 2′-deoxycoformycin in the treatment of cutaneous T-cell lymphoma. Blood 61:279-282, 1983
26. Cummings FJ, Kim K, Neiman RS, Comis RL, Oken MM, Weitzman SA, et al: Phase II trial of pentostatin in refractory lymphomas and cutaneous T-cell disease. J Clin Oncol 9:565-571, 1991
27. Ho AD, Thaler J, Willemze R, Lauria F, Mandelli F, Stryckmans P, et al: Pentostatin (2′-deoxycoformycin) for the treatment of lymphoid neoplasms. Cancer Treat Rev 17:213-215, 1990
28. Ho AD, Suciu S, Stryckmans P, De Cataldo F, Willemze R, Thaler J, et al: Pentostatin in T-cell malignancies—A phase II trial of the EORTC Leukemia Cooperative Group. Ann Oncol 10:1493-1498, 1999
29. Greiner D, Olsen EA, Petroni G: Pentostatin (2′-deoxycoformycin) in the treatment of cutaneous T-cell lymphoma. J Am Acad Dermatol 36:950-955, 1997
30. Grever MR, Leiby JM, Kraut EH, Wilson HE, Neidhart JA, Wall RL, et al: Low-dose deoxycoformycin in lymphoid malignancy. J Clin Oncol 3:1196-1201, 1985
31. Mercieca J, Matutes E, Dearden C, MacLennan K, Catovsky D: The role of pentostatin in the treatment of T-cell malignancies: Analysis of response rate in 145 patients according to disease subtype. J Clin Oncol 12:2588-2593, 1994
32. Dearden C, Matutes E, Catovsky D: Deoxycoformycin in the treatment of mature T-cell leukaemias. Br J Cancer 64:903-906, 1991
33. Kurzrock R, Pilat S, Duvic M: Pentostatin therapy of T-cell lymphomas with cutaneous manifestations. J Clin Oncol 17:3117-3121, 1999
34. Tsimberidou AM, Giles F, Duvic M, Fayad L, Kurzrock R: Phase II study of pentostatin in advanced T-cell lymphoid malignancies: Update of an M.D. Anderson Cancer Center series. Cancer 100:342-349, 2004
35. Braiteh F, Ng C, Kurzrock R: Refractory Hodgkin's lymphoma responds to pentostatin (2′ deoxycoformycin). Leuk Lymphoma 47:373-375, 2006
36. Foss FM, Ihde DC, Breneman DL, Phelps RM, Fischmann AB, Schechter GP, et al: Phase II study of pentostatin and intermittent high-dose recombinant interferon alfa-2a in advanced mycosis fungoides/Sezary syndrome. J Clin Oncol 10:1907-1913, 1992
37. Saven A, Carrera CJ, Carson DA, Beutler E, Piro LD: 2-Chlorodeoxyadenosine: An active agent in the treatment of cutaneous T-cell lymphoma. Blood 80:587-592, 1992
38. O'Brien S, Kurzrock R, Duvic M, Kantarjian H, Stass S, Robertson LE, et al: 2-Chlorodeoxyadenosine therapy in patients with T-cell lymphoproliferative disorders. Blood 84:733-738, 1994
39. Kuzel TM, Hurria A, Samuelson E, Tallman MS, Roenigk HH Jr, Rademaker AW, et al: Phase II trial of 2-chlorodeoxyadenosine for the treatment of cutaneous T-cell lymphoma. Blood 87:906-911, 1996
40. Ravandi F, O'Brien S: Infections associated with purine analogs and monoclonal antibodies. Blood Rev 19:253-273, 2005
41. Tam CS, Wolf MM, Januszewicz EH, Grigg AP, Prince HM, Westerman D, et al: A new model for predicting infectious complications during fludarabine-based combination chemotherapy among patients with indolent lymphoid malignancies. Cancer 101:2042-2049, 2004
42. Ravandi F, O'Brien S: Alemtuzumab. Expert Rev Anticancer Ther 5:39-51, 2005
43. Dearden CE, Matutes E, Cazin B, Tjonnfjord GE, Parreira A, Nomdedeu B, et al: High remission rate in T-cell prolymphocytic leukemia with CAMPATH-1H. Blood 98:1721-1726, 2001
44. Gautschi O, Blumenthal N, Streit M, Solenthaler M, Hunziker T, Zenhausern R: Successful treatment of chemotherapy-refractory Sezary syndrome with alemtuzumab (Campath-1H). Eur J Haematol 72:61-63, 2004
45. Kennedy GA, Seymour JF, Wolf M, Januszewicz H, Davison J, McCormack C, et al: Treatment of patients with advanced mycosis fungoides and Sezary syndrome with alemtuzumab. Eur J Haematol 71:250-256, 2003
46. Lundin J, Hagberg H, Repp R, Cavallin-Stahl E, Freden S, Juliusson G, et al: Phase 2 study of alemtuzumab (anti-CD52 monoclonal antibody) in patients with advanced mycosis fungoides/Sezary syndrome. Blood 101:4267-4272, 2003
47. Ginaldi L, De Martinis M, Matutes E, Farahat N, Morilla R, Dyer MJ, et al: Levels of expression of CD52 in normal and leukemic B and T cells: Correlation with in vivo therapeutic responses to Campath-1H. Leuk Res 22:185-191, 1998
48. Ravandi F, Faderl S: Complete response in a patient with adult T-cell leukemia (ATL) treated with combination of alemtuzumab and pentostatin. Leuk Res, 30:103-105, 2006
49. Rook AH, Kuzel TM, Olsen EA: Cytokine therapy of cutaneous T-cell lymphoma: Interferons, interleukin-12, and interleukin-2. Hematol Oncol Clin North Am 17:1435-1448, 2003
50. Marolleau JP, Baccard M, Flageul B, Rybojad M, Laroche L, Verola O, et al: High-dose recombinant interleukin-2 in advanced cutaneous T-cell lymphoma. Arch Dermatol 131:574-579, 1995
51. Piekarz RL, Robey R, Sandor V, Bakke S, Wilson WH, Dahmoush L, et al: Inhibitor of histone deacetylation, depsipeptide (FR901228), in the treatment of peripheral and cutaneous T-cell lymphoma: A case report. Blood 98:2865-2868, 2001
52. Knox S, Hoppe RT, Maloney D, Gibbs I, Fowler S, Marquez C, et al: Treatment of cutaneous T-cell lymphoma with chimeric anti-CD4 monoclonal antibody. Blood 87:893-899, 1996

Seminars in
HEMATOLOGY

The Role of Purine Analogues in Low-Intensity Regimens With Allogeneic Hematopoietic Stem Cell Transplantation

Francine M. Foss

Host conditioning prior to allogeneic bone marrow transplantation (BMT) has traditionally involved the use of high-dose, myeloablative chemotherapy and irradiation, focusing on maximal tumor cytoreduction as well as adequate immunosuppression to allow engraftment of allogeneic stem cells. High-dose chemoradiation conditioning regimens have been associated with a significant incidence of organ toxicity and acute and chronic graft-versus-host disease (GVHD). Recent efforts to diminish the acute transplant-associated toxicities have focused on the development of relatively nontoxic, nonmyeloablative, or less myeloablative conditioning regimens, with the emphasis being predominantly on induction of immunosuppression to enable engraftment. Without ablative chemotherapy, disease control in these regimens is largely relegated to the graft-versus-leukemia/lymphoma (GVL) effect. While the evolution these regimens has resulted in successful engraftment of allogeneic stem cells with minimal toxicity, acute and chronic GVHD occurs in 20% to 50% of patients and remains a major cause of transplant-associated morbidity. Strategies to lower the incidence of acute GVHD have primarily focused on more precise molecular donor/recipient matching, alternative stem cell sources, and T-cell depletion of the graft. While successful in lowering the frequency and severity of GVHD, T-cell–depleted grafts have been associated with compromised the graft-versus-disease effect. Recent studies have suggested that, in addition to T-effector cells within the graft, donor and host dendritic cells may play a role in GVHD. Purine analogues have been evaluated as part of these regimens. While fludarabine and cladribine have been shown to be effective, these agents have been associated with an increased incidence of serious infection and severe acute GVHD. Pentostatin has a different mechanism of action and was also investigated as part of these preparative regimens. Regimens using pentostatin/extracorporeal photopheresis (ECP)/total body irradiation (TBI) have been shown to be well tolerated and associated with early full donor engraftment with a predominance of donor dendritic cell (DC)2 cells and a low incidence of acute GVHD. Further investigation evaluating this preparative regimen is warranted.
Semin Hematol 43(suppl 2):S35-S43

Allogeneic bone marrow transplantation (BMT) remains the most commonly performed transplantation in patients with hematologic disorders. Preparative regimens for allogeneic transplantation must address the two immunologic barriers to establish successful hematopoietic engraftment: the host-versus-graft effect (HVG), and the graft-versus-host (GVH) effect. High-dose chemotherapy combined with sublethal doses of radiation therapy has been used to immune suppress the host sufficiently to prevent rejection of donor cells. Although effective in most patients, the myeloablative regimens are toxic to nonhematopoietic tissues and are associated with high transplant-associated morbidity and mortality, limiting the potential of this curative treatment to younger patients without underlying end-organ dysfunction. Further, conventional ablative regimens require long-term immunosuppression to control graft-versus-host disease (GVHD), with resulting immune compromise and toxicity related to these agents.

With the recognition that the graft-versus-disease effect is responsible for many of observed cures following allogeneic transplantation, less intensive and nonmyeloablative prepar-

Department of Medical Oncology, Yale Cancer Center, New Haven, CT.
Address correspondence to Francine M. Foss, MD, Yale Cancer Center, Department of Medical Oncology, 333 Cedar St, New Haven, CT 06520. E-mail: Francine.foss@yale.edu

doi:10.1053/j.seminhematol.2005.12.007

ative regimens have been developed that rely on the graft-versus-disease effect while lessening the myeloablative effect of the transplant. Compared to conventional marrow toxic conditioning regimens in which host hematopoiesis is fully ablated, mini-transplant or nonmyeloablative regimens utilize immunosuppressive strategies, including low-dose total body irradiation (TBI) and T-cell–depleting agents to create marrow space for engraftment of allogeneic stem cells, in many instances establishing mixed donor/host lymphohematopoietic chimerism. The goals in the development of these strategies have been twofold: to facilitate engraftment of allogeneic stem cells with minimal end-organ toxicity, and to modulate graft-host alloreactivity in the direction of graft-versus-leukemia/lymphoma (GVL) while minimizing GVHD. In some instances, donor lymphocyte infusions (DLI) have been implemented in nonmyeloablative regimens to enhance donor chimerism and to provide effector T cells to augment GVL effect. This use of this nonmyeloablative regimens have gained wide acceptance over the last several years.[1] While the evolution of nonmyeloablative or less intensive conditioning regimens has resulted in successful engraftment of allogeneic stem cells with minimal toxicity, acute and chronic GVHD occur in 20% to 50% of patients and remains a major cause of transplant-associated morbidity.[2] The purpose of this review is to update the latest advancements in the use of reduced intensity conditioning regimens, highlighting the role of purine analogues as a part of this regimen.

Alternative Conditioning Regimens for Allogeneic Stem Cell Transplantation

The definition of a nonablative regimen is one that can be given without stem cell support, with neutrophil recovery within 28 days, and in which mixed chimerism can be routinely detected early after transplantation.[3,4] There have been a variety of alternative conditioning regimens evaluated and some are minimally myelosuppressive so can be classified as nonablative. However, many regimens cannot be safely given without stem cell support so these regimens are referred to as "reduced-intensity" regimens. Reduced-intensity regimens involve the use of agents that are toxic to the stem and tumor cells just in reduced doses compared to the doses used in conventional transplant regimens, which may extend the application of transplantation to older patients.[5,6] The regimens usually involve the combination of a purine analog with an alkylating agent.[7] de Lima et al[8] compared the outcomes of a truly nonablative regimen (120 mg/m^2 fludarabine, 4 mg/m^2 cytarabine, and 36 mg/m^2 idarubicin [FAI]) to a more myelosuppressive reduced intensity regimen (100 to 150 mg/m^2 fludarabine and 140 or 180 mg/m^2 melphalan [FM]) in patients with acute myeloid leukemia (AML) and high-risk myelodysplastic syndrome (MDS). Disease recurrence was more frequent in patients who received the FAI regimen, suggesting that myelosuppressive intensity of cytotoxic agents is import for disease control as well as establishment of long-term donor chimerism. Other investigators have also reported similar findings.[9] The FM regimen was significantly associated with a higher degree of donor cell engraftment, higher cumulative incidence of treatment-related mortality, and lower cumulative incidence or relapse-related mortality. The investigators concluded that the reduced-intensity regimen provided superior disease control but at the cost of higher morbidity and treatment-related mortality.[8] Sorror et al[6] also reported that nonablative conditioning, even though patients had significantly higher pretransplantation comorbidities, experienced less toxicity, had a lower incidence of acute GVHD, and lower non-relapse mortality than patients who receive high-dose ablative hematopoietic cell transplants.

Preclinical studies have demonstrated that mixed chimerism can be established in mice following low-dose TBI (300 cGy) or cyclophosphamide (200 mg/kg), monoclonal anti–T-cell antibody therapy, thymic irradiation, and cyclosporine.[10] Canine studies have demonstrated that mixed lymphohematopoietic chimerism could be established using as little as 200 cGy of TBI followed by post-transplant immunosuppression with mycophenolate mofetil and cyclosporine A.[11-16] In these studies, it was demonstrated that 200 cGy was the threshold below which engraftment could not be maintained with this immunosuppression regimen.[17]

Based on the preclinical data indicating that stable mixed chimerism could be established with nonmyeloablative doses of TBI along with T-cell–depleting agents, a number of fludarabine-based regimens were initiated. Khori et al[18] treated 15 patients with fludarabine 30mg/m^2 × 3 days and either cyclophosphamide 300 mg/m^2/d × 3 days, or cisplatin 25 mg/m^2/d × 4 days and cytosine arabinoside (ara-c) 500 mg/m^2/d × 2. Eleven of 15 patients had at least 50% donor engraftment, four had no engraftment, and five developed acute GVHD. Eight had a complete response. Reduced-intensity conditioning using TBI (8 cGy), fludarabine (30 mg/m^2 × 4), cyclophosphamide (40 mg/kg), and anti-thymocyte globulin (ATG) (20 mg/kg) has also shown benefit in early transplantation (within 1 year of diagnosis) in high-risk patients.[19] Giralt et al[20] reported 15 patients treated with either fludarabine 30mg/m^2/d × 4 and idarubicin 12 mg/m^2/d × 3 or high-dose melphalan 140mg/m^2/d, or cladribine 12 mg/m^2/d × 5 days and ara-c 1,000 mg/m^2/d × 5 days. Thirteen patients demonstrated engraftment, seven had 90% donor hematopoiesis by day 30, and three had acute GVHD. Giralt et al[21] provided a more recent report of 78 patients receiving a combination of fludarabine (30 mg/m^2/d × 4 days) and melphalan (180 mg/m^2, n = 66, or 140 mg/m^2, n = 12) or eight patients who received cladribine 12 mg/m^2 by continuous infusion for 5 days with melphalan 180 mg/m^2. These purine analog/melphalan combinations produced between 80% and 100% donor cell engraftment by day 30 in 93% of patients. Non-relapse mortality for the fludarabine-based combination was 37.4% and 87.5% for the cladribine-based regimen. The main cause of death prior to day 100 in patients who received the fludarabine combination was infection and GVHD. Some investigators have shown that the fludarabine/melphalan combination is an aggressive regimen and the clinical pattern of a transplantation using this regimen is not dissimilar to that of a conventional myeloablative regimen.[22]

Slavin et al[7] treated 22 patients with busulfan 8 mg/kg and fludarabine 180 mg/m^2 with ATG and granulocyte colony-stimulating factor (G-CSF)–mobilized peripheral stem cells and reported donor engraftment in all patients and acute GVHD in 12 of 26. In another small cohort of patients the addition of ATG (15 mg/kg/d on days −4 to −1) to low-dose TBI (200 cGy on day −5) and fludarabine (30 mg/m^2/day on days −4 to −2) resulted in greater than 80% donor engraftment; however, a high incidence of relapse was reported.[23] Childs et al[24] treated 15 patients, including three with renal cell carcinoma and four with melanoma, with a regimen of cyclophosphamide 60 mg/kg/d × 4 days and fludarabine 25 mg/kg/d × 5 days in the setting of human leukocyte antigen (HLA)-matched or single mismatched donor peripheral blood stem cells and reported stable engraftment in 14 of 15 patients and acute GVHD in all seven patients who had established 100% donor T-cell chimerism by day 30. More recently, Childs and Barrett[25] reported successful T and myeloid donor engraftment in 19 patients with metastatic renal cell carcinoma using this regimen. In this study, 53% of patients developed acute GVHD, but the occurrence of GVHD was associated with disease response. A recent phase I study showed that fludarabine (30 mg/m^2/d from days −4 to −2) and TBI (2 cGy) in combination with cyclosporine and mycophenolate mofetil can induce durable donor chimerism in 88% of matched or partially mismatched unrelated donor patients with a 8% incidence of grade III acute GVHD and 13% grade IV acute GVHD.[26] In summary, fludarabine-based regimens have enabled engraftment of allogeneic stem cells without significant regimen-related toxicity, but the incidence of acute and chronic GVHD has remained clinically significant with these regimens.

Another approach to induce mixed chimerism has involved the use of low-dose cyclophosphamide, thymic irradiation, and ATG. Sykes et al[27] reported establishment of stable mixed chimerism in 20 of 23 HLA-matched and seven of 10 mismatched recipients. This platform was based on the establishment of graft tolerance in the setting of mixed chimerism, with later use of DLI to augment GVL. Many of the patients were converted to full donor chimerism by DLI without significant GVHD and had complete remission of their disease, suggesting that significant GVL effect could be achieved without significant GVHD. Recently, Dey et al[28] reported similar results in 13 patients with a regimen of cyclophosphamide 150 to 200 mg/kg, ATG, and thymic irradiation along with a short course of cyclosporine for GVHD prophylaxis. Seven patients with no acute GVHD had DLI beginning 5 to 6 weeks after transplant to convert mixed to full donor chimerism and augment GVL. In this study, seven patients had a complete disease response with a median disease-free survival (DFS) probability at 2 years of 37.5%, but, disappointingly, grade II to IV acute GVHD related to DLI occurred in most of the patients.

More recently, the anti-CD52 antibody (alemtuzumab) has been used in up-front conditioning at a dose of 20 mg on days −8 to −4, along with a 30 mg/m^2 fludarabine on days −7 to −3 and 150 mg/m^2 melphalan on day −2. Using this regimen, which has been shown to deplete both host lymphoid and dendritic cell populations, the incidence of grade II to IV acute GVHD remained similar to other regimens at 21% in 45 evaluable patients, but the incidence of life-threatening grade IV GVHD was low.[29,30] Of 34 patients who were evaluated for chimerism at 1 month, 29 (85%) had achieved full donor chimerism; at 5 months, five of these patients had converted to mixed chimerism. While this regimen was well tolerated and associated with a low incidence of life-threatening acute GVHD, the incidence of serious infections related to alemtuzumab-associated immunosuppression was 64%, with *Cytomegalovirus*(CMV) viremia necessitating preemptive antiviral therapy in 22 patients. Since CAMPATH-1H has a half-life of 15 to 21 days, it is likely that the infused donor stem cells were exposed to the antibody, thereby T-cell–depleting the stem cell product, which could be relevant when comparing these results to other strategies using drugs with short half-lives, such as fludarabine or pentostatin, for host T-cell immunomodulation.

The use of rituximab-BEAM (carmustine, etoposide, ara-c, melphalan)-alemtuzumab reduced-intensity conditioning regimen for allogeneic hematopoietic stem cell transplantation was evaluated in five patients with follicular lymphoma.[31] BEAM has been used for autologous transplantation in lymphoma and has shown efficacy with a lower toxicity profile. At the mean follow-up time of 521 days, four of the five patients were alive and three were in complete molecular remission. There was a high incidence of CMV reactivation, with three of the five patients requiring preemptive therapy. This was a small study with a relatively short follow-up time, but this regimen appears safe and induces molecular remissions. However, further study will be necessary.

Similarly, Faulkner et al[32] evaluated the conditioning regimen BEAM-alemtuzumab in reduced-intensity allogeneic stem cell transplantation in patients with lymphoproliferative diseases. A total of 65 patients (57 sibling donor; eight matched unrelated donor) were evaluated. Sustained donor engraftment occurred in 97% of patients. In the patients with chimerism studies (n = 56), 63% had full donor chimerism. The incidence of acute GVHD was 17% but only grades I/II. The 1-year transplantation-related mortality was estimated to be 8%. Age at transplantation (<46 years) and histologic diagnosis (mantle cell lymphoma or high-grade non-Hodgkin's lymphoma) were significantly associated with higher relapse risk and worse event-free survival (EFS). Overall it was concluded that this was an acceptable regimen alternative.[32]

Recently, the use of fludarabine, busulphan, and alemtuzumab (FBC) conditioning in hematopoietic stem cell transplantation has been evaluated in patients with MDS and AML.[33] Although longer follow-up will be necessary to evaluate any survival advantage of this regimen, this regimen did produce durable donor engraftment (86% achieved full donor chimerism) and a low incidence of acute GVHD (9% for matched unrelated donor recipients; 0% sibling recipients).

In summary, host conditioning with sublethal doses of TBI and/or combinations of cytotoxic agents and T-cell–depleting therapies, such as ATG and purine analogs, even across HLA barriers, can establish engraftment and stable mixed chimerism. Despite the rapid kinetics of engraftment and the relatively modest toxicities associated with these regimens, the incidence of acute GVHD may be as high as 40% and is augmented by the need for DLI to establish full donor chimerism.

Recent Strategies Using Purine Analogues in Reduced-Intensity Regimens

Nonmyeloablative and alternative preparative regimens have taken advantage of selective T-cell–depleting agents, such as ATG, alemtuzumab, and purine analogues. While studies using fludarabine and cladribine for immunosuppression prior to allogeneic stem cell engraftment have demonstrated that these agents are effective in creating marrow space for the graft, studies have reported a significant incidence of infections post-transplant as well as moderately severe acute GVHD, which occurred in 20 of 56 patients treated in three studies Recent studies using CAMPATH-1H "in the bag" for T-cell depletion of the graft along with administration of CAMATH-1H to the transplant recipient for immunosuppression have demonstrated a high rate of engraftment with minimal toxicity but with prolonged immunosuppression related to the long half-life of the antibody.[34]

Pentostatin has a different mechanism of action than other purine analogs in that it is a reversible inhibitor of adenosine deaminase (ADA).[35-37] Pentostatin has been shown to induce profound and prolonged T-cell depletion lasting years after completion of therapy in patients with hairy cell leukemia.[38] Conventional dosing schedules for pentostatin have been daily for 3 consecutive days in patients with hairy cell leukemia or non-Hodgkin's lymphoma, and the toxicities at the highest dose of 10 mg/m^2/d were nausea and vomiting, bone marrow suppression, and renal insufficiency.[39-41] Only one study has explored the use of continuous infusion pentostatin. (S O'Brien, personal communication). In this study of refractory lymphoma patients, the maximum tolerated dose was 1 mg/m^2/d × 7 days, with reversible hepatic and renal toxicity at higher doses. In our pilot study, we used a continuous infusion of pentostatin over 48 hours at a dose of 4 mg/m^2/d in an attempt to maximize the AUC with respect to T-cell exposure and to minimize toxicity. This dose was based on our previous demonstration that doses of 3 mg/m^2/day by intravenous bolus were necessary to inhibit ADA activity by greater than 95% in plasma and buffy coat mononuclear cells.

Our group recently reported the results of 55 high-risk patients who received extracorporeal photopheresis (ECP) (days −7 and −6), pentostatin 4 mg/m^2 by continuous infusion (days −5 and −4), and TBI 600 cGy in three fractions (days −3 and −2) followed by unmanipulated allogeneic stem cell transplant.[42] The patients enrolled in this phase I/II trial were otherwise ineligible to undergo a conventional ablative conditioning regimen due to age greater than 50 years, intercurrent medical conditions, or lack of a matched related donor. For GVHD prophylaxis, all patients received adjusted-dose continuous infusion cyclosporine A (CSA) administered through an indwelling catheter starting on day −1 and continuing until day +30 or until the patient could start oral CSA to maintain a plasma concentration of 475 to 525 ng/mL.[43] Oral CSA was administered at a dose of 5 mg/kg twice daily as tolerated and tapered over the next 6 months. All patients received methotrexate (MTX) administered as a bolus intravenous infusion on day +1 (15 mg/m^2) and day +3 (10 mg/m^2). Mycophenolate mofetil was administered from day 180 to 365 for chronic GVHD prophylaxis.

The overall documented disease response was 86% (72% complete responders and 14% partial responders) and the median EFS was 15 months. Engraftment failure occurred in six patients with AML with circulating blasts at the time of the transplants. This conditioning regimen was well tolerated even in this high-risk group of patients. There was no regimen-related grade III–IV liver, renal, or CNS toxicity and no mucositis. A univariate analysis of factors influencing survival included sex, age at transplant (≥50 years *v* <50 years), time from diagnosis to transplant (≥15 months *v* <15 months), sex-mismatched transplant, donor and recipient CMV status, type of transplant (allogeneic *v* matched unrelated donor), and risk group (high-high risk defined as prior transplant or ≥3 prior courses of chemotherapy *v* intermediate-high risk defined as <3 prior courses of chemotherapy). Risk group assignment was made based on prior transplant or three or more courses of chemotherapy (high-high risk) or others (intermediate-high risk). Risk group assignment (51% for high-high *v* 79% for the intermediate-high risk group, P = .03) and time from diagnosis to transplant (83% for greater than 15 months *v* 44%, P = .04) were significant predictors of survival. The overall survival and EFS were significantly different in the two risk groups. The 1-year overall survival was 62% in the high-high risk group versus 71% for the intermediate-high risk group (P=0.05). Similarly the one-year DFS was 52% for the high-high risk group and 64% for the intermediate-high risk group (P = .04) (see Fig 1).[42]

The most significant outcome of this trial was the low incidence of acute and chronic GVHD in the setting of a preserved graft-versus-disease effect. Based on the risk factors of the population (age >50, mismatched donors, prior transplant, refractory disease, CMV$^+$ donor/recipient), the expected incidence of serious acute GVHD with a standard ablative conditioning regimen for this group of patient would be 40%. Only 9% had grade III–IV acute GVHD, while 43% developed chronic GVHD (extensive in 12% and limited in 31%). Univariate analysis demonstrated an association between donor type (unrelated *v* related) and incidence of acute GVHD (P = .01), but no association with age (<50 *v* >50), prior transplant, donor/recipient sex mismatch, or underlying disease status. The only variable predictive of severe chronic GVHD was presence of acute GVHD, with age, prior transplant, and donor status being not significant. Likewise, there was no correlation between chronic GVHD and disease relapse, suggesting no correlation between GVHD and GVL effect in this group of patients.[42]

To determine the kinetics of the achievement of full donor

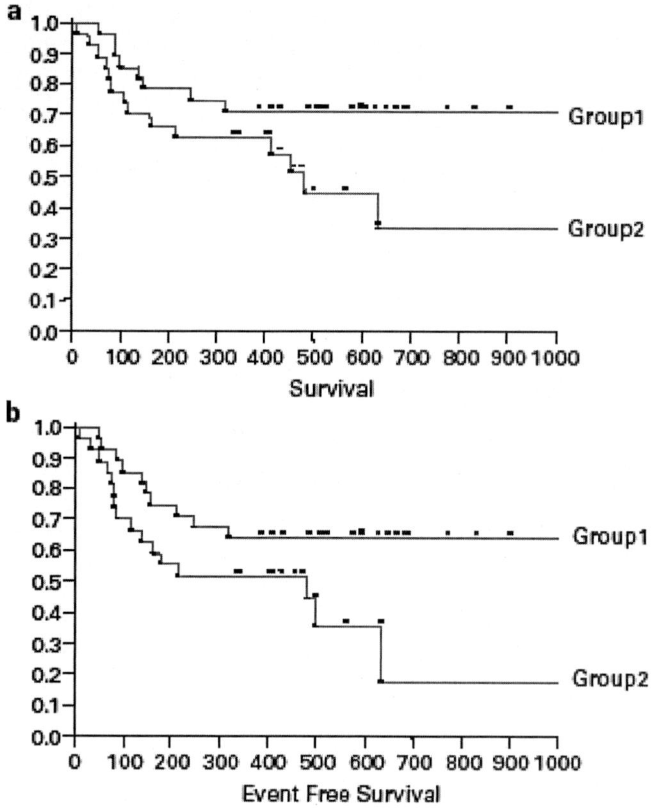

Figure 1 Kaplan-Meier curves illustrating overall survival and event-free survival based upon risk groups. Group 1 represents the high-high risk group and Group 2 represents the intermediate-high risk group. Patients received a pentostatin-based reduced-intensity conditioning regimen. Reprinted by permission from Macmillan Publishers Ltd: *Bone Marrow Transplantation*,[42] © 2004.

chimerism and whether chimerism status correlated with GVHD, the host/donor origin of circulating T cells and dendritic cell (DC) populations were examined at days 30, 60, and 100 by restriction fragment length polymorphisms.[44] Of the first 23 patients, 10 were sex-mismatched and 13 were sex-matched. T-cell donor hematopoiesis in sex-mismatched transplants was 100% at day 30 and was durable through day 100. Of 13 sex-matched patients, 11 were available for assessment. Ten of these patients had full donor T-cell chimerism by day 30, and one patient failed to engraft. In patients who underwent a conventional preparative regimen with high-dose cyclophosphamide and 1,200 cGy TBI as a comparison, all achieved full T-cell donor chimerism in their peripheral blood. One had no acute GVHD or chronic GVHD, one who received marrow from a matched unrelated donor had only grade 1 acute GVHD but developed extensive chronic GVHD of the skin and liver, and one developed grade 4 acute GVHD and extensive chronic GVHD of the skin and gut.[44]

DC chimerism was determined from DC precursors cultured in vitro in the presence of growth factors as described above. Of 21 patients treated with the ECP-based regimen, all 18 patients with only grade 0 or 1 acute GVHD and limited or no chronic GVHD had a complete absence of host DCs, indicating that the circulating DCs were all of donor origin. The one patient with severe acute GVHD and extensive chronic GVHD had only host DC bands but donor lymphocytes, suggesting the persistence of host DCs and the absence of donor DC. The two patients who failed to engraft and developed autologous bone marrow reconstitution had only host DC bands at day +100 as expected. In the three patients who underwent ablative conditioning, DC chimerism at day +100 followed the same pattern. The one patient with no GVHD showed an absence of host DCs and the presence of only donor DCs and donor T cells. In the two patients with severe chronic GVHD, only host DC bands were present, along with donor lymphocytes.[44]

Pavletic et al[45] reported the results of a pilot study evaluating the kinetics of lymphodepletion and safety of a pentostatin-based conditioning regimen. Twelve patients (related donors = 4; unrelated donors = 8) received pentostatin 4 mg/m^2 (days −21, −20, and −19) and 200 cGy TBI (day −1) followed by CSA and mycophenolate mofetil. ADA activity was assessed in peripheral blood mononuclear cells prior to and within 30 minutes after pentostatin administration in nine patients. Median ADA activity decreased from 132.87 pmol/h/μg on day −21 to 19.19 pmol/h/μg on day −19. Following the initiation of pentostatin a 49% reduction in baseline T cells (CD3$^+$) (nadir, 14 days), 55% in natural killer cells (nadir, 7 days), and a 92% reduction of B cells (CD19$^+$) (nadir, 20 days) was reported. CD4$^+$ cells were depressed more than CD8$^+$ cells, while neutrophils and monocytes were minimally affected by pentostatin. Posttransplant peripheral white blood cell chimerism studies demonstrated rapid establishment of donor chimerism in most patients with a median of 90% chimerism at day +28 and 95% chimerism at day +70. Hematologic toxicity of pentostatin was minimal with lymphocytes being the cell type most affected. Nonhematologic-related toxicities were mild and the engraftment rate was high (72% achieved disease-free status). The overall incidence of GVHD was insignificant. Based on these results, this group of investigators hypothesized that the optimal time for transplantation may be as early as 7 days after initiation of pentostatin.[45]

Sandmaier et al[46] administered pentostatin prior to DLI in patients with low (<50%) donor CD3 chimerism and at risk for graft failure following reduced-intensity conditioning for hematopoietic cell transplant. The conditioning regimen consisted of 2 cGy TBI ± fludarabine and both host and donor were given CSA and mycophenolate mofetil. Eight patients were treated with pentostatin 4 mg/m^2 2 days before DLI (10^7 CD3 cells/kg). Five patients developed neutropenia with a median number of 11 days (range, 0 to 36) and an absolute neutrophil count less than 500. Fifty percent of the patients showed increased of donor CD3 chimerism of 63% to 100% and all of these patients developed acute GVHD (two grade II, two grade III) and two developed extensive chronic GVHD. In the remaining four patients, donor chimerism remained low at 5% to 25% following DLI. From these preliminary results, it appears that using pentostatin followed by DLI is more effective for conversion to full donor chimerism than DLI alone in patients at high risk of graft rejection after a nonmyeloablative hematopoietic cell transplant.

Strategies to Reduce GVHD by Graft Manipulations

To date, strategies to lower the incidence of acute GVHD have primarily focused on more precise molecular donor/recipient matching, alternative stem cell sources, and T-cell depletion of the graft in vitro or in vivo by administering T-cell–depleting monoclonal antibodies to the patient. While successful in lowering the frequency and severity of GVHD, T-cell–depleted grafts have been associated with compromised graft-versus-disease effect and higher relapse rates.[47-51] Early studies by Dicke et al demonstrated that irradiated mice engrafted with T-cell–depleted splenocytes had a significantly attenuated incidence of acute GVHD and prolonged survival compared to those given fractions containing increasing numbers of T cells. This led to the development of techniques to remove T cells from allogeneic stem cells prior to reinfusion. Early studies of T-cell depletion used monoclonal antibodies (ATG) with or without complement. More recently, CAMPATH-1H, which is immunoreactive against both T and B cells and which can fix both human and rabbit complement, has been used to T-deplete stem cells.

T-cell depletion has facilitated alternative donor and mismatched donor transplants, with the incidence of acute GVHD decreased 34% to 38% in T-cell–depleted compared to non–T-cell–depleted matched related transplants in the International Bone Marrow Transplant Registry (IBMTR).[52] The incidence of post-transplant pulmonary complications has been significantly less in T-cell–depleted than in non-depleted patients, with a study by Breuer et al[53] showing fatal interstitial pneumonitis in 7.5% of patients, compared to up to 33% in patients receiving MTX and cyclosporine. Similarly, the incidence of venoocclusive disease has been reported to be only 1.2% after T-cell–depleted marrow.[33]

Despite the lower incidence of organ toxicity and acute GVHD, the mortality after T-cell depletion is not necessarily lower among studies. Transplant-associated mortalities have been reported to range from 20% to 32%, with deaths due to graft failure and infections.[46,47] In a review of the IBMTR data of more than 3,000 patients, T-cell depletion was associated with a ninefold increase of graft failure.[54] In a number of retrospective studies analyzing risk of graft failure, donor-recipient disparity, male donor gender, donor over age 25 years, absence of post-transplant immunosuppression, and T-cell depletion are significant risks. Graft failure after T-cell depletion can occur due to failure of initial engraftment, partial engraftment with later graft failure, or delayed engraftment months after BMT. Graft failure in the setting of T-cell depletion is believed to result from rejection of the graft by host lymphoid elements that have survived the conditioning regimen. Supporting this is the identification of host cytotoxic T cells exhibiting donor-specific cytotoxicity at the time of rejection.[55] Another contributing factor may be the induction of mixed chimerism after T-cell depletion. When mixed chimerism is present, host lymphoid tolerance of the graft may be attenuated and lead to graft failure. Because graft failure is believed to mediated by residual host T cells that escaped myeloablation, strategies to intensify conditioning regimens have been applied to T-cell–depleted grafts. Among these include the use of ATG or CAMPATH 1-H to in vivo deplete host T cells prior to allogeneic stem cell infusion.[47] Using CAMPATH for simultaneous host and donor T-cell depletion has led to an incidence of graft failure of only 10%.

The Emerging Role of Dendritic Cells in Allogeneic Stem Cell Transplantation

DCs form a complex network of antigen presenting cells that play a vital role in the induction of primary immunity as well as the modulation of tolerance. DCs are the most potent antigen-presenting cells and are uniquely able to induce primary immune responses against novel antigens through the rich expression of costimulatory and adhesion molecules. DCs generated from non-myeloid lineages or in an immature state may mediate immune tolerance and direct T-cell responses towards a TH2 phenotype. DCs isolated from patients with malignancy demonstrate functional deficiencies that potentially contribute to lack of tumor recognition by host immunity. Little is known about DC engraftment or phenotypic and functional characteristics after allogeneic transplantation. The interactions of DCs with effector populations is likely to be unique following nonmyeloablative conditioning given the presence of mixed donor/recipient chimerism that may characterize the post-transplant period.

A study by Aufferman-Gretzinger et al[56] in patients who underwent conventional and nonmyeloablative conditioning regimens showed that DC reconstitution occurs early, with 80% of the circulating DCs of donor origin on day 14, increasing to 93% by day 28 for patients undergoing both conventional and nonmyeloablative transplants. DCs have been purported to play a role in engraftment, GVL, and acute and chronic GVHD. A role for DCs in establishment of GVHD was defined by Shlomchik et al[57] in a murine HLA-matched allogeneic transplant model, in which GVHD was driven by persistence of functional host antigen-presenting cells after allogeneic stem cell infusion. These results suggested that incidence and severity of GVHD might be influenced by the quality of host/donor DC chimerism achieved after engraftment. In this model, host DCs capable of presenting minor histocompatibility antigens to infused donor T cells would initiate T-cell activation and a Th-1 cytokine cascade implicated in the pathogenesis of acute GVHD.

In addition to chimerism status, functional characteristics of DCs have been implicated in GVHD and graft-versus-disease effect. Distinct DC populations have been identified in peripheral blood, which are differentiated by the presence of myeloid (CD11c) or plasmacytoid (CD123) markers. DC2 (plasmacytoid) cells are characterized by expression of type 2 cytokines and thus initiate a Th-2 response, whereas DC1 (myeloid) cells initiate Th-1 cytokine response.[58] Bone marrow contains monocytes and lineage-negative DC precursors that are capable of differentiating into DC1/DC2 cells in the presence of cytokines. Polarization of DC populations in vivo by G-CSF priming prior to stem cell collection has been demonstrated.[59] Increased numbers of DC2 cells in G-CSF–mobilized peripheral blood stem cells was shown to be associated with an decrease in GVHD but an increased incidence of relapse and impact on survival.[60,61] The impact of DC chimerism, patterns of reconstitution, and presence of DC1 and DC2 populations following nonmyeloablative allogeneic transplant has not been well studied in terms of its effect on transplant outcomes, particularly GVHD and the GVL effect.

In light of the emerging role of DCs in GVHD, the impact of alternative conditioning strategies on donor/recipient chimerism patterns for different aspects of cellular immunity and its implications for immune reconstitution and GVHD remain to be defined. We recently reported that ECP modulated DC function in patients with chronic GVHD and subsequently initiated a pilot study to explore the impact of prophylactic use of ECP as part of a conditioning regimen on the incidence of acute GVHD. Studies of the effects of this regimen on host DCs and on reconstitution of immune effector populations demonstrated that ECP modulated host DC number prior to the infusion of allogeneic stem cells and that this regimen was associated with rapid establishment of full donor DC chimerism in the majority of patients.[44] Of four patients who demonstrated mixed DC chimerism, all had grade II to IV acute GVHD. Immunophenotypic analysis of circulating DC populations revealed a predominance of plasmacytoid (DC2) DCs after engraftment. We hypothesize that our significantly low incidence of acute GVHD with preserved GVL effect using this conditioning regimen is due to early engraftment and establishment of donor DC chimerism as well as a predominance of DC2 versus DC1 cells, or tolerance phenotype, resulting in attenuation of Th1-mediated cytokine production and subsequently, acute GVHD without adversely affecting donor T-cell–mediated GVL.[57,62]

Conclusions

Significant advancements have been made in developing preparative regimens for allogeneic transplantation. The traditional myeloablative regimens used previously were effective; however, toxicity limited these regimens to otherwise healthy younger patients. With the recognition that GVL may be responsible of many of the cures reported following allogeneic transplantation, less intensive nonmyeloablative preparative regimens have been investigated. Purine analogues have played a central role in these regimens. We have evaluated pentostatin-based regimens and demonstrated that the pentostatin/ECP/TBI regimen is well tolerated and is associated with early full donor engraftment with a predominance of donor DC2 cells and a low incidence of acute GVHD in a population of high-risk patients. The early recovery of donor-derived DC function is likely to be correlated with improved cellular immunity, restoration of T-cell repertoire, and decreased risk of infectious complications. Further investigation is needed to explore the effects of regimens themselves as well as the various components of a regimen on host DC subpopulations and to determine whether these immunologic parameters correlate with clinical outcome overall or in subgroups of patients.

References

1. Gratwohl A, Baldomero H, Passweg J, Urbano-Ispizua A: Increasing use of reduced intensity conditioning transplants: Report of the 2001 EBMT activity survey. Bone Marrow Transplant 30:813-831, 2002
2. Lazarus HM, Gale RP: Blood cell and bone marrow transplants. Bone Marrow Transplant 18:839-841, 1996
3. Giralt S, Khouri I, Champlin R: Non myeloablative "mini transplants." Cancer Treat Res 101:97-108, 1999
4. Champlin R, Khouri I, Shimoni A, Gajewski J, Kornblau S, Molldrem J, et al: Harnessing graft-versus-malignancy: Non-myeloablative preparative regimens for allogeneic haematopoietic transplantation, an evolving strategy for adoptive immunotherapy. Br J Haematol 111:18-29, 2000
5. Wong R, Giralt SA, Martin T, Couriel DR, Anagnostopoulos A, Hosing C, et al: Reduced-intensity conditioning for unrelated donor hematopoietic stem cell transplantation as treatment for myeloid malignancies in patients older than 55 years. Blood 102:3052-3059, 2003
6. Sorror ML, Maris MB, Storer B, Sandmaier BM, Diaconescu R, Flowers C, et al: Comparing morbidity and mortality of HLA-matched unrelated donor hematopoietic cell transplantation after nonmyeloablative and myeloablative conditioning: Influence of pretransplantation comorbidities. Blood 104:961-968, 2004
7. Slavin S, Nagler A, Naparstek E, Kapelushnik Y, Aker M, Cividalli G, et al: Nonmyeloablative stem cell transplantation and cell therapy as an alternative to conventional bone marrow transplantation with lethal cytoreduction for the treatment of malignant and nonmalignant hematologic diseases. Blood 91:756-763, 1998
8. de Lima M, Anagnostopoulos A, Munsell M, Shahjahan M, Ueno N, Ippoliti C, et al: Nonablative versus reduced-intensity conditioning regimens in the treatment of acute myeloid leukemia and high-risk myelodysplastic syndrome: Dose is relevant for long-term disease control after allogeneic hematopoietic stem cell transplantation. Blood 104: 865-872, 2004
9. Anderlini P, Saliba R, Acholonu S, Okoroji GJ, Donato M, Giralt S, et al: Reduced-intensity allogeneic stem cell transplantation in relapsed and refractory Hodgkin's disease: Low transplant-related mortality and impact of intensity of conditioning regimen. Bone Marrow Transplant 35:943-951, 2005
10. Pelot MR, Pearson DA, Swenson K, Zhao G, Sachs J, Yang YG, et al: Lymphohematopoietic graft-vs.-host reactions can be induced without graft-vs.-host disease in murine mixed chimeras established with a cyclophosphamide-based nonmyeloablative conditioning regimen. Biol Blood Marrow Transplant 5:133-143, 1999
11. Storb R, Raff RF, Appelbaum FR, Deeg HJ, Graham TC, Schuening FG, et al: Fractionated versus single-dose total body irradiation at low and high dose rates to condition canine littermates for DLA-identical marrow grafts. Blood 83:3384-3389, 1994
12. Deeg HJ, Anasetti C, Petersdorf E, Storb R, Doney K, Hansen JA, et al: Cyclophosphamide plus ATG conditioning is insufficient for sustained hematopoietic reconstitution in patients with severe aplastic anemia transplanted with marrow from HLA-A, B, DRB matched unrelated donors. Blood 83:3417-3418, 1994
13. Storb R, Yu C, Wagner JL, Deeg HJ, Nash RA, Kiem HP, et al: Stable mixed hematopoietic chimerism in DLA-identical littermate dogs given sublethal total body irradiation before and pharmacological immunosuppression after marrow transplantation. Blood 89:3048-3054, 1997
14. Wagner JL, Storb R: Preclinical large animal models for hematopoietic stem cell transplantation. Curr Opin Hematol 3:410-415, 1996
15. Yu C, Seidel K, Nash RA, Deeg HJ, Sandmaier BM, Barsoukov A, et al: Synergism between mycophenolate mofetil and cyclosporine in preventing graft-versus-host disease among lethally irradiated dogs given

DLA-nonidentical unrelated marrow grafts. Blood 91:2581-2587, 1998
16. Storb R, Yu C, Barnett T, Wagner JL, Deeg HJ, Nash RA, et al: Stable mixed hematopoietic chimerism in dog leukocyte antigen-identical littermate dogs given lymph node irradiation before and pharmacologic immunosuppression after marrow transplantation. Blood 94:1131-1136, 1999
17. Storb R, Yu C, Sandmaier B, McSweeney P, Georges G, Nash R, et al: Mixed hematopoietic chimerism after hematopoietic stem cell allografts. Transplant Proc 31:677-678, 1999
18. Khouri IF, Keating M, Korbling M, Przepiorka D, Anderlini P, O'Brien S, et al: Transplant-lite: Induction of graft-versus-malignancy using fludarabine-based nonablative chemotherapy and allogeneic blood progenitor-cell transplantation as treatment for lymphoid malignancies. J Clin Oncol 16:2817-2824, 1998
19. Weisser M, Schleuning M, Ledderose G, Rolf B, Schnittger S, Schoch C, et al: Reduced-intensity conditioning using TBI (8 Gy), fludarabine, cyclophosphamide and ATG in elderly CML patients provides excellent results especially when performed in the early course of the disease. Bone Marrow Transplant 34:1083-1088, 2004
20. Giralt S, Estey E, Albitar M, van Besien K, Rondon G, Anderlini P, et al: Engraftment of allogeneic hematopoietic progenitor cells with purine analog-containing chemotherapy: Harnessing graft-versus-leukemia without myeloablative therapy. Blood 89:4531-4536, 1997
21. Giralt S, Thall PF, Khouri I, Wang X, Braunschweig I, Ippolitti C, et al: Melphalan and purine analog-containing preparative regimens: reduced-intensity conditioning for patients with hematologic malignancies undergoing allogeneic progenitor cell transplantation. Blood 97: 631-637, 2001
22. Ritchie DS, Morton J, Szer J, Roberts AW, Durrant S, Shuttleworth P, et al: Graft-versus-host disease, donor chimerism, and organ toxicity in stem cell transplantation after conditioning with fludarabine and melphalan. Biol Blood Marrow Transplant 9:435-442, 2003
23. Grosskreutz C, Ross V, Scigliano E, Fruchtman S, Isola L: Low-dose total body irradiation, fludarabine, and antithymocyte globulin conditioning for nonmyeloablative allogeneic transplantation. Biol Blood Marrow Transplant 9:453-459, 2003
24. Childs R, Clave E, Contentin N, Jayasekera D, Hensel N, Leitman S, et al: Engraftment kinetics after nonmyeloablative allogeneic peripheral blood stem cell transplantation: Full donor T-cell chimerism precedes alloimmune responses. Blood 94:3234-3241, 1999
25. Childs R, Barrett J: Nonmyeloablative stem cell transplantation for solid tumors: Expanding the application of allogeneic immunotherapy. Semin Hematol 39:63-71, 2002
26. Niederwieser D, Maris M, Shizuru JA, Petersdorf E, Hegenbart U, Sandmaier BM, et al: Low-dose total body irradiation (TBI) and fludarabine followed by hematopoietic cell transplantation (HCT) from HLA-matched or mismatched unrelated donors and postgrafting immunosuppression with cyclosporine and mycophenolate mofetil (MMF) can induce durable complete chimerism and sustained remissions in patients with hematological diseases. Blood 101:1620-1629, 2003
27. Sykes M, Preffer F, McAfee S, Saidman SL, Weymouth D, Andrews DM, et al: Mixed lymphohaemopoietic chimerism and graft-versus-lymphoma effects after non-myeloablative therapy and HLA-mismatched bone-marrow transplantation. Lancet 353:1755-1759, 1999
28. Dey BR, McAfee S, Sackstein R, Colby C, Saidman S, Weymouth D, et al: Successful allogeneic stem cell transplantation with nonmyeloablative conditioning in patients with relapsed hematologic malignancy following autologous stem cell transplantation. Biol Blood Marrow Transplant 7:604-612, 2001
29. Kottaridis PD, Milligan DW, Chopra R, Chakraverty RK, Chakrabarti S, Robinson S, et al: In vivo CAMPATH-1H prevents graft-versus-host disease following nonmyeloablative stem cell transplantation. Blood 96:2419-2425, 2000
30. Chakrabarti S, Mackinnon S, Chopra R, Kottaridis PD, Peggs K, O'Gorman P, et al: High incidence of cytomegalovirus infection after nonmyeloablative stem cell transplantation: Potential role of Campath-1H in delaying immune reconstitution. Blood 99:4357-4363, 2002
31. Ho AY, Devereux S, Mufti GJ, Pagliuca A: Reduced-intensity rituximab-BEAM-CAMPATH allogeneic haematopoietic stem cell transplantation for follicular lymphoma is feasible and induces durable molecular remissions. Bone Marrow Transplant 31:551-557, 2003
32. Faulkner RD, Craddock C, Byrne JL, Mahendra P, Haynes AP, Prentice HG, et al: BEAM-alemtuzumab reduced-intensity allogeneic stem cell transplantation for lymphoproliferative diseases: GVHD, toxicity, and survival in 65 patients. Blood 103:428-434, 2004
33. Ho AY, Pagliuca A, Kenyon M, Parker JE, Mijovic A, Devereux S, et al: Reduced-intensity allogeneic hematopoietic stem cell transplantation for myelodysplastic syndrome and acute myeloid leukemia with multilineage dysplasia using fludarabine, busulphan, and alemtuzumab (FBC) conditioning. Blood 104:1616-1623, 2004
34. McLaughlin P: Biotherapy for lymphoma. Curr Oncol Rep 2:157-162, 2000
35. Major PP, Agarwal RP, Kufe DW: Clinical pharmacology of deoxycoformycin. Blood 58:91-96, 1981
36. Mitchell BS, Sidi Y, Hershfield M, Koller CA: Biochemical consequences of adenosine deaminase inhibition in vivo. Differential effects in acute and chronic T cell leukemia. Ann N Y Acad Sci 451:129-137, 1985
37. Carson DA, Kaye J, Seegmiller JE: Differential sensitivity of human leukemic T cell lines and B cell lines to growth inhibition by deoxyadenosine. J Immunol 121:1726-1731, 1978
38. Steis RG, Urba WJ, Kopp WC, Alvord WG, Smith JW 2nd, Longo DL: Kinetics of recovery of $CD4^+$ T cells in peripheral blood of deoxycoformycin-treated patients. J Natl Cancer Inst 83:1678-1679, 1991
39. Grever MR, Siaw MF, Jacob WF, Neidhart JA, Miser JS, Coleman MS, et al: The biochemical and clinical consequences of 2′-deoxycoformycin in refractory lymphoproliferative malignancy. Blood 57:406-417, 1981
40. Foss FM: Combination therapy with purine nucleoside analogs. Oncology (Williston Park) 14:31-35, 2000
41. Foss FM: Activity of pentostatin (Nipent) in cutaneous T-cell lymphoma: Single-agent and combination studies. Semin Oncol 27:58-63, 2000
42. Miller KB, Roberts TF, Chan G, Schenkein DP, Lawrence D, Sprague K, et al: A novel reduced intensity regimen for allogeneic hematopoietic stem cell transplantation associated with a reduced incidence of graft-versus-host disease. Bone Marrow Transplant 33:881-889, 2004
43. Miller KB, Schenkein DP, Comenzo R, Erban JK, Fogaren T, Hirsch CA, et al: Adjusted-dose continuous-infusion cyclosporin A to prevent graft-versus-host disease following allogeneic bone marrow transplantation. Ann Hematol 68:15-20, 1994
44. Chan GW, Gorgun G, Miller KB, Foss FM: Persistence of host dendritic cells after transplantation is associated with graft-versus-host disease. Biol Blood Marrow Transplant 9:170-176, 2003
45. Pavletic SZ, Bociek RG, Foran JM, Rubocki RJ, Kuszynski CA, Wisecarver JL, et al: Lymphodepleting effects and safety of pentostatin for nonmyeloablative allogeneic stem-cell transplantation. Transplantation 76:877-881, 2003
46. Sandmaier B, Maloney D, Maris M, Chauncey T, Pulsipher M, Bethge W, et al: Conversion of low donor chimerism following nonmyeloablative conditioning for hematopoietic cell transplantation (HCT) using pentostatin and donor lymphocyted infusion (DLI). Blood 103:186, 2004 (abstr)
47. Hale G, Cobbold S, Waldmann H: T cell depletion with CAMPATH-1 in allogeneic bone marrow transplantation. Transplantation 45:753-759, 1988
48. Martin PJ, Hansen JA, Buckner CD, Sanders JE, Deeg HJ, Stewart P, et al: Effects of in vitro depletion of T cells in HLA-identical allogeneic marrow grafts. Blood 66:664-672, 1985
49. Martin PJ, Hansen JA, Storb R, Thomas ED: T cell depletion of donor marrow for prevention of acute graft-versus-host disease. Haematol Blood Transfus 29:42-43, 1985
50. Starobinski M, Roosnek E, Hale G, Roux E, Helg C, Chapuis B: T cell depletion of allogeneic peripheral blood stem cells. Bone Marrow Transplant 21:429-430, 1998
51. Ho VT, Soiffer RJ: The history and future of T-cell depletion as graft-versus-host disease prophylaxis for allogeneic hematopoietic stem cell transplantation. Blood 98:3192-3204, 2001

52. Champlin RE, Passweg JR, Zhang MJ, Rowlings PA, Pelz CJ, Atkinson KA, et al: T-cell depletion of bone marrow transplants for leukemia from donors other than HLA-identical siblings: Advantage of T-cell antibodies with narrow specificities. Blood 95:3996-4003, 2000
53. Breuer R, Or R, Lijovetzky G, Naparstek E, Engelhard D, Lafair J, et al: Interstitial pneumonitis in T cell-depleted bone marrow transplantation. Bone Marrow Transplant 3:625-630, 1988
54. Marmont AM, Horowitz MM, Gale RP, Sobocinski K, Ash RC, van Bekkum DW, et al: T-cell depletion of HLA-identical transplants in leukemia. Blood 78:2120-2130, 1991
55. Champlin R, Giralt S, Gajewski J: T cells, graft-versus-host disease and graft-versus-leukemia: Innovative approaches for blood and marrow transplantation. Acta Haematol 95:157-163, 1996
56. Auffermann-Gretzinger S, Lossos IS, Vayntrub TA, Leong W, Grumet FC, Blume KG, et al: Rapid establishment of dendritic cell chimerism in allogeneic hematopoietic cell transplant recipients. Blood 99:1442-1448, 2002
57. Shlomchik WD, Couzens MS, Tang CB, McNiff J, Robert ME, Liu J, et al: Prevention of graft versus host disease by inactivation of host antigen-presenting cells. Science 285:412-415, 1999
58. Liu YJ, Kanzler H, Soumelis V, Gilliet M: Dendritic cell lineage, plasticity and cross-regulation. Nat Immunol 2:585-589, 2001
59. Arpinati M, Green CL, Heimfeld S, Heuser JE, Anasetti C: Granulocyte-colony stimulating factor mobilizes T helper 2-inducing dendritic cells. Blood 95:2484-2490, 2000
60. Waller EK, Rosenthal H, Sagar L: DC2 effect on survival following allogeneic bone marrow transplantation. Oncology (Williston Park) 16:19-26, 2002
61. Waller EK, Rosenthal H, Jones TW, Peel J, Lonial S, Langston A, et al: Larger numbers of CD4(bright) dendritic cells in donor bone marrow are associated with increased relapse after allogeneic bone marrow transplantation. Blood 97:2948-2956, 2001
62. Alcindor T, Gorgun G, Miller KB, Roberts TF, Sprague K, Schenkein DP, et al: Immunomodulatory effects of extracorporeal photochemotherapy in patients with extensive chronic graft-versus-host disease. Blood 98:1622-1625, 2001

ELSEVIER

Seminars in
HEMATOLOGY

Purine Analogue-Based Chemotherapy Regimens for Second-Line Therapy in Patients With Chronic Lymphocytic Leukemia

Nicole Lamanna and Mark A. Weiss

A dramatic change has occurred in the management of chronic lymphocytic leukemia (CLL) over the past 20 years. The use of newer therapies, including the purine analogues, has resulted in higher frequencies of response. Combination therapy with purine analogues, alkylators, and/or monoclonal antibodies represents a promising new approach to the treatment of patients with CLL. The most commonly studied regimens have utilized fludarabine, but severe myelosuppression and immunosuppression of these combinations require close attention to dosing and schedule. Of the purine analogues that show activity in CLL, pentostatin appears to be the least myelosuppressive. These combination strategies are associated with high-quality responses in the majority of patients and may one day lead to improved survival or possibly even a cure for patients with CLL.
Semin Hematol 43(suppl 2):S44-S49

Chronic lymphocytic leukemia (CLL) is the most common leukemia in adults, accounting for 22.3% of cases.[1] The long-term survival in these patients is poor. It is a clonal disorder that involves proliferation and accumulation of mature B lymphocytes. Traditionally, patients with CLL have been treated in a palliative fashion. Conventional therapy with oral alkylating agents with or without corticosteroids produced clinical improvement but rarely produced complete responses (CRs) and patients usually succumbed to progressive resistant disease. The introduction of the purine analogues has renewed interest in developing more aggressive therapies, which may result in durable responses for these patients.

Overview of Chronic Lymphocytic Leukemia

CLL is primarily a disease of older individuals, with 90% of patients greater than 50 years of age at the time of diagnosis.[2] Recently, the incidence of CLL has increased thought to be due to the increase in initial diagnosis upon annual physical examinations. The incidence in men is twice that of women.[1] Diehl et al[1] published an epidemiologic study of CLL from the National Cancer Data Base. The 5-year relative survival rates were 69.5%, 72.2%, 63.1%, and 41.7% for age groups <40, 40–59, 60–79, and 80+ years, respectively. These data indicate that patients are dying as a result of the disease and not comorbid conditions.[1]

In general, CLL is a slowly progressive disease manifested by the accumulation of mature-appearing lymphocytes in the blood, bone marrow, spleen, and lymph nodes. The B cells are phenotypically characterized by coexpression of the B-cell markers CD19, CD20, CD21, CD5, CD24, and CD23.[3] Common chromosomal abnormalities identified using fluorescence-in-situ hybridization (FISH) analysis includes del(17p) (7%), del (11q22-23) (17%), trisomy 12 (14%), and del(13q14) (36%).[4] These genetic aberrations have important implications as predictors of disease progression and survival. Patients who have del(17p) and del (11q22-23) have more advanced disease and a shorter treatment-free interval than those in the other groups.[4] Differential diagnosis of CLL should include mantle cell leukemia/lymphoma, prolymphocytic leukemia (PLL), and hairy cell leukemia (HCL). Diagnostic distinction of mantle cell leukemia/lymphoma includes CD23 negativity, presence of t(11;14), and intracellular cyclin D1 expression. HCL and PLL are morphologically different than CLL and also lack expression of CD5.

The clinical features of this disease are progressive bone marrow failure manifested by anemia, neutropenia, thrombocytopenia, lymphadenopathy, splenomegaly, and hepato-

Department of Medicine, Leukemia Service, Memorial Sloan-Kettering Cancer Center, New York, NY.

Address correspondence to Mark A. Weiss, MD, Department of Medicine, Leukemia Service, Memorial Sloan-Kettering Cancer Center, 1275 York Ave, New York, NY 10021.E-mail: weissm@mskcc.org

 0037-1963/06/$-see front matter
doi:10.1053/j.seminhematol.2005.12.009

Table 1 Staging and Risk Stratification for Chronic Lymphocytic Leukemia

Rai Staging[5]	Median Survival (mo)	Binet Staging[6]	Median Survival (yr)
0 = Bone marrow/blood lymphocytosis	>150	A = Hgb ≥10 g/dL, platelets ≥100,000/μL <3 areas involved*	>10
1 = Lymphocytosis with enlarged nodes	101		
2 = Lymphocytosis with enlarged spleen and/or liver	71	B = Hgb ≥10 g/dL, platelets ≥100,000/μL ≥3 areas involved*	7
3 = Lymphocytosis with Hgb <11 g/dL	19	C = Hgb <10 g/dL, platelets <100,000/μL or both (independent of areas involved)	2
4 = Lymphocytosis with platelets <100,000/μL	19		
High-risk stratification[45]			
Rai stage 3 or 4			
CD38 expression >30% lymphocytes			
ZAP70 expression in >30% lymphocytes			
Unmutated IgV_H gene			
Doubling of lymphocyte count <12 months			
Cytogenetic abnormalities (14q changes, 11q changes, 17p deletion, trisomy 12, absence of 13q changes)			

Abbreviations: Hgb, hemoglobin; NR, not reported.
*Areas involved include one of the following: axillary, cervical, inguinal, lymph nodes, whether unilateral or bilateral, spleen, and liver.

megaly. Frequently there is hypogammaglobulinemia with a resultant increased risk of infection. Infections may in fact be a common cause of death in these patients. Diagnostic criteria of CLL includes lymphocyte counts greater than 5 × 10^9/L and bone marrow lymphocyte counts greater than 30%. Several risk classification schemes have been reported. Rai et al[5] described the earliest system with stage 0 to 4 based on lymphadenopathy, splenomegaly, anemia, and thrombocytopenia. Binet et al[6] simplified the staging system to stages A to C based on the numbers of enlarged lymph nodes and the presence of anemia and thrombocytopenia. Table 1 describes the two staging systems. Since CLL displays an indolent course, it is essential to identify patients who are at high risk for disease progression so appropriate therapeutic intervention may be instituted. All of the features that have been associated with high-risk disease are listed in Table 1.

Treatment Strategies of Chronic Lymphocytic Leukemia and the Role of Purine Analogues

Patients with CLL do not always require treatment at the time of diagnosis. Early chemotherapeutic intervention has not been shown to alter the natural history of the disease.[7,8] The National Cancer Institute Working Group developed criteria for institution of therapy and evaluation of responses in patients with CLL.[9] Indications for therapeutic intervention include extreme fatigue, fevers greater than 100.5°F for longer than 2 weeks, loss of more than 10% body weight, night sweats, autoimmune cytopenias poorly responsive to steroids, massive splenomegaly, progressive marrow failure, massive adenopathy, and progressive lymphocytosis with a doubling time less than 6 months.[9]

Traditionally, therapy for patients with CLL has been mainly palliative since it is considered to be an incurable disease. The alkylating agents, chlorambucil and cyclophosphamide with or without steroids, have been considered the cornerstone in the management of CLL. In general, these agents rarely induced CRs and these responses were not durable, with patients ultimately dying from progressive resistant disease. However, the treatment of CLL has changed significantly over the past 10 years. The introduction of the purine analogues (pentostatin, fludarabine, and cladribine) has renewed interest in aggressive therapy in patients with CLL. The first evidence that purine analogues possessed anti-CLL properties came in the late 1980s.[10] Since that time there has been a progressive trend towards the use of these agents as first-line therapy, which was further substantiated following the publication of a trial comparing fludarabine to chlorambucil.[11] This was a large American study showing superiority of fludarabine over chlorambucil based on CR rate (20% *v* 4%), duration of remission (25 *v* 14 months, median), and frequency of remission (63% *v* 37%). However, a higher rate of toxicity was noted, including severe infections and neutropenia in the patients treated with fludarabine.[11] Other investigators suggested that the dose of chlorambucil used in this trial was not sufficient and have reported increased responses using higher doses.[12] Nonetheless, results from three other clinical trials[13-15] confirm the superior activity of the purine analogues as initial therapy for CLL.

Rationale for Purine Analogue Therapy

The purine nucleoside analogues, fludarabine (Fludara; Berlex Laboratories, Richmond, CA), cladribine (Leustatin; Ortho Biotech, Bridgewater, NJ), and 2′-deoxycoformycin (pentostatin, Nipent®; Supergen, Dublin, CA), represent a class of cytotoxic agents with novel mechanisms of action, such as induction of apoptosis, and exhibit a high degree of activity against hematologic malignancies, including CLL.[16] The agents are similar in chemical structure but differ in their mechanism of interaction with the enzymes involved in adenosine and deoxyadenosine metabolism. Fludarabine and cladribine are taken up into cells then phosphorylated by deoxycytidine kinase to the equivalent nucleotide triphosphate prior to incorporation into DNA causing interference with DNA synthesis. Lymphocytes have high levels of deoxycytidine kinase, which helps explain the specificity of these agents for these cells. Pentostatin is an irreversible inhibitor of adenosine deaminase (ADA). It blocks the deamination of adenosine to inosine and deoxyadenosine to deoxyinosine, resulting in accumulation of deoxyadenosine triphosphate. These metabolites block DNA synthesis through the inhibition of ribonucleotide reductase.[17] ADA is present in virtually all tissues, but its activity is the greatest in lymphoid cells. Pentostatin was thought to be beneficial in treating lymphoproliferative disorders since patients who are congenitally deficient in ADA have profound defects in lymphocyte function resulting in the syndrome of severe combined immunodeficiency disease.[18] Purine analogues also show synergistic cytotoxic activity with other agents, especially alkylating agents. The DNA damage produced by alkylating agents increases the opportunities for incorporation of therapeutic nucleosides into DNA.[19]

Historical Perspective of Purine Analogue Therapy in Chronic Lymphocytic Leukemia

Numerous studies have been conducted evaluating purine analogues in CLL. Fludarabine is the most extensively studied agent in this class. Fludarabine was first studied as single-agent therapy in patients with relapsed or refractory CLL.[20] These studies reported overall response rates between 12% and 44%; however, CR rates were only 3% to 15%.[20] Further retrospective analysis reported higher response rates in patients with earlier stage disease, normal serum albumin levels, and minimal prior therapy.[21,22] The observation that purine analogues are active in previously treated patients led to trials of these agents in previously untreated patients. In previously untreated patients, fludarabine induced responses in the majority of patients and CRs in a significant minority.[23] This led to evaluations of fludarabine as first-line therapy compared to standard therapeutic regimens. Fludarabine was shown to be superior to chlorambucil,[11] and combination regimens including CVP (cyclophosphamide, vincristine, prednisone) and CHOP (cyclophosphamide, doxorubicin, vincristine, prednisone).[13] Superiority was demonstrated as higher response rates and longer disease-free intervals. However, despite this, no improvement in survival was reported. A possible explanation for the lack of survival benefit is the lack of high-quality responses induced by fludarabine. Nonetheless, fludarabine is quite active in CLL and this initial work led to the investigation of combination regimens, which might further improve the frequency of complete response.

The early combination studies with fludarabine and corticosteroids[21] or chlorambucil[24,25] were disappointing due to combined toxicities, which limited the dose intensity and thus any improvement in response frequency. More recently, combination studies with fludarabine have shown significant activity with acceptable toxicity. O'Brien et al[26] evaluated 128 patients (34 previously untreated and 94 previously treated) with CLL treated with fludarabine (30 mg/m^2/d for 3 days) and cyclophosphamide. An initial cohort of 12 patients received the initial cyclophosphamide dosing schedule of 500 mg/m^2/d for 3 days; however, toxicity led to dose reductions to 350 mg/m^2/d for 3 days (n = 27) initially, and then to 300 mg/m^2/d for 3 days (n = 22). This regimen exhibited marked activity with an overall response rate of 74%. The most impressive response rates were reported in patients who were previously untreated (88%) while less impressive activity was reported in fludarabine-refractory patients (39%). Increased myelosuppression was observed with this combination with 40% of patients experiencing grade 3 or 4 infections.[26] This same group of investigators at M.D. Anderson Cancer Center added rituximab to this combination and reported results of this combination in 177 previously treated CLL patients.[27] Adding rituximab to this regimen increased the frequency of CRs (25%) but not overall responses (73%). Unfortunately, myelosuppression was more pronounced, with 81% of patients developing grade 3 or 4 neutropenia and 47% with grade 3 or 4 infections and/or fever. These toxicities prohibited the administration of this combination to all patients, with only 38% of patients who were able to receive the full course of therapy.[27]

Another combination of fludarabine (20 mg/m^2/d for 5 days) and cyclophosphamide (600 mg/m^2 on day 1 administered in conjunction with growth factors) was studied in 17 previously untreated patients at the Johns Hopkins University Oncology Center.[28] The overall response rate was 100%, with 47% of patients achieving CR. The combination was generally well tolerated but did result in one death from pneumocystis pneumonia and one case of cryptococcal pneumonia. At the completion of therapy, three cases of herpes zoster infection were observed.[28]

We have also evaluated the combination of fludarabine and cyclophosphamide using a sequential approach to allow for administration of full-dose fludarabine (25 mg/m^2/d for 5 days every 4 weeks for six cycles) followed by dose-intense consolidation with cyclophosphamide (3,000 mg/m^2 every 2 to 3 weeks for three cycles with growth factor support).[29] A total of 25 patients were evaluated with a 76% overall response rate (32% CR). Six patients (24%) were treatment failures. Consolidation therapy with cyclophosphamide was shown to improve the quality of responses in 48% of patients as evidenced by the following: ability to achieve CR (8% following fludarabine *v* 32% following cyclophosphamide), ability to achieve a flow-cytometric CR (8% following fludarabine *v* 36% following cyclophosphamide), and the likelihood of testing polymerase chain reaction–negative (0% following fludarabine *v* 12% following cyclophosphamide).

Table 2 Activity of Purine Analogues Combined With Alkylator Therapy for Patients With Previously Treated Chronic Lymphocytic Leukemia

Selected Reference	Agents	N	ORR (%)	CR (%)
O'Brien et al [26]	Fludarabine + cyclophosphamide	94	73	14
Montillo et al [33]	Cladribine + cyclophosphamide	29	28	14
Weiss et al [44]	Pentostatin + cyclophosphamide	22	74	17

Abbreviations: ORR, overall response rate; CR, complete response rate.

This is clinically important because consolidation with high-dose cyclophosphamide increased the proportion of patients achieving a nodular response or CR threefold and the projected 6-year survival for patients achieving a CR or nodular response was 91% compared to 41% for all others (P = .012).[29] We have also added rituximab (375 mg/m^2 once weekly for 4 weeks) to this regimen as a second consolidation therapy.[30] Sequential therapy with these agents produces a high frequency of CR and appears to enhance the quality of responses.

Cladribine has also been studied in several small trials.[15,31-33] Robak et al[15] reported results of a randomized trial of cladribine (0.12 mg/kg/d for 5 days) with prednisone (30 mg/m^2/d for 5 days) compared with chlorambucil (12 mg/m^2/d for 7 days) and prednisone (30 mg/m^2/d for 7 days) in 229 previously untreated patients with CLL. The likelihood of achieving a response was superior in the cladribine group compared to chlorambucil (87% *v* 57%, P = .001), as was the likelihood of achieving a CR (47% *v* 12%, P = .001). Unfortunately, the improvement in response was offset by the increased toxicity observed in the cladribine-treated patients. The incidence of myelosuppression was 23% in the cladribine group compared to 11% in the chlorambucil group (P = .02) and the incidence of infection was 56% versus 40% (P = .02). Survival at 2 years was comparable for the two groups (78% *v* 82%).[15]

Pentostatin Combinations for Previously Treated Chronic Lymphocytic Leukemia

During the 1980s, case reports first suggested that pentostatin exhibited significant activity in CLL patients who had relapsed following treatment with alkylating agents.[34,35] Pentostatin was investigated as single-agent therapy in several studies using a dose of 4 mg/m^2 every 1 to 2 weeks in patients with advanced stage and refractory CLL.[36-38] The overall frequency of response ranged from 18% to 29% with CR rates of 0% to 8%.

In an effort to improve the response rates, combination therapy with pentostatin was explored. In vitro data support a synergistic effect when combined with alkylating agents.[39] The use of pentostatin in combination regimens is appealing since pentostatin has the least myelosuppressive properties of the purine analogue class, with cladribine being the most myelosuppressive. Since myelosuppression is often the dose-limiting toxicity of alkylating agents, it is postulated that pentostatin would be the best purine analogue to combine with an alkylating agent to take advantage of the synergy seen with this combination. The differences in mechanism of action of these compounds, as previously described, may account for the differences in myelosuppression seen. Drug-related myelosuppression has been reported in some patients treated with pentostatin, primarily in those with bone marrow involvement. These data were derived from analysis encountered in previous studies where 90% of patients with HCL developed grade 3 or 4 myelosuppression[40] and none of the patients with mycosis fungoides treated with pentostatin developed grade 3 or 4 myelosuppression.[41]

The combination of pentostatin, prednisone (80 mg/d), and chlorambucil (30 mg/m^2) was studied in a phase II trial of 55 previously untreated patients.[42] The purpose of this study was to evaluate the dose of pentostatin that could be combined with these agents. The pentostatin dose was 2 mg/m^2 on day 1 for the first six patients; 3 mg/m^2 on day 1 for the next six patients; and 4 mg/m^2 on day 1 for the last set of six patients. Due to increasing toxicity with no improvement in clinical efficacy on escalation of the pentostatin dose, 2 mg/m^2 was chosen as the phase II dose, with 43 patients treated using this dose. The overall response rate was 87%, including a 44% CR rate. Unfortunately, this trial was associated with significant toxicity, particularly opportunistic infections (31%). To reduce the incidence of infectious complications, a trial has been initiated omitting prednisone and combining chlorambucil and pentostatin with growth factors.[43]

At Memorial Sloan-Kettering Cancer Center, we have investigated a combination of pentostatin and cyclophosphamide in pretreated patients with CLL.[44] We treated 23 patients with a fixed dose of pentostatin (4 mg/m^2) in combination with either cyclophosphamide 600 mg/m^2 or 900 mg/m^2 given once every 3 weeks for six cycles. High-risk disease was present in 71% of patients and median number of prior treatments was three (range, one to five), primarily refractory to fludarabine and alkylating agents. Despite the high-risk status of these patients, there were responses in 74% including 17% with CRs and 57% with partial responses (PRs). In patients who were fludarabine-refractory, there was a 77% response rate. In addition, the toxicity profile with this regimen was acceptable. Grade 3 or 4 neutropenia and thrombocytopenia was seen in 35% and 30% of patients, respectively, while grade 3 or 4 infections were seen in only 9% of patients.[44] Based on these promising findings, we are currently evaluating the combination of rituximab, pentostatin, and cyclophosphamide. We anticipate the results of this study to be published soon.

Conclusions

We have entered an exciting era in the treatment of CLL. With the introduction of newer therapies, the treatment goals for patients with CLL have shifted from palliative to curative. More effective therapy with purine analogues has led to better response rates than that reported with traditional alkylator therapy. CRs are associated with longer duration of response and prolonged progression-free survival. Newer combination therapies with purine analogues show promise for more CRs along with molecular responses. The introduction of improved diagnostic techniques will also assist in identifying patients who will likely benefit from aggressive therapy.

References

1. Diehl LF, Karnell LH, Menck HR: The American College of Surgeons Commission on Cancer and the American Cancer Society. The National Cancer Data Base report on age, gender, treatment, and outcomes of patients with chronic lymphocytic leukemia. Cancer 86:2684-2692, 1999
2. O'Brien S, del Giglio A, Keating M: Advances in the biology and treatment of B-cell chronic lymphocytic leukemia. Blood 85:307-318, 1995
3. Zwiebel JA, Cheson BD: Chronic lymphocytic leukemia: Staging and prognostic factors. Semin Oncol 25:42-59, 1998
4. Dohner H, Stilgenbauer S, Benner A, Leupolt E, Krober A, Bullinger L, et al: Genomic aberrations and survival in chronic lymphocytic leukemia. N Engl J Med 343:1910-1916, 2000
5. Rai KR, Sawitsky A, Cronkite EP, Chanana AD, Levy RN, Pasternack BS: Clinical staging of chronic lymphocytic leukemia. Blood 46:219-234, 1975
6. Binet JL, Auquier A, Dighiero G, Chastang C, Piguet H, Goasguen J, et al: A new prognostic classification of chronic lymphocytic leukemia derived from a multivariate survival analysis. Cancer 48:198-206, 1981
7. Dighiero G, Maloum K, Desablens B, Cazin B, Navarro M, Leblay R, et al: Chlorambucil in indolent chronic lymphocytic leukemia. French Cooperative Group on Chronic Lymphocytic Leukemia. N Engl J Med 338:1506-1514, 1998
8. The French Cooperative Group on Chronic Lymphocytic Leukemia: Effects of chlorambucil and therapeutic decision in initial forms of chronic lymphocytic leukemia (stage A): Results of a randomized clinical trial on 612 patients. Blood 75:1414-1421, 1990
9. Cheson BD, Bennett JM, Grever M, Kay N, Keating MJ, O'Brien S, et al: National Cancer Institute-sponsored Working Group guidelines for chronic lymphocytic leukemia: Revised guidelines for diagnosis and treatment. Blood 87:4990-4997, 1996
10. Keating MJ, Kantarjian H, Talpaz M, Redman J, Koller C, Barlogie B, et al: Fludarabine: A new agent with major activity against chronic lymphocytic leukemia. Blood 74:19-25, 1989
11. Rai KR, Peterson BL, Appelbaum FR, Kolitz J, Elias L, Shepherd L, et al: Fludarabine compared with chlorambucil as primary therapy for chronic lymphocytic leukemia. N Engl J Med 343:1750-1757, 2000
12. Summerfield GP, Taylor PR, Mounter PJ, Proctor SJ: High-dose chlorambucil for the treatment of chronic lymphocytic leukaemia and low-grade non-Hodgkin's lymphoma. Br J Haematol 116:781-786, 2002
13. Leporrier M, Chevret S, Cazin B, Boudjerra N, Feugier P, Desablens B, et al: Randomized comparison of fludarabine, CAP, and ChOP in 938 previously untreated stage B and C chronic lymphocytic leukemia patients. Blood 98:2319-2325, 2001
14. Johnson S, Smith AG, Loffler H, Osby E, Juliusson G, Emmerich B, et al: Multicentre prospective randomised trial of fludarabine versus cyclophosphamide, doxorubicin, and prednisone (CAP) for treatment of advanced-stage chronic lymphocytic leukaemia. The French Cooperative Group on CLL. Lancet 347:1432-1438, 1996
15. Robak T, Blonski JZ, Kasznicki M, Blasinska-Morawiec M, Krykowski E, Dmoszynska A, et al: Cladribine with prednisone versus chlorambucil with prednisone as first-line therapy in chronic lymphocytic leukemia: Report of a prospective, randomized, multicenter trial. Blood 96:2723-2729, 2000
16. Robak T: The role of nucleoside analogues in the treatment of chronic lymphocytic leukemia—Lessons learned from prospective randomized trials. Leuk Lymphoma 43:537-548, 2002
17. Brogden RN, Sorkin EM: Pentostatin. A review of its pharmacodynamic and pharmacokinetic properties, and therapeutic potential in lymphoproliferative disorders. Drugs 46:652-677, 1993
18. Giblett ER, Anderson JE, Cohen F, Pollara B, Meuwissen HJ: Adenosine-deaminase deficiency in two patients with severely impaired cellular immunity. Lancet 2:1067-1069, 1972
19. Johnson SA, Thomas W: Therapeutic potential of purine analogue combinations in the treatment of lymphoid malignancies. Hematol Oncol 18:141-153, 2000
20. Grever MR, Kopecky KJ, Coltman CA, Files JC, Greenberg BR, Hutton JJ, et al: Fludarabine monophosphate: A potentially useful agent in chronic lymphocytic leukemia. Nouv Rev Fr Hematol 30:457-459, 1988
21. O'Brien S, Kantarjian H, Beran M, Smith T, Koller C, Estey E, et al: Results of fludarabine and prednisone therapy in 264 patients with chronic lymphocytic leukemia with multivariate analysis-derived prognostic model for response to treatment. Blood 82:1695-1700, 1993
22. Keating MJ, O'Brien S, Lerner S, Koller C, Beran M, Robertson LE, et al: Long-term follow-up of patients with chronic lymphocytic leukemia (CLL) receiving fludarabine regimens as initial therapy. Blood 92:1165-1171, 1998
23. Keating MJ, Kantarjian H, O'Brien S, Koller C, Talpaz M, Schachner J, et al: Fludarabine: A new agent with marked cytoreductive activity in untreated chronic lymphocytic leukemia. J Clin Oncol 9:44-49, 1991
24. Elias L, Stock-Novack D, Head DR, Grever MR, Weick JK, Chapman RA, et al: A phase I trial of combination fludarabine monophosphate and chlorambucil in chronic lymphocytic leukemia: A Southwest Oncology Group study. Leukemia 7:361-365, 1993
25. Weiss M, Spiess T, Berman E, Kempin S: Concomitant administration of chlorambucil limits dose intensity of fludarabine in previously treated patients with chronic lymphocytic leukemia. Leukemia 8:1290-1293, 1994
26. O'Brien SM, Kantarjian HM, Cortes J, Beran M, Koller CA, Giles FJ, et al: Results of the fludarabine and cyclophosphamide combination regimen in chronic lymphocytic leukemia. J Clin Oncol 19:1414-1420, 2001
27. Wierda W, O'Brien S, Wen S, Faderl S, Garcia-Manero G, Thomas D, et al: Chemoimmunotherapy with fludarabine, cyclophosphamide, and rituximab for relapsed and refractory chronic lymphocytic leukemia. J Clin Oncol 23:4070-4078, 2005
28. Flinn IW, Byrd JC, Morrison C, Jamison J, Diehl LF, Murphy T, et al: Fludarabine and cyclophosphamide with filgrastim support in patients with previously untreated indolent lymphoid malignancies. Blood 96:71-75, 2000
29. Weiss MA, Glenn M, Maslak P, Rahman Z, Noy A, Zelenetz A, et al: Consolidation therapy with high-dose cyclophosphamide improves the quality of response in patients with chronic lymphocytic leukemia treated with fludarabine as induction therapy. Leukemia 14:1577-1582, 2000
30. Lamanna N: Advances in the treatment of chronic lymphocytic leukemia. Curr Oncol Rep 7:333-338, 2005
31. Robak T, Blonski JZ, Kasznicki M, Gora-Tybor J, Dwilewicz-Trojaczek J, Stella-Holowiecka B, et al: Cladribine combined with cyclophosphamide is highly effective in the treatment of chronic lymphocytic leukemia. Hematol J 3:244-250, 2002
32. Saven A, Emanuele S, Kosty M, Koziol J, Ellison D, Piro L: 2-Chloro-

deoxyadenosine activity in patients with untreated, indolent non-Hodgkin's lymphoma. Blood 86:1710-1716, 1995

33. Montillo M, Tedeschi A, O'Brien S, Di Raimondo F, Lerner S, Ferrajoli A, et al: Phase II study of cladribine and cyclophosphamide in patients with chronic lymphocytic leukemia and prolymphocytic leukemia. Cancer 97:114-120, 2003
34. Grever MR, Siaw MF, Jacob WF, Neidhart JA, Miser JS, Coleman MS, et al: The biochemical and clinical consequences of 2′-deoxycoformycin in refractory lymphoproliferative malignancy. Blood 57:406-417, 1981
35. Dillman RO, Yu AL, Qiao CN: Repeated pentostatin (2′deoxycoformycin)-induced remissions in a patient with advanced chronic lymphocytic leukemia. West J Med 148:334-337, 1988
36. Dillman RO, Mick R, McIntyre OR: Pentostatin in chronic lymphocytic leukemia: A phase II trial of Cancer and Leukemia Group B. J Clin Oncol 7:433-438, 1989
37. Ho AD, Thaler J, Stryckmans P, Coiffier B, Luciani M, Sonneveld P, et al: Pentostatin in refractory chronic lymphocytic leukemia: A phase II trial of the European Organization for Research and Treatment of Cancer. J Natl Cancer Inst 82:1416-1420, 1990
38. Johnson SA, Catovsky D, Child JA, Newland AC, Milligan DW, Janmohamed R: Phase I/II evaluation of pentostatin (2′-deoxycoformycin) in a five day schedule for the treatment of relapsed/refractory B-cell chronic lymphocytic leukaemia. Invest New Drugs 16:155-160, 1998
39. Johnston JB, Verburg L, Shore T, Williams M, Israels LG, Begleiter A: Combination therapy with nucleoside analogues and alkylating agents. Leukemia 8:S140-S143, 1994 (suppl 1)
40. Spiers AS, Moore D, Cassileth PA, Harrington DP, Cummings FJ, Neiman RS, et al: Remissions in hairy-cell leukemia with pentostatin (2′-deoxycoformycin). N Engl J Med 316:825-830, 1987
41. Grever MR, Bisaccia E, Scarborough DA, Metz EN, Neidhart JA: An investigation of 2′-deoxycoformycin in the treatment of cutaneous T-cell lymphoma. Blood 61:279-282, 1983
42. Oken MM, Lee S, Kay NE, Knospe W, Cassileth PA: Pentostatin, chlorambucil and prednisone therapy for B-chronic lymphocytic leukemia: A phase I/II study by the Eastern Cooperative Oncology Group study E1488. Leuk Lymphoma 45:79-84, 2004
43. Waselenko JK, Grever MR, Beer M, Lucas MA, Byrd JC: Pentostatin (Nipent) and chlorambucil with granulocyte-macrophage colony-stimulating factor support for patients with previously untreated, treated, and fludarabine-refractory B-cell chronic lymphocytic leukemia. Semin Oncol 27:44-51, 2000
44. Weiss MA, Maslak PG, Jurcic JG, Schenberg DA, Aliff TB, Lamanna N, et al: Pentostatin and cyclophosphamide: An effective new regimen in previously treated patients with chronic lymphocytic leukemia. J Clin Oncol 21:1278-1284, 2003
45. Abbott BL: Advances in the diagnosis and treatment of chronic lymphocytic leukemia. Hematol Oncol 23:34-40, 2005

Seminars in HEMATOLOGY

Purine Analogue-Based Chemotherapy Regimens for Patients With Previously Untreated B-Chronic Lymphocytic Leukemia

Neil E. Kay

B-cell chronic lymphocytic leukemia (B-CLL) is a clonal malignancy characterized by the expansion of small B lymphocytes and accumulation of CLL cells. This disease is the most common form of leukemia in the Western hemisphere and is currently not considered to be curable using currently available therapies. Published reports have suggested that purine analogues have activity in B-CLL and superior to alkylating agents. Even though responses have been observed with purine analogues that are used as single agents, these responses were not durable. The use of combination purine analogue therapy with alkylating agents and/or monoclonal antibodies was then explored in order to take advantage of synergistic actions of these agents to improve the quality of clinical responses. Both fludarabine and pentostatin have shown improved responses when combined with alkylating agents and even higher overall and complete responses (CRs) when combined with monoclonal antibodies.
Semin Hematol 43(suppl 2):S50-S54 © 2006 Elsevier Inc. All rights reserved.

Significant advances have been made over the last several years in the way we manage B-cell chronic lymphocytic leukemia (B-CLL). Historically, B-CLL has been treated with alkylating agents either alone or combined with corticosteroids; however, several studies now suggest that higher remission rates can be achieved when purine analogues are used as initial therapy.[1,2] When used alone, purine analogues induced responses, although very few were complete responses (CRs) nor durable. Purine analogues have been shown to be synergistic with many agents, including alkylating agents and monoclonal antibodies. Therefore, the use of combinations of these agents may provide more effective therapy for both previously untreated and relapsed/refractory CLL patients. The focus of this review is to highlight the advances that have been made in regards to the use of purine analogue combinations in B-CLL patients who are previously untreated with other chemotherapeutic regimens and to briefly mention key data in patients who were previously treated.

Overview of B-Cell Chronic Lymphocytic Leukemia

B-CLL is the most common adult leukemia in the United States, representing 25% of all leukemia cases. Despite a substantial population of patients who live greater than 10 years, the median survival of B-CLL is 5 to 7 years and is heavily influenced by clinical stage.[3-5] Clinical staging systems are valuable for classifying B-CLL patients into broad prognostics groups, but they do not take into account the molecular pathology of the disease. More recently, novel prognostic parameters including certain fluorescence-in-situ hybridization (FISH) defects and their immunoglobulin (Ig) heavy (H) chain variable (V) region (ie, IgV_H) status have been found to strongly predict risk of disease progression.[6,7] The stratification of B-CLL patients using these newer molecular markers is becoming more feasible albeit not universally available. Future studies will be needed to determine the best use of both the novel and the classical prognostic factors in counseling of CLL patients. Table 1 presents a risk stratification scheme proposed by Montillo et al.,[7] including both classical and novel markers. With the development of these newer diagnostic methods, our ability to detect higher risk patients with early-stage disease is increasing. In the future this may represent a group of patients, which are currently not being treated or entered into clinical trials, that may require earlier therapeutic intervention in order to change the natural history of the disease.

Brief History of Treatments for B-CLL

There are widely accepted guidelines for the initiation of chemotherapy in B-CLL patients.[8] In general, therapy should

Department of Internal Medicine, Mayo Clinic, Rochester, MN.
Address correspondence to Neil E. Kay, MD, Mayo Clinic, Stabile 628, 200 First St SW, Rochester, MN 55905. E-mail: kay.neil@mayo.edu

 0037-1963/06/$-see front matter © 2006 Elsevier Inc. All rights reserved.
doi:10.1053/j.seminhematol.2005.12.011

Table 1 Risk Stratification Scheme of B-CLL Patients Based on Prognostic Factors

Parameter	Low Risk	High Risk
Traditional markers		
Binet clinical staging system	A	B, C
Bone marrow infiltration	Non-diffuse	Diffuse
Atypical morphology	No	Yes
Lymphocyte doubling time	≤12 months	>12 months
Newer molecular and biologic markers		
Serum markers	Normal	Increased
Cytogenetics	Normal, del(13q) isolated	del(11q), del (17p)
CD38	≤30%	>30%
IgV_H	Mutated	Unmutated
ZAP70	Negative	Positive

Abbreviations: del(13q), chromosome 13q deletion; del (11q), chromosome 11q deletion; del (17p), chromosome 17p deletion; CD38, cell differentiation antigen CD38; IgV_H, immunoglobulin heavy-chain variable-region gene; ZAP70, zeta-chain (TCR)-associated protein kinase 70 kd.
Adapted with permission.[7]

not be initiated in patients who have early-stage disease. Once there are signs of disease progression, treatment is initiated. The disease-related symptoms that are considered criteria for initiation of treatment include fever; body weight loss, increasing bone marrow failure, autoimmune anemia and/or thrombocytopenia responding poorly to corticosteroids; massive or progressive splenomegaly and/or lymphadenopathy, progressive lymphocytosis; and recurrent infections.[8]

The original therapeutic approach to treating patients primarily included the use of alkylating agents, chlorambucil or cyclophosphamide, either alone or in combination with prednisone. These agents when given at adequate doses for sufficient durations frequently yield total response rates greater than 70%, although CRs were only in the range of 5% to 10%.[9-13] Since then, the purine analogues fludarabine (Fludara; Berlex Laboratories, Richmond, CA), pentostatin (Nipent®; Supergen, Dublin, CA), and cladribine (Leustatin; Ortho Biotech, Bridgewater, NJ) have all demonstrated activity in B-CLL. While very similar in structure, there are subtle differences that likely play a role in the clinical differences observed with these agents. Initial clinical work with the purine nucleosides in B-CLL has been dominated by the use of fludarabine as a single drug with objective responses in up to 60% of alkylator resistant B-CLL patients and 80% in previously untreated patients. [2,14] More recently, several reports have found that combination therapy has substantial activity in both previously untreated and treated B-CLL.[15-22]

Purine Analogue-Based Combinations as First-Line Therapy

Significant improvement has been made in treating patients with B-CLL and combination therapy with purine analogues has been a cornerstone in these advancements. In general, the combination of a monoclonal antibody (ie, rituximab) with purine nucleosides and/or cyclophosphamide has generated significantly increased levels of clinical responses compared to using these agents alone. The rationale for combining these agents is linked to independent functions that seem to at least generate additive if not synergistic outcomes with respect to B-CLL. Several studies have suggested that rituximab sensitized cells to the cytotoxicity of many chemotherapeutic agents, including fludarabine and cyclophosphamide.[23] Rituximab can down-regulate certain key anti-apoptotic proteins such as Mcl-1 or Bcl-2 and fludarabine can down-modulate the complement-resistant proteins CD46, CD55, and CD59 in leukemia cells. These actions could theoretically then make the B-CLL cell more vulnerable to cell death. Synergistic cytotoxicity has also been reported with purine analogues and alkylating agents. The enhancement of DNA damage produced by alkylating agents increases the opportunities for incorporation of purine analogues into DNA.[24] Table 2 contains a summary of the studies presented below which have been conducted using purine analogue combinations in patients with previously untreated B-CLL.

Fludarabine Combinations

Fludarabine in combination with cyclophosphamide (FC) is the best-characterized regimen as initial therapy in previously untreated B-CLL patients (see Table 2). Two single-center studies assessing this combination reported improved remission rates with the combination.[16,25] O'Brien et al[16] reported a greater than 80% response rate in previously untreated patients, along with a 35% CR rate. Residual disease assessed by flow cytometry occurred in only 8% of patients.[16] Weiss et al[25] evaluated sequential administration of fludarabine followed by three courses of high-dose cyclophosphamide and reported similar response rates including molecular responses. The patients who received consolidation therapy had an improved quality of response (threefold increase in nodular responses or CRs) compared to that achieved alone with fludarabine.[25]

The use of fludarabine, cyclophosphamide, and rituximab (FCR) has been tested in large numbers of patients with previously untreated CLL.[26] There were 224 patients reported with previously untreated CLL but progressive disease. The overall response rate was 95%, with a 70% CR rate, including a 10% nodular partial response (nPR) and 15% PR rate. However, this study had a large percentage of Rai stage 0–2 patients (149/224) with only 33 % having Rai stage 3–4. The CR rate for stage 0–2 patients was 74% compared to 52% for Rai stage 3–4. These investigators also found that patients under the age of 70 had a higher rate CR compared to older patients (72 % *v* 47%). Based on flow cytometry, 78% of CR

Table 2 Summary of Combination Therapies With Purine Analogues for Previously Untreated B-CLL Patients

Reference	N	Regimen	ORR (%)	CR (%)
Fludarabine combinations				
O'Brien et al[16]	34	F 30 mg/m²/d × 3 d + C 300–500 mg/m²/d × 3 d	88	35
Weiss et al[25]	25	F 25 mg/m²/d × 5 d every 4 wks + C 1.5–4 g/m² every 4wks + G-CSF 5 μg/kg/d days 3–12	76	32
Byrd et al[27]	51 (concurrent)	F 25 mg/m² d 1–5 every 28 d × 6 cycles + R 375 mg/m² d 1 (×2) and 4 (cycle 1) and 375 mg/m² d 1 (cycles 2–6)	90	47
	53 (sequential)	F 25 mg/m² d1–5 every 28 d × 6 cycles R 375 mg/m² d 1 (×2) and 4 (cycle 1) and 375 mg/m² d 1 (cycles 2–6)	77	28
Keating et al[26]	224	F* 25 mg/m²/d days 2–4+ C 250 mg/m² days 2–4+ R 375 mg/m² day 1 (1st cycle then 500 mg/m² for cycles 2–6)	95	70
Pentostatin combinations				
Oken et al[22]	36	P 2 mg/m² day1 + Cb 30 mg/m² Prednisone 80 mg days 1–5 every 2 wks	87	45
Kay et al[28]	33	P 2 mg/m² + C 600 mg/m² + R 375 mg/m² every 3 wks × 6	94	48

Abbreviations: ORR, overall response rate; CR, complete response rate; F, fludarabine; C, cyclophosphamide; R, rituximab; P, pentostatin; Cb, chlorambucil.

*The dose of fludarabine and cyclophosphamide were reduced from 30 mg/m² and 300 mg/m², respectively, after the first nine patients were enrolled due to significant tumor lysis.

patients had less than 1% $CD5^+/CD19^+$ B cells in their bone marrow aspirate. Of interest, even with nPR or PR patients, 24% and 47%, respectively, had less than 1% $CD5^+/CD19^+$ B cells. Finally, grade 3–4 neutropenia was seen in 52% of the FCR treatment courses and 33% had at least one infection, with major infections seen in 2%.[26]

A recent trial for previously untreated B-CLL compared simultaneous administration of rituximab with fludarabine versus fludarabine followed by rituximab.[27] Patients were randomized to receive either 6 monthly courses of fludarabine concurrently with rituximab followed 2 months later by 4 weekly doses of rituximab for consolidation therapy or sequential fludarabine alone followed 2 months later by rituximab consolidation therapy. The overall response (OR) rate with the concurrent regimen was 90%, with a 47% CR rate and a 43% PR rate compared to a 77% OR rate, a 28% CR rate, and 49% PR rate with the sequential regimen. At a follow-up of 23 months, the median response duration and survival were still not reached for either combination approach. The toxicity for this concurrent regimen during induction was worse with more grade 3 or 4 neutropenia and grade 3 or 4 infusion-related toxicity compared to the sequential protocol. The frequency of infections was similar in the two treatments, with eight opportunistic infections in the concurrent and 14 in the sequential treatment. Most of the opportunistic infections were viral but tissue site–restricted, while two patients experienced *Pneumocystis carinii* pneumonia.[27]

Pentostatin Combinations

Based on the high response rates seen with the FC and FCR combination regimens and the promising activity and toxicity profile of pentostatin, studies were initiated evaluating combinations with this agent. Pentostatin is of interest due to the lack of reported bone marrow suppression, ease of dosing schedule, and individual antitumor activity in B-CLL.

The combinations of pentostatin and cyclophosphamide[18] and pentostatin and chlorambucil[22] have been found to generate excellent clinical response rates in pretreated B-CLL patients. Use of pentostatin and cyclophosphamide in heavily pretreated B-CLL patients generated a 74% response rate with four CRs in 23 patients.[18] Importantly, the PR rate was 50% and a "best response" rate of 41% was reported. This latter response category refers to the combination of pentostatin and cyclophosphamide generating the best clinical response when compared to multiple prior therapies for a given patient. The marrow suppression of this regimen was very acceptable as evidence by the low rate of platelet transfusions.[18]

Oken et al[22] treated 55 B-CLL patients with a combination of pentostatin, chlorambucil, and prednisone (see Table 2). Thirty-six of these patients were previously untreated. CRs were seen in 45% of patients and the overall response rate was 87%. The median duration of response was 33 months and the median survival was 5 years. The median time to treatment failure was 32 months while severe infections were reported in 31% of the population. The authors concluded that while this regimen was extremely effective, the significantly high infection rate was unacceptable and they thus recommended omitting prednisone from future investigation and adding viral and bacterial prophylaxis.[22]

We are currently evaluating the efficacy of pentostatin, cyclophosphamide, and rituximab (PCR) for previously untreated B-CLL patients. Our interest in this combination was sparked by the very high response rates reported with FCR. Eligible patients receive a regimen consisting of pentostatin (2 mg/m^2) on day 1, cyclophosphamide (600 mg/m^2), and rituximab (375 mg/m^2) given intravenously on day 1. This is a 21-day, six-cycle regimen with a planned enrollment of 65 patients. Prophylactic co-trimoxazole and acyclovir were given to all patients for 1 year starting on the first cycle of therapy. Granulocyte colony-stimulating factor (G-CSF) was given on day 3 of each PCR cycled for 10 consecutive days or until the total neutrophil count was greater than 1,000/mL for 2 consecutive days. With this clinical trial we plan to answer a series of critical questions: (1) Does the use of a PCR regimen generate reversible immune system changes in responding patients?; (2) Can we predict which B-CLL patients, stratified by novel prognostic parameters, will respond differentially to PCR?; and (3) Can B-CLL patients who achieved clinical responses and also reach minimal residual disease achieve a more prolonged response time compared to those who do not?

We have currently enrolled 65 patients into this clinical trial but have formally analyzed the first 33 for this discussion.[28] The patients enrolled to date are considered to be very high risk based on the following features: Rai intermediate status ($n = 13$) and Rai high-risk status ($n = 17$), 80% were IgV_H nonmutated, and 28 patients had FISH defects that are considered high-risk defects (ie, trisomy 12, 11q or complex defects). In addition, approximately one third were $CD38^+$ using a 30% cutoff and a third were ZAP-70^+ using a 20% cutoff. To define the extent of clinical response we used the National Cancer Institute (NCI) Working Group criteria[8] and performed a bone marrow aspirate and biopsy 2 months after the initiation of cycle 6 of treatment. Overall 16 of the 33 patients had a complete clinical response (48%) and 16 patients (48%) experienced a CR, nine patients (28%) had a nPR, and seven patients had a PR to treatment. Only one patient did not achieve any response and had stable disease prior to dying on study after one treatment cycle. The median time to first documentation of any response was 47 days (95% confidence interval, 33 to 84). At this time we cannot comment on median disease-free interval time in the 32 responding patients due to the short follow-up period of 2 years.[28] The responding patients in CR or nPR can also have negative minimal residual disease using flow or molecular analysis (data not shown). In addition, achieving a CR or NPR was independent of the presence of high risk factors such as complex FISH defects or nonmutated IgV_H status.

In general, this PCR regimen was well tolerated with the most common toxicity grade 3+ neutropenia (55%) and grade 3+ (18%) thrombocytopenia. Despite these toxicities none of the patients required red blood cell or platelet transfusions during their treatment courses. The G-CSF was typically given for only 2 days before cessation of the drug based on neutrophil counts. No serious infections were noted and not cytomegalovirus activation was documented. We continue to conduct analysis of the data in order to answer not only the clinical efficacy questions but the critical questions discussed above.

Toxicity of Combinations

The increased efficacy of purine analogue combinations may be obtained at the cost of increased toxicity. The major side effects of purine analogues are myelosuppression and $CD4^+$ T-cell depletion leading to an increase risk of opportunistic infections. Fludarabine and cladribine have been associated with significant toxicity, consisting of myelosuppression and infection.[16,29,30] O'Brien et al[16] reported neutropenia in 48% of patients and severe infections in 25% of patients treated with fludarabine combinations. While cladribine combinations have a higher reported incidence of complications (42% severe infections and 58% dose-limiting cytopenias),[30] pentostatin is thought to be less myelosuppressive; therefore, this agent is currently being extensively studied in B-CLL patients. We and others have seen that there is a reduced incidence of significant infectious complications and a reduced need for transfusion support with the use of pentostatin-based combinations compared to that reported for fludarabine and cladribine.[18,28]

Conclusions

Treatment of B-CLL has seen significant advancements over the last few years. The nucleoside analogues have shown clinical activity in B-CLL patients who were previously untreated. In an effort to increase the quality of responses, combination therapy protocols were initiated in these patients. Fludarabine has been the most extensively studied and has clear clinical activity; however, it is associated with significant bone marrow suppression. We are currently evaluating the PCR combination in these patients and have reported encouraging results. An additional benefit is that to date we have not seen significant marrow toxicity or serious infections that compromised the clinical course of our patients. We also used a risk stratification scheme for our cohort of patients and have reported responses even in patients who have high-risk features such as complex FISH or trisomy 12 defects or the presence of unmutated IgV_H type clones. Future work that will evaluate the combination of PCR with follow-up drugs to eliminate residual disease may be contemplated.

References

1. Rai KR, Peterson B, Elias L: A randomized comparison of fludarabine and chlorambucil for patients with previously untreated chronic lymphocytic leukemia. A CALGB, SWOG, CTG/NCI-C and ECOG intergroup study. Blood 88:141a, 1996 (abstr)
2. Keating MJ, Kantarjian H, O'Brien S, Koller C, Talpaz M, Schachner J, et al: Fludarabine: A new agent with marked cytoreductive activity in untreated chronic lymphocytic leukemia. J Clin Oncol 9:44-49, 1991
3. Rai KR, Sawitsky A, Cronkite EP, Chanana AD, Levy RN, Pasternack BS:

Clinical staging of chronic lymphocytic leukemia. Blood 46:219-234, 1975

4. Binet JL, Catovsky D, Chandra P: Chronic lymphocytic leukemia: Proposals for a revised prognostic staging system. Br J Haematol 48:365-367, 1981
5. Hansen MM: Chronic lymphocytic leukaemia. Clinical studies based on 189 cases followed for a long time. Scand J Haematol 18:3-286, 1973 (suppl)
6. Shanafelt TD, Geyer SM, Kay NE: Prognosis at diagnosis: integrating molecular biologic insights into clinical practice for patients with CLL. Blood 103:1202-1210, 2004
7. Montillo M, Hamblin T, Hallek M, Montserrat E, Morra E: Chronic lymphocytic leukemia: Novel prognostic factors and their relevance for risk-adapted therapeutic strategies. Haematologica 90:391-399, 2005
8. Cheson BD, Bennett JM, Grever M, Kay N, Keating MJ, O'Brien S, et al: National Cancer Institute-sponsored Working Group guidelines for chronic lymphocytic leukemia: revised guidelines for diagnosis and treatment. Blood 87:4990-4997, 1996
9. Raphael B, Andersen JW, Silber R, Oken M, Moore D, Bennett J, et al: Comparison of chlorambucil and prednisone versus cyclophosphamide, vincristine, and prednisone as initial treatment for chronic lymphocytic leukemia: Long-term follow-up of an Eastern Cooperative Oncology Group randomized clinical trial. J Clin Oncol 9:770-776, 1991
10. Han T, Ezdinli EZ, Shimaoka K, Desai DV: Chlorambucil vs. combined chlorambucil-corticosteroid therapy in chronic lymphocytic leukemia. Cancer 31:502-508, 1973
11. Keller JW, Knospe WH, Raney M, Huguley CM Jr, Johnson L, Bartolucci AA, et al: Treatment of chronic lymphocytic leukemia using chlorambucil and prednisone with or without cycle-active consolidation chemotherapy. A Southeastern Cancer Study Group trial. Cancer 58:1185-1192, 1986
12. Hansen MM, Andersen E, Birgens H: CHOP versus chlorambucil + prednisolone in chronic lymphocytic leukemia. Leuk Lymphoma 5:97-100, 1991
13. Dighiero G, Maloum K, Desablens B, Cazin B, Navarro M, Leblay R, et al: Chlorambucil in indolent chronic lymphocytic leukemia. French Cooperative Group on Chronic Lymphocytic Leukemia. N Engl J Med 338:1506-1514, 1998
14. Keating MJ: Fludarabine phosphate in the treatment of chronic lymphocytic leukemia. Semin Oncol 17:49-62, 1990
15. Robak T, Blonski JZ, Kasznicki M, Gora-Tybor J, Dwilewicz-Trojaczek J, Stella-Holowiecka B, et al: Cladribine combined with cyclophosphamide is highly effective in the treatment of chronic lymphocytic leukemia. Hematol J 3:244-250, 2002
16. O'Brien SM, Kantarjian HM, Cortes J, Beran M, Koller CA, Giles FJ, et al: Results of the fludarabine and cyclophosphamide combination regimen in chronic lymphocytic leukemia. J Clin Oncol 19:1414-1420, 2001
17. Hallek M, Schmitt B, Wilhelm M, Busch R, Krober A, Fostitsch HP, et al: Fludarabine plus cyclophosphamide is an efficient treatment for advanced chronic lymphocytic leukaemia (CLL): Results of a phase II study of the German CLL Study Group. Br J Haematol 114:342-348, 2001
18. Weiss MA, Maslak PG, Jurcic JG, Scheinberg DA, Aliff TB, Lamanna N, et al: Pentostatin and cyclophosphamide: an effective new regimen in previously treated patients with chronic lymphocytic leukemia. J Clin Oncol 21:1278-1284, 2003
19. Wierda W, O'Brien S, Albitar M, Lerner S, Plunkett W, Giles FJ, et al: Combined fludarabine, cyclophosphamide, and rituximab achieves a high complete remission rate as initial treatment for chronic lymphocytic leukemia. Blood 98:771a, 2001 (abstr)
20. Wierda W, O'Brien S, Wen S, Faderl S, Garcia-Manero G, Thomas D, et al: Chemoimmunotherapy with fludarabine, cyclophosphamide, and rituximab for relapsed and refractory chronic lymphocytic leukemia. J Clin Oncol 23:4070-4078, 2005
21. Schiavone EM, De Simone M, Palmieri S, Annunziata M, Pocali B, Copia C, et al: Fludarabine plus cyclophosphamide for the treatment of advanced chronic lymphocytic leukemia. European Journal of Haematology 71:23-28, 2003
22. Oken MM, Lee S, Kay NE, Knospe W, Cassileth PA: Pentostatin, chlorambucil and prednisone therapy for B-chronic lymphocytic leukemia: A phase I/II study by the Eastern Cooperative Oncology Group study E1488. Leuk Lymphoma 45:79-84, 2004
23. Demidem A, Lam T, Alas S, Hariharan K, Hanna N, Bonavida B: Chimeric anti-CD20 (IDEC-C2B8) monoclonal antibody sensitizes a B cell lymphoma cell line to cell killing by cytotoxic drugs. Cancer Biother Radiopharm 12:177-186, 1997
24. Johnson SA, Thomas W: Therapeutic potential of purine analogue combinations in the treatment of lymphoid malignancies. Hematol Oncol 18:141-153, 2000
25. Weiss MA, Glenn M, Maslak P, Rahman Z, Noy A, Zelenetz A, et al: Consolidation therapy with high-dose cyclophosphamide improves the quality of response in patients with chronic lymphocytic leukemia treated with fludarabine as induction therapy. Leukemia 14:1577-1582, 2000
26. Keating MJ, O'Brien S, Albitar M, Lerner S, Plunkett W, Giles F, et al: Early results of a chemoimmunotherapy regimen of fludarabine, cyclophosphamide, and rituximab as initial therapy for chronic lymphocytic leukemia. J Clin Oncol 23:4079-4088, 2005
27. Byrd JC, Peterson BL, Morrison VA, Park K, Jacobson R, Hoke E, et al: Randomized phase 2 study of fludarabine with concurrent versus sequential treatment with rituximab in symptomatic, untreated patients with B-cell chronic lymphocytic leukemia: Results from Cancer and Leukemia Group B 9712 (CALGB 9712). Blood 101:6-14, 2003
28. Kay N, Geyer SM, Lin T, Byrd JC: Combination chemotherapy with pentostatin, cyclophosphamide and rituximab induces high rate of remissions including complete responses and achievement of minimal residual disease in previoulsy untreated B-chronic lymphocytic leukemia. Blood 104:100a, 2004 (abstr 339)
29. Robak T, Blonski JZ, Kasznicki M, Blasinska-Morawiec M, Krykowski E, Dmoszynska A, et al: Cladribine with prednisone versus chlorambucil with prednisone as first-line therapy in chronic lymphocytic leukemia: Report of a prospective, randomized, multicenter trial. Blood 96:2723-2729, 2000
30. Van Den Neste E, Michaux L, Layios N, Costantini S, Francart J, Lambert C, et al: High incidence of complications after 2-chloro-2′-deoxyadenosine combined with cyclophosphamide in patients with advanced lymphoproliferative malignancies. Ann Hematol 83:356-363, 2004

Vol 43, No 2, Suppl 3 April 2006

Supplement to

Seminars in HEMATOLOGY

Neal S. Young · Photis Beris
Editors

Management of Hemophilia in the Midst of Emerging Pathogens: A Societal Perspective

Steven Pipe
Guest Editor

W.B. Saunders

Seminars in HEMATOLOGY

Neal S. Young · Photis Beris
Editors

Peter A. Miescher, *Founding Editor* Ernst R. Jaffé, *Co-Editor Emeritus*

Editorial correspondence should be addressed to Photis Beris, MD, Division d'Hématologie, Hôpital Cantonal Universitaire, 25 rue Micheli-du-Crest, 1211 Geneve 14, Switzerland, or Neal S. Young, MD, 4400 17th Street, NW, Washington, DC 20011.

Business correspondence (subscriptions, change of address) should be addressed to the Publisher, Elsevier, 6277 Sea Harbor Dr, Orlando, FL 32887-4800; Email elspcs@elsevier.com.

Change of address notices, including both the old and new addresses of the subscriber, should be sent at least one month in advance.

Customer Service: 1-800-654-2452; outside the United States and Canada, (407) 345-4000.

Yearly subscription rates: United States and possessions: individual, $169.00; institution, $267.00; single issues, $81.00. All other countries: individual, $239.00; institution, $339.00; single issues, $81.00. Student and resident: United States and possessions, and Canada: $85.00; all other countries: $122.00. To receive student/resident rate, orders must be accompanied by name of affiliated institution, date of term, and the *signature* of program/residency coordinator on institution letterhead. Orders will be billed at individual rate until proof of status is received. Current prices are in effect for back volumes and back issues. Single issues, both current and back, exist in limited quantities and are offered for sale subject to availability. Back issues sold in conjunction with a subscription are on a prorated basis. Prices are subject to change without notice. *Checks* should be made payable to Elsevier and sent to *Seminars in Hematology*, Elsevier, Periodicals Department, PO Box 628239, Orlando, FL 32862-8239.

The contents of *Seminars in Hematology* are indexed in *Index Medicus* and *MEDLINE, Current Contents/Clinical Medicine, Current Contents/Life Sciences*, Science Citation Index, and *EMBASE/* Excerpta Medica.

The *Seminars in Hematology* home page is located at *www.seminhematol.org*.

W.B. Saunders **Philadelphia, PA**

Seminars in
HEMATOLOGY

Vol 43, No 2, Supplement 3, April 2006

Management of Hemophilia in the Midst of Emerging Pathogens: A Societal Perspective

Steven Pipe
Guest Editor

Introduction: Management of Hemophilia in the Midst of Emerging Pathogens: A Societal Perspective S1
Steven Pipe

Infectious Disease in the Blood Supply and the Public Health Response S4
Bruce Evatt

The Precautionary Principle and Emerging Biologic Risks: Lessons From Human Immunodeficiency Virus in Blood Products S10
Michael A. Stoto

A Patient's Perspective on Hemophilia S13
Ellis Sulser

The Need for Continuing Vigilance: Addressing the Threat for Transmission of Blood-Borne Infectious Disease S17
Samuel L. Stanley, Jr

Consideration in Hemophilia Therapy Selection S23
Steven Pipe

Seminars in HEMATOLOGY

Management of Hemophilia in the Midst of Emerging Pathogens: A Societal Perspective

Steven Pipe

Guest Editor

This supplement was made possible by an unrestricted educational grant from Baxter BioScience.

The opinions or views expressed in this professional education supplement are those of the authors and do not necessarily reflect the opinions or recommendations of Baxter BioScience.

The guest editors, authors, and publisher have tried to ensure that recommended measures and drug dosages discussed in this supplement are accurate and conform to the standards that prevailed at the time of publication. The reader is advised, however, to check the product information available for any product discussed in this supplement to be familiar with any changes in the dosage schedule, techniques of use, or contraindications. Because of the uniqueness of each patient, physicians should use this information only as a general guide in determining the best treatment for each patient. For approved product information, consult the manufacturer's prescribing information.

ELSEVIER

Seminars in HEMATOLOGY

Volume 43, Number 2, Supplement 3 **April 2006**

Introduction
Management of Hemophilia in the Midst of Emerging Pathogens: A Societal Perspective

The rapid increase in the number of biologic therapies entering the medical marketplace has exacerbated spiraling healthcare costs and drawn keen attention from public and private third-party payers who are developing cost-containment policies. The hemophilia community currently enjoys generally unhampered access to a full range of factor therapies and services, each with its own unique value. This combination of therapies and services is costly, but its use reduces the need for more costly hospital stays, transfusions, and rehabilitation. As a result, management models developed for and successfully applied to other disease states do not translate well for the management of hemophilia, and the application of these models to hemophilia care could have a negative impact on its quality in the near future, and even result in increases in costs over the long term. Hemophilia treatment is clearly expensive, but there are no cheaper alternatives currently available, either for therapy or support services, that offer the same quality of care or degree of safety and efficacy. The stakes are high given that the community has had to confront the threat of pathogen infection in the blood supply and in factor therapies for many years.

A clear argument needs to be made so that reimbursement policies continue to ensure that the highest levels of patient care are maintained while the risks to the hemophilia community are minimized. Instead of price competition and formulary restrictions, open access to treaters and a range of clotting factor therapies should be a critical goal in the formulation of policy. Failure could result in a loss of the long-term treatment improvements achieved thus far.

In May 2005, in an effort to promote such an understanding, an interdisciplinary working group assembled to discuss several issues regarding the management of hemophilia, with a special focus on the ongoing threat of emerging pathogens. The forum, entitled "Management of Hemophilia in the Midst of Emerging Pathogens: A Societal Perspective," took place over 1.5 days and featured individual presentations and extended periods for discussion. It drew upon the experience of experts in the fields of epidemiology, infectious disease, medical ethics, hemophilia, public policy, and managed care communities, and the experience of a person with hemophilia who is also a patient advocate.

The forum participants joining me included Drs Bruce Evatt, Michael Stoto, and Samuel Stanley and Mr Ellis Sulser. Dr Bruce Evatt is the retired chief of the hematologic diseases branch of the Division of AIDS, STD, and TB Laboratory Research of the Centers for Disease Control and Prevention who helped recognize that acquired immune deficiency syndrome (AIDS) is a blood-borne disease and was affecting persons with hemophilia and blood-transfusion recipients. Dr Michael Stoto is an epidemiologist and statistician who is an associate director for public health in the RAND Center for Domestic and International Health Security and one of the authors of the Institute of Medicine report *HIV and the Blood Supply*. Dr Samuel Stanley, an infectious disease expert, is a professor in the department of Medicine at Washington University School of Medicine and a principle investigator and director of the Midwest Regional Center of Excellence for Biodefense and Emerging Infectious Diseases Research. Ellis Sulser, who has hemophilia and is coinfected with human immunodeficiency virus (HIV) and hepatitis C virus (HCV), is the president of Factor Support Network Pharmacy and an advocate for maintaining a safe, affordable, and available choice of therapies for the care for bleeding disorders. As an associate professor in the department of Pediatrics and Communicable Diseases and the pediatric medical director of the Hemophilia and Coagulation Disorders Program at the University of Michigan, I provided the group with the perspective of a practicing clinician.

The principal goal of this collaborative effort was to develop presentations on various aspects of a paramount concern in current hemophilia therapy management—choice of and access to the highest quality of care—and then to develop ways of communicating the concerns to the public and private third-party payers, medical directors, formulary deci-

doi:10.1053/j.seminhematol.2006.02.006

sion-makers, and healthcare policy makers to help guide their discussions on hemophilia and its treatment.

During the forum we explored a number of factors that affect choice of and access to hemophilia care. Two of the issues raised at the meeting but not discussed elsewhere in the supplement are the potential impact of new management strategies and the role of the advocate in shaping policies for hemophilia care. As mentioned previously, the cost-containment strategies that have been implemented or are planned for private and public healthcare programs are of considerable concern. Under the established model, hospital stays, physician visits, and related expenses are all covered and patients have access to a variety of ancillary education and support programs.[1] Some newer models cover only the cost of the clotting factor therapy plus a small dispensing fee, offer only a small group of in-network providers and require far greater co-pays for out-of-network providers, and limit or eliminate access to some individual therapies.[2] In some cases, therapies are stratified by cost and the least expensive (generally plasma-derived therapies) must be prescribed and found ineffective before authorization is forthcoming for the next most expensive therapy. New patients treated under this "step therapy" model would almost certainly be treated with one of the less expensive, plasma-derived therapies.[3] This would be in opposition to medical policies established by most hemophilia care providers in the developed world, including those adopted by governments supporting socialized national health care programs. All of these cost-limiting strategies have the potential to imperil the traditional physician-patient relationship, in which people with hemophilia, their clinicians, and their caregivers are free to jointly choose the most appropriate therapy and management plan.

Limitations such as a preferred drug list are problematic for a number of reasons. First, there are no generic clotting factor concentrates and these biologic therapies are not equivalent. Each therapy has a unique formulation and manufacturing process, which differs in modes of action, protein structure, glycosylation, stabilizer content, trace components, and purification methods. As with step therapy and other private healthcare practices, preferred drug lists limit the ability of a physician, in consultation with the patient or caregiver, to choose the most appropriate therapy. Given that the differences between therapies and in patients' responses to them may have very real clinical consequences for efficacy, tolerability, the risk of developing inhibitors, and for the level of risk or elimination of infectious agents, preventing a person with hemophilia from accessing the most appropriate treatment could result in severe complications.

With the trend for third-party payers to regulate the reimbursement of biologic therapies, the hemophilia community now needs to focus its considerable advocacy power on securing access to a full range of therapeutic options, which could be limited or denied by new restrictive reimbursement policies. These policies have also been considered for state- and federal-funded healthcare plans. Recently, government agencies regulating these plans have been responding to efforts by hemophilia organizations and advocates to maintain access to a full range of therapeutic agents. Participation by people who have a personal stake in the hemophilia community is a vital means to guide decision-makers in formulating policies that support the highest levels of care. The hemophilia community has been central to efforts to change public policy before. In the early 1990s, members of the hemophilia community went to Washington, DC, to request a Congressional investigation into the HIV tragedy. The outcome of their lobbying efforts was the 1994 Institute of Medicine (IOM) hearings, which proved to be critical in subsequent HIV and hemophilia policy making and, ultimately, influential in determining liability.

Fourteen recommendations emerged from the 1995 publication of the IOM hearings.[4] A number of these recommendations stipulated the government's role in guaranteeing the safety of the nation's blood supply. Another described a no-fault compensation plan for those who were harmed by tainted blood products. Several recommendations urged the review of previous policies in light of new data and made the ongoing review of scientific evidence of safety or risk related to the use of blood and blood-derived products a priority. Others stressed the importance of clear communication between the government and the blood products industry, as well as between physicians and their patients, regarding the risks involved in using blood-derived products. Finally, two other recommendations concerned the importance of equal representation between commercial and non-commercial interests and necessity for voluntary organizations to avoid conflicts of interests in recommending commercial blood products.

The recommendations of the IOM still provide hemophilia advocates with a roadmap for future policy development and the clear mandate that safety must always supersede reimbursement considerations. The need expressed in the IOM recommendations for ongoing vigilance to maintain the safety and purity of the blood supply also remains undiminished. Given that many people with hemophilia still rely on blood or blood-derived therapies, any blood-borne pathogen that emerges or other problem in the blood supply will likely affect the hemophilia community first. Safety is critical, and so it is appropriate that consumers of blood therapies continue to advocate for safety and drive those policy decisions.

The effects of hemophilia advocacy are long lasting and far reaching. The IOM recommendations resulted in the formation of the Blood Safety Council (later the Advisory Committee on Blood Safety and Availability), which in turn has adhered to the IOM recommendations by investigating new emerging pathogens, developing flexible partial solutions when called for, and regularly re-evaluating decisions and policies as new data have emerged. As an example, the Food and Drug Administration Transmissible Spongiform Encephalopathy Advisory Committee was established in response to concern about the then little-known variant Creutzfeldt-Jakob disease, a disease in humans caused by the same pathogen that manifests in cows as bovine spongiform encephalopathy, or "mad cow" disease. The committee studied variant Creutzfeldt-Jakob disease, as well as classical Creutzfeldt-Jakob disease, and went on to make policy decisions, which have since been evaluated and then re-evaluated. The processes that emerged following the IOM meetings are robust and continually improving, and can result in policies to help prevent infection and to meet the needs of those already infected. These processes are definite improvements over those demonstrated during the AIDS crisis.

As public and private third-party payers' cost containment investigations become more extensive, it becomes even more important for the hemophilia community to ensure that payers understand the impact of such policies on the continuity of care, the reality of threats posed by emerging pathogens, and the complex considerations underlying optimal treatment of hemophilia. This supplement is intended to provide a comprehensive exposition of these issues for professional hemophilia treaters. We hope that each article may, from its individual perspective, help to raise awareness among clinicians and formulary and reimbursement decision-makers of the impact that a changing environment for hemophilia reimbursement may have on the management of hemophilia, including the ability of the hemophilia community to deal with the threat of emerging pathogens.

In a review of the devastating consequences of the HIV epidemic on the hemophilia community Dr Bruce Evatt details the identification of, and reaction to, HIV contamination of the blood supply that took place among public health organizations in the early 1980s, and assesses the impact of those strategies on people with hemophilia. A synopsis of an article previously published by Dr Michael Stoto describes a risk management approach to public health crises, illustrated by the HIV scenario. In his article he encourages the application of the precautionary principle to all major policy and clinical decisions regarding blood and blood products. Dr Samuel Stanley presents an overview of the worldwide experience of emergence of infectious pathogens in recent years. He outlines the rationale for believing that new pathogens will continue to emerge, and argues that continued and increased vigilance over the safety of the blood supply will be crucial to preventing future epidemics. Ellis Sulser provides a patient's perspective on the current threats to the hemophilia community, including the threat of emerging pathogens, and potential changes in public and private reimbursement coverage for hemophilia therapies. Finally, in my article I identify the complex issues affecting all hemophilia therapy selections, emphasizing the importance of a proactive and cooperative approach to ensuring the best standard of care for patients with hemophilia.

Indeed, the hemophilia community may need to launch and support substantial effort in order to retain its freedom of choice—choice of regimen, provider, and therapy. The overarching message from the interdisciplinary forum is that incorporation of multiple insights—from epidemiology, hematology, infectious disease, public policy, patient, and medical ethics perspectives—will be critical to the formulation of a sound hemophilia healthcare policy that protects and values the patient.

Steven Pipe, MD
Pediatric Medical Director
Hemophilia and Coagulation Disorders Program
University of Michigan
Ann Arbor, MI
Guest Editor

References

1. Parent Empowerment Newsletter, vol 15, issue 2. Georgetown, MA, LA Kelley Communications, May 2005
2. Parent Empowerment Newsletter, vol 14, issue 4. Georgetown, MA, LA Kelley Communications, November 2004
3. Parent Empowerment Newsletter, vol 15, issue 1. Georgetown, MA, LA Kelley Communications, February 2005
4. Leveton LB, Sox HC, Stoto MA: HIV and the Blood Supply: An Analysis of Crisis Decisionmaking. Committee to Study HIV Transmission Through Blood and Blood Products, Division of Health Promotion and Disease Prevention, Institute of Medicine. Washington, DC, National Academy Press, 1995

ELSEVIER

Seminars in
HEMATOLOGY

Infectious Disease in the Blood Supply and the Public Health Response

Bruce Evatt

The consistent improvements in hemophilia care seen in the years 1960 to 1980 halted when human immunodeficiency virus (HIV) appeared in the blood supply. In the early 1980s, before HIV virulence was fully understood, a complacent blood therapy industry and its regulators waffled on an appropriate response. As a result, the period between the appearance of HIV and its effective elimination from the blood supply was lengthy and many recipients of blood therapies became infected, with devastating impact on their quality of life, quality of care, and longevity. As the decade wore on, even as they began to better understand the threat, industry and public health officials continued to stall, in part because development of interventions was costly and cumbersome. In order to protect the safety of the blood supply and blood-derived therapies, it must be recognized that new pathogens will continue to emerge. Agencies' and companies' decision-making processes in this regard must therefore be proactive rather than reactive, and should preferably implement a formalized risk-management approach. The ongoing safety of blood therapies and the blood supply will also depend on continued vigilance and research. Finally, the hemophilia community must be allowed to play an active and educated role in their own care.
Semin Hematol 43(suppl 3):S4-S9

The consistent improvement in quality of life, quality of care, and longevity for patients with hemophilia seen in the years 1960 to 1980 halted unequivocally when human immunodeficiency virus (HIV) appeared in the blood supply in the 1980s. Prior to the extreme morbidity and mortality of the acquired immunodeficiency syndrome (AIDS) epidemic, improvement in the prognosis for patients with hemophilia had been very encouraging. For example, until the 1960s, hemophilia usually disabled patients before they reached the age of 20. In the time period 1941 through 1960, when the standard of care was blood transfusion, the median life expectancy of a 12-month-old male with severe hemophilia was 39.7 years. In the years 1961 through 1970, following the availability of clotting-factor therapies isolated from human plasma, such as cryoprecipitate, that life expectancy had climbed to 53.8 years, as illustrated in Figure 1.[1]

In the mid 1970s, care for patients with hemophilia improved further with the availability of freeze-dried concentrates, which were more convenient to use than the frozen precipitates, and the Congressional passage of legislation to establish and fund comprehensive hemophilia treatment centers (HTCs); the treatment centers substantially enhanced the quality and consistency of medical care for patients with hemophilia.[2] A 2000 review of records of 2,950 patients with hemophilia in six states demonstrated that patients who were cared for at an HTC had a significantly decreased risk of death compared with patients who did not receive treatment at such facilities (relative risk 0.6, $P = .002$).[3] The combination of these plasma-derived blood clotting therapies and better management through HTCs measurably improved the length and quality of life for persons with hemophilia.

The Public Health Crisis of the 1980s

By the early 1980s, the preceding years' advances had led to a general complacency about the safety of treatment options for patients with hemophilia. Yet cause for concern remained: all clotting-factor therapies available at that time were derived from the pooled blood products of up to 20,000 donors. Procedures for donor screening, infective agent testing, and inactivation for endemic chronic diseases like hepatitis were in their infancy. As a result, patients who received multiple treatments were likely to be exposed to and become infected with hepatitis and other diseases. Studies conducted

Chief (Retired), Hematologic Diseases Branch, National Center for Infectious Diseases, Centers for Disease Control and Prevention, Atlanta, GA.
Address correspondence to Bruce Evatt, MD, Chief (Retired), Hematologic Diseases Branch, National Center for Infectious Diseases, Centers for Disease Control and Prevention, 2094 Valiant Dr NE, Atlanta, GA 30345. E-mail: ble2@mindspring.com

 0037-1963/06/$-see front matter
doi:10.1053/j.seminhematol.2006.02.001

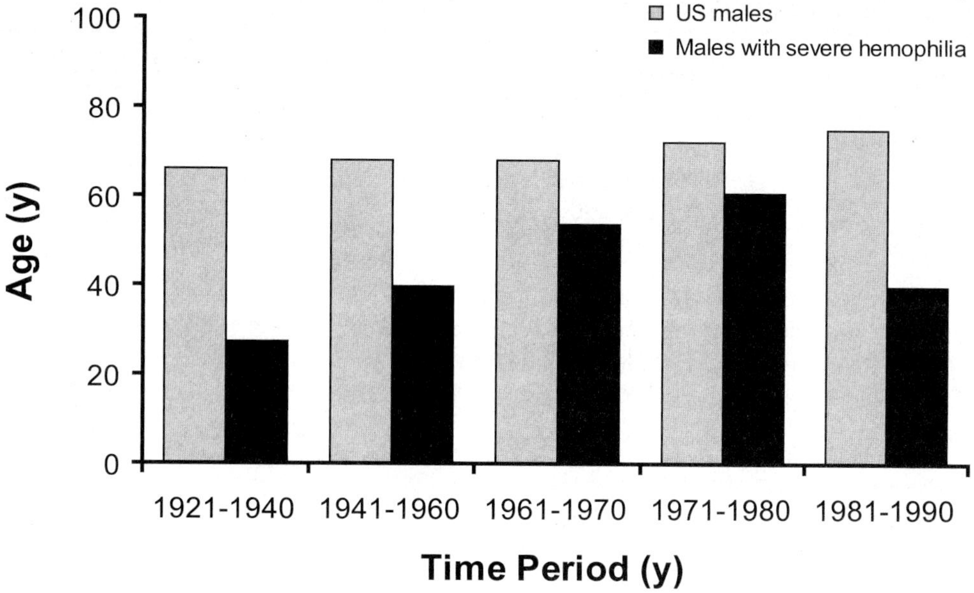

Figure 1 Median life expectancy at age 1 year.[1]

in the years 1972 to 1991 consistently showed infectivity rates of hepatitis B (HBV) and hepatitis C (HCV) higher than 60% in people with hemophilia.[4] However, in light of hemophilia patients' enhanced quality of life and increased longevity at the time, this risk of exposure and infection was deemed acceptable. In addition, in 1982, therapies containing blood-clotting factors were widely thought to be reasonably safe due to the development of antigen screening tests against HBV and the eventual introduction of an HBV vaccine.[5] Unfortunately, the hemophilia community was not provided with adequate information in order to accurately assess the health risks of using these clotting-factor concentrates.[6] The tragic inadequacy of these early safety efforts and the lack of effective communication between hemophilia treaters and patients were soon demonstrated.

By the summer of 1982, three cases of AIDS had been identified,[7] but health professionals from many sectors remained skeptical of this previously unheard of diagnosis and response to protect the blood supply was slow or ineffectual. The debate about the origins of infection and its control was further complicated by the following:

- Preconceptions about the status of infectious disease
- Unusual presentation of the disease
- Rapid movement of the epidemic
- Long incubation period of the virus
- Affected population(s) unwilling to acknowledge their target group status

Regarding the last point, there was concern about stigmatizing already marginalized populations of patients—homosexuals, intravenous drug users, and black immigrants from Haiti—who presented with this new disease.

Meanwhile, throughout the early to mid 1980s, patients with hemophilia were being infected at an increasingly alarming rate. For example, a Centers for Disease Control and Prevention (CDC) analysis estimated that by 1987, 63% of the 15,500 patients with hemophilia in the United States had been infected with HIV through the use of contaminated blood therapies.[8] In addition, many patients with hemophilia and HIV were coinfected with HBV and HCV. In one study of US patients with hemophilia A and B (N = 727) seen during 1987 and 1988, 53% were HIV-positive and 47% were HIV-negative. Of those infected with HIV (n = 382), most were coinfected with HCV or HBV: 24% were seropositive for HCV and 65% were seropositive for both HCV and HBV. Of the patients with hemophilia not infected with HIV (n = 345), 20% had no viral hepatitis markers, 46% were seropositive for HCV, and 30% were coinfected with HBV and HCV.[3]

As a result of these infectious diseases, the life expectancy of patients with hemophilia plummeted from a high of 60.5 years during the period of 1971 to 1980 to a low of 39.8 years during the 1980s.[1] From 1979 to 1998—the worst years of the HIV epidemic—71% of the deaths of patients with hemophilia A were attributed to HIV.[9] For patients with hemophilia, the impact of the HIV epidemic was devastating.

Early Efforts to Stop the Spread of HBV and HIV

Before the virulence of HIV was fully understood, the blood therapy industry and its regulators vacillated on an appropriate response.[6] As a result, the period of time between the appearance of HIV and its effective elimination from the blood supply was lengthy and many recipients of blood therapies became infected.

The plasma industry first tackled the problem of HBV, and in 1983 they introduced the first heat-treated clotting factor for protection against HBV. Yet even after regulatory approval, some hemophilia treaters and patients were concerned that heat treatment might diminish the effectiveness of the active factor protein, as well as increase costs of therapy

Table 1 Testing Performed on Each Unit of Donated Blood in the United States[15]

Disease	Test	Implemented	Discontinued
HIV/AIDS	HIV-I antibody test	1985	
	HIV-1/2 antibody test	1992	
	HIV-I p24 antigen test	1996	2003
Hepatitis B	Hepatitis B surface antigen	1971	
	Hepatitis B core antibody	1987	
Hepatitis C	Anti-HCV	1990	
Hepatitis	ALT	1986	2003
Syphilis	Serologic test for syphilis—TP or RPR	1948	
Human T-cell lymphotrophic virus (HTLV)	HTLV-I antibody test	1989	
	HTLV-I/II antibody test	1998	
Hepatitis C and HIV/AIDS	Nucleic acid testing (NAT)	1999	
West Nile virus	Nucleic acid testing (WNV-NAT)	2003	

Abbreviations: ALT, alanine aminotransferase; RPR, rapid plasma reagin; TP, *Treponema pallidum*.

by requiring the use of larger amounts of active factor protein to compensate for decreased efficacy.[6] Also of growing concern in the mid 1980s was that heat treatment of active clotting factor might alter its labile proteins and foster the creation of new antigens, which in turn could promote inhibitor development.[10,11]

Two factors contributed to the cessation of new HIV infections in patients with hemophilia: (1) the universal adoption of heat-treated concentrates in early 1985 as the result of the publication of studies showing HIV was extremely sensitive to heat inactivation,[12] and (2) the licensing by the Food and Drug Administration (FDA) of the first enzyme-linked immunosorbent assay (ELISA) test for HIV in March 1985 that was used on all blood for transfusions and plasma therapies beginning in May of the same year.[13] From 1981, when the first case of AIDS was reported, until January 1985, thousands of patients with hemophilia became unnecessarily infected with HIV; however, no hemophilia patients born in 1985 or later were infected.[14] Had concerned parties—including the plasma industry, blood banks, the FDA, and other government agencies—worked harder to develop viral inactivation processes in earlier years, despite the high costs and complicated, lengthy approval processes, much morbidity and mortality would surely have been avoided.

Blood Screening Comes of Age

From 1985 through 2003, a number of screening tests were developed to reduce the risk of infectious disease transmissions in the US blood supply and in an effort to ensure that another HIV/AIDS-like tragedy did not recur. These assay tests screen for serologic markers such as antibodies and proteins that indicate the presence of an infectious agent; infected donations are then destroyed and donors are notified of the results. Today, each individual unit and pool of blood undergoes a number of tests to identify and eliminate donations infected with the known virulent pathogens (Table 1).[15] The effects of such screening tests used from 1985 through 2001 on the risk for infection are illustrated in Figure 2.[16]

A person may be infected with a disease-causing agent but donate blood before the development of detectable antibodies; this period of time is called the "window period." Further testing innovations came in 2001 in the form of nucleic acid amplification testing (NAT), which amplifies the nucleic acid sequences in a donation to allow for the detection of infections more quickly than with other tests. NAT performed on minipools (16 to 20 units) of blood has been shown to significantly reduce the window period for selected diseases: 11 days for HIV, 59 days for HCV, and 25 days for HBV.[17]

The Reliability of Modern Viral Inactivation

Despite slow early adoption by the community, viral inactivation has proven to be very effective at eliminating lipid-enveloped viruses such as HIV, HBV, and HCV. Viral inactivation is used for most clotting-factor therapies and usually includes both heating and exposure to an organic solvent and detergent.[18] For the removal of non–lipid-enveloped viruses, which are insensitive to treatment with heat or solvents, other techniques such as nanofiltration are being used and refined, although with currently limited success.[19] Additionally, some recombinant factors VIII and IX concentrates are now produced without the use of any human or animal plasma protein additives, making the risk of viral transmission through these therapies exceedingly low.[20,21]

Management Strategies to Protect the Blood Supply

Outside of the laboratory, a number of strategies have been developed and implemented to reduce the threat of infection of the blood supply and resulting blood therapies. These include:

- Self-deferral (donor indicates that he or she presents a potential blood risk)
- Deferral by center
- Donor retesting

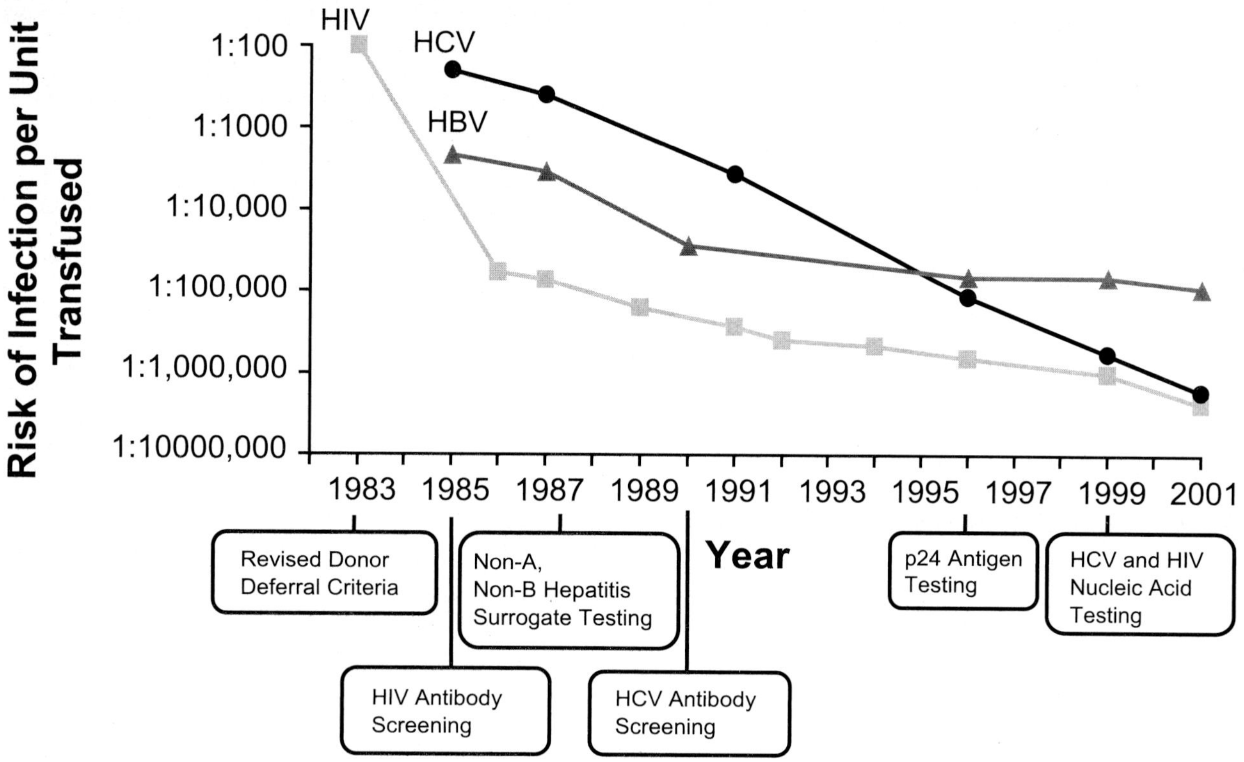

Figure 2 Risks for HIV, HBV, and HCV transfusion transmission in the US from 1983 through 2001. Adapted with permission.[16]

Careful donor selection is critical to maintaining blood safety. For example, one study has demonstrated that voluntary unpaid donors have a lower incidence of infection than paid donors.[22] Persons are also ineligible to be blood donors if they are members of high-risk populations, such as those identified in Table 2.[5]

Table 2 Population at High Risk of Infection, Who Are Not Eligible to Donate Blood[5]

- Anyone who has ever used intravenous drugs (illegal IV drugs)
- Men who have had sexual contact with other men since 1977
- Anyone who has ever received clotting factor concentrates
- Anyone with a positive test for HIV (AIDS virus)
- Men and women who have engaged in sex for money or drugs since 1977
- Anyone who has had hepatitis since his or her eleventh birthday
- Anyone who has had babesiosis or Chagas disease
- Anyone who has taken Tegison for psoriasis
- Anyone who has risk factors for Creutzfeldt-Jakob disease (CJD) or who has an immediate family member with CJD
- Anyone who has risk factors for vCJD
- Anyone who spent three months or more in the United Kingdom from 1980 through 1996
- Anyone who has spent 5 years in Europe from 1980 to the present

Current Safety of Blood and Blood Therapies

While the infection rate per transfusion unit has dropped dramatically since the outbreak of the HIV crisis, it should be noted that the blood supply is still vulnerable to infectious agents. This is particularly true regarding blood donated during the window period. For persons with hemophilia who must rely on cryoprecipitate—where exposure to risk is cumulative—blood therapy free of infectious agents is key. Many of those patients live outside the United States and viral contamination is a greater risk. For example, researchers developed a model comparing the lifetime risk of exposure to HIV in Venezuela versus the risk of exposure to the disease in the United States. The model showed that a hemophilia population in Venezuela receiving monthly infusions of cryoprecipitate from 15 donors had a 40% risk of exposure to HIV, compared with the risk of exposure to HIV in the United States, which was estimated to be only 2% over a 60-year life span.[23]

Stringent state-of-the-art procedures have made the blood supply in the developed countries of the world very safe. However, the risk of exposure to infectious agents has not been entirely eliminated in those countries; pathogens continue to emerge and their potential impact on the blood supply and factor therapies requires ongoing evaluation.[24] For example, in 2004 in the United Kingdom, one possible transmission of variant Creutzfeldt-Jakob disease (vCJD) occurred through transfusion of red blood cells.[25,26] As a result, the

British blood industry and public health officials are carefully monitoring persons who become infected with vCJD and the UK government is implementing sweeping measures to limit the spread of the disease. These measures include halting the use of blood clotting therapies derived from UK-sourced plasma, educating patients who are at risk based on their prior use of these therapies, and preventing the reuse of medical instruments that might become contaminated with vCJD.[27,28] Unfortunately, to date there is still only a limited understanding of how this disease can be controlled or eliminated. Consequently, the actual impact of prion diseases on the blood supply cannot easily be predicted.[29]

Lessons Learned From the HIV Crisis

An analysis of the events in the 1980s surrounding the emergence of HIV, the contamination of the blood supply, and the infection of patients with hemophilia reveals the devastating impact of a slow and reactive decision-making process in a time of crisis.[6] Very early in the 1980s, the magnitude of the threat of HIV was not clear, the infectious agent had not yet been fully identified, and its impact could only be surmised. However, as the decade progressed, inaction became less and less defensible. This was clearly spelled out in the 1995 Institute of Medicine (IOM) report on the decision-making process related to the HIV epidemic. In the report, the authors note that "preference for the status quo under the prevailing conditions of uncertainty and danger led decisionmakers to underestimate the threat of AIDS for blood recipients." In other words, even as industry and public health officials began to better understand the threat, they continued to stall and procrastinate, in part because development of interventions were costly and cumbersome.[6]

Patients with hemophilia are dependent on clotting-factor therapies for their survival and quality of life. In order to protect the safety of therapies developed from blood products, it must be recognized that pathogens will continue to emerge. In the face of these potential threats to the blood supply, the decision-making process of agencies and companies must be proactive rather than reactive, and a formalized risk-management approach should be considered. Only through continued vigilance and ongoing research will the safety of blood therapies and the blood supply be maintained. Lastly, the hemophilia community must play an active and educated role in decision making about their own treatments.

References

1. Jones PK, Ratnoff OD: The changing prognosis of classic hemophilia (factor VIII "deficiency"). Ann Intern Med 114:641-648, 1991
2. Public Health Service Act. Section 606 of P.L. 94-63 amended Title XI of the Public Health Service Act, 1975
3. Soucie JM, Nuss R, Evatt B, Abdelhak A, Cowan L, Hill H, et al: Mortality among males with hemophilia with source of medical care. Blood 96:437-442, 2000
4. Troisi CL, Hollinger FB, Hoots WK, Contant C, Gill J, Ragni M, et al: A multicenter study of viral hepatitis in the United States hemophilic population. Blood 81:412-418, 1993
5. American Association of Blood Banks: Frequently Asked Questions. Available at: http://www.aabb.org/All_About_Blood/FAQs/aabb_faqs.htm, accessed December 2005
6. Leveton LB, Sox HC Jr, Stoto MA, eds: HIV and the Blood Supply: An Analysis of Crisis Decisionmaking. Washington, DC, National Academy Press, 1995
7. Centers for Disease Control and Prevention: Epidemiologic notes and reports Pneumocystis carinii pneumonia among persons with hemophilia A. MMWR Morb Mortal Wkly Rep 31:365-367, 1982
8. Centers for Disease Control and Prevention: Human immunodeficiency virus infection in the United States: A review of current knowledge. MMWR Morb Mortal Wkly Rep 36:1-20, 1987
9. Chorba TL, Holman RC, Clarke MJ, Evatt BL: Effects of HIV infection on age and cause of death for persons with hemophilia A in the United States. Am J Hematol 66:229-240, 2001
10. Department of Health and Human Services, Food and Drug Administration, Center for Biologics Evaluation and Research: Workshop on factor VIII inhibitors: Proceedings of the Food and Drug Administration International Association of Biologicals Workshop on Factor VIII Inhibitors; November 21, 2003; Bethesda, MD. Available at www. fda.gov/cber/minutes/fctrviii112103t.pdf, accessed December 2005
11. Josić D, Buchacher A, Kannicht C, Lim YP, Loster K, Pock K, et al: Degradation products of factor VIII which can lead to increased immunogenicity. Vox Sang 77:90-99, 1999 (suppl 1)
12. McDougal JS, Martin LS, Cort SP, Mozen M, Heldebrant CM, Evatt BL: Thermal inactivation of the acquired immunodeficiency syndrome virus, human T lymphotropic virus-III/lymphadenopathy-associated virus, with special reference to antihemophilic factor. J Clin Invest 76: 875-877, 1985
13. Food and Drug Administration: FDA Approves First Nucleic Acid Test (NAT) Systems to Screen Plasma for Human Immunodeficiency Virus (HIV) and Hepatitis C Virus (HCV). Rockville, MD, National Press Office, September 21, 2001. Talk Paper T01-42
14. Soucie JM, Richardson LC, Evatt BL, Linden JV, Ewenstein BM, Stein SF, et al: Risk factors for infection with HBV and HCV in a large cohort of hemophiliac males. Transfusion 41:338-343, 2001
15. American Red Cross: How blood is tested. Available at http://www.pleasegiveblood.org/education/blood_tested.php, accessed December 2005
16. Busch MP, Kleinman SH, Nemo GJ: Current and emerging infectious risks of blood transfusions. JAMA 289:959-962, 2003
17. Schreiber GB, Busch MP, Kleinman SH, Korelitz JJ, the Retrovirus Epidemiology Donor Study: The risk of transfusion-transmitted viral infections. N Engl J Med 336:1685-1690, 1996
18. Teitel JM: Viral safety of haemophilia treatment products. Ann Med 32:485-492, 2000
19. Burnouf T, Radosevich M: Nanofiltration of plasma-derived biopharmaceutical products. Haemophilia 9:24-37, 2003
20. Ananyeva N, Khrenov A, Darr F, Summers R, Sarafanov A, Saenko E: Treating haemophilia A with recombinant blood factors: A comparison. Expert Opin Pharmacother 5:1061-1070, 2004
21. Schlesinger KW, Ragni MV: Safety of the new generation recombinant factor concentrates. Expert Opin Drug Saf 1:213-223, 2002
22. Van der Poel CL, Siefried E, Schaasberg WP: Paying for blood donations: Still a risk? Vox Sang 83:385–293, 2002
23. Evatt BL, Austin H, Leon G, Ruiz-Saez A, De Bosch N: Predicting the long-term risk of HIV exposure by cryoprecipitate. Haemophilia 6:128-132, 2000 (suppl 1)
24. Dodd RY: Emerging infections, transfusion safety, and epidemiology. N Engl J Med 349:1205-1206, 2003
25. Llewelyn CA, Hewitt PE, Knight RS, Amar K, Cousens S, Mackenzie J, et al: Possible transmission of variant Creutzfeldt-Jakob disease by blood transfusion. Lancet 363:417-421, 2004
26. Peden AH, Head MW, Ritchie DL, Bell JE, Ironside JW: Preclinical vCJD after blood transfusion in a PRNP codon 129 heterozygous patient. Lancet 364:527-529, 2004
27. Department of Health: Assessing the risk of vCJD transmission via

surgery: An interim review. March 2005. Available at: http://www.dh.gov.uk/assetRoot/04/11/35/42/04113542.pdf, accessed December 2005
28. Department of Health: Guidance on local reporting by clinicians of Creutzfeldt-Jakob Disease (CJD) and local action by consultants in communicable disease control (CsCDC). November 2003. Available at: http://www.cjd.ed.ac.uk/guidance.htm, accessed December 2005
29. Department of Health: Assessing the implications for blood donors if recipients are infected with vCJD. July 2005. Available at: http://www.dh.gov.uk/assetRoot/04/11/53/12/04115312.pdf, accessed December 2005

ELSEVIER

Seminars in
HEMATOLOGY

The Precautionary Principle and Emerging Biologic Risks: Lessons From Human Immunodeficiency Virus in Blood Products

Michael A. Stoto

In times of crisis, such as during the early 1980s when acquired immune deficiency syndrome (AIDS) was first recognized as a threat to the blood supply, it can be difficult to find reliable evidence upon which to base appropriate public health policies. Unreliable evidence produces substantial scientific uncertainty. Yet despite ambiguity and unanswered questions, decisions must be made and policy established to protect people's health. The precautionary principle provides important guidelines for public health policy decision making that are of particular value in times of crisis, such as the emergence of a new pathogen: be open and honest about scientific uncertainty; communicate with the public; and consider immediate, adaptable policy decisions. Ongoing research into the important uncertainties and review of policies in light of the data that emerge are crucial to the development of good public policy.
Semin Hematol 43(suppl 3):S10-S12

This article explores the precautionary principle's overall capacity to assess and manage risk, with a focus on how its application might have reduced the amount of human immunodeficiency virus (HIV) contamination in the nation's blood supply and the incidence of transmission. The account of the early years of the HIV crisis is drawn from published reports by the Department of Heath and Human Services, in particular a report of the Institute of Medicine, *HIV and the Blood Supply*.[1] Lessons learned from the HIV tragedy are discussed here to enable decision makers to recognize opportunities to avoid similar tragedies in the future.

The Precautionary Principle Versus the Standard Risk Management Model

The precautionary principle has many definitions, but most incorporate three essential principles:

- consideration of public health and the environment should take precedence over economic gain and decision making should involve public participation in order to offset the influence of industry,
- the appropriate burden of proof for deciding whether to make changes or maintain the status quo must be determined, and
- there must be explicit recognition of scientific uncertainty in policy making.

The standard risk management model addresses two fundamental questions: How robust is the evidence of risk, and how potentially serious is that risk? Some regulatory processes focus on the qualitative level of risk, shown as the horizontal axis in Figure 1. If a risk is perceived as high, for example if a fatality risk exceeds one in a million people exposed, the associated product or activity would be restricted.[2] Other processes focus on the strength of the evidence, depicted as the vertical axis in Figure 1. Even if the magnitude of risk is small, the product or activity associated with that risk would be restricted if the evidence of that risk was strong.

Central to the concept of the precautionary principle is a balancing of risks and benefits that recognizes that zero risk is generally not achievable and its cost almost always prohibitive. The precautionary principle helps calculate how acceptable a risk is given its known benefits. It takes into account both the strength of evidence that something is harmful and the level of risk that that something will occur. As shown in

RAND Health, Arlington, VA.

Summary of Stoto MA: The precautionary principle and emerging biological risks: lessons from swine flu and HIV in blood products. Public Health Rep 117:546-52, 2002. Adapted with permission from Michael A. Stoto and Public Health Reports (2002;117:546-52). Copyright 2002, Association of Schools of Public Health.

Address correspondence to Michael A. Stoto, PhD, RAND Health, 1200 S Hayes St, Arlington, VA 22202. E-mail: mstoto@rand.org

 0037-1963/06/$-see front matter © 2006 Elsevier Inc. All rights reserved.
doi:10.1053/j.seminhematol.2006.02.003

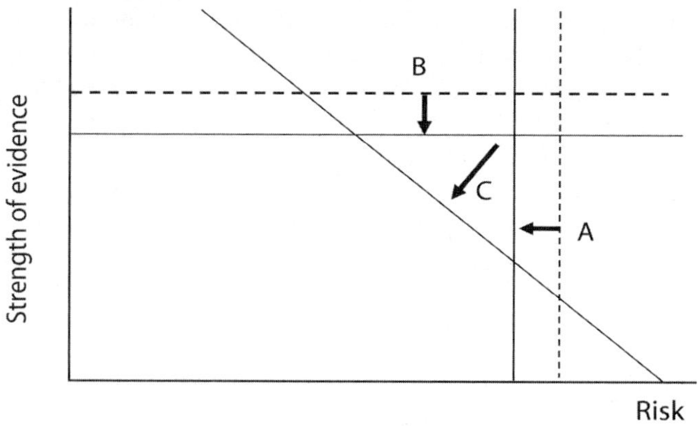

Figure 1 Standard regulatory risk management models are formulated in terms of the estimated magnitude of risk (horizontal axis) or the strength of the evidence (vertical axis). The precautionary principle can be interpreted as lowering the threshold for decision-making in terms of risk (A), strength of evidence (B), or when the apparent risk is high, the standard of scientific proof should be lower (C).

Figure 1, if the level of risk is very high, the action threshold for the strength of the evidence might be lowered. Conversely, if the evidence is very strong, reducing the action threshold for the magnitude of risk could be appropriate.

The HIV Crisis

The first cases of what would later be classified as acquired immunodeficiency syndrome (AIDS) were reported in homosexual men in mid 1981. The following year cases of the disease were identified in intravenous drug users and in people with hemophilia. By the end of 1982 the disease was recognized in an infant who had received a transfusion, strongly supporting the epidemiologic theory that the transmission patterns were similar to those of hepatitis B, and reinforcing suspicions that blood and blood products transmitted this new disease. At that time, the standard of care for hemophilia was transfusions of blood coagulation products (antihemophilic factor [AHF] concentrate) derived from large pools of plasma from many donors.

Early in 1983 the Centers for Disease Control and Prevention (CDC) convened a public meeting to identify strategies to prevent AIDS from spreading. A serum test for HIV would not be developed until 2 years later, and at that point in time it was not even known that AIDS was caused by a virus. Present at the meeting were the major Public Health Service agencies, including the US Food and Drug Administration (FDA), as well as members of the Red Cross and the blood services industry. Two strategies for urgent action were suggested:

- blood banks should question donors explicitly about relevant sexual behavior, and
- collection agencies should perform surrogate marker tests—specifically assays for hepatitis B core antibodies—on all blood donations.

The suggestions were not embraced. Both gay activists and spokespersons for blood banks around the country made the case that questions explicitly identifying homosexual sex as unsafe were discriminatory. Blood banks were also concerned that requiring potential donors to divulge information about sexual behavior would serve as a significant donor deterrent and diminish the nation's blood supply. The plasma industry recommended donor education and self-deferral programs for high-risk groups, basically putting the burden of responsibility for perception of risk on the high-risk donors themselves; this recommendation was formally issued by the US Public Health Service (USPHS) a couple of months later.

The second CDC recommendation, for surrogate marker tests, was also rejected. Although a high correlation between HIV infection and the presence of the selected surrogate marker—hepatitis B core antibodies—had been found in one study, the plasma industry recommended against the use of the surrogate marker tests pending further assessment, owing to the study's small size and weak methodology. In response, USPHS recommended undertaking additional studies to evaluate surrogate testing, including laboratory tests and physical examinations, rather than immediately implementing the surrogate marker testing recommended by the CDC. Attempts were made later in the same year by the Blood Products Advisory Committee (BPAC) of the FDA to review and recommend the use of surrogate marker tests, but each time the costs projected by the blood product industry for safety measures were deemed too high and evidence about the risk of the disease was downplayed. By the middle of 1983, the plasma industry stated that the risk for acquiring AIDS from plasma appeared to be one per 1 million patients transfused, implying that donation deferral programs might seriously interrupt the blood supply and would still not be effective. No data were provided to support either claim.

One month later, the BPAC considered the safety of AHF concentrate lots in light of the potential for the plasma of one donor with AIDS to infect an entire plasma lot. The BPAC issued guidelines that recommended the withdrawal of lots that, following a case-by-case evaluation of evidence, were deemed likely to contain plasma from an infected donor. Again, blood industry representatives on the BPAC expressed uncertainty about the risk of AHF concentrate contamination as well as concern about limiting the supply of AHF concentrate.

At the end of 1983, the BPAC again reviewed the case for surrogate marker testing and ultimately recommended against its use on the basis that it:

- would eliminate noninfected donors and deplete the blood supply,
- could not differentiate high-risk men who have sex with men from other male homosexual donors, and
- could defer too many Asians and others with a high prevalence of the surrogate marker as potentially infected with HIV.

While representatives of government agencies, blood banks, and the plasma industry met, patient groups and hemophilia treaters also worked to lessen the potential for the transmission of AIDS. Early in 1983, the National Hemophilia Foundation (NHF) made recommendations to clinicians that they use cryoprecipitate rather than AHF concentrate in infants, newly diagnosed patients, and mild cases. (Cryoprecipitate, a less effective treatment for hemophilia, is not derived from pooled plasma.) The NHF also stated that there was insufficient evidence to develop specific recommendations on blood-clotting therapy use in the treatment of severe hemophilia. The NHF was, however, largely silent with regard to the other strategies discussed by the blood supply community that might have limited the spread of AIDS in the hemophilia community, such as restricting the prophylactic use of AHF or practicing safe sex. Nor did the NHF inform patients of their recommendations or of the risks associated with hemophilia therapies. Similarly, physicians did not share with their patients the concerns raised about the safety of their hemophilia therapies, in part because they had high confidence in factor concentrates and were not convinced that AIDS was transmitted through them, and also because they believed that such disclosure would unnecessarily burden their patients with difficult decisions.

Lessons Learned

In retrospect, it is clear that many opportunities to prevent further HIV infection were lost during the early years of the AIDS crisis. Looking at this experience through the lens of the precautionary principle, three lessons become clear.

First, it is important to probe assumptions and explore uncertainty. Decisions were made on the basis of weak evidence that AIDS is a blood-borne disease, as well as a number of uncertain estimates regarding the risk per transfusion or per use of blood product; the performance of potential screening methods; the impact of screening on amount of blood and blood products available; and the availability of alternatives for blood and blood products. If studies and other efforts had been undertaken in 1983 to clear up some of these uncertainties, it might have been possible to make better decisions by the end of that year.

Second, these experiences show the importance of open communication between all potentially affected individuals, particularly in the face of uncertainty. Involving patients in decision making concerning their therapy options and warning them of the risks to their sexual partners would have saved lives. Learning about the potential for AIDS to be transmitted via blood would have prompted some patients to reduce their use of AHF concentrate and others to practice safer sex with their partners.

Third, uncertainty and the restrictions of limited data should be explicitly recognized in and accommodated by the use of intermediate options. The outcomes might have been improved at least marginally by implementing self-deferral and studying the impact on blood supply; warning people with hemophilia of risks to themselves and their sexual partners; involving patients in decision making about their own care and behavior; and ceasing the prophylactic use of AHF concentrate.

European Union Guidelines for Applying the Precautionary Principle

Application of the precautionary principle to science, medicine, and public health policy issues is expanding rapidly. Following international summits on the application of the precautionary principle in health sciences, the European Union (EU) has issued guidelines urging proactive initiatives, even in the face of scientific uncertainty, to address the complexity of contemporary health risks.[3]

EU guidelines support regulatory action that is "proportional to the chosen level of protection." This recommendation promotes the adoption of the least restrictive option that still meets public health needs—an important principle in public health law and public health ethics. This recognizes that any kind of legal or regulatory approach puts limits and restrictions into play. The least restrictive options that still meet public health goals and are capable of producing the most optimal outcomes are those that need to be seriously considered and potentially promoted. In the case of HIV and the patient with hemophilia, this might have resulted in a policy under which providers and clinicians routinely warned each patient of the potential for HIV transmission to himself and his sexual partners, and that enabled patients to help make educated decisions about their own care.

Another guideline advises that regulatory actions be "based on examination of the potential benefits and costs of action or lack of action," recognizing that lack of action can be a viable decision as well. For example, in the case of HIV and the blood supply, a potential reduction in risk for HIV would be weighed against a potential reduction in the availability of blood and blood therapies.

In addition, the EU guidelines also recommend that regulations "be subject to review in the light of new data" and "capable of assigning responsibility for producing the scientific evidence for risk assessment." In the case of HIV in the blood supply, policy makers following this recommendation would have reconsidered the various levels of risk for acquiring HIV associated with distinct therapies and uses, as well as the impact of screening alternatives on that risk and the availability of blood and blood therapies.

Conclusion

The precautionary principle provides important guidelines for public health policy decision making that are of particular value in times of crises such as the emergence of a new pathogen: be open and honest about scientific uncertainty; communicate with the public; and consider immediate, adaptable policy decisions. Crucial to the development of good public policy are ongoing research into the important uncertainties and review of policies in the light of the data that emerge.[2]

References

1. Leveton LB, Sox HC, Stoto MA (eds): HIV and the Blood Supply: An Analysis of Crisis Decisionmaking. Washington, DC, National Academy Press, 1995
2. Funtowicz SO, Ravetz JR: Three types of risk assessment and the emergence of post-normal science, in Krimsky S, Golding D (eds): Social Theories of Risk. New York, NY, Praeger, 1992, pp 251-273
3. Commission of the European Communities: Communication From the Commission on the Precautionary Principle, Report Number COM (2000) 1. Brussels, Belgium, Commission on the European Communities, 2000

ELSEVIER

Seminars in
HEMATOLOGY

A Patient's Perspective on Hemophilia

Ellis Sulser

People with hemophilia play a central role in partnering with their physicians to achieve the best possible clinical and economic outcomes. To make informed choices regarding a hemophilia therapy, patients and their caregivers must assess four basic areas: safety, purity, cost, and convenience—where safety is the number one concern. Access to information, including informed consent on issues affecting choice of therapy, treater, regimen, and point of service, ancillary, and comprehensive care services, is of fundamental importance when choosing a therapy. Hemophilia treaters are often the primary source for information and also play a large part in therapy decisions based on possible inhibitor formation, patients' lifetime insurance caps, and therapy availability. In order to help optimize a patient's outcomes, hemophilia treaters must also periodically re-evaluate and modify disease management techniques. Given the devastation of the hemophilia community during the worst years of the acquired immune deficiency syndrome (AIDS) epidemic, physicians, government agencies, and industry must complement policy decisions with medical ethics, psychosocial, and quality-of-life considerations—and patients must remain vigilant about the safety of their therapy. It is imperative that standards of care ensure access to the safest therapies available and enable those with hemophilia to live a life only minimally disrupted by their disease.
Semin Hematol 43(suppl 3):S13-S16 © 2006 Elsevier Inc. All rights reserved.

Progress in hemophilia management has traditionally focused on broadening the understanding of this rare genetic bleeding disorder and improving the safety and convenience of the pharmaceutical therapies available. In the process, researchers and clinicians have developed a broad consensus with respect to the complications and definitions of clinical success in treating patients with hemophilia. Validation of standardized instruments to enable meaningful comparisons among available therapies is also taking place. These advances are encouraging but must be coupled with patient choice and ongoing availability of hemophilia therapies, both new and established. The patient has a central role to play in partnering with his or her physician to achieve the best possible clinical and economic outcomes. In sum, therapeutic developments in hemophilia should enhance overall patient outcomes and quality of life, manage and mitigate inhibitor development, maintain patient acceptance of and adherence to therapy, reduce disease complications and attendant costs, and provide an essential element of protection against future epidemics of infectious disease.

Although younger patients may lack the acute sensitivity to the special history of the hemophilia community and cannot imagine disease management without the blood clotting factor therapies now available, even newly diagnosed patients, their families, and caregivers are usually well educated regarding the management of the disease. In making informed choices regarding a hemophilia therapy, patients and their caregivers assess four basic areas: safety, purity, cost, and convenience, where safety is the number one concern. Patient awareness of treatment risks and benefits is critical to making informed therapy choices in each of these four key domains.

Factor Support Network Pharmacy, Inc, Camarillo, CA.
Address correspondence to Ellis Sulser, President, Factor Support Network Pharmacy, Inc, 900 Avenida Acaso, Suite A, Camarillo, CA 93012-8749. E-mail: ellissulser@factorsupport.com

Safety and Purity

As consumers, people with hemophilia are generally well informed on the history of blood clotting therapies, the potential drawbacks of specific therapies, and the strength and integrity of published studies to support claims of therapeutic safety and effectiveness. Patients considering a new therapy seek the experience of others to judge the therapy's benefits and drawbacks.

Purity is another key to therapy choice. Degree of purity will limit or increase a hemophilia patient's immune system to exposure to foreign protein. This is important for three crucial reasons: those patients with hemophilia who continue to use plasma-derived clotting therapies pooled from multi-

0037-1963/06/$-see front matter © 2006 Elsevier Inc. All rights reserved.
doi:10.1053/j.seminhematol.2006.02.005

ple blood donations are reliant on the purity of the blood supply; persons who already have a significantly compromised immune system are particularly vulnerable; and the presence of foreign protein may exacerbate the formation of inhibitors to blood clotting factor therapies.

Inhibitor Formation

Inhibitors are pathologic circulating antibodies that result from an immune response identification of factor VIII (FVIII) as a foreign antigen, and which may develop following the administration of one or many infusions of either plasma-derived or recombinant clotting factor therapy. Inhibitors may diminish or entirely eliminate the hemostatic activity of the FVIII molecule. The likelihood of inhibitor development in any one patient is fundamentally unpredictable; the fear of inhibitor development is often a major complication in patient care.

What Is the Cost of Fear?

Although pathogen infection of the blood supply is always a risk that must be managed, it is fair to say the blood supply has never been safer; it is also accurate to claim that it could be safer with additional resources for better education and more stringent selection of donors, further testing for infectious disease markers, more sophisticated viral inactivation techniques, and more conservative transfusion practices. However, it is clear that no amount of testing for infectious disease markers or increases in the sophistication of viral inactivation or elimination techniques can offer sure protection against the infectious pathogens of the future, about which we now know nothing and against which we may find ourselves, at first, defenseless. Because of this fundamental uncertainty, and because, currently, the nation's blood supply is reliably safe, additional viral inactivation and other processes to prevent viral transmission through the blood supply are likely to only slightly improve safety and may be considered a poor use of finite resources. Such is the perspective of policy makers as they debate the cost-effectiveness of achieving zero or near zero risk with respect to the safety of the nation's blood supply. Patients with hemophilia or others who are completely reliant upon a safe blood supply, on the other hand, may look at the issue differently. The devastating effect of human immunodeficiency virus (HIV) contamination of the blood supply is still etched in the collective memory of the hemophilia community: application of pure cost-effectiveness analysis to ensure the safety of blood therapies is an emotionally and politically charged issue. Hemophilia spokespersons have argued that achieving peace of mind through pathogen risk reduction should be recognized as a component in economic evaluations, however difficult that calculation may be. Physicians are in a unique position to address the understandable fears in hemophilia patients while at the same time keeping administrators and decision makers abreast of the most effective use of resources that will yield the safest blood and blood-derived therapies possible. Careful explanation by physicians will help patients understand risk and associated cost. This discussion will not be easy, but it is essential if the concerns of the patient are to be fairly and adequately addressed.[1]

Cost and Convenience

Cost is also a critical consideration—especially in the context of lifetime reimbursement caps that may be imposed by third-party payers—and can significantly complicate a patient's treatment decisions. Treating hemophilia is not inexpensive and patients reasonably worry about being able to pay for the therapies they need. Exceeding lifetime caps is not infrequent, especially at the $1 million dollar level, among patients with severe hemophilia. The cost burden can force patients or their caregivers to change jobs, move to different locations, or deliberately impoverish themselves so that Medicaid coverage can be invoked. Lower-cost therapies, such as those that are plasma derived, may enable a person with hemophilia or the caregiver to remain employed and privately insured. The main issue is whether or not the plasma-derived therapies will adequately manage the disease while providing an optimal level of safety. Whenever a change to a safer—and more expensive—therapy is prescribed, informed patients will understand the ramifications of that change relative to increasing immediate costs as well as to more quickly exceeding their lifetime caps.

As more clotting factor therapies enter the marketplace, convenience becomes a factor. Storage and a patient's ability to travel without concern about temperature are key considerations. Early factor clotting therapy concentrates had to be refrigerated and kept in containers of dry ice, presenting a significant inconvenience to patients when they traveled. Now, small vials can be placed in a container and transported at room temperature. Additionally, in the past, 60 mL was a required volume of injection that took 30 or 40 minutes to infuse. Today, in some cases volumes are down to 2.5 mL and are injected in 5 minutes.

Ongoing Management of the Disease

Daily management of hemophilia has changed dramatically over the past 30 years, due in large part to the introduction of new treatment modalities. Advanced therapeutic options have had a generally positive impact on quality of life for patients living with hemophilia and have led to considerable improvements in patients' functional status.

Prior to the availability of today's blood clotting factor therapies, patients with hemophilia were routinely advised to curtail their physical activities to a minimum to reduce risk for injury and bleeds. Today, such restrictions are generally unnecessary, because modern blood clotting factor therapies can correct factor levels quickly. This enables the average patient with hemophilia to live a more active and normal life.

Psychosocial Impact of Safety Concerns in Hemophilia Treatment

Patients with hemophilia have two ever-present worries: the potential for accident or trauma resulting in serious bleeding and the safety of the blood clotting factors that they must use to prevent such a scenario. The historic HIV tragedy still lingers as a specter in the minds of many patients with hemophilia. Therefore, it is not surprising that the potential for future pathogen infection in the blood supply, such as that currently seen with variant Creutzfeldt-Jakob disease (vCJD), has a strong psychosocial impact. In light of recent cases of vCJD transmission via blood transfusions,[2,3] this fatal disease is of substantial concern within the hemophilia population. Uncertainty regarding the epidemiology of the disease has led the UK government to institute precautionary measures aimed at minimizing vCJD risk.[4] The Canadian government has also conducted a consensus conference to determine the cost-effectiveness of developing a diagnostic test for vCJD. Although the incidence of this disease in Canada is virtually zero, its epidemiologic potential is taken very seriously. Consequently, characteristics of a potential epidemic are closely watched and a commitment has been made to be continually vigilant.[5]

All the current evidence points to the need for further studies before patients and their physicians can make fully informed choices regarding the risk posed by the vCJD pathogen. These choices will need to include alternatives to plasma therapies, such as recombinant factor concentrates, and take into consideration the potential risks to supply owing to an over-reliance on one form of therapy.[6,7] In the aftermath of the HIV tragedy, it is understandable that today's patient with hemophilia will demand reliable, unbiased information and stay self-educated on the risk for emerging pathogens.

Patients usually turn for such information to physicians and other caregivers. The clinician community bears the onus of appropriate communications that fully disclose risk while weighing and individually assessing benefit for each patient—not easily accomplished, especially given the psychological history of this disorder.

This can present the following conundrum. On the one hand, patients deserve unbiased, unfiltered information about risks and benefits of treatment. But full disclosure is viewed by some providers and patients as potentially, and possibly unnecessarily, alarmist.

The Need for Patient Advocacy Groups

During the HIV epidemic, patients with hemophilia and their advocates felt that organizations such as the National Hemophilia Foundation (NHF), the American Association of Blood Banks, the Council of Community Blood Centers, the American Red Cross, and even the Food and Drug Administration were entities that represented manufacturers, health care providers, and then, finally, the consumers. Members of the hemophilia community expressed serious doubt about the reliability of information received from these organizations concerning the epidemic. The perception of a lack of representation, along with skepticism about disseminated information, spawned creation of consumer advocacy organizations such as the Committee of Ten Thousand, PEER Association, Hemophilia Federation of America, and LA Kelley Communications.

Now, manufacturers are working with advocacy groups to provide information to physicians and patients that will keep them abreast of developments in hemophilia treatment options. The NHF also disseminates information through consumer or chapter-level meetings, which have been effectively sponsored by a number of manufacturers. Hotlines and websites have been established to provide patients and clinicians with the latest available data, which today is viewed with general trust and confidence by those who use it to make important treatment decisions.

Being Born Today With Hemophilia

A person born today with hemophilia should have little concern about the risk for pathogen infections of the blood supply, that is, assuming blood clotting factor therapies with optimal safety margins remain available and the safety of these therapies remains uncompromised. But a relaxing of vigilance, such as deciding to use a therapy with higher vulnerability to infectious pathogens, could be dangerous. To the degree that some current recombinant clotting factor concentrates contain traces of human or animal proteins, the risk of transmission of infectious pathogens remains. Among the different generations of FVIII clotting therapies, varying levels of vulnerability to emerging pathogens exist, and this differential risk should play a role in formulary decisions that determine patient's access to certain therapies.

However, given the "cost-savings" mentality of private and public third-party payers, there may be slow uptake of newer therapies or shifts in selection to less costly ones, which, unfortunately, may result in greater exposure to emerging pathogens. Patients with hemophilia and members of their advocacy groups need to have representation when healthcare providers and payers review safety and efficacy profiles of blood clotting factor concentrates being considered for availability and reimbursement. Without a voice in the decision, patients are likely to be skeptical about how and why a therapy choice has been determined. Fortunately, a few patients with hemophilia have advocated successfully for the entire community. These advocates have a generally high profile when it comes to interactions with those who make the drug benefit decisions that ultimately determine quality of care for all patients with hemophilia.

Ensuring the least possible exposure to pathogens and the highest quality of care are two of the most critical reasons for hemophilia patients to continue to educate themselves about potential risk on the one hand and optimal outcomes on the other. Advocacy from the hemophilia community will continually remind and compel providers and payers to develop and institute the best standards of care for all hemophilia patients.

Conclusion

In optimizing a hemophilia patient's outcomes, many decision-making elements must be in alignment. Hemophilia treaters must periodically re-evaluate and modify disease management techniques. The physician plays a large part in therapy decisions based on possible inhibitor formation, patients' lifetime insurance caps, and availability of therapies.

In order to select optimal therapy, a patient's right to information is critical. This includes informed consent on issues affecting choice of factor replacement therapy, treater, regimen, point of service, ancillary, and comprehensive care services.

During the nationwide devastation of the acquired immune deficiency syndrome (AIDS) epidemic, the transmission of HIV through transfusions of blood and blood products resulted in additional, and unnecessary, loss of life and loss of trust throughout the hemophilia community. Given this history, policy decisions should always be complemented by medical ethics and quality-of-life considerations. In addition, patients themselves must avoid complacency in order to prevent another HIV-like tragedy. It is imperative to develop standards of care that will ensure access to the safest therapies available and enable those with hemophilia to live a life that is only minimally disrupted by their disease.

References

1. AuBuchon JP, Birkmeyer JD, Busch MP: Safety of the blood supply in the United States. Ann Intern Med 127:904-909, 1997
2. Llewelyn CA, Hewitt, PE, Knight RSG, Amar K, Cousens S, Mackenzie J, et al: Possible transmission of variant Creutzfeldt-Jakob disease by blood transfusion. Lancet 363:417-421, 2004
3. Peden AH, Head MW, Ritchie DL, Bell JE, Ironside JW: Preclinical vCJD after blood transfusion in a PRNP codon 129 heterozygous patient. Lancet 364:527-529, 2004
4. Ironside JW. The spectrum of safety: variant Creutzfeldt-Jakob disease in the United Kingdom. Semin Hematol 40:16-22, 2003 (suppl 3)
5. McCullough J, Anderson D, Brookie D, Bouchard JP, Fergusson D, Joly J, et al: Consensus conference on vCJD screening of blood donors: report of the panel. Transfusion 44:675-683, 2004
6. Farraguia A: Risk of variant Creuzfeldt-Jakob disease from factor concentrates: current perspectives. Haemophilia 3:230-235, 2002
7. Evatt BL, Farrugia A, Shapiro AD, Wilde JT: Haemophilia 2002: Emerging risks of treatment. Haemophilia 3:221-229, 2002

ELSEVIER

Seminars in
HEMATOLOGY

The Need for Continuing Vigilance: Addressing the Threat for Transmission of Blood-Borne Infectious Disease

Samuel L. Stanley, Jr

As international travel and human encroachment into previously isolated areas have increased, so too has the potential for the emergence of new infectious diseases. Populations likely to be susceptible to new infectious diseases have also increased in size. The past three decades have seen outbreaks of diseases caused by parvoviruses, Nipah virus, circoviruses, and prions. Infectious pathogens such as these are formidable opponents; they can adapt to new hosts or cause variant diseases within new hosts. Many are also resistant to current inactivation techniques. In order to prevent or contain outbreaks, pathogens that emerge must be identified quickly and efficiently; research and ongoing global surveillance are therefore of primary importance. To effectively protect the blood supply and blood-based therapies, this research should include investigations into improved techniques for detection, screening, and viral inactivation, as well as into ways to reduce patient exposure to infectious pathogens via therapeutic agents. The proactive devotion of appropriate resources to infectious disease containment and prevention prior to an epidemic should be perceived as both essential public health policy and cost effective.
Semin Hematol 43(suppl 3):S17-S22

In the wake of the significant strides in vaccines and antibiotics that followed World War II, most of the public health community believed that infectious diseases could be effectively controlled. By the 1990s, however, as new infectious pathogens emerged, public health experts could no longer believe that the threat of infectious diseases had receded.[1] In fact, the potential for the emergence of new infectious diseases was increasing, a result of commonplace and extensive international travel and steady human encroachment into previously isolated areas.

Infectious diseases are categorized as "emerging" based on either their documented increased incidence in humans over the past two decades or on evidence of their potential to increase in the near future.[1] Such evidence would include reports of a pathogen's demonstrated ability to increase its host range by jumping species to infect new populations. Emerging infectious pathogens in recent decades have included human immunodeficiency virus (HIV), avian/variant influenza, severe acute respiratory syndrome (SARS) virus, West Nile virus, dengue fever, monkeypox, parvovirus, Nipah virus, Ebola virus, and variant Creuzfeldt-Jakob disease (vCJD). Not all infectious diseases are a threat to the blood supply, because the clinical presentation associated with many infectious diseases is severe enough that infected patients are not likely to be blood donors. For example, the Ebola virus is blood-borne, but infected persons are not likely to donate blood because they become ill very quickly. However, other infectious diseases, such as HIV and vCJD, have long latent infectious periods during which persons can donate blood with no knowledge that they are infected. These latter types of infectious diseases as well as others with mild clinical sequelae have the potential to infect the blood supply through donation and be transmitted to the hemophilia community and other persons through blood products (Figure 1).

There are multiple arguments to support a belief in the inevitability of the emergence of additional infectious diseases, principally reflecting the following five factors:

- Adaptability of viruses allows for viral mutations that enable defensive or aggressive adaptation to new environments, promoting development of drug resistance or achievement of cross-species transmission[2]
- Human encroachment into previously unexplored habitats increases exposure to new agents[2]

Departments of Medicine and Molecular Microbiology, Washington University School of Medicine, St Louis, MO.
Address correspondence to Samuel L. Stanley Jr, MD, Professor, Departments of Medicine and Molecular Microbiology, Washington University School of Medicine, 660 S Euclid Ave, St Louis, MO 63110. E-mail: sstanley@wustl.edu

0037-1963/06/$-see front matter
doi:10.1053/j.seminhematol.2006.02.004

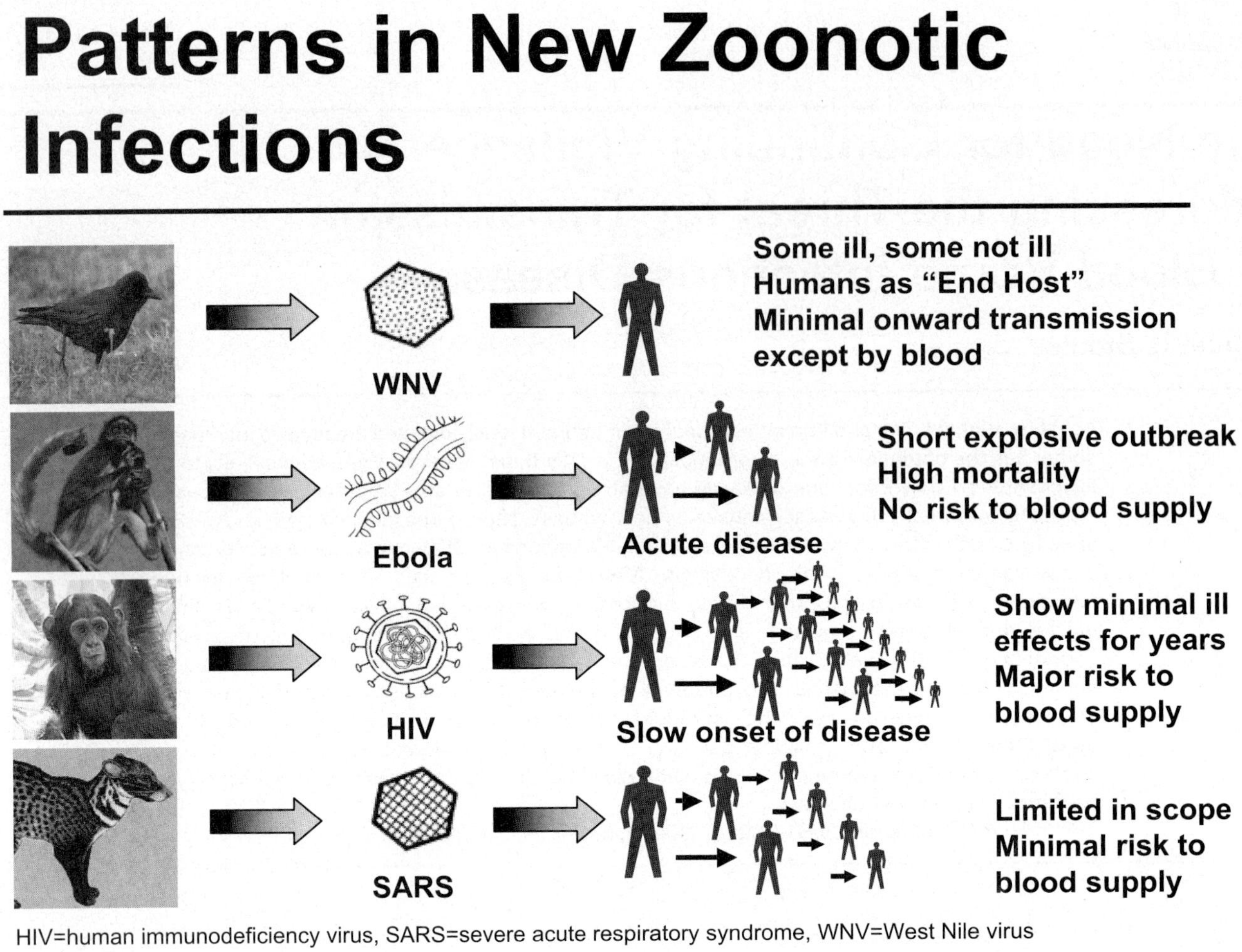

Figure 1 Infectious diseases have different potential impact on the blood supply. Figure courtesy of Dr David Onions.

- Increases in the numbers of susceptible hosts (eg, elderly, HIV-infected, or chemotherapy patients) offer greater opportunities for infectious pathogen disease transmission[2]
- Advances in pathogen screening technologies have resulted in increased sensitivity and, as a result, better detection of novel (or previously unrecognized) pathogens
- Currently unknown biological factors that may become evident in the future (referred to as the "X-factor").

Specific Pathogen Threats

Parvoviruses

Parvoviruses are non–lipid-enveloped, single-stranded DNA viruses that prefer to infect and lyse rapidly dividing cells, and are a continuous viral threat.[3] Currently, parvovirus B19 (PVB19) is the only known pathogenic parvovirus in humans,[4] in whom it is capable of causing several diseases. PVB19 typically causes a self-limiting febrile illness, *erythema infectiosum*, also called slapped cheek syndrome or Fifth disease.[5] However, in patients with immunosuppression or hematologic disorders, PVB19 can cause aplastic crises.[5]

Parvoviruses are potential threats to human health and safety because they can alter their host-specific proteins and effect cross-species transmission. Feline parvovirus (FPLV), for example, which causes feline panleukopenia disease (ie, feline distemper), altered its host specificity, and in the mid to late 1970s there was an outbreak of a new disease in dogs with symptoms similar to feline distemper, including a high mortality rate.[3,6,7] The most widely accepted hypothesis is that mutations in FPLV (or a closely related virus infecting mink or foxes) caused the emergence of a new virus, canine parvovirus (CPV-2)[3]; essentially, FPLV jumped species. There was no natural resistance to CPV-2 in dogs and the result was a rapid global epidemic[3] stopped within a year only by the development of a new vaccine for dogs and the use of the previously available cat vaccine.[7]

The ability of parvoviruses or related viruses to mutate and cross to humans is particularly alarming because they are difficult to eliminate. Parvovirus and other non–lipid-enveloped viruses are highly resistant to the multiple viral inactivation protocols used in blood product processing, eg, pasteurization, heat treatment, and solvent/detergent techniques, that are effective against lipid-enveloped viruses.[8,9] Parvovirus contamination has been extensively documented in animal products such as trypsin, used in the preparation of recombinant factors and serum.[10] PVB19 can also be transmitted from asymptomatic blood donors and there are numerous reports of transmission through transfusion of virus-inactivated or purified clotting factor concentrates. Many of these cases have serious clinical consequences.[11–14] PVB19 DNA has been found in virally attenuated plasma-derived clotting factors VIII (FVIII) and IX (FIX) and in first-generation recombinant FVIII (rFVIII) therapies.[11,15,16] Contaminated human albumin used as a stabilizer was the most likely source for PVB19 DNA in these clotting factor therapies.[16] PVB19 has also infected a patient who received a contaminated intravenous immune globulin infusion.[5] Purification techniques, involving polymerase chain reaction (PCR) screening and removal of infected blood, reduce the presence of parvovirus in blood products but do not eliminate it entirely.[8,17] As of yet, there have been no reports of the development of parvovirus disease subsequent to transfusion with any recombinant preparation, but the possibility has not been eliminated. Until more effective elimination techniques can be developed, there will always be the concern that animal- or human-derived products could serve as a source of transmission.

Nipah, Zoonoses

Malaysia, between September 1998 and June 1999, suffered a sudden outbreak of encephalitis, with more than 50% of those affected exhibiting reduced consciousness and brain stem dysfunction.[2,18] Authorities determined that the epicenter of the outbreak was a Nipah river village in which all 27 of the initial cases had had contact with pigs infected with a respiratory disease. The disease spread throughout Malaysia as farmers sold their pigs across the country. The resultant epidemic caused 265 cases of acute encephalitis and 105 deaths, a mortality of approximately 40%.[18] The new virus, identified as belonging to the Paramyxovirus family (measles and mumps),[19] was named Nipah for the village of origin.[18]

Evidence suggests that the viral reservoir for Nipah is the fruit bat in whose urine Nipah has been isolated. It is conjectured that bats feeding on fruit in an orchard adjacent to a piggery in Nipah urinated and defecated onto the fruit; the pigs then ate the fruit and contracted the virus. The close proximity of the pigs in the piggery fostered pig-to-pig transmission.[18] The Nipah virus was transmitted to humans primarily through direct contact with infected pigs or contaminated pig tissue.[2] Pigs also transferred the Nipah virus to cats, dogs, and horses.[18] There have been epidemics of Nipah in Bangladesh in 2001, 2003, and 2004[20]; although the source of the virus was unclear, Nipah-positive bats were found.[21] The evolution of the Nipah virus emphasizes the real threat of cross-species transmission.

Circoviruses, Viral Plasticity

Circoviruses are non–lipid-enveloped, single-stranded circular DNA viruses that can be pathogenic within animal hosts and could become pathogenic within humans.[22,23] Circoviruses have extraordinarily small genomes (3,750 to 3,900 bases) and are some of the smallest viruses known. The circovirus family includes porcine circovirus (PCV), chicken anemia virus (CAV), and TT virus (TTV), which affects humans, although at this time TTV's ability to cause disease is unclear. Blood-borne TTV displays substantial genetic diversity and it is unknown whether genetic variability could lead to an increased potential to cause disease. Detection rates for TTV DNA in humans are very high and TTV infection may be universal[23]; in fact, some individuals are infected with multiple genotypes of TTV. Although the potential repercussions of such infection are unknown,[24] TTV can be transmitted both by blood and by fecal–oral routes and there is debate about mother–infant transmission.[22,23,25] TTV is a particular concern because circoviruses demonstrate a high degree of plasticity, and animal circoviruses can cause severe disease in their respective hosts. In addition, circoviruses, which are non–lipid-enveloped and have small genomes, are very resistant to standard inactivation methods, including irradiation.

Prions

Prions are insoluble cellular protein particles that lack nucleic acid and, therefore, do not depend on genes or other factors for transmission of their traits. In humans, the prion protein gene (*PRNP*) on chromosome 20 usually encodes for a normal prion protein. In some instances, a post-translational conformational change occurs that creates an abnormal and transmissible particle, PrP^{Sc}, termed a prion.[26] Believed to be responsible in humans for at least five clinical diseases (Kuru, Gerstmann-Straussler-Scheinker disease, fatal familial insomnia, Creutzfeldt-Jakob disease [CJD], and variant CJD [vCJD]), prions are also present in other species. In animals prions cause scrapie, bovine spongiform encephalopathy (BSE or "mad cow" disease), chronic wasting disease, or feline encephalopathy.[27] While prion diseases can develop spontaneously, they are more likely to be transmitted by dietary or blood-borne contamination[26]; vCJD may be transmitted through consumption of contaminated meat or blood transfusion, while classical CJD has been transmitted by contaminated human pituitary hormones, dura matter drafts, corneal grafts, and surgical instruments.[28] Given the characteristics of prions and their transmission, vCJD-associated prions present an alarming and real concern for all patients reliant on blood products, including patients with hemophilia.

As of December 2005, there have been 159 cases of vCJD reported worldwide.[29] Although a majority of the cases have occurred in the United Kingdom, vCJD has also been identified in France, Ireland, Italy, the United States, and Canada.[26,30] Patients with vCJD initially present with psychiatric symptoms such as depression, withdrawal, anxiety, cognitive impairment, and persistent painful sensory symptoms[26]; eventually the symptoms progress to dementia and death. The median age at death is 28 years old, indicating that vCJD most frequently occurs in young people.[26–30]

Susceptibility to vCJD, clinical symptoms of the disease, and the time to appearance of symptoms are determined by a polymorphism at codon 129 of the PRNP. Individuals who are heterozygous at codon 129 may be infected but still in the incubation period and, as a case report (detailed later) demonstrates, vCJD can be transmitted while the patient is in the incubation period.[31] Therefore, though the incidence of vCJD has been decreasing worldwide since 2000,[30] latent infection may still be present, and the threat for transmission remains.

Blood transfusions are possibly responsible for two known cases of vCJD.[28,31] In one case, a 62-year-old patient received a transfusion of red cells during surgery in 1996. One unit of the transfused blood was donated by a 24-year-old, who developed symptoms of vCJD 3 years and 4 months after the blood donation and died in 2000. In 2002, 6.5 years after the transfusion, the recipient manifested clinical symptoms of vCJD and died 13 months later.[28] In the second case, an elderly patient received a transfusion of red blood cells in 1999. The blood donor developed symptoms of vCJD 18 months after the donation and died in 2001; vCJD was confirmed at autopsy. The recipient patient died 5 years after the transfusion, but showed no evidence of a neurologic disease. Nonetheless, postmortem, the patient was shown to be positive for vCJD.[31]

In response to the vCJD threat, the United Kingdom announced that patients with hemophilia and other congenital bleeding disorders were at risk for vCJD,[32] an announcement that has had notable financial and psychological impact, since patients with hemophilia and other congenital bleeding disorders who might be infected with vCJD are now considered capable of transmitting it to others. Therefore, the United Kingdom has implemented a new standard of care that includes disposal of those instruments used on patients with hemophilia that cannot be easily disinfected (eg, endoscopes, some dental equipment).[32] This new standard of care is very costly, and some dentists are refusing to treat patients with hemophilia.

Other countries are also being forced to confront the spread of prion diseases. In October 2004, the French health ministry announced that a blood donor, who is still alive, had developed vCJD, and within a month French authorities announced discovery of blood donations by another individual later diagnosed with vCJD. The Belgian Red Cross used French-sourced plasma (from one infected donor) to produce factor VIII and IX in 1995 and 2002.[33] Although as of yet there have been no reports of vCJD transmission in any person with hemophilia,[33] it is clear that continued vigilance is necessary.

Vigilance Is Expensive

Interventions to improve blood safety can be expensive. By comparing the cost of an intervention to the benefit given, the quality-adjusted-life year (QALY) can be calculated. To improve blood safety, the HIV antibody testing was developed and introduced in the mid 1980s. With 16 million transfusions each year in the United States, and an estimated prevalence of HIV of one in 10,000 blood donors, the cost per QALY for this intervention is calculated at $3,600.[34] By contrast, the cost per QALY for p24 antigen testing for HIV is estimated at $2.3 million and for HIV NAT at $2.0 million. This difference in cost-effectiveness reflects the decreasing

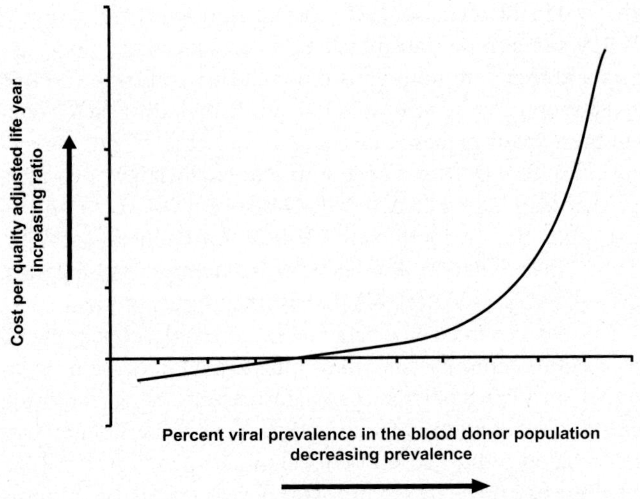

Figure 2 Hypothetical relationship between cost-effectiveness and viral prevalence. As the prevalence of blood donor disease decreases, the costs of blood screening increases because there is little health benefit for the general population. Conversely, when disease prevalence is high, blood screening is cost effective because it prevents spread of disease. Reprinted from Custer et al,[35] © 2004, with permission from Elsevier.

prevalence of HIV in the blood donor population.[35] However, new defensive interventions could be very cost effective if (and when) a new blood-borne pathogen enters the blood supply (Figure 2).[35] The costs of pathogen screening techniques must be considered in relation to the potential future costs for disease treatments in those who become infected. The medical costs associated with treatment of viral infections can be substantial: the costs involved in treating a patient with hemophilia co-infected with HIV are nearly 1.5 times greater than costs for those without co-infection.[36]

Cost-effectiveness and cost-utility analyses are important for developing resource allocation decisions and many resources are used to ensure that transfusions of donated blood carry nearly "zero risk."[35] Economic evaluations of techniques for ensuring blood safety show that interventions may not be cost effective, but these conclusions have limited impact on developing blood policy decisions; society appears to accept that the value of protecting a nation's blood supply from pathogen infection could transcend standard cost considerations. In addition, lessons appear to have been absorbed from the HIV epidemic, in which economics-based decisions could not control, and in fact inadvertently contributed to, the spread of the epidemic. Finally, policymakers fear litigation if their decisions with respect to infectious disease control are later shown to be irresponsible.[37]

Continued vigilance may present a major financial burden, but is currently considered to be worthwhile in the face of the continuous emergence of new pathogens potentially transmissible through blood and blood products. It is important that this attitude be reinforced in the years to come, when the incidence of emerging pathogens is unlikely to diminish while the costs of pathogen control are likely to increase.

Addressing the Threat

Vigilance requires the establishment of a public health infrastructure that can operate appropriately in response to a crisis. This will need to include improved surveillance, constantly reviewed and updated to respond to emerging diseases. Since emerging pathogens occur worldwide, effective surveillance must be global.[2] Currently the Centers for Disease Control and Prevention collaborates with the World Health Organization on surveillance and reporting of emerging infectious disease.

To ensure that emerging pathogens are identified quickly and efficiently, research into new technology is of primary importance. To be effective in protecting the blood supply and blood products these techniques should include improvement in detection, blood screening, and viral inactivation processes, as well as reducing exposure of patients to animal proteins capable of transmitting infectious pathogens.

Conclusion

Currently available hemophilia therapies have varying levels of exposure and vulnerability to contamination by blood-borne pathogens, reflecting the degree to which they incorporate components of human- or animal-derived plasma or albumin. Wherever possible, levels of vulnerability should be reduced, and those therapies with the least exposure to human- or animal-derived proteins, and therefore the lowest levels of vulnerability, should be made widely available.

Continued vigilance over the nation's—and the world's—blood supply is critical as long as infectious disease is a possibility, which is to say, far into the foreseeable future. Infectious pathogens are formidable opponents; they have the ability to change their genetic blueprint to adapt to new hosts or to cause variant diseases within new hosts. Globalization is increasing risks for pathogen emergence, and populations likely to be susceptible to new infectious diseases are growing in size. To proactively devote appropriate resources to infectious disease containment and prevention prior to an epidemic should be perceived as both essential public health policy and cost-effective.

References

1. Centers for Disease Control and Prevention (CDC): Preventing Emerging Infectious Diseases: A Strategy for the 21st Century. US Department of Health and Human Services. Atlanta, GA, Centers for Disease Control and Prevention, October 1998
2. Smolinski MS, Hamburg MA, Lederberg J (eds): Microbial Threats to Health: Emergence, Detection, and Response. National Institutes of Health. Washington, DC, National Academies Press, 2003
3. Ikeda Y, Nakamura K, Miyazawa T, Tohya Y, Takahashi E, Mochizuki M: Feline host range of canine parvovirus: Recent emergence of new antigenic types in cats. Emerg Infect Dis 8:341-346, 2002
4. Azzi A, Morfini M, Mannucci PM: The transfusion-associated transmission of parvovirus B19. Transfus Med Rev 13:194-204, 1999
5. Hayakawa F, Imada K, Towatari M, Saito H: Life-threatening human parvovirus B19 infection transmitted by intravenous immune globulin. Br J Haematol 118:1187-1189, 2002
6. Carpenter JL: Feline panleukopenia: Clinical signs and differential diagnosis. J Am Vet Med Assoc 158:857-859, 1971
7. Michigan Society for Medical Research (MISMR): Disease brochures. Canine Parvo Virus. Available at: http://www.mismr.org/educational/parvo.html, accessed December 2005
8. Weimer T, Streichert S, Watson C, Gröner A: High-titer screening PCR: A successful strategy for reducing the parvovirus B19 load in plasma pools for fractionation. Transfusion 41:1500-1504, 2001
9. Morfini M, Azzi A, Mannucci PM: B19 parvovirus withstands "super heating" in antihemophilic concentrates. Thromb Haemost 76:821, 1996 (letter)
10. Croghan DL, Matchett A, Koski TA: Isolation of porcine parvovirus from commercial trypsin. Appl Microbiol 26:431-433, 1973
11. Coumau E, Peynet J, Harzic M, Beal G, Castaigne S, Leverger G, et al: Severe parvovirus B19 infection in an immunocompetent child with hemophilia A. Arch Pediatr 3:35-39, 1996
12. Yee TT, Cohen BJ, Pasi KJ, Lee CA: Transmission of symptomatic parvovirus B19 infection by clotting factor concentrate. Br J Haematol 93:457-459, 1996
13. Matsui H, Sugimoto M, Tsuji S, Shima M, Giddings J, Yoshioka A: Transient hypoplastic anemia caused by primary human parvovirus B19 infection in a previously untreated patient with hemophilia transfused with a plasma-derived, monoclonal antibody-purified factor VIII concentrate. J Pediatr Hematol Oncol 21:74-76, 1999
14. Koenigbauer UF, Eastlund T, Day JW: Clinical illness due to parvovirus B19 infection after infusion of solvent/detergent-treated pooled plasma. Transfusion 40:1203-1206, 2000
15. Eis-Hubinger AM, Sasowski U, Brackmann HH, Kaiser R, Matz B, Schneweis KE: Parvovirus B19 DNA is frequently present in recombinant coagulation factor VIII products. Thromb Haemost 76:1120, 1996 (letter)
16. Eis-Hubinger AM, Sasowski U, Brackmann HH: Parvovirus B19 DNA contamination in coagulation factor VIII products. Thromb Haemost 81:476-477, 1999
17. Abe H, Sugawara H, Hirayama J, Ihara H, Kato T, Ikeda H, et al: Removal of parvovirus B19 from hemoglobin solution by nanofiltration. Artif Cells Blood Substit Immobil Biotechnol 28:375-383, 2000
18. Wong KT, Shieh WJ, Zaki SR, Tan CT: Nipah virus infection, an emerging paramyxoviral zoonosis. Springer Semin Immunopathol 24:215-228, 2002
19. Chua KB, Goh KJ, Wong KT, Kamarulzaman A, Tan PS, Ksiazek TG, et al: Fatal encephalitis due to Nipah virus among pig farmers in Malaysia. Lancet 354:1257-1259, 1999
20. World Health Organization: Weekly Epidemiological Record 79:161-172, 2004
21. Choi C: Nipah's return: The lethal "flying fox" virus may spread between people. Scientific American.com [serial online]. September 13, 2004. Available at: http://www.sciam.com/article.cfm?articleID=0006321E-8ECD-111B-87CB83414B7F0000&sc=I100322, accessed December 2005
22. Tawara A, Akahane Y, Takahashi M, Nishizawa T, Ishikawa T, Okamoto H: Transmission of human TT virus of genotype 1a to chimpanzees with fecal supernatant or serum from patients with acute TTV infection. Biochem Biophys Res Commun 278:470-476, 2000
23. Simmonds P: TT virus infection: A novel virus-host relationship. J Med Microbiol 51:455-458, 2002
24. Ball JK, Curran R, Berridge S, Grabowska AM, Jameson CL, Thomson BJ, et al: TT virus sequence heterogeneity in vivo: Evidence for co-infection with multiple genetic types. J Gen Virol 80:1759-1768, 1999
25. Ohto H, Ujiie N, Takeuchi C, Sato A, Hayashi A, Ishiko H, et al: TT virus infection during childhood. Transfusion 42:892-898, 2002
26. Knight RSG, Will RG: Prion diseases. J Neurol Neurosurg Psychiatry 75:i36-i42, 2004 (suppl 1)
27. Prusiner SB: Prion diseases and the BSE crisis. Science 278:245-251, 1997
28. Llewelyn CA, Hewitt, PE, Knight RSG, Amar K, Cousens S, Mackenzie

J, et al: Possible transmission of variant Creutzfeldt-Jakob disease by blood transfusion. Lancet 363:417-421, 2004
29. The National Creutzfeldt-Jakob Disease Surveillance Unit: CJD statistics. Available at: http://www.cjd.ed.ac.uk/figures.htm, accessed December 2005
30. Health Protection Agency Communicable Disease Surveillance Centre: Incidence of Variant Creutzfeldt-Jakob Disease Onsets and Deaths in the UK: January 1994-December 2004. Quarterly Report, January 19, 2005
31. Peden AH, Head MW, Ritchie DL, Bell JE, Ironside JW: Preclinical vCJD after blood transfusion in a PRNP codon 129 heterozygous patient. Lancet 364:527-529, 2004
32. World Federation of Hemophilia (WFH): TSE Task Force bulletin on vCJD risk in U.K.-sourced plasma products. September 2004. Available at: http://www.hemophilia.ca/en/4.2.1.php, accessed December 2005
33. World Federation of Hemophilia (WFH): Update on vCJD and plasma products produced in France. December 14, 2004.
34. AuBuchon JP, Birkmeyer JD, Busch MP: Cost-effectiveness of expanded human immunodeficiency virus-testing protocols for donated blood. Transfusion 37:45-51, 1997
35. Custer B: Economic analyses of blood safety and transfusion medicine interventions: A systematic review. Transfus Med Rev 18:127-143, 2004
36. Aledort LM: Economic aspects of haemophilia care. Haemophilia 5:216-219, 1999
37. Weinberg PD, Hounshell J, Sherman LA, Godwin J, Ali S, Tomori C, et al. Legal, financial, and public health consequences of HIV contamination of blood and blood products in the 1980s and 1990s. Ann Intern Med 136:312-319, 2002

ELSEVIER

Seminars in
HEMATOLOGY

Consideration in Hemophilia Therapy Selection

Steven Pipe

The risk of pathogen transmission via clotting factor therapies has been reduced over the last two decades through the development of effective and progressively more sensitive pathogen screening and inactivation methods and the introduction of recombinant clotting factors for hemophilia, beginning with recombinant factor VIII (FVIII) in 1992. However, new understanding about the potential for transmission of an emerging infectious agent through blood and blood products has renewed concerns about vulnerabilities that remain in plasma-derived and some recombinant clotting therapies that still use plasma components during some stages of the manufacturing process. In the 1980s, patients with hemophilia became "canaries in the coal mine" for human immunodeficiency virus (HIV) and hepatitis C virus (HCV) in the blood supply. Moving forward, healthcare providers must continue to take a proactive role in educating themselves about new information regarding emerging pathogens and develop approaches to discussing this risk with their patients as part of their therapy selection process.
Semin Hematol 43(suppl 3):S23-S27

The development of recombinant clotting factors therapies, for which protein is synthesized in mammalian cell culture instead of extracted from blood, in the past 15 years was fueled by several issues of concern to the hemophilia community. The need to increase the capacity of supply of clotting factor therapies, concerns regarding the vulnerabilities of plasma-derived clotting factors to infectious disease risk, and the demand for increased affordability and availability in the developing world all contributed to the development of these new therapies.[1] Although only some of these issues have been addressed adequately in this new era of recombinant therapies, recombinant clotting factors have been embraced in the developed world and have proven to be highly effective and safe in on-demand and prophylactic regimens, with similar risks for inhibitor development as plasma-derived concentrates.

This review will address healthcare providers' responsibility in the selection of a clotting factor replacement therapy, and the issues that they should discuss with patients as a part of the decision-making process. Clinical considerations include the progress in pathogen screening and inactivation, the risks of pathogen transmission that remain in some therapies, and the fear of developing inhibitors that makes many patients reluctant to change therapies.

Hemophilia and Coagulation Disorders Program, University of Michigan, Ann Arbor, MI.

Address correspondence to Steven Pipe, MD, Pediatric Medical Director, Hemophilia and Coagulation Disorders Program, University of Michigan, Room L2110 Women's Hospital, 1500 E Medical Center Dr, Ann Arbor, MI 48109. E-mail: ummdswp@med.umich.edu

Increasing Use of Recombinant Therapies

In 2004, the US Centers for Disease Control and Prevention (CDC) reported on the distribution of clotting factor therapies among the nearly 14,000 persons with clotting disorders who had registered in the CDC's Universal Data Collection surveillance program, beginning in 1998.[2] In the 12 months preceding entry into the surveillance program, the majority of patients with hemophilia A (62.7%) and hemophilia B (56.1%) had used a recombinant therapy (Table 1).[2] This is reflective of similar trends in Europe, where in some cases recombinant therapy is used exclusively, particularly in pediatric patients.[3-5]

The Healthcare Provider's Responsibilities in Therapy Selection

The hemophilia community has developed deep beliefs and concerns about its access to treatment options and the appropriate conditions for making therapy selections. Patients with hemophilia have embraced the concept of "patient choice" to allow both their unrestricted access to all therapy choices and their right to full participation in the final decision on therapy choice. The steady trend detected among private third-party payers to reduce patient therapy options through formulary limitations is cause for major concern for members of the hemophilia community.

0037-1963/06/$-see front matter
doi:10.1053/j.seminhematol.2006.02.002

Table 1 Blood and Factor Replacement Options Used by People in the 12 Months Preceding Their Enrollment in the CDC Universal Data Collection Program Between May 1998 Through December 2003

Therapy	Hemophilia A (n = 8,365)		Hemophilia B (n = 2,284)		von Willebrand Disease (n = 2,981)	
	n	%	n	%	n	%
Recombinant factor	5243	62.7	1281	56.1	13	0.4
Monoclonal FVIII	1426	17.1	3	0.1	4	0.1
Other human factor FVII	182	2.2	2	0.1	581	19.5
Porcine FVIII	10	0.1	0	-	0	-
Purified FIX	6	0.1	464	20.3	0	-
Prothrombin complex	32	0.4	26	1.1	0	-
Activated prothrombin	290	3.5	22	1.0	0	-
Cryoprecipitate of FFP	50	0.6	6	0.3	38	1.3
Desompressin	680	8.1	9	0.4	1250	41.9
None	973	11.6	520	22.8	1136	38.1

NOTE: Individuals may have used more than one type of treatment product.
Abbreviation: FFP, fresh-frozen plasma.

The availability of recombinant clotting factor therapies and the extensive donor deferral and viral inactivation procedures for plasma-derived therapies have allayed many practitioners' concerns about blood-borne infectious disease transmission: many practitioners who treat hemophilia believe that the safety of current therapies is sufficient.[5,6] For pediatric hemophilia treaters, cases of patients infected with human immunodeficiency virus (HIV) and hepatitis C virus (HCV) are no longer common. However, the mainstream media cover reports of new emerging pathogens, both airborne and blood-borne, as frequently as scientific journals. Recent reports in the medical literature have linked some of these pathogens to transfusion and blood-derived therapies. As a result, hemophilia treaters need to be able to clearly and knowledgably respond to their patients' questions and concerns about the most effective and safe treatments for their individual circumstances.

Overview of Hemophilia Therapy Selection Criteria

In order to comprehensively and appropriately guide patient selection in hemophilia therapy, it is necessary to consider all the following criteria:

- Safety and efficacy
- Potential for inhibitor development
- Convenience
- Consistency of supply
- Company reputation
- Cost-benefit ratio
- Reimbursement
- Patient preference

Safety and efficacy are, as with most therapies, the most important criteria in therapy selection, but the choice in hemophilia therapy is substantially complicated by fear of inhibitor development. Convenience is also of great importance for patients, particularly for those on prophylaxis, because they may receive infusions up to three times per week. As evidenced by the therapy shortages experienced worldwide in 2001 as a result of manufacturing and documentation problems, availability and consistency of a therapy's supply are also important.[6,7] Because efficacy among therapies is generally equivalent and many safety risks are still theoretical, cost-benefit ratios still play a role in a patient's choice of therapy.[3-7] Absolute cost concerns are complicated by the realities of a patient's reimbursement situation, particularly as formulary restrictions imposed by private third-party payers become more common.

Discussing new therapies with patients may be difficult because the clinician needs to maintain trust by being honest about potential risks while minimizing fear and anxiety.[8,9] This can lead to seemingly contradictory situations. For example, patients with hemophilia A or B are generally encouraged to select recombinant therapies over plasma derivatives because recombinant therapies have reduced vulnerabilities to emerging pathogens. Yet patients with von Willebrand disease, for which there is no recombinant factor therapy, must be reassured that treatment with screened and virally inactivated plasma derivatives is the safest available option. In this scenario, potential risk to the patient is to be balanced with the need to treat with an effective product.

In the next section, we will look more closely at two of these selection criteria, safety and the potential for inhibitor development.

Selection Criteria: Safety From Blood-Borne Pathogens

Safety and efficacy have long been the most important considerations in selection of factor replacement therapy.[5,6,10,11] Safety with regard to infectious pathogen risk has been enhanced through effective and progressively more sensitive pathogen screening of blood products and their derivatives. Most known blood-borne pathogens are identifiable, but a high degree of sensitivity in their identification is less common.

Pathogen Screening

Presently, each unit of blood donated in the United States is routinely screened for seven pathogens with a series of 10 tests.[12] Three types of tests are utilized: serologic (antibody), antigen (viral protein), and nucleic acid amplification technology (NAT). A screening test for syphilis has been part of routine laboratory testing on every unit of blood (or blood component) for transfusion for nearly 60 years. Testing for hepatitis B virus (HBV) became mandatory in 1972. Today there are two different tests: a hepatitis B surface antigen test (HBsAg) and a serologic test for antibodies to the hepatitis B core protein (anti-HBc). Serologic testing for two rare retroviruses, human T-lymphotropic virus (HTLV)-I and HTLV-II, began in 1989.

Significant progress in HIV testing has been achieved over the past two decades. This progress reflects not only improvements in the development of more sensitive assays and better molecular biology techniques to detect the virus but also a greater understanding of the viral life cycle. The first tests to detect HIV infection were serologic-based tests.[13] Despite this giant leap forward, it was soon recognized that a "window" period existed. Defined as the time between infection and detectable seroconversion, this period could extend from 22 days up to 6 months; thus, a high percentage of blood from infected donors tested negative for HIV. To reduce the window period, more stringent detection methods were developed to measure HIV protein (viremia), and in 1996 the HIV p24 antigen testing of donated blood was approved by the US Food and Drug Administration (FDA). However, this assay only shortened the window to approximately 16 days. With the advent of polymerase chain reaction testing to detect genetic material (RNA/DNA), a new NAT test became available. This further reduced the preseroconversion window to about 11 days. Furthermore, the NAT test has a specificity of 99.5% and sensitivity of detection of 99.5% for samples containing HIV-1 RNA at $\geq$100 copies/mL.[13] The FDA indicated in an industry guidance letter issued in October 2004 that all blood collection and processing organizations would need to fully implement HIV-1 NAT testing procedures by mid 2005.[14]

Similarly, testing for other infectious agents has also progressed. Serologic testing for HCV (previously referred to as non-A, non-B hepatitis) started in 1990, and the FDA approved a NAT test for HCV in 2002 and a NAT test for West Nile virus (WNV) in December 2005. Prior to the approval of the WNV test, it was used on an investigational basis, and blood centers implemented supplementary precautionary measures to protect the blood supply, including stockpiling frozen blood components before the start of mosquito season. Currently, there is no commercially available test for prions, the agents responsible for variant Creutzfeldt-Jakob disease (vCJD).[12]

Ongoing pathogen threats to the blood supply often reflect not the difficulty of identifying the pathogen but rather the difficulty of developing a test with high sensitivity. Thus, many years may elapse between the detection, isolation, and sequencing of a new pathogen and the development, rigorous testing, FDA approval, and wide dissemination of a highly sensitive test. For example, almost 20 years elapsed between 1984, when HIV was first identified as the cause of acquired immunodeficiency syndrome (AIDS), and approval by the FDA in 2002 of an HIV NAT test. Yet, once developed and proven, the impact of a highly sensitive screening test can be enormous: the current safety evaluations on HIV in the blood supply estimate that fewer than one in 1,900,000 blood components are capable of transmitting HIV undetected by NAT testing.[12] And with the advent of testing for genetic material, less time elapsed between the identification of WNV in 1999 and the development of a responsive NAT test in 2003.[15]

Pathogen Inactivation

Clotting factor concentrate safety has also been enhanced through improved viral inactivation processes. Physical and chemical reduction techniques are employed during the manufacturing process to reduce and inactivate viruses. The effectiveness of such procedures concerning individual pathogens directly reflects the physical characteristics of the pathogen in question.

Of the currently known blood-borne pathogens, HIV, HBV, HCV, WNV, and severe acquired respiratory syndrome (SARS) are all lipid-enveloped[16,17] and can contain double-stranded RNA or DNA. Non–lipid-enveloped viruses include hepatitis A virus (HAV) and parvovirus B19 (PVB19).[18] This group also includes members of the reovirus, adenovirus, polyomavirus, papillomavirus, and (in pigs) circovirus families, and can contain double- or single-stranded RNA or DNA. PrP^{Sc} and PrP^{Res}, abnormal forms of the soluble protein particle (prion) PrP^{C}, have been implicated in transmissible spongiform encephalopathies in humans (eg, vCJD)[19] and animals (eg, "mad cow" disease), respectively.

All licensed plasma products and human/animal protein-added recombinant products use validated methods to detect and eliminate HCV, HBV, HIV, and all other enveloped viruses. The presence of a lipid envelope to protect a virus's genetic material enables modern manufacturing processing methods to efficiently eliminate and inactivate that virus. These procedures ensure a very high margin of safety with respect to the likelihood of viral transmission.

Techniques needed to inactivate non–lipid-enveloped viruses are less reliable than those used for lipid-enveloped viruses.[20,21] Inactivation of non–lipid-enveloped viruses by vapor heating, solvent/detergent, and gamma irradiation in lyophilized products is either not at all or only partly effective. In addition, systematic inactivation of non–lipid-enveloped viruses requires a physicochemical environment that compromises factor VIII (FVIII) activity.[22] Finally, the small size of some non–lipid-enveloped viruses—notably PVB19—requires filter sizes generally not practical for the successful large-scale filtration of commercial blood products.[23]

As effective blood product screening and inactivation procedures have been implemented, the incidence of viruses in therapies, in particular lipid-enveloped viruses such as HIV, HBV, and HCV, has dropped dramatically.[24] As a result, it is tempting to feel confident and become complacent about the safety of the nation's blood supply. Figure 2 of Bruce Evatt's article in this issue shows the evolution of residual risk of infection per unit transfused in the United States from 1985 to 2001. However, as reported in other articles in this supplement, new understanding about the potential for transmission of an emerging infectious agent (eg, WNV or PrP^{Sc}) through blood and blood products has renewed concerns about vulnerabilities that remain in both recombinant and plasma-derived clotting therapies.

Proactive Measures to Protect Clotting Factor Concentrates

Since the approval of the first generation of recombinant FVIII clotting therapies in 1992, most patients with hemophilia have switched from plasma-derived to recombinant therapies.[25,26] In 1994, the majority of Canadian patients with hemophilia A were prescribed recombinant FVIII.[27] This decision was made by the Canadian Blood Agency at the advice of the Association of Hemophilia Clinic Directors of Canada, which considered recombinant FVIII to be the safest replacement therapy available. This proactive decision was made despite the fact that there have been no documented transmissions of HIV, HBV, or HCV with any of the plasma-derived therapies currently available,[28] based on the theory that previously unrecognized pathogens may gain access to the blood donor pool.

It is important to note that some recombinant therapies are not completely free of human- or animal-derived protein additives, and thus they remain capable of transmitting blood-borne infectious agents. A number of hemophilia organizations, including the National Hemophilia Foundation,[28] The United Kingdom Haemophilia Centre Doctors' Organisation,[29] and the Association of Hemophilia Clinic Directors of Canada,[30] recommended that every effort be made to remove all human- and animal-derived proteins from blood therapies. As a result, human albumin used in the final formulation of the original recombinant therapies has been replaced by sucrose in later recombinant FVIII therapies.[31] In 2003, an advanced generation of recombinant FVIII was approved for use by the FDA.[32] In this therapy, animal- and human-derived protein have been eliminated from all stages of processing, including from the cell culture medium and the final formulation.

Selection Criteria: Concerns About Inhibitor Development

In addition to issues of product safety and efficacy, patients with hemophilia are concerned about the potential for inhibitor development. Inhibitors that develop in a patient in response to one FVIII clotting therapy will not only make that therapy but all FVIII clotting therapies ineffective. Up to 30% of previously untreated patients[33] and approximately 1% of previously treated patients[34] develop inhibitors. No particular therapy is associated with increased inhibitor development: ongoing research and debate have identified no notable difference in inhibitor development among currently available therapies. Randomized trials comparing the incidence of inhibitor development in previously untreated patients receiving recombinant clotting factors to those receiving plasma-derived clotting factors have not been done, but the available literature suggests that they are very similar.[35-37] However, the likelihood for inhibitor development following any individual patient's treatment with any given therapy is currently unpredictable.

Understandably, patients for whom one therapy has been effective are reluctant to relinquish that security by changing therapies. Even when they thought another therapy was safer, patients have been resistant to switching to new products.[3,8] Concerns may include a perceived potential to increase inhibitor development, increased costs or reduced efficacy. In addition, many patients prefer to postpone adoption of a newly approved therapy that has only limited clinical exposure in order to see if the therapy will continue to be found safe and effective in larger numbers of patients.[3]

Although there was a mass adoption of heat-treated products in the 1980s, in that case the willingness to switch was informed by the knowledge that the heat-treated therapies eliminated HIV, as well as other pathogens, from the blood supply.[38] This situation reflected the extreme circumstances of that time; similar crisis decision-making has also impacted recent policies in the UK in response to transfusion-associated vCJD.[39-41] However, as seen in Canada in 1994, government agencies have made the proactive decision to transition patients to the use of recombinant therapies, without evidence of an imminent threat to the blood supply and despite concerns over increased costs and the potential for increased inhibitor formation.

Conclusion

Patients with hemophilia have expressed that, historically, they have been the "canaries in the coal mine" for HIV in the blood supply. Healthcare providers, government, and industry have an ongoing responsibility to be proactive about threats to patient safety, even when levels of acceptable risk are hard to define. Clinicians should work closely with patients to choose the safest and most appropriate hemophilia therapy, especially when the criteria for selection are complex and competitive.

References

1. Hilgartner MW: The need for recombinant factor VIII: Historical background and rationale. Semin Hematol 28:6-9, 1991 (suppl 1)
2. Centers for Disease Control and Prevention: Report on the Universal Data Collection Program, 6 (No. 2), 2004. Available at http://www.cdc.gov/ncbddd/hbd/documents/UDC6(2).pdf, accessed November 2005
3. Mauser-Bunschoten EP, Roosendaal G, van den Berg HM: Product choice and haemophilia treatment in the Netherlands. Haemophilia 7:96-98, 2001

4. Mantovani LG, Monzini MS, Mannucci PM, Scalone L, Villa M, Gringeri A: Differences between patients', physicians' and pharmacists' preferences for treatment products in haemophilia: A discrete choice experiment. Haemophilia 11:589-597, 2005
5. Brown SA, Aledort LM, Lee CA: Issues in making a therapeutic choice: Recombinant and/or human-derived products. Haemophilia 6:125-129, 2000
6. Aledort LM: Making a therapeutic choice: Human versus recombinant fractions—Can we do it? Haemophilia 7:1-3, 2001 (suppl 1)
7. Farrugia A: Evolving perspectives in product safety for haemophilia. Haemophilia 8:236-243, 2002
8. Miller R: The responsibility of separating truth from myth to patient and family. Haemophilia 7:91-95, 2001
9. Magli-Barioz D, Ounnoughene N, Paugy P, Quarre MC, Vassilief D, Lopez I, et al: Evaluation of the impact of information about treatment-related risks in patients receiving blood-derived or recombinant medications. Haemophilia 10:572-581, 2004
10. Giangrande PL: Treatment of hemophilia: Recombinant factors only? Yes. J Thromb Haemost 1:214-215, 2003
11. Kasper CK: Concentrate safety and efficacy. Haemophilia 8:161-165, 2002
12. AABB: All About Blood. Available at: http://www.aabb.org/All_About-_Blood/FAQs/aabb_faqs.htm, accessed December 2005
13. Giachetti C, Linnen JM, Kolk DP, Dockter J, Gillotte-Taylor K, Park M, et al: Highly sensitive multiplex assay for detection of human immunodeficiency virus type 1 and hepatitis C virus RNA. J Clin Microbiol 40:2408-2419, 2002
14. Food and Drug Administration: Guidance for Industry: Use of Nucleic Acid Tests on Pooled and Individual Samples from Donors of Whole Blood and Blood Components (including Source Plasma and Source Leukocytes) to Adequately and Appropriately Reduce the Risk of Transmission of HIV-1 and HCV. Rockville, MD, US Department of Health and Human Services, Food and Drug Administration, Center for Biologics Evaluation and Research, 2004
15. Centers for Disease Control and Prevention: Update: West Nile Virus screening of blood donations and transfusion-associated transmission—United States, 2003. MMWR Morb Mortal Wkly Rep 53:281-284, 2004
16. Rajcani J: Molecular mechanisms of virus spread and virion components as tools of virulence. A review. Acta Microbiol Immunol Hung 50:407-431, 2003
17. Klempner MS, Shapiro DS: Crossing the species barrier—One small step to man, one giant leap to mankind. N Engl J Med 350:1171-1172, 2004
18. Chandran K, Farsetta DL, Nibert ML: Strategy for nonenveloped virus entry: A hydrophobic conformer of the reovirus membrane penetration protein micro 1 mediates membrane disruption. J Virol 76:9920-9933, 2002
19. Knight RS, Will RG: Prion diseases. J Neurol Neurosurg Psychiatry 75:i36-i42, 2004 (suppl 1)
20. Jakubik JJ, Vicik SM, Tannatt MM, Kelley BD: West Nile virus inactivation by the solvent/detergent steps of the second and third generation manufacturing processes for B-domain deleted recombinant factor VIII. Haemophilia 10:69-74, 2004
21. Goodnough LT: Risks of blood transfusion. Crit Care Med 31:678-686, 2003 (suppl 12)
22. Miekka SI, Busby TF, Reid B, Pollock R, Ralston A, Drohan WN: New methods for inactivation of lipid-enveloped and non-enveloped viruses. Haemophilia 4:402-408, 1998
23. Yokoyama T, Murai K, Murozuka T, Wakisaka A, Tanifuji M, Fujii N, et al: Removal of small non-enveloped viruses by nanofiltration. Vox Sang 86:225-229, 2004
24. Soucie JM, Richardson LC, Evatt BL, Linden JV, Ewenstein BM, Stein SF, et al: Risk factors for infection with HBV and HCV in a large cohort of hemophiliac males. Transfusion 41:338-343, 2001
25. Chambost H, Ljung R: Changing pattern of care of boys with haemophilia in western European centres. Haemophilia 11:92-99, 2005
26. Giangrande P. Haemophilia B: Christmas disease. Expert Opin Pharmacother 6:1517-1524, 2005
27. Giles AR, Rivard GE, Teitel J, Walker I: Surveillance for factor VIII inhibitor development in the Canadian Hemophilia A population following the widespread introduction of recombinant factor VIII replacement therapy. Transfus Sci 19:139-148, 1998
28. National Hemophilia Foundation: MASAC recommendations concerning the treatment of hemophilia and other bleeding disorders. MASAC Document #151, Nov 2003. Available at: www.hemophilia.org/research/masac/masac151.pdf, accessed July 2004
29. United Kingdom Haemophilia Centre Doctors' Organisation: Guidelines on the selection and use of therapeutic products to treat haemophilia and other hereditary bleeding disorders. Haemophilia 9:1-23, 2003
30. Association of Hemophilia Clinic Directors of Canada: Clinical Practice Guidelines: Hemophilia and von Willebrand's Disease (2. Management; Update 2). July 7, 1999. Available at http://www.ahcdc.ca/Management.htm, accessed December 2005
31. Abshire TC, Brackmann HH, Scharrer I, Hoots K, Gazengel C, Powell JS, et al: Sucrose formulated recombinant human antihemophilic factor VIII is safe and efficacious for treatment of hemophilia A in home therapy—International Kogenate-FS Study Group. Thromb Haemost 83:811-816, 2000
32. Mitterer A, Mundt W, Bjornson E, Dorner F: Development of an advanced category recombinant FVIII, anti-hemophilic factor (recombinant) plasma/albumin-free method (rAHF-PFM). J Thromb Haemost 1:P1652, 2003 (suppl 1, abstr)
33. Lusher JM: First and second generation recombinant factor VIII concentrates in previously untreated patients: Recovery, safety, efficacy, and inhibitor development. Semin Thromb Hemost 28:273-276, 2002
34. Gringeri A, Tagliaferri A, Tagariello G, Morfini M, Santagostino E, Mannucci P, for the ReFacto-AICE Study Group: Efficacy and inhibitor development in previously treated patients with haemophilia A switched to a B domain-deleted recombinant factor VIII. Br J Haematol 126:398-404, 2004
35. Lusher JM: Hemophilia treatment. Factor VIII inhibitors with recombinant products: Prospective clinical trials. Haematologica 85:2-5, 2000 (suppl 10)
36. Mauser-Bunschoten EP, van der Bom JG, Bongers M, Twijnstra M, Roosendaal G, Fischer K, et al: Purity of factor VIII product and incidence of inhibitors in previously untreated patients with haemophilia A. Haemophilia 7:364-368, 2001
37. Scharrer I, Bray GL, Neutzling O: Incidence of inhibitors in haemophilia A patients—A review of recent studies of recombinant and plasma-derived factor VIII concentrates. Haemophilia 5:145-154, 1999
38. Mannucci PM, Schimpf K, Abe T, Aledort LM, Anderle K, Brettler DB, et al: Low risk of viral infection after administration of vapor-heated factor VIII concentrate. International Investigator Group. Transfusion 32:134-138, 1992
39. Ironside JW: The spectrum of safety: Variant Creutzfeldt-Jakob disease in the United Kingdom. Semin Hematol 40:16-22, 2003
40. Ironside JW, Head MW: Variant Creutzfeldt-Jakob disease: Risk of transmission by blood and blood products. Haemophilia 10:64-69, 2004 (suppl 4)
41. Dunstan RA, Alpers MP: Variant Creutzfeldt-Jakob disease: implications for the health care system. Aust NZ J Public Health 29:308-312, 2005

ELSEVIER
SAUNDERS
email: reprints@elsevier.com

Vol 43, No 2, Suppl 4 April 2006

Supplement to

Seminars in HEMATOLOGY

Neal S. Young · Photis Beris
Editors

Current Opinion on Management of Inhibitor Therapy

Cindy A. Leissinger
Guest Editor

W.B. Saunders

Seminars in HEMATOLOGY

Neal S. Young · Photis Beris
Editors

Peter A. Miescher, *Founding Editor* Ernst R. Jaffé, *Co-Editor Emeritus*

Editorial correspondence should be addressed to Photis Beris, MD, Division d'Hématologie, Hôpital Cantonal Universitaire, 25 rue Micheli-du-Crest, 1211 Geneve 14, Switzerland, or Neal S. Young, MD, 4400 17th Street, NW, Washington, DC 20011.

Business correspondence (subscriptions, change of address) should be addressed to the Publisher, Elsevier, 6277 Sea Harbor Dr, Orlando, FL 32887-4800; Email elspcs@elsevier.com.

Change of address notices, including both the old and new addresses of the subscriber, should be sent at least one month in advance.

Customer Service: 1-800-654-2452; outside the United States and Canada, (407) 345-4000.

Yearly subscription rates: United States and possessions: individual, $169.00; institution, $267.00; single issues, $81.00. All other countries: individual, $239.00; institution, $339.00; single issues, $81.00. Student and resident: United States and possessions, and Canada: $85.00; all other countries: $122.00. To receive student/resident rate, orders must be accompanied by name of affiliated institution, date of term, and the *signature* of program/residency coordinator on institution letterhead. Orders will be billed at individual rate until proof of status is received. Current prices are in effect for back volumes and back issues. Single issues, both current and back, exist in limited quantities and are offered for sale subject to availability. Back issues sold in conjunction with a subscription are on a prorated basis. Prices are subject to change without notice. *Checks* should be made payable to Elsevier and sent to *Seminars in Hematology*, Elsevier, Periodicals Department, PO Box 628239, Orlando, FL 32862-8239.

Other correspondence (copyediting, production) should be addressed to Elsevier, 1600 John F. Kennedy Blvd, Ste 1800, Philadelphia, PA 19103-2899.

Reprints: For 100 or more copies of an article in this publication, please contact the Commercial Reprints Department, Elsevier, 360 Park Ave South, New York, NY 10010-1710. Telephone (212) 633-3813, fax (212) 633-3820; e-mail, reprints@elsevier.com.

Advertising Representative: Cunningham Associates, PO Box 308, Park Ridge, NJ 07656. Telephone (201) 767-4170.

The contents of *Seminars in Hematology* are indexed in *Index Medicus* and *MEDLINE, Current Contents/Clinical Medicine, Current Contents/Life Sciences,* Science Citation Index, and *EMBASE/* Excerpta Medica.

The *Seminars in Hematology* home page is located at *www.seminhematol.org.*

W.B. Saunders **Philadelphia, PA**

Seminars in HEMATOLOGY

Vol 43, No 2, Supplement 4, April 2006

Current Opinion on Management of Inhibitor Therapy

Cindy A. Leissinger
Guest Editor

Inhibitor Development in Patients With Hemophilia: An Overview S1
Cindy A. Leissinger

Overview of Inhibitors S3
Jan Astermark

Current Opinion on Inhibitor Treatment Options S8
Prasad Mathew

Inhibitor Economics S14
Jerome Teitel

Surgery in Patients With Hemophilia and Inhibitors: A Review of the Norwegian Experience With FEIBA S18
Geir E. Tjønnfjord

Seminars in
HEMATOLOGY

Current Opinion on Management of Inhibitor Therapy

Cindy A. Leissinger

Guest Editor

The articles in this supplement are based on presentations made during the 2004 World Federation of Hemophilia Congress in Montreal, Québec, Canada.

This supplement was made possible by an unrestricted educational grant from Baxter Healthcare SA.

ELSEVIER

Seminars in
HEMATOLOGY

Volume 43, Number 2, Supplement 4 **April 2006**

Inhibitor Development in Patients With Hemophilia: An Overview

The development of inhibitors in patients with hemophilia is a serious complication that results in limited or no response to standard therapy with factor VIII (FVIII) or factor IX (FIX) concentrates. Inhibitors are antibodies that can occur as a result of exposure to exogenous FVIII or FIX concentrates; the antibodies bind to and neutralize the activity of factor concentrates, thus reducing their efficacy.[1,2] Inhibitors develop more frequently in patients with severe hemophilia and are more prevalent in patients with hemophilia A than in patients with hemophilia B.[3] The reported cumulative incidence of inhibitors in patients with severe hemophilia A typically ranges from 20% to 30%; for hemophilia B the incidence is much lower, 5% or less.[2]

Although improvements have been made in the therapeutic regimens available to patients with hemophilia, the risk for severe bleeding complications in patients with inhibitors remains higher than in those without inhibitors.[4] Patients with inhibitors often develop repetitive, poorly controlled joint bleeds that can lead to arthropathy and cause permanent disability.[5] Until the 1990s, increased mortality rates were observed in patients with inhibitors[6]; however, with the introduction of new and more aggressive treatment strategies, mortality rates do not appear to be as high as previously reported.[7]

Inhibitor eradication with immune tolerance induction (ITI) is the most effective long-term strategy for patients with high-responding inhibitors; however, approximately 30% to 40% of all patients who undergo ITI will fail therapy,[8,9] and older patients with longstanding inhibitors are not considered candidates for ITI due to their very high failure rate. In addition, ITI is extremely costly, and thus unavailable for much of the world. Nevertheless, ITI remains the only known strategy capable of eliminating inhibitors and remains a standard of care.

For patients with inhibitors, whether undergoing ITI or not, treatment of bleeding episodes remains a major therapeutic focus. For patients with low-titer inhibitors (<5 Bethesda units [BU]), increased doses of FVIII or FIX concentrates can be used to overcome the inhibitor, especially for patients who have low-responding inhibitors that do not anamnestically rise after exposure to the deficient clotting factor. For patients with high-responding or high-titer inhibitors, bleeds are treated with bypassing agents that circumvent the effects of the inhibitor to achieve hemostasis.[10] The two bypassing agents currently available include activated prothrombin complex concentrates (aPCCs) (Factor Eight Inhibitor Bypassing Activity, Anti-Inhibitor Coagulant Complex, Vapor Heated [FEIBA; Baxter AG, Vienna, Austria]) and activated recombinant factor VII (rFVIIa; NovoSeven, Novo Nordisk A/S, Bagsvaerd, Denmark).[10]

Several factors will determine the most appropriate treatment strategy for patients with inhibitors. Patients with high-responding inhibitors of recent onset should be considered for ITI when possible. However, some patients with FIX inhibitors may not be appropriate candidates for ITI due to anaphylactic reactions to FIX and/or development of nephrotic syndrome while on FIX.[11,12] For all inhibitor patients, the choice of bypassing agents for treatment of bleeds may be influenced by a variety of factors, including the agent's duration of action, the ability to give frequent infusions, and a patient's previous experiences with the agent. Since rFVIIa has a short half-life and duration of action, it is generally dosed more frequently than FEIBA. However, FEIBA, unlike rFVIIa, contains trace amounts of FVIII, as well as large amounts of FIX. While the risk of anamnesis should be considered as a possibility in some patients on FEIBA,[13] the efficacy of FEIBA is not diminished by an anamnestic response.

Finally, the cost of therapy is a major concern when treating patients with inhibitors. Factor concentrates account for the majority of the cost associated with treating patients with hemophilia.[14] The cost of treating patients with inhibitors is generally higher than the cost of treating patients without inhibitors since bypassing agents are more expensive than FVIII or FIX concentrates. However, there is evidence suggesting that much of the cost associated with treating patients with inhibitors can be attributed to a minority of patients[15]

Address correspondence to Cindy A. Leissinger, MD, Section of Hematology/Oncology, Box SL-78, Tulane University School of Medicine, 1430 Tulane Ave, New Orleans, LA 70112. E-mail: cleissi@tulane.edu

doi:10.1053/j.seminhematol.2006.03.002

who experience serious, prolonged bleeding episodes that are difficult to control.

The development of inhibitors in patients with hemophilia is a major complication that forces physicians to make difficult choices regarding the most appropriate therapy to use, while also considering the cost of therapy. Therapeutic decisions become even more problematic when patients develop complications following treatment. The obstacles facing physicians who treat patients with inhibitors are a testament to the fact that inhibitor development continues to challenge existing treatment strategies. Despite these challenges, physicians are able to use currently available therapeutic regimens to successfully treat bleeding episodes in nearly all patients with inhibitors, while continuing to seek newer, better therapeutic options to enhance quality of life in these patients.

The content of the following supplement is based in part on the proceedings from an educational symposium entitled "Current Opinion on Management of Inhibitor Therapy" that was held at the World Federation of Hemophilia World Congress 2004 in Bangkok, Thailand. Support for the symposium and manuscripts was provided by Baxter Healthcare Corporation.

FEIBA is a trademark of Baxter Healthcare SA.

Cindy A. Leissinger
Tulane University
New Orleans, LA
Guest Editor

References

1. Evans GL, Morgan RA: Genetic induction of immune tolerance to human clotting factor VIII in a mouse model for hemophilia A. Proc Natl Acad Sci U S A 95:5734-5739, 1998
2. Kasper CK: Diagnosis and Management of Inhibitors to Factors VIII and IX. An Introductory Discussion for Physicians. Treatment of Hemophilia Monograph Series, No. 34. Montreal, Québec, Canada, World Federation of Hemophilia, 2004
3. Scharrer I, Bray GL, Neutzling O: Incidence of inhibitors in haemophilia A patients—A review of recent studies of recombinant and plasma-derived factor VIII concentrates. Haemophilia 5:145-154, 1999
4. Key NS: Inhibitors in congenital coagulation disorders. Br J Haematol 127:379-391, 2004
5. Young G, McDaniel M, Nugent DJ: Prophylactic recombinant factor VIIa in haemophilia patients with inhibitors. Haemophilia 11:203-207, 2005
6. DiMichele D, Rivard G, Hay C, Antunes S: Inhibitors in haemophilia: Clinical aspects. Haemophilia 10:140-145, 2004 (suppl 4)
7. Darby SC, Keeling DM, Spooner RJ, Wan Kan S, Giangrande PL, Collins PW, et al: The incidence of factor VIII and factor IX inhibitors in the hemophilia population of the UK and their effect on subsequent mortality, 1977-99. J Thromb Haemost 2:1047-1054, 2004
8. DiMichele D: Immune tolerance therapy dose as an outcome predictor. Haemophilia 9:382-386, 2003
9. DiMichele DM, Kroner BL, North American Immune Tolerance Study Group: The North American Immune Tolerance Registry: Practices, outcomes, outcome predictors. Thromb Haemost 87:52-57, 2002
10. DiMichele D: Inhibitors: Resolving diagnostic and therapeutic dilemmas. Haemophilia 8:280-287, 2002
11. Hay CR, Baglin TP, Collins PW, Hill FG, Keeling DM: The diagnosis and management of factor VIII and IX inhibitors: A guideline from the UK Haemophilia Centre Doctors' Organization (UKHCDO). Br J Haematol 111:78-90, 2000
12. Warrier I, Ewenstein BM, Koerper MA, Shapiro A, Key N, DiMichele D, et al: Factor IX inhibitors and anaphylaxis in hemophilia B. J Pediatr Hematol Oncol 19:23-27, 1997
13. Green D: Complications associated with the treatment of haemophiliacs with inhibitors. Haemophilia 5:11-17, 1999 (suppl 3)
14. Ross-Degnan D, Soumerai SB, Avorn J, Bohn RL, Bright R, Aledort LM: Hemophilia home treatment. Economic analysis and implications for health policy. Int J Technol Assess Health Care 11:327-344, 1995
15. Chang H, Sher GD, Blanchette VS, Teitel JM: The impact of inhibitors on the cost of clotting factor replacement therapy in haemophilia A in Canada. Haemophilia 5:247-252, 1999

ELSEVIER

Seminars in
HEMATOLOGY

Overview of Inhibitors

Jan Astermark

Inhibitory antibodies that develop in patients with hemophilia render standard therapy with factor concentrates ineffective. Several factors may influence inhibitor incidence, including genetics, the type of factor concentrate, and environment. A higher incidence of inhibitors in siblings compared to extended relatives, and in African Americans compared to Caucasians, suggests that genetics may play an important role in inhibitor development; however, genetic markers that indicate a predisposition for inhibitor development have yet to be identified. In addition, the appearance of inhibitors in immunologically challenged patients points to the role of the immune response system in the development of inhibitor antibodies, an area that warrants further study. Thus, the medical community faces the difficult task of developing new, improved therapies to combat inhibitors in patients with hemophilia, a task that will require careful consideration of the roles of environmental factors, the immune system, and genetics in inhibitor development.
Semin Hematol 43(suppl 4):S3-S7

The development of inhibitory antibodies is a serious complication in hemophilia that occurs in some patients in response to routine administration of exogenous factor VIII (FVIII) or factor IX (FIX).[1] In these cases, the replacement factor is recognized as a foreign protein by the body. In response, antibodies develop that neutralize the activity of the clotting factor. Inhibitors may be detected during routine screening, but are generally discovered when a patient whose bleeding was previously well controlled presents with increased frequency of bleeding or inadequate bleed control.[2] Until the 1990s, inhibitors were associated with an increased risk of death from major bleeding episodes; however, recent improvements in therapeutic regimens for patients with inhibitors have reduced the risk of mortality.[3]

FVIII inhibitory antibodies are polyclonal and generally of the immunoglobulin G (IgG) 4 subtype,[4] although antibodies of the IgG1 subtype also exist. Most antibodies bind to the A_2 domain and the C-terminal part of the FVIII molecule, inhibiting normal function of factor Xase complex and normal binding of phospholipids and von Willebrand factor (VWF) (Fig 1).[5] However, epitopes in the A_3 domain are also recognized.[5] Inhibitory antibodies in the plasma are quantified using the Bethesda assay, which was first described by Kasper and colleagues in 1975.[6] One Bethesda unit (BU) is defined as the amount of antibody that neutralizes 50% of FVIII or FIX in normal plasma. Since the introduction of the Bethesda assay, modifications have been made to the assay to improve the specificity and reliability of the results obtained, in order to better distinguish between inhibitor-positive and inhibitor-negative samples.[7] Despite these modifications, variability still exists in the Bethesda titer when measured by different laboratories, ranging from 30% to 80%. In addition, different cut-off levels used by laboratories to distinguish between inhibitor-positive and inhibitor-negative patients have made measurements of inhibitor incidence across different cohorts problematic.

The prevalence of inhibitors is defined as the proportion of patients with inhibitors at a given time, whereas the incidence of inhibitors is defined as the number of new cases in a defined period.[8] Overall, inhibitor incidence is much higher than inhibitor prevalence. Cumulative inhibitor incidence in patients with hemophilia ranges from 3.6% to 52% and typically varies from 20% to 30% in patients with severe hemophilia A.[1,9] The incidence in patients with hemophilia B is lower and usually less than 5%, although higher figures have been reported in some cohorts.[1,10] The variation between inhibitor prevalence, which is usually in the range of 5% to 7%,[8] and inhibitor incidence figures is attributed to the sudden disappearance of low-titer inhibitors (transient inhibitors) and the eradication of inhibitors with immune tolerance induction (ITI) therapy.

University of Lund, Malmö, Sweden.

This article is based in part on the proceedings from an educational symposium held at the World Federation of Hemophilia World Congress 2004 in Bangkok, Thailand. Both the symposium and this manuscript were supported by Baxter Healthcare Corporation.

Address correspondence to Jan Astermark, MD, PhD, Department of Hematology and Coagulation Disorders, Malmö University Hospital, SE-205 02 Malmö, Sweden. E-mail: Jan.astermark@med.lu.se

Factors Contributing to Inhibitor Development

Several factors may influence the risk of inhibitor development, such as the type of factor replacement regimen used,

0037-1963/06/$-see front matter
doi:10.1053/j.seminhematol.2006.03.006

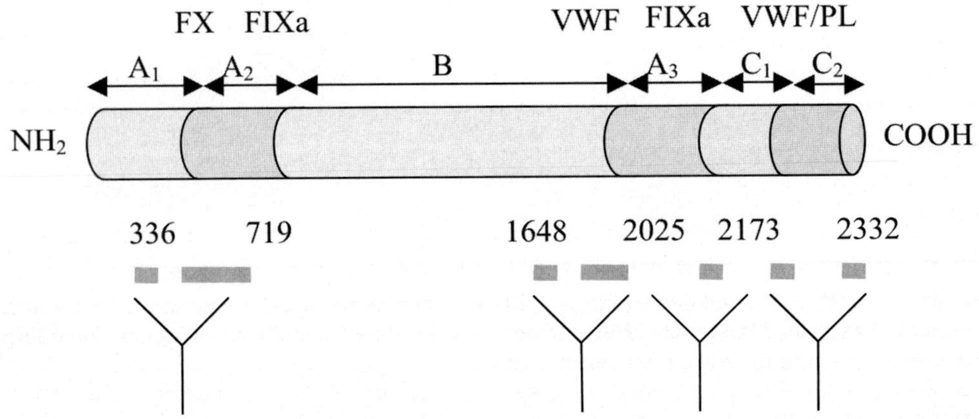

Figure 1 FVIII inhibitor binding sites. FX indicates factor X; FIXa, activated factor IX; VWF, von Willebrand factor; PL, phospholipid; A_1, A_1 domain (poorly immunogenic); A_2, A_2 domain; B, B domain (poorly immunogenic); A_3, A_3 domain; C_1, C_1 domain; C_2, C_2 domain; NH_2, amino terminal; COOH, carboxyl terminal; inhibitory antibodies and corresponding inhibitory epitopes on the FVIII protein that are assigned to specific regions are indicated at the bottom of the figure. Reprinted with permission from Blackwell Publishing.[5]

environmental factors, and genetics (Fig 2). The number of exposure days to factor concentrates and a patient's age at the time of exposure may play a role. The risk for the development of new inhibitors is typically greatest shortly after the first exposure to factor concentrates. The median number of factor exposure days before development of inhibitory antibodies is reportedly 9 to 12 days, and the inhibitors generally develop within the first 50 days following factor exposure.[2] Antibodies are less likely to develop after 200 days of treatment with factor concentrate.[2,11–13] The influence of age at treatment initiation on inhibitor development is still a matter of debate. Studies conducted by Lorenzo et al[14] and van der Bom et al[15] suggested that treatment with factor concentrates early in life, particularly before the age of 6 months, increased the incidence of inhibitor development. Lorenzo et al[14] found that the cumulative incidence of inhibitors at 3 years of age in patients with hemophilia A first treated with factor concentrates prior to the age of 6 months, between 6 and 12 months of age, or after 1 year of age was 41%, 29%, and 12%, respectively. van der Bom et al[15] reported a similar trend in the incidence of inhibitors. After 100 exposure days to factor concentrates, cumulative inhibitor incidence in patients with hemophilia A beginning therapy before 6 months of age, between 6 months and 1 year, between 1 and 1.5 years, or after 1.5 years was 34%, 20%, 13%, and 0%, respectively. However, not all cohorts appear to show this trend in inhibitor development, and the sample sizes studied to date have been small. Recently, no association was seen between inhibitors and treatment started before the age of 11 months after adjusting for genetic factors. Furthermore, patients receiving early prophylactic treatment exhibited a reduced risk for inhibitor development compared to patients treated on demand.[16] Therefore, careful follow-up studies of these preliminary data are needed.

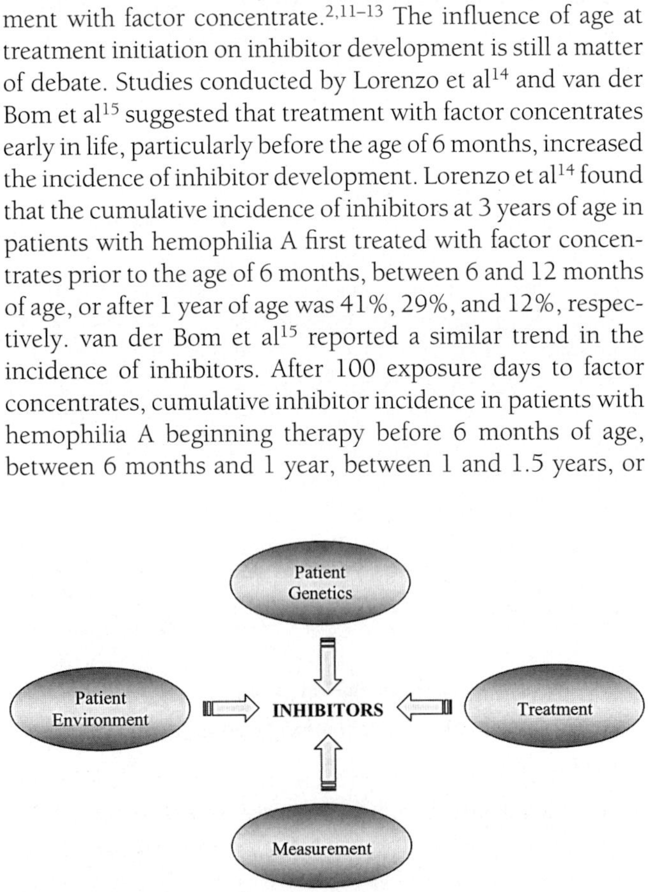

Figure 2 Potential factors of importance for inhibitor formation.

Continuous infusion (CI) of factor concentrates may induce inhibitor development in some patients with mild hemophilia who are generally at a lower risk for inhibitor development. CI of factor concentrates is advocated since it allows for the maintenance of a particular factor concentration, eliminates the peak and trough concentrations associated with periodic bolus injections, and usually reduces the amount of factor consumed and, hence, the cost.[17] However, some studies suggest that CI is associated with an increased risk for inhibitor development, particularly in adult patients. Sharathkumar et al[17] noted that inhibitor incidence in patients with mild hemophilia A was 14% for any exposure to FVIII, compared to 57% for exposure to FVIII via CI. The development of inhibitors in some patients following treatment via CI may be attributed to an immunogenic response induced by systemic factor concentrate exposure in a setting of major bleeds associated with tissue damage and inflammation.[17] These findings also suggest that various immunologic challenges can promote inhibitor development. Inflammatory processes that occur in response to infections, surgery, or major bleeds activate the immune system and can potentially increase the risk of inhibitor development if these processes occur during initiation of therapy with factor concentrates. Similarly, immunizations given to children with hemophilia may stimulate the immune system and possibly increase the risk for inhibitor development. However, definitive risk factors for inhibitor development that may be associated with immunologic challenges have not yet been established, and future studies in this area are warranted.

In the past, plasma-derived factor concentrates were associated with viral transmission, which led to the development of improved manufacturing techniques to reduce the risk of viral contamination. Plasma-derived factor products now undergo viral inactivation and purification procedures during manufacturing; however, these improvements may be associated with potential drawbacks. Inhibitors have been observed in multi-transfused patients with hemophilia who were switched from one type of factor concentrate to another during the course of their treatment, suggesting that use of new or modified factor concentrates in multi-transfused patients could induce inhibitors.[18–20] Studies have also shown that viral inactivation procedures can affect antigenicity[21] by inducing structural changes in the C_2 domain of the FVIII molecule, thus promoting inhibitor development in previously treated patients.[22] Thus, additional testing for inhibitors is recommended in patients who are being switched from one type of factor concentrate to another.[20] In vitro studies have shown that certain FVIII and FIX products can depress immune function which, in part, may be due to the presence of contaminants.[23] It is also speculated that VWF protects against neutralizing antibodies by masking areas of the FVIII molecule.[23–25] However, the implications of these results with respect to in vivo immune function in patients with hemophilia still need to be addressed.

The amplified role of immune response genes during an inflammatory response, coupled with genetic mutations in FVIII or FIX, can affect the development of inhibitory antibodies.[5,26] The prevalence of inhibitors in patients with severe FVIII genetic defects (eg, large deletions, nonsense mutations, and intron 22 inversions) is seven to 10 times higher than the prevalence of inhibitors in patients with less severe genetic defects (eg, missense mutations, small deletions, and splice site mutations) (Fig 3).[5] Mutations resulting in no circulating antigen (ie, null mutations) are especially prone to increase the risk for inhibitor development. In addition, genes within the human leukocyte antigen (HLA) gene complex are thought to affect the immune response.[27,28] Studies of patients with hemophilia A and the intron 22 inversion demonstrated that certain HLA class I and II alleles appeared to be more frequent in patients with inhibitors than in those without, corresponding to relative risks in the range of 1.9 to 4.0 (Table 1).[27,28] Conversely, other alleles seemed protective and were rarely identified in inhibitor patients (relative risk of 0.1 to 0.2). The associations were, however, weak and have not yet been settled. Ethnicity also appears to influence inhibitor development; in African Americans, the susceptibility to inhibitor development is reportedly twice that in white patients.[9,29–31] In a meta-analysis, inhibitor incidence was noted to be 51.9% in African Americans with severe hemophilia A, compared to 25.8% in Caucasians.[31] The genetic profiles of patients of African descent need to be characterized to explore why patients of African descent seem to be at an increased risk for inhibitor development. Overall, the data suggest that a genetic predisposition for inhibitor development exists,[4,30,32] and the correlation between various types

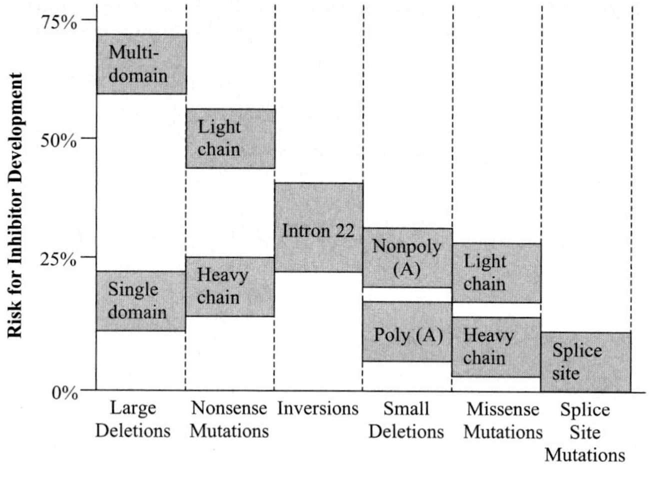

Figure 3 FVIII mutation type as predictor of FVIII inhibitor development. Adapted with permission from Blackwell Publishing.[5]

of genetic mutations and polymorphisms and the development of inhibitors will need to be addressed in future studies.

Inhibitors in Patients With Hemophilia B

The incidence of inhibitors is lower in patients with hemophilia B than in patients with hemophilia A,[1] and inhibitor development is generally associated with the absence of FIX antigen due to large deletions or major derangements of the FIX gene.[26] The lower incidence of inhibitors in patients with hemophilia B has been attributed to the relatively high frequency of low-risk missense or point mutations in these patients compared with patients with hemophilia A.[33] In addition, the structural similarity of FIX to other vitamin K–dependent coagulation factors (ie, factor VII, prothrombin, and factor X)[34] may also confer tolerance and protect against inhibitor development. However, treating bleeding episodes in patients with FIX inhibitors can be a challenge due to the potential risk for allergic reactions to FIX products, a complication that is more common in patients with hemophilia B than in patients with hemophilia A treated with factor VIII concentrates.[35] Anaphylaxis may occur at the time of inhibitor development,[35] and it is speculated that the lower molecular weight and higher normal plasma concentration of FIX compared to FVIII may contribute to the development of anaphylactic reactions.[35,36] The molecular weight of FIX is 55 kd, and the molecule readily diffuses into extravascular spaces.[35] In comparison, the molecular weight of FVIII is 265 kd, without carbohydrates.[37] In addition, the higher normal plasma concentration of FIX (5 μg/mL) compared to FVIII (0.1 μg/mL) causes patients to be exposed to higher amounts of exogenous FIX antigen with administration of a standard dose, and this may induce hypersensitivity.[35]

The success rate of ITI in patients with hemophilia B is usually lower than for patients with hemophilia A, and high doses of FIX replacement during ITI may be associated with

Table 1 HLA Alleles and Inhibitor Development in Patients With Severe Hemophilia A and Intron 22 Inversion[27,28]

	Alleles Class I	Alleles Class II	Relative Risk of Inhibitor Development
High frequency in inhibitor patients	A3, B7, C7	DQA0102, DQB0602, DR15	1.9–4.0
Lower frequency in inhibitor patients ("protective alleles")	C2	DQA0103, DQB0603, DR13	0.1–0.2

Abbreviation: HLA, human leukocyte antigen.

nephrotic syndrome.[33,35] Common characteristics that may be observed in patients who develop nephrotic syndrome include a history of anaphylactic reactions, the presence of proteinuria during ITI with FIX concentrates, and gene deletions.[38] This has prompted clinicians to suggest routine urine tests for proteinuria in patients who develop anaphylactic reactions and in patients undergoing ITI.[38] Thus, although the incidence of inhibitors in patients with hemophilia B is lower than the incidence observed in patients with hemophilia A, physicians are faced with overcoming additional challenges (eg, anaphylaxis and nephrotic syndrome) when treating bleeding episodes in patients with hemophilia B and inhibitors.

Conclusions and Future Issues to Address in the Area of Inhibitor Development

Future studies will need to address some key questions regarding the relationship between genetics and inhibitor development. The patient population with hemophilia A and severe gene mutations or null mutations exhibits an inhibitor prevalence of greater than 30%.[5] However, not all patients with null mutations develop inhibitors. In the case of intron 22 inversions, approximately 20% to 35% of the patients with this type of mutation develop inhibitors, while the majority of patients remain inhibitor-free.[5,39] The reason for inhibitor development in only a select population exhibiting intron 22 inversions is unknown. Family studies have also reported a higher inhibitor concordance in siblings than expected, based on the available data of unrelated patients, and a higher incidence of inhibitors in siblings (~50%) compared to extended relatives with hemophilia (~10%).[4,31] These findings may be attributed to genetic variations in the immune system (ie, major histocompatibility complex classes and polymorphic genes) rather than genetic defects of the FVIII gene since genetic defects in FVIII would purportedly be similar in siblings and extended relatives.[32] Finally, the success of ITI may also be influenced by genetic factors; therefore, establishing whether there is a correlation between genetics and the outcome of ITI can be an important consideration when assessing therapeutic regimens available to patients with hemophilia. Clearly, the genetic basis for the development of inhibitors in certain individuals with hemophilia warrants further investigation in order to identify markers that delineate a predisposition for inhibitor development.

It is evident that various mechanisms are involved in the formation of antibodies, and it is not yet established how these mechanisms work together to determine the formation of antibodies to FVIII or FIX, including those directed against nonfunctional epitopes. It is also not known whether the immune response to FVIII or FIX differs in patients with high-responding inhibitors versus low-responding inhibitors and in patients with severe hemophilia and inhibitors versus patients with mild or moderate hemophilia and inhibitors. The interactions between dendritic cells, T cells, and B cells, including cofactors and cytokines involved in the immune response to FVIII and FIX concentrates, could potentially be determinants for a dysfunctional immune system and contribute to the development of inhibitors. Memory B cells are responsible for mounting the antibody response to antigen re-exposure, and inhibition of the restimulation process may also represent a new avenue to explore.[40]

The development of future therapeutic regimens for patients with hemophilia may require the modification of factor concentrates in order to reduce the potential for inhibitor development. Genetic markers may need to be identified in order to individualize treatment. Gene therapy in patients with hemophilia seems feasible, and future prospects for gene therapy may include modification of genes involved in the immunologic response and gene transfer using vector delivery systems, the goal of which would be to produce a long-term therapeutic coagulant protein without inducing an immune response.[33] In addition, the use of stem cells to genetically correct hemophilia is being considered.[33] Still other novel ideas for gene therapy are on the forefront, suggesting that gene therapy may, in time, become a viable therapeutic option for patients with hemophilia.

References

1. Kasper CK: Diagnosis and Management of Inhibitors to Factors VIII and IX. An Introductory Discussion for Physicians. Treatment of Hemophilia Monograph Series, No. 34. Montreal, Québec, Canada, World Federation of Hemophilia, 2004
2. DiMichele D: Inhibitors: Resolving diagnostic and therapeutic dilemmas. Haemophilia 8:280-287, 2002
3. DiMichele D, Rivard G, Hay C, Antunes S: Inhibitors in haemophilia: Clinical aspects. Haemophilia 10:140-145, 2004 (suppl 4)

4. Gill JC: The role of genetics in inhibitor formation. Thromb Haemost 82:500-504, 1999
5. Oldenburg J, El-Maarri O, Schwaab R: Inhibitor development in correlation to factor VIII genotypes. Haemophilia 8:23-29, 2002 (suppl 2)
6. Kasper CK, Aledort L, Aronson D, Counts R, Edson JR, van Eys J, et al: Proceedings: A more uniform measurement of factor VIII inhibitors. Thromb Diath Haemorrh 34:612, 1975
7. Verbruggen B, Novakova I, Wessels H, Boezeman J, van den Berg M, Mauser-Bunschoten E: The Nijmegen modification of the Bethesda assay for factor VIII:C inhibitors: Improved specificity and reliability. Thromb Haemost 73:247-251, 1995
8. Wight J, Paisley S: The epidemiology of inhibitors in haemophilia A: A systematic review. Haemophilia 9:418-435, 2003
9. Scharrer I, Bray GL, Neutzling O: Incidence of inhibitors in haemophilia A patients—A review of recent studies of recombinant and plasma-derived factor VIII concentrates. Haemophilia 5:145-154, 1999
10. Ljung R, Petrini P, Tengborn L, Sjörin E: Haemophilia B mutations in Sweden: A population-based study of mutational heterogeneity. Br J Haematol 113:81-86, 2001
11. Addiego J, Kasper C, Abildgaard C, Hilgartner M, Lusher J, Glader B, et al: Frequency of inhibitor development in haemophiliacs treated with low-purity factor VIII. Lancet 342:462-464, 1993
12. Bray GL, Gomperts ED, Courter S, Gruppo R, Gordon EM, Manco-Johnson M, et al: A multicenter study of recombinant factor VIII (Recombinate): Safety, efficacy, and inhibitor risk in previously untreated patients with hemophilia A. The Recombinate Study Group. Blood 83:2428-2435, 1994
13. de Biasi R, Rocino A, Papa ML, Salerno E, Mastrullo L, De Blasi D: Incidence of factor VIII inhibitor development in hemophilia A patients treated with less pure plasma derived concentrates. Thromb Haemost 71:544-547, 1994
14. Lorenzo JI, Lopez A, Altisent C, Aznar JA: Incidence of factor VIII inhibitors in severe haemophilia: The importance of patient age. Br J Haematol 113:600-603, 2001
15. van der Bom JG, Mauser-Bunschoten EP, Fischer K, van den Berg HM: Age at first treatment and immune tolerance to factor VIII in severe hemophilia. Thromb Haemost 89:475-479, 2003
16. Santagostino E, Mancuso ME, Rocino A, Mancuso G, Mazzucconi MG, Tagliaferri A, et al: Environmental risk factors for inhibitor development in children with haemophilia A: A case-control study. Br J Haematol 130:422-427, 2005
17. Sharathkumar A, Lillicrap D, Blanchette VS, Kern M, Leggo J, Stain AM, et al: Intensive exposure to factor VIII is a risk factor for inhibitor development in mild hemophilia A. J Thromb Haemost 1:1228-1236, 2003
18. Peerlinck K, Arnout J, Gilles JG, Saint-Remy JM, Vermylen J: A higher than expected incidence of factor VIII inhibitors in multitransfused haemophilia A patients treated with an intermediate purity pasteurized factor VIII concentrate. Thromb Haemost 69:115-118, 1993
19. Peerlinck K, Arnout J, Di Giambattista M, Gilles JG, Laub R, Jacquemin M, et al: Factor VIII inhibitors in previously treated haemophilia A patients with a double virus-inactivated plasma derived factor VIII concentrate. Thromb Haemost 77:80-86, 1997
20. Rosendaal FR, Nieuwenhuis HK, van den Berg HM, Heijboer H, Mauser-Bunschoten EP, van der Meer J, et al: A sudden increase in factor VIII inhibitor development in multitransfused hemophilia A patients in The Netherlands. Dutch Hemophilia Study Group. Blood 81: 2180-2186, 1993
21. Josic D, Buchacher A, Kannicht C, Lim YP, Loster K, Pock K, et al: Degradation products of factor VIII which can lead to increased immunogenicity. Vox Sang 77:90-99, 1999 (suppl 1)
22. Saenko E, Josic D, Stadler M, Sarafanov A, Lim Y, Shima M, et al: Molecular modifications in factor VIII concentrates produced from different plasma pools. Thromb Res 101:501-511, 2001
23. Astermark J, Ekman M, Berntorp E: No effect of a new second-generation B-domain-deleted recombinant product on lymphocyte transformation in vitro: A study of plasma-derived and recombinant products. Br J Haematol 99:289-294, 1997
24. Grosset AB, McGregor JR, Samlowski WE, Rodgers GM: Immunosuppressive effects of factor IX products: An in vitro study. Haemophilia 5:416-425, 1999
25. Auerswald G, Spranger T, Brackmann HH: The role of plasma-derived factor VIII/von Willebrand factor concentrates in the treatment of hemophilia A patients. Haematologica 88:EREP05, 2003
26. Warrier I, Ewenstein BM, Koerper MA, Shapiro A, Key N, DiMichele D, et al: Factor IX inhibitors and anaphylaxis in hemophilia B. J Pediatr Hematol Oncol 19:23-27, 1997
27. Hay CR, Ollier W, Pepper L, Cumming A, Keeney S, Goodeve AC, et al: HLA class II profile: A weak determinant of factor VIII inhibitor development in severe haemophilia A. UKHCDO Inhibitor Working Party. Thromb Haemost 77:234-237, 1997
28. Oldenburg J, Picard JK, Schwaab R, Brackmann HH, Tuddenham EG, Simpsom E: HLA genotype of patients with severe haemophilia A due to intron 22 inversion with and without inhibitors of factor VIII. Thromb Haemost 77:238-242, 1997
29. Addiego JE Jr, Kasper C, Abildgaard C, Lusher J, Hilgartner M, Glader B, et al: Increased frequency of inhibitors in African American hemophilia A patients. Blood 1:239a, 1994 (suppl, abstr)
30. Astermark J, Berntorp E, White GC, Kroner BL, MIBS Study Group: The Malmö International Brother Study (MIBS): Further support for genetic predisposition to inhibitor development in hemophilia patients. Haemophilia 7:267-272, 2001
31. Saint-Remy J-MR, Lacroix-Desmazes S, Oldenburg J: Inhibitors in haemophilia: Pathophysiology. Haemophilia 10:146-151, 2004 (suppl 4)
32. Astermark J, Oldenburg J, Escobar M, White GC II, Berntorp E, Malmö International Brother Study study group: The Malmö International Brother Study (MIBS). Genetic defects and inhibitor development in siblings with severe hemophilia A. Haematologica 90:924-931, 2005
33. Rick ME, Walsh CE, Key NS: Congenital bleeding disorders. Hematology (Am Soc Hematol Educ Program) 559-574, 2003
34. McKenna R: Factor IX. 2005. Available at: http://www.emedicine.com/MED/topic364.htm. Accessed August 2, 2005
35. Warrier I, Lusher JM: Development of anaphylactic shock in haemophilia B patients with inhibitors. Blood Coagul Fibrinolysis 9:S125-S128, 1998 (suppl 1)
36. Dahlbäck B: Blood coagulation and its regulation by anticoagulant pathways: Genetic pathogenesis of bleeding and thrombotic diseases. J Intern Med 257:209-223, 2005
37. MRC haemostasis and thrombosis database resource sites. The molecular pathology of haemophilia A. 2003. Available at: http://europium.csc.mrc.ac.uk/WebPages/Database/Review/Review_txt.html. Accessed December 20, 2005
38. Tengborn L, Hansson S, Fasth A, Lübeck P-O, Berg A, Ljung R: Anaphylactoid reactions and nephrotic syndrome—A considerable risk during factor IX treatment in patients with haemophilia B and inhibitors: A report on the outcome in two brothers. Haemophilia 4:854-859, 1998
39. Oldenburg J, Schröder J, Brackmann HH, Müller-Reible C, Schwaab R, Tuddenham E: Environmental and genetic factors influencing inhibitor development. Semin Hematol 41:82-88, 2004 (suppl 1)
40. Hausl C, Ahmad RU, Schwarz HP, Muchitsch EM, Turecek PL, Dorner F, et al: Preventing restimulation of memory B cells in hemophilia A: A potential new strategy for the treatment of antibody-dependent immune disorders. Blood 104: 115-122, 2004

ELSEVIER

Seminars in
HEMATOLOGY

Current Opinion on Inhibitor Treatment Options

Prasad Mathew

Inhibitor development in patients with hemophilia complicates hemostatic management. Currently, high doses of factor concentrates are used to override low-titer, low-responding inhibitors during acute bleeding episodes. Bypassing agents, such as the activated prothrombin complex concentrate (aPCC), Factor Eight Inhibitor Bypassing Activity, Anti-Inhibitor Coagulant Complex, Vapor Heated (FEIBA; Baxter AG, Vienna, Austria), and activated recombinant factor VII (rFVIIa; NovoSeven, Novo Nordisk A/S, Bagsvaerd, Denmark), are commonly used to treat acute bleeding episodes in patients with high-titer, high-responding inhibitors, whereas long-term therapeutic options include inhibitor eradication using immune tolerance induction. Neither FEIBA nor rFVIIa can be monitored with a laboratory assay, making it difficult to establish optimal dosages. Comparative studies evaluating the efficacy of FEIBA and rFVIIa for bleed control have been sparse, prompting investigators to initiate crossover comparison studies to assess the efficacy and cost of aPCC and rFVIIa in the treatment of joint hemorrhages. Both the cost of therapy and the outcome of therapy will need to be considered in the development of future hemostatic agents for patients with inhibitors.
Semin Hematol 43(suppl 4):S8-S13

Patients with hemophilia require replacement therapy with factor concentrates (eg, factor VIII [FVIII] or factor IX [FIX]) to promote hemostasis; however, inhibitor antibodies that neutralize the activity of FVIII and FIX can develop in response to the exogenous introduction of FVIII and FIX.[1] These inhibitor antibodies are generally detected during routine screening (when symptoms are absent) or when there is a lack of response to factor replacement.[2] The cumulative incidence of inhibitors in previously untreated patients ranges from a mean of 25.9% (range, 20.3% to 33%) in those receiving multiple FVIII plasma products to a mean of 37.5% (range, 36% to 38.7%) in those receiving a single recombinant factor VIII (rFVIII) product.[3] The incidence of new inhibitor development in previously treated patients using rFVIII products is up to 3%.[4] Anti-FVIII and anti-FIX antibodies in the plasma are quantified using the Bethesda assay. One Bethesda unit (BU) represents the amount of antibody that neutralizes 50% of FVIII or FIX in normal plasma.[2,5]

Inhibitors are classified as either high or low responding. High-responding inhibitors are defined by a peak historical titer greater than 5 BU (high-titer) and a risk of anamnesis (ie, spike in antibody production) with factor re-exposure.[2,6] Patients with high-responding, high-titer inhibitors are generally treated with bypassing agents. Low-responding inhibitors are defined by a peak historical titer of less than 5 BU (low-titer) and a lack of anamnesis in response to factor re-exposure.[2,6] Patients with low-responding, low-titer inhibitors can be treated with high doses of specific factor concentrates. Transient inhibitors, defined as low-titer antibodies that occur and subsequently disappear over no defined period in patients who are not receiving regular factor infusions, have also been known to develop.[2,7] The disappearance of transient inhibitors suggests that natural tolerance to exogenic clotting factors is possible, and understanding the mechanism of this process is important to the future design of inhibitor therapeutic options.[2]

Inhibitors complicate treatment and make hemostatic management more difficult. Alternate treatments that are available to patients with inhibitors may not be as effective as the standard factor replacement therapy that is used in patients without inhibitors.[8] Patients with inhibitors are also liable to have more complications, such as hemophilic arthropathy, that can lead to permanent disability.[9] Additionally, treatment costs are generally greater for patients with inhibitors, as are the amounts of medical resources required to improve quality of life.[10] Until the 1990s, inhibitors were associated with a high mortality rate; however, the high mortality rate previously associated with inhibitors is no longer

This article is based in part on the proceedings from an educational symposium held at the World Federation of Hemophilia World Congress 2004 in Bangkok, Thailand. Both the symposium and the manuscript were supported by Baxter Healthcare Corporation.
Address correspondence to Prasad Mathew, MD, University of New Mexico, Department of Pediatrics, MSC 10 5590, 1 University of New Mexico, Albuquerque, NM, 87113. E-mail: PMathew@salud.unm.edu

 0037-1963/06/$-see front matter
doi:10.1053/j.seminhematol.2006.03.005

evident,[11] indicating that advances in medicine have contributed to a prolonged life expectancy.[10] For example, mortality rates in the United Kingdom for patients with severe hemophilia and inhibitors were reported as 20.3 per 1,000 years (95% confidence interval, 12.9 to 27.8) from 1977 to 1984, compared to 11.9 per 1,000 years (95% confidence interval, 4.5 to 19.3) from 1993 to 1999 ($P = .16$).[11]

Thus, the medical community faces a number of dilemmas when managing bleeding episodes in patients with hemophilia and inhibitors, including the type of hemostatic agent to use and the cost of therapy. The development of lower-cost therapeutic agents that can better manage hemostasis in patients with inhibitors needs to be addressed.

Current Therapeutic Options and Strategies for Managing Inhibitors

A number of therapeutic options are currently available to treat acute bleeds in patients with inhibitors. In patients with low-titer, low-responding inhibitors, factor replacement can be used to override the inhibitor; high doses of recombinant or plasma-derived FVIII or FIX can be administered to patients with low-responding inhibitors.[12] In the past, porcine FVIII has also been used to treat inhibitor patients, although it is currently unavailable. A recombinant version of this product is being tested in clinical trials.

In patients for whom factor replacement is not an option, bypassing agents can be used to circumvent the inhibitor. Since the 1970s, prothrombin complex concentrates (PCCs) and activated prothrombin complex concentrates (aPCCs) have been available to treat patients with high-titer inhibitors.[2] PCCs were used initially, before the introduction of aPCCs,[13] but are now not as commonly used as aPCCs, such as Factor Eight Inhibitor Bypassing Activity, Anti-Inhibitor Coagulant Complex, Vapor Heated (FEIBA; Baxter AG, Vienna, Austria). PCCs have been reported to be effective in 50% of bleeding episodes, whereas aPCCs have been reported to be effective in approximately 62% to 96% of bleeds.[14–16] Activated recombinant factor VII (rFVIIa; NovoSeven, Novo Nordisk A/S, Bagsvaerd, Denmark) was recently introduced and has been reported to restore hemostasis in 60% to 100% of bleeding episodes in patients with inhibitors.[13] In addition, there are a number of studies demonstrating the beneficial use of bypassing agents being used for prophylaxis in patients with inhibitors.[17–21]

Finally, the option to eliminate or eradicate the inhibitor exists,[2,22] using immune tolerance induction (ITI) or immunosuppression. ITI is commonly used to eliminate inhibitors in patients with hemophilia; however, the best method for inducing immune tolerance and the length of time required before an ITI attempt is considered a failure are still under debate. ITI involves treatment with factor concentrates over an extended period of time,[23] with most dosing intervals ranging from twice per day to every other day.[22] In some cases, extracorporeal immunoadsorption, a procedure that temporarily lowers inhibitor titers,[24] can be used to lower high-titer inhibitors before initiating ITI. Concomitant immunosuppression with ITI has also been described, generally involving treatment with cyclophosphamide, high-dose immunoglobulin, and protein A immunoadsorption.[23] Thus, a number of factors must be assessed when determining the most appropriate therapeutic regimen for a patient, and algorithms have been developed to assist with choosing the best options available to treat a patient with an inhibitor (Fig 1).

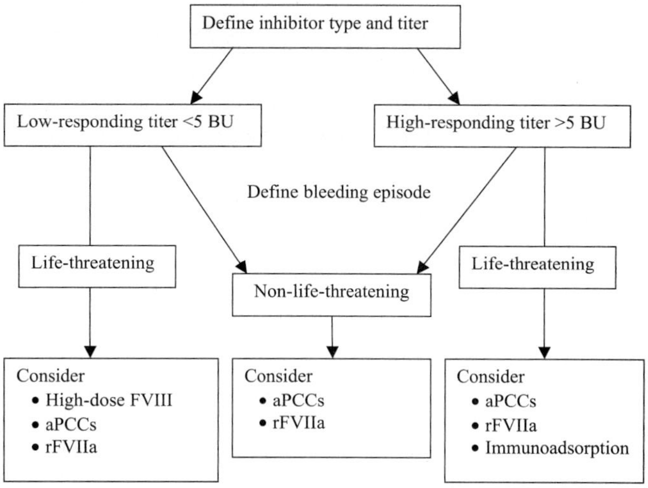

Figure 1 Algorithm for acute treatment strategies. BU indicates Bethesda unit; FVIII, factor VIII; aPCCs, activated prothrombin complex concentrates; rFVIIa, activated recombinant factor VII.

Bypassing Agents

When determining which bypassing agent to use, the advantages and disadvantages associated with each agent must be weighed against a patient's current needs and clinical status. FEIBA has been used for the past 30 years and can be administered at home and over long dosing intervals of 6 to 12 hours,[25] making it a more suitable choice for prophylactic therapy.[9] FEIBA has been shown to be effective in controlling acute bleeds occurring at home, bleeds occurring during surgery, and bleeds associated with acquired hemophilia (Fig 2).[15,16,26,27] Hilgartner and Knatterud[26] reported an efficacy rate of 93% using FEIBA to treat 165 bleeding episodes occurring in joints, mucous membranes, muscles and soft tissues, and bleeding associated with emergencies. Hilgartner et al[27] later reported bleed control in 88% of bleeding episodes using FEIBA when treating 106 bleeding episodes, including joint hemorrhage, muscle and soft tissue bleeding, mucous membrane hemorrhage, intraoperative or perioperative hemorrhage, and central nervous system hemorrhage. Similar efficacy rates were reported by Négrier et al[15] using FEIBA to treat 433 bleeding episodes, including minor and major surgical procedures. Three hundred fifty-two of 433 bleeding episodes (81.3%) were rated as excellent or good, and all surgical procedures using FEIBA as the unique substitution product were reported to have favorable outcomes. Yet another study was conducted by Négrier and the French FEIBA

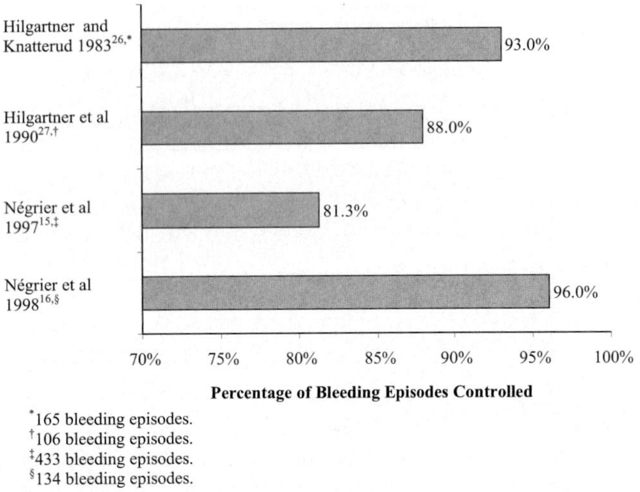

Figure 2 Reported efficacy of FEIBA in a variety of bleeding episodes.[15,16,26,27]

Study Group,[16] which demonstrated an efficacy rate of 96% and showed that FEIBA could safely provide patients with treatment comparable to that provided with factor concentrates in a home setting. One hundred thirty-four bleeding episodes, including hemarthroses, hematomas, soft tissue bleeding, and others, were treated, and hemostasis was achieved in 83.6% of cases within 1 day of treatment. Furthermore, it has been suggested that the expense associated with the use of FEIBA may potentially be less than the expense associated with using rFVIIa, due to the longer dosing intervals allowed by FEIBA administration.[25]

FEIBA has demonstrated efficacy in controlling a variety of bleeding episodes, yet, as with all bypassing agents, the hemostatic efficacy of FEIBA can be unpredictable, and there is no laboratory assay to monitor efficacy or determine an optimal FEIBA dose.[9,28] Additionally, FEIBA contains trace amounts of FVIII, which may produce an anamnestic response; nevertheless, there is no impact on efficacy if an anamnestic response does occur.[28] Since FEIBA is a product derived from human plasma that has undergone viral inactivation, a potential for viral transmission exists[9]; however, to date, there have been no confirmed reports of human immunodeficiency virus, hepatitis A, hepatitis B, or hepatitis C transmission with commercially available FEIBA.[29] In view of the multiple coagulation factors in FEIBA, very large or repeated doses that exceed recommended doses may be associated with a risk for thromboembolic events,[9] particularly in patients with known risk factors, including obesity and lipid abnormalities.[30]

The introduction of rFVIIa has provided physicians with an alternate bypassing agent to treat patients with inhibitors. Due to its recombinant nature, there is no risk of human viral transmission.[31] In addition, there is no risk for an anamnestic response since the concentrate does not contain any amounts of FVIII or FIX. rFVIIa has been shown to be effective in controlling acute bleeds (including those occurring at home) and bleeding during surgery.[2,31] In a study using rFVIIa in a home setting to treat mild to moderate joint, muscle, and mucocutaneous bleeding episodes, hemostasis was rated effective in 92% (566 of 614) of evaluable bleeds (Fig 3).[32] In addition, hemostasis was maintained in 95% (538 of 566) of the effective cases 24 hours after the initial successful response.[32] Like with FEIBA, hemostatic efficacy with rFVIIa is unpredictable, and there is no laboratory assay to monitor efficacy or establish an optimal dose of rFVIIa.[9] In some cases, higher doses than recommended (90 μg/kg) may be required due to individual differences in efficacy and clearance.[13] The short half-life ($t_{1/2}$) of rFVIIa makes frequent dosing necessary; thus, rFVIIa is less likely to be used prophylactically when compared to FEIBA[9] and, as a result, may also be more costly to use.[25] Although low, a risk of thrombic events associated with the use of rFVIIa or FEIBA still exists.[33]

Bypassing agents have proven valuable in the treatment of patients with hemophilia and inhibitors. While aPCCs and rFVIIa share some disadvantages, comparative studies evaluating their efficacy in the treatment of bleeding episodes have been lacking. Currently, an investigator-initiated crossover comparison study (the FEIBA–NovoSeven Comparative [FENOC] study) is in progress to assess the efficacy and cost of aPCCs and rFVIIa in the treatment of joint hemorrhages.

Removal or Eradication of Inhibitors Using ITI Therapy

Use of ITI can improve quality of life and reduce morbidity in patients with inhibitors. The International ITI Study that was established to evaluate the best approach to inducing immune tolerance is currently ongoing. The success rate for ITI therapy is reportedly 60% to 80% in patients with hemophilia A and 36% in patients with hemophilia B.[2] Success rates of 60% to 100% have been reported using the Bonn, van Creveld, and Malmö ITI protocols.[22] With ITI, tolerance can be achieved in 1 to 3 years, but at a very high cost.[8] Results from 50 hemophilia care centers worldwide showed that successful ITI could be achieved in 90% of patients in approximately 2 years, with relapses occurring in 4.3% of cases; the risk of relapse after 15 years of follow-up was approximately 15%.[34] However, ITI is not always successful, and combined

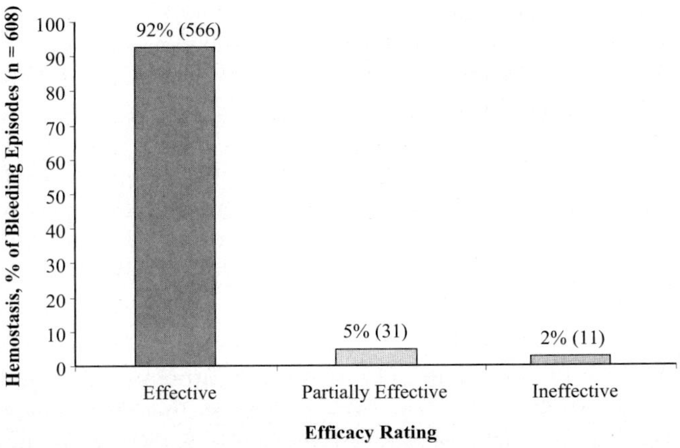

Figure 3 Effectiveness of open-label treatment with rFVIIa at home in patients with hemophilia A or B with inhibitors.[32]

Table 1 Success Rate of Immune Tolerance Regimens for FVIII Inhibitors[35]

	International	North America	Combined
Success	167 (67%)	136 (77%)	303 (71%)
Failure	82 (33%)	41 (23%)	123 (29%)

international and North American registries indicate an approximate 29% failure rate (Table 1).[35] To complicate matters further, ideal factor dosages have not yet been established. A randomized clinical trial is currently in progress to assess the efficacy of a number of regimens.[8] Prophylactic therapy with factor concentrates after successful ITI is a viable consideration as it prevents bleeding episodes and reduces morbidity associated with hemophilic arthropathy, enabling patients to lead more normal lives. For patients in whom ITI is unsuccessful, bypassing agents are often used to manage acute bleeds.[8]

Role of von Willebrand Factor in Inhibitor Eradication

von Willebrand factor (VWF) is speculated to play a role in inhibitor eradication.[36] In patients with inhibitors, VWF may protect FVIII against neutralizing antibodies, enabling increased activity of FVIII following replacement therapy with VWF-containing FVIII concentrates.[36] Inhibitor antibodies with A_2 plus light chain reactivity were found to be less inhibitory to FVIII/VWF products.[37] In addition, anti-C_2 antibodies that can prevent binding of FVIII to VWF have been shown to be less inhibitory to FVIII/VWF concentrates.[38] Over a median of 4 months, 90% eradication was observed in patients with the use of intermediate purity concentrate containing high amounts of VWF; success rates fell when FVIII products without VWF were used.[22,36] For some physicians, use of FVIII/VWF complex concentrates has become the treatment of choice in patients with inhibitors when ITI with FVIII products fails.[36]

Use of aPCC (FEIBA) and rFVIIa for Prophylaxis During ITI

Use of FEIBA for prophylaxis during ITI has been investigated in a prospective study involving 22 pediatric patients with high-responding inhibitors.[17] In this study, the ITI success rate was 82% (18 of 22) after 0.5 to 42 months of treatment. The median annual number of joint bleeding episodes was 1 (range, 0 to 6) using FEIBA prophylaxis. World Federation of Hemophilia radiologic (scale of 0 to 78) and orthopedic (scale of 0 to 90) scores were used to assess joint status; in six of eight patients with joint evaluations the scores were 0, indicating the absence of joint damage. No thrombotic complications or serious adverse events were observed, and FEIBA appeared to be well tolerated. These results were comparable to those observed in patients with severe hemophilia without inhibitors who were treated prophylactically with FVIII, suggesting that FEIBA can be used effectively as prophylaxis during ITI to prevent bleeding episodes and hemophilic arthropathy.

The safety and efficacy of FEIBA for long-term prophylaxis in patients with inhibitors is currently being evaluated. Preliminary results from a prospective study in five pediatric patients with maximum inhibitor titers of 118 to 4,342 BU have been presented.[18] The treatment period for these patients ranged from 0.7 to 12.3 years, and the median annual number of joint bleeds was 2.5 (range, 0 to 6). No life-threatening bleeding episodes or thrombotic complications were observed, and severe hemophilic arthropathy was prevented; FEIBA was well tolerated, joint bleeding episodes were infrequent, and there were no thrombotic events despite the administration of FEIBA over an extended period of time. These results suggest that prophylactic use of FEIBA can be effective in preventing life-threatening hemorrhage in patients with high-responding inhibitors who are unresponsive to ITI.

Despite its short $t_{1/2}$ and the requirement for frequent dosing, use of rFVIIa for prophylaxis is also being considered. Young et al[19] treated two patients with 200 μg/kg rFVIIa every 6 to 12 hours. One patient (15 years old) with hemophilia B had been experiencing frequent bleeds and had previously failed ITI. This patient responded well to a prophylactic regimen of 200 μg/kg rFVIIa every 12 hours, with a reduction in bleeding episodes from an average of 2.2 per month to 0.8 per month.[19] The other patient, a 3-year-old child, was treated for a total of 14 months, during which time no bleeds occurred over a 6-month period of prophylactic therapy with rFVIIa (200 μg/kg every 6 hours, followed by every 8 hours), and a decrease in inhibitor titer was also observed.[19] In other cases, 90 μg/kg per day rFVIIa given to a 5-year-old patient for 21 weeks decreased bleeding episodes and appeared to stop bleeding in a target joint,[20] and 300 μg/kg rFVIIa given three times per week to a 9-year-old patient over 4 months reduced bleeding episodes.[21] These cases demonstrate that use of rFVIIa as prophylaxis can be an option in reducing bleeding episodes and complications related to bleeding episodes in patients with inhibitors.[19]

Future Considerations in the Management of Patients With Inhibitors

The medical community faces some difficult decisions when treating patients with inhibitors, including how to best utilize expensive resources to treat this small population of patients and how to ensure that the best outcome and quality of life are achieved. Our understanding of inhibitor development must continue to be improved. More effective immunomodulatory strategies should be developed. There have been reports of anti-idiotypic antibodies reacting with FVIII inhibitors, and they are thought to contribute to the reduction in inhibitor levels and the inhibition of antibody binding to the FVIII molecule.[39–41] Anti-idiotypic antibodies have been detected in plasma from patients who had both successful and unsuccessful treatment with ITI, and these antibodies are thought to occur in any patient with hemophilia who receives factor replacement therapy.[39] Studies suggest that anti-idiotypic antibodies can play both a passive and an active role in the elimination of inhibitor antibodies, characteristics that may be advantageous in the development of new therapeutic options. Passive therapy would involve the infusion of anti-idiotypic antibodies that can neutralize the activity of inhibitors, whereas active therapy would involve injecting patients with autologous FVIII and anti-FVIII antibody complexes to increase levels of anti-idiotypic antibodies.[40]

Oral tolerance is yet another method that is being considered as a simpler and less expensive option for inducing immune tolerance.[42] Although results were not conclusive, one study noted a drop in inhibitor titer from 42 BU/mL to 11 BU/mL in one patient receiving oral FVIII, suggesting that oral tolerance may be effective in reducing inhibitor levels and could potentially be used with other therapies to enhance response to treatment.[42] In addition, the disappearance of transient inhibitors, a phenomenon that occurs in some patients with low-titer antibodies, suggests that natural tolerance to factor concentrates can occur. Understanding the mechanisms involved in the induction of natural tolerance can be beneficial in the development of future therapeutic regimens that may prevent inhibitor development.[2]

CD20 antibody treatment with rituximab (Rituxan, IDEC Pharmaceutical Corp, San Diego, CA, and Genentech, San Francisco, CA) is also being explored. Rituximab is known to rapidly eliminate circulating B cells, suggesting that it could be effective in the treatment of autoantibody-mediated disorders, such as hemophilia, where autoantibodies develop against coagulation factors.[43] Rituximab appears to be effective in treating patients with acquired hemophilia exhibiting both low-titer and high-titer inhibitors, with patients remaining in remission for several months following discontinuation of treatment.[43] Combination therapy with rituximab and prednisone may improve response to treatment in some patients.[43] Its efficacy in patients with congenital hemophilia who develop inhibitors awaits further study. Finally, hybrid human/porcine factor molecules may be useful in identifying inhibitor domain specificity and the regions of the FVIII molecule that inhibitors act upon.[44] Additionally, studies suggest that a hybrid human/porcine FVIII molecule that lacks immunogenic porcine epitopes may be a more favorable therapeutic option than porcine FVIII.[44]

Conclusions

The treatment of patients with hemophilia who develop inhibitors is one of the most challenging aspects of the disorder facing the medical community. Several therapeutic regimens are currently available to treat patients with inhibitors; however, these therapies are generally costly, forcing physicians to weigh the financial burden of treating patients with inhibitors against the available therapeutic options that will achieve the best outcome and quality of life. Thus, it is imperative that research in the development of newer, improved, and possibly less costly therapies for patients with inhibitors continues to forge ahead, seeking other avenues to explore in an attempt to overcome the challenges associated with treating these patients.

FEIBA is a trademark of Baxter Healthcare SA.

References

1. Kasper CK: Diagnosis and Management of Inhibitors to Factors VIII and IX. An Introductory Discussion for Physicians. Treatment of Hemophilia Monograph Series, No. 34. Montreal, Québec, Canada, World Federation of Hemophilia, 2004
2. DiMichele D: Inhibitors: Resolving diagnostic and therapeutic dilemmas. Haemophilia 8:280-287, 2002
3. Wight J, Paisley S: The epidemiology of inhibitors in haemophilia A: A systemic review. Haemophilia 9:418-435, 2003
4. Kessler CM: New perspectives in hemophilia treatment. Hematology (Am Soc Hematol Educ Program):429-435, 2005
5. Kasper CK, Aledort L, Aronson D, Counts R, Edson JR, van Eys J, et al: Proceedings: A more uniform measurement of factor VIII inhibitors. Thromb Diath Haemorrh 34:612, 1975
6. White GC II, Rosendaal F, Aledort LM, Lusher JM, Rothschild C, Ingerslev J, Factor VII and Factor IX Subcommittee: Definitions in hemophilia. Recommendation of the scientific subcommittee on factor VIII and factor IX of the scientific and standardization committee of the International Society on Thrombosis and Haemostasis. Thromb Haemost 85:560, 2001
7. Rothschild C, Gill J, Scharrer I, Bray G: Transient inhibitors in the Recombinate PUP study. Thromb Haemost 84:145-146, 2000
8. DiMichele D, Rivard G, Hay C, Antunes S: Inhibitors in haemophilia: Clinical aspects. Haemophilia 10:140-145, 2004 (suppl 4)
9. Lessinger CA: Prevention of bleeds in hemophilia patients with inhibitors: Emerging data and clinical direction. Am J Hematol 77:187-193, 2004
10. Gringeri A, Mantovani LG, Scalone L, Mannucci PM, COCIS Study Group: Cost of care and quality of life for patients with hemophilia complicated by inhibitors: The COCIS Study Group. Blood 102:2358-2363, 2003
11. Darby SC, Keeling DM, Spooner RJ, Wan Kan S, Giangrande PL, Collins PW, et al: The incidence of factor VIII and factor IX inhibitors in the hemophilia population of the UK and their effect on subsequent mortality, 1977-99. J Thromb Haemost 2:1047-1054, 2004
12. Rodriguez-Merchan EC, Rocino A: Literature review of surgery management in inhibitor patients. Haemophilia 10:22-29, 2004 (suppl 2)
13. Ananyeva NM, Lacroix-Desmazes S, Hauser CA, Shima M, Ovanesov MV, Khrenov AV, et al: Inhibitors in hemophilia A: Mechanisms of inhibition, management and perspectives. Blood Coagul Fibrinolysis 15:109-124, 2004
14. Lusher JM, Blatt PM, Penner JA, Aledort LM, Levine PH, White GC, et al: Autoplex versus proplex: A controlled, double-blind study of effectiveness in acute hemarthroses in hemophiliacs with inhibitors to factor VIII. Blood 62:1135-1138, 1983
15. Négrier C, Goudemand J, Sultan Y, Bertrand M, Rothschild C, Lauroua P: Multicenter retrospective study on the utilization of FEIBA in France in patients with factor VIII and factor IX inhibitors. French FEIBA Study Group. Factor Eight Bypassing Activity. Thromb Haemost 77: 1113-1119, 1997
16. Négrier C, French FEIBA Study Group: FEIBA VH in home treatment—A 3-year prospective experience. Presented at the XXIII International Congress of the World Federation of Hemophilia in The Hague, The Netherlands. Haemophilia 4:238, 1998 (abstr 330)
17. Kreuz W, Ettingshausen CE, Mentzer D, Martinez Saguer I, Becker S, Stoll H, et al: Immune tolerance induction (ITI) and factor VIII inhibitor bypass activity (FEIBA) for prophylaxis in patients with high responding inhibitors. Ann Hematol 80:A38, 2001 (suppl 1, abstr 138)
18. Kreuz W, Ettingshausen CE, Martinez I, Mentzer D, Figura S, Klarmann: Efficacy and safety of factor VIII inhibitor bypass activity (Feiba) for long-term prophylaxis in patients with high-responding inhibitors. Blood 96:265a, 2000 (abstr 1140)
19. Young G, McDaniel M, Nugent DJ: Prophylactic recombinant factor

VIIa in haemophilia patients with inhibitors. Haemophilia 11:203-207, 2005
20. Saxon BR, Shanks D, Jory CB, Williams V: Effective prophylaxis with daily recombinant factor VIIa (rFVIIa-Novoseven) in a child with high titre inhibitors and a target joint. Thromb Haemost 86:1126-1127, 2001
21. Bryant PC, Carr ME, Martin EJ, Sutton JF: High dose recombinant activated factor VII in a pediatric patient with factor VIII deficiency and high titer inhibitor. Blood 102:104b, 2003 (abstr 4128)
22. Kreuz W, Ettingshausen CE, Auerswald G, Saguer IM, Becker S, Funk M, et al: Epidemiology of inhibitors and current treatment strategies. Haematologica 88:17-20, 2003
23. Hay CRM, Baglin TP, Collins PW, Hill FGH, Keeling DM: The diagnosis and management of factor VIII and IX inhibitors: A guideline from the UK Haemophilia Centre Doctors' Organization (UKHCDO). Br J Haematol 111:78-90, 2000
24. Uehlinger J, Button GR, McCarthy J, Forster A, Watt R, Aledort LM: Immunoadsorption for coagulation factor inhibitors. Transfusion 31: 265-269, 1991
25. Teitel JM: Recombinant factor VIIa versus aPCCs in haemophiliacs with inhibitors: Treatment and cost considerations. Haemophilia 5:43-49, 1999 (suppl 3)
26. Hilgartner MW, Knatterud GL: The use of factor eight inhibitor bypassing activity (FEIBA immuno) product for treatment of bleeding episodes in hemophiliacs with inhibitors. Blood 61:36-40, 1983
27. Hilgartner M, Aledort L, Andes A, Gill J: Efficacy and safety of vapor-heated anti-inhibitor coagulant complex in hemophilia patients. FEIBA Study Group. Transfusion 30:626-630, 1990
28. Wilde JT: Evidence for the use of activated prothrombin complex concentrates (aPCCs) in the treatment of patients with haemophilia and inhibitors. Pathophysiol Haemost Thromb 32:9-12, 2002 (suppl 1)
29. Luu H, Ewenstein B: FEIBA safety profile in multiple modes of clinical and home-therapy application. Haemophilia 10:10-16, 2004 (suppl 2)
30. Ehrlich HJ, Henzl MJ, Gomperts ED: Safety of factor VIII inhibitor bypass activity (FEIBA): 10-year compilation of thrombotic adverse events. Haemophilia 8:83-90, 2002
31. Shapiro AD, Gilchrist GS, Hoots WK, Cooper HA, Gastineau DA: Prospective, randomised trial of two doses of rFVIIa (NovoSeven) in haemophilia patients with inhibitors undergoing surgery. Thromb Haemost 80:773-778, 1998
32. Key NS, Aledort LM, Beardsley D, Cooper HA, Davignon G, Ewenstein BM, et al: Home treatment of mild to moderate bleeding episodes using recombinant factor VIIa (Novoseven) in haemophiliacs with inhibitors. Thromb Haemost 80:912-918, 1998
33. Aledort LM: Comparative thrombotic event incidence after infusion of recombinant factor VIIa versus factor VIII inhibitor bypass activity. J Thromb Haemost 2:1700-1708, 2004
34. Mariani G, Kroner B, Immune Tolerance Study Group (ITSG): Immune tolerance in hemophilia with factor VIII inhibitors: Predictors of success. Haematologica 86:1186-1193, 2001
35. DiMichele DM, Kroner BL, North American Immune Tolerance Study Group: The North American Immune Tolerance Registry: Practices, outcomes, outcome predictors. Thromb Haemost 87:52-57, 2002
36. Auerswald G, Spranger T, Brackmann HH: The role of plasma-derived factor VIII/von Willebrand factor concentrates in the treatment of hemophilia A patients. Haematologica 88:21-25, 2003
37. Gensana M, Altisent C, Aznar JA, Casaña P, Hernàndez F, Jorquera JI, et al: Influence of von Willebrand factor on the reactivity of human factor VIII inhibitors with factor VIII. Haemophilia 7:369-374, 2001
38. Berntorp E: Variation in factor VIII inhibitor reactivity with different commercial factor VIII preparations: Is it of clinical importance? Haematologica 88:13-16, 2003
39. Sakurai Y, Shima M, Tanaka I, Fukuda K, Yoshida K, Yoshioka A: Association of anti-idiotypic antibodies with immune tolerance induction for the treatment of hemophilia A with inhibitors. Haematologica 89:696-703, 2004
40. Gilles JG, Vanzieleghem B, Saint-Remy J-MR: Natural autoantibodies and anti-idiotypes. Semin Thromb Hemost 26:151-155, 2000
41. Gilles JG, Saint-Remy JM: Healthy subjects produce both anti-factor VIII and specific anti-idiotypic antibodies. J Clin Invest 94:1496-1505, 1994
42. Terada K, Yagi Y, Niizuma T, Kataoka N: Is oral tolerance therapy possible for haemophilia with inhibitors? Vox Sang 80:61-62, 2001
43. Wiestner A, Cho HJ, Asch AS, Michelis MA, Zeller JA, Peerschke EIB, et al: Rituximab in the treatment of acquired factor VIII inhibitors. Blood 100:3426-3428, 2002
44. Barrow RT, Healey JF, Gailani D, Scandella D, Lollar P: Reduction of the antigenicity of factor VIII toward complex inhibitory antibody plasmas using multiply-substituted hybrid human/porcine factor VIII molecules. Blood 95:564-568, 2000

Seminars in
HEMATOLOGY

Inhibitor Economics

Jerome Teitel

The majority of direct costs associated with caring for patients with hemophilia are attributed to replacement therapy with clotting factor concentrates (CFC). For patients who develop high-titer inhibitors, CFC are ineffective and bypassing therapy is used to achieve hemostasis, thus changing the direct costs associated with treatment. As bypassing agents are less predictably effective than CFC (often necessitating more frequent dosing) and are more costly on a per-unit basis, treatment costs for patients with inhibitors are usually much higher than those for patients without inhibitors. In addition, the immune tolerance induction protocols used to eradicate inhibitors are costly due to the frequent dosing of CFC over prolonged periods. It is estimated that the cost of hemostatic therapy for patients with inhibitors can be 2.5 times higher than the cost for patients without inhibitors. However, some studies have reported an outlier effect caused by a small percentage of inhibitor patients who require a disproportionate amount of treatment. These outliers magnify overall treatment costs, making cost assessments for hemostatic therapy less predictable in patients with inhibitors than in those without inhibitors.
Semin Hematol 42(suppl 4):S14-S17

The majority of the direct costs of hemophilia care are due to the clotting factor concentrates (CFC) used as replacement therapy. In the mid 1990s, CFC were estimated to account for 50% to 80% of total direct costs,[1] and this proportion has probably increased since then.

Patients who develop high-titer inhibitors (anti-factor VIII [FVIII] antibodies complicating therapy for hemophilia A or anti-factor IX [FIX] antibodies in the case of hemophilia B) generally cannot be treated with specific replacement therapy. For acute bleeding episodes, they are most commonly treated with bypassing agents, either activated prothrombin complex concentrates (aPCCs), such as Factor Eight Inhibitor Bypassing Activity, Anti-Inhibitor Coagulant Complex, Vapor Heated (FEIBA; Baxter AG, Vienna, Austria) or activated recombinant factor VII (rFVIIa; NovoSeven, Novo Nordisk A/S, Bagsvaerd, Denmark).

For several reasons, it is generally assumed that treatment costs for hemophilia patients with inhibitor antibodies are considerably greater than for those without inhibitors. Bypassing agents are more costly than most FVIII concentrates on a per-treatment basis, and more doses of bypassing agents (especially rFVIIa) than of replacement concentrates may be required to control a bleeding episode. This phenomenon is partly due to less predictable efficacy of bypassing agents than of regular factor replacement therapy, and partly due to the unavailability of laboratory monitoring, both of which can lead practitioners to err on the side of over-treatment. Furthermore, although inhibitors most commonly develop in patients with severe hemophilia, when they occur in individuals with less severe disease, FVIII activity usually falls to undetectable levels, resulting in the need for more frequent and intensive component therapy. Finally, attempts are generally made to eradicate newly recognized inhibitors by immune tolerance induction (ITI); these protocols can be very costly as they entail frequent high doses of factor concentrate, often given for a prolonged period of time. An Italian longitudinal study found that bypassing agents and CFC accounted for nearly 99% of the total cost of treating patients with inhibitors, illustrating the impact of the cost of treating bleeding episodes in these patients.[2] Thus, it is important to treat patients with the most appropriate product at an optimal dose from the moment bypassing agents are deemed necessary, in order to minimize costs associated with their use.

The Cost of Bypassing Agents

Early studies confirmed the assumptions about the high cost of treating patients with hemophilia and inhibitors. Aledort et al[3] analyzed product costs covering the period of introduc-

University of Toronto, Toronto, Ontario, Canada.
This article is based in part on the proceedings from an educational symposium held at the World Federation of Hemophilia World Congress 2004 in Bangkok, Thailand. Both the symposium and the manuscript were supported by Baxter Healthcare Corporation.
Address correspondence to Jerome Teitel, MD, St. Michael's Hospital, Suite 2-065, 30 Bond St, Toronto, Ontario, Canada M5B 1W8. E-mail: TEITELJ@smh.toronto.on.ca

 0037-1963/06/$-see front matter
doi:10.1053/j.seminhematol.2006.03.004

Table 1 Retrospective Study of Factor VIII Bypassing Therapy Treatment Costs[5]

	Annual Cost (€)		
	1988–1995	1996–1998*	Ratio
Inhibitor	56,262	186,482	3.31
Noninhibitor	43,234	59,887	1.39
Ratio	1.30	3.11	. . .

NOTE. Ellipses indicate not applicable.
*rFVIIa introduced in France in 1996.

Table 2 Retrospective Case-Control Study of Nine Inhibitor and Nine Matched Control Patients in Toronto[6]

	Patients With Inhibitors	Controls	Inhibitor: Control
Total cost (C$)	3,030,091	1,346,188	2.25
Mean cost (C$)	336,677	149,576	2.25
Median cost (C$)	150,686	133,342	1.13

tion of aPCCs, the first highly effective anti-inhibitor bypassing agent. In 1981 the only product available to treat bleeding in patients with inhibitors was nonactivated PCCs, and the authors calculated that the average annual treatment cost for these patients was approximately $18,000. This was twice the estimated annual CFC cost of $8,900 for treating patients without inhibitors. In the following year, aPCCs became available, and the average cost to treat patients with inhibitors almost doubled to $33,000.

A survey carried out in Canada, covering the years 1988 to 1993, identified 33 patients with inhibitors who were treated with the aPCC, FEIBA, at an annualized cost (in Canadian dollars) of C$107,513.[4] This compared to an annualized CFC cost of C$37,670 for patients without inhibitors, an estimate based on the number of patients with severe hemophilia in Canada at that time and on the total amount of FVIII concentrate issued across the country. Therefore, the cost of providing hemostatic therapy for patients with inhibitors was approximately 2.85-fold greater than for those without inhibitors. The relative costs may have changed since that time as a more expensive product, rFVIIa, has become widely used in Canada and many other countries.

In 1999, another opportunity for a cost comparison arose with the introduction of rFVIIa, the second highly effective FVIII bypassing agent. The high per-treatment cost of rFVIIa and its unfavorable pharmacokinetic profile, which necessitates repeated doses as often as every 2 hours during acute bleeding episodes, raised concern about further cost escalation in the treatment of patients with inhibitors. The impact of rFVIIa on overall treatment costs for hemophilia patients with inhibitors was addressed in a retrospective cohort study from a single institution in France (Table 1).[5] This cohort included 17 patients with high-responding inhibitors and 103 patients without inhibitors treated over two periods of time, one preceding the introduction of rFVIIa (1988 to 1995) and one following its introduction (1996 to 1998). The mean annual cost of all FVIII bypassing treatments for patients with high-responding inhibitors more than tripled from €56,262 in the first time period to €186,482 in the second. By comparison, CFC treatment costs for patients without inhibitors increased by only 39% across the two time periods, from €43,234 to €59,887. Thus, it cost 30% more to treat patients with high-responding inhibitors than patients without inhibitors before the introduction of rFVIIa, and over 200% more in the years immediately following its availability.

The Outlier Effect

The clinical severity of bleeding in hemophiliacs is highly variable, no less among patients with inhibitors than among those without inhibitors. Analyses of total costs to treat cohorts of patients with inhibitors may mask this variability. The effect of high-cost outlier patients was highlighted in a retrospective analysis that we performed in our hemophilia treatment center in the years 1993 to 1997 (Table 2).[6] CFC utilization was compared for nine patients with inhibitors and nine matched control patients without inhibitors. We were surprised to find that, in six of the nine pairs, CFC costs were lower for the inhibitor patient. The median costs for treating patients with inhibitors and those without inhibitors were very similar, approximately C$151,000 and C$133,000, respectively. However, two high-cost outlier patients with inhibitors skewed the overall results, such that the *mean* cost to treat patients with inhibitors was approximately C$337,000, roughly 2.25 times greater than the mean cost of CFC for treatment of controls (approximately C$150,000). A much larger Japanese case-control study involving 136 patient pairs showed very similar results for average treatment costs.[7] In this study, bypassing agents for treating patients with inhibitors cost ¥10.9 million, which was approximately 2.5-fold greater than the cost of CFC for treating patients without inhibitors (¥4.3 million).

Other investigators have observed the same outlier effect. Bohn et al[8] conducted a retrospective cohort study in two US hemophilia treatment centers, involving 12 patients with inhib-

Table 3 Retrospective Case-Control Study of 12 Inhibitor and 28 Matched Control Patients[8]

	Patients With Inhibitors	Controls	Inhibitor: Control
Mean cost ($)	141,000	80,000	1.76
Median cost ($)	55,853	58,300	0.96
Median hospital stay (days)	3.5	3.75	. . .

NOTE. Ellipses indicate not applicable.

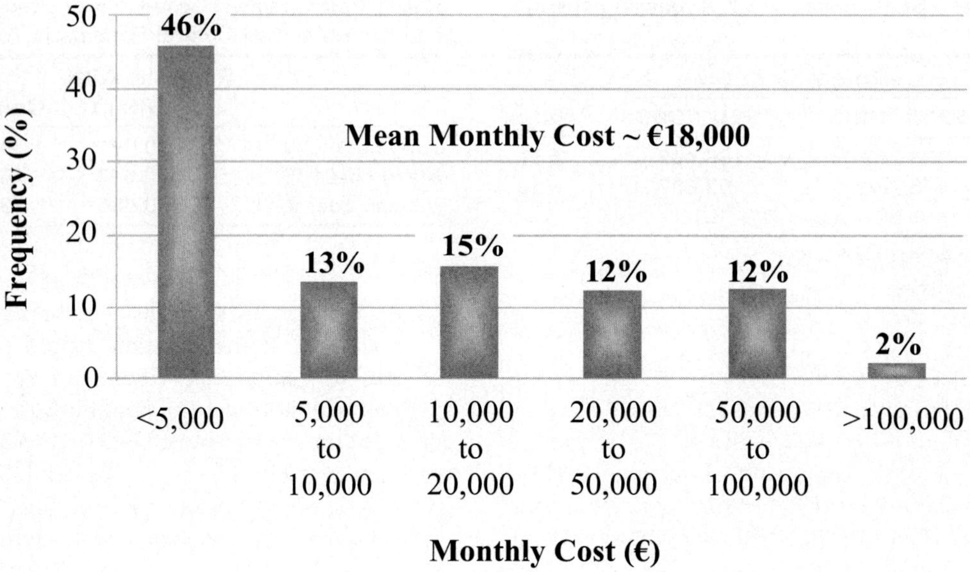

Figure 1 Distribution of anti-inhibitor concentrate costs in 52 patients followed up for 18 months in Italy. Copyright 2003 by the American Society of Hematology. Reprinted with permission.[2]

itors and 28 controls (Table 3). As observed in our study,[6] there was little difference between the median costs for the two groups ($55,853 and $58,300 per year, respectively, for patients with inhibitors and controls). However, they observed the same outlier effect; two patients with inhibitors skewed the total results, such that the mean costs were $141,000 for patients with inhibitors and $80,000 for controls, a ratio of 1.76. The Italian longitudinal study cited above[2] also demonstrated the distorting effect of a small number of high-cost patients (Fig 1). The mean cost of inhibitor treatment products for 52 patients was approximately €18,000 per month, but approximately three quarters of patients consumed less than this amount, and almost half (46%) consumed less than €5,000 worth of products.[2] The highest costs were related to patients who required joint replacement surgery.

Cost Considerations Versus Quality of Life

Surgery is especially problematic in patients with inhibitors, owing to the unpredictable and variable efficacy of bypassing agents and the lack of validated assays for laboratory monitoring. A survey of hospital inpatient costs for patients with hemophilia was performed at six hemophilia treatment centers in France for the years 1997 to 1999.[9] As part of this survey, the cost of performing major surgery in patients with and without inhibitors was analyzed. The cost of major surgical procedures was several times greater for patients with inhibitors than for those without inhibitors when expressed as mean or median values (Table 4). There was an even greater discrepancy when costs were compared for inpatient management of major nonsurgical bleeding episodes.

Cost considerations need to be balanced by a measure of effectiveness in which the value of a health intervention is expressed in a nonmonetary natural unit, such as the quality adjusted life year (QALY). Colowick et al[10] modeled the effectiveness of ITI as a long-term strategy for inhibitor management. They concluded that successful ITI in a 5-year-old child would result in a lifetime reduction of CFC costs from $4.6M to $2.9M. In addition, successful ITI increased life expectancy by 4.6 years. The cost savings reflected the incremental expense of treating bleeding with aPCCs and plasma-derived porcine FVIII (an inhibitor treatment product that is no longer being produced). In another analysis based on consensus assumptions from a group of German hemophilia experts, the cost of a successful 12-month ITI regimen was calculated as varying from approximately €1.15M in a young child with a high-responding inhibitor to €5.75M in an adult with a high-responding inhibitor.[11] Extrapolating from the authors' estimated annual treatment costs for patients with and without inhibitors, one may crudely estimate from their data that it would take 20 to 25 years of ongoing CFC treatment to recoup the cost of the successful ITI regimen.

Table 4 Hospital Inpatient Cost Comparison for Major Surgery and Major Nonsurgical Bleeding in Hemophilia Patients With and Without Inhibitors[9]

	Major Surgery		Major Bleeding	
	Noninhibitor	Inhibitor	Noninhibitor	Inhibitor
Median cost (€)	21,409	79,286	13,877	106,844
Mean cost ± SD (€)	32,058 ± 26,970	156,193 ± 160,072	20,149 ± 20,750	227,956 ± 317,589

Models are exquisitely sensitive to their underlying assumptions, and they can only answer the questions asked by the modelers. An intricate cost-effectiveness model compared several regimens of hemostatic therapy and ITI for patients with inhibitors.[12] This analysis showed that the aggressive Malmö ITI regimen was less costly and gave better quality of life than three other modeled inhibitor treatment regimens (two of these regimens involved ITI therapy; and one, on-demand therapy). Analysis of other ITI protocols showed benefit with respect to quality of life but at an increased cost. In another model analyzing treatment of patients for whom ITI was not an option, the investigators found a small reduction in lifetime costs for a child with an inhibitor whose treatment regimen consisted exclusively of rFVIIa, as opposed to a regimen in which an aPCC was given as first-line treatment for minor bleeding, and rFVIIa was used in all other circumstances. The lifetime difference was approximately £208,000, representing approximately 10% of total lifetime costs.[12]

The modeled treatment regimens may also not be a very accurate reflection of the typical sequential therapeutic approaches used by physicians with expertise in treating hemophilia. Another decision-analysis model using different assumptions (presented in abstract form and as a poster at the Hemophilia 2004 World Congress) found that the average cost for treatment and control of bleeding was approximately twice as high with rFVIIa as with aPCCs.[13] The higher cost was likely attributable to the short half-life ($t_{1/2}$) of rFVIIa, which makes frequent dosing necessary.[14] Other studies have demonstrated a similar increase in cost associated with the use of rFVIIa.[2,15] In one case, the availability of rFVIIa resulted in a decline in FEIBA and porcine factor VIII use and a subsequent increase in hemostatic product expenses for patients with inhibitors, from 1% of the total factor concentrate budget to 3% of the budget, over a 2-year period.[6] However, these results are very sensitive to assumptions about relative efficacy, which will remain questionable until direct comparative data for aPCCs and rFVIIa are available. Comparative studies thus far have been sparse. However, results of an investigator-initiated crossover comparison study (the FEIBA–NovoSeven Comparative [FENOC] study) to compare the efficacy of aPCCs and rFVIIa in the treatment of joint hemorrhages were recently presented in abstract form.[16] Among the 48 patients evaluated in an intention-to-treat analysis, 76.1% of bleeding episodes were reported to have resolved at 6 hours after treatment with FEIBA, compared with 65.2% after rFVIIa, although the overall subjective efficacy ratings of the two treatments at 6 hours were 80.9% and 78.7%, respectively. The authors concluded that FEIBA and rFVIIa may have similar efficacy in treating these bleeding episodes, but that there was variability among patients.

Conclusions

In summary, owing to the rarity of hemophilia and the high cost of replacement products, small numbers of patients who require a disproportionate amount of treatment can have a profound effect on overall costs within any given jurisdiction or cost center. In the subset of hemophilia patients with high-titer inhibitors, both of these complicating factors (rarity of the disorder and expense of treatment products) are further magnified. Although many patients with inhibitors do not bleed excessively and do not consume large amounts of bypassing products, others are heavily treated in the context of life- or limb-threatening bleeding, surgery, or ITI regimens. The effect of these outliers is such that the overall cost of delivering hemostatic treatment to patients with inhibitors is high and difficult to predict.

FEIBA is a trademark of Baxter Healthcare SA.

References

1. Ross-Degnan D, Soumerai SB, Avorn J, Bohn RL, Bright R, Aledort LM: Hemophilia home treatment. Economic analysis and implications for health policy. Int J Technol Assess Health Care 11:327-344, 1995
2. Gringeri A, Mantovani LG, Scalone L, Mannucci PM, COCIS Study Group: Cost of care and quality of life for patients with hemophilia complicated by inhibitors: The COCIS Study Group. Blood 102:2358-2363, 2003
3. Aledort LM, Cohen M, Hilgartner M, Lipton R: Treatment of hemophiliacs with inhibitors: Cost and effect on blood resources, in Hoyer L (ed): Factor VIII Inhibitors. New York, NY, Liss, 1984, pp 353-365
4. Rivard GE, Vick S: Factor VIII inhibitor treatment. Economics of inhibitor treatment in Canada. Semin Hematol 31:41-43, 1994 (2 suppl 4)
5. Goudemand J: Hemophilia. Treatment of patients with inhibitors: Cost issues. Haemophilia 5:397-401, 1999
6. Chang H, Sher GD, Blanchette VS, Teitel JM: The impact of inhibitors on the cost of clotting factor replacement therapy in Haemophilia A in Canada. Haemophilia 5:247-252, 1999
7. Honda K, Nagao T, Kamiya T, Yoshioka A, Miyazaki T, Takeda T, et al: Prospective matched control study concerning the treatment and quality of life of hemophiliacs with inhibitors [in Japanese]. Rinsho Ketsueki 39:416-421, 1998
8. Bohn RL, Aledort LM, Putnam KG, Ewenstein BM, Mogun H, Avorn J: The economic impact of factor VIII inhibitors in patients with haemophilia. Haemophilia 10:63-68, 2004
9. Gautier P, D'Alche-Gautier MJ, Coatmelec B, Marques-Verdier A, Bertrand MA, Dieval J, et al: Cost related to replacement therapy during hospitalization in haemophiliacs with or without inhibitors: Experience of six French haemophilia centres. Haemophilia 8:674-679, 2002
10. Colowick AB, Bohn RL, Avorn J, Ewenstein BM: Immune tolerance induction in hemophilia patients with inhibitors: Costly can be cheaper. Blood 96:1698-1702, 2000
11. Auerswald G, von Depka Prondzinski M, Ehlken B, Kreuz W, Kurnik K, Lenk H, et al: Treatment patterns and cost-of-illness of severe haemophilia in patients with inhibitors in Germany. Haemophilia 10:499-508, 2004
12. Knight C, Paisley S, Wight J, Jones ML: Economic modelling of different treatment strategies for haemophilia A with high-responding inhibitors. Haemophilia 9:521-540, 2003
13. Chung K, Berger A, Edelsberg J, Neufeld E, Oster J: Cost-effectiveness of FEIBA vs. NovoSeven as initial therapy for the treatment of mild-to-moderate bleeds in hemophilia patients with inhibitors. Haemophilia 10:30, 2004 (suppl 3, abstr)
14. Hay CR, Baglin TP, Collins PW, Hill FG, Keeling DM: The diagnosis and management of factor VIII and IX inhibitors: A guideline from the UK Haemophilia Centre Doctors' Organization (UKHCDO). Br J Haematol 111:78-90, 2000
15. Berger A, Edelsberg J, Neufeld E, Chung K, Oster G: Cost-effectiveness of FEIBA VH vs NovoSeven as initial therapy for the treatment of mild-to-moderate bleeds in hemophilia patients with inhibitors. Presented at the Hemophilia 2004 World Congress, Bangkok Thailand, October 17-21, 2004 (abstr 114E)
16. Berntorp E, Donfield S, Waters J, Mattson E, DiMichele D, Gringeri A, et al: The FEIBA NovoSeven Comparative Study (FENOC)—A randomization evaluation of by-passing agents in hemophilia complicated by inhibitors. Blood 106:324, 2005 (abstr)

ELSEVIER

Seminars in
HEMATOLOGY

Surgery in Patients With Hemophilia and Inhibitors: A Review of the Norwegian Experience With FEIBA

Geir E. Tjønnfjord

Surgical interventions in patients with hemophilia and inhibitors have often been postponed as long as possible due to difficulties in maintaining intra- and postoperative hemostatic control. Nonactivated and activated prothrombin complex concentrates have been successful in controlling acute bleeding in patients with inhibitors and have been useful in the surgical setting. At the Rikshospitalet–Radiumhospitalet University Hospital in Oslo, Norway, 17 minor and seven major surgical procedures were performed in nine patients with congenital hemophilia A and two patients with acquired hemophilia. Patients are generally treated according to the following dosing regimen, with changes made on a case-by-case basis: a preoperative loading dose of 100 U/kg of Factor Eight Inhibitor Bypassing Activity, Anti-Inhibitor Coagulant Complex, Vapor Heated (FEIBA; Baxter AG, Vienna, Austria), followed by 200 U/kg per day for 3 days. The dose is then tapered to 150 U/kg per day and subsequently to 100 U/kg per day. Hemostatic control was attained in all cases and only 1 major adverse event was observed. A 69-year-old patient experienced a non-ST-elevation myocardial infarction 3 days after undergoing a sigmoidectomy. He continued on FEIBA therapy and was stabilized with nitrates, opioid analgesia, and diuretics without clinical signs of heart failure.
Semin Hematol 43(suppl 4):S18-S21

Surgical procedures are approached with great caution in patients with bleeding disorders. In patients with hemophilia, bleed management can be further complicated by the development of inhibitory antibodies to coagulation factors.[1] These antibodies can render factor replacement, the mainstay therapy for hemophilia, ineffective. As a result, until recently, surgery was generally avoided in hemophilia patients with inhibitors unless deemed absolutely necessary, even though elective surgery may have led to an improved quality of life.

Activated prothrombin complex concentrates (aPCCs), specifically Factor Eight Inhibitor Bypassing Activity, Anti-Inhibitor Coagulant Complex, Vapor Heated (FEIBA; Baxter AG, Vienna, Austria), and activated recombinant factor VII (rFVIIa; NovoSeven, Novo Nordisk A/S, Bagsvaerd, Denmark) have been successful in controlling bleeding episodes in patients with inhibitors.[2,3] Moreover, there are a growing number of studies demonstrating the successful use of these inhibitor bypassing agents in the surgical management of patients with hemophilia and inhibitors.[4–15]

The use of rFVIIa in surgery was first described by Hedner et al[8] in 1988, where rFVIIa was successfully used during a synovectomy. Since then, several studies have reported the use of rFVIIa during surgery.[13,15] In 2002, Hvid and Rodriguez-Merchan[11] summarized the experience of rFVIIa in 53 elective orthopedic surgeries reported in the literature. All reported patients survived, and efficacy was considered excellent in most cases; however, six patients experienced moderate bleeding complications.[11] Similar to rFVIIa, there are a number of studies describing the successful use of aPCCs for surgeries in patients with hemophilia and inhibitors.[4–6] Prior to the use of rFVIIa, Hilgartner and Knatterud[5] first described the use of FEIBA in four surgical procedures in 1983. More recently, Negrier et al[6] and Rodriguez-Merchan et al[14] reported studies describing the successful use of FEIBA in surgical procedures involving inhibitor patients. In the study by Negrier et al,[6] FEIBA was administered to cover four major and 19 minor surgical procedures in patients with inhibitors. All outcomes were rated favorably, with one complication of excessive bleeding in a knee arthroscopy procedure. Similar results were reported by Rodriguez-Merchan et al, [14] where

Medical Department, Division of Hematology, Rikshospitalet–Radiumhospitalet University Hospital, University of Oslo, Oslo, Norway.
This manuscript is based in part on the proceedings from an educational symposium held at the World Federation of Hemophilia World Congress 2004 in Bangkok, Thailand. Both the symposium and this manuscript were supported by Baxter Healthcare Corporation.
Address correspondence to Geir E. Tjønnfjord, MD, PhD, Medical Department, Division of Hematology, Rikshospitalet–Radiumhospitalet University Hospital, N-0027 Oslo, Norway. E-mail: geir.tjonnfjord@rikshospitalet.no

 0037-1963/06/$-see front matter
doi:10.1053/j.seminhematol.2006.03.003

FEIBA was used in four major and 47 minor elective orthopedic surgeries without any complications.

Since 1996, due to a change in policy at our center, FEIBA has been used as first-line treatment in bleed management and surgeries in adult hemophilia patients with inhibitors. Here, we present and review our experience with the use of FEIBA during surgery and invasive diagnostic and therapeutic procedures performed in adult hemophilia patients with high-titer factor VIII (FVIII) or factor IX (FIX) inhibitors.

Patients

In Norway, all elective surgical interventions on patients with hemophilia and inhibitors are performed at the Rikshospitalet–Radiumhospitalet University Hospital in Oslo. Since January 1996, 24 surgical procedures have been performed on 11 patients with hemophilia and high-titer inhibitors. Of these patients, nine had congenital hemophilia A and two had acquired hemophilia. Of the two patients with acquired hemophilia, one had developed inhibitory antibodies to FVIII and the other to FIX. The 11 patients had a mean age of 54 years (range, 22 to 79 years), with five patients above 60 years of age, and a mean weight of 81 kg (range, 50 to 130 kg). All of the patients had peak inhibitor titers over 10 Bethesda units (BU). The mean peak titer was 235 BU (range, 13 to 1,350 BU).

Treatment Regimen

At our center, the treatment regimen is generally as follows: a preoperative loading dose of 100 U/kg of FEIBA, followed by 200 U/kg per day for 3 days. The dose is then tapered to 150 U/kg per day and subsequently to 100 U/kg per day. Changes in this dosing regimen are made on a case-by-case basis. In the current study, antifibrinolytics (tranexamic acid) were not used systemically, but were applied locally when possible; in patients with dental extractions, a dilute solution was used as a mouth rinse four times per day for 1 week postoperatively, and for patient no. 3, dressings containing tranexamic acid were applied daily for 1 week following circumcision.

Surgical Experience

A total of 24 surgical procedures using FEIBA have been performed on patients with inhibitors in Norway since 1996 (Table 1). Of these, 17 were minor procedures and seven were major procedures. The minor procedures included five dental extraction procedures, three cataract surgeries with lens implantation, and one each of the following: trephine biopsy, Hickman line insertion (Hickman Single-Lumen CV Catheter, BARD Access Systems, BARD Medical Systems, Norden AB, Helsingborg, Sweden), circumcision, telangiectasia laser coagulation, cystoscopy/pyelography, endoscopic treatment of an esophageal ulcer, excision of prepatellar bursa, exchange of pacemaker batteries, and excision of a toenail. The major procedures included three knee arthroplasties, one hip arthroplasty, one wound rupture repair, one nephrectomy/splenectomy, and one sigmoidectomy.

Hemostatic efficacy was judged to be excellent in all 17 minor procedures, with no blood loss following the procedures. Hemostatic efficacy was also rated excellent without complications in three of seven major procedures. Hemostatic efficacy was rated as good in the remaining four major procedures. Patient no. 6 underwent a left-sided nephrectomy for renal carcinoma and subsequently became hemodynamically unstable. The hemostatic instability was due to a subcapsular splenic hemorrhage that resulted from splenic trauma during the nephrectomy, and was not attributed to poor efficacy of FEIBA. The patient required a splenectomy, but experienced no further bleeding complications. Hemostatic efficacy of FEIBA was rated as good for this procedure. Patient no. 5 experienced blood loss (750 mL) after a total knee arthroplasty and a subsequent drop in hemoglobin concentration, but did not require transfusion with packed red blood cells (PRBCs). The same patient also underwent a hip arthroplasty and again experienced a decrease in hemoglobin concentration. On this occasion, the patient was transfused with 2 units of PRBCs. Patient no. 8 also experienced a decrease in hemoglobin concentration after a total knee arthroplasty and was transfused with 2 units of PRBCs. The blood loss in these procedures was within the range reported in literature for similar orthopedic procedures performed on noninhibitor patients. However, since the blood loss was in the upper range of what we experienced in our center with noninhibitor patients, the hemostatic efficacies were judged to be good.

Adverse Events

Tolerance to FEIBA during infusion was excellent. There were no reports of disseminated intravascular coagulation, thromboembolism, fever, chills, or rash associated with FEIBA administration. However, there was one report of a major adverse event. Patient no. 7, a 69-year-old man, experienced a non-ST-elevation myocardial infarction following a sigmoidectomy. On postoperative day 3, the patient complained of chest pain and dyspnea. He had no history of coronary artery disease, but was a smoker and was wheelchair-bound for many years due to hemophilic arthropathy. Details regarding his triglyceride and cholesterol levels were not available, and coronary angiography was not performed. The patient was managed with nitrates, opiate analgesia, and diuretics. There was no progression of the non-ST-elevation myocardial infarction, and FEIBA administration was continued after some consideration. The patient showed no clinical signs of heart failure.

Discussion

Although inhibitors complicate the treatment of bleeding episodes in some patients with hemophilia, a number of treatment options exist for these patients.[2,3,5,6,16–18] Available therapeutic options have been applied in a surgical setting in many studies.[7–15,19] Using FEIBA, the Norwegian experience

Table 1 Surgical Procedures and Outcomes

Patient No.	Hemophilia Type	Peak Inhibitor Titer (BU)	Age (yr)	Procedure Type	FEIBA Dose	Hemostatic Outcome	Adverse Events
1	Acquired (anti-FIX)	37	58	Minor; trephine biopsy	55 U/kg per day × 1 d	Excellent	None
2	Acquired (anti-FVIII)	1350	64	Minor; Hickman line insertion	253 U/kg per day × 1 d	Excellent	None
				Minor; dental extraction	115 U/kg per day × 1 d	Excellent	None
3	A	488	71	Minor; cataract with lens implantation	267 U/kg per day × 1 d	Excellent	None
				Minor; cataract with lens implantation	186 U/kg per day × 1 d	Excellent	None
				Minor; circumcision (phimosis)	186 U/kg per day × 1 d	Excellent	None
				Minor; telangiectasia laser coagulation	50 U/kg per day × 1 d	Excellent	None
4	A	100	64	Minor; cataract with lens implantation	162 U/kg per day × 1 d	Excellent	None
				Minor; dental extraction	112 U/kg per day × 3 d	Excellent	None
				Minor; exchange pacemaker batteries	135 U/kg per day × 4 d	Excellent	None
5	A	76	48	Minor; cystoscopy/pyelography	47 U/kg per day × 1 d	Excellent	None
				Minor; endoscopic treatment of esophageal ulcer	165 U/kg per day × 1 d	Excellent	None
				Major; arthroplasty of knee	167 U/kg per day × 9 d	Good	None
				Major; arthroplasty of hip	180 U/kg per day × 9 d	Good	None
6	A	28	41	Major; nephrectomy/splenectomy—splenic hemorrhage intraoperatively	127 U/kg per day × 17 d	Good	None
				Major; wound rupture revision	156 U/kg per day × 5 d (rFVIIa used subsequently due to FEIBA shortage)	Excellent	None
7	A	13	69	Major; sigmoidectomy	104 U/kg per day × 13 d	Excellent	Non-ST-elevation myocardial infarction
8	A	270	26	Minor; excision of prepatellar bursa	132 U/kg per day × 5 d	Excellent	None
				Major; arthroplasty of knee	127 U/kg per day × 14 d	Good	None
9	A	77	79	Minor; dental extraction	212 U/kg per day × 3 d	Excellent	None
				Minor; dental extraction	146 U/kg per day × 1 d	Excellent	None
10	A	124	22	Minor; paronychia/toenail excision	156 U/kg per day × 5 d	Excellent	None
				Major; arthroplasty of knee	139 U/kg per day × 23 d	Excellent	None
11	A	26	54	Minor; dental extraction	167 U/kg per day × 4 d	Excellent	None

Abbreviations: BU, Bethesda unit; FEIBA, factor eight inhibitor bypassing activity; FIX, factor IX; FVIII, factor VIII; rFVIIa, activated recombinant factor VII.

has demonstrated that minor and major surgical procedures may be performed with a low risk of bleeding complications in patients with hemophilia and inhibitors, with a high expectation of success. None of the patients experienced bleeding complications due to ineffective hemostatic treatment with FEIBA. One patient became hemodynamically unstable as a result of splenic trauma during a nephrectomy procedure. This was attributed to intraoperative trauma and not to ineffective hemostatic treatment. Patients no. 5 and 8 did experience significant blood loss postoperatively, but overall hemostatic control was still considered to be sufficient and FEIBA efficacy was rated as good. Overall, FEIBA was well tolerated, with no adverse events reported in any of the patients, except patient no. 7. This patient suffered a non-ST-elevation myocardial infarction on the third day following a sigmoidectomy. He was managed with nitrates, opiate analgesia, and diuretics. He was continued on FEIBA therapy, after some consideration, and experienced no further complications. He recovered without any clinical signs of heart failure.

The treatment of patients with high-titer inhibitors is often further complicated by the lack of a reliable laboratory assay to monitor bypassing efficacy. Measurements of prothrombin time (PT) are useful indicators of procoagulant activity but do not provide the information necessary to establish a minimum effective dose or determine dosing frequency. Having a reliable laboratory assay would also help reduce hospital costs, which may be four to five times higher in patients with inhibitors than in patients without inhibitors.[19] A thrombin generation assay is currently under investigation and may prove to be a useful tool in monitoring the efficacy of bypassing agents.

Establishing a minimum effective dose would also be important in reducing cost and preventing overdosing of bypassing agents, which have been associated with severe thrombotic complications. Thrombotic complications are a well-known risk associated with the use of both rFVIIa and FEIBA. In patients with inhibitors, the major clinical manifestation of thrombotic complications is myocardial infarction.[19] While it is uncertain whether an established minimum effective dose could have prevented the occurrence of a non-ST-elevation myocardial infarction in patient no. 7 (evaluated in the Norwegian experience), the risk of such a complication could have been minimized.

Conclusions

Surgical experience in patients with hemophilia and inhibitors has shown that FEIBA can be used safely to maintain perioperative hemostatic control and minimize the risk of major bleeding complications in both major and minor surgical procedures. An accurate method of measuring efficacy is still required and would allow both the establishment of a minimum effective dose and a reduction in the cost of care.

References

1. Ehrenforth S, Kreuz W, Scharrer I, Linde R, Funk M, Güngör T, et al: Incidence of development of factor VIII and factor IX inhibitors in haemophiliacs. Lancet 339:594-598, 1992
2. Sjamsoedin LJM, Heijnen L, Mauser-Bunschoten EP, van Geijlswijk JL, van Houwelingen H, van Asten P, et al: The effect of activated prothrombin-complex concentrate (FEIBA) on joint and muscle bleeding in patients with hemophilia A and antibodies to factor VIII. A double-blind clinical trial. N Engl J Med 305:717-721, 1981
3. Bech RBM, Nielsen L, Falch JF, Glazer S, Hedner U: Evaluation of efficacy of recombinant factor VIIa in 149 patients treated for critical bleeds. Blood 84:68a, 1994 (abstr 262)
4. Rodriguez-Merchan EC, Rocino A: Literature review of surgery management in inhibitor patients. Haemophilia 10:22-29, 2004 (suppl 2)
5. Hilgartner MW, Knatterud GL: The use of factor eight inhibitor bypassing activity (FEIBA immuno) product for treatment of bleeding episodes in hemophiliacs with inhibitors. Blood 61:36-40, 1983
6. Negrier C, Goudemand J, Sultan Y, Bertrand M, Rothschild C, Lauroua P: Multicenter retrospective study on the utilization of FEIBA in France in patients with factor VIII and factor IX inhibitors. French FEIBA Study Group. Factor Eight Bypassing Activity. Thromb Haemost 77: 1113-1119, 1997
7. Faradji A, Bonnomet F, Lecocq J, Grunebaum L, Desprez D, Kern O, et al: Knee joint arthroplasty in a patient with haemophilia A and high inhibitor titre using recombinant factor VIIa (NovoSeven): A new case report and review of the literature. Haemophilia 7:321-326, 2001
8. Hedner U, Glazer S, Pingel K, Alberts KA, Blombäck M, Schulman S, et al: Successful use of recombinant factor VIIa in patient with severe haemophilia A during synovectomy. Lancet 2:1193, 1988
9. Heisel MA, Gomperts ED, McComb JG, Hilgartner M: Use of activated prothrombin complex concentrate over multiple surgical episodes in a hemophilic child with an inhibitor. J Pediatr 102:951-954, 1983
10. Hutchinson RJ, Penner JA, Hensinger RN: Anti-inhibitor coagulant complex (Autoplex) in hemophilia inhibitor patients undergoing synovectomy. Pediatrics 71:631-633, 1983
11. Hvid I, Rodriguez-Merchan EC: Orthopaedic surgery in haemophilic patients with inhibitors: An overview. Haemophilia 8:288-291, 2002
12. Ingerslev J: Efficacy and safety of recombinant factor VIIa in the prophylaxis of bleeding in various surgical procedures in hemophilic patients with factor VIII and factor IX inhibitors. Semin Thromb Hemost 26:425-432, 2000
13. O'Marcaigh AS, Schmalz BJ, Shaughnessy WJ, Gilchrist GS: Successful hemostasis during a major orthopedic operation by using recombinant activated factor VII in a patient with severe hemophilia A and a potent inhibitor. Mayo Clin Proc 69:641-644, 1994
14. Rodriguez-Merchan EC, Wiedel JD, Wallny T, Hvid I, Berntorp E, Rivard G-E, et al: Elective orthopaedic surgery for inhibitor patients. Haemophilia 9:625-631, 2003
15. Schulman S, Lindstedt M, Alberts KA, Agren PH: Recombinant factor VIIa in multiple surgery. Thromb Haemost 71:154, 1994
16. Blatt PM, White GC II, McMillan CW, Roberts HR: Treatment of anti-factor VIII antibodies. Thromb Haemost 38:514-523, 1977
17. Blatt PM, Menache D, Roberts HR: A survey of the effectiveness of prothrombin complex concentrates in controlling hemorrhage in patients with hemophilia and anti-factor VIII antibodies. Thromb Haemost 44:39-42, 1980
18. Penner JA: Treatment of inhibitor patients with activated prothrombin complex concentrates. Prog Clin Biol Res 150:291-308, 1984
19. Tjønnfjord GE, Brinch L, Gedde-Dahl T, Brosstad FR: Activated prothrombin complex concentrate (FEIBA) treatment during surgery in patients with inhibitors to FVIII/IX. Haemophilia 10:174-178, 2004

ELSEVIER
SAUNDERS
email: reprints@elsevier.com

Vol 43, No 3 July 2006

Seminars in HEMATOLOGY

Neal S. Young · Photis Beris
Editors

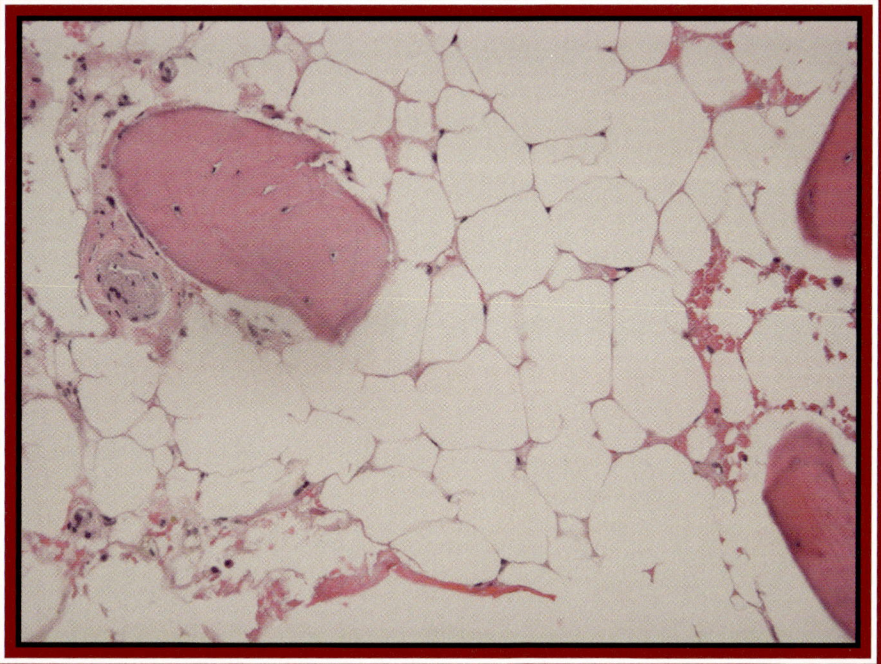

Constitutional Marrow Failure

Grover C. Bagby
Guest Editor

W.B. Saunders

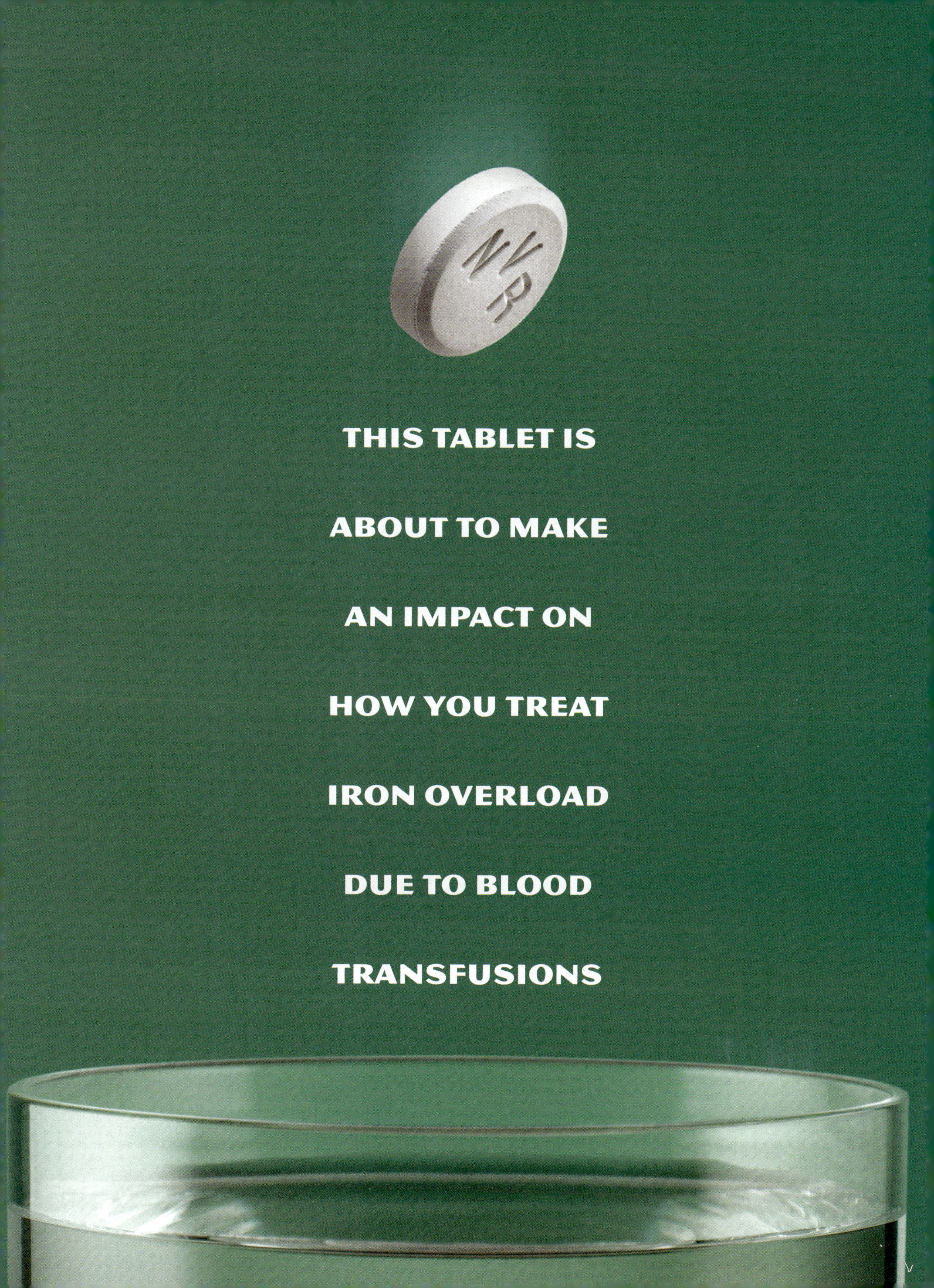
NVR
THIS TABLET IS
ABOUT TO MAKE
AN IMPACT ON
HOW YOU TREAT
IRON OVERLOAD
DUE TO BLOOD
TRANSFUSIONS

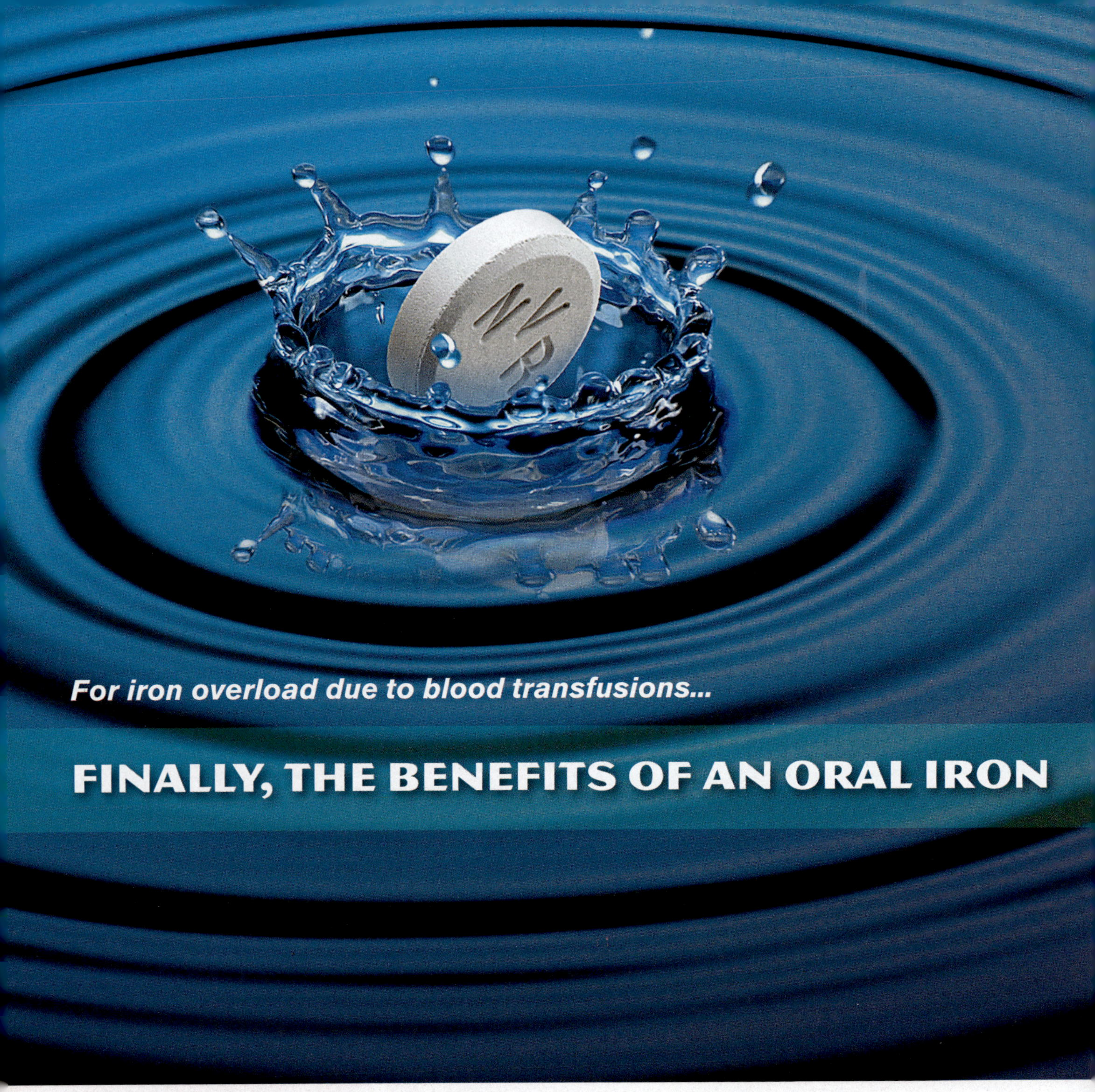

Important safety information

EXJADE is contraindicated in patients with hypersensitivity to deferasirox or to any other component of EXJADE.

Non-progressive increases in serum creatinine have been noted in 38% of EXJADE-treated patients, compared to 15% of deferoxamine-treated patients, and appear to be dose-related. These increases were within the normal range in 94% of patients. Since dose adjustments were made where necessary to manage serum creatinine, serum creatinine should be assessed before initiating therapy and should be monitored monthly thereafter, to determine if dose modification or discontinuation is necessary.

Intermittent proteinuria (urine protein/creatinine ratio >0.6 mg/mg) occurred in 18.6% of EXJADE-treated patients, compared to 7.2% of deferoxamine-treated patients in Study 1 and monitoring is recommended.

Liver function should be monitored monthly, and if there is an unexplained, persistent, or progressive increase in serum transaminase levels, treatment with EXJADE should be interrupted or discontinued. In Study 1, seventeen (5.7%) of patients developed elevations in SGPT/ALT levels >5 times the upper limit of normal at 2 consecutive visits.

Auditory (high frequency hearing loss, decreased hearing) and ocular (lens opacities, cataracts, elevations in intraocular pressure, and retinal disorders) disturbances have been reported with EXJADE therapy in less than 1% of patients in clinical trials. Auditory and ophthalmic testing (including slit lamp examinations and dilated fundoscopy) are recommended before the start of EXJADE treatment and thereafter at regular intervals (every 12 months). If disturbances are noted, dose reduction or interruption should be considered.

Skin rashes may occur during treatment with EXJADE. For rashes of mild to moderate severity, EXJADE may be continued without dose adjustment, since the rash often

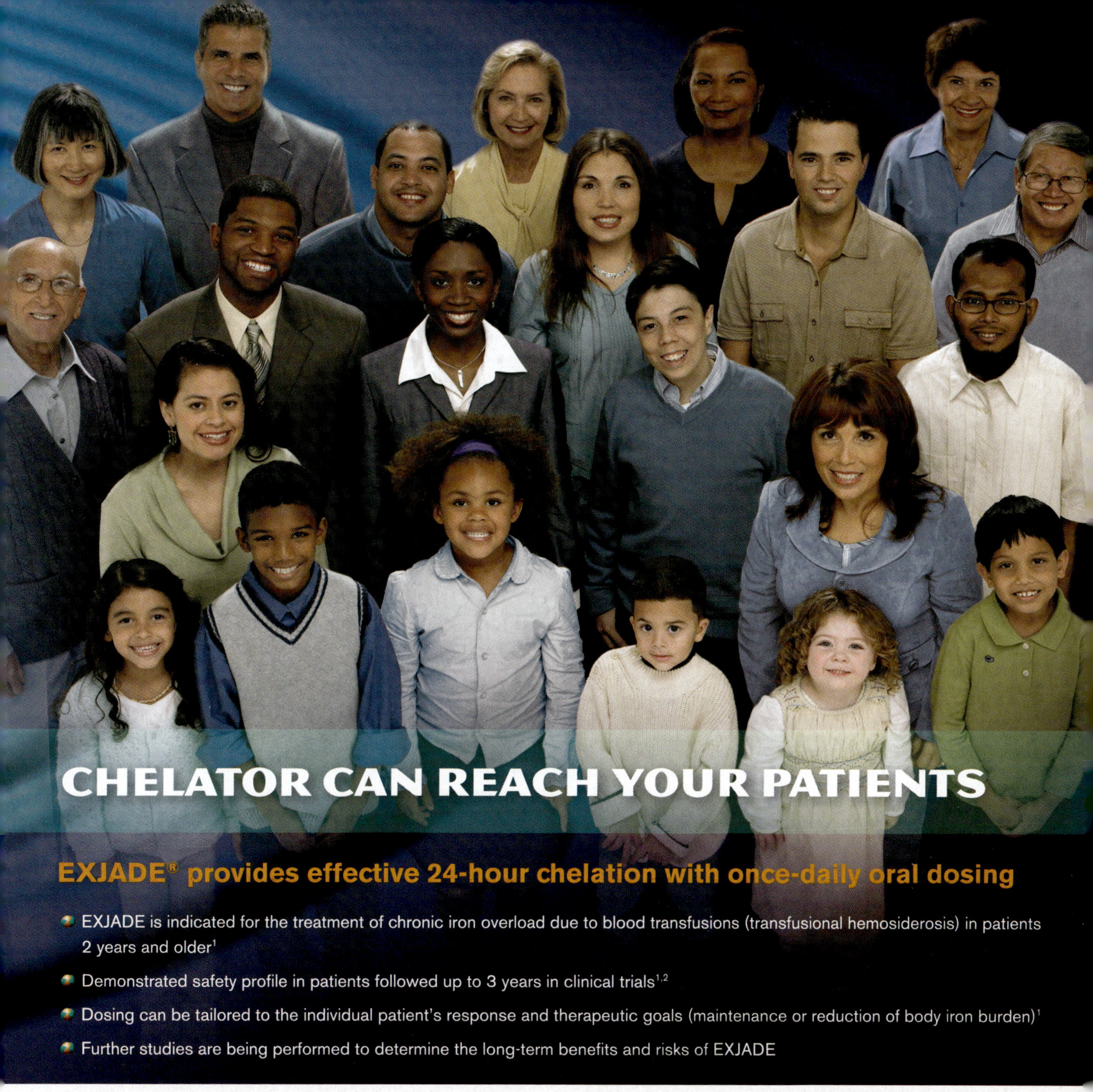

resolves spontaneously. For more severe rash where interruption of treatment may be necessary, EXJADE may be reintroduced at a lower dose and gradually escalated after resolution of the rash. Reintroduction of EXJADE at a lower dose with escalation may be considered in combination with a short period of oral steroid administration.

The most frequently occurring adverse events considered possibly related to EXJADE, included dose-related gastrointestinal disturbances (mainly nausea, vomiting, diarrhea, or abdominal pain), increases in serum creatinine, and skin rash. These commonly reported adverse events were predominantly mild to moderate in severity with limited serious adverse events reported in 9.1% of patients in the EXJADE arm and 8.6% of patients in the deferoxamine arm.

Please see brief summary of prescribing information on adjacent page.

References: 1. EXJADE prescribing information. East Hanover, NJ: Novartis Pharmaceuticals Corporation; 2005. **2.** Data on file, Novartis Pharmaceuticals Corporation, East Hanover, NJ.

EXJADE™

Tablets for Oral Suspension (deferasirox)

ONCE A DAY. EVERY DAY.

EXJADE®

(deferasirox)

Tablets for Oral Suspension

Rx only

BRIEF SUMMARY: Please see package insert for full prescribing information.

INDICATIONS AND USAGE

EXJADE® (deferasirox) is indicated for the treatment of chronic iron overload due to blood transfusions (transfusional hemosiderosis) in patients 2 years of age and older.

CONTRAINDICATIONS

Use of EXJADE® (deferasirox) is contraindicated in patients with hypersensitivity to deferasirox or to any other component of EXJADE.

WARNINGS

Renal

EXJADE® (deferasirox)-treated patients experienced dose-dependent increases in serum creatinine. These increases occurred at a greater frequency compared to deferoxamine-treated patients (38% vs. 15%, respectively) in Study 1. Most of the creatinine elevations remained within the normal range. Serum creatinine should be assessed before initiating therapy and should be monitored monthly thereafter. Dose reduction, interruption, or discontinuation should be considered for elevations in serum creatinine. In the clinical trials, for increases of serum creatinine on two consecutive measures (>33% in patients >15 years of age or >33% and greater than the age-appropriate upper limit of normal in patients <15 years of age), the daily dose of EXJADE was reduced by 10 mg/kg. Patients with serum creatinine above the upper limit of normal were excluded from clinical trials.

In clinical trials, urine protein was measured monthly. Intermittent proteinuria (urine protein/creatinine ratio >0.6 mg/mg) occurred in 18.6% of EXJADE-treated patients compared to 7.2% of deferoxamine-treated patients in Study 1. Although no patients were discontinued from EXJADE in clinical trials up to 1 year due to proteinuria, close monitoring is recommended. The mechanism and clinical significance of the proteinuria are uncertain.

Hepatic

In Study 1, 4 patients discontinued EXJADE because of hepatic abnormalities (drug-induced hepatitis in 2 patients and increased serum transaminases in 2 additional patients). Liver function tests should be monitored monthly during EXJADE treatment and dose modifications considered for severe or persistent elevations.

Special Senses

Auditory disturbances (high frequency hearing loss, decreased hearing), and ocular disturbances (lens opacities, cataracts, elevations in intraocular pressure, and retinal disorders) have been reported at a frequency of <1% with EXJADE therapy in the clinical trials. Auditory and ophthalmic testing (including slit lamp examinations and dilated fundoscopy) are recommended before the start of EXJADE treatment and thereafter at regular intervals (every 12 months). If disturbances are noted, dose reduction or interruption should be considered.

PRECAUTIONS

General

Skin rashes may occur during EXJADE® (deferasirox) treatment. For rashes of mild to moderate severity, EXJADE may be continued without dose adjustment, since the rash often resolves spontaneously. In severe cases, EXJADE may be interrupted. Reintroduction at a lower dose with escalation may be considered in combination with a short period of oral steroid administration.

Information for Patients

EXJADE should be taken once daily on an empty stomach at least 30 minutes prior to food, preferably at the same time every day. The tablets should not be chewed or swallowed whole. The tablets should first be completely dispersed in water, orange juice, or apple juice, and the resulting suspension drunk immediately. After swallowing the suspension, any residue should be resuspended in a small volume of the liquid and swallowed.

Patients should be cautioned not to take aluminum-containing antacids and EXJADE simultaneously.

Because auditory and ocular disturbances have been reported with EXJADE, patients should have auditory and ophthalmic testing before starting EXJADE treatment and thereafter at regular intervals. *(See WARNINGS, Special Senses.)*

Patients experiencing dizziness should exercise caution when driving or operating machinery *(see ADVERSE REACTIONS)*.

Laboratory Tests

Serum ferritin should be measured monthly to assess response to therapy and to evaluate for the possibility of overchelation of iron. If the serum ferritin falls consistently below 500 mcg/L, consideration should be given to temporarily interrupting therapy with EXJADE. *(See DOSAGE AND ADMINISTRATION.)*

In the clinical studies, the correlation coefficient between the serum ferritin and LIC was 0.63. Therefore, changes in serum ferritin levels may not always reliably reflect changes in LIC.

Laboratory monitoring of renal and hepatic function should be performed. *(See WARNINGS.)*

Drug Interactions

The concomitant administration of EXJADE and aluminum-containing antacid preparations has not been formally studied. Although deferasirox has a lower affinity for aluminum than for iron, EXJADE should not be taken with aluminum-containing antacid preparations.

In healthy volunteers, EXJADE had no effect on the pharmacokinetics of digoxin. The effect of digoxin on EXJADE pharmacokinetics has not been studied.

The concomitant administration of EXJADE and vitamin C has not been formally studied. Doses of vitamin C up to 200 mg were allowed in clinical studies without negative consequences.

The interaction of EXJADE with hydroxyurea has not been formally studied. No inhibition of deferasirox metabolism by hydroxyurea is expected based on the results of an *in vitro* study.

EXJADE should not be combined with other iron chelator therapies as safety of such combinations has not been established.

Drug/Food Interactions

The bioavailability (AUC) of deferasirox was variably increased when taken with a meal. Deferasirox should be taken on an empty stomach 30 minutes before eating.

EXJADE tablets for oral suspension can be dispersed in water, orange juice, or apple juice.

Carcinogenicity/Mutagenesis/Impairment of Fertility

A 104-week oral carcinogenicity study in Wistar rats showed no evidence of carcinogenicity from deferasirox at doses up to 60 mg/kg per day (about 0.48 times the recommended human oral dose based on body surface area). A 26-week oral carcinogenicity study in p53 (+/-) transgenic mice has shown no evidence of carcinogenicity from deferasirox at doses up to 200 mg/kg per day (about 0.81 times the recommended human oral dose based on body surface area) in males and 300 mg/kg per day (about 1.21 times the recommended human oral dose based on body surface area) in females.

Deferasirox was negative in the Ames test and chromosome aberration test with human peripheral blood lymphocytes. It was positive in 1 of 3 *in vivo* oral rat micronucleus tests.

Deferasirox at oral doses up to 75 mg/kg per day (about 0.6 times the recommended human oral dose based on body surface area) was found to have no adverse effect on fertility and reproductive performance of male and female rats.

Pregnancy, Teratogenic Effects: Pregnancy Category B

Reproduction studies have been performed in pregnant rats at oral doses up to 100 mg/kg per day (about 0.8 times the recommended human oral dose based on body surface area) and in pregnant rabbits at oral doses up to 50 mg/kg per day (about 0.8 times the recommended human oral dose based on body surface area). These studies have revealed no evidence of impaired fertility or harm to the fetus due to deferasirox. There are, however, no adequate and well-controlled studies in pregnant women. Because animal reproduction studies are not always predictive of human response, deferasirox should be used during pregnancy only if clearly needed.

Nursing Mothers

It is not known whether deferasirox is excreted in human milk. Deferasirox and its metabolites were excreted in breast milk of rats following a 10 mg/kg dose (about 0.08 times the recommended human oral dose based on body surface area). Because many drugs are excreted in human milk, caution should be exercised when deferasirox is administered to a nursing woman.

Pediatric Use

Of the 700 patients who received EXJADE during clinical trials, 292 were pediatric patients 2 to <16 years of age with various congenital and acquired anemias, including 52 patients age 2 to <6 years, 121 patients age 6 to <12 years and 119 patients age 12 to <16 years. Seventy percent of these patients had β-thalassemia. Children between the ages of 2 to <6 years have a systemic exposure to EXJADE approximately 50% of that of adults *(see CLINICAL PHARMACOLOGY)*. However, the safety and efficacy of EXJADE in pediatric patients was similar to that of adult patients, and younger pediatric patients responded similarly to older pediatric patients. The recommended starting dose and dosing modification are the same for children and adults. *(See CLINICAL STUDIES, INDICATIONS AND USAGE, and DOSAGE AND ADMINISTRATION.)*

During the 1 year study, the growth and development were within normal limits.

Geriatric Use

EXJADE did not include sufficient numbers of subjects aged 65 and over to determine whether they respond differently from younger subjects. Thirty patients ≥65 years of age were included in clinical trials of EXJADE. The majority of these patients had myelodysplastic syndrome (MDS, n=27; other anemias, n=3). In general, caution should be used in elderly patients due to the greater frequency of decreased hepatic, renal, or cardiac function, and of concomitant disease or other drug therapy.

ADVERSE REACTIONS

A total of 700 patients were treated with EXJADE® (deferasirox) in therapeutic studies lasting for 48 weeks in adult and pediatric patients. These 700 patients included 469 with β-thalassemia, 99 with rare anemias, and 132 with sickle cell disease. Of these patients, 45% were male, 70% were Caucasian and 292 patients were <16 years of age. In the sickle cell disease population, 89% of patients were Black. Four hundred sixty-nine patients (403 β-thalassemia and 66 rare anemias) were entered into extensions of the original clinical protocols. In ongoing extension studies, median durations of treatment were 85 to 143 weeks.

The most frequently occurring adverse events in the therapeutic trials of EXJADE were diarrhea, vomiting, nausea, headache, abdominal pain, pyrexia, cough, and an increase in serum creatinine. Gastrointestinal symptoms, increases in serum creatinine, and skin rash were dose related.

Table 1 displays adverse events occurring in >5% of patients in either treatment group in Study 1. Abdominal pain, nausea, vomiting, diarrhea, and skin rashes were the most frequent adverse events reported with a suspected relationship to EXJADE.

Table 1
Adverse Events Occurring in >5% of β-Thalassemia Patients in Study 1

Preferred Term	EXJADE® N=296 n (%)	Deferoxamine N=290 n (%)	Preferred Term	EXJADE® N=296 n (%)	Deferoxamine N=290 n (%)
Pyrexia	56 (18.9)	69 (23.8)	Bronchitis	27 (9.1)	32 (11.0)
Headache	47 (15.9)	59 (20.3)	Rash	25 (8.4)	9 (3.1)
Abdominal Pain	41 (13.9)	28 (9.7)	Abdominal Pain Upper	23 (7.8)	15 (5.2)
Cough	41 (13.9)	55 (19.0)	Pharyngitis	23 (7.8)	30 (10.3)
Nasopharyngitis	39 (13.2)	42 (14.5)	Arthralgia	22 (7.4)	14 (4.8)
Diarrhea	35 (11.8)	21 (7.2)	Acute Tonsillitis	19 (6.4)	15 (5.2)
Creatinine Increased*	33 (11.1)	0 (0)	Fatigue	18 (6.1)	14 (4.8)
Influenza	32 (10.8)	29 (10.0)	Rhinitis	18 (6.1)	22 (7.6)
Nausea	31 (10.5)	14 (4.8)	Back Pain	17 (5.7)	32 (11.0)
Pharyngolaryngeal Pain	31 (10.5)	43 (14.8)	Ear Infection	16 (5.4)	7 (2.4)
Vomiting	30 (10.1)	28 (9.7)	Urticaria	11 (3.7)	17 (5.9)
Respiratory Tract Infection	28 (9.5)	23 (7.9)			

*Includes 'blood creatinine increased' and 'blood creatinine abnormal' which were reported as adverse events. *Also see Table 2.*

In Study 1, 113 patients treated with EXJADE had increases in serum creatinine >33% above baseline on 2 separate occasions (Table 2). Twenty-five patients required dose reductions. Increases in serum creatinine appeared to be dose related. *(See WARNINGS, Renal.)* Seventeen patients developed elevations in SGPT/ALT levels >5 times the upper limit of normal at 2 consecutive visits. Two patients had liver biopsy proven drug-induced hepatitis and both discontinued EXJADE therapy. *(See WARNINGS, Hepatic.)* Two additional patients, who did not have elevations in SGPT/ALT >5 times the upper limit of normal, discontinued EXJADE because of increased SGPT/ALT. Increases in transaminases did not appear to be dose related.

Table 2
Number (%) of Patients with Increases in Serum Creatinine or SGPT/ALT in Study 1

Laboratory Parameter	EXJADE® N=296 n (%)	Deferoxamine N=290 n (%)
Serum Creatinine		
Creatinine >33% and <ULN at ≥2 consecutive post-baseline visits	113 (38.2)	41 (14.1)
Creatinine increase >33% and >ULN at ≥2 consecutive post-baseline visits	7 (2.4)	1 (0.3)
SGPT/ALT		
SGPT/ALT >5 x ULN at ≥2 post-baseline visits	25 (8.4)	7 (2.4)
SGPT/ALT >5 x ULN at ≥2 consecutive post-baseline visits	17 (5.7)	5 (1.7)

Adverse events that led to discontinuations included abnormal liver function tests (2 patients) and drug-induced hepatitis (2 patients), skin rash, glycosuria/proteinuria, Henoch Schönlein purpura, hyperactivity/insomnia, drug fever, and cataract (1 patient each).

In the overall population of 700 patients, uncommon adverse reactions (0.1% to 1%) included gastritis, edema, sleep disorder, pigmentation disorder, dizziness, anxiety, maculopathy, cholelithiasis, pyrexia, fatigue, pharyngolaryngeal pain, early cataract and hearing loss *(see PRECAUTIONS)*. Adverse events which most frequently led to dose interruption or dose adjustment were rash, gastrointestinal disorders, infections, increased serum creatinine, and increased serum transaminases.

OVERDOSAGE

There have been no reports of acute overdose with EXJADE® (deferasirox). Single doses up to 80 mg/kg in iron overloaded β-thalassemic patients have been tolerated with nausea and diarrhea noted. In healthy volunteers, single doses of up to 40 mg/kg were tolerated. There is no specific antidote for EXJADE. In case of overdose, induce vomiting and gastric lavage.

DOSAGE AND ADMINISTRATION

It is recommended that therapy with EXJADE® (deferasirox) be started when a patient has evidence of chronic iron overload, such as the transfusion of approximately 100 mL/kg of packed red blood cells (approximately 20 units for a 40 kg patient) and a serum ferritin consistently >1000 mcg/L.

Starting Dose

The recommended initial daily dose of EXJADE is 20 mg/kg body weight.

Maintenance

After commencing initial therapy, it is recommended that serum ferritin be monitored every month and the dose of EXJADE adjusted if necessary every 3 to 6 months based on serum ferritin trends. Dose adjustments should be made in steps of 5 or 10 mg/kg and should be tailored to the individual patient's response and therapeutic goals (maintenance or reduction of body iron burden). If the serum ferritin falls consistently below 500 mcg/L, consideration should be given to temporarily interrupting therapy with EXJADE. Doses of EXJADE should not exceed 30 mg/kg per day since there is limited experience with doses above this level.

Administration Instructions

EXJADE should be taken once daily on an empty stomach at least 30 minutes before food, preferably at the same time each day. Tablets should not be chewed or swallowed whole. EXJADE should not be taken with aluminum-containing antacid products. Doses (mg/kg) should be calculated to the nearest whole tablet. Tablets should be completely dispersed by stirring in water, orange juice, or apple juice until a fine suspension is obtained. Doses of <1 g should be dispersed in 3.5 ounces of liquid and doses of >1 g in 7.0 ounces of liquid. After swallowing the suspension, any residue should be resuspended in a small volume of liquid and swallowed.

Storage

Store at 25°C (77°F). Excursions permitted to 15-30°C (59-86°F) [see USP Controlled Room Temperature]. Protect from moisture.

T2005-65
NOVEMBER 2005 PRINTED IN U.S.A. 5000546

Manufactured by:
Novartis Pharma Stein AG
Stein, Switzerland

Distributed by:
Novartis Pharmaceuticals Corporation
East Hanover, New Jersey 07936

NOVARTIS
ONCOLOGY

Seminars in HEMATOLOGY

Neal S. Young · Photis Beris
Editors

Peter A. Miescher, *Founding Editor* Ernst R. Jaffé, *Co-Editor Emeritus*

Seminars in Hematology (ISSN 0037-1963) is published quarterly by Elsevier Inc, 360 Park Avenue South, New York, NY 10010-1710. Months of issue are January, April, July and October. Business and Editorial Office: 1600 John F. Kennedy Blvd., Ste. 1800, Philadelphia, PA 19103-2899. Customer Service Office: 6277 Sea Harbor Drive, Orlando, FL 32887-4800. Periodicals postage paid at New York, NY and additional mailing offices.

POSTMASTER: Send address changes to *Seminars in Hematology*, Elsevier Customer Service, 6277 Sea Harbor Drive, Orlando, FL 32887-4800.

Editorial correspondence should be addressed to Photis Beris, MD, Division d'Hématologie, Hôpital Cantonal Universitaire, 25 rue Micheli-du-Crest, 1211 Geneve 14, Switzerland, or Neal S. Young, MD, 4400 17th Street, NW, Washington, DC 20011.

Business correspondence (subscriptions, change of address) should be addressed to the Publisher, Elsevier, 6277 Sea Harbor Dr, Orlando, FL 32887-4800; Email elspcs@elsevier.com.

Change of address notices, including both the old and new addresses of the subscriber, should be sent at least one month in advance.

Customer Service: 1-800-654-2452; outside the United States and Canada, (407) 345-4000.

Yearly subscription rates: United States and possessions: individual, $169.00; institution, $267.00; single issues, $81.00. All other countries: individual, $239.00; institution, $339.00; single issues, $81.00. Student and resident: United States and possessions, and Canada: $85.00; all other countries: $122.00. To receive student/resident rate, orders must be accompanied by name of affiliated institution, date of term, and the *signature* of program/residency coordinator on institution letterhead. Orders will be billed at individual rate until proof of status is received. Current prices are in effect for back volumes and back issues. Single issues, both current and back, exist in limited quantities and are offered for sale subject to availability. Back issues sold in conjunction with a subscription are on a prorated basis. Prices are subject to change without notice. *Checks* should be made payable to Elsevier and sent to *Seminars in Hematology*, Elsevier, Periodicals Department, PO Box 628239, Orlando, FL 32862-8239.

Other correspondence (copyediting, production) should be addressed to Elsevier, 1600 John F. Kennedy Blvd, Ste 1800, Philadelphia, PA 19103-2899.

Reprints: For 100 or more copies of an article in this publication, please contact the Commercial Reprints Department, Elsevier, 360 Park Ave South, New York, NY 10010-1710. Telephone (212) 633-3813, fax (212) 633-3820; e-mail, reprints@elsevier.com.

Advertising Representative: Cunningham Associates, 180 Old Tappan Rd, Old Tappan, NJ 07675. Telephone: (201) 767-4170; fax: (201) 767-8065; email: kdunn@cunnasso.com.

The contents of *Seminars in Hematology* are indexed in *Index Medicus* and *MEDLINE, Current Contents/Clinical Medicine, Current Contents/Life Sciences,* Science Citation Index, and *EMBASE/* Excerpta Medica.

The *Seminars in Hematology* home page is located at *www.seminhematol.org*.

W.B. Saunders **Philadelphia, PA**

Seminars in HEMATOLOGY

Vol 43, No 3, July 2006

Constitutional Marrow Failure

Grover C. Bagby
Guest Editor

Constitutional Marrow Failure: Introduction 145
Grover C. Bagby

Fanconi Anemia 147
Grover C. Bagby and Blanche P. Alter

Dyskeratosis Congenita 157
Tom Vulliamy and Inderjeet Dokal

Diamond Blackfan Anemia: New Paradigms for a "Not So Pure" Inherited Red Cell Aplasia 167
Jeffrey M. Lipton

Shwachman-Diamond Syndrome 178
Akiko Shimamura

Severe Congenital Neutropenia 189
Karl Welte, Cornelia Zeidler, and David C. Dale

Inherited Thrombocytopenia: Congenital Amegakaryocytic Thrombocytopenia and Thrombocytopenia With Absent Radii 196
Amy E. Geddis

Erratum 204

Cover Illustration: Hematoxylin and eosin–stained bone marrow biopsy from a pancytopenic patient with severe acquired aplastic anemia (courtesy of Dr K. Gatter, OHSU School of Medicine, Department of Pathology).

Seminars in HEMATOLOGY

Previous Issues

2005

Vol 42, No 1, January — **von Willebrand Factor in Hemostasis and Thrombosis**
Pier M. Mannucci, Guest Editor

Vol 42, No 2, April — **Immune Hemolytic Anemia**
George Garratty, Guest Editor

Vol 42, No 3, July — **Transplant Immunobiology**
Effie W. Petersdorf, Guest Editor

Vol 42, No 4, October — **Chronic Myeloproliferative Disorders**
Radek Skoda and Josef T. Prchal, Guest Editors

2004

Vol 41, No 1, January — **Thrombotic Thrombocytopenic Purpura: Advances in Pathophysiology, Diagnosis, and Treatment**
Bernhard Lämmle and James N. George, Guest Editors

Vol 41, No 2, April — **Erythrocyte Membrane Proteins and Their Diseases**
Narla Mohandas, Guest Editor

Vol 41, No 3, July — **Chronic Lymphocytic Leukemia**
Kanti R. Rai and Jacques Louis Binet, Guest Editors

Vol 41, No 4, October — **Gene Therapy in Hematology**
Cynthia E. Dunbar, Guest Editor

2003

Vol 40, No 1, January — **Management of Chronic Myeloid Leukemia**
John M. Goldman, Guest Editor

Vol 40, No 2, April — **Herpesvirus in Hematology**
Giovanna Tosato, Guest Editor

Vol 40, No 3, July — **Hematologic Malignancies of Cytotoxic Cells**
Thomas P. Loughran Jr, Guest Editor

Vol 40, No 4, October — **Genomics in Hematology**
Louis M. Staudt, Guest Editor

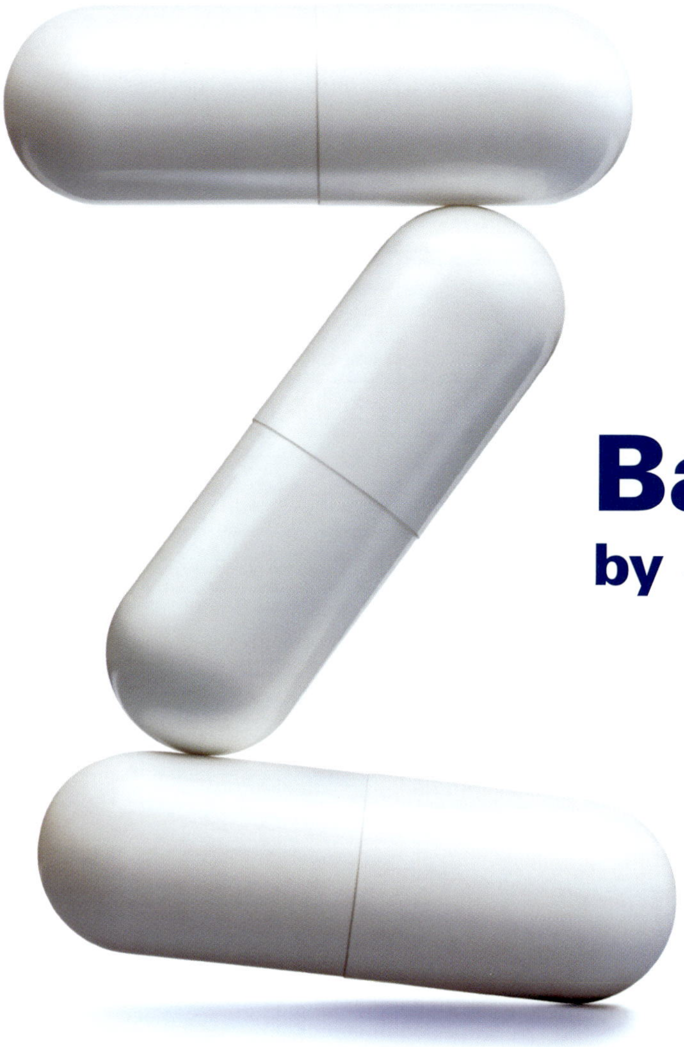

For adults with mild-to-moderate ***type 1 Gaucher disease*** *for whom enzyme replacement therapy is not an option*

Balance
by Substrate Reduction

Substrate Reduction Therapy (SRT) With Zavesca Provides Important Benefits

- Liver and spleen volume reductions seen as early as month 6—continued reductions over 24 months
- Hemoglobin concentration and platelet count improvements seen as early as month 6—significant improvements seen at 24 months

Zavesca Maintained Benefits of Long-Term Enzyme Replacement Therapy (ERT)

- In patients on ERT for a mean of 5.6 years, liver and spleen volume, as well as hemoglobin concentration and platelet count, were maintained after 6 months of Zavesca monotherapy

Important Safety Information

- Peripheral neuropathy has been reported in patients receiving Zavesca
- Zavesca may cause fetal harm if administered to a pregnant woman
- There is a risk of impaired fertility in men

Convenient Oral Dosing

- Recommended at 100 mg tid
- May be taken with or without food

Zavesca may be prescribed only by physicians knowledgeable in the management of Gaucher disease

- **Visit www.ZAVESCA.com or call 1.866.228.3546**

ZAVESCA® 100mg
(miglustat) capsules

Please see brief summary of full prescribing information on following page.

ACTELION

ZAVESCA® [miglustat] Capsules, 100mg

ZAVESCA 100mg
(miglustat) capsules

Brief Summary: Please see package insert for full prescribing information.

INDICATION AND USAGE: ZAVESCA® is indicated for the treatment of adult patients with mild to moderate type 1 Gaucher disease for whom enzyme replacement therapy is not a therapeutic option (e.g., due to constraints such as allergy, hypersensitivity, or poor venous access).

CONTRAINDICATIONS: ZAVESCA® is contraindicated in patients who have demonstrated hypersensitivity to the active substance or any of the excipients. Pregnancy Category X. Miglustat may cause fetal harm when administered to a pregnant woman. ZAVESCA® is contraindicated in women who are or may become pregnant. If this drug is administered to a woman with reproductive potential, the patient should be apprised of the potential hazard to a fetus.

WARNINGS: Cases of peripheral neuropathy have been reported in patients treated with ZAVESCA®. All patients undergoing ZAVESCA® treatment should undergo baseline and repeat neurological evaluations at approximately 6-month intervals. Patients who develop symptoms such as numbness and tingling should have a careful re-assessment of the risk/benefit of ZAVESCA® therapy and cessation of treatment may be considered.

PRECAUTIONS: *Tremor:* Approximately 30% of patients have reported tremor or exacerbation of existing tremor on treatment. Tremor usually began within the first month of therapy and in many cases resolved between 1 to 3 months during treatment. Dose reduction may ameliorate the tremor usually within days but discontinuation of treatment may sometimes be required. *Diarrhea and Weight Loss:* Diarrhea and weight loss were common in clinical studies of patients treated with ZAVESCA®, approximately 85% and up to 65% of treated patients, respectively, reporting these conditions. Diarrhea appears to be the result of the disaccharidase inhibitory activity of ZAVESCA®, with a resultant osmotic diarrhea. It is unclear if weight loss results from the diarrhea and associated gastrointestinal complaints, a decrease in food intake, or a combination of these or other factors. The incidence of diarrhea was noted to decrease over time with continued ZAVESCA® treatment, and was noted to result in an increase in the use of anti-diarrheal medications, most commonly loperamide. Patients may be instructed to avoid high carbohydrate content foods during treatment with ZAVESCA® if they present with diarrhea. The incidence of weight loss was most evident in the first 12 months of treatment. *Male Fertility:* Male patients should maintain reliable contraceptive methods while taking ZAVESCA®. Studies in the rat have shown that miglustat adversely affects spermatogenesis and sperm parameters, thereby reducing fertility. Until further information is available, it is advised that before seeking to conceive, male patients should cease ZAVESCA® and maintain reliable contraceptive methods for 3 months thereafter.

Information for patients: Patients are advised to consult the ZAVESCA® Patient Information section in the full prescribing information on the safe use of ZAVESCA®. Patients should be informed of the potential risks and benefits of ZAVESCA® and of alternative modes of therapy. Patients should be advised that diarrhea, gastrointestinal complaints, and weight loss are common side effects of ZAVESCA® therapy, and to adhere to dietary instructions. Patients should also be advised to promptly report any numbness, pain, or burning in the hands and feet, and the development of tremor or worsening in an existing tremor.

Drug Interactions: While co-administration of ZAVESCA® appeared to increase the clearance of Cerezyme® (imiglucerase) by 70%, these results are not conclusive because of the small number of subjects studied and because patients took variable doses of Cerezyme. Combination therapy with Cerezyme and ZAVESCA® is not indicated. Miglustat does not inhibit or induce various substrates of CYP450 enzymes; consequently significant interactions are unlikely with drugs that are substrates of CYP450 enzymes. Concomitant therapy with loperamide during clinical trials did not appear to significantly alter the pharmacokinetics of ZAVESCA®.

Carcinogenesis, Mutagenesis, and Impairment of Fertility: Long-term studies in animals to evaluate the carcinogenic potential of miglustat have not been conducted. Miglustat was not mutagenic or clastogenic in a battery of *in vitro* and *in vivo* assays including the bacterial reverse mutation (Ames), chromosomal aberration (in human lymphocytes), gene mutation in mammalian cells (Chinese hamster ovary), and mouse micronucleus assays. Male rats, given 20 mg/kg/day miglustat by oral gavage 14 days prior to mating, had decreased spermatogenesis with altered sperm morphology and motility and decreased fertility. Decreased spermatogenesis was reversible following 6 weeks of drug withdrawal. A higher dose of 60 mg/kg/day resulted in seminiferous tubule and testicular atrophy/degeneration. Female rats were given oral gavage doses of 20, 60, 180 mg/kg/day beginning 14 days before mating and continuing through gestation. Effects observed at 20 mg/kg/day included decreased corpora lutea, increased post implantation loss, and decreased live births.

Pregnancy: Category X. There are no adequate and well-controlled studies of miglustat in pregnant women. ZAVESCA® should not be used during pregnancy.

SPECIAL POPULATIONS: *Labor and Delivery:* Studies in pregnant rats exposed to ZAVESCA® during gestation through lactation are associated with dystocia and delayed parturition at systemic exposure 2 times the human therapeutic systemic exposure, based on body surface area comparisons. *Nursing Mothers:* It is not known whether miglustat is excreted in human milk. ZAVESCA® should not be used in nursing mothers unless the potential benefit justifies the potential risk to the infant. A decision should be made whether to discontinue nursing or discontinue the drug, taking into account the importance of the drug to the lactating woman. *Pediatric Use:* The safety and effectiveness of ZAVESCA® have not been evaluated in patients under the age of 18. The effects of ZAVESCA® on growth and development in children have not been evaluated. *Geriatric Use:* Clinical studies of ZAVESCA® did not include sufficient numbers of patients aged 65 and over. Other reported clinical experience has not identified differences in responses between elderly and younger patients. In general, dose selection for an elderly patient should be cautious, usually starting at the low end of the dosing range, reflecting the greater frequency of decreased hepatic, renal, and cardiac function and of concomitant disease or other drug therapy. *Renal Impairment:* Miglustat is known to be substantially excreted by the kidney, and the risk of adverse reactions to this drug may be greater in patients with impaired renal function. As a result of this, dose reductions are recommended for those patients with mild to moderate renal impairment, the reduction being dependent upon the level of their creatinine clearance adjustment. For those patients with severe renal impairment, treatment with miglustat is not recommended. Since elderly patients are more likely to have decreased renal function, care should be taken in dose selection, and it may be useful to monitor renal function.

ADVERSE REACTIONS: The safety and tolerability of ZAVESCA® have been evaluated in 80 adult type 1 Gaucher disease patients in two open-label uncontrolled and one open-label active controlled trials. All 80 patients in the combined dataset from the clinical studies reported at least one adverse event during their treatment period. *Open-Label Uncontrolled Monotherapy Trials:* In two trials in adult type 1 Gaucher disease patients treated with ZAVESCA® at a starting dose of 100 mg three times daily for 12 months in 28 patients [Study 1], or at a dose of 50 mg three times daily for 6 months in 18 patients [Study 2], gastrointestinal events were observed in more than 80% of patients either at the outset of treatment, or intermittently during treatment. Diarrhea was observed in approximately 85% of patients. Weight loss has been observed in up to 65% of patients. In the two open-label, uncontrolled monotherapy trials, the Adverse Reactions by WHO body system and preferred term occurring with an incidence of ≥5%, are presented in the following table.

Adverse Reactions in ≥5% of Patients in Two Open-Label, Uncontrolled Monotherapy Trials of ZAVESCA®

	Incidence of Adverse Reaction	
	Study 1 (starting dose of 100 mg TID)	Study 2 (50 mg TID)
Patients Entered in Study (n)	28	18
Body System—Preferred Term	% of patients reporting	% of patients reporting
Gastrointestinal System		
Diarrhea	89	89
Flatulence	29	44
Abdominal pain	18	50
Nausea	14	22
Vomiting	4	11
Bloating	0	6
Anorexia	7	0
Dyspepsia	7	0
Epigastric pain not food related	0	6
Metabolic and Nutritional Disorders		
Weight decrease	39	67
Central and Peripheral Nervous System		
Headache	21	22
Tremor	11	11
Dizziness	0	11
Cramps legs	4	11
Paresthesia	7	0
Migraine	0	6
Vision Disorders		
Visual disturbance	0	17
Musculoskeletal Disorders		
Cramps	0	11
Platelet, Bleeding, and Clotting Disorders		
Thrombocytopenia	7	6
Reproductive Disorders, Female		
Menstrual disorder	0	6

Open-Label Active-Controlled Study: In an open-label, active-controlled study, 36 adult type 1 Gaucher disease patients were treated with ZAVESCA®, Cerezyme, or ZAVESCA® + Cerezyme (Study 3). Gastrointestinal adverse events and weight loss were commonly seen in patients exposed to ZAVESCA®. The Adverse Reactions by WHO body system and preferred term occurring with an incidence of ≥5%, are presented in the following table.

Adverse Reactions in ≥5% of Patients in Open-Label Active-Controlled Study

	Incidence of Adverse Reaction		
	ZAVESCA® alone	Cerezyme alone	ZAVESCA® + Cerezyme
Patients Entered in Study (n)	12	12	12
Body System – Preferred Term	% of patients reporting	% of patients reporting	% of patients reporting
Gastrointestinal System			
Diarrhea	100	0	83
Abdominal pain	67	0	58
Flatulence	50	0	42
Constipation	8	0	25
Nausea	8	0	8
Mouth dry	8	0	0
Body as a Whole			
Influenza-like symptoms	0	0	8
Pain	0	8	8
Pain legs	0	0	8
Weakness generalized	17	0	8
Abdominal distension	8	0	8
Back pain	8	0	0
Abdominal distension gaseous	8	0	0
Chills	0	0	8
Heaviness in limbs	8	0	0
Metabolic and Nutritional Disorders			
Weight decrease	67	0	42
Central and Peripheral Nervous System			
Tremor	17	0	33
Dizziness	8	0	25
Cramps legs	8	0	0
Gait unsteady	8	0	0
Numbness localized	0	0	8
Shaking	0	0	8
Psychiatric Disorders			
Appetite absent	0	0	8
Jitteriness	0	0	8
Memory loss	8	0	0
Vision Disorders			
Eye abnormality	0	0	8
Visual disturbance	0	0	8
Reproductive Disorders, Female			
Menstrual irregularity	0	0	8

OVERDOSAGE: In the clinical development program for ZAVESCA®, no patient experienced an overdose of study drug. However, ZAVESCA® has been administered at doses of up to 3000 mg/day (approximately 10 times the recommended starting dose administered to Gaucher patients) for up to six months in HIV-positive patients. Adverse events observed in the HIV studies included granulocytopenia, dizziness, and paresthesia. Leukopenia and neutropenia have also been observed in a similar group of patients receiving 800 mg/day or above.

DOSAGE AND ADMINISTRATION: Therapy should be directed by physicians who are knowledgeable in the management of Gaucher disease. The recommended dose for the treatment of adult patients with type 1 Gaucher disease is one 100 mg capsule administered orally three times a day at regular intervals. It may be necessary to reduce the dose to one 100 mg capsule once or twice a day in some patients for adverse effects, such as diarrhea or tremor. In patients with mild renal impairment (adjusted creatinine clearance 50–70 mL/min/1.73 m^2), ZAVESCA® administration should commence at a dose of 100 mg twice per day. In patients with moderate renal impairment (adjusted creatinine clearance of 30–50 mL/min/1.73 m^2), ZAVESCA® administration should commence at a dose of one 100 mg capsule per day. Use of ZAVESCA® in patients with severe renal impairment (creatinine clearance of <30 mL/min/1.73 m^2) is not recommended.

HOW SUPPLIED: ZAVESCA® is supplied in hard gelatin capsules containing 100 mg miglustat. ZAVESCA® 100 mg capsules are white opaque with "OGT 918 " printed in black on the cap and "100 " printed in black on the body. ZAVESCA® 100 mg capsules are packed in blister cards. Five blister cards of 18 capsules are supplied in each carton. NDC 66215-201-90: carton containing 90 capsules. NDC 66215-201-18: blister card containing 18 capsules.

Rx only

STORAGE: Store at 20°C to 25°C (68°F to 77°F). Brief exposure to 15°C to 30°C (59°F to 86°F) permitted (see USP Controlled Room Temperature).

ACTELION

Seminars in
HEMATOLOGY

Future Topics

Vol 43, No 4, October	**Treatment of Diffuse Large B-Cell Lymphomas** *Richard I. Fisher, Guest Editor*
Vol 44, No 1, January	**Transfusion Medicine in the Early 21st Century** *Harvey Klein, Guest Editor*
Vol 44, No 2, April	**Inherited Thrombophilias** *Michael Greaves, Guest Editor*
Vol 44, No 3, July	**Hematopoietic Growth Factors** *Arnold Ganser, Guest Editor*

Seminars in HEMATOLOGY

Forthcoming Issue
October 2006

Treatment of Diffuse Large B-Cell Lymphomas
Richard I. Fisher, *Guest Editor*

Role of ASCT of Advanced Stage Diffuse Large B-Cell Lymphomas — *Stephen J. Forman*

Diffuse Aggressive Histologies of Non-Hodgkin Lymphoma: Treatment and Biology of Limited Disease — *Thomas P. Miller, Catherine M. Spier, and Lisa Rimsza*

Standard Treatment of Advanced Stage Diffuse Large B-Cell Lymphomas — *Bertrand Coiffier*

Dose-Intensified Treatment of Advanced Stage Diffuse Large B-Cell Lymphomas — *Gerhard Held, Joerg Schubert, Marcel Reiser, and Michael Pfreundschuh*

Drug Resistance in Diffuse Large B-Cell Lymphomas — *Wyndham H. Wilson*

New Drugs for the Treatment of Advanced Stage Diffuse Large Cell Lymphomas — *Owen A. O'Connor and Paul Hamlin*

ELSEVIER

Seminars in
HEMATOLOGY

Volume 43, Number 3 July 2006

Constitutional Marrow Failure: Introduction

Many decades ago, before stem cells and progenitor cells could be counted or transplanted, all discussions on the pathogenesis of aplastic states were theoretical. Some hematologists argued that marrow injury was a reflection of external environmental factors. Others thought that it might reflect some inherent defect in tolerance of hematopoietic stem cells or progenitor cells to microenvironmental or intrinsic regulatory factors. In the past 20 years much has been clarified and the answer is: *all of the above*. Many of the recent revelations have been developed in studies on inherited or "constitutional" bone marrow failure states. These are rare conditions, but many are diagnosed initially in adulthood and, most importantly, patients with these types of conditions must be treated differently than one would treat patients with acquired aplastic anemia. For example, treatment of patients with Fanconi anemia or dyskeratosis congenita with routine conditioning regimens for stem cell transplantation will result in excessive morbidity and mortality. Therefore, when hematologists meet pancytopenic patients whose bone marrow biopsy looks like the one on the cover of this issue of *Seminars in Hematology*, these diagnoses must be considered in the interest of the patient and his or her family.

In some cases, studies on acquired aplastic anemia have informed studies on the inherited ones. Since Mathé first observed that some patients transplanted for aplastic anemia recovered with autologous (not donor) hematopoietic cells, a phenomenon attributed to the immunosuppressive conditioning prior to the stem cell infusion, strong evidence has emerged that acquired aplastic anemia is more often than not an autoimmune syndrome mediated by T lymphocytes that release cytokines that induce apoptotic responses in stem cells and progenitors. These studies and clinical observations by Lyle Sensenbrenner on the unusual intensity of graft-versus-host disease (GVHD) in Fanconi anemia (FA) patients informed the design of our own studies on marrow cells from FA patients and FA knockout mice. Today the results from a number of centers indicate that FA hematopoietic progenitor cell populations are apoptotic in the ground state and that the pro-apoptotic state reflected an inherent hypersensitivity of these cells to precisely the same cytokines (eg, tumor necrosis factor-alpha and interferon-gamma) that were over-produced in patients with acquired aplastic anemia (and in GVHD). The role played by some of the FA proteins in normal cells to control these responses is being clarified in a number of centers. More importantly, it is clear that hematopoietic cells from patients with most of the constitutional marrow failure syndromes share the common feature of high apoptotic rates.

Two marrow failure states are truly limited to one lineage. In one the cause is intuitively obvious. Congenital amegakaryocytic thrombocytopenia is clearly associated with mutations of c-MPL, the receptor for thrombopoietin. However, in severe congenital neutropenia, the genotype–phenotype relationship is a bit more mysterious. In this disorder, the mutant protein, neutrophil elastase (ELA-2) seems to ignite an unfolded protein response (and apoptosis) in cells of this lineage. Some surprising molecular convergence points are emerging around ribosomal biogenesis and protein synthesis. Cells from patients with dyskeratosis congenita, Diamond-Blackfan anemia, and Shwachman-Diamond syndrome, for example, share the common features of disordered ribosome biogenesis and/or mRNA translation. Moreover, inactivation of certain of the FA genes as well as ELA-2 suppresses translation. How these commonalities lead to a holistic picture of hematopoietic control will be the subject of intense investigation over the next few years for three reasons.

First, understanding hematopoietic control from a molecular genetic standpoint is inherently important for individuals investigating stem cell biology, stem cell transplantation, and gene therapy. Second, while these disorders can be considered to be "orphan" diseases, the "reach" of research on these disorders includes cancer research in general. Specifically, not only do some of these syndromes predispose patients to epithelial malignancies, it is increasingly clear that the genes mutated in some of these disorders (eg, FA) can be inactivated somatically in neoplastic cells (leading to genetic instability and progression) and overexpressed somatically in others (leading to a drug-resistant phenotype). Therefore these genes can influence the progression of cancer in patients who have not inherited a mutant allele. Third, patients with some of these diseases reliably evolve to acute leukemia and in some the relative risk is nearly 1,000. We are obligated to use this tragic clinical circumstance as a window to identify the very first genetic alterations that occur in a stem cell that set it on a course to acute myelogenous leukemia.

doi:10.1053/j.seminhematol.2006.04.007

How does a rapidly expanding clone evolve from an empty marrow? I think the Darwinian notion of "fitness" is the most reasonable starting point. Intuitively, the AML stem cell has an advantage over the inherently unfit population of stem cells in the marrow of patients in the hypoplastic phase. To become more fit, somatic mutations must occur in a stem cell that interdict precisely the apoptotic pathways ignited in that stem cell population by virtue of the inherited mutation (eg, loss of a FA protein or loss of ELA-2). Given the high apoptotic index of cells lacking the new trait, progeny of cells with the new trait will be selectable. Whether the process involves the selection of a clone that arose stochastically or whether the somatic change meets a geneticist's standard for an "adaptive" mutation is less important than the idea that the successful stem cell clones have adapted, one way or the other.

Three things can happen to an FA stem cell and two of them are bad. First, they can die. Second they can adapt by somatic mutation. Third, they can maladapt by somatic mutation. The least common mutations are those that correct the specific FA mutation in some way. These are "reversions" and are perfect adaptations because many patients with revertant hematopoietic stem cells have good blood counts and improved bone marrow cellularity. All other cells of these patients still have the FA phenotype and genotype, but failure of the marrow no longer represents the leading life-threatening condition for them. The incidence of AML in such cases may be reduced as well, and if this is confirmed, it will validate the key role of damage as a seminal selective force and would also suggest that gene therapy might prevent AML in this setting.

Another type of somatic mutation in FA is probably best categorized as maladaptive. Rather than directly correcting the inherited genetic lesion (which in FA would correct the genetic instability and signal transduction abnormalities at the same time), stem cells might inactivate a related apoptotic pathway, rendering the cells more "fit." However, because not all of the functions of the multifunctional mutant protein are restored, cells may survive that really ought to die (because they are genetically unstable, for example). Naturally this would result in the failure of a genetically unstable clone to respond at all to apoptotic cues—a recipe for additional oncogenic mutations. Now that the functions of the proteins encoded by the genes involved in these disorders are being identified, the signaling pathways that might be targets of maladaptive somatic change will be revealed and this intuitively appealing model of "damage–adaptation–clonal evolution" can be formally tested.

Thought leaders who think day and night about these diseases, the patients afflicted by them, and their families, have written the chapters in this issue. I am confident that readers will find, as I have, that the advances described are exciting and contain lessons of importance not only for practicing hematologists involved in the care of patients with bone marrow failure but for scientists focusing on basic and applied research on hematopoiesis, development, signal transduction, apoptosis, genetic instability, and carcinogenesis. These diseases may be orphan diseases but the clinical consequences of ignoring them diagnostically can be devastating and the overall impact of understanding them at a molecular level will be enormous.

Acknowledgment

I thank Dr Ken Gatter, Department of Pathology, OHSU, and Portland VA Medical Center, for providing the cover image and Lyle Sensenbrenner for sharing his insights on the complexities of GVHD in patients with Fanconi anemia.

Grover C. Bagby, MD
OHSU Cancer Institute
Oregon Health and Science University
and
Portland VA Medical Center
Portland, OR
Guest Editor

Seminars in
HEMATOLOGY

Fanconi Anemia

Grover C. Bagby[a] and Blanche P. Alter[b]

Fanconi anemia (FA) is a rare hereditary disease characterized by bone marrow failure and developmental anomalies; a high incidence of myelodysplasia (MDS), acute nonlymphocytic leukemia (AML), and solid tumors; and cellular hypersensitivity to cross-linking agents. The genetic basis of FA is mutations in any one of the known FA genes. The function of the proteins is largely unknown, but many form complexes with each other, and in one canonical "pathway," eight of the known FA proteins bind together in a complex and monoubiquitinate FANCD2, a protein not present in the core complex. Monoubiquitinated FANCD2 translocates to damage-induced nuclear foci containing BRCA1, BRCA2, and Rad51, thereby protecting the genome. Because hypersensitivity to genotoxic stress is a feature of all somatic cells, this aspect of FA protein function cannot account for the nearly universal development of bone marrow failure. There is strong in vitro and in vivo evidence that at least some of the FA proteins promote survival signaling pathways in hematopoietic cells by forming complexes with signaling molecules. Because associations with heat shock proteins occur in this context, we suggest that these proteins function as co-chaperones and scaffolds that organize proper responses to a wide variety of extracellular cues, some global, and some specific for hematopoietic cells.
Semin Hematol 43:147-156

Seventy-nine years ago, Dr Guido Fanconi reported three siblings who exhibited both congenital defects and aplastic anemia.[1] We now know this disease is largely autosomal recessive (FANCB is X-linked) and rare, with a prevalence of 1 to 5 per million[2] and that it is characterized by life-threatening bone marrow failure and extraordinary risks of myelodysplasia, acute nonlymphocytic leukemia (AML), and certain epithelial malignancies.[3,4] Known as a disorder of cytogenetic instability in which somatic cells are consistently hypersensitive to bifunctional alkylating agents,[5] the diagnostic tests for Fanconi anemia (FA) consist of in vitro culture of replicative cells (usually phytohemagglutinin [PHA]-stimulated peripheral blood lymphocytes or primary skin fibroblasts) in the presence of low doses of either mitomycin C (MMC) or diepoxybutane (DEB) followed by examination of metaphase spreads for evidence of chromosomal breaks and radial chromosomes.[6] Classic clinical features such as growth retardation, small head size, café-au-lait spots, and radial ray defects can be strong diagnostic clues, but FA can occur in patients without congenital defects and may only be ascertained in some cases in adulthood. Consequently, FA should be considered in the differential diagnosis of hypoplastic or aplastic anemias, MDS, and AML in young adults as well as in children, and specific types of solid tumors in young adults (especially head and neck or gynecologic squamous cell carcinomas [SCC]).

Genetic Heterogeneity

Biallelic inactivation of any of 11 known genes causes FA. These genes are termed FANCA, -B,[7] -C, -D1 (BRCA2), -D2, -E, -F, -G (XRCC9), -J (BACH1/BRIP1),[8,9] -L (PHF9),[10] and -M (Hef) (Table 1).[11] The proteins they encode have no strong homologies to one another or to any other known protein (except BRCA2, for which some truncating mutations appear to account for FA-D1).[12] Studies on the function of the FA proteins indicate (1) that they function to protect against genotoxic stress by forming complexes with each other,[13-15] and (2) that they protect some somatic cells from apoptotic cues by both suppressing apoptotic signaling pathways and enhancing signaling pathways ignited by survival factors.[16-18] This second role, at least in the case of FANCC,

[a]OHSU Cancer Institute, Departments of Medicine and Molecular and Medical Genetics, Oregon Health and Science University, Portland, OR.
[b]Clinical Genetics Branch, Division of Cancer Epidemiology and Genetics, National Cancer Institute, National Institutes of Health, Department of Health and Human Services, Bethesda, MD.
Supported in part by grants from the National Heart Lung and Blood Institute, the Department of Veteran's Affairs, and the Fanconi Anemia Research Fund (G.C.B.). Supported in part by the Intramural Research Program of the National Institutes of Health and the National Cancer Institute (B.P.A.).
Address correspondence to Grover C. Bagby, MD, OHSU Cancer Institute, CR145, 3181 SW Sam Jackson Park Rd, Portland, OR 97239. E-mail: grover@ohsu.edu

0037-1963/06/$-see front matter
doi:10.1053/j.seminhematol.2006.04.005

Table 1 The Fanconi Anemia Genes

Gene	Approximate Incidence Among FA Patients (%)	Chromosomal Location	Exon No.	Amino Acid Residues
FANCA	70*	16q24.3	43	1,455
FANCB	1	Xp22.31	10	859
FANCC	10	9q22.3	14	558
FANCD1/BRCA2†	1	13q12.3	27	3,418
FANCD2	2	3p25.3	44	1451
FANCE	5	6p21.3	10	536
FANCF	2	11p15	1	374
FANCG/XRCC9	10	9p13	14	622
FANCJ/BACH1/BRIP1	1	21q22.11	4	736
FANCL	1	2p16.1	11	373
FANCM/Hef	1	14q21.3	23	2,048

*There are more than 100 mutant FANCA alleles, about 40% of which are large intragenic deletions.
†Although a BRCA2 null genotype is an embryonic lethal phenotype, certain biallelic BRCA2 mutations that lead to C-terminal truncations result in FA of the D1 complementation group.

appears not to require the formation of the canonical nuclear core complex.[19]

FA Protein Complex Formation

With the exceptions of FANCD2, FANCJ, and BRCA2, most of the FA proteins are believed to function to protect the genome by forming a single large multi-protein nuclear complex. FANCD2, BRCA1, and Rad51 form complexes in S phase as well, an observation of functional relevance with recent evidence that FA proteins prevent the accumulation of DNA breaks that arise during replication.[20] Most of the FA proteins are clearly nuclear in localization, as is the core complex, and patient-derived inactivating mutations of FANCA, FANCC, FANCE, and FANCG proteins reduce assembly, stability, and/or nuclear translocation of the multi-subunit FA protein complex.[21,22] However, the proteins and complexes of them can also be found in the cytoplasm[23,24] and while not formally demonstrated, it is likely that some of the signaling functions of these molecules take place there.

Function of the Fanconi Protein Complex

There is a clear relationship between Fanconi proteins and some functions of BRCA1, BRCA2, and Rad51. First, certain biallelic BRCA2 mutations can result in FA (FA-D1)[12] and the mutations result in failure of Rad51 to localize in damage-induced nuclear foci.[25] Second, mutations of any one of the genes that encode FA core complex partners interdict formation of the complete FA complex, one consequence of which is reduced ubiquitinylation and BRCA1-colocalizing capacity of the nuclear FA protein FANCD2 (Fig 1).[14] For BRCA1 and Rad51 to accumulate in damage-induced foci, ubiquitinylated FANCD2 is required, and for that post-translational modification to occur, an intact FANCA, -B, -C, -E, -F, -G, and -L, complex is needed. The biochemical mechanisms involved in establishing these requirements are entirely unknown.

The convergence of the BRCA and Fanconi systems is a coherent narrative that has informed the respective fields of study. The proteins are known to protect cells from cross-linking agent and oxidation-induced genotoxicity.[25-29] These proteins are likely effectors of DNA repair (because of their known function in transcription-coupled and homologous recombination repair[26,29]), but biochemical studies are not as yet confirmatory. Moreover, like the FA proteins, BRCA1 and BRCA2 exhibit other activities, including direct participation in transcriptional control,[30-33] cytoplasmic signal transduction,[34] and regulation of differentiation.[35,36] Further experimental investigation is required to clarify the FA–BRCA1 functional relationship, particularly in tissues most affected by dysfunction of these proteins, specifically epithelial cells from the ovary and breast in the case of BRCA1 and BRCA2 and hematopoietic tissues in the case of the Fanconi proteins.

Other Functions of FA Proteins

In murine FA gene knockout models, the most consistent FA phenotype is hypogonadism,[37-39] but in humans the early life-threatening feature of FA is hematopoietic failure that results from excessive apoptosis in stem and progenitor cells.[11] Programmed cell death responses of FA cells exposed to certain extracellular apoptotic cues (interferon gamma [IFN-γ], tumor necrosis factor-alpha [TFN-α], mip-1α, fas ligand, and double-stranded RNA [dsRNA]) are exaggerated.[16,17,40] If the nuclear complex "pathway" accounted for the hematopoiesis-specific anti-apoptotic function of FA proteins, the complex might serve to govern the expression of genes that encode intra- or extracellular survival factors for hematopoietic cells. An alternative view, better supported by current experimental evidence, is that the Fanconi proteins have functions independent of their capacity to form a nuclear complex.[19]

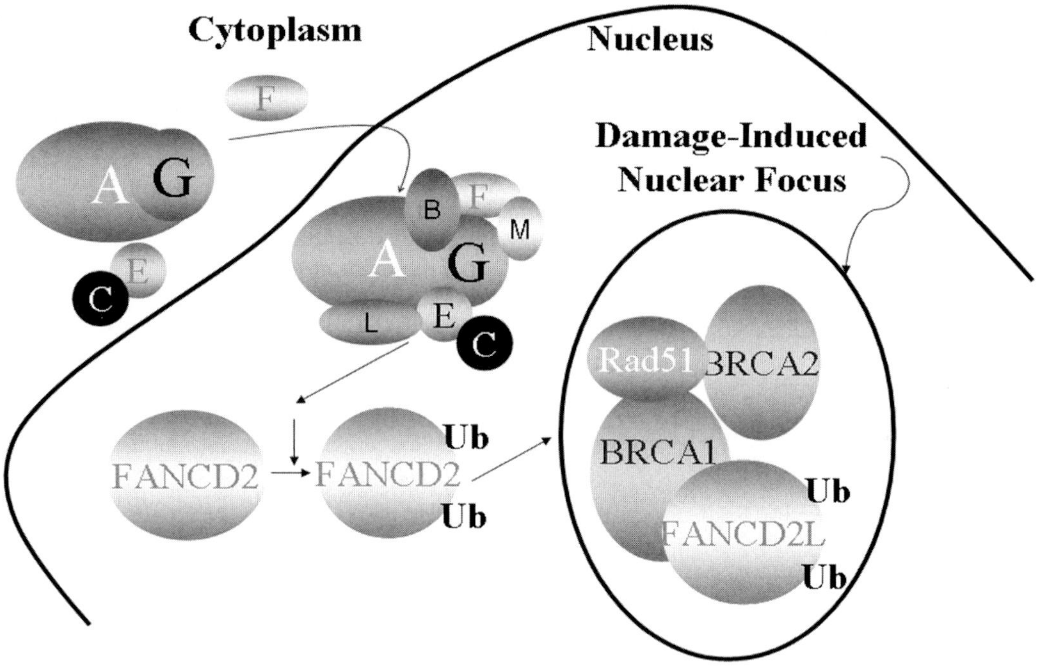

Figure 1 The FA/BRCA/Rad51 pathway in normal cells. In response to bifunctional cross-linking agents, Rad51, ubiquitinylated FANCD2, BRCA2, and BRCA1 colocalize in "damage-induced nuclear foci." Although these foci are thought to be niches involved in DNA repair, the possibility that they are also involved in damage-prevention has not yet been excluded. The characteristic hypersensitivity to cross-linking agents exhibited by FA cells results in part from the incomplete formation of these foci. FA alleles of BRCA2 result in failure of Rad51 to move to foci. Mutations of FANCD2 result in failure of FANCD2 to colocalize with BRCA1 and 2 in such foci. Mutations of FANCA, FANCB, FANCC, FANCE, FANCF, FANCG, FANCL, and FANCM result in failure of the multimeric FA complex to form in the nucleus and, as a result (although the mechanism by which it occurs is unknown), FANCD2 is not monoubiquitinylated ("Ub"). Because mono-ubiquitinylated FANCD2 is required for it to move to damage-induced foci, failure of the multimeric FA complex has the same end result as do inactivating mutations of FANCD2. The role played by this linear pathway in maintaining survival of hematopoietic cells is unclear. In fact, this pathway may play no role at all in promoting tissue-specific survival of hematopoietic progenitors and stem cells apart from protecting them from cross-linking agents.

Non-FA Binding Partners of FA Proteins

Deduction of the functionality of FA proteins by determination of their non-FA binding partners has been effective in identifying the components of the nuclear complex. Some non-canonical protein-protein interactions have been instructive as well (Table 2), and three in particular have led to important molecular insights.

STATS

FANCC and STAT1 physically interact in cells stimulated with cytokines. This interaction is reduced in FA-C mutant cells: STAT1 activation in response to cytokines is suppressed in deficient hematopoietic cells and embryonic fibroblasts (Fig 2). The activation of the JAK family member Tyk2 is supported by FANCC.[41] Work in progress in our laboratory (G.B.) has revealed that STAT5 activation in H_2O_2-stimulated normal cells protects them from apoptosis, but FA cells so exposed do not activate STAT5 and die. We have also found that H_2O_2 induced formation of complexes between FANCD2, FANCC, and STAT5. Thus, some of the intolerance of FA cells to oxidative stress might involve the STAT pathway.

Heat Shock Molecules

Heat shock proteins serve several anti-apoptotic functions of relevance to the FA phenotype.[42-44] Hsp70 binds to FANCC and modulates the activity of the dsRNA-dependent protein kinase, PKR,[17] a well recognized pro-apoptotic serine threonine kinase activated in normal cells by a variety of stimuli, including combinations of dsRNA and IFN-γ or IFN-γ and TNF-α.[45] PKR functions to induce apoptotic responses, in part by inducing phosphorylation of translation initiation factor eIF-2α, resulting in translational inhibition and apoptosis. PKR and eIF-2α are excessively activated in FANCC cells in response to inductive stimuli and are also active in the ground state (Fig 3).[46] Moreover, the apoptotic response characteristic of FA-C cells can be complemented by either FANCC cDNA or a dominant negative mutant of PKR.[46] Suppression of hsp70 expression sensitizes normal cells to IFN-γ and TNF-α but does not further sensitize FA-C cells—they are already sensitized by the failure of hsp70 to associate with FANCC.[17]

Table 2 Non-FA Binding Partners of FA Proteins

FA Protein	Non-FA Binding Partner	Functional Relevance
BRCA2	Rad51[86]	Experiments demonstrating that FANCD1 mutant cells exhibited aberrant damage-induced Rad51 nuclear focus formation led to identification of *BRCA2* as a FA-D1 complementing gene. Mutations of *BRCA2* that lead to FA disrupt the Rad51 binding region.
FANCC	STAT1	FANCC facilitates activation of STATs by cytokines and probably promotes survival of hematopoietic cells by doing so.
FANCC	hsp70	FANCC/hsp70 binding suppresses PKR* activation and thereby promotes survival of hematopoietic and embryonal cells.
FANCC	NADPH cytochrome p450 reductase	Unknown.
FANCC	FAZF	Unknown. Possible chromatin-remodeling function. The relevance of FAZF is suggested by its consistent expression in primitive hematopoietic cells.
FANCC	GRP94	Unknown. GRP94 has anti-apoptotic activity and FANCC may facilitate that function.
FANCC	cdc2	Unknown
FANCA	BRG1	Unknown. Possible chromatin remodeling function (BRG1 is a subunit of the chromatin-remodeling SWI/SNF complex).

NOTE. The FA proteins not only bind to each other in a nuclear complex but also associate with a wide variety of other proteins in multimeric complexes.

GSTP1

A fundamental defect of FA cells has long appeared to be intolerance to oxidative stress.[47,48] In support, Buchwald's group recently reported that FANCC enhances the function of GSTP1 in cells exposed to inducers of apoptosis. GSTP1 is an enzyme that detoxifies byproducts of redox stress and xenobiotics.[49] While FANCC does not directly interact with GSTP1, its influence on this molecule may play a central role in tolerance of extracellular cues of many kinds.

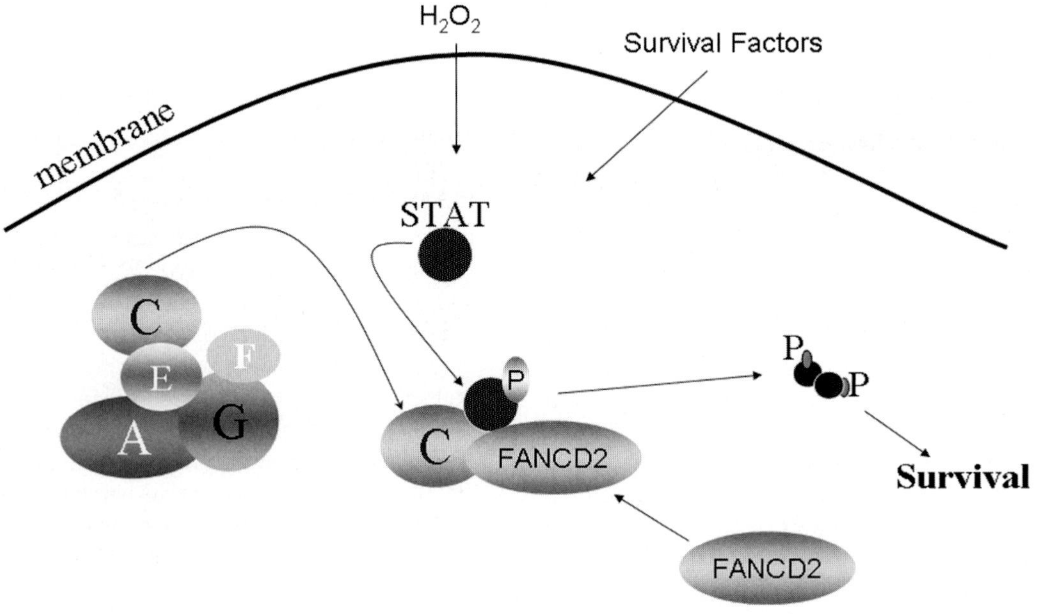

Figure 2 Survival signaling functions of FANCC. In cytokine stimulated and H2O2 -stimulated cells, FANCC and FANCD2 form multimeric high molecular weight complexes with STAT molecules (including STATs 1, 3, and 5). This complex is required for optimal phosphorylation of STATs which then can translocate to the nucleus to govern transcriptional responses that effect cell survival. Mutations of FANCC prevent its association with STAT and the association of FANCD2 with STAT as well. Fewer STAT molecules are phosphorylated and fewer of them appear in the nucleus of FA-C cells.

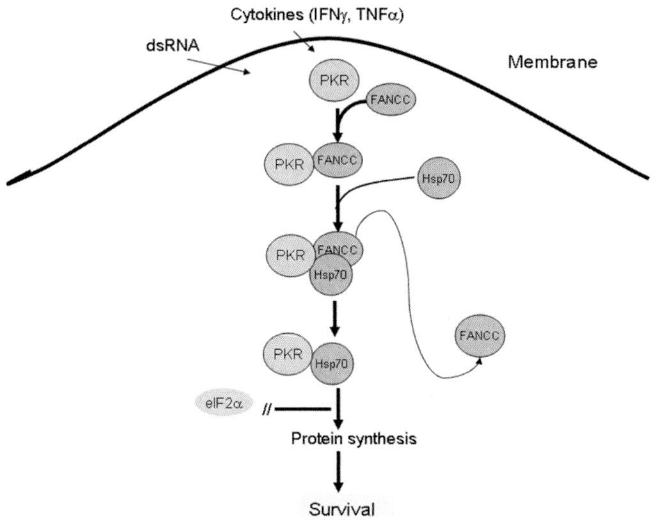

Figure 3 FANCC facilitates anti-apoptotic function of hsp70. FANCC associates with PKR and hsp70 (a PKR activation inhibitor) in hematopoietic cells and embryonic fibroblasts exposed to either combinations of TNF and IFN-γ or dsRNA and IFN-γ. Hsp70 cannot bind to PKR in the absence of a fully functional FANCC molecule. We believe that once hsp70 is brought to PKR by FANCC, FANCC leaves the PKR/hsp70 complex leaving PKR in an inactive configuration (monomeric and unphosphorylated), interdicting its capacity to phosphorylate eIF-2α. Mutant FANCC molecules fail to associate with hsp70 and, as a result, FA-C cells have excessive PKR activation (homodimerization and autophosphorylation on serines) and excessive apoptosis. The pivotal role of PKR in transducing death signals in FA-C cells is best demonstrated by the capacity of dominant-negative mutants of PKR to abrogate the excessive apoptotic responses of FA-C cells to TNF and IFN-γ or dsRNA and IFNγ.

Structural Evidence of Molecular Multifunctionality

Site-directed Ala-substitution mutants of FANCC were used to confirm the multifunctionality of that molecule. Two mutants of the highly conserved middle domain of FANCC facilitate ubiquitination of FANCD2 and induce resistance to mitomycin C in FA-C cells, but they were unable to correct STAT activation defects or interact with hsp70 to suppress PKR activation in the same cells (Fig 4). Conversely, a FANCC mutation, 322delG, known to lead to a more mild hematopoietic phenotype, is incapable of complementing in MMC assays but does complement in apoptosis assays.[50] This particular mutation is reported to result in a truncated protein by translational reinitiation at methionine 55,[51] but it does contain an intact conserved middle domain.

Clinical Diagnosis

Classic clinical features such as growth retardation, small head size, café-au-lait spots, radial ray defects, and renal structural abnormalities can be strong diagnostic clues, but FA may occur in patients without congenital defects and can be diagnosed in adulthood. Increases of fetal hemoglobin (HbF) and macrocytosis are commonly noted but their absence does not exclude disease. Safest is to consider FA in all young adults and children with one or more of hypoplastic or aplastic anemia or cytopenias, unexplained macrocytosis, MDS, AML, epithelial malignancies, or characteristic physical anomalies. There is a correlation between the number of important congenital anomalies and early onset bone marrow failure as the first adverse outcome.[52]

Understanding of the relation between genotype and phenotype is still evolving. For example, a specific mutation in FANCC (IVS4+4A→T) is associated with multiple birth defects and early-onset hematologic problems in Ashkenazi Jews,[53] while the same mutation results in a mild phenotype in Japanese.[54] In the most compelling analysis of genotype/phenotype, patients with null mutations were more severely affected than those with hypomorphic mutations, independent of the gene involved.[55] The correlations between genotype, phenotype, and adverse outcomes such as aplastic anemia, leukemia, and cancer will be better defined in the future, as specific mutations (not just the complementation groups) are identified for the majority of the patients. However, it must be emphasized that we now only study the patients known to us. There are individuals with biallelic mutations in FA genes who are unaware of this diagnosis. Many may be healthy, but some may have leukemia or cancer. Indeed, in a series of patients with FA and either cancer and leukemia, 25% were diagnosed only after they had presented with their malignancy.[56]

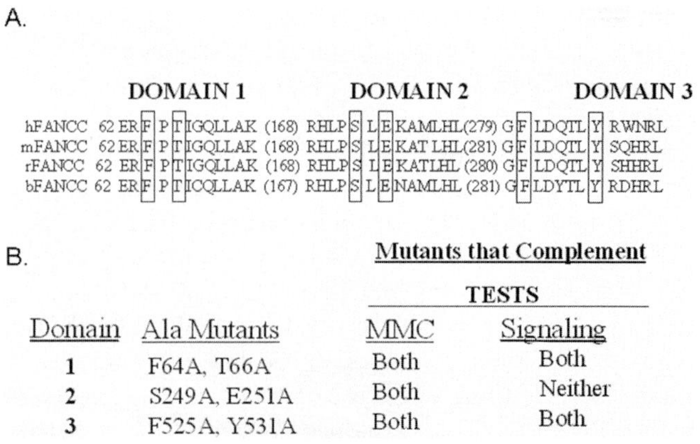

Figure 4 FANCC is multifunctional. There exist many highly conserved domains in FANCC three of which are shown here as amino acid sequences of human, murine, rat, and bovine *FANCC*. We introduced Ala mutations at two positions in each domain and used these cDNAs to complement FA-C cells using retroviral mediated gene transfer. In these experiments we asked whether the aberrant responses of FA-C cells to MMC and to apoptotic cytokines (AA Signaling) might be structurally distinguished. We found that while both domain 2 mutants were capable of complementing in the MMC assay neither complemented in the apoptotic signaling assays (Signaling), demonstrating structurally that FANCC has more than one function.

Laboratory Diagnosis

The standard for diagnosis of FA is the MMC or DEB chromosomal breakage test. This assay should be performed in laboratories with substantial prior experience. The methods involve culturing replicative cells (usually PHA-stimulated peripheral blood T lymphocytes or skin fibroblasts) in the presence of low doses of either MMC or DEB, followed by examination of metaphase spreads for evidence of chromosomal breaks and radial chromosomes. If the test is negative in lymphocytes and yet the clinical setting is highly suspicious, skin fibroblasts must be assessed because some patients are mosaics in whom hematopoietic somatic mutations have corrected the molecular defect in a single hematopoietic stem cell.[57,58] For his reason, in practice, when young patients present with specific solid tumors, the diagnosis of FA should be considered even if blood counts are normal or only minimally decreased.[59]

If chromosomes from patients in the proper clinical setting are "breakage-positive," the mutant gene should be sought, provided that the patient and family are fully informed, counseled, and provide written consent. Mutated genes can be identified by retroviral complementation studies, by direct sequencing, or by denaturing high-performance liquid chromatography (DHCLP) heteroduplex analysis.

Complementation Group Screening

Immunoblotting

The resources required for broad genomic sequencing or mutation analysis by DHPLC can be time-consuming and expensive, so we prefer to screen cells using Western blot as described by Shimamura et al.[60] Immunoblotting for FANCD2 can distinguish the ubiquitinylated and non-ubiquitinylated forms (Fig 5) of FANCD2 so the method can be used to predict the function of the members of the core complex. In the context of an unambiguous FA phenotype (by MMC-chromosomal breakage assays in the appropriate clinical setting), FANCD2 mutations could be presumed if no full-length FANCD2 is detected, inactivating mutations of one of the core complex proteins if FANCD2 exists but is not ubiquitinylated in response to MMC, and BRCA2 or FANCJ mutations if FANCD2 is ubiquitinylated after exposure to MMC (Fig 5). In the latter case, immunoblotting for BRCA2 and FANCJ should show reduced or absent levels or truncated versions of the protein. Once the most likely protein is discovered, sequencing experiments can be performed for the specific gene.

Retroviral-Mediated Gene Transfer Methods

The introduction of normal FANCA cDNA into FA-A cells rectifies their hypersensitivity to MMC and DEB; of course, the introduction of FANCC into FA-A cells will not complement their MMC defect. A practical screening method has been developed in which primary peripheral blood-derived FA T cells are transduced with oncoretroviral vectors that expressed specific FA genes in order to correct cytogenetic instability.[61] As FA cells exposed to alkylating agents arrest in the G_2 phase of the cell cycle, for retrovirally transduced cells exposed first to an alkylating agent, the fraction of cells dwelling in G_2/M can be quantified by flow cytometry.[62] The transduced gene that reduces G_2/M arrested cells to the greatest extent is the presumptive mutant gene.

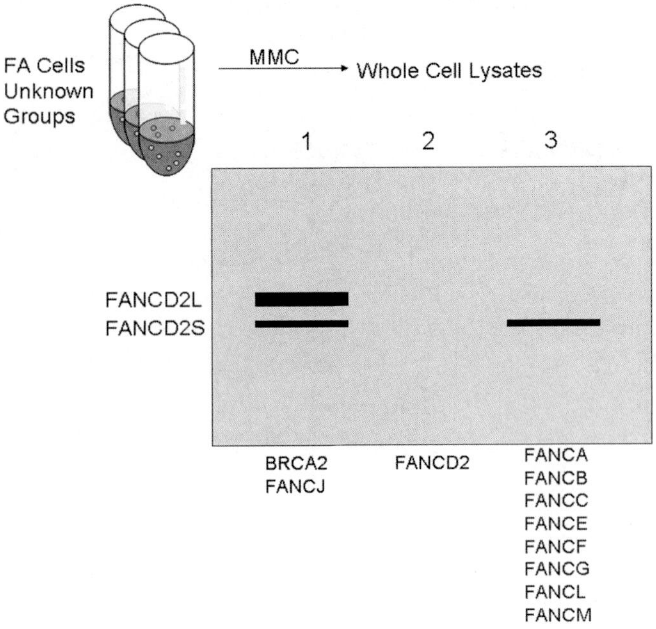

Figure 5 FANCD2 immunoblotting helps to screen primary cells for FA defects. Cells from patients whose fibroblasts or lymphocytes test positive in the MMC chromosomal breakage test are exposed to MMC or radiation, after which lysates are prepared for FANCD2 immunoblotting. In lane 1 both the long ubiquitinylated form (FANCD2L) and the non-ubiqutininylated short form (FANCD2L) are detected. This would be consistent with a mutation of BRCA2 or FANCJ. In lane 2, no protein is detected, consistent with a mutation of FANCD2. In lane 3, only FANCD2S is detected, compatible with a mutation of any one of the FA proteins in the nuclear core complex (FANCA, FANCB, FANCC, FANCE, FANCF, FANCG, FANCL, or FANCM).

Clinical Diagnostics: FA Without MMC Hypersensitivity?

Can inherited aplastic anemia be due to a mutation in one of the FA genes that disrupts survival function of the protein without interdicting the function of the protein the nuclear core complex? No effort to ascertain such cases has been made because the disease is rare and the effort would be expensive. Our observations on differentially functional domains in FANCC and the likelihood that most of the FA proteins will be as multifunctional as FANCC, indicate such cases are likely to exist. The responsible mutations would score as "negative" in the MMC/DEB tests. We now test primary marrow cells from children and young adults with aplastic anemia, MDS, and AML using clonal assays for both MMC and cytokine hypersensitivity (TNF-α and IFN-γ).

There are patients who have been described as having an autosomal recessive marrow failure syndrome who might fit this model.[63]

Clinical Management

The median survival of patients with FA is approximately 30 years but prognosis is highly variable.[3] The life-threatening early event in most complementation groups is bone marrow failure (patients with biallelic BRCA2 mutations, who seem to have early-onset AML, brain tumors, and Wilm's tumors, may be exceptions), so management of bone marrow failure is the primary concern.

Transplantation

Stem cell transplantation is the only option to establish normal hematopoiesis (for a comprehensive discussion, readers are referred to a recent review[64]). Patients with significant pancytopenia (absolute neutrophil count $<1{,}000/\mu L$, hemoglobin ≤ 8 g/dL, or platelet count ≤ 40–$50{,}000/\mu L$) who are (1) otherwise healthy, and (2) have an available human leukocyte antigen (HLA)-matched sibling donor are excellent candidates for hematopoietic stem cell transplantation. Therefore, all probands and siblings should be HLA-typed early and sibling cord blood samples should be preserved. In vitro fertilization and pre-implantation genetic diagnosis (both to exclude FA and to determine an HLA match) have been employed, and in at least one instance cord blood stem cells of the sibling were used successfully to transplant the proband.[65]

As patients are extremely sensitive to the chemotherapy and radiation ordinarily used to condition non–Fanconi anemia recipients, the doses of conditioning agents must be reduced to avoid fatal toxicities.[66] Even with such reductions, there is retrospective evidence that long-term survivors are at high risk of epithelial cancers of the head and neck.[67] Nonmyeloablative preparative regimens for transplant have been attempted to avoid this complication. Five-year survival of patients receiving stem cells from HLA-identical siblings approaches 75% and in some centers 5-year survival is 58% even with matched unrelated stem cell donors.[68]

Androgens

Not all patients are candidates for transplantation. Apart from supportive measures, androgen therapy frequently induces meaningful responses in pancytopenic patients,[3] but male sex hormones usually are reserved for transfusion-dependent patients or patients with platelet and neutrophil counts that confer a high risk of bleeding and infection. Androgen administration requires surveillance for deterioration of liver function or development of adenomas, hepatomas, and peliosis hepatica; these complications rarely develop in FA patients who have not been treated with androgens.[69]

Gene Therapy

Gene therapy for FA patients is a theoretically appealing option and there is strong, albeit circumstantial evidence that were one hematopoietic stem cell corrected, it might suffice to repopulate the bone marrow of an FA patient.[57] The apoptotic phenotype of the uncorrected cells provides a perfect opportunity for the selective emergence of transduced cells. However, it is this very apoptotic state that complicates the technique: FA cells tend to undergo programmed cell death in vitro, even during the short ex vivo transduction periods required for efficient gene transfer.

Some selective pressure also might be required in recipients of genetically modified stem cells. MMC treatment has little appeal because all somatic FA cells are hypersensitive to MMC and, like all bifunctional alkylating agents, MMC is a carcinogen, hardly a desirable agent for selection of transduced cells. Models of selection that utilize biological agents that suppress only hematopoietic activity might be less toxic to nonhematopoietic cells than MMC, and such an approach has been successful in murine models of FA.[70]

Standard Monitoring

For patients with stable disease ineligible for transplantation, annual surveillance examinations and bone marrow aspiration (with cytogenetic studies) and biopsy are suggested, but their value is not strongly evidence-based. For patients with complex cytogenetic abnormalities or MDS, closer periodic evaluations are warranted.

Development of Malignancies

In a competing risk analysis, after accounting for severe bone marrow failure, the development of solid tumors is the adverse outcome with the highest risk. The cumulative incidence of leukemia appeared to plateau at 10% by age 20, while the incidence of solid tumors approached 30% by age 45 and did not appear to reach a stable plateau. The risks of AML, or of squamous cell carcinoma of the head and neck, esophagus, or vulva were, respectively, approximately 800-, 700-, 2,000-, and 4,000-fold increased over the expected rates.[71] Stem cell transplantation also increased the risk and reduced the age of onset of head and neck squamous cell cancer. Chronic graft-versus-host disease was highly predictive of this complication.[72]

Treatment of Malignancies

Neoplasia is a major challenge in the care of FA patients. The treatment of malignancies that develop in FA is extraordinarily difficult, particularly those for which standard care involves radiation or alkylating agents (such as cisplatin), as not only the tumor but normal tissues are hypersensitive to these agents. If FA patients are treated with full doses of alkylating agents or radiation, the morbidity may be extreme and iatrogenic mortality rates high.[73] Treatment of such malignancies should be in collaboration with specialized centers and should focus on novel targeted therapies that are not uniquely toxic to the somatic cells of patients with this difficult disease. The best option would be to develop rational strategies for disease prevention, including vaccines. Since human papilloma virus (HPV) has been implicated in both gynecologic and head and neck cancer in the general population and because a vaccine will be available soon, immunization might provide an important measure of risk reduction.[74,75] There are two caveats in designing vaccine trials for FA patients. First, the role of HPV in FA cancers is unclear (one group reported an 84% incidence,[76] another found none[77]). Second, subtle immune defects may exist in FA patients[41,78] that could reduce the effectiveness of vaccines.

The Future

Prevention

There exist no strategies for prevention of marrow failure, leukemia, or cancer in FA patients other than the avoidance of exposure to cross-linking agents. For development of such strategies in the future, preclinical models of bone marrow failure in FA would be of value, but the current murine models lack this critical clinical feature. Although a state of chronic bone marrow failure can be induced by exposing knockout mice to MMC,[79,80] they do not develop bone marrow failure spontaneously. If pharmacologic approaches to bone marrow failure in FA patients were to be developed based on current knowledge of the apoptotic pathways involved, a reasonable first approach would be to focus on key tissue-specific effectors of programmed cell death.

For example, in the case of FA-C, one approach could be to suppress the high ground-state activation of PKR in hematopoietic cells, without affecting the induced activation of the enzyme (PKR is an essential component of the antiviral response). Therefore, to precisely target therapies, one requirement is a complete understanding of the molecular mechanisms by which PKR is specifically activated in FA cells, so that ground state activation of PKR can be inhibited while inducible PKR function is preserved. Whether inhibiting PKR in FA cells is sufficient to overcome all of the defects in cellular signaling remains to be tested directly.

Molecular Pathogenesis of Clonal Evolution Through the FA Window

MDS and AML are major predictors of clinical outcome in children with FA.[81] In the context of a mutator phenotype (a marker of which is MMC hypersensitivity), the cytokine hypersensitivity of many FA cells (linked to cytoplasmic and/or nuclear survival signaling pathways) may create selective pressure for adaptive mutations that result in outgrowth of cytokine-resistant clones.[82] To date, all progenitor cells we have tested from FA MDS/AML bone marrow samples exhibit substantial resistance to certain extracellular cues, including IFN-γ and TNF-α, to which non MDS/AML progenitors from FA patients are exquisitely hypersensitive, supporting the hypothesis of selective pressure and clonal adaptation.[82] A multi-institutional FA transcriptome consortium has been organized to seek genome wide confirmation of the clonal adaptation model of MDS. Preliminary results of the study will be broadly shared with the scientific community.

Alkylating agents are known to cause MDS and AML in adults who do not have FA. The non-random cytogenetic defects seen in the neoplastic clones in such patients are precisely the same as those in children with FA who have evolved to MDS and AML.[83-85] Consequently, findings in studies on FA MDS/AML samples may also reveal molecular correlates of clonal evolution in secondary AML/MDS.

Eleven of the FA genes now have been identified, and the elucidation of the FA nuclear complex model by Garcia-Higuera et al[14] has been extraordinarily useful in describing a unified model of how mutations of these disparate proteins can lead to the same aberrant response to MMC. The hematopoietic defects in this disease are not likely related to that canonical pathway. It is clear that the FA proteins are part of a cluster of survival signaling molecules, most of which function in complexes with other proteins. With emerging evidence that FA proteins both affiliate with critically important tumor-suppressor genes, and participate in survival signaling pathways in hematopoietic cells, studies on the function of these gene products will occupy scientists interested in mammalian development, cellular responses to viral infections, carcinogenesis, hematopoiesis, and the immune response.

References

1. Fanconi G: Familiare infantile perniziosaartige anaemia (perniziöses blutbild und konstitution). Jahrb Kinderhilkd 117:257-280, 1927
2. Joenje H, Patel KJ: The emerging genetic and molecular basis of Fanconi anaemia. Nat Rev Genet 2:446-459, 2001
3. Alter BP: Inherited bone marrow failure syndromes, in Nathan DG, Orkin SH, Ginsburg D, Look AT (eds): Hematology of Infancy and Childhood. Philadelphia, PA, Saunders, 2003, pp 280-365
4. Kutler DI, Singh B, Satagopan J, Batish SD, Berwick M, Giampietro PF, et al: A 20-year perspective on the International Fanconi Anemia Registry (IFAR). Blood 101:1249-1256, 2003
5. Sasaki MS, Tonomura A: A high susceptibility of Fanconi's anemia to chromosome breakage by DNA cross-linking agents. Cancer Res 33: 1829-1836, 1973
6. Auerbach AD, Adler B, Chaganti RS: Prenatal and postnatal diagnosis and carrier detection of Fanconi anemia by a cytogenetic method. Pediatrics 67:128-135, 1981
7. Meetei AR, Levitus M, Xue Y, Medhurst AL, Zwaan M, Ling C, et al: X-linked inheritance of Fanconi anemia complementation group B. Nat Genet 36:1219-1224, 2004
8. Levitus M, Waisfisz Q, Godthelp BC, Vries YD, Hussain S, Wiegant WW, et al: The DNA helicase BRIP1 is defective in Fanconi anemia complementation group J. Nat Genet 37:934-935, 2005
9. Levran O, Attwooll C, Henry RT, Milton KL, Neveling K, Rio P, et al: The BRCA1-interacting helicase BRIP1 is deficient in Fanconi anemia. Nat Genet 37:931-933, 2005
10. Meetei AR, de Winter JP, Medhurst AL, Wallisch M, Waisfisz Q, van de Vrugt HJ, et al: A novel ubiquitin ligase is deficient in Fanconi anemia. Nat Genet 35:165-170, 2003
11. Bagby GC: Genetic basis of Fanconi anemia. Curr Opin Hematol 10: 68-76, 2003
12. Howlett NG, Taniguchi T, Olson S, Cox B, Waisfisz Q, Die-Smulders C, et al: Biallelic inactivation of BRCA2 in Fanconi anemia. Science 297: 606-609, 2002
13. Garcia-Higuera I, Kuang Y, Naf D, Wasik J, D'Andrea, AD: Fanconi anemia proteins FANCA, FANCC, and FANCG/XRCC9 interact in a functional nuclear complex. Mol Cell Biol 19:4866-4873, 1999
14. Garcia-Higuera I, Taniguchi T, Ganesan S, Meyn MS, Timmers C, Hejna J: Interaction of the Fanconi anemia proteins and BRCA1 in a common pathway. Mol Cell 7:249-262, 2001
15. Medhurst AL, Huber PA, Waisfisz Q, de Winter J, Mathew CG: Direct interactions of the five known Fanconi anaemia proteins suggest a common functional pathway. Hum Mol Genet 10:423-429, 2001
16. Pang Q, Fagerlie S, Christianson TA, Keeble W, Faulkner G, Diaz J, et al: The Fanconi anemia protein FANCC binds to and facilitates the

activation of STAT1 by gamma interferon and hematopoietic growth factors. Mol Cell Biol 20:4724-4735, 2000
17. Pang Q, Keeble W, Christianson TA, Faulkner G, Bagby GC: FANCC interacts with hsp70 to protect hematopoietic cells from IFNγ/TNFα-mediated cytotoxicity. EMBO J 20:4478-4489, 2001
18. Pang QS, Christianson TA, Keeble W, Koretsky T, Bagby GC: The anti-apoptotic function of Hsp70 in the interferon-inducible double-stranded RNA-dependent protein kinase-mediated death signaling pathway requires the Fanconi anemia protein, FANCC. J Biol Chem 277:49638-49643, 2002
19. Fagerlie S, Lensch MW, Pang Q, Bagby GC: The Fanconi anemia group C gene product. Signaling functions in hematopoietic cells. Exp Hematol 29:1371-1381, 2001
20. Sobeck A, Stone S, Costanzo V, de Graaf B, Reuter T, de Winter J, et al: Fanconi anemia proteins are required to prevent accumulation of replication-associated DNA double-strand breaks. Mol Cell Biol 26:425-437, 2006
21. Kupfer GM, Näf D, Suliman A, Pulsipher M, D'Andrea AD: The Fanconi anaemia proteins, FAA and FAC, interact to form a nuclear complex. Nat Genet 17:487-490, 1997
22. Näf D, Kupfer GM, Suliman A, Lambert K, D'Andrea AD: Functional activity of the Fanconi anemia protein FAA requires FAC binding and nuclear localization. Mol Cell Biol 18:5952-5960, 1998
23. Hoatlin ME, Christianson TA, Keeble WW, Hammond AT, Zhi Y, Heinrich MC, et al: The Fanconi anemia group C gene product is located in both the nucleus and cytoplasm of human cells. Blood 91:1418-1425, 1998
24. Thomashevski A, High AA, Drozd M, Shabanowitz J, Hunt DF, Grant PA, et al: The Fanconi anemia core complex forms 4 different sized complexes in different subcellular compartments. J Biol Chem 79: 26201-26209, 2004
25. Godthelp BC, Artwert F, Joenje H Zdienicka MZ: Impaired DNA damage-induced nuclear Rad51 foci formation uniquely characterizes Fanconi anemia group D1. Oncogene 21:5002-5005, 2002
26. Xia F, Taghian DG, DeFrank JS, Zeng ZC, Willers H, Iliakis G, et al: Deficiency of human BRCA2 leads to impaired homologous recombination but maintains normal nonhomologous end joining. Proc Natl Acad Sci U S A 98:8644-8649, 2001
27. Davies AA, Masson J, McIlwraith MJ, Stasiak AZ, Stasiak A, Venkitaraman AR, et al: Role of BRCA2 in control of the RAD51 recombination and DNA repair protein. Mol Cell 7:273-282, 2001
28. Gowen LC, Avrutskaya AV, Latour AM, Koller BH, Leadon SA: BRCA1 required for transcription-coupled repair of oxidative DNA damage. Science 281:1009-1012, 1998
29. Moynahan ME, Pierce AJ, Jasin M: BRCA2 is required for homology-directed repair of chromosomal breaks. Mol Cell 7:263-272, 2001
30. Aprelikova O, Pace AJ, Fang B, Koller BH, Liu ET: BRCA1 is a selective co-activator of 14-3-3 sigma gene transcription in mouse embryonic stem cells. J Biol Chem 276:25647-25650, 2001
31. Siddique H, Zou JP, Rao VN, Reddy ESP: The BRCA2 is a histone acetyltransferase. Oncogene 16:2283-2285, 1998
32. Yarden RI, Brody LC: BRCA1 interacts with components of the histone deacetylase complex. Proc Natl Acad Sci U S A 96:4983-4988, 1999
33. Zhang HB, Somasundaram K, Peng Y, Tian H, Zhang HX, Bi DK, et al: BRCA1 physically associates with p53 and stimulates its transcriptional activity. Oncogene 16:1713-1721, 1998
34. Gao B, Shen XN, Kunos G, Meng QH, Goldberg ID, Rosen EM, et al: Constitutive activation of JAK-STAT3 signaling by BRCA1 in human prostate cancer cells. FEBS Lett 488:179-184, 2001
35. Kubista M, Rosner M, Kubista E, Bernaschek G, Hengstschlager M: Brca1 regulates in vitro differentiation of mammary epithelial cells. Oncogene 21:4747-4756, 2002
36. Zheng L, Li S, Boyer TG, Lee WH: Lessons learned from BRCA1 and BRCA2. Oncogene 19:6159-6175, 2000
37. Nadler JJ, Braun RE: Fanconi anemia complementation group C is required for proliferation of murine primordial germ cells. Genesis 27:117-123, 2000
38. Koomen M, Cheng NC, van de Vrugt HJ, Godthelp BC, Der Valk MA, Oostra AB, et al: Reduced fertility and hypersensitivity to mitomycin C characterize Fancg/Xrcc9 null mice. Hum Mol Genet 11:273-281, 2002
39. Cheng NC, van de Vrugt HJ, Van der Valk MA, Oostra AB, Krimpenfort B, de Vries Y, et al: Mice with a targeted disruption of the Fanconi anemia homolog Fanca. Hum Mol Genet 9: 1805-1811, 2000
40. Rathbun RK, Faulkner GR, Ostroski MH, Christianson T, Hughes G, Jones G, et al: Inactivation of the Fanconi anemia group C (FAC) gene augments interferon-gamma-induced apoptotic responses in hematopoietic cells. Blood 90:974-985, 1997
41. Fagerlie SR, Koretsky T, Torok-Storb B, Bagby GC: Impaired type-I IFN-induced Jak/STAT signaling in FA-C cells and abnormal $CD4^+$ Th cell subsets in $Fancc^{-/-}$ mice. J Immunol 173:3863-3870, 2004
42. Beere HM, Wolf BB, Cain K, Mosser DD, Mahboubi A, Kuwana T, et al: Heat-shock protein 70 inhibits apoptosis by preventing recruitment of procaspase-9 to the Apaf-1 apoptosome. Nat Cell Biol 2:469-475, 2000
43. Beere HM, Green DR: Stress management–Heat shock protein-70 and the regulation of apoptosis. Trends Cell Biol 11:6-10, 2001
44. Jaattela M, Wissing D, Kokholm K, Kalunki T, Egeblad M: Hsp70 exerts its anti-apoptotic function downstream of caspase-3-like proteases. EMBO J 17:6124-6134, 1998
45. Williams BR: PKR; a sentinel kinase for cellular stress. Oncogene 18: 6112-6120, 1999
46. Pang Q, Keeble W, Diaz J, Christianson T, Fagerlie S, Rathbun K, et al: Role of double-stranded RNA-dependent protein kinase in mediating hypersensitivity of Fanconi anemia complementation group C cells to interferon gamma, tumor necrosis factor-alpha, and double-stranded RNA. Blood 97:1644-1652, 2001
47. Pagano G: Mitomycin C and diepoxybutane action mechanisms and FANCC protein functions: Further insights into the role for oxidative stress in Fanconi's anaemia phenotype. Carcinogenesis 21:1067-1068, 2000
48. Clarke AA, Philpott NJ, Gordon-Smith EC, Rutherford TR: The sensitivity of Fanconi anaemia group C cells to apoptosis induced by mitomycin C is due to oxygen radical generation, not DNA crosslinking. Br J Haematol 96:240-247, 1997
49. Cumming RC, Lightfoot J, Beard K, Youssoufian H, O'Brien PJ, Buchwald M: Fanconi anemia group C protein prevents apoptosis in hematopoietic cells through redox regulation of GSTP1. Nat Med 7:814-820, 2001
50. Pang Q, Christianson TA, Keeble W, Diaz J, Faulkner G, Reifsteck C, et al: The Fanconi anemia complementation group C gene product: structural evidence of multifunctionality. Blood 98:1392-1401, 2001
51. Yamashita T, Wu N, Kupfer G, Corless C, Joenje H, Grompe M, et al: Clinical variability of Fanconi anemia (type C) results from expression of an amino terminal truncated Fanconi anemia complementation group C polypeptide with partial activity. Blood 87:4424-4432, 1996
52. Rosenberg PS, Huang Y, Alter BP: Individualized risks of first adverse events in patients with Fanconi anemia. Blood 104:350-355, 2004
53. Verlander PC, Lin JD, Udono MU, Zhang Q, Gibson RA, Mathew CG, et al: Mutation analysis of the Fanconi anemia gene FACC. Am J Hum Genet 54:595-601, 1994
54. Futaki M, Yamashita T, Yagasaki H, Toda T, Yabe M, Kato S, et al: The IVS4+4 A to T mutation of the Fanconi anemia gene FANCC is not associated with a severe phenotype in Japanese patients. Blood 95: 1493-1498, 2000
55. Faivre L, Guardiola P, Lewis CM, Dokal I, Ebell W, Zatterale A, et al: Association of complementation group and mutation type with clinical outcome in Fanconi anemia. Blood 96:4064-4070, 2000
56. Alter BP: Cancer in Fanconi anemia, 1927-2001. Cancer 97:425-440, 2003
57. Mankad A, Taniguchi T, Cox B, Akkari Y, Rathbun RK, Lucas L, et al: Natural gene therapy in monozygotic twins with Fanconi anemia. Blood 107:3084-3090, 2006
58. Gregory JJ, Wagner JE, Verlander PC, Levran O, Batish SD, Eide CR, et al: Somatic mosaicism in Fanconi anemia: Evidence of genotypic reversion in lymphohematopoietic stem cells. Proc Natl Acad Sci U S A 98:2532-2537, 2001
59. Alter BP, Joenje H, Oostra AB, Pals G: Fanconi anemia: Adult head and

neck cancer and hematopoietic mosaicism. Arch Otolaryngol Head Neck Surg 131:635-639, 2005
60. Shimamura A, Montes DO, Svenson JL, Haining N, Moreau LA, Nathan DG, et al: A novel diagnostic screen for defects in the Fanconi anemia pathway. Blood 100: 4649-4654, 2002
61. Hanenberg H, Batish SD, Pollok KE, Vieten L, Verlander PC, Leurs C, et al: Phenotypic correction of primary Fanconi anemia T cells with retroviral vectors as a diagnostic tool. Exp Hematol 30:410-420, 2002
62. Chandra S, Levran O, Jurickova I, Maas C, Kapur R, Schindler D, et al: A Rapid method for retrovirus-mediated identification of complementation groups in Fanconi anemia patients. Mol Ther 12:976-984, 2005
63. Giampietro PF, Auerbach AD, Elias ER, Gutman A, Zellers NJ, Davis JG: New recessive syndrome characterized by increased chromosomal breakage and several findings which overlap with Fanconi anemia. Am J Med Genet 78:70-75, 1998
64. Vlachos A, Lipton JM: Hematopoietic stem cell transplant for inherited bone marrow failure syndromes, in Mehta P (ed): Pediatric Stem Cell Transplantation, Sudbury, MA, Jones and Barlett, 2004, pp 281-311
65. Grewal SS, Kahn JP, MacMillan ML, Ramsay NKC, Wanger JE: Successful hematopoietic stem cell transplantation for Fanconi anemia from an unaffected HLA-genotype-identical sibling selected using preimplantation genetic diagnosis. Blood 103:1147-1151, 2004
66. Gluckman E: Radiosensitivity in Fanconi anemia: Application to the conditioning for bone marrow transplantation. Radiother Oncol 18:88-93, 1990 (suppl 1)
67. Alter BP: Fanconi's anemia, transplantation, and cancer. Pediatr Transplant 9:81-86, 2005 (suppl 7)
68. Boyer MW, Gross TG, Loechelt B, Leehuis T, Filipovich A, Harris RE: Low risk of graft-versus-host disease with transplantation of CD34 selected peripheral blood progenitor cells from alternative donors for Fanconi anemia. J Pediatr Hematol Oncol 25:890-895, 2003
69. Velazquez I, Alter BP: Androgens and liver tumors: Fanconi's anemia and non-Fanconi's conditions. Am J Hematol 77:257-267, 2004
70. Li X, Yang Y, Yuan J, Hong P, Freie B, Orazi A, et al: Continuous in vivo infusion of Interferon-gamma (IFN-{gamma}) preferentially reduces myeloid progenitor numbers and enhances engraftment of syngeneic wildtype cells in Fancc-/- mice. Blood 104:1204-1209, 2004
71. Rosenberg PS, Greene MH, Alter BP: Cancer incidence in persons with Fanconi anemia. Blood 101:822-826, 2003
72. Rosenberg PS, Socie G, Alter BP, Gluckman E: Risk of head and neck squamous cell cancer and death in patients with Fanconi anemia who did and did not receive transplants. Blood 105:67-73, 2005
73. Alter BP: Radiosensitivity in Fanconi's anemia patients. Radiother Oncol 62:345-347, 2002
74. Herrero R, Hildesheim A, Bratti C, Sherman ME, Hutchinson M, Morales J, et al: Population-based study of human papillomavirus infection and cervical neoplasia in rural Costa Rica. J Natl Cancer Inst 92:464-474, 2000
75. Gillison ML, Shah KV: Chapter 9: Role of mucosal human papillomavirus in nongenital cancers. J Natl Cancer Inst Monogr 31:57-65, 2003
76. Kutler DI, Wreesmann VB, Goberdhan A, Ben Porat L, Satagopan J, Ngai I, et al: Human papillomavirus DNA and p53 polymorphisms in squamous cell carcinomas from Fanconi anemia patients. J Natl Cancer Inst 95:1718-1721, 2003
77. van Zeeburg HJ, Snijders PJ, Joenje H, Barkenhoff RH: Re: Human papillomavirus DNA and p53 polymorphisms in squamous cell carcinomas from Fanconi anemia patients. J Natl Cancer Inst 96:968-969, 2004
78. Fagerlie SR, Bagby GC: Immune defects in Fanconi anemia. Crit Rev Immunol 26:81-96, 2006
79. Carreau M, Gan OI, Liu L, Doedens M, McKerlie C, Dick JE, et al: Bone marrow failure in the Fanconi anemia group C mouse model after DNA damage. Blood 91:2737-2744, 1998
80. Otsuki T, Wang J, Demuth I, Digweed M, Liu JM: Assessment of mitomycin C sensitivity in Fanconi anemia complementation group C gene (Fac) knock-out mouse cells. Int J Hematol 67:243-248, 1998
81. Alter BP, Caruso JP, Drachtman RA, Uchida T, Velagaleti GVN, Elghetany MT: Fanconi anemia: Myelodysplasia as a predictor of outcome. Cancer Genet Cytogenet 117:125-131, 2000
82. Lensch MW, Rathbun RK, Olson SB, Jones GR, Bagby GC: Selective pressure as an essential force in molecular evolution of myeloid leukemic clones: A view from the window of Fanconi anemia. Leukemia 13:1784-1789, 1999
83. Rubin CM, Arthur DC, Woods WG, Lange BJ, Nowell PC, Rowley JD, et al: Therapy-related myelodysplastic syndrome and acute myeloid leukemia in children: Correlation between chromosomal abnormalities and prior therapy. Blood 78:2982-2988, 1991
84. Whang-Peng J, Young RC, Lee EC, Longo DL, Schecter GC, DeVita VT: Cytogenetic studies in patients with secondary leukemia/dysmyelopoietic syndrome after different treatment modalities. Blood 71:403-414, 1988
85. Luna-Fineman S, Shannon KM, Lange BJ: Childhood monosomy 7: Epidemiology, biology, and mechanistic implications. Blood 85:1985-1999, 1995
86. Marmorstein LY, Ouchi T, Aaronson SA: The BRCA2 gene product functionally interacts with p53 and RAD51. Proc Natl Acad Sci U S A 95:13869-13874, 1998

ELSEVIER

Seminars in
HEMATOLOGY

Dyskeratosis Congenita

Tom Vulliamy and Inderjeet Dokal

Dyskeratosis congenita (DC) is a rare inherited multi-system disorder. Although DC is classically characterized by mucocutaneous features, the vast majority of patients develop hematologic abnormalities, and in its occult form the disease can present as aplastic anemia. The gene responsible for the X-linked form of the disease encodes a protein involved in ribosome biogenesis and in stabilizing the telomerase complex, while the autosomal dominant form is caused by mutations in the core RNA component of telomerase. It has been suggested that DC is primarily a disease of defective telomere maintenance. Premature shortening of telomeres resulting in a limited proliferative potential of stem cells would explain the pathology observed in DC, as the affected tissues are those that require constant renewal.
Semin Hematol 43:157-166

In the early years of the last century, Zinsser, Engman, and Cole described an inherited condition characterized by the mucocutaneous features of nail dystrophy, oral leukoplakia, and reticular pigmentation of the skin. Their observations established a classical definition of the disease that has become known as dyskeratosis congenita (DC). In subsequent years, it became apparent that these symptoms and signs are closely associated with bone marrow failure and that other somatic abnormalities are often present.[1-3] A recent review of these anomalies shows that in order of prevalence they involve the eye epithelia, neurological, pulmonary, skeletal, dental and gastrointestinal systems, hair loss or greying, and the genitourinary tract[4] (Table 1). From the recent identification of genes underlying DC, it has also become clear that patients may not necessarily present with physical features.

In classical DC, nail dystrophy and abnormal skin pigmentation present first, often in the first decade of life. Bone marrow failure develops later but in more than 80% of cases is present by the third decade. This complication is the primary cause of death in DC, through increased susceptibility to infection or haemorrhage. Notably, patients also have a predisposition to malignancy, present in nearly 10% of all cases, and pulmonary complications (present in 20% of cases) can prove fatal. However, it is important to stress that considerable clinical heterogeneity exists, sometimes even within the same family. A patient may have diverse combinations of somatic abnormalities, while others live into their fourth decade with only a moderate nail dystrophy and mild blood abnormalities.

At the other extreme is a severe disease previously recognized as the Hoyeraal-Hreidaarson (HH) syndrome.[5] HH syndrome is characterized by severe growth retardation, bone marrow failure, and neurologic abnormalities, often presenting in the first years of life and with a very poor prognosis. Several male cases of this syndrome have now been shown to be allelic to X-linked DC.[6] The disorder is also characterized by a severe "T+B -NK" immunodeficiency[7]; immunologic abnormalities are more variable in other DC patients. Female cases of the HH syndrome are also recognized.

That manifestations of bone marrow failure in DC can precede the appearance of diagnostic mucocutaneous features has been known for some time.[8] In some kindreds, an affected individual has died from aplastic anemia without a diagnosis of DC, which was only made subsequently as a result of other family members surviving to present with classical features. Rarely, individuals diagnosed with idiopathic or acquired aplastic anemia are shown to have occult DC.

Currently, little can be offered for the treatment of the somatic features of this disease. While some improvement in hematopoietic function can be obtained in many with the anabolic steroid oxymetholone, and successful responses to granulocyte-macrophage colony-stimulating factor, granulocyte colony-stimulating factor, and erythropoetin have been reported,[9,10] the main treatment option for severe bone marrow failure is stem cell transplantation (SCT). However, there have been serious early and late vascular and pulmonary complications following SCT in DC, presumably due to the

Department of Haematology, Division of Investigative Science, Faculty of Medicine, Imperial College, Hammersmith Hospital, London, UK.
Supported in part by the Wellcome Trust.
Address correspondence to Tom Vulliamy, PhD, Department of Haematology, Imperial College London, Commonwealth Building, Hammersmith Hospital, London W12 ONN, UK. E-mail: t.vulliamy@imperial.ac.uk

0037-1963/06/$-see front matter
doi:10.1053/j.seminhematol.2006.04.001

Table 1 Prevalence of Clinical Features in Patients With Classical DC

Disease Feature	~% of Patients*
Diagnostic mucocutaneous triad	
Abnormal skin pigmentation	89
Nail dystrophy	88
Leucoplakia	78
Bone marrow failure	86
Other somatic abnormalities	
Epiphora	31
Learning difficulties/developmental delay/ mental retardation	25
Pulmonary disease	20
Short stature	20
Extensive dental caries/loss	17
Oesophageal stricture	17
Premature hair loss/greying/sparse eyelashes	16
Hyperhiderosis	15
Malignancy	10
Intrauterine growth retardation	8
Liver disease/peptic ulceration/enteropathy	7
Ataxia/cerebellar hypoplasia	7
Hypogonadism/undescended testes	6
Microcephaly	6
Urethral stricture/phimosis	5
Osteoporosis/aseptic necrosis/scoliosis	5
Deafness	1

*These numbers are based on patients that were entered into the DC Registry at the Hammersmith Hospital on the basis of a clinical diagnosis. It does not include patients who have been shown to have DC on the basis of mutational analysis alone. When the latter are included, it is likely that these percentages will change.[4]

increased sensitivity of the host cells to the conditioning regimens employed.[11-13] While agents that are associated with pulmonary toxicity such as busulfan and radiotherapy should be avoided, SCT remains the only curative option. There have been recently encouraging reports of low-intensity fludarabine-based protocols for SCT in DC.[7,14,15]

The study of the bone marrow failure syndrome Fanconi anemia has been aided by the diagnostic test for an increased frequency of chromosomal breaks in response to clastogenic agents. While some reports have suggested that a similar hypersensitivity exists in DC,[16] others have found no significant difference in the frequency of chromosomal breakage between DC and normal lymphocytes with or without the use of bleomycin, diepoxybutane, mitomycin-C, and γ-irradiation.[17] No clear laboratory test therefore exists for DC, and with a wide range of clinical presentations, the diagnosis is often problematic.

Genetics

DC is genetically heterogeneous: although primarily an X-linked disorder (MIM305000), autosomal recessive (MIM 224230) and autosomal dominant (MIM 127550) patterns of inheritance have been recognized. In the DC Registry, which has been assembled at the Hammersmith Hospital since 1995, the vast majority of families (158/228) have only a single affected individual (123 male, 35 female) and it is not possible to infer a pattern of inheritance.[18] Only 22 of the families show clear X-linked inheritance; in a further 19 there are two affected male siblings (Table 2). In 11 families the disease follows an autosomal dominant pattern of inheritance and in 18 it appears to be autosomal recessive.

In 1986, by linkage analysis in one large family, the gene responsible for the X-linked form of the disease was assigned to band Xq28.[19] Through screening cDNAs in a candidate region that had been refined by recombination events to 1.4 Mb,[20] the gene mutated in X-linked DC was identified,[21] therefore providing an unambiguous genetic test for DC. The gene, *DKC1*, comprises 15 exons, encodes a protein of 514 amino acids named dyskerin, and is expressed in all tissues of the body, indicating an essential housekeeping function consistent with the multi-system phenotype of DC. Targeted knock-out of the *Dkc1* locus in mice is embryonically lethal.[22]

Homology searches showed that dyskerin is a highly conserved protein that localizes to the nucleolus.[23,24] Of functional interest, dyskerin shares 83% identity with the rat nucleolar-associated protein (NAP57)[25] and 69% identity with the yeast centromere/microtubule-binding factor (Cbf5p).[26] Like NAP57 and Cbf5p, dyskerin contains a TruB domain that shows homology to members of a family of bacterial tRNA pseudouridine synthases, as well as a PUA domain named after the pseudouridine synthase and archeosine-specific transglycosylases that have a putative RNA-binding

Table 2 Number of Families With Different Patterns of Inheritance and Mutations in the DC Registry

Pattern of Inheritance	*DKC1* Mutated	*TERC* Mutated	No Mutation Identified	Total
X-linked	21	0	1	22
Two affected male sibs	11	1	7	19
Sporadic affected male	40	3	80	123
Autosomal dominant	0	7*	4	11*
Autosomal recessive	0	0	18	18
Sporadic affected female	0	0	35	35
All	72	11	145	228

Data are from the number of families in each group in the DC Registry at the Hammersmith Hospital.
*Includes two families in which both parents are asymptomatic and which were initially thought to show autosomal recessive inheritance but are now known to have autosomal dominant DC due to *TERC* mutations.[18]

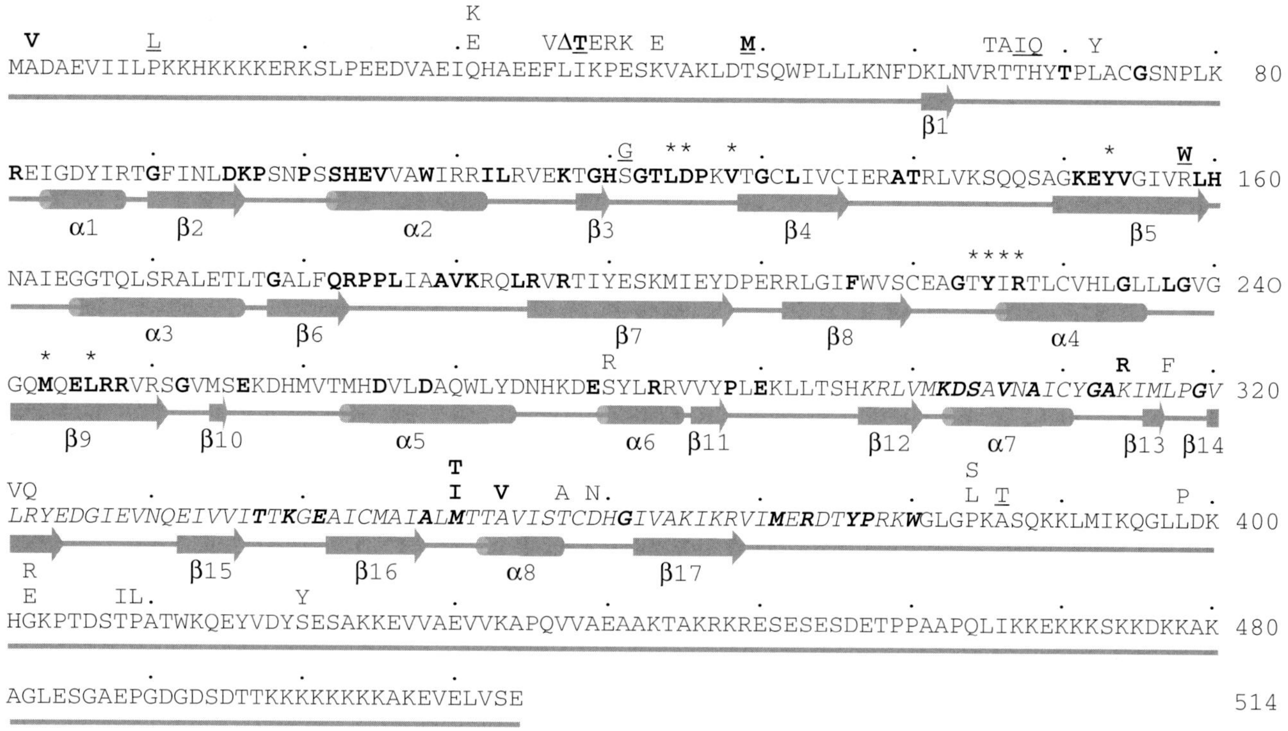

Figure 1 Dyskerin: amino acid sequence and substitutions in DC. The amino acid sequence of dyskerin is shown with residue numbers to the right and intervals of 10 marked with a dot. Highly conserved residues are shown in bold type. Amino acid substitutions seen in DC patients are given above the sequence. Those that cause HH are underlined; those that are seen repeatedly are shown in bold type. Δ represents a deletion. Below the sequence, the secondary structure is shown with β-sheets as arrows and α-helices as cylinders, as inferred from the three-dimensional structure of the archea Cbf5-Nop10 complex.[34] Residues that comprise the conserved core of the 3′ PUA domain are shown in italics. Asterisks are drawn above residues that line the active site in the catalytic domain. The first ~80 N-terminal amino acids form a tail, which surrounds the PUA domain.[35]

function.[27] In yeast and rats, Cbf5p and NAP57 associate with other nucleolar proteins (GAR 1, NHP2, and NOP10) and small nucleolar RNAs that have a hairpin-hinge-hairpin-ACA (H/ACA) motif to form a ribonucleoprotein complex.[28-30] The H/ACA RNAs act as guides, bringing the complex to specific uridine residues in ribosomal RNA, which are then modified to pseudouridine. This essential step in the maturation of ribosomal RNA is a prerequisite for ribosome biogenesis, and it has been suggested that the pathology in X-linked DC may be linked to impaired ribosome production.[31] Yeast cbf5 mutants have a pronounced defect in ribosomal RNA biosynthesis and are deficient in cytoplasmic ribosomal subunits.[32] Immunoprecipitation studies in rat have shown that the NOP10/NAP57 interaction is primary and that the NAP57-NOP10-NHP2 core trimer specifically recognizes H/ACA RNAs, while in yeast, Cbf5p can form a complex with Gar1p and Nop10p in the absence of Nhp2.[33]

The crystal structure of the archeal Cpf5-Nop10[34] and the Cbf5-Nop10-Gar1[35] complexes have recently been solved. Cbf5 alone was only modestly soluble and biochemically unstable. It has two major structural domains: the main catalytic domain, comprised of a six-stranded β-sheet with several α-helixes and loops on one surface, and the PUA domain, which protrudes from one corner of the catalytic domain. Nop10 and Gar1 surround the catalytic domain, where they may act to facilitate and stabilize RNA-binding. Highly conserved, positively charged surfaces of Cbf5 that are involved in this RNA-binding lie in a 20-Å wide trough that opens out from the active site both in the main domain and into the PUA domain,[34] where sequence-specific interaction with the guide RNA and anchoring of the target RNA are thought to occur.[35] As discussed below, it is of interest that the N-terminal tail of Cbf5 encircles the entire PUA domain.

Dyskerin Mutations

X-linked DC is almost entirely caused by missense mutations in dyskerin (36 of the 42 mutations described to date) (Fig 1). With only one exception (M350T or I), the resulting amino acid substitutions do not impact on highly conserved residues. The only significant deletion identified removes the last exon. Three splicing mutations and a promoter mutation also have been identified in DC patients. These findings suggest that a null mutation would not be viable. Amino acid substitutions do seem to cluster into two regions of the protein, one throughout the PUA domain and another toward the N-terminal (Fig 1). Whether these mutations affect protein function through reducing catalytic activity, decreasing protein stability, impairing correct folding, or disrupting protein-

protein or protein-RNA interactions has not been established.

Considerable insight has been gained from a model of the three-dimensional structure of dyskerin that was based on the crystal structure of the archeal protein.[35] The N-terminal and C-terminal clusters of amino acids mutated in DC both localize to one side of the PUA domain. The most plausible conclusion from this striking observation is that most of the amino acid substitutions in DC cause a reduction of the ability of dyskerin to bind its cognate RNAs. Two notable exceptions to this localization of mutations (S121G and R158W), which lie in the catalytic domain in closer proximity to the active site (N125), both cause a severe DC phenotype, resembling the HH syndrome. An artificial mutation to this catalytic residue in other species abolished pseudouridylation activity and significantly reduced H/ACA RNA association.[36]

In the DC Registry, dyskerin mutations have been identified in about one third of all families (Table 2) and most are private mutations. Quite remarkably, one amino acid substitution (A353V) has been seen in 30 different families from disparate parts of the world. In 11 cases, the mutation has arisen de novo. Although the mutation is a favoured CpG→TpG transition, this aspect alone cannot explain its extraordinary prevalence; it may be the only such mutation that can cause a DC-inducing amino acid substitution that also maps to the trough surface of the PUA domain. There is a considerable range of disease severity of subjects with the A353V mutation, with four cases manifesting with the severe HH syndrome, while eight patients did not present until more than 15 years of age.[18]

The Link to Telomerase

Telomerase is a specialized ribonucleoprotein reverse transcriptase complex that is expressed in germ cells and some stem cells, where it is responsible for maintaining the telomeric ends of chromosomes, which in most other somatic cells shorten with each cell division.[37,38] The complex has two core components: an RNA molecule (TERC) that acts as a template for the synthesis of the telomeric repeat sequence and a reverse transcriptase (TERT). TERC is comprised of three conserved structural elements,[39] the pseudoknot (responsible for positioning of the RNA template with respect to the catalytic site of TERT), the CR4-CR5 domain, and the scaRNA domain (essential for RNA 3′-end processing and stability). TERT has an amino-terminal domain involved in RNA binding and localization to the nucleolus, an RT domain, essential for catalytic activity and conserved among all reverse transcriptases, and a C-terminal domain, which binds other telomerase-associated proteins and contains a nuclear export signal.[40]

TERC contains an H/ACA motif[41] and dyskerin, GAR1, NHP2, and NOP10 are also components of the telomerase complex.[42,43] In cell lines from DC patients with dyskerin mutations, the level of TERC was reduced while there was no significant defect in ribosomal RNA processing or site-specific psuedouridylation.[44] Furthermore, telomere lengths were shorter in DC lymphoblastoid cell lines than in age-matched normal individuals, a difference confirmed in the analysis of peripheral blood telomere lengths.[45] Patients with the most severe form of DC have significantly shorter telomeres than do those with a relatively mild presentation.[18] In one patient with a Q31E substitution in dyskerin, a reduction in the level of telomerase RNA in peripheral blood was demonstrated.[46] Telomerase activity, induced by overexpression of TERT in an X-linked DC fibroblast cell line, was reduced compared to similarly treated cell lines from DC carriers,[44] but a similar reduction was not apparent in peripheral blood mononuclear cells.[45]

These observations indicated that DC might be a disorder of telomerase function rather than of ribosome production. Further studies on X-linked DC lymphoblastoid cell lines are supportive, suggesting that the reduced expansion and increased levels of apoptosis that characterizes these cells is caused by premature telomere shortening.[47,48] Evidence from murine models is more ambiguous. In a mouse model in which dyskerin expression levels were reduced by an insertional event at the 3′ end of the gene, impaired ribosomal RNA pseudouridylation appeared to be important in the initiation of the disease phenotpye, and telomere shortening, occurring only in later generations, acted to modify and/or exacerbate the symptoms.[49] Mouse embryonic stem cells harboring dyskerin missense mutations observed in DC patients show destabilization of telomerase RNA and reduced telomerase activity, and also decreased accumulation of a subset of H/ACA small nucleolar RNAs, resulting in reduced pseudouridylation activity.[50]

Mutations in the RNA Component of Telomerase

The hypothesis that DC is primarily a disorder of telomere maintenance was strengthened by the discovery that some families with autosomal dominant inheritance of DC have heterozygous mutations in the TERC gene.[51] In two families, large deletions were identified, removing either the 5′ end (to nucleotide 316) or the 3′ end of the gene (from nucleotide 378). Aberrant transcripts were not detected in individuals with the 3′ deletion, and therefore the disease arises through haploinsufficiency. In other autosomal dominant DC families, point mutations or small internal deletions have been identified.[51,52]

Some kindreds with autosomal dominant DC do not have mutations in TERC,[18] and the families with TERC mutations do not necessarily present as autosomal dominant DC.[53-55] A small number of patients who have presented with apparently acquired aplastic anemia have been shown, by large-scale mutation screening, to have mutations in TERC. In these families, the inherited nature of the disease is not always apparent and the mucocutaneous features of DC are absent. These cases may represent cryptic DC with a relatively mild course in which only the most proliferative tissue of the body, the hematopoietic system, is affected. In one patient with aplastic anemia and paroxysmal nocturnal hemoglobinuria, a promoter mutation in TERC disrupted bind-

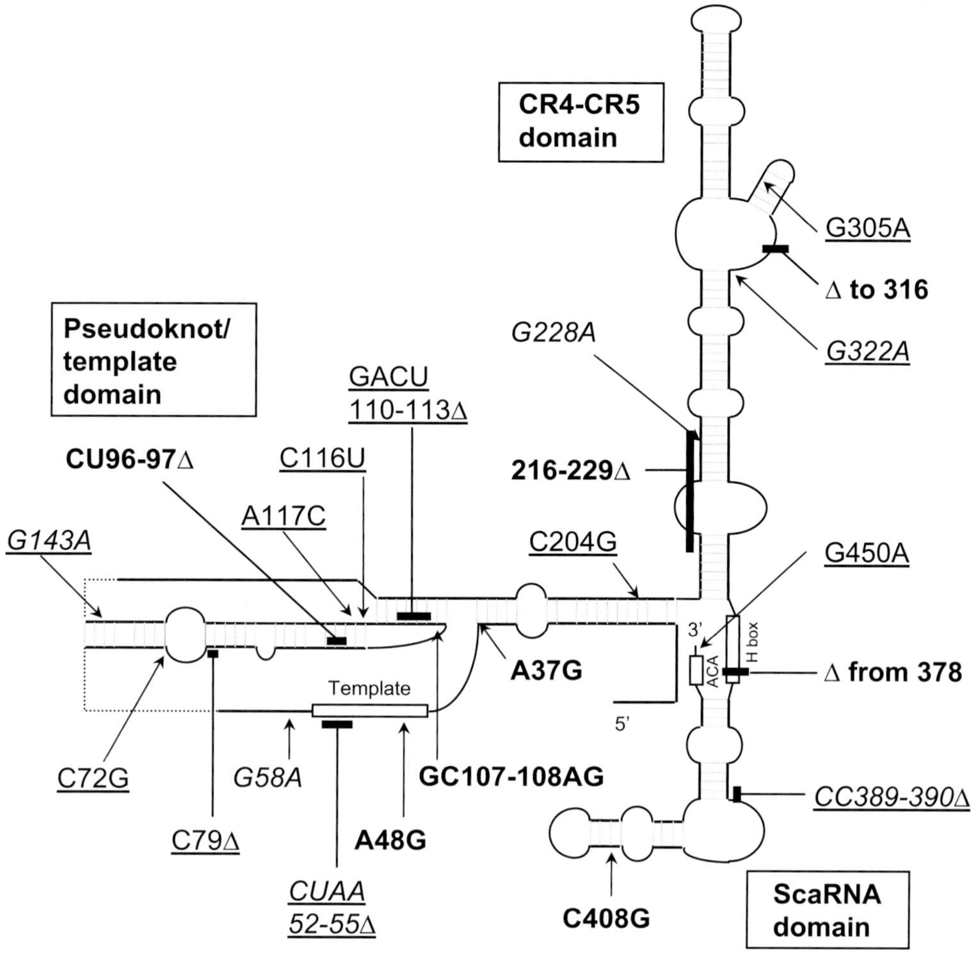

Figure 2 Sequence changes in TERC. The locations of sequence changes found in TERC in patients with DC (bold type), aplastic anemia (underlined), myelodysplastic syndrome or essential thrombocythemia (underlined and italics), and in normal individuals (italics) are shown on the structure of the molecule (from reference 39). Point mutations are shown by arrows; deletions are indicated by bars.

ing of the transcription factor Sp1.[56] A germ-line mutation in TERC was also identified in a patient who presented with essential thrombocythemia, which is considered to be an acquired clonal disorder.[57] Especially intriguing is the finding of TERC mutations in the form of myelodysplasia.[52,55] Myelodysplasia patients also tend to have short telomeres,[58] but their marrow cellularity is usually increased with marked abnormalities in morphology. As with aplastic anemia, the primary pathology of this stem cell disorder remains unknown.

In addition to the two large deletions that remove the 5′ and 3′ ends of TERC, point mutations and small deletions have been found in all domains of the molecule (Fig 2). Predominantly they appear to cause disruption of base pairing and destabilization of the pseudoknot domain. One mutation (GC1078→AG) perturbs an equilibrium between two different conformational forms that exist for the domain; the switch between these two states is important for telomerase activity.[59,60]

The functional consequences of several mutations have been investigated in vitro, either in a cell-free reconstitution assay or after introduction into a cell line (W138VA13) that does not express telomerase. Using these methods, it has been possible to assess whether TERC mutations seen in autosomal dominant DC and aplastic anemia reduce telomerase activity (Table 3).[57,61-63] TERC mutations fall into three main categories:

(1) Those that clearly reduce activity in both the cell-free system and in the cell line, and presumably therefore cause a catalytic defect, as occurs for all of the disease-causing pseudoknot mutations.
(2) Mutations that reduce telomerase activity only in the cell line, as with the C408G mutation that disrupts base pairing in the scaRNA domain,[61,62] resulting in impaired RNA accumulation and stability due to a reduction of TERC in dimer formation.[64] The only other disease-causing mutation in the scaRNA domain (del 389-390) completely abolished telomerase activity but had no apparent effect on the stability of the RNA.[57]
(3) Mutations that do not apparently cause a reduction of telomerase activity in these assays, as for two mutations that have been identified in patient samples

Table 3 Location and Consequence of Sequence Changes in *TERC*

Sequence Change	Location	Disease	Activity*
Δ~2Kb to 316	5′ UTR & 5′ of TERC	DC	ND
C-99G	5′UTR	AA, PNH	ND
C-21T	5′UTR	WT	ND
A37G	Pseudoknot stem P1b	DC	+++
A48G	Template	DC	ND
CTAA52-55Δ	Template	MDS/DC	ND
G58A	Near template	WT	++ or +++
C72G	Pseudoknot stem P2a.1	CAA	+
C79Δ	Pseudoknot stem P2a	CAA	ND
CT96-97Δ	Pseudoknot stem P2b	DC	−
GC107-108AG	Pseudoknot stem P3	DC	+
GACT110-113Δ	Pseudoknot stem P3	CAA	−
C116T	Pseudoknot stem P2b	SAA	−
A117C	Pseudoknot stem P2b	SAA	−
G143A	Pseudoknot stem P2a.1	MDS/DC	ND
C204G	Pseudoknot stem P1a	NSAA	−
216-229Δ	Hyper-variable paired region P4	DC	−
G228A	CR4-5 domain stem P4.1	WT	+++
G305A	CR4-5 domain stem P6.1	NSAA	+
G322A	CR4-5 domain stem P5	MDS	+
Δ3783→′	H/ACA & CR7 domain and 3′ flanking	DC	+
CC389-90Δ	CR7 domain stem P7b	ET	−
C408G	CR7 domain stem P8b	DC	+ or ++
G450A	H/ACA domain	SAA	+++

Abbreviations: ND, not determined; PNH, paroxysmal nocturnal haemoglobinuria; CAA, constitutional aplastic anemia; SAA, severe aplastic anemia; NSAA, non-severe aplastic anemia; MDS, myelodysplastic syndrome; ET, essential thrombocythemia; Δ, deletion.

*Activity as determined through telomeric repeat amplification protocol (TRAP) assays of transient expression in telomerase-negative cell lines (−, undetectable; + low activity [1–5%]; ++, moderate activity [5–25%]; +++, near normal activity). Where alternatives are given, the results come from independent studies.[51-57, 62, 63]

(A37G and G450A) and also for a polymorphism, G228A.

Analysis of another polymorphic change among individuals of African origin (G58A) has shown discrepant results, either a mild reduction or no reduction in telomerase activity.[61,62] In vitro experiments have also clarified two other important aspects of TERC mutations. First, mixing together mutant and wild-type molecules in the same cell does not reduce the level of wild-type telomerase activity[57,61-63,65]; thus there is no evidence of a significant dominant negative effect of the mutant allele. Instead, as suggested by the presence of large deletions in some families, it appears that disease results by haploinsufficiency for TERC. By implication, the levels of TERC are finely regulated, and reduction by half is sufficient to cause suboptimal function of the telomerase complex as a whole. Second, for some of the mutations that disrupt the stem structure of TERC, their effect on secondary structure rather than primary sequence determines their functional consequences.[57,62,66]

A recurring pattern in the families with TERC mutations is presentation of an affected individual whose parents are both asymptomatic, or occult DC that appears as an acquired aplastic anemia. In large pedigrees, symptoms and death due to disease occur at a younger age with each succeeding generation.[52,67] Disease anticipation is associated with progressive telomere shortening through the generations.[52] In $Terc^{-/-}$ mice, telomere shortening and the clinical features similar to those of DC require several generations to manifest.[68] Heterozygous $Terc^{+/-}$ mice, which are defective in their ability to elongate telomeres,[69] also show reduced tissue-renewal ability in bone marrow, intestines, and testes in later generations.[70] Furthermore, the wild-type mice derived from late-generation $Terc^{+/-}$ mice also had short telomeres and germ cell defects, implying that it is telomere length rather than telomerase activity that determines this phenotype.[70] In a large autosomal dominant DC family, although no symptoms were reported by the children of affected parents who have a normal TERC genotype, two generations appear to be necessary to restore telomere length.[67]

TERT Mutations in Aplastic Anemia and DC

In a substantial majority of families with DC (144/228 in the DC Registry), no mutation has been identified in either the *DKC1* or *TERC* gene (Table 2). A study of a subset of these families has failed to reveal mutations in the other components of the dyskerin complex (GAR1, NOP10, and NHP2).[71] However, in a screen of 200 patients with aplastic anemia, eight different amino acid substitutions were identified in the reverse transcriptase component on telomerase, TERT.[72]

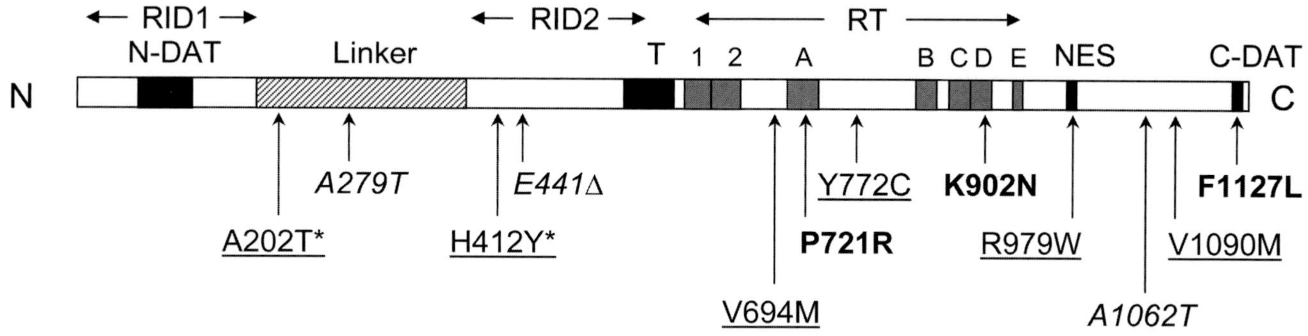

Figure 3 Amino acid substitutions in TERT. Amino acid substitutions that have been observed in TERT are shown on a linear representation of the protein. Those in bold type are seen in patients with DC or HH, those underlined are seen in patients with AA; those seen in more than one patient are shown with an asterisk, and those seen in normal individuals are shown in italics. Domains of the TERT protein are shown as follows: the N- and C-terminal domains that dissociate the activities of telomerase (N-DAT and C-DAT), a nuclear export signal (NES), and the telomerase specific domain (T) are shown as black boxes; motifs (1, 2, A-E) in the reverse transcriptase (RT) domain are shown as grey boxes; an N-terminal linker domain is shown as a hatched box and the extent of the RNA interaction domains (RID1 and RID2) is indicated.

Two were clearly polymorphic, one was seen in one patient and one normal subject, but five were observed only in patient samples (Fig 3). These heterozygous mutations were associated with variable degrees of telomere shortening, and four could be demonstrated to cause a dramatic reduction in telomerase activity when expressed from plasmids in a telomerase-negative cell line. No evidence of a dominant negative effect was observed in mixing experiments, suggesting a mechanism of haploinsufficiency.[72]

In another survey of TERT mutations in 74 families with DC and 56 patients with aplastic anemia, three additional TERT missense mutations have been identified[18,73] (Fig 3). However, one striking feature of these TERT mutations is their failure to consistently segregate with disease, particularly noticeable for the A202T substitution, which lies in a nonessential linker domain of the protein. In one family, three siblings and one daughter of the proband are also heterozygous for the mutation, and although they have shortened telomeres, they do not have any hematologic abnormalities.[72] In another family, the A202T substitution was present in an asymptomatic boy, while his cousins with aplastic anemia/myelodysplasia did not carry the mutation.[73] TERT mutations therefore appear to act as risk factors for marrow failure.

Recently, a family with autosomal dominant DC has been described in which a heterozygous TERT mutation segregated with the disease in seven affected and three unaffected members in three generations.[74] The mutation causes the substitution of a residue (K902N) that lies in motif D of the RT domain of TERT and is conserved among all reverse transcriptase families. In vitro expression and mixing experiments showed that the mutant enzyme had essentially no telomerase activity and were consistent with a mechanism of haploinsufficiency. Although the number of individuals available in this one family is small, disease anticipation was inferred from an increased proportion of short telomeres in the younger generation. Possibly the severity of this mutation distinguishes it from others in being directly disease-causing rather than predisposing to disease. The range of the phenotypes observed in patients with TERT mutations may be further confounded by the disease anticipation observed, with telomeres shortening only over several generations to the critical length that impairs stem cell function. Analogies with knock-out alleles in mice are not as clear for TERT as they are for TERC. Data are conflicting: in a recent study, $Tert^{+/-}$ heterozygotes, in contrast to $Terc^{+/-}$ heterozygotes, had no detectable defect in telomere elongation.[75]

Autosomal Recessive DC

Considered originally to be a rare exception to this predominantly X-linked disorder, a significant proportion of DC families may represent the autosomal recessive form of the disease. In the DC Registry, 18 families currently show this inheritance pattern and there are 35 sporadic female cases.[18] There is a wide range of clinical features within this genetic subtype, with a number of young girls presenting with HH while in other autosomal recessive families the affected individuals present at a later age, sometimes with only the mucocutaneous features of DC in the absence of any evidence of bone marrow failure.

The search for a genetic locus responsible for disease in autosomal recessive DC has focused on families in which there is a consanguineous marriage. To date, autosomal recessive DC appears genetically heterogeneous, with no single area of homozygosity being shared by affected individuals in different consanguineous families.[76] These loci are of interest to establish the extent to which they are related in a pathway that leads to telomerase dysfunction and/or perturbation of the assembly of other small nucleolar or Cajal body ribonucleoprotien complexes. For DC as for Fanconi's anemia,[77] multiple genes may be involved in a unified phenotype, and some of the involved genes may be mutated in only a few families.

Conclusion

The clinical manifestations of DC involve tissues that require constant renewal. When the product of the gene responsible for the X-linked form of the disease (dyskerin) was identified and found to be homologous to proteins involved in the processing of ribosomal RNAs, a plausible explanation of the pathology was that stem cell function was impaired by defective ribosome biogenesis. This intriguing connection between bone marrow failure and the ribosome was strengthened when it was established that some cases of Diamond-Blackfan anemia were due to mutations in a structural component of the ribosome (RPS19). Although the function of the Shwachman-Bodian-Diamond protein (SBDS) is less clear, it is also be likely to be involved in RNA metabolism.

The emphasis on the underlying pathophysiology of DC has shifted since dyskerin was identified as a component of the telomerase complex and patients with the autosomal dominant form of the disease were discovered to have mutations in TERC, a critical component of the telomerase complex with no other described function. A telomerase defect would easily result in a reduced proliferative potential of the stem cell pool. That mutations in dyskerin and TERC can result in such a similar phenotype supports the idea that the primary pathology of DC in humans is due to telomere dysfunction. Although pseudouridylation is defective in mouse models of DC, no such evidence has come from affected human cells, which show clear defects in telomerase function.

However, the other known core components of the telomerase are not or only very rarely mutated in DC, while a large number of patients remain uncharacterized. The identification of other genes in DC will provide further insight into how the activity, transport and stability of telomerase and perhaps other ribonucleoprotein complexes impact on hematopoietic stem cell function.

References

1. Sirinavin C, Trowbridge AA: Dyskeratosis congenita: Clinical features and genetic aspects. Report of a family and review of the literature. J Med Genet 12:339-354, 1975
2. Drachtman RA, Alter BP: Dyskeratosis congenita. Dermatol Clin 13:33-39, 1995
3. Knight S, Vulliamy T, Copplestone A, Gluckman E, Mason PJ, Dokal I: Dyskeratosis Congenita (DC) Registry: Identification of new features of DC. Br J Haematol 103:990-996, 1998
4. Dokal I, Vulliamy T: Telomerase deficiency and human disease, in de Lange T, Lundblad V, Blackburn E (eds): Telomeres. Cold Spring Harbor, NY, Cold Spring Harbor Laboratory Press, 2006, pp 139-161
5. Aalfs CM, van den Berg H, Barth PG, Hennekam RC: The Hoyeraal-Hreidarsson syndrome: The fourth case of a separate entity with prenatal growth retardation, progressive pancytopenia and cerebellar hypoplasia. Eur J Pediatr 154:304-308, 1995
6. Knight SW, Heiss NS, Vulliamy TJ, Aalfs CM, McMahon C, Richmond P, et al: Unexplained aplastic anaemia, immunodeficiency, and cerebellar hypoplasia (Hoyeraal-Hreidarsson syndrome) due to mutations in the dyskeratosis congenita gene, DKC1. Br J Haematol 107:335-339, 1999
7. Cossu F, Vulliamy TJ, Badiali M, Cao A, Dokal I: Bone marrow transplantation in an infant with Hoyerall-Hreidarrson syndrome associated with severe combined immune deficiency (T+B-NK- SCID) and a novel *DKC1* mutation. Br J Haematol 119:765-768, 2002
8. De Boeck K, Degreef H, Verwilghen R, Corbeel L, Casteels-Van Daele M: Thrombocytopenia: First symptom in a patient with dyskeratosis congenita. Pediatrics 67:898-903, 1981
9. Russo CL, Glader BE, Israel RJ, Galasso F: Treatment of neutropenia associated with dyskeratosis congenita with granulocyte-macrophage colony-stimulating factor. Lancet 336:751-752, 1990
10. Alter BP, Gardner FH, Hall RE: Treatment of dyskeratosis congenita with granulocyte colony-stimulating factor and erythropoietin. Br J Haematol 97:309-311, 1997
11. Rocha V, Devergie A, Socie G, Ribaud P, Esperou H, Parquet N, et al: Unusual complications after bone marrow transplantation for dyskeratosis congenita. Br J Haematol 103:243-248, 1998
12. M'kacher R, Laithier V, Valent A, Delhommeau F, Violot D, Deutsch E, et al: Sensitivity to radiation and alkylating agent of peripheral lymphocytes and fibroblasts in a Hoyeraal-Hreidarsson syndrome patient. Pediatr Hematol Oncol 20:651-656, 2003
13. Cengiz M, Celebioglu B, Ozyar E, Atahan L: Unusual hypersensitivity to radiation therapy in a patient with dyskeratosis congenita syndrome Oral Oncol 40:758-759, 2004
14. Dror Y, Freedman MH, Leaker M, Verbeek J, Armstrong CA, Saunders FE: Low-intensity hematopoietic stem-cell transplantation across human leucocyte antigen barriers in dyskeratosis congenita. Bone Marrow Transplant 31:847-850, 2003
15. Gungor T, Corbacioglu S, Storb R, Seger RA: Nonmyeloablative allogeneic hematopoietic stem cell transplantation for treatment of dyskeratosis congenita. Bone Marrow Transplant 31:407-410, 2003
16. Pai GS, Yan Y, DeBauche DM, Stanley WS, Paul SR: Bleomycin hypersensitivity in dyskeratosis congenita fibroblasts, lymphocytes, and transformed lymphoblasts. Cytogenet Cell Genet 52:186-189, 1989
17. Coulthard S, Chase A, Pickard J, Goldman J, Dokal I: Chromosomal breakage analysis in dyskeratosis congenita peripheral blood lymphocytes. Br J Haematol 102:1162-1164, 1998
18. Vulliamy TJ, Marrone M, Knight S, Walne A, Mason PJ, Dokal I: Mutations in dyskeratosis congenita: Their impact on telomere length and the diversity of clinical presentation. Blood 107:2680-2685, 2006
19. Connor JM, Gatherer D, Gray FC, Pirrit LA, Affara NA: Assignment of the gene for dyskeratosis congenita to Xq28. Hum Genet 72:348-351, 1986
20. Knight SW, Vulliamy TJ, Heiss N, Matthijs G, Devriendt K, Connor JM, et al: 1.4Mb candidate region for X-linked dyskeratosis congenita defined by combined haplotype and X-chromosome inactivation analysis. J Med Genet 35:993-996, 1998
21. Heiss NS, Knight SW, Vulliamy TJ, Klauk SM, Wiemann S, Mason PJ, et al: X-linked dyskeratosis congenita is caused by mutations in a highly conserved gene with putative nucleolar functions. Nat Genet 19:32-38, 1998
22. He J, Navarrete S, Jasinski M, Vulliamy T, Dokal I, Bessler M, et al: Targeted disruption of Dkc1, the gene mutated in X-linked dyskeratosis congenita, causes embryonic lethality in mice. Oncogene. 21:7740-7744, 2002
23. Heiss NS, Girod A, Salowsky R, Wiemann S, Pepperkok R, Poustka A: Dyskerin localizes to the nucleolus and its mislocalization is unlikely to play a role in the pathogenesis of dyskeratosis congenita. Hum Mol Genet 8:2515-2524, 1999
24. Youssoufian H, Gharibyan V, Qatanani M: Analysis of epitope-tagged forms of the dyskeratosis congenital protein (dyskerin): Identification of a nuclear localization signal. Blood Cells Mol Dis 25:305-309, 1999
25. Meier UT, Blobel G: NAP57, a mammalian nucleolar protein with a putative homolog in yeast and bacteria. J Cell Biol 127:1505-1514, 1994
26. Jiang W, Middleton K, Yoon HJ, Fouquet C, Carbon J: An essential yeast protein, CBF5p, binds in vitro to centromeres and microtubules. Mol Cell Biol 13:4884-4893, 1993
27. Aravind L, Koonin EV: Novel predicted RNA-binding domains associated with the translation machinery. J Mol Evol 48:291-302, 1999
28. Tollervey D, Kiss T: Function and synthesis of small nucleolar RNAs. Curr Opin Cell Biol 9:337-342, 1997
29. Wang C, Meier UT: Architecture and assembly of mammalian H/ACA

small nucleolar and telomerase ribonucleoproteins. EMBO J 23:1857-1867, 2004
30. Meier UT: The many facets of H/ACA ribonucleoproteins. Chromosoma 114:1-14, 2005
31. Luzzatto L, Karadimitris A: Dyskeratosis and ribosomal rebellion. Nat Genet 19:6-7, 1998
32. Cadwell C, Yoon HJ, Zebarjadian Y, Carbon J: The yeast nucleolar protein Cbf5p is involved in rRNA biosynthesis and interacts genetically with the RNA polymerase I transcription factor RRN3. Mol Cell Biol 17:6175-6183, 1997
33. Henras AK, Capeyrou R, Henry Y, Caizergues-Ferrer M: Cbf5p, the putative pseudouridine synthase of H/ACA-type snoRNPs, can form a complex with Gar1p and Nop10p in absence of Nhp2p and box H/ACA snoRNAs. RNA 10:1704-1712, 2004
34. Hamma T, Reichow SL, Varani G, Ferre-D'Amare AR: The Cbf5-Nop10 complex is a molecular bracket that organizes box H/ACA RNPs. Nat Struct Mol Biol 12:1101-1107, 2005
35. Rashid R, Liang B, Baker DL, Youssef OA, He Y, Phipps K, et al: Crystal structure of a Cbf5-Nop10-Gar1 complex and implications in RNA-guided pseudouridylation and dyskeratosis congenita. Mol Cell 21: 249-260, 2006
36. Zebarjadian Y, King T, Fournier MJ, Clarke L, Carbon J. Point mutations in yeast CBF5 can abolish in vivo pseudouridylation of rRNA. Mol Cell Biol 19:7461-7472, 1999
37. Blackburn EH: Telomeres and telomerase: Their mechanisms of action and the effects of altering their functions. FEBS Lett 579:859-862, 2005
38. Shay JW, Wright WE: Senescence and immortalization: Role of telomeres and telomerase. Carcinogenesis 26:867-874, 2005
39. Chen JL, Greider CW: Telomerase RNA structure and function: Implications for dyskeratosis congenita. Trends Biochem Sci 29:183-192, 2004
40. Nakamura TM, Morin GB, Chapman KB, Weinrich SL, Andrews WH, Lingner J, et al: Telomerase catalytic subunit homologs from fission yeast and human. Science 277:955-959, 1997
41. Mitchell JR, Cheng J, Collins K: A box H/ACA small nucleolar RNA-like domain at the human telomerase RNA 3′ end. Mol Cell Biol 19:567-576, 1999
42. Dez C, Henras A, Faucon B, Lafontaine D, Caizergues-Ferrer M, Henry Y: Stable expression in yeast of the mature form of human telomerase RNA depends on its association with the box H/ACA small nucleolar RNP proteins Cbf5p, Nhp2p and Nop10p. Nucleic Acids Res 29:598-603, 2001
43. Pogacic V, Dragon F, Filipowicz W: Human H/ACA small nucleolar RNPs and telomerase share evolutionarily conserved proteins NHP2 and NOP10. Mol Cell Biol 20:9028-9040, 2000
44. Mitchell JR, Wood E, Collins K: A telomerase component is defective in the human disease dyskeratosis congenita. Nature 402:551-555, 1999
45. Vulliamy TJ, Knight SW, Mason PJ, Dokal I: Very short telomeres in the peripheral blood of patients with X-linked and autosomal dyskeratosis congenita. Blood Cells Mol Dis 27:353-357, 2001
46. Wong JM, Kyasa MJ, Hutchins L, Collins K: Telomerase RNA deficiency in peripheral blood mononuclear cells in X-linked dyskeratosis congenita. Hum Genet 115:448-455, 2004
47. Montanaro L, Chilla A, Trere D, Pession A, Govoni M, Tazzari PL, et al: Increased mortality rate and not impaired ribosomal biogenesis is responsible for proliferative defect in dyskeratosis congenita cell lines. J Invest Dermatol 118:193-198, 2002
48. Montanaro L, Tazzari PL, Derenzini M: Enhanced telomere shortening in transformed lymphoblasts from patients with X linked dyskeratosis. J Clin Pathol 56:583-586, 2003
49. Ruggero D, Grisendi S, Piazza F, Rego E, Mari F, Rao PH, et al: Dyskeratosis congenita and cancer in mice deficient in ribosomal RNA modification. Science 299:259-262, 2003
50. Mochizuki Y, He J, Kulkarni S, Bessler M, Mason PJ: Mouse dyskerin mutations affect accumulation of telomerase RNA and small nucleolar RNA, telomerase activity, and ribosomal RNA processing. Proc Natl Acad Sci U S A 101:10756-10761, 2004
51. Vulliamy T, Marrone A, Goldman F, Dearlove A, Bessler M, Mason PJ, et al: The RNA component of telomerase is mutated in autosomal dominant dyskeratosis congenita. Nature 413, 432-435, 2001
52. Vulliamy T, Marrone A, Szydlo R, Walne A, Mason PJ, Dokal I: Disease anticipation is associated with progressive telomere shortening in families with dyskeratosis congenita due to mutations in *TERC*. Nature Genetics 36:447-449, 2004
53. Vulliamy TJ, Marrone A, Dokal I, Mason PJ: Association between aplastic anaemia and mutations in telomerase RNA. Lancet 359:2168-2170, 2002
54. Fogarty PF, Yamaguchi H, Wiestner A, Baerlocher GM, Sloand E, Zeng WS, et al: Late presentation of dyskeratosis congenita as apparently acquired aplastic anaemia due to mutations in telomerase RNA. Lancet 362:1628-1630, 2003
55. Yamaguchi H, Baerlocher GM, Lansdorp PM, Chanock SJ, Nunez O, Sloand E, et al: Mutations of the human telomerase RNA gene (TERC) in aplastic anemia and myelodysplastic syndrome. Blood 102:916-918, 2003
56. Keith WN, Vulliamy T, Zhao J, Cem A, Erzik C, Bilsland A, et al: A mutation in a functional Sp1 binding site of the telomerase RNA gene (hTERC) promoter in a patient with paroxysmal nocturnal haemoglobinuria. BMC Blood Disorders 4:3-7, 2004
57. Ly H, Calado RT, Allard P, Baerlocher GM, Lansdorp PM, Young NS, et al: Functional characterization of telomerase RNA variants found in patients with hematologic disorders. Blood 105:2332-2339, 2005
58. Boultwood J, Fidler C, Kusec R, Rack K, Elliott PJ, Atoyebi O, et al: Telomere length in myelodysplastic syndromes. Am J Hematol 56:266-271, 1997
59. Comolli LR, Smirnov I, Xu L, Blackburn EH, James TL: A molecular switch underlies a human telomerase disease. Proc Natl Acad Sci U S A 99:16998-7003, 2002
60. Theimer CA, Finger LD, Trantirek L, Feigon J: Mutations linked to dyskeratosis congenita cause changes in the structural equilibrium in telomerase RNA. Proc Natl Acad Sci U S A 100:449-454, 2003
61. Fu D, Collins K: Distinct biogenesis pathways for human telomerase RNA and H/ACA small nucleolar RNAs. Mol Cell 11:1361-1372, 2003
62. Marrone A, Stevens D, Vulliamy T, Dokal I, Mason PJ: Heterozygous telomerase RNA mutations found in dyskeratosis congenita and aplastic anemia reduce telomerase activity via haploinsufficiency. Blood 104: 3936-3942, 2004
63. Ly H, Schertzer M, Jastaniah W, Davis J, Yong SL, Ouyang Q, et al: Identification and functional characterization of 2 variant alleles of the telomerase RNA template gene (TERC) in a patient with dyskeratosis congenita. Blood 106:1246-1252, 2005
64. Ren X, Gavory G, Li H, Ying L, Klenerman D, Balasubramanian S: Identification of a new RNA.RNA interaction site for human telomerase RNA (hTR): Structural implications for hTR accumulation and a dyskeratosis congenita point mutation. Nucleic Acids Res 31:6509-6515, 2003
65. Cerone MA, Ward RJ, Londono-Vallejo JA, Autexier C: Telomerase RNA mutated in autosomal dyskeratosis congenita reconstitutes a weakly active telomerase enzyme defective in telomere elongation. Cell Cycle 4:585-589, 2005
66. Ly H, Blackburn EH, Parslow TG: Comprehensive structure-function analysis of the core domain of human telomerase RNA. Mol Cell Biol 23:6849-6856, 2003
67. Goldman F, Bouarich R, Kulkarni S, Freeman S, Du HY, Harrington L, et al: The effect of TERC haploinsufficiency on the inheritance of telomere length. Proc Natl Acad Sci U S A 102:17119-17124, 2005
68. Blasco MA, Lee HW, Hande MP, Samper E, Lansdorp PM, DePinho RA, et al: Telomere shortening and tumor formation by mouse cells lacking telomerase RNA. Cell 91:25-34, 1997
69. Hathcock KS, Hemann MT, Opperman KK, Strong MA, Greider CW, Hodes RJ: Haploinsufficiency of mTR results in defects in telomere elongation. Proc Natl Acad Sci U S A 99:3591-3596, 2002
70. Hao LY, Armanios M, Strong MA, Karim B, Feldser DM, Huso D, et al: Short telomeres, even in the presence of telomerase, limit tissue renewal capacity. Cell 16:1121-1131, 2005
71. Marrone A, Mason PJ: Dyskeratosis congenita. Cell Mol Life Sci 60:507-511, 2003
72. Yamaguchi H, Calado RT, Ly H, Kajigaya S, Baerlocher GM, Chanock

SJ, et al: Mutations in TERT, the gene for telomerase reverse transcriptase, in aplastic anemia. N Engl J Med 352:1413-1424, 2005
73. Vulliamy TJ, Walne A, Baskaradas A, Mason PJ, Marrone A, Dokal I: Mutations in the reverse transcriptase component of telomerase (TERT) in patients with bone marrow failure. Blood Cells Mol Dis 34:257-263, 2005
74. Armanios M, Chen JL, Chang YP, Brodsky RA, Hawkins A, Griffin CA, et al: Haploinsufficiency of telomerase reverse transcriptase leads to anticipation in autosomal dominant dyskeratosis congenita. Proc Natl Acad Sci U S A 102:15960-15964, 2005
75. Chiang YJ, Hemann MT, Hathcock KS, Tessarollo L, Feigenbaum L, Hahn WC, et al: Expression of telomerase RNA template, but not telomerase reverse transcriptase, is limiting for telomere length maintenance in vivo. Mol Cell Biol 24:7024–3701, 2004
76. Walne A, Vulliamy T, Marrone A, Dokal I: Genome wide linkage analysis suggests genetic heterogeneity in autosomal recessive dyskeratosis congenita, with one locus on chromosome 15. Blood 106:307a, 2005 (abstr)
77. Bagby GC Jr, Alter B: Fanconi anemia. Semin Hematol 43:147–156, 2006

ELSEVIER

Seminars in
HEMATOLOGY

Diamond Blackfan Anemia: New Paradigms for a "Not So Pure" Inherited Red Cell Aplasia

Jeffrey M. Lipton

Diamond Blackfan anemia (DBA) is a genetically and clinically heterogeneous disorder characterized by erythroid failure, congenital anomalies, and a predisposition to cancer. Faulty ribosome biogenesis is hypothesized to be the underlying defect, leading to erythroid failure due to accelerated apoptosis in affected erythroid progenitors/precursors. Since first observed in DBA, pro-apoptotic hematopoiesis has been recognized as a common mechanism for hematopoietic failure in virtually all of the inherited bone marrow failure syndromes. Inherited as an autosomal dominant trait, one of what appears to be multiple DBA genes, coding for ribosomal protein RPS19, has been cloned. The discovery of additional genes will no doubt clarify the molecular pathophysiology of this disorder. Even within families, individuals may vary dramatically as to the degree of anemia, treatment response, and the presence of congenital anomalies. The study of DBA has been facilitated by the creation of international patient registries that provide more reliable information regarding clinical presentation, genetics, and outcome, as well as descriptions of congenital malformations and cancer predisposition, than can be culled from the literature. Analysis of registry data has led to improvements in clinical care and provides patients and research specimens for clinical and laboratory investigations.
Semin Hematol 43:167-177

Diamond Blackfan anemia (DBA; OMIM #205900) is one of a rare group of genetic disorders, known as the inherited bone marrow failure syndromes.[1] These disorders have in common pro-apoptotic hematopoiesis, bone marrow failure, birth defects,[2] and a predisposition to cancer.[3] Interest in these disorders has grown dramatically as the study of each has clarified, or revealed for the first time, new molecular events in development or cellular function.

Diamond Blackfan anemia was first reported in 1936[4] and more completely described by Diamond and Blackfan in 1938.[5] The diagnostic criteria for DBA published in 1976 are: presentation of anemia prior to the first birthday with near normal or slightly decreased neutrophil counts, variable platelet counts, reticulocytopenia, macrocytosis, and normal marrow cellularity with a paucity of red cell precursors. These criteria have, until recently, remained the accepted standard.[6] Careful analysis of DBA-affected pedigrees for the presence of members with macrocytosis, elevated fetal hemoglobin (HbF) levels, and/or increased erythrocyte adenosine deaminase (eADA) activity (elevated in 85% of patients with DBA) and congenital anomalies strongly suggested a greater number of autosomal dominant cases than previously expected.[7] With the discovery of the first gene mutated in DBA,[8,9] it has become evident that the penetrance of autosomal dominant DBA is quite variable for both hematologic and nonhematologic manifestations. Indeed, the estimate of 10% to 15% of DBA cases being familial has increased to around 45% as a consequence of mutation analysis of family members of probands.[10]

A combination of laboratory and clinical investigations has begun to reveal the relationships between the moribund erythron, biology, and nonhematologic manifestations of DBA. Moreover, recent advances in the understanding of DBA, in part as a result of data from international Diamond Blackfan anemia registries,[4,10-13] are resulting in more sophisticated diagnostic criteria and improvements in clinical care.[14]

Division of Pediatric Hematology/Oncology and Stem Cell Transplantation, Schneider Children's Hospital, Albert Einstein College of Medicine, Long Island Jewish Medical Center, New Hyde Park, NY; and the Feinstein Institute for Medical Research, Manhasset, NY.

Supported by grants from the Daniella Maria Arturi Foundation, Diamond Blackfan Anemia Foundation, Pediatric Cancer Foundation, National Institutes of Health RO1 HL 079571, and the Feinstein Institute for Medical Research at the NSLIJ General Clinical Research Center MO1 RR018535.

Address correspondence to Jeffrey M. Lipton, MD, PhD, Schneider Children's Hospital, 269-01 76th Ave, New Hyde Park, NY 11040. E-mail: jlipton@lij.edu

0037-1963/06/$-see front matter
doi:10.1053/j.seminhematol.2006.04.002

Pathophysiology and Genetics: Is DBA a Disorder of Ribosome Biosynthesis?

A number of theories regarding the pathophysiology of DBA have been proposed and discarded.[15-18] Widely accepted is that the disorder results from an intrinsic cellular defect in which erythroid progenitors and precursors are highly sensitive to death by apoptosis.[19-22] Familial DBA appears to be inherited as an autosomal dominant. No instance of autosomal recessive inheritance has been confirmed, and apparent recessive inheritance is likely a consequence of non-penetrance[2] or, rarely, gonadal mosaicism.[23] The first DBA gene, *DBA1*, located at chromosome 19q13.2 and mutated in approximately 25% of patients, has been cloned and is identified as *RPS19*, which codes for a ribosomal protein.[8,9] The exact function of this protein in ribosome biogenesis is only poorly understood. The yeast homolog of RPS19 is required for the maturation of the 3′ end of 18S rRNA, failure of which results in the accumulation of faulty pre-40S ribosome subunits.[24] Extra-ribosomal functions have been ascribed to RPS19: in addition to the post-apoptotic mediation of monocyte chemotaxis,[25] RPS19 has been shown to interact with a novel nucleolar protein S19–binding protein (S19BP),[26] fibroblast growth factor 2,[27] and the PIM-1 oncoprotein.[28] The role of these proteins in erythropoiesis, birth defects, or oncogenesis has not been established, but a role for the disruption of these extraribosomal functions in the pathogenesis of DBA cannot be excluded.

Current evidence suggests that, in patients for whom *RPS19* is mutated, disease results from RPS19 protein haplo-insufficiency. This hypothesis is supported in DBA by the demonstration of two classes of *RPS19* mutations (Fig 1). Quantitative defects resulting from nonsense mutations, insertions, deletions, and splice site mutations causing frameshifts, premature stop codons, and mRNA decay scattered over the entire allele result in no protein. In contrast, hotspot mutations are postulated to lead to major loss of function.[29] When *RPS19* is knocked down in cellular models,[30-32] defective erythropoiesis results. In addition, the repair of defective hematopoiesis follows gene transfer by increased RPS19 protein expression in both RPS19-deficient and DBA patient-derived erythroid cells.[33] In yeast, the introduction of *RPS19* mutations found in DBA results in a defect in the processing of pre-rRNA similar to that observed in cells with decreased expression of *RPS19*.[24] In the hematologically normal *RPS19*$^{+/-}$ knockout mouse model, compensatory transcriptional upregulation of RPS19 expression may result in normal erythropoiesis, but RPS19 protein levels in early erythroid cells have not been reported.[34] There is evidence in DBA that non-erythroid cells may compensate at the protein level for *RPS19* haplo-insufficiency, whereas erythroid cells do not.[29] In recent reviews, Ellis and Massey[35] and Liu and Ellis[36] hypothesize that, in addition to compensatory mechanisms needed to explain normal function in mutated cells, some components necessary for ribosome assembly are rate-limiting, presumably in some tissues but not others and in certain tissues at different stages of development—accounting for the relatively selective red cell failure and the presence of characteristic congenital anomalies.

A disorder of craniofacial morphogenesis, Treacher Collins syndrome (TCS; OMIM #154500), provides additional evidence that DBA results from defective ribosome synthesis. TCS is classically characterized by "bilateral downslanting palpebral fissures, frequently accompanied by colobomas of the lower eyelids and a paucity of eyelashes medial to the defect, abnormalities of the external ears, atresia of the external auditory canal and bilateral conductive hearing loss, hypoplasia of the zygomatic complex and mandible and cleft palate."[37] As in DBA, the disorder is inherited as an autosomal dominant trait, with a high spontaneous mutation rate of about 60%. The incidence is of the same order of magnitude, about one in 50,000 live births for TCS[38] and one in 100,000 for DBA.[11] Case ascertainment of mild phenotypes in both disorders is clearly a cause for under-reporting. Additional similarities between TCS and DBA exist. Orofacial clefts have been reported in 3% of cases of DBA in the literature[39] and in 5.7% of cases from the Diamond Blackfan Anemia Registry.[7] First cousins, male children of sisters, with bilateral microtia and cleft palate consistent with TCS, but with hematologic abnormalities consistent with DBA have been described.[2] The proband had been enrolled in the Diamond Blackfan Anemia Registry of North America (DBAR), a database of more than 400 patients,[7,40] while his cousin with similar facial anomalies had not developed classic DBA at the time of the report. The cousin's relevant hematologic parameters were significant for macrocytosis, elevated HbF level, and increased eADA activity, consistent with a nonclassical hematologic DBA phenotype. Physical and hematologic evaluations of the patients' mothers were normal. Therefore, both mothers appear to be obligate heterozygotes for this dominantly inherited disorder, with neither demonstrating any hematologic evidence of DBA or even minimal congenital anomalies. This multiplex family demonstrates the extremely variable penetrance and expressivity of this DBA gene. In all, the described proband and two other of the 21 patients with DBA and a cleft palate reported to the DBAR were originally diagnosed with "classical" TCS (Fig 2); none of these three had mutations at *TCOF1* (5q32-q33.1), the gene mutated in 90% of patients with TCS.[41] All patients met the criteria for a diagnosis of DBA, but none with craniofacial anomalies had *RPS19* mutations.[42] In addition, the DBAR[42] and other investigators[10,43] have identified no patients with cleft palate/microtia and an *RPS19* mutation. Thus, although not yet statistically significant, a possible genotype-phenotype correlation is suggested in which the "TCS-like" phenotype in DBA is not associated with mutations in *RPS19*.[42] The other patients with DBA and craniofacial anomalies were not evaluated for *TCOF1* mutations, nor have extensive hematologic evaluations of patients with TCS been reported.

TCOF1 encodes the nucleolar phosphoprotein treacle,[41,43,44] mutated in TCS. Analogous to RPS19 in DBA, TCS results most likely from treacle haplo-insufficiency.[45] Treacle

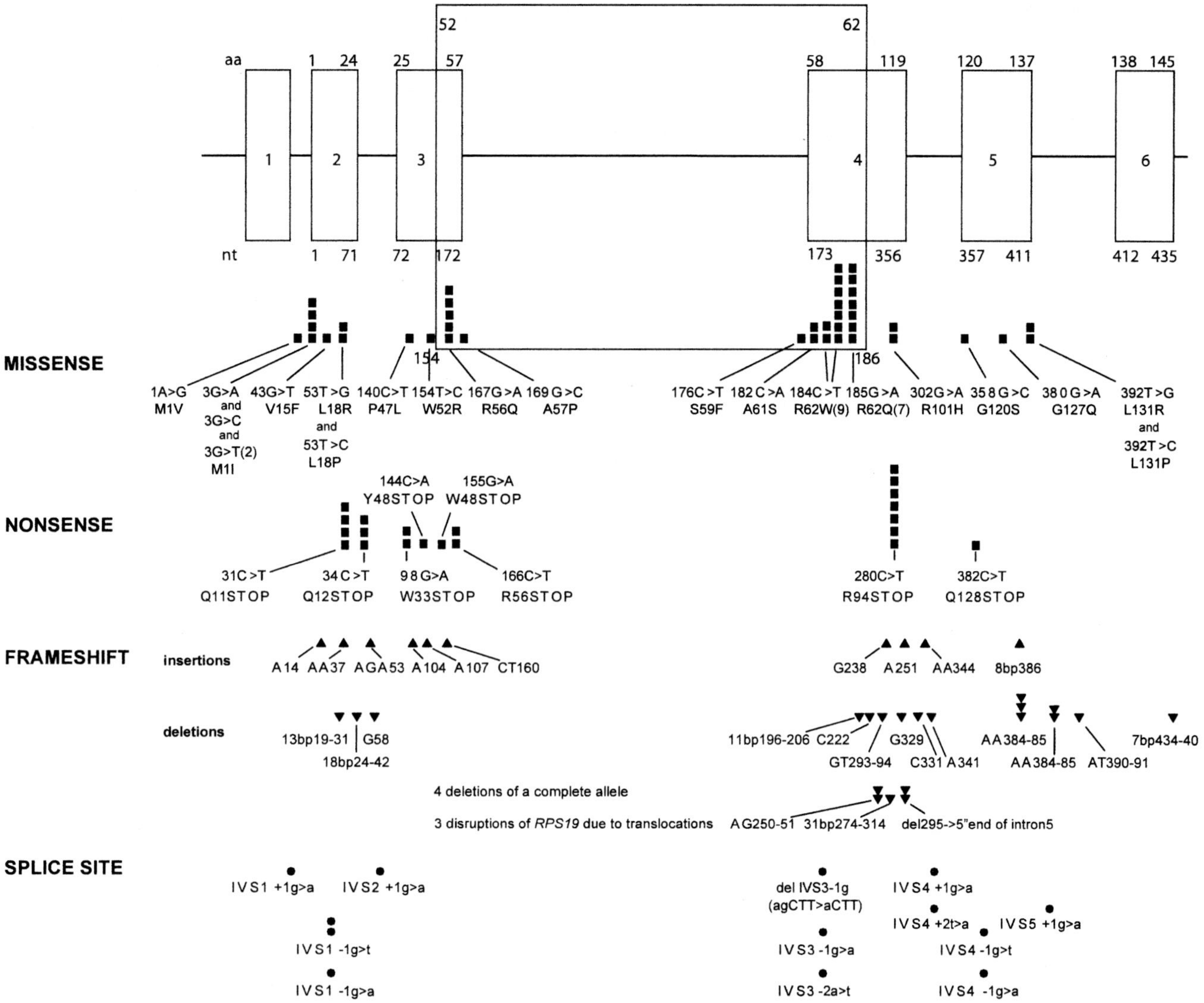

Figure 1 Distribution of *RPS19* mutations in DBA (kindly provided by Hanna Gazda, MD). Summary of the reported.[9,11,12,23,29,79-82] *RPS19* mutations in unrelated DBA index patients. Sixty-two unique mutations (nonsense, missense, frameshift, and splice site) in coding region of *RPS19* have been reported in 106 unrelated probands. In addition, four deletions of an entire allele and three disruptions of *RPS19* due to translocations were identified for a total of 113 mutations in 457 studied unrelated probands (25%). Patients whose mutations are reported in more than one article are included only once in the summary.

interacts with upstream binding factor (UBF), a known transcription regulator of RNA polymerase I (Pol I), which participates in the initiating event in ribosomal DNA (rDNA) transcription, generating the 47S pre-ribosomal RNA (pre-rRNA).[46] Treacle is involved in other early steps in ribosome synthesis, linking rDNA transcription to pre-rRNA post-transcriptional methylation.[47] Treacle haplo-insufficiency would inhibit early events in the biosynthetic pathway, with a profound effect on ribosome synthesis. Comparable to pro-apoptotic erythropoiesis in DBA, the mechanism for the disruption of craniofacial structures in TCS appears to be increased apoptosis in the neural crest cells of the prefusion neural folds just prior to fusion during embryogenesis.[48]

Although DBA patients with *RPS19* mutations do not have craniofacial abnormalities, the similarities between the known disorder of ribosome biogenesis, TCS and DBA, strongly suggest that the remaining DBA mutations will affect ribosome assembly or function. In Fanconi anemia[49] and dyskeratosis congenita,[50] the discovery of additional defects or deficiencies in gene products that cooperate in a common pathway or function has led to a clearer understanding of the pathophysiology of these disorders. Likely, the discovery of abnormalities in the structure or function of additional gene products will clarify the role of defective ribosome biogenesis in the pathophysiology of DBA. As *RPS19* (*DBA1*) mutations account for only 20% to 25% of both sporadic and familial cases, the search for additional "DBA genes" is active in a number of laboratories. An analysis using well-characterized multiplex families ascertained through international DBA patient registries has provided statistical evidence that a second gene, *DBA2*, is present on 8p23-22, but no DBA gene has yet been described within this 8.1-cM region.[51]

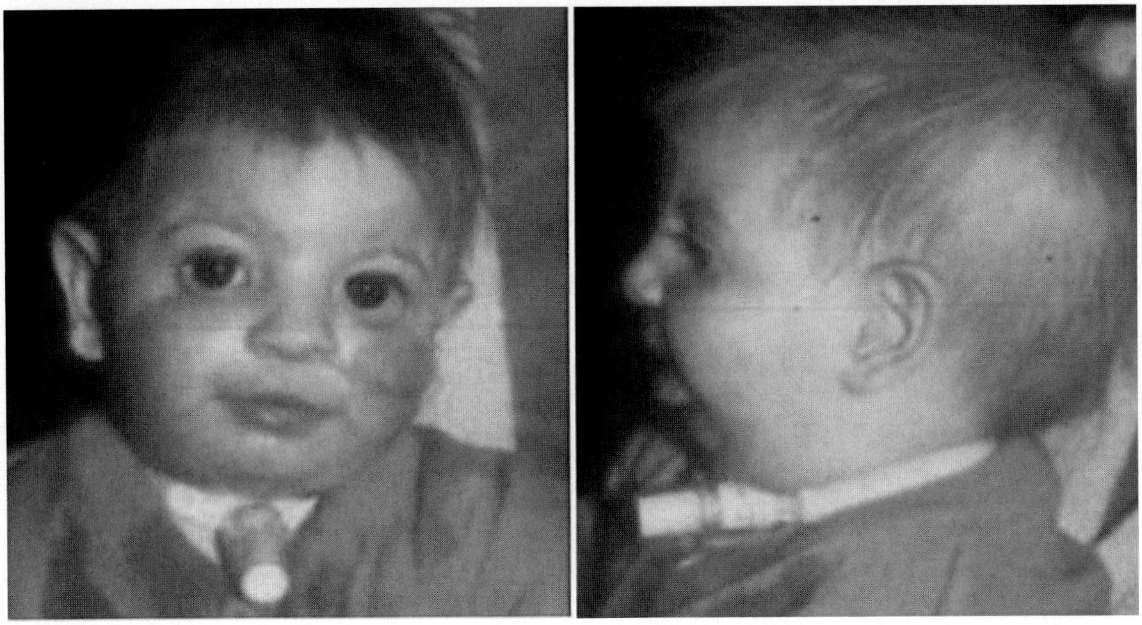

Figure 2 Patient with Diamond Blackfan anemia originally diagnosed with Treacher Collins syndrome. Parental consent provided to publish photographs.

Making the Diagnosis of Diamond Blackfan Anemia

The median age at presentation and diagnosis of classical DBA are 8 weeks (range, birth to 6 years) and 12 weeks (range, birth to 26 years), respectively.[40] Ninety-three percent of DBA patients present in the first year of life, but as in the other inherited bone marrow failure syndromes, DBA may present in adulthood,[52] when it is often misdiagnosed. The differential diagnosis of DBA in children presenting with red cell failure, anemia, reticulocytopenia, and decreased or absent marrow erythroid precursors is limited. In adults the diagnosis is less common and the differential diagnosis includes a vast array of conditions, many of which rarely, if ever, occur in children (Table 1). With awareness that mild DBA phenotypes may be missed in children and even more obvious cases misdiagnosed in adults, maintaining an index of suspicion is important. In the presence of a family history and in particular when a mutation is identified, the diagnosis of nonclassical DBA may be simple. Isolated macrocytosis, for example, should not be dismissed after more obvious etiologies (folate or B_{12} deficiencies) are excluded. Of importance is that patients with characteristic birth defects must be carefully evaluated for DBA and other inherited bone marrow failure syndromes.

In children, the more common disorder of transient erythroblastopenia of childhood (TEC) must be excluded. TEC is an acquired, short-lived failure of red cell production usually of about a month in duration. As in DBA, children with TEC often present with profound anemia. TEC, which is usually a post-infectious, transient autoimmune IgG-mediated disorder,[53] characteristically occurs in older children, probably from infections acquired through contact with playmates. As more infants are placed in daycare settings, TEC is appearing more often in children younger than 1 year of age. Table 2 summarizes the salient features distinguishing the two disorders. Most important, neither a positive family history nor congenital anomalies are typical of TEC. Elevated HbF levels and macrocytosis, common presenting features in DBA, are only seen in TEC upon recovery with "stress erythropoiesis." Macrocytosis is often obscured in the newborn period by residual fetal erythrocytes and can be masked by concomitant thalassemia minor or iron deficiency. Although the mechanism is unknown, an elevated eADA activity is found in about 85% of patients with DBA but in none with TEC.[54,55] Thus, the two disorders can usually be distinguished. The use of limited packed red cell transfusions to achieve a hemoglobin level that will not inhibit erythroid recovery is recommended, particularly when the diagnosis is unclear. With a correct diagnosis, treatment for DBA can commence.

When DBA is clinically diagnosed or in equivocal cases, *RPS19* mutation analysis should be performed; it will confirm the diagnosis in the 25% of cases in which the mutation is found. All immediate family members of the proband should be evaluated with a history and physical examination, seeking evidence of a transient or mild to moderate chronic anemia and birth defects. In addition, a complete blood cell count with red cell indices, HbF levels, and eADA activity may disclose a mild phenotype. When the proband is mutated at *RPS19*, the family, even if their evaluations are normal, should be similarly tested as it will provide information of value with regard to reproductive choices and in the consideration of family members as potential hematopoietic stem cell donors. In the future, the identification of a specific mutation may direct cancer-screening strategies or other clinical decisions.

Table 1 Classification of Pure Red Cell Aplasia

Inherited
Diamond Blackfan anemia
Acquired PRCA
Primary
Autoimmune (includes transient erythroblastopenia of childhood [TEC])
Pearson syndrome
Preleukemic
Idiopathic
Secondary, associated with:
Thymoma
Hematologic malignancies
Chronic lymphocytic leukemia
Large granular lymphocytic leukemia (Tγ lymphoproliferative disorder)
Chronic myelocytic leukemia
Acute lymphoblastic leukemia
Hodgkin's disease
Non-Hodgkin's lymphomas
Multiple myeloma
Waldenström's macroglobulinemia
Myelofibrosis with myeloid metaplasia
Essential thrombocythemia
Solid tumors
Carcinoma of the stomach
Adenocarcinoma of the breast
Adenocarcinoma of bile duct
Squamous cell carcinoma of the lung
Epidermoid carcinoma of the skin
Carcinoma of the thyroid
Renal cell carcinoma
Carcinoma of unknown primary site
Kaposi sarcoma
Infections
Human B19 parvovirus
Human immunodeficiency virus (HIV)
T-cell leukemia-lymphoma virus
Epstein-Barr virus (infectious mononucleosis)
Viral hepatitis
Mumps
Cytomegalovirus
Atypical pneumonia
Meningococcemia
Staphylococcemia
Leishmaniasis
Chronic hemolytic anemias (usually associated with B19 parvovirus)
Collagen vascular diseases
Systemic lupus erythematosus
Rheumatoid arthritis
Mixed Connective Tissue disease
Sjögren syndrome
Drugs and chemicals
Pregnancy
Severe renal failure
Severe nutritional deficiencies
Miscellaneous
Post-ABO incompatible bone marrow transplantation
Angioimmunoblastic lymphadenopathy
Autoimmune multiple endocrine gland insufficiency
Autoimmune hypothyroidism
Autoimmune chronic hepatitis
Anti-erythropoietin antibodies post-treatment with erythropoietin

Modified with permission from Dessypris EN, Lipton, JM: Red cell aplasia, in Wintrobe's Clinical Hematology, (ed 11). Greer, JP; Foerster, J; Lukens, JN; Rogers, GM; Paraskevas, F; Glader BE (eds): Philadelphia, Lippincott, Williams & Wilkins, PA, 2003, pp 1421–1437.

NOTE. The differential diagnoses more commonly described in children are highlighted in bold.

A Clinically Heterogeneous Syndrome: More Than Just Red Cell Failure

Congenital Anomalies

Birth defects have long been known to be a feature of DBA. A distinct facial appearance and triphalangeal thumbs have been classically described in DBA as the Cathie facies[56] and Aase syndrome,[57] respectively. A cute snub nose and wide-spaced eyes, as originally described by Cathie, and other craniofacial anomalies, some as already discussed quite severe, are the most common physical anomalies of DBA. Abnormal thumbs are classic.[58] In all, congenital anomalies were found in 30% to 47% of the patients in the Italian,[12] French,[11] UK,[10] and North American registries.[40] Additional anomalies of the upper limb and hand, genitourinary system, and heart each are described in as many as 30% to 40 % of patients.[40] The prevalence of genitourinary and cardiac anomalies may be underestimated if abdominal/pelvic and cardiac ultrasonography are not routinely performed in asymptomatic patients. More than one anomaly is described in about a quarter of all patients. Short stature is clearly constitutional in many patients. An accurate assessment of linear growth retardation is complicated in patients who may be anemic, iron-overloaded, or on corticosteroid therapy, all from a very young age. A representative table of malformations has been published.[11]

As described, a number of patients with unequivocal DBA have a phenotype indistinguishable from TCS.[3,59] In some, the hematologic abnormalities are extremely mild and likely there are individuals, heterozygous for a dominant-acting *DBA* gene, with a mild to no hematologic phenotype. Indeed, in a recent survey of patients who were diagnosed or had undergone repair of common DBA-associated anomalies, congenital heart disease (atrial septal defect, ventricular septal defect, coarctation of the aorta, and multiple defects), radial ray anomalies (bifid, subluxed, triphalangeal, or hypoplastic thumbs and flat thenar muscles), and orofacial clefts, approximately 2% to 3% had otherwise unexplained macrocytosis. Unrecognized DBA and perhaps other inherited bone marrow failure syndromes likely exist undiagnosed in the general population.[60]

Table 2 Differential Diagnosis of DBA Versus TEC

	Diamond Blackfan Anemia (DBA)	Transient Erythroblastopenia of Childhood (TEC)
Pure red cell aplasia	Present	Present
Age	Younger than 1 year	Older than 1 year
Inheritance	Sporadic and dominant inheritance Mutation analysis available for *DBA1* (*RPS19*)	Not inherited
Congenital anomalies	Present	Absent
Mean corpuscular volume (MCV)	Elevated	Normal (may be elevated upon recovery)
Fetal hemoglobin	Elevated	Normal (may be elevated upon recovery)
i RBC antigen	Present	Absent (may be present upon recovery)
Erythrocyte adenosine deaminase (eADA) activity	Elevated	Normal

NOTE. All red blood cell (RBC) characteristics except eADA activity are helpful only when tested in a reticulocytopenic child. During recovery from TEC, a transient wave of fetal-like erythropoiesis with elevated MCV, fetal hemoglobin, and i RBC antigen may be detected.
Modified with permission from Dessypris EN, Lipton JM: Red cell aplasia, in Wintrobe's Clinical Hematology, (ed 11). Greer P, Foerster J, Lukens JN, Rogers GM, Paraskevas F, Glader BE, (eds): Philadelphia, PA, Lippincott, Williams & Wilkins, 2003, pp 1421–1437.

Cancer: Is DBA a Cancer Predisposition Syndrome?

At least 26 cases of cancer in patients with DBA have been reported in the literature. Sixteen were hematopoietic malignancies: 10 acute myeloid leukemia (AML), two myelodysplastic syndrome (MDS), two Hodgkin disease, one non-Hodgkin lymphoma, and one acute lymphoblastic leukemia. Ten solid tumors have been reported: three osteogenic sarcoma, two breast cancer, two hepatocellular carcinoma, and one each of gastric carcinoma, vaginal melanoma, and malignant fibrous histiocytoma.[3] A number of cases have been reported from international registries and a large institutional cohort.[11,40,61] Of the 420 patients registered in the DBAR at the time of the most recent analysis, there were eight patients who had solid tumors, hematopoietic malignancies, or MDS (some of these patients also appear as case reports in the literature). Three patients were diagnosed with osteogenic sarcoma (total of five known cases) and one each with AML, MDS and myelofibrosis with myeloid metaplasia, colon cancer, and soft tissue sarcoma. (One individual, a DBA-affected relative of a registered patient with melanoma, is not yet enrolled in the DBAR.) Although cancer is relatively rare in DBA as compared to Fanconi anemia, the incidence appears to be well in excess of what would be expected for the age group represented. In particular, cases of breast and colon cancer have been described in very young adults.[3,11] The prognosis for patients with DBA and cancer is extremely poor, due in part to severe chemotherapy-induced myelosuppression.[3] The presence of these malignancies and the young age at diagnosis of many of these cancers appears to define DBA as a cancer predisposition syndrome. Before a true cancer incidence is determined, data from international DBA registries will need the same careful analysis as has been applied to Fanconi anemia[62] and severe congenital neutropenia.[63]

A mechanism leading to AML and MDS in Fanconi anemia has been postulated.[64,65] In this model, the existence of pro-apoptotic hematopoiesis exerts a selective pressure on the myeloid compartment, resulting in the emergence of clones with apoptosis-contravening mutations and ultimately in leukemia. The predisposition to solid tumors, in particular osteogenic sarcoma,[3,11] is not at all understood. Although at least some patients mutated at *RPS19* are known to have developed cancer, insufficient data exist to predict a cancer genotype, and a putative role for *RPS19* as an oncogene has not been explored. Recently, heterozygous mutations in 11 different ribosomal proteins in zebrafish have been found in fish with tumors; the majority of these dominantly inherited mutations seem to result in loss of function. Rather than acting as oncogenes, these ribosomal protein gene mutations were postulated to behave as tumor suppressors.[66]

Treatment and Outcomes: Where Are We Now?

Corticosteroids and Red Cell Transfusions

Corticosteroids and red cell transfusions are the mainstays of therapy for DBA. Since 1951,[67] it has been known that the anemia of DBA can be ameliorated by corticosteroids. The initial suggestion to use corticosteroids was based on the theory that DBA was an "allergic" disorder. The response to corticosteroids further perpetuated the erroneous notion of DBA as an autoimmune disease, even when only miniscule doses were required to maintain adequate erythropoiesis. The almost unlimited use of corticosteroids in the clinic, even when toxic doses were required, continued into the early 21st century, due largely to the persistent fear, in patients and physicians, of transfusion-acquired human immunodeficiency virus and hepatitis C, as well as the difficulty encountered in the almost daily subcutaneous administration of the iron chelator, deferoxamine (Desferal; Novartis Pharmaceuticals, East Hanover, NJ).[68] Data from international registries have clarified the efficacy and toxicity of corticosteroid therapy. Analysis from the DBAR is representative[40]: as has been reported in the literature, 79% of patients were initially responsive to corticosteroids, 17% were nonresponsive, and

4% of patients were never treated with corticosteroids. Unpredicted was the high incidence of significant untoward effects. Not surprising, nearly half of the patients had developed cushingoid features, but in addition 22% and 12% of patients ever treated with corticosteroids had developed pathologic fractures and cataracts, respectively. The use of corticosteroids is now being modified. Currently, 37% of the patients are receiving corticosteroids and 31% red cell transfusions. Of the transfusion-dependent patients, 35% were never corticosteroid-responsive, 22% became corticosteroid-refractory over time, and 33% could not be weaned to an acceptable dose. Five percent never received corticosteroid therapy and 5% are being transfused for unknown reasons. Although too soon to statistically validate, there appears to be a recent increase in the number of cases judged as "unweanable," as well as more patients who never received steroids. The ability to reduce the corticosteroid dose is dependent on the side effects that the patient and the physician are willing to tolerate. In general, a corticosteroid dose-equivalent of 0.5 mg/kg/d of prednisone is suggested as a maximum "maintenance" dose after an initial dose of 2 mg/kg/d.[14] Patients who fail to respond within a month are considered refractory. The recognition that the blood supply is safe combined with the recent availability of the oral iron chelator Deferasirox (ICL670, Exjade; Novartis)[69] has allowed for the more liberal use of packed red cell transfusions in patients rather than toxic doses of corticosteroids. The number of patients never on corticosteroids has increased, reflecting the older and safer age at which corticosteroid treatment is being commenced.[40]

Although remissions had been reported in DBA, the fraction of patients who were able to sustain erythropoiesis for over 6 months without treatment has been unclear. The DBAR has provided some actuarial data.[40] About 20% of patients will enter remission, the majority sustained; about 75% do so prior to their 10th birthday. These data may reflect the bias to a younger age of patients in the DBAR as anecdotal observations suggest a surge in remissions in adolescent males. Proportionally, an equal number of patients remit from both transfusion and steroid therapy. However, there are very few remitters who had never responded to corticosteroids. Pregnancy[70] and the use of birth control pills contribute to relapse.

Stem Cell Transplant

Although curative in DBA,[11,71,72] hematopoietic stem cell transplantation remains the most controversial aspect of therapy. A recent series from the International Bone Marrow Transplant Registry[73] and a compilation from the literature are consistent with findings from the DBAR.[74] In this database, 36 patients have undergone stem cell transplant (SCT): 21 human leukocyte antigen (HLA)-matched related and 15 alternative donor SCT. The major indication for SCT was transfusion dependence. In addition, two patients developed severe aplastic anemia and one had significant thrombocytopenia. Two patients transplanted using a nonmyeloablative conditioning regimen, one receiving a matched related umbilical cord and one receiving unrelated bone marrow, are alive and well. The majority of alternative donor transplants were performed using total body irradiation for conditioning, whereas busulfan/cyclophosphamide-containing regimens were typical of the matched-related transplants. Sixteen of the 21 HLA-matched sibling donor transplants are alive and red cell transfusion–independent. Of the 15 alternative donor SCTs, two patients received mismatched related bone marrow, four unrelated cord blood, eight unrelated bone marrow, and one unrelated peripheral blood stem cells. Four of these 15 patients are alive. Of the 16 deaths, 15 were related to infection, graft-versus-host disease, and/or veno-occlusive disease of the liver, with only one death, in the alternative donor group, as a consequence of graft failure. In contrast to Fanconi anemia, dyskeratosis congenita, and Shwachman Diamond syndrome, deaths do not appear to be the consequence of intolerance to typical transplant conditioning regimens. Survival for allogeneic sibling versus alternative donor transplant is 72.7% ± 10.7% versus 19.1% ± 11.9% at greater than 5 years from SCT ($P = .01$) or 17.1% ± 10.8% (including a patient diagnosed with osteogenic sarcoma post-transplant, $P = .012$) (Fig 3). The survival rate for patients under the age of 10 years receiving matched related SCT is greater than 90%. This success has led to an increase in preimplantation genetic diagnosis (PGD) with in vitro fertilization to "create" HLA-matched, non–*RPS19*-mutated sibling donors, and a number of patients worldwide have been successfully transplanted using umbilical cord–derived stem cells from donors produced in this way. A discussion of the complicated religious, ethical, and economic questions generated by this approach is beyond the scope of this review.[75,76]

Outcomes

Of the 36 deaths reported to the DBAR, 25 (70%) were treatment-related: five from infections (two *Pneumocystis jiroveci* pneumonia, one varicella pneumonia, one pseudomonas pneumonia/sepsis, one unknown infection), five from complications of iron overload, one from cardiac tamponade secondary to a vascular access device complication, and 14 from SCT complications. Only three of the deaths related to SCT were in patients with life-threatening cytopenias. Just eight deaths were directly related to DBA: one from severe aplastic anemia and seven from malignancy (two of whom also received a SCT), and three deaths were from undetermined causes. Thus, although SCT is potentially curative and reduces the risk of aplastic anemia, AML, and MDS, the poor outcomes for unrelated donor SCT suggest restraint in the use of this modality. The probability of remission must also be taken in to account when high-risk SCT is being considered.

The overall actuarial survival at greater than 40 years of age is 75% ± 4.8%; 100% for those in sustained remission, 87% ± 7.0% for corticosteroid-maintainable patients and 57% ± 8.9% for transfusion-dependent patients (Fig 4).[40] There is a trend to increased survival in patients with sustained remission versus corticosteroid-maintained patients ($P = .08$) and

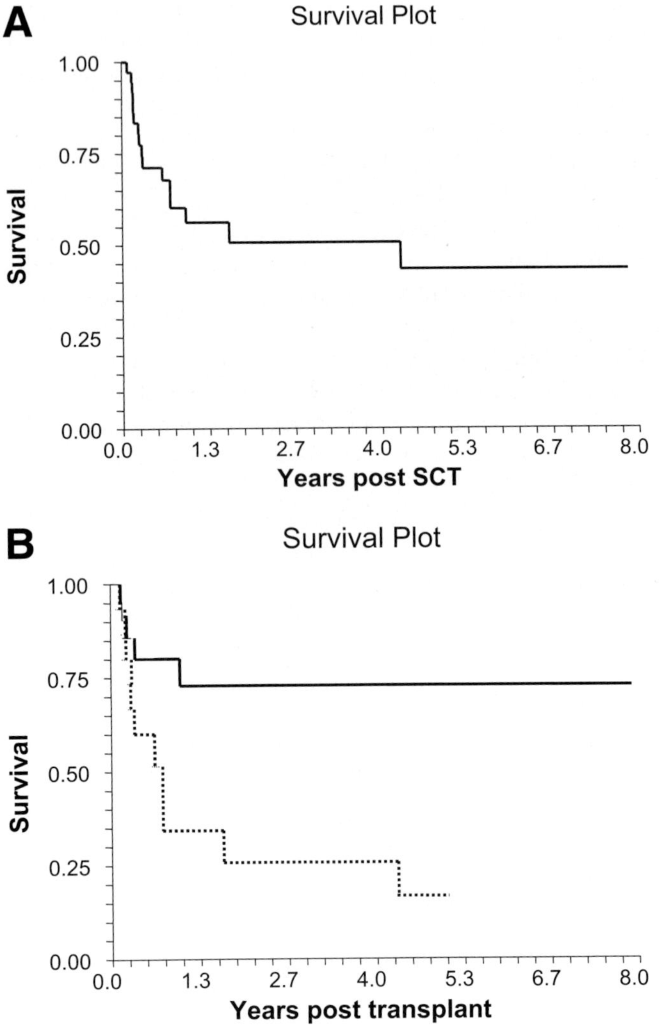

Figure 3 Kaplan-Meier analysis of (A) overall survival for DBA patients who underwent SCT, and (B) survival of DBA patients undergoing matched related (—), 72.7% (confidence limits, 51.7–93.8), versus unrelated or mismatched SCT (▪▪▪▪), 19.1% (confidence limits, 0.0–42.3) (P = .011). Reprinted with permission from Lipton et al.[40]

a statistically significant survival advantage for steroid-maintainable as compared to transfusion-dependent patients (P = .007). Seven transfusion-dependent patients died as a consequence of SCT-related complications.

Conclusions: Where Are We Going?

Progress in the understanding of the inherited bone marrow failure syndromes and in particular DBA has resulted from the combination of clinical and research laboratory science. Patient registries have permitted the more precise description of congenital anomalies, suggesting a possible connection between DBA and TCS; similarities between them strongly support their classification as disorders of ribosome biosynthesis. Other disorders have been postulated to involve defects in ribosome assembly and or function—cartilage hair hypoplasia, Shwachman Diamond syndrome[36]—a new nosology of human disease is emerging.

DBA as a disorder of variable penetrance and expressivity provides a model for influence of non-mutated genes and the environment on the clinical phenotype of dominantly inherited disorders. The investigation of this variable penetrance and expressivity of both hematologic and nonhematologic phenotypes will be facilitated by the use of gene array hybridization technology.[31]

A number of laboratories are using patient databases for DBA gene discovery; the complete genotyping awaits the discovery of the majority of the remaining DBA genes. Ultimately, the availability of a genetically based DBA diagnosis in the remaining 75% of patients not mutated at *RPS19* will

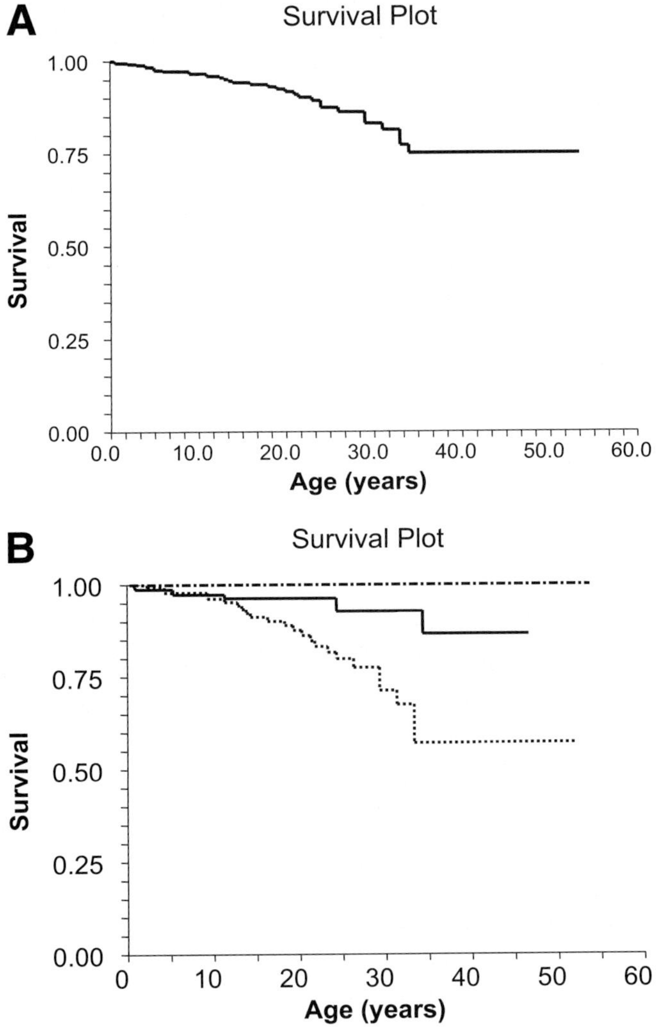

Figure 4 Kaplan-Meier analysis of survival in DBA patients. (A) Overall survival and (B) survival by treatment response; survival of patients in sustained remission (▪-▪-▪) are shown, along with survival of patients maintainable on corticosteroids (—) and survival of transfusion-dependent patients (▪▪▪▪). There is a trend to increased survival in sustained remitters as compared to cortico-steroid-maintainable DBA patients (P = .08). There is a statistically significant increase in survival among steroid-maintainable patients as compared to transfusion-dependent patients (P = .007). Reprinted with permission from Lipton et al.[40]

allow the diagnosis of previously undetectable mild phenotypes, facilitating reproductive choices, SCT donor selection,[77,78] and perhaps cancer screening strategies. The patient substrate provided by these registries will also allow for genotype-phenotype correlations that will be scientifically interesting and also suggest treatment and surveillance strategies. Within a few years, an accurate cancer risk assessment will be available and perhaps a cancer genotype will emerge. Registries have provided a clearer understanding of the epidemiology of DBA. Treatment options are already being modified based on new information regarding the natural history of DBA. Prolonged use of corticosteroids, starting in infancy, has been curtailed as a result. Packed red cell transfusions, rather than corticosteroids, are now used to avoid corticosteroid-related growth retardation, developmental delay, pathologic fractures, cataracts, and other toxicities. Analyses of outcomes reveal that the vast majority of patients succumb to complications that may be avoidable. There are extremely poor results with alternative donor hematopoietic stem cell transplantation. A greater than expected incidence of remission and a lower than expected incidence of aplastic anemia, MDS, and hematopoietic malignancy strongly support restraint in the use of high-risk therapies. In contrast, allogeneic matched sibling SCT appears to have an acceptable outcome, justifying its use as frontline therapy. In such a rare disease as DBA, controlled SCT clinical trials are virtually impossible to perform. Thus, emerging therapies such as SCT using reduced-intensity conditioning regimens in high-risk DBA patients must be captured by the registries to provide a reasonable evaluation of efficacy. As data mature, the predisposition to nonhematopoietic malignancy in the context of SCT will also become known. The availability of tumor specimens, obtained from well-characterized patients, will allow for an investigation of the molecular biology of tumorigenesis in DBA. The recognition of nonclassical occult phenotypes strongly suggests that patients with characteristic birth defects, certain cancers, or unexplained macrocytosis may have DBA. Clarification of these issues is critical with regard to patient follow-up, genetic counseling, and reproductive strategies. With the cloning of at least one DBA gene, preliminary work for gene therapy trials is being planned. The study of DBA, since its first description 70 years ago, has yielded extraordinary opportunities to understand the biology of hematopoiesis, oncogenesis, and morphogenesis. Significant improvements in patient care have emerged and should continue with a greater knowledge of disease mechanism.[74]

Acknowledgment

The progress described in this review is testament to the commitment of the patients with DBA, their families, clinicians who care for the patients, and the dedicated scientists, clinical and laboratory-based, with whom I have the privilege to work. The author would also like to thank Adrianna Vlachos, MD, Johnson Liu, MD, Hanna Gazda, MD, and Eva Atsidaftos, MA, for their invaluable advice and assistance.

References

1. Young NS, Alter BP: Inherited bone marrow failure syndromes: Introduction, in Aplastic Anemia Acquired and Inherited. Philadelphia, PA, Saunders, 1994, pp 271-274
2. Gripp KW, McDonald-McGinn DM, La Rossa D, McGain D, Federman N, Vlachos A, et al: Bilateral microtia and cleft palate in cousins with Diamond-Blackfan anemia. Am J Med Genet 101:268-274, 2001
3. Lipton JM, Federman N, Khabbaze Y, Schwartz CL, Hilliard LM, Clark JI, et al: Osteogenic sarcoma associated with Diamond-Blackfan anemia: A report from the Diamond-Blackfan Anemia Registry. J Pediatr Hematol Oncol 23:39-44, 2001
4. Josephs HW: Anemia of infancy and early childhood. Medicine 15:307-451, 1936
5. Diamond LK, Blackfan KD: Hypoplastic anemia. Am J Dis Child 56: 464-467, 1938
6. Diamond LK, Wang WC, Alter BP: Congenital hypoplastic anemia. Adv Pediatr 22:349-378, 1976
7. Vlachos A, Klein GW, Lipton JM: The Diamond Blackfan Anemia Registry: Tool for investigating the epidemiology and biology of Diamond-Blackfan anemia. J Pediatr Hematol Oncol 23:377-382, 2001
8. Gustavsson P, Willig TN, van Haeringen A, Tchernia G, Dianzani I, Donner M, et al: Diamond-Blackfan anaemia: Genetic homogeneity for a gene on chromosome 19q13 restricted to 1.8 Mb. Nat Genet 16:368-371, 1997
9. Draptchinskaia N, Gustavsson P, Andersson B, Pettersson M, Willig TN, Dianzani I, et al: The ribosomal protein S19 gene is mutated in Diamond-Blackfan anemia. Nat Genet 21:169-175, 1999
10. Orfali KA, Ohene-Abuakwa Y, Ball SE: Diamond Blackfan anaemia in the UK: Clinical and genetic heterogeneity. Br J Haematol 125: 243-252, 2004
11. Willig TN, Niemeyer CM, Leblanc T, Tiemann C, Robert A, Budde J, et al: Identification of new prognosis factors from the clinical and epidemiologic analysis of a registry of 229 Diamond-Blackfan anemia patients. Pediatr Res 46:553-561, 1999
12. Campagnoli MF, Garelli E, Quarello P, Carando P, Varotto S, Nobili B, et al: Molecular basis of Diamond-Blackfan anemia: New findings from the Italian registry and a review of the literature. Haematologica 89: 480-489, 2004
13. Ohga S, Mugishima H, Ohara A, Kojima S, Fujisawa K, Yagi K, et al: Diamond-Blackfan anemia in Japan: Clinical outcomes of prednisolone therapy and hematopoietic stem cell transplantation. Int J Hematol 79:22-30, 2004
14. Vlachos A, Ball S, Dahl N, Alter BP, Sheth S, Ramenghi U, et al: Diagnosing and treating Diamond Blackfan anemia: Results of an international consensus conference. (in preparation)
15. Hoffman R, Zanjani ED, Vila J, Zalusky R, Lutton JD, Wasserman LR: Diamond-Blackfan syndrome: Lymphocyte-mediated suppression of erythropoiesis. Science 193:899-900, 1976
16. Ershler WB, Ross J, Finlay JL, Shahidi NT: Bone-marrow microenvironment defect in congenital hypoplastic anemia. N Engl J Med 302: 1321-1327, 1980
17. Ortega JA, Shore NA, Dukes PP, Hammond D: Congenital hypoplastic anemia inhibition of erythropoiesis by sera from patients with congenital hypoplastic anemia. Blood 45:83-89, 1975
18. Sawada K-I, Koyanagawa Y, Sakurama S, Nakagawa S, Konno T: Diamond-Blackfan syndrome: A possible role of cellular factors for erythropoietic suppression. Scand J Haematol 35:158-165, 1985
19. Lipton JM, Kudisch M, Gross R, Nathan DG: Defective erythroid progenitor differentiation system in congenital hypoplastic (Diamond-Blackfan) anemia. Blood 67:962-968, 1986
20. Tsai P, Arkin S, Lipton JM: An intrinsic progenitor defect in Diamond-Blackfan anemia. Br J Haematol 73:112-120, 1989
21. Perdahl EB, Naprstek BL, Wallace WC, Lipton JM: Erythroid failure in Diamond-Blackfan anemia is characterized by apoptosis. Blood 83: 645-650, 1994
22. Ohene-Abuakwa Y, Orfali KA, Marius C, Ball SE: Two-phase culture in Diamond Blackfan anemia: Localization of erythroid defect. Blood 105: 838-846, 2005
23. Cmejla R, Blafkova J, Stopka T, et al: Ribosomal protein S19 gene

mutations in patients with Diamond-Blackfan anemia and identification of ribosomal protein S19 pseudogenes. Blood Cells Mol Dis 26:124-132, 2000
24. Leger-Silvistre I, Caffrey JM, Dawaliby , et al: Specific role for yeast homologs of Diamond Blackfan anemia-associated Rps19 protein in ribosome synthesis. J Biol Chem 280:38177-38185, 2005
25. Yamamoto T: Molecular mechanism of monocyte predominant infiltration in chronic inflammation: Mediation by a novel monocyte chemotactic factor, S19 ribosomal protein dimer. Pathol Int 50:863-871, 2000
26. Maeda N, Toku S, Kenmochi N, Tanaka T: A novel nucleolar protein interacts with ribosomal protein S19. Biochem Biophys Res Commun 339:41-46, 2006
27. Soulet F, Saati TA, Roga S, Amalric F, Bouche G: Fibroblast growth factor-2 interacts with free ribosomal protein S19. Biochem Biophys Res Commun 289:591-596, 2001
28. Chiocchetti A, Gibello L, Carando A, Aspesi A, Secco P, Garelli E, et al: Interactions between RPS19, mutated in Diamond-Blackfan anemia, and the PIM-1 oncoprotein. Haematologica 90:1453-1462, 2005
29. Gazda HT, Zhong R, Long L, Niewiadomska E, Lipton JM, Plosynksa A, et al: RNA and protein evidence for haplo-insufficiency in Diamond-Blackfan anaemia patients with RPS19 mutations. Br J Haematol 127: 105-113, 2004
30. Flygare J, Kiefer T, Miyake K, Utsugisawa T, Hamaguchi I, DaCosta L, et al: Deficiency of ribosomal protein S19 in CD34+ cells generated by siRNA blocks erythroid development and mimics defects seen in Diamond-Blackfan anemia. Blood 105:4627-4634, 2005
31. Ebert BL, Lee MM, Pretz JL, Subramanian A, Mak R, Golub TR, et al: An RNA interference model of RPS19 deficiency in Diamond-Blackfan anemia recapitulates defective hematopoiesis and rescue by dexamethasone: Identification of dexamethasone-responsive genes by microarray. Blood 105:4620-4626, 2005
32. Çeliker MY, Arkin S, Çeliker I, Atsidaftos E, Lipton JM, et al: The role RPS-19 in differentiation and survival of UT-7/Epo cells: A potential in vitro model for erythropoiesis. J Pediatr Hematol Oncol 42:513, 2004 (abstr)
33. Hamaguchi I, Ooka A, Brun A, Richter J, Dahl N, Karlsson S: Gene transfer improves erythroid development in ribosomal protein S19-deficient Diamond-Blackfan anemia. Blood 100:2724-2731, 2002
34. Mattson H, Davey EJ, Fröjmark AS, Miyake K, Utsugisawa T, Flygare J, et al: Erythropoiesis in the *Rps19* disrupted mouse: Analysis of erythropoietin response and biochemical markers for Diamond-Blackfan anemia. Blood Cells Mol Dis (in press)
35. Ellis SR, Massey AT: Diamond Blackfan anemia: A paradigm for a ribosome-based disease. Med Hypotheses 66:643-648, 2006
36. Liu JM, Ellis SR: Ribosomes and marrow failure: Coincidental association or molecular paradigm. Blood First Edition Paper, January 28, 2006. DOI 10.1182/blood-2005-12-4831
37. Teber OA, Gillessen-Kaesbach G, Fischer S, Böhringer S, Albrecht B, Albert A, et al: Genotyping in 46 patients with tentative diagnosis of Treacher Collins syndrome revealed unexpected phenotypic variation. Eur J Hum Genet 12:879-890, 2004
38. Fazen LE, Elmore J, Nadler HL: Mandibulo-facial dysostosis (Treacher-Collins syndrome). Am J Dis Child 113:405-410, 1967
39. Lipton JM, Alter BP: Diamond Blackfan anemia, in Feig SA, Freedman MH (eds): Clinical Disorders and Experimental Models of Erythropoietic Failure. Boca Raton, FL, CRC Press, 1993, pp 39-67
40. Lipton JM, Atsidaftos E, Zyskind I, Vlachos A: Improving clinical care and elucidating the pathophysiology of Diamond Blackfan anemia: an update from the Diamond Blackfan Anemia Registry. Pediatr Blood Cancer (in press)
41. Wise CA, Chiang LC, Paznekas WA, Sharma M, Musy MM, Ashley JA, et al: *TCOF1* gene encodes a putative phosphoprotein that exhibits mutations in Treacher Collins syndrome throughout its coding region. Proc Natl Acad Sci U S A 94:3110-3115, 1997
42. Vlachos A, Klein GW, Avarello JT, Rivera RD, Atsidaftos E, Gripp KW, et al: Diamond Blackfan anemia (DBA) and associated orofacial clefts (OFC): A Diamond Blackfan Anemia Registry (DBAR) analysis. J Pediatr Hematol Oncol 24:1426, 2002 (abstr)
43. So RB, Gonzales B, Henning D, Dixon J, Dixon MJ, Valdez BC: Another face of the Treacher Collins syndrome (*TCOF1*) gene: Identification of additional exons. Gene 328:49-57, 2004
44. Dixon J, Edwards SJ, Anderson I, Brass A, Scambler PJ, Dixon MJ: Identification of the complete coding sequence and genomic organization of the Treacher Collins syndrome gene. Genome Res 7:223-234, 1997
45. Dixon MJ: Treacher Collins syndrome. Hum Mol Genet 5:1391-1396, 1997
46. Valdez BC, Henning D, So RB, Dixon J, Dixon MJ: The Treacher Collins syndrome (*TCOF1*) gene product is involved in ribosomal DNA gene transcription by interacting with upstream binding factor. Proc Natl Acad Sci U S A 101:10709-10714, 2004
47. Gonzales B, Henning D, So RB, Dixon J, Valdez BC: The Treacher Collins syndrome (*TCOF1*) gene product is involved in pre-rRNA methylation. Hum Mol Genet 14:2035-2043, 2005
48. Dixon J, Brakebush C, Fässler R, Dixon MJ: Increased levels of apoptosis in the prefusion neural folds underlie the craniofacial, Treacher Collins syndrome. Hum Mol Genet 9:1473-1480, 2000
49. D'Andrea AD, Grompe M: The Fanconi anaemia/BRCA pathway. Nat Rev Cancer 3:23-34, 2003
50. Marrone A, Dokal I: Dyskeratosis congenita: Molecular insights into telomerase function, ageing and cancer. Expert Rev Mol Med 6:1-23, 2004
51. Gazda H, Lipton JM, Willig TN, Ball S, Niemeyer CM, Tchernia G, et al: Evidence for linkage of familial Diamond-Blackfan anemia to chromosome 8p23.3-p22 and for non-19q non-8p disease. Blood 97:2145-2150, 2001
52. Balaban EP, Buchanan GR, Graham M, Frenkel EP: Diamond-Blackfan syndrome in adult patients. Am J Med 78:533-538, 1985
53. Dessypris EN, Kranz SB, Roloff JS, Lukens JN: Mode of action of the IgG inhibitor of erythropoiesis in transient erythroblastopenia of childhood. Blood 59:114-123, 1982
54. Glader BE, Backer K, Diamond LK: Elevated erythrocyte adenosine deaminase activity in congenital hypoplastic anemia. N Engl J Med 309:1486-1490, 1983
55. Glader BE: Personal communication, January 2006.
56. Cathie IAB: Erythrogenesis imperfecta. Arch Dis 25:313-324, 1950
57. Aase JM, Smith D: Congenital anemia and triphalangeal thumbs: A new syndrome. J Pediatr 74:471-472, 1969
58. Alter BP: Thumbs and anemia. Pediatr 62:613-614, 1978
59. Hasan R, Inoue S: Diamond-Blackfan anemia associated with Treacher-Collins syndrome. J Pediatr Hematol Oncol 10:261-265, 1993
60. Zyskind I, Atsidaftos E, Vlachos A, Lipton JM: Search for macrocytosis as a marker of an inherited bone marrow failure syndrome (IBMFS) in congenital heart disease and cleft palate: A provocative first look. J Pediatr Hematol Oncol 42:542, 2004 (abstr)
61. Janov AJ, Leong T, Nathan DG, Guinan EC: Diamond-Blackfan anemia. Natural history and sequelae of treatment. Medicine (Baltimore) 75:77-78, 1996
62. Rosenberg PS, Greene MH, Alter BP: Cancer incidence in persons with Fanconi anemia. Blood 101:822-826, 2003
63. Rosenberg PS, Alter BP, Bolyard AA, Bonilla MA, Boxer LA, Cham B, et al: The incidence of leukemia and mortality from sepsis in patients with severe congenital neutropenia receiving long-term G-CSF therapy. Blood 106:669, 2005 (abstr)
64. Lensch MW, Rathbun RK, Olson SB, Jones GR, Bagby GC Jr: Selective pressure as an essential force in molecular evolution of myeloid leukemia clones: A view from the window of Fanconi anemia. Leukemia 13:1784-1789, 1999
65. Lipton JM: Inherited childhood bone marrow failure syndromes. From the clinic to the laboratory and back again, in Fischer EP, Klose S (eds): The Diagnostic Challenge. Knowledge for Health. Munchen, Germany, Piper, 1998, pp 39-87
66. Amsterdam A, Sadler KC, Lai K, Farrington S, Bronson RT, Lees JA, et al: Many ribosomal protein genes are cancer genes in zebrafish. Plos Biol 2:690-698, 2004
67. Gasser C: Aplastische anämie (cronische erythroblastophthise) und cortison. Schhhweiz Med Wochenschr 81:1241-1242, 1951

68. Olivieri NF, Brittenham GM: Iron-chelating therapy and the treatment of thalassemia. Blood 89:739-761, 1997
69. Nisbet-Brown E, Olivieri NF, Giardina PJ, Grady RW, Neufeld EJ, Sechaud R, et al: Effectiveness and safety of ICL670 in iron-loaded patients with thalassaemia: A randomised, double-blind, placebo-controlled, dose-escalation trial. Lancet 361:1597-1602, 2003
70. Alter BP, Kumar M, Lockhart LL, Sprinz PG, Rowe TF: Pregnancy in bone marrow failure syndromes: Diamond-Blackfan anaemia and Shwachman-Diamond syndrome. Br J Haematol 107:49-54, 1999
71. Vlachos A, Federman N, Reyes-Haley C, Abramson, J, Lipton, JM: Hematopoietic stem cell transplantation for Diamond Blackfan anemia: A report from the Diamond Blackfan Anemia Registry. Bone Marrow Transplant 27:381-386, 2001
72. Vlachos A, Atsidaftos E, Lipton JM: Matched related vs alternative donor stem cell transplantation (SCT) for Diamond Blackfan anemia: A report of the Diamond Blackfan Anemia Registry. Blood 106:2063, 2005 (abstr)
73. Roy V, Perez WS, Eapen M, Marsh JC, Pasquini M, Mustafa MM, et al: Bone marrow transplantation for Diamond-Blackfan anemia. Biol Blood Marrow Transplant 11:600-608, 2005
74. Alter BP: Bone marrow transplant in Diamond-Blackfan anemia. Bone Marrow Transplant 21:965-966, 1998 (letter)
75. Kuliev A, Rechitsky S, Tur-Kaspa I, Verlinsky Y: Preimplantation genetics. Improving access to stem cell therapy. Ann NY Acad Sci 1054: 223-227, 2005
76. Wagner JE, Kahn JP, Wolf SM, Lipton, JM: Preimplantation testing to produce an HLA-matched donor infant JAMA 292:803-804, 2004 (letter)
77. Orfali RF, Wynn RF, Stevens R, Chopra R, Ball SE: Failure of red cell production following allogenic BMT for Diamond Blackfan anaemia (DBA) illustrates functional significance of high erythrocyte adenosine deaminase (eADA) activity in the donor. Blood 94:41832, 1999 (abstr)
78. Wynn RF, Grainger JD, Carr TF, Eden OB, Stevens RF, Will AM: Failure of allogeneic bone marrow transplantation to correct Diamond-Blackfan anemia despite haemopoietic stem cell engraftment. Bone Marrow Transplant 24:803-805, 1999
79. Matsson H, Klar J, Draptchinskaia N, Gustavsson P, Carlsson B, Bowers D, et al: Truncating ribosomal protein S19 and variable clinical expression in Diamond-Blackfan anemia. Hum Genet 105:496-500, 1999
80. Ramenghi U, Campagnoli MF, Garelli E, Carando A, Brusco A, Bagnara GP, et al: Diamond-Blackfan anemia: Report of seven mutations in the RPS19 gene and evidence of mutation heterogeneity in the Italian population. Blood Cells Mol Dis 26:417-422, 2000
81. Proust A, Da Costa L, Rince P, Landois A, Tamary H, Zaizov R, et al: SHIP Working Group on DBA: Ten novel Diamond-Blackfan anemia mutations and three polymorphisms within the rps19 gene. Hematol J 4:132-136, 2003
82. Orfali KA, Ohene-Abuakwa Y, Ball SE: Diamond Blackfan anemia in the UK: Clinical and genetic heterogeneity. Br J Haematol 125:243-252, 2004

ELSEVIER

Seminars in HEMATOLOGY

Shwachman-Diamond Syndrome

Akiko Shimamura

Shwachman-Diamond syndrome (SDS) is an autosomal recessive marrow failure syndrome associated with exocrine pancreatic insufficiency and leukemia predisposition. Bone marrow failure typically manifests with neutropenia, but anemia, thrombocytopenia, or aplastic anemia may also develop. Additional organ systems, such as liver or bone, may also be affected. Clonal cytogenetic abnormalities, particularly those involving chromosome 7 such as monosomy 7 or isochromosome 7, may develop. Mutations in the *SBDS* gene are found in approximately 90% of patients meeting clinical diagnostic criteria. *SBDS* is a highly conserved gene of unknown function. Studies of the yeast orthologue YLR022c and structurally related proteins suggest a role in RNA metabolism. In human cells, the SBDS protein localizes to both the cytoplasm and the nucleus, and shuttles in and out of the nucleolus in a cell cycle-dependent manner. A discussion of diagnostic workup, medical management, and treatment is presented.
Semin Hematol 43:178-188

A cohort of pediatric patients with hypoproductive hematologic cytopenias and exocrine pancreatic insufficiency was first described in 1964 by Shwachman, Diamond, and colleagues[1] and shortly thereafter by Bodian et al.[2] This disorder, subsequently known as Shwachman-Diamond syndrome (SDS), is an autosomal recessive disease associated with leukemia predisposition. Additional features, such as short stature and liver and skeletal abnormalities, may also be present. The recent discovery of the gene mutated in the majority of patients with SDS has revealed new insights into the molecular pathogenesis of this disorder. This review will describe the clinical features of SDS, discuss recent molecular studies, and explore issues surrounding clinical management and treatment.

Genetics

Approximately 90% of patients meeting clinical criteria for the diagnosis of SDS harbor mutations in the *SBDS* gene (Shwachman-Bodian-Diamond syndrome). *SBDS* maps to the 7q11 centromeric region of chromosome 7.[3,4] The carrier frequency has been estimated at 1/110.[3] The gene consists of five exons encompassing 7.9 kb. A highly conserved pseudogene with 97% transcript identity to *SBDS* is located 5.8 mB distally on chromosome 7.[4] This pseudogene is transcribed, but its corresponding mRNA contains deletions and point mutations that preclude proper protein translation. Gene conversion mutations between the *SBDS* gene and the adjacent pseudogene account for 89% of *SBDS* mutations, with 60% of patients containing two converted alleles. The most common mutation arising from gene conversion, 258+2T→C, results in a donor splice-site mutation in the second intron predicted to result in a frameshift mutation with premature protein truncation. Another common gene mutation, 183-184TA→CT, is also found in the pseudogene and introduces a premature stop codon (K62X). The majority of mutations studied to date result in marked reduction of SBDS protein expression.[5,6] So far, no patient carrying two truncating deletion or nonsense mutations has been identified.[4,5,7,8] It has been postulated that, as observed in yeast,[9] complete abrogation of SBDS protein expression might be lethal. In this case, the IVS2 splice-site mutation may still allow a small level of correct splicing to occur, and missense mutations might represent hypomorphic alleles.[6,10] *SBDS* encodes a unique protein of unknown function, further discussed below.

Clinical Presentation

In addition to case reports, several large cohort studies[11-15] have summarized the clinical features associated with SDS. With the advent of genetic testing, our understanding of the clinical phenotype of SDS may be subject to future revision.

Department of Hematology, Children's Hospital Boston, Boston, MA.
Address correspondence to Akiko Shimamura, MD, PhD, Children's Hospital Boston, Department of Hematology, Karp Research Laboratories, Room 08214, 300 Longwood Ave, Boston, MA 02115. E-mail: akiko.shimamura@childrens.harvard.edu

 0037-1963/06/$-see front matter
doi:10.1053/j.seminhematol.2006.04.006

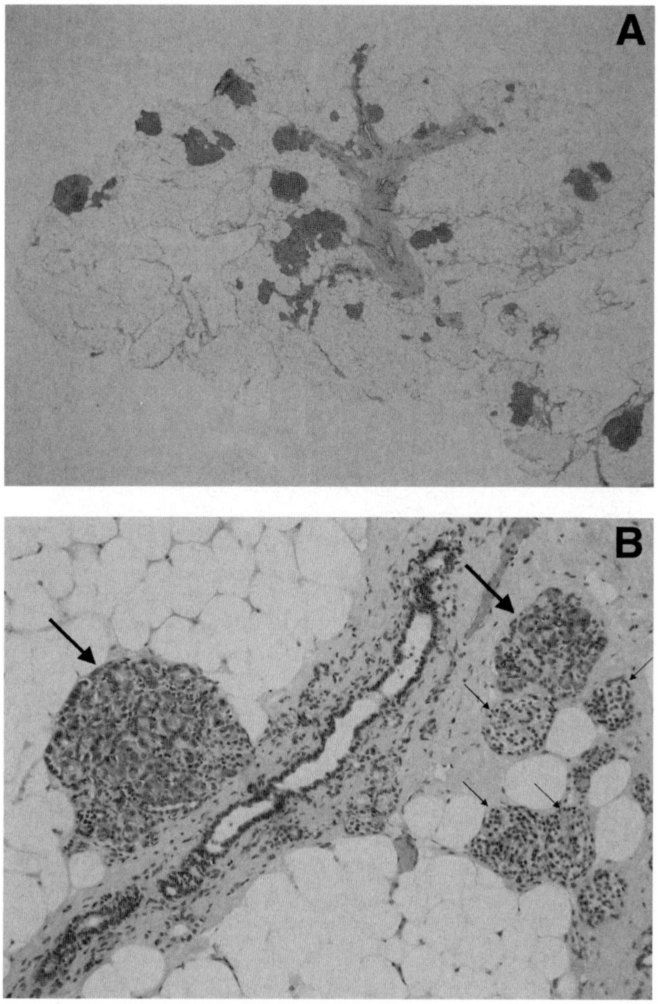

Figure 1 A pancreatic duct is shown (center). Pancreas histology in SDS. (A) Pancreatic biopsy in a 6-year-old boy with SDS shows extensive replacement of the exocrine pancreas by adipose tissue with remaining small islands of parenchyma. (B) Extensive fat surrounding acini (large arrows) with poorly granulated exocrine cells and naked islets (small arrows). Figure courtesy of Dr Harry Kozakewich, Department of Pathology, Children's Hospital, Boston, MA.

Gastrointestinal Features

Pancreas

Patients with SDS classically present in early infancy with steatorrhea and failure to thrive. Levels of fat-soluble vitamins (A, D, E, and K) may be diminished. Pathologic examination reveals fatty replacement of the pancreatic tissue with few pancreatic acini, and relative sparing of the pancreatic ducts and pancreatic islets (Fig 1). The ducts appear of normal caliber without mucous distention. Pancreatic islets of Langerhans appear normal and their function is generally intact as evidenced by normal glucose tolerance tests, although a few cases of insulin-dependent diabetes mellitus have been reported in patients with SDS.[11] Sweat chloride testing is normal. Exocrine pancreatic function may improve with increasing patient age, and overt clinical symptoms may be absent. While fat maldigestion was commonly documented in patients below the age of 2 years, symptoms may resolve in about 50% of older patients.[12,14] Of note, only a small fraction of exocrine pancreatic function (between 2% to 10%) is sufficient to render the patient functionally replete with respect to clinical symptoms.[14] The mechanisms underlying improvement in fat absorption remain unknown.

Exocrine pancreatic insufficiency has been demonstrated through pancreatic stimulation testing, showing low pancreatic enzyme secretion in response to stimulation testing. Increased fecal fat excretion in the absence of intestinal pathology or cholestatic liver disease may be seen. Imaging studies with ultrasound or computed tomography (Fig 2) typically reveal fatty replacement of pancreatic tissue.

The serum enzymes trypsinogen and isoamylase are useful markers for exocrine pancreatic insufficiency in patients with SDS.[16] In normal control subjects, serum trypsinogen showed little variation with age; in patients with SDS below the age of 3 years, serum trypsinogen values were low. Serum trypsinogen was less useful in patients over age 3, since trypsinogen levels increased to normal levels in a subset of SDS patients. Serum isoamylase levels remain low in SDS patients at all ages, with the oldest patient in the reported series being older than 30 years; however, the utility of this test below the age of 3 is limited by the low isoamylase levels found in normal control subjects in this lower age range. Thus, for patients over the age of 3 with normal serum trypsinogen levels, isoamylase measurements are useful.

Liver

Hepatomegaly with elevated liver transaminases typically ranging from two- to threefold higher than the normal range[12] is often seen in young patients with SDS. Histologic abnormalities reported on liver biopsies of 13 patients included microvesicular and macrovesicular steatosis, periportal and portal inflammation, bridging fibrosis, and glycogenosis, in most but not all patients.[2,11,12,15,17] Elevated liver enzymes were most common in patients less than 2 years of age and typically normalized with age.[12,14,18]

Hematologic Features

Neutropenia, typically defined as a neutrophil count less than $1{,}500 \times 10^9$/L, is the most common manifestation of bone marrow failure in SDS and is found in 88% to 100% of patients. Neutropenia is intermittent in about two thirds of all patients, chronic in the remaining one third. Neutrophil counts may range from normal to severely depressed. The total white blood cell count may also be depressed. Although two case reports[17,19] mentioned cyclic neutropenia in three patients with SDS, no data or discussion of the periodicity of the neutropenia were available, leaving it unclear whether the neutrophil counts followed the regular rhythmic cycling pattern currently associated with typical cyclic neutropenia.

In addition to decreased neutrophil numbers, neutrophil chemotaxis is decreased in vitro.[20] Improvement in neutrophil mobility in response to lithium has been reported.[21] Although general neutrophil motility appears to be intact, a diminished ability of neutrophils from SDS patients to orient towards a gradient of N-formyl-methionyl-leucyl-phenylalanine (fMLP) has been described.[22] Aberrant concanavalin A distribution on the neutrophil surfaces of SDS patients has been noted.[23] The

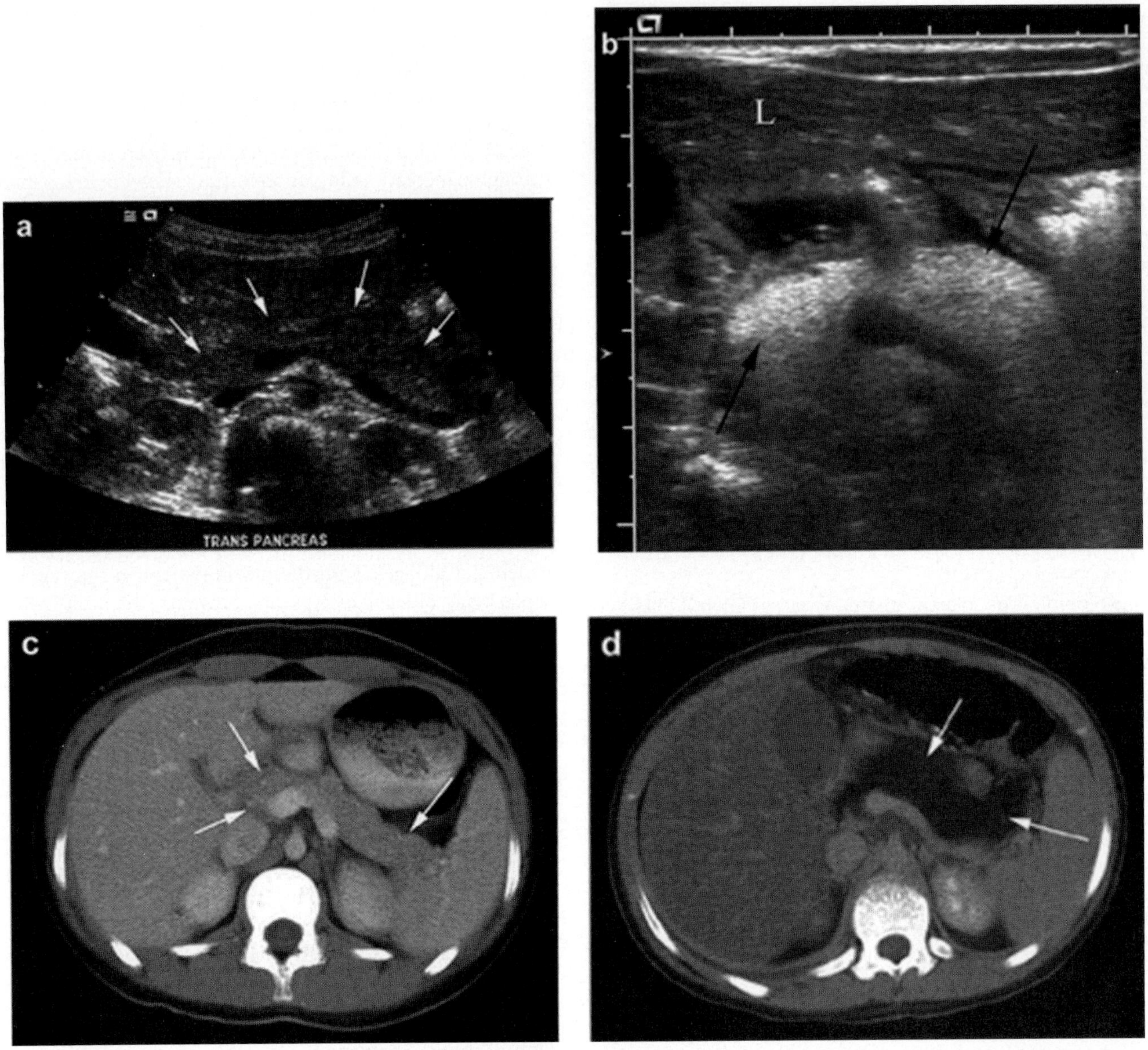

Figure 2 Pancreatic imaging in SDS. (A) Normal pancreas in a 7-year-old girl. A transverse sonogram of the upper abdomen shows the normal pancreas (arrows), which is isoechoic to liver. (B) SDS in a 3-year-old boy. Transverse sonogram of the upper abdomen reveals an enlarged, diffusely echogenic pancreas (arrows) due to fatty infiltration. Note normal adjacent liver (L). (C) Normal pancreas in a 16-year-old girl. A transverse computed tomography image demonstrates a normal pancreas. The density of the pancreas (arrows) is similar to liver. (D) SDS in a 5-year-old boy. Transverse contrast-enhanced computed tomography image shows diffuse fatty infiltration of the pancreas (arrowheads). Similar computed tomography findings can be seen with cystic fibrosis. Reproduced with kind permission of Springer Science and Business Media. From: Nijs E, Callahan MJ, Taylor GA: Disorders of the pediatric pancreas: Imaging features. Pediatr Radiol 35:358-373, 2005.

clinical significance of these chemotactic defects with respect to infection risk remains to be ascertained. One study described similar chemotactic defects in neutrophils from parents of SDS patients,[20] but no increased infection risk has been described in carriers of this disease. In contrast to the clinical presentation of some other leukocyte chemotaxis disorders, neutrophil recruitment into abscesses or empyemas occurs in patients with SDS.[24]

Additional cytopenias may also be present. Anemia has been reported in 42% to 66% of patients. The reticulocyte count is typically not elevated. Red blood cells may be normocytic or macrocytic. Elevation in hemoglobin F levels, a common feature of many of the inherited marrow failure syndromes, is often present. Thrombocytopenia, typically defined as less than 150×10^9/L, occurs in 24% to 60% of patients. Fatal bleeding in the setting of thrombocytopenia has been reported.[25] Pancytopenia developed in 10% to 44% of patients in these series, with progression to aplastic anemia also reported[11,26]; in one case aplastic anemia at birth was the presentation of SDS.[27]

Although cytopenias are typically seen at an early age, they also may have a later onset. One patient presented with exocrine pancreatic insufficiency in infancy, short stature, and metaphyseal dysostosis, and was monitored with serial complete blood cell count evaluations; he did not develop cytopenias until the age of 10 and subsequently M0 acute myeloid leukemia (AML) was diagnosed at age 23.[28] There is no relationship between severity of hematologic abnormalities and *SBDS* genotype recognized.[29]

There are no pathognomonic bone marrow features in SDS, and the bone marrow examination serves the primary function of excluding alternative diagnoses and monitoring for marrow aplasia and for the emergence of clonal disease. The bone marrow may be hypercellular, hypocellular, or normocellular; cellularity does not necessarily correlate with the degree of peripheral cytopenia. The marrow myeloid ratio may be normal, decreased, or increased; myeloid maturation arrest has also been reported. As seen in many other inherited marrow failure syndromes, marrow precursors may exhibit dysplastic features in all three hematopoietic lineages. Such baseline dysplasia must be carefully distinguished from myelodysplastic syndrome (MDS).

The development of aplastic anemia in patients with SDS suggests that the hematopoietic defect may reside at the level of an early hematopoietic stem cell. Bone marrow progenitor cultures show reduced numbers of both granulocyte-macrophage and erythroid progenitor colonies.[30,31] Increased Fas-mediated apoptosis has been described in marrow cells derived from SDS patients,[32] but it is unclear whether this apoptosis represents a primary pathogenic defect or a compensation to delete abnormal, possibly pre-leukemic cells. This distinction carries important clinical implications: the former would suggest that interventions designed to inhibit apoptosis might be therapeutic, whereas the latter would imply that inhibition of apoptosis might prove detrimental by allowing abnormal cells to propagate. As with other marrow failure states, leukocytes from patients with SDS contain abnormally short telomeres.[33] Whether this accelerated telomeric shortening represents a primary cellular defect or merely reflects the high proliferative rate of the few remaining stem cells is not known. An in vitro defect in marrow stromal cells has been described,[31] although no significant elevation in engraftment failure following hematopoietic stem cell transplant (HSCT) has been noted.

There is an increased frequency of clonal cytogenetic abnormalities in SDS, but estimates of the incidence of cytogenetic abnormalities in SDS patients are difficult to ascertain from a review of case reports. In a cohort study,[15] six of 88 patients developed clonal cytogenetic abnormalities. Five of 12 patients had clonal abnormalities in another study[13]; a third longitudinal prospective study of 14 patients with SDS with up to 5 years of follow-up (range, 0 to 5) found clonal marrow cytogenetic abnormalities consisting of i(7q) or del(20q) in four of 14 patients.[34] Abnormalities of chromosome 7, such as monosomy 7 or isochromosome 7q, are common: 44% of the cytogenetic abnormalities in SDS patients involved i(7q) in a recent review.[25] Other chromosome 7 abnormalities included monosomy 7, combined i(7q) and monosomy 7, and deletion or translocations involving 7q, and accounted for 33% of the reported cytogenetic abnormalities in these patients.[25] Del20(q12) was the next most common chromosomal abnormality reported in 16% of cases. These same cytogenetic abnormalities are found in MDS and leukemias in the general population.

Although clonal cytogenetic abnormalities are typical in MDS and AML associated with SDS, the clinical significance of many of these cytogenetic abnormalities, such as the isochromosome 7 or del(20q) clonal populations, arising in the absence of morphologic MDS is unclear. In Fanconi anemia, morphologic evidence of MDS may be a more important prognostic factor than are clonal cytogenetic abnormalities.[35] In a prospective study,[34] none of the patients with clonal cytogenetic abnormalities involving i(7q) or del(20q) developed symptomatic cytopenias or leukemias and there was no correlation between severity of peripheral cytopenia and the development of clonal abnormalities. Although activating *Ras* mutations may be associated with monosomy 7 and malignant transformation in patients with congenital neutropenia,[36] no associated mutations in *Ras* were noted in this patient cohort. p53 levels have been elevated in SDS bone marrow,[37] but no p53 mutations were found in association with the clonal cytogenetic abnormalities. In one patient, the cytogenetic clone was no longer detected after two years of follow-up. Patients with a persistent isochromosome 7q clone for 5 years[38] or 9 years[39] without evidence of progression to MDS have been reported. A second clone with del20q was also intermittently noted in one of these patients.[39] Clonal populations have been observed to fluctuate or even become undetectable over time in SDS patients.[34,40] No progression to AML has been reported among SDS patients presenting with i(7q) abnormalities.[25] In contrast, 42% of patients with other chromosome 7 abnormalities either presented with or progressed to advanced MDS or AML.[25] Four cases of monosomy 7 were observed among 26 patients with SDS followed in the Severe Chronic Neutropenia Registry (SCNIR), and transformation to AML was seen in two of these patients.[41] Three patients died, while one was alive 56 months after a matched unrelated donor bone marrow transplant. No evidence of cytogenetic abnormalities or leukemic transformation was observed in 11 additional SDS patients treated with granulocyte colony-stimulating factor (G-CSF) for 1 to 103 months.[41]

Current data suggest that chromosome 7 abnormalities may contribute to, but are not sufficient for, leukemic progression.[42] While monosomy 7 is a common cytogenetic abnormality in patients with other inherited bone marrow failure disorders, isochromosome 7q is a relatively uncommon finding in other marrow failure disorders or in AML, MDS, and acute lymphocytic leukemia (ALL) in general.[43] The molecular mechanisms leading to isochromosome formation are not clear. One hypothesis is that isochromosomes result from abnormal centromeric division, leading to transverse rather than longitudinal separation, together with a chromosomal recombination event.[43] Another possibility is that chromosomal translocation or unequal chromatid exchange might result in the formation of isochromosomes.[43] Isochromosome 7q involves the duplication of the q arm of chromosome 7 with corresponding loss of the 7p arm, thus effectively resulting in trisomy of 7q and monosomy of 7p. In contrast, chromosome 7 deletions associated with MDS and AML typically involve loss of regions of the 7q arm but maintenance of two copies of 7p. Monosomy 7 results in the retention of one copy of 7p and 7q. Thus, neither a tumor-suppressor model of loss of heterozygosity involving chromosome 7 nor a model invoking haploinsufficiency uniformly encompasses all three chromosome 7 abnormalities associated with leukemias, unless monosomy of either 7p or 7q could contribute to leukemic progression. Since i(7q) does not appear to associate with progression to MDS or AML, in contrast to the other chromosome 7 abnormalities, the molecular implications of these two categories of chromosome 7 abnormalities may require separate consideration. Chromosome 7 abnormalities might merely be markers for underlying chromosomal instability or acquired genotoxic stress. In such a model, chromosome 7 abnormalities might either confer a growth or survival advantage, or simply represent a chromosome whose loss is readily promoted or tolerated.

The role of acquired *SBDS* gene mutations in leukemogenesis in the general population remains to be fully addressed. One study of 77 AML patients did not find any associated *SBDS* mutations.[44] Whether *SBDS* mutations contribute to leukemogenesis in a specific subset of AML patients remains to be ascertained.

Malignancy

Fifty-five SDS patients in the French Severe Chronic Neutropenia Registry were followed prospectively for a median of 8 years (range, 0.3 to 35.6 years). Age at diagnosis ranged from birth to 23 years. Seven patients developed MDS or AML, with an estimated risk of 19% at 20 years and 36% at 30 years. Complex cytogenetic abnormalities were noted in all cases. i7q was noted in two cases and monosomy 7 in three. MDS and AML developed at an older age, with a median age at diagnosis of 19 years. In contrast, in severe congenital neutropenia, the median age for MDS/AML was almost 11 years. Only one patient from the MDS/AML group was still alive after having received a bone marrow transplant for MDS 4 years previously. Causes of death were disease-related in four cases and bone marrow transplant–related in two.

A recent review of the literature tabulated an additional 26 reported cases of leukemia in SDS patients.[25] There was a striking male predominance, with 23 male patients and two female patients, and one not specified. In 10 cases, antecedent MDS was observed prior to the development of AML. AML subtypes included AML-M0,[28] AML-M1,[45] AML-M4,[46-48] AML-M5,[49], and AML-M6.[50,51] AML-M6 was the most frequently noted subtype. ALL[52,53] and JMML[54] also have been reported.

MDS and leukemias typically presented with complex clonal cytogenetics, often involving abnormalities of chromosome 7. A similarity has been drawn between leukemias in SDS patients and those arising in patients who had received prior treatment with alkylating agents. Prognosis of leukemia in SDS is poor: 24 of 29 reported patients with AML died of refractory disease or treatment-related toxicity.[25,55] The remaining five patients were alive 2 to 4 years following treatment with chemotherapy or HSCT. One of the three patients with ALL was alive 1 year after diagnosis. The patient with JMML died of complications of treatment.

The mechanism underlying this tendency towards malignant transformation is unknown. Spontaneous chromosomal instability has been reported in two patients[56,57] but not in others.[58,59] We have not observed consistently elevated spontaneous chromosomal breakage in five patients tested (Lisa Moreau and Akiko Shimamura, unpublished observations).

The role of G-CSF in malignant myeloid transformation also is unclear. In theory, G-CSF might support the proliferation or survival of malignant clones to promote to leukemogenesis. Activating G-CSF receptor mutations have been associated with leukemic progression in severe congenital neutropenia (see Welte et al in this issue). In the absence of randomized clinical trials, it is difficult to separately evaluate the risk of G-CSF from the risks conferred by disease severity, since patients with the lowest neutrophil counts or highest infectious complications tend to have the highest G-CSF exposures. Thus, it is possible that the most severely affected patients are at the highest risk for AML and that G-CSF is merely a marker of disease severity. Alternatively, G-CSF may promote longer survival, allowing patients to live long enough to develop AML. To date, there is no direct evidence linking G-CSF to leukemic transformation in SDS patients.

Growth

Patients with SDS tend to be below the age-adjusted medians for the general population, with approximately half of patients exhibiting growth parameters below the third percentile.[15,60] Diminished growth was observed despite the prompt administration of pancreatic enzyme supplementation and likely represents an intrinsic growth defect. Growth velocity was lowest during the first 6 months of life and normalized thereafter to parallel normal growth curves.[60] The growth phenotype is variable, and patients with normal height and weight were also observed.[15,60]

Skeletal Abnormalities

Skeletal dysplasia is a variable feature described in association with SDS in a subset of patients. Metaphyseal dysostosis, most commonly of the femoral head, is frequently found[11] and was present in 46% of a total of 61 patients evaluated[15] (Fig 3); other affected sites include the knees, humeral heads, wrists, ankles, and vertebrae. The metaphyseal lesions typically are detected after the age of 1 year. Abnormally short ribs with flared anterior ends also have been reported. A recent study of 15 SDS patients (mean age, 9.7 years) with documented *SBDS* gene mutations found skeletal abnormalities in al[61]; there was no correlation between genotype and skeletal phenotype. Bone abnormalities included delayed secondary ossification, variable widening and irregularity of the metaphyses followed by thickening and irregularity of the growth plates, and generalized osteopenia. The epiphyseal

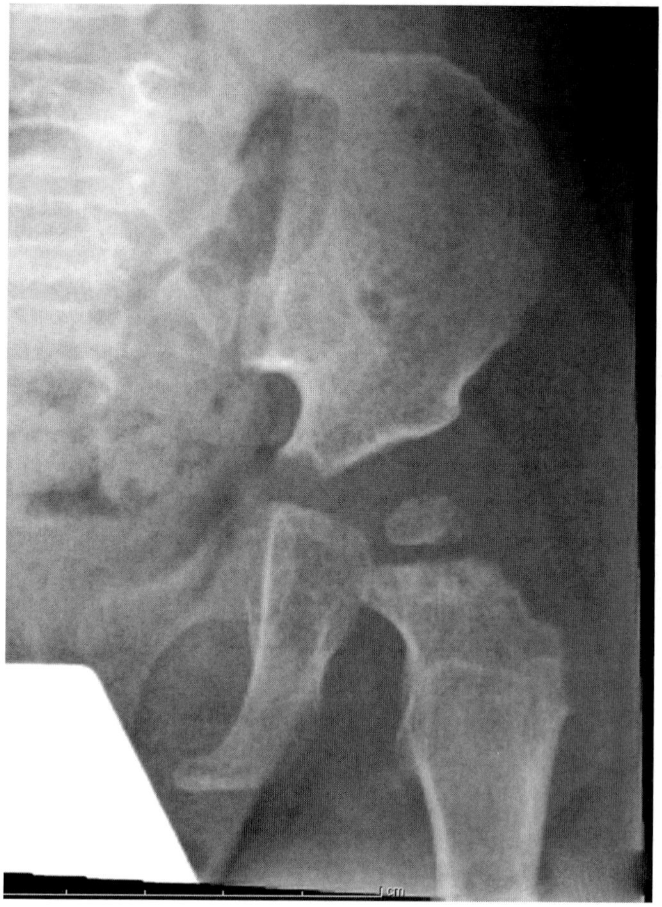

Figure 3 Metaphyseal dysostosis in a 13-month-old boy with SDS. Figure courtesy of D. George Taylor, Department of Radiology, Children's Hospital, Boston, MA.

maturation defects and metaphyseal changes tended to improve with age.

Infection

As for neutropenia in general, patients with SDS are susceptible to recurrent bacterial infections, particularly of the upper respiratory tract, oropharynx, and skin. A recent literature review[24] found that the most common infections reported in SDS patients were pneumonia (33%), recurrent otitis media (29%), and acquired skin infections and/or abscesses (15%). Additional infections included meningitis, osteomyelitis, and urinary tract infections. Bacterial causes of infection included gram-positive, gram-negative, and enteric organisms. Viral infections also occur, including cytomegalovirus, parvovirus, and measles. A literature review found no reports of fungal infections in SDS outside of HSCT.[24] Patients are at risk for life-threatening sepsis, and deaths from infection can occur.

Immune Abnormalities

In addition to neutropenia, defects in B-cell and T-cell function also have been observed: variable degrees of immunologic abnormalities, including low IgG or IgG subclasses, low numbers of circulating B cells, decreased in vitro B-lymphocyte proliferation, and lack of specific antibody production against both protein and polysaccharide antigens.[18,20,62,63] Whether this combination of hematological and immunologic abnormalities results from a defect in an early pluripotent hematopoietic stem cell giving rise to both lymphoid and myeloid lineages or from stromal defects affecting both cell lineages has not been established.[63]

Additional Features

Endocrine abnormalities in SDS include insulin-dependent diabetes,[11,60] growth hormone deficiency,[64] hypogonadotropic hypogonadism,[65] and hypothyroidism (Akiko Shimamura, unpublished observation). Cardiomyopathies have been noted in some cases.[19] Psychomotor delay of varying severity,[11,14,15] urinary tract anomalies, renal tubular acidosis, cleft palate, and dental abnormalities also occur.[11,15]

Molecular Pathogenesis

The *SBDS* gene is highly conserved throughout evolution.[4] It is widely expressed throughout human tissues at both the mRNA[4] and protein[6] levels. *SBDS* encodes a predicted protein of 28.8 kd, and lacks any recognizable functional domain. Endogenous SBDS was found to be localized to both the nucleus and the cytoplasm in human patient primary fibroblast cells, but shuttled in and out the nucleolus in a cell cycle–dependent fashion.[6] The significance of this nucleolar shuttling is currently unclear. One possibility is that SBDS functions in the nucleolus, which is a primary site of rRNA processing (see below); the nucleolus also contains many additional proteins,[66] so alternative functions are not excluded. The nucleolus also might serve as a site of SBDS sequestration, while its primary activity is in the nucleoplasm during S-phase.

Based on suggestive evidence in orthologues, Boocock et al proposed that the SBDS protein might function in RNA metabolism. Archael orthologues are found within operons for RNA-processing genes.[67] Orthologues in *Arabidopsis thaliana* and partial sequences from *Populus balsamifera* and *Gossypium arboreum* have extended carboxy-termini containing RNA-binding motifs.[4] Broad screening assays primarily in yeast suggest that SBDS might function in RNA metabolism. An analysis of the literature on SBDS orthologues revealed that the yeast orthologue clusters with genes involved in RNA processing by expression array analysis.[68] *Ylr022c*, the yeast orthologue of *SBDS* also known as *Sdo1*, scored positive in a screen of mutant yeast strains probed for rRNA biogenesis defects using microarrays to assess noncoding RNAs.[69] Spectral analysis to identify topologic features of protein-protein interactions also predicted that YLR022c might function in rRNA processing.[70]

Crystal structure analysis of the archaeal SBDS orthologue was reported by two groups[10,71] (Fig 4). The SBDS protein crystal structure revealed three domains. The amino terminus (domain I) forms a novel three-dimensional structure, which was subsequently named the FYSH domain (for Fungal, Yhr087wp, Shwachman) since this domain shares struc-

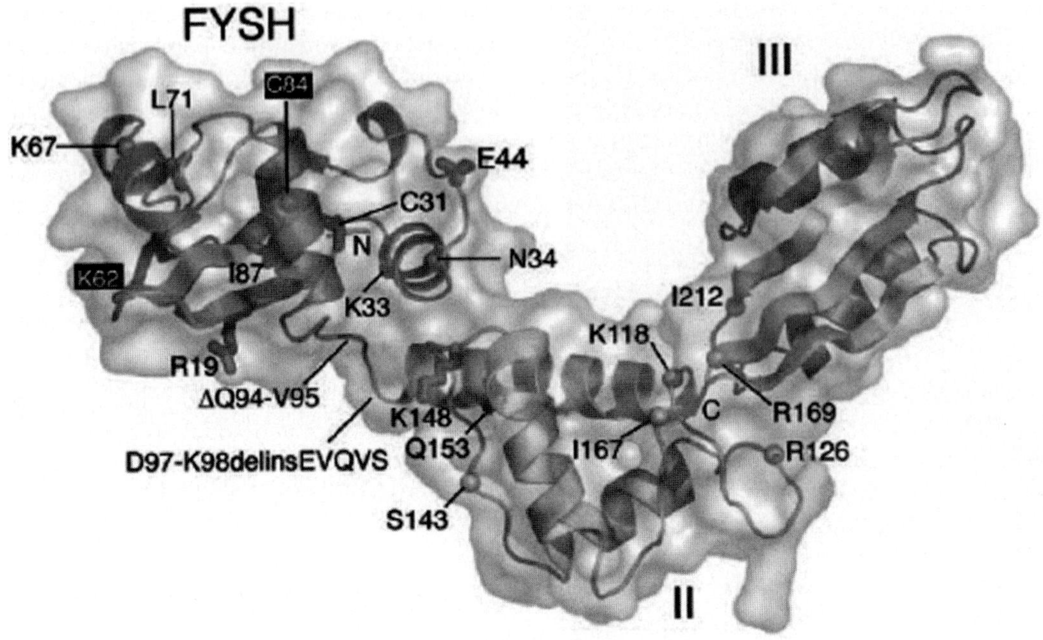

Figure 4 Crystal structure of the Archaeoglobus fulgidus SBDS protein orthologue. Ribbon representation of Archaeoglobus fulgidus AF0491 SBDS orthologue. Domains I (FYSH), II and III are indicated. The positions of disease-related mutations are indicated. Reproduced with permission from: Shammas C, Menne TF, Hilcenko C, Michell SR, Goyenechea B, Boocock GRB, et al: Structural and mutational analysis of the SBDS protein family. J Biol Chem 280:19221-19229, 2005.

tural homology to YHR087wp, a single-domain protein from *Saccharomyces cerevisiae* that belongs to a small protein family found in fungi.[10] The central domain (domain II) consists of a three-α helical structure with an intervening conserved proline-rich loop that appears structurally related to the C-terminal domain of *Escherichia coli* RuvA, a protein involved in Holliday junction recognition.[10] The C-terminal domain (domain III) consists of four antiparallel β-sheets with two α-helices against one side, forming a structure similar to a ferredoxin-like fold ($\beta\alpha\beta\beta\alpha\beta$). Although this type of motif is similar to that observed in some RNA-binding proteins, including hnRNPs (heterogeneous nuclear ribonucleoproteins) and snRNPs (small nuclear ribonucleoproteins),[10] this motif is not specific and its function cannot be easily inferred.[71]

TAP-tagged YLR022c was purified by tandem affinity chromatography and associated proteins identified by mass spectrometry included proteins linked to rRNA processing and components of the 60S ribosomal subunit. Since mutations in *YHR087W* are not lethal to yeast, these mutant strains were crossed with other strains carrying mutations in genes implicated in RNA metabolism. Crosses between *YHR087W* mutants with strains mutant for the *NATB* complex (*MDM20/NAT3*), *NSR1*, *NPL3*, or *YRA2* were lethal.[71] The NatB complex functions in ribosomal protein acetylation. Nsr1 functions in rRNA synthesis. Npl3 is involved in rRNA processing and RNA nuclear export. Yra2 associates with RNP complexes.

Although studies in yeast suggest a role in RNA metabolism, how this function relates to disease pathogenesis, such as exocrine pancreatic insufficiency, marrow failure, and leukemia, remains obscure. Additional functions of SBDS have yet to be explored in yeast, human patients, and animal models.

Clinical Management and Treatment

Diagnosis

As with any rare disease, there is a paucity of controlled clinical trials to guide clinical management. A summary statement from the First International Scientific meeting on SDS described the general consensus of the meeting attendants on the management of SDS.[72]

Prior to the advent of genetic testing for SDS, the diagnosis was based on the clinical constellation of exocrine pancreatic insufficiency and bone marrow failure. Exocrine pancreatic insufficiency may be demonstrated by one of the following: (1) low serum trypsinogen in patients under the age of 3 or low serum isoamylase testing in patients over the age of 3; and (2) elevated fecal fat excretion following a 72-hour collection in the absence of concomitant intestinal or cholestatic liver disease with imaging studies showing a small or fatty pancreas.[16,72] Low levels of pancreatic enzymes may be seen following pancreatic stimulation testing with intravenous pancreozymin with/without secretin, but this invasive procedure is less commonly used with the advent of serum markers. Bone marrow dysfunction may be demonstrated by: (1) neutropenia, which may be chronic or intermittent, with an absolute neutrophil count less than 1,500/μL documented at least three times over a minimum of 3 months; (2) hemoglobin below age-adjusted norms; (3) platelet count less than

150,000/μL; (4) pancytopenia; or (5) MDS documented on bone marrow examination. Alternative etiologies of cytopenias must be excluded. Additional features variably associated with Shwachman-Diamond syndrome, such as short stature, metaphyseal dysostosis, or hepatic abnormalities, are not required for diagnosis. Although patients are typically small for age, normal height and weight does not exclude the diagnosis of SDS.[12,15]

The diagnosis of SDS may be elusive, particularly in older patients as the symptoms of steatorrhea may have resolved and the neutropenia may be mild and intermittent. The role of *SBDS* genetic testing in diagnosis has yet to be defined, particularly in the asymptomatic patient who lacks the clinical manifestations of SDS and has no family history of SDS. *SBDS* gene testing may help to provide corroboration for a patient in whom the diagnosis is suspected on clinical grounds and may be useful in testing family members of an affected patient. A negative test for *SBDS* gene mutations does not exclude the diagnosis, since up to 10% of patients with the clinical features of SDS lack *SBDS* mutations.[4] Extensive gene conversion mutations may be missed with standard primers against the *SBDS* gene.[8] The lack of *SBDS* mutations does not appear to result from alternative mutations that might not be observed in an exon-directed sequencing approach, such as promoter mutations or large gene deletions or inversions, since SBDS protein expression remains intact.[5,6] It is currently unclear whether patients lacking *SBDS* mutations might harbor mutations in an additional gene(s) responsible for SDS or represent a separate distinct disorder.

Assessment of height, weight, growth patterns, congenital anomalies, and family history are important in the initial evaluations. Alternative causes of exocrine pancreatic insufficiency such as cystic fibrosis or Pearson syndrome should be sought. Cystic fibrosis may be excluded with a sweat chloride test; Pearson syndrome typically manifests with sideroblastic anemia, vacuolization of erythroid and myeloid marrow precursors, exocrine pancreatic dysfunction, and deletions of mitochondrial DNA. Cartilage-hair hypoplasia presents with metaphyseal dysostosis, cytopenias, immune deficiencies, and fine sparse hair; it is associated with mutations in the RNA component of RNase MRP. Alternative marrow failure syndromes should also be considered as clinically indicated. Fanconi anemia may be excluded by a MMC/DEB chromosomal breakage test (see Bagby and Alter in this issue). Genetic testing is available for some of the other marrow failure syndromes. As with any inherited disease, all siblings of the proband should be tested for SDS. An outline for the workup of SDS is listed in Table 1.

Exocrine Pancreatic Insufficiency

Referral to a pediatric gastroenterologist is indicated for patients with SDS. Clinically significant exocrine pancreatic insufficiency is treated with oral pancreatic enzyme supplements. Regular assessments are recommended to monitor exocrine pancreatic function since it may improve over time. Steatorrhea resolves in about 50% of patients, usually by 4 years of age. To assess a need for continued pancreatic enzyme supplementation, a fecal fat measurement is helpful. This test is done by first discontinuing enzyme supplementation for 48 hours then collecting a 72-hour fecal specimen. Since vitamin deficiencies may accompany fat malabsorption, assessment of vitamin A, D, E, and K levels are recommended, with vitamin supplementation as appropriate. Prolongation of the prothrombin time (PT) and the partial thromboplastin time (aPTT) may accompany vitamin K deficiency. Serial measurements of growth, both height and weight, should be monitored.

Hematology

Patients with SDS should be monitored by a pediatric hematologist. Regular blood counts every 4 months are recommended to monitor for cytopenias. If cytopenias are noted, alternative treatable causes should considered and, if persistent, may require assessment of the bone marrow to determine the presence of clonal disease or aplastic anemia. The heightened risk of developing aplastic anemia, MDS, or acute leukemia makes it reasonable to perform periodic assessment of the bone marrow for evidence of progressive clonal disease or early signs of MDS or leukemia. Annual bone marrow examinations have been suggested for these patients, with more frequent aspirations if clinically indicated.[72] Marrow cellularity must be assessed in the context of the peripheral cell counts since cellularity may be patchy and subject to sampling variability.

Fever and neutropenia should be evaluated expeditiously with clinical examination, cultures of any potential infectious sources including blood cultures, and prompt institution of broad-spectrum antibiotics as indicated. For neutropenic patients with repeated infections or serious life-threatening infections, G-CSF administration may be considered. In the French Neutropenia Registry, neutrophil responses to G-CSF were seen in 12 of 15 patients treated; the remaining three patients either failed to respond or later developed resistance.[55] No clear association between G-CSF use and subsequent AML risk has been demonstrated to date, but the potential risks of treatment should be carefully weighed against the clinical benefits.

Currently the only curative therapy for bone marrow failure is a HSCT. Transfusion support for anemia and thrombocytopenia may be required. A chronic red blood cell transfusion regimen demands attention to total body iron load with appropriate institution of iron chelation therapy. Isolated case reports of improvements in blood counts have been reported with other medical interventions. A transient partial response, primarily in the red cell and platelet lineages, was reported in one patient treated with nandrolone decanoate,[73] while no response to oxymethalone was noted in two other cases.[26] One transient trilineage response within several weeks of initiating prednisone was seen in a patient who subsequently developed leukemia.[53] One case of a transient trilineage response to cyclosporin has been reported.[74]

Leukemia

Treatment of leukemias with chemotherapy is often associated with significant treatment-related toxicities, most com-

Table 1 Suggested Workup for Shwachman-Diamond Syndrome[71,72]

Diagnostic studies
Exocrine pancreatic function
Trypsinogen (age < 3 yr) or isoamylase (age > 3 yr)
or
Elevated 72-hour fecal fat measurement with pancreatic lipomatosis demonstrated by imaging studies such as ultrasound
or
Diminished pancreatic enzyme secretion documented by endoscopic pancreatic stimulation testing
Bone marrow function:
Blood counts including reticulocyte count, MCV, and blood smear
Bone marrow aspirate and biopsy with cytogenetics and iron stain
SBDS mutation analysis (note: currently a negative result does not rule out SDS)
Supportive studies (not necessary for diagnosis)
X-rays studies to evaluate metaphyseal dysostosis or rib abnormalities
Liver enzymes (AST, ALT)
Immunoglobulin levels and T and B cell subsets
Differential Diagnosis (as clinically indicated)
Sweat chloride test to rule out cystic fibrosis
Chromosomal breakage test for Fanconi anemia
Mitochondrial DNA sequencing to rule out Pearson syndrome
Consultations
Hematology
Gastroenterology
Endocrinology
Genetics
Developmental assessment (as clinically indicated)
Dental evaluation (as clinically indicated)

Abbreviations: MCV, mean corpuscular volume; AST, aspartate aminotransferase; ALT, alanine aminotransferase.

monly prolonged pancytopenia with marrow aplasia but also pulmonary, renal, and cardiac toxicities. Chemotherapy outcomes for SDS patients with AML are poor. One patient with ALL was still alive 12 months after diagnosis,[53] while a second patient with ALL died of complications of prolonged marrow aplasia following chemotherapy.[52]

Hematopoietic Stem Cell Transplant

The only potentially curative therapy currently available for bone marrow failure or MDS is hematopoietic stem cell transplant. A review of the literature revealed 58 patients who had undergone HSCT.[45,51,75] Most of the published literature consists of case reports and small case series. Table 2 tabulates results from those cases for which sufficient information regarding diagnosis and transplant donor are provided. Patient numbers are small and must be interpreted with caution since follow up time was often short. Stem cell transplants for marrow failure generally carried a more favorable prognosis than those performed for MDS or AML,[45,51,75] although the patients transplanted for marrow failure tended to be younger than those transplanted for MDS or AML. Risk of graft failure does not appear to be significantly elevated. Numerous reports suggest an increased risk of transplant-related end-organ toxicities,[76-78] although this is not seen in every patient.[79] The single reported surviving case of a patient receiving an unrelated donor transplant for AML and achieving full engraftment (34-month follow-up) used a reduced-intensity conditioning regimen.[45]

Additional Medical Issues

Referral to an endocrinologist is recommended to exclude additional treatable causes of short stature. The use of growth hormone is generally reserved for those patients with growth hormone deficiency. Because of the increased risk of osteopenia, monitoring of thyroxine (T4), thyroid-stimulating hormone (TSH), thyroxine binding globulin (TBGI), calcium, phosphorus, magnesium, parathyroid hormone (PTH), vitamin D (25D, 1,25D), spot urine for calcium, phosphorus,

Table 2 Summary of HSCT Literature for Patients With Shwachman-Diamond Syndrome

Indication	Sibling Donor*	Unrelated Donor*	Unspecified*	Total*
Marrow failure	1/2	7/7	13/16	21/25
MDS	5/9	1/5		6/14
Leukemia	0/2	2†/4		2/6

Abbreviations: HSCT, hematopoietic stem cell transplantation; MDS, myelodysplastic syndrome.
*Number of patients surviving at time of report/total number of patients transplanted.
†One patient failed to fully engraft

and creatinine with calculation of urine calcium/urine creatinine ratio may be helpful, as well as nutritional history to ensure adequate calcium intake. Careful attention to dental hygiene is important, particularly for patients with chronic neutropenia in order to prevent infections and to protect against gingivitis and tooth loss. Early developmental assessment should be pursued as clinically indicated.

Future Directions

With the advent of genetic testing, the full clinical spectrum of SDS will be ascertained. Since a subset of patients lack *SBDS* gene mutations, further investigation may reveal additional genes responsible for this syndrome. Molecular and cellular studies and the development of animal models will continue to shed light on the aberrant biological pathways of this syndrome. The elucidation of affected molecular pathways may identify potential therapeutic targets to prevent or treat marrow failure and leukemia; additional investigation into the apparent sensitivity of these patients to cytotoxic therapies is warranted. The potential role of acquired somatic *SBDS* mutations in leukemogenesis in the general population remains to be fully explored.

References

1. Shwachman H, Diamond LK, Oski FA, Khaw KT: The syndrome of pancreatic insufficiency and bone marrow dysfunction. J Pediatr 65: 645-663, 1964
2. Bodian M, Sheldon W, Lightwood R: Congenital hypoplasia of the exocrine pancreas. Acta Paediatr 53:282-293, 1964
3. Goobie S, Popovic M, Morrison J, Ellis L, Ginzberg H, Boocock GR, et al: Shwachman-Diamond syndrome with exocrine pancreatic dysfunction and bone marrow failure maps to the centromeric region of chromosome 7. Am J Hum Genet 68:1048-1054, 2001
4. Boocock GR, Morrison JA, Popovic M, Richards N, Ellis L, Durie PR, et al: Mutations in SBDS are associated with Shwachman-Diamond syndrome. Nat Genet 33:97-101, 2003
5. Woloszynek JR, Rothbaum RJ, Rawls AS, Minx PJ, Wilson RK, Mason PJ, et al: Mutations of the SBDS gene are present in most patients with Shwachman-Diamond syndrome. Blood 104:3588-3590, 2004
6. Austin KM, Leary RJ, Shimamura A: The Shwachman-Diamond SBDS protein localizes to the nucleolus. Blood 106:1253-1258, 2005
7. Nakashima E, et al: Novel SBDS mutations caused by gene conversion in Japanese patients with Shwachman-Diamond syndrome. Hum Genet 114:345-348, 2004
8. Nicolis E, Bonizzato A, Assael BM, Cipolli M: Identification of novel mutations in patients with Shwachman-Diamond syndrome. Hum Mutat 25:410, 2005
9. Winzeler EA, Shoemaker DD, Astromoff A, Liang H, Anderson K, Andre B, et al: Functional characterization of the S. cerevisiae genome by gene deletion and parallel analysis. Science 285:901-906, 1999
10. Shammas C, Menne TF, Hilcenko C, Michell SR, Goyenechea B, Boocock GR, et al: Structural and mutational analysis of the SBDS protein family. Insight into the leukemia-associated Shwachman-Diamond syndrome. J Biol Chem 280:19221-19229, 2005
11. Aggett PJ, Cavanagh NP, Matthew DJ, Pincott JR, Sutcliffe J, Harries JT, et al: Shwachman's syndrome. A review of 21 cases. Arch Dis Child 55:331-347, 1980
12. Mack DR, Forstner GG, Wilschanski M, Freedman MH, Durie PR: Shwachman syndrome: Exocrine pancreatic dysfunction and variable phenotypic expression. Gastroenterology 111:1593-1602, 1996
13. Smith OP, Hann IM, Chessells JM, Reeves BR, Milla P: Haematological abnormalities in Shwachman-Diamond syndrome. Br J Haematol 94: 279-284, 1996
14. Cipolli M, D'Orazio C, Delmarco A, Marchesini C, Miano A, Mastella G: Shwachman's syndrome: Pathomorphosis and long-term outcome. J Pediatr Gastroenterol Nutr 29:265-272, 1999
15. Ginzberg H, Shin J, Ellis L, Morrison J, Ip W, Dror Y, et al: Shwachman syndrome: Phenotypic manifestations of sibling sets and isolated cases in a large patient cohort are similar. J Pediatr 135:81-88, 1999
16. Ip WF, Dupuis A, Ellis L, Beharry S, Morrison J, Stormon MO, et al: Serum pancreatic enzymes define the pancreatic phenotype in patients with Shwachman-Diamond syndrome. J Pediatr 141:259-265, 2002
17. Brueton MJ, Mavromichalis J, Goodchild MC, Anderson CM: Hepatic dysfunction in association with pancreatic insufficiency and cyclical neutropenia. Shwachman-Diamond syndrome. Arch Dis Child 52:76-78, 1977
18. Maki M, Sorto A, Hallstrom O, Visakorpi JK: Hepatic dysfunction and dysgammaglobulinaemia in Shwachman-Diamond syndrome. Arch Dis Child 53:693-694, 1978
19. Savilahti E, Rapola J: Frequent myocardial lesions in Shwachman's syndrome. Eight fatal cases among 16 Finnish patients. Acta Paediatr Scand 73:642-651, 1984
20. Aggett PJ, Harries JT, Harvey BA, Soothill JF: An inherited defect of neutrophil mobility in Shwachman syndrome. J Pediatr 94:391-394, 1979
21. Azzara A, Carulli G, Petrini M: Lithium effects on neutrophil motility in Shwachman-Diamond syndrome: Evaluation by computer-assisted image analysis. Br J Haematol 123:369-370, 2003
22. Stepanovic V, Wessels D, Goldman FD, Geiger J, Soll DR: The chemotaxis defect of Shwachman-Diamond syndrome leukocytes. Cell Motil Cytoskel 57:158-174, 2004
23. Rothbaum RJ, Williams DA, Daugherty CC: Unusual surface distribution of concanavalin A reflects a cytoskeletal defect in neutrophils in Shwachman's syndrome. Lancet 2:800-801, 1982
24. Grinspan ZM, Pikora CA: Infections in patients with Shwachman-Diamond syndrome. Pediatr Infect Dis J 24:179-181, 2005
25. Dror Y: Shwachman-Diamond syndrome. Pediatr Blood Cancer 45: 892-901, 2005
26. Woods WG, Krivit W, Lubin BH, Ramsay NK: Aplastic anemia associated with the Shwachman syndrome. In vivo and in vitro observations. Am J Pediatr Hematol Oncol 3:347-351, 1981
27. Kuijpers TW, Nannenberg E, Alders M, Bredius R, Hennekam RC: Congenital aplastic anemia caused by mutations in the SBDS gene: A rare presentation of Shwachman-Diamond syndrome. Pediatrics 114: e387-e391, 2004
28. Lesesve JF, Dugue F, Gregoire MJ, Witz F, Dror Y: Shwachman-Diamond syndrome with late-onset neutropenia and fatal acute myeloid leukaemia without maturation: A case report. Eur J Haematol 71:393-395, 2003
29. Kuijpers TW, Alders M, Tool AT, Mellink C, Roos D, Hennekam RC, et al: Hematologic abnormalities in Shwachman Diamond syndrome: Lack of genotype-phenotype relationship. Blood 106:356-361, 2005
30. Suda T, Mizoguchi H, Miura Y, Kubota K, Ikuta K, Sasaki H, et al: Hemopoietic colony-forming cells in Shwachman's syndrome. Am J Pediatr Hematol Oncol 4:129-133, 1982
31. Dror Y, Freedman MH: Shwachman-Diamond syndrome: An inherited preleukemic bone marrow failure disorder with aberrant hematopoietic progenitors and faulty marrow microenvironment. Blood 94:3048-3054, 1999
32. Dror Y, Freedman MH: Shwachman-Diamond syndrome marrow cells show abnormally increased apoptosis mediated through the Fas pathway. Blood 97:3011-3016, 2001
33. Thornley I, Dror Y, Sung L, Wynn RF, Freedman MH: Abnormal telomere shortening in leucocytes of children with Shwachman-Diamond syndrome. Br J Haematol 117:189-192, 2002
34. Dror Y, Durie P, Ginzberg H, Herman R, Banerjee A, Champange M, et al: Clonal evolution in marrows of patients with Shwachman-Diamond syndrome: A prospective 5-year follow-up study. Exp Hematol 30:659-669, 2002
35. Alter BP, Caruso JP, Drachtman RA, Uchida T, Velagaleti GV, Elghetany MT: Fanconi anemia: Myelodysplasia as a predictor of outcome. Cancer Genet Cytogenet 117:125-131, 2000

36. Kalra R, Dale D, Freedman M, Bonilla MA, Weinblatt M, Ganser A, et al: Monosomy 7 and activating RAS mutations accompany malignant transformation in patients with congenital neutropenia. Blood 86: 4579-4586, 1995
37. Elghetany MT, Alter BP: p53 protein overexpression in bone marrow biopsies of patients with Shwachman-Diamond syndrome has a prevalence similar to that of patients with refractory anemia. Arch Pathol Lab Med 126:452-455, 2002
38. Mellink CH, Alders M, van der Lelie H, Hennekam RH, Kuijpers TW: SBDS mutations and isochromosome 7q in a patient with Shwachman-Diamond syndrome: No predisposition to malignant transformation? Cancer Genet Cytogenet 154:144-149, 2004
39. Smith A, Shaw PJ, Webster B, Lammi A, Gaskin K, Diaz S, et al: Intermittent 20q- and consistent i(7q) in a patient with Shwachman-Diamond syndrome. Pediatr Hematol Oncol 19:525-528, 2002
40. Smith OP: Shwachman-Diamond syndrome. Semin Hematol 39:95-102, 2002
41. Dale DC, Cottle TE, Fier CJ, Bolyard AA, Bonilla MA, Boxer LA, et al: Severe chronic neutropenia: treatment and follow-up of patients in the Severe Chronic Neutropenia International Registry. Am J Hematol 72: 82-93, 2003
42. Luna-Fineman S, Shannon KM, Lange BJ: Childhood monosomy 7: Epidemiology, biology, and mechanistic implications. Blood 85:1985-1999, 1995
43. Mertens F, Johansson B, Mitelman F: Isochromosomes in neoplasia. Genes Chromosomes Cancer 10:221-230, 1994
44. Majeed F, Jadko S, Freedman MH, Dror Y: Mutation analysis of SBDS in pediatric acute myeloblastic leukemia. Pediatr Blood Cancer 45:920-924, 2005
45. Mitsui T, Kawakami T, Sendo D, Katsuura M, Shimizu Y, Hayasaka K: Successful unrelated donor bone marrow transplantation for Shwachman-Diamond syndrome with leukemia. Int J Hematol 79:189-192, 2004
46. Huijgens PC, van der Veen EA, Meijer S, Muntinghe OG: Syndrome of Shwachman and leukaemia. Scand J Haematol 18:20-24, 1977
47. Seymour JF, Escudier SM: Acute leukemia complicating bone marrow hypoplasia in an adult with Shwachman's syndrome. Leuk Lymphoma 12:131-135, 1993
48. Arseniev L, Diedrich H, Link H: Allogeneic bone marrow transplatation in a patient with Shwachman-Diamond syndrome. Ann Hematol 72: 83-84, 1996
49. Smith OP, Chan MY, Evans J, Veys P: Shwachman-Diamond syndrome and matched unrelated donor BMT. Bone Marrow Transplant 16:717-718, 1995
50. Dokal I, Rule S, Chen F, Potter M, Goldman J: Adult onset of acute myeloid leukaemia (M6) in patients with Shwachman-Diamond syndrome. Br J Haematol 99:171-173, 1997
51. Donadieu J, Michel G, Merlin E, Bordigoni P, Monteux B, Beaupain B, et al: Hematopoietic stem cell transplantation for Shwachman-Diamond syndrome: Experience of the French neutropenia registry. Bone Marrow Transplant 36:787-792, 2005
52. Strevens MJ, Lilleyman JS, Williams RB: Shwachman's syndrome and acute lymphoblastic leukaemia. Br Med J 2:18, 1978
53. Woods WG, Roloff JS, Lukens JN, Krivit W: The occurrence of leukemia in patients with the Shwachman syndrome. J Pediatr 99:425-428, 1981
54. Caselitz J, Kloppel G, Delling G, Gruttner R, Holdhoff U, Stern M: Shwachman's syndrome and leukaemia. Virchows Arch A Pathol Anat Histol 385:109-116, 1979
55. Donadieu J, Leblanc T, Bader Meunier B, Barkaoui M, Fenneteau O, Bertrand Y, et al: Analysis of risk factors for myelodysplasias, leukemias and death from infection among patients with congenital neutropenia. Experience of the French Severe Chronic Neutropenia Study Group. Haematologica 90:45-53, 2005
56. Tada H, Ri T, Yoshida H, Ishimoto K, Kaneko M, Yamashiro Y, et al: A case of Shwachman syndrome with increased spontaneous chromosome breakage. Hum Genet 77:289-291, 1987
57. Hershkovits BS, Dagan J, Freier S: Increased spontaneous chromosomal breakage in Shwachman syndrome. J Pediatr Gastroenterol Nutr 28:449-450, 1999
58. Fraccaro M, Scappaticci S, Arico M: Shwachman syndrome and chromosome breakage. Hum Genet 79:194, 1988
59. Koiffmann CP, Gonzalez CH, Souza DH, Romani EG, Kim CA, Wajntal A: Is Shwachman syndrome (McKusick 26040) a chromosome breakage syndrome? Hum Genet 87:106-107, 1991
60. Mack DR: Shwachman-Diamond syndrome. J Pediatr 141:164-165, 2002
61. Makitie O, Ellis L, Durie PR, Morrison JA, Sochett EB, Rommens JM, et al: Skeletal phenotype in patients with Shwachman-Diamond syndrome and mutations in SBDS. Clin Genet 65:101-112, 2004
62. Hudson E, Aldor T: Pancreatic insufficiency and neutropenia with associated immunoglobulin deficit. Arch Intern Med 125:314-316, 1970
63. Dror Y, Ginzberg H, Dalal I, Cherepanov V, Downey G, Durie P, et al: Immune function in patients with Shwachman-Diamond syndrome. Br J Haematol 114:712-717, 2001
64. Kornfeld SJ, Kratz J, Diamond F, Day NK, Good RA: Shwachman-Diamond syndrome associated with hypogammaglobulinemia and growth hormone deficiency. J Allergy Clin Immunol 96:247-250, 1995
65. Raj AB, Bertolone SJ, Barch MJ, Hersh JH: Chromosome 20q deletion and progression to monosomy 7 in a patient with Shwachman-Diamond syndrome without MDS/AML. J Pediatr Hematol Oncol 25:508-509, 2003
66. Andersen JS, Lam YW, Leung AK, Ong SE, Lyon CE, Lamond AI, et al: Nucleolar proteome dynamics. Nature 433:77-83, 2005
67. Koonin EV, Wolf YI, Aravind L: Prediction of the archaeal exosome and its connections with the proteasome and the translation and transcription machineries by a comparative-genomic approach. Genome Res 11:240-252, 2001
68. Wu LF, Hughes TR, Davierwala AP, Robinson MD, Stoughton R, Altschuler SJ: Large-scale prediction of Saccharomyces cerevisiae gene function using overlapping transcriptional clusters. Nat Genet 31:255-265, 2002
69. Peng WT, Robinson MD, Mnaimneh S, Krogan NJ, Cagney G, Morris Q, et al: A panoramic view of yeast noncoding RNA processing. Cell 113:919-933, 2003
70. Bu D, Zhao Y, Cai L, Xue H, Zhu X, Lu H, et al: Topological structure analysis of the protein-protein interaction network in budding yeast. Nucleic Acids Res 31:2443-2450, 2003
71. Savchenko A, Krogan N, Cort JR, Evdokimova E, Lew JM, Yee AA, et al: The Shwachman-Bodian-Diamond syndrome protein family is involved in RNA metabolism. J Biol Chem 280:19213-19220, 2005
72. Rothbaum R, Perrault J, Vlachos A, Cipolli M, Alter BP, Burroughs S, et al: Shwachman-Diamond syndrome: Report from an international conference. J Pediatr 141:266-270, 2002
73. Barrios NJ, Kirkpatrick DV: Successful cyclosporin A treatment of aplastic anaemia in Shwachman-Diamond syndrome. Br J Haematol 74:540-541, 1990
74. Barrios N, Kirkpatrick D, Regueira O, Wuttke B, McNeil J, Humbert J: Bone marrow transplant in Shwachman Diamond syndrome. Br J Haematol 79:337-338, 1991
75. Cesaro S, Oneto R, Messina C, Gibson BE, Buzyn A, Steward C, et al: Haematopoietic stem cell transplantation for Shwachman-Diamond disease: A study from the European Group for Blood and Marrow Transplantation. Br J Haematol 131: 231-236, 2005
76. Tsai PH, Sahdev I, Herry A, Lipton JM: Fatal cyclophosphamide-induced congestive heart failure in a 10-year-old boy with Shwachman-Diamond syndrome and severe bone marrow failure treated with allogeneic bone marrow transplantation. Am J Pediatr Hematol Oncol 12: 472-476, 1990
77. Okcu F, Roberts WM, Chan KW: Bone marrow transplantation in Shwachman-Diamond syndrome: Report of two cases and review of the literature. Bone Marrow Transplant 21:849-851, 1998
78. Ritchie DS, Angus PW, Bhathal PS, Grigg AP: Liver failure complicating non-alcoholic steatohepatitis following allogeneic bone marrow transplantation for Shwachman-Diamond syndrome. Bone Marrow Transplant 29:931-933, 2002
79. Hsu JW, Vogelsang G, Jones RJ, Brodsky RA: Bone marrow transplantation in Shwachman-Diamond syndrome. Bone Marrow Transplant 30:255-258, 2002

ELSEVIER

Seminars in
HEMATOLOGY

Severe Congenital Neutropenia

Karl Welte,[a] Cornelia Zeidler,[a] and David C. Dale[b]

Severe congenital neutropenia (CN) includes a variety of hematologic disorders characterized by severe neutropenia, with absolute neutrophil counts (ANC) below 0.5 × 10⁹/L, and associated with severe systemic bacterial infections from early infancy. One subtype of CN, Kostmann syndrome, is an autosomal recessive disorder, characterized histopathologically by early-stage maturation arrest of myeloid differentiation. CN with similar clinical features occurs as an autosomal dominant disorder and many sporadic cases also have been reported. This genetic heterogeneity suggests that several pathophysiological mechanisms may lead to this common clinical phenotype. Recent studies on the genetic bases of CN have detected inherited or spontaneous point mutations in the neutrophil elastase gene (*ELA 2*) in about 60% to 80% of patients and, less commonly, mutations in other genes. Acquisition of additional genetic defects during the course of the disease, for example, granulocyte colony-stimulating factor (G-CSF) receptor gene mutations and cytogenetic aberrations, indicates an underlying genetic instability as a common feature for all congenital neutropenia subtypes. Data on more than 600 patients with CN collected by the Severe Chronic Neutropenia International Registry (SCNIR) demonstrate that, regardless of the particular CN subtype, more than 95% of these patients respond to recombinant human (rHu)G-CSF with ANCs that can be maintained above 1.0 × 10⁹/L. Adverse events include mild splenomegaly, osteoporosis, and malignant transformation into myelodysplasia (MDS)/leukemia. If and how G-CSF treatment impacts on these adverse events is not fully understood. In recent analyses the influence of the G-CSF dose required to achieve neutrophil response (ANC >1,000/μL) in the risk of developing acute myeloid leukemia (AML) has been reported. Hematopoietic stem cell transplantation (HSCT) is still the only treatment available for patients who are refractory to G-CSF treatment.
Semin Hematol 43:189-195

In 1956 the Swedish physician Rolf Kostmann described an autosomal recessive hematologic disorder with severe neutropenia with an absolute neutrophil count (ANC) less than 0.2×10^9/L and early onset of severe bacterial infections.[1,2] Most children died because of these infections despite antibiotic treatment. The underlying genetic defect of Kostmann syndrome is largely unknown, but genetic analyses in autosomal dominant and sporadic cases of severe congenital neutropenia (CN) indicate that 60% of cases are attributable to mutations in the gene for neutrophil elastase (*ELA 2*). Current knowledge on the pathophysiology of severe CN implicates that the clinical diagnosis of CN includes a heterogeneous group of disorders following different patterns of inheritance (Table 1).

Bone marrow transplantation (BMT) was previously the only curative treatment option for patients with human leukocyte antigen (HLA)-compatible donors[3]. The availability of recombinant human granulocyte colony-stimulating factor (rHuG-CSF) in 1987[4] dramatically changed both the prognosis of CN and the quality of life of patients with CN.[5,6] Since the establishment of the Severe Chronic Neutropenia International Registry (SCNIR) in 1994, data on 611 patients with CN have been collected to monitor the clinical course, treatment, and disease outcomes. More than 90% of patients in clinical trials responded to rHuG-CSF treatment with an increase in ANCs to greater than 1.0×10^9/L. All responding patients required significantly fewer antibiotics and fewer days of hospitalization.[6-10]

Hematopoietic stem cell transplantation (HSCT) remains the only currently available treatment for patients who are refractory to rHuG-CSF treatment and continue to have severe and life-threatening bacterial infections and when the disease has transformed into myelodysplasia (MDS)/leukemia.[11]

[a]Department of Pediatric Hematology/Oncology, Medical School Hannover, Hannover, Germany.
[b]Department of Medicine, University of Washington, Seattle, WA.
Address correspondence to Karl Welte, MD, PhD, Department for Pediatric Hematology/Oncology, Medizinische Hochschule Hannover, Carl-Neuberg-Str. 1, 30625 Hannover, Germany. E-mail: Welte.Karl.H@mh-hannover.de

0037-1963/06/$-see front matter © 2006 Elsevier Inc. All rights reserved.
doi:10.1053/j.seminhematol.2006.04.004

Table 1 Genetic Aberrations Causing Congenital Neutropenia

Disorder	Genetic Defect	Recessive (R-CN)	Dominant (D-CN)	Neutropenia Plus:
Congenital neutropenia with *ELA 2* mutations*	*ELA2*	–	+	Preleukemic syndrome
Congenital neutropenia with *GFI-1* mutation	*GFI-1*	–	+	B-/T-cell deficiency
WHIM syndrome	*CXCR4*	–	+	Myelokathexis, IgG deficiency, warts
Shwachman-Diamond syndrome	*SBDS*	+	–	Exocrine pancreas insufficiency
Glycogen storage disease, type Ib	*Glucose-6-phosphate-Translocase*	+	–	Hypoglycemia, lactic acidosis
Hyper IgM	*CD40-L*	X-linked	–	IgG, IgA, IgE deficiency
Barth syndrome (3-methylglutaconic aciduria)	*Taz 1*	X-linked		Dilatative cardiomyopathy, skeletal myopathy, short stature,
Congenital neutropenia with WASP mutation	*WASP*	X-linked	–	Monocytopenia, platelets normal
Hermansky-Pudlak syndrome	*AP3B1*	+	–	Partial albinism, short stature, IgG deficiency, platelet dysfunction
Congenital neutropenia with p14 (MAPBPIP) mutation	*P14/MAPBPIP*	+	–	Partial albinism, short stature, IgG deficiency
Griscelli syndrome	*Rab27a*	+	–	Partial albinism, hemophagocytosis
Chediak-Higashi syndrome	*LYST (CHS1)*	+	–	Partial albinism, T-/natural killer cytotoxicity and chemotaxis defect
Congenital neutropenia (unclassified)	Not known	+	?	Elevated IgG levels

*Congenital neutropenia with *ELA 2* mutations comprises approximately 60% of patients.

Pathophysiologic Mechanisms

The underlying genetic defect of CN is still only partially understood. The original hypotheses for this disorder included defective production of G-CSF or defective response of the neutrophilic precursors to G-CSF or other hematopoietic growth factors. We showed, however, that serum from patients with CN contains normal or increased levels of G-CSF[12] with normal biological activity of endogenous G-CSF and that G-CSF receptors are expressed on myeloid cells from CN patients in normal or increased numbers.[13]

Linkage analyses of inherited forms of the disease and sequencing of candidate genes provided alternative approaches to understanding the pathogenesis of CN. The identification of mutations within the *ELA 2* gene as the cause of cyclic neutropenia[14] led to similar studies in patients diagnosed with CN.[15-19] Heterozygous *ELA 2* mutations were found in 60% of these cases. Analysis of CN families with autosomal dominant inheritance of elastase mutation and a case with mosaic expression of mutant *ELA 2*[15] provided the strongest evidence to implicate *ELA 2* mutations in the etiology of CN.

The precise cellular mechanisms by which mutant *ELA 2* causes neutropenia are uncertain and the search for the role of the altered elastase protein in the pathophysiologic mechanism of CN continues to be investigated.[15-17,19-21] We proposed that mutant *ELA 2* triggers accelerated apoptosis of developing neutrophil precursors, a concept now supported by several lines of evidence.[16] We recently demonstrated that the mutation in the elastase protein leads to cytoplasmic accumulation of a nonfunctional protein, disturbance of intracellular trafficking, and activation of unfolded protein response in neutrophils from patients with CN.[21]

In addition to *ELA 2* mutations, a number of genetic aberrations have been identified in patients with disorders associated with severe CN. Genes that were mutated in minor subgroups of patients with CN included GFI-1, CXCR4, SBDS, WASP, Glucose-6-phophatase-translocase, Taz-1, AP3B1, and others (Table 1). However, these gene mutations in patients with CN are associated with additional symptoms such as pancreas insufficiency in patients with SBDS mutations (Shwachman-Bodian-Diamond syndrome), glycogen-storage disease type Ib, glucose-6-phosphatase-translocase mutations, cardiomyopathy in patients with Taz-1 mutations, and partial albinism and short stature in patients with AP3B1 or p14 mutations (Table 1). A common feature of CN patients is an increase in immunoglobulin levels, a finding that may be secondary to recurrent infections or perhaps suggests a gene defect affecting both myelopoiesis and lymphopoiesis. Myeloid cells from all patients with congenital neutropenia have reduced expression of LEF-1 transcription factor (known to regulate expression of cyclin D1, c-myc, and c/EBP-alpha), suggesting that a LEF-1 defect may be a common downstream defect.[22] That myeloid cells from patients with CN demonstrate an increased degree of apoptosis[16] suggests that defective or increased expression or mutation of one of the apoptosis-regulating genes could be the cause of neutropenia in some cases. Thus, current data suggest that CN is a multi-gene disorder. Mutations in *ELA 2* are the most common genetic abnormality and, along with other genetic or acquired abnormalities, may have a common functional

Table 2 Time Course of the Acquisition of G-CSF Receptor Point Mutations in a Patient With Congenital Neutropenia

	Diagnosis			
	CN	CN	CN	CN/AML
Age (yr)	7	13	15	16
G-CSF receptor mutation at nucleotide	2362	2362 2414	2363 2414	2363 2414 2390

outcome: reduced survival of myeloid progenitor cells leading to granulopoietic failure.

Among CN patients who developed leukemia, acquired G-CSF receptor mutations affecting the cytoplasmic domain have been present in most patients tested,[23-29] indicating that such mutations may play a role in leukemogenesis. These G-CSF receptor mutations have not been identified at birth, which suggests they are not responsible for the neutropenia and develop as somatic mutations in a small subgroup of patients, most likely caused by genetic instability. G-CSF receptor analyses cannot be used to diagnose the underlying disease, but might be helpful to screen for the risk of leukemia. The time-course between acquisition of a G-CSF receptor mutation(s) and the development of leukemia varies considerably (Table 2). In a few patients, a G-CSF receptor gene mutation is only present in the leukemic cells, while in others single or multiple mutations of the G-CSF receptor gene predate leukemic transformation by several years.[29] In the majority of patients, the G-CSF receptor gene mutations affect only one allele and are most frequently located between nucleotide 2342 and 2522 of the G-CSF receptor gene (Fig 1), coding for a critical region within the cytoplasmic portion of the G-CSF receptor protein. Even in the face of a G-CSF receptor mutation there seems to be no change in the responsiveness of patients' cells to G-CSF. In some instances of acute myeloid leukemia (AML), reductions in blast counts can occur if G-CSF is discontinued.[30]

Diagnosis

CN is a rare condition with an estimated frequency of approximately one to two cases per million with equal distribution for gender. The disease is usually detected in infancy after fever or signs of a severe infection develop. CN patients suffer from severe chronic neutropenia with ANCs continuously below 200/μL; in many cases, peripheral blood neutrophils are completely absent. With infection, there may be a transient increase in neutrophils, but counts rarely increase to normal levels. The diagnosis of Kostmann syndrome is sometimes used to categorize sporadic cases of CN, children with no known affected family member. We prefer the term "severe congenital neutropenia" or "congenital neutropenia" for this heterogeneous patient population. For diagnosis during the first months of life, testing for anti-neutrophil antibodies is helpful to exclude autoimmune neutropenia of infancy. In CN cases, the results are usually (but not always) negative.

Blood Values

Repeated differential blood counts indicating persistent ANCs within a range of 0 to 0.2 × 109/L are required for diagnosis. Blood counts often indicate mild anemia and thrombocytosis. There is usually a two- to fourfold increase in blood monocytes and an increase in the blood eosinophil count is common. IgG levels are elevated in the majority of patients, independent of their infectious status (unpublished data). The specific immunologic competence after vaccination is normal. Blood chemistry is within the normal, age-dependent range for electrolytes and kidney and liver function.

Bone Marrow

The bone marrow usually shows a maturation arrest of neutrophil precursors at an early stage (promyelocyte/myelocyte level) with few cells of the neutrophilic series beyond the promyelocyte stage (Fig 2). Promyelocytes often have morphologically atypical nuclei and vacuolization of the cytoplasm. The absolute number of promyelocytes is slightly increased.[9] Marrow eosinophilia and monocytosis are common and do not change during treatment. Cellularity is usually normal or slightly decreased. Megakaryocytes are normal in number and morphology. In vitro growth of granulocyte-macrophage progenitor cells is defective, with few colonies formed and evidence for "maturation arrest."

Cytogenetic Evaluation and Molecular Testing

Cytogenetics at the time of diagnosis of CN are almost always normal. Bone marrow cytogenetics may change during the course of the disease, with monosomy 7 being the most frequent aberration in about 50% of abnormal cytogenetic results. The interval from the original finding of normal cytogenetics to the appearance of an abnormality is often several years. Abnormal cytogenetics are often associated with morphologic changes of the bone marrow indicating the development of MDS or leukemia (see below) and may occur with the development of cytopenias or refractoriness to G-CSF treatment.

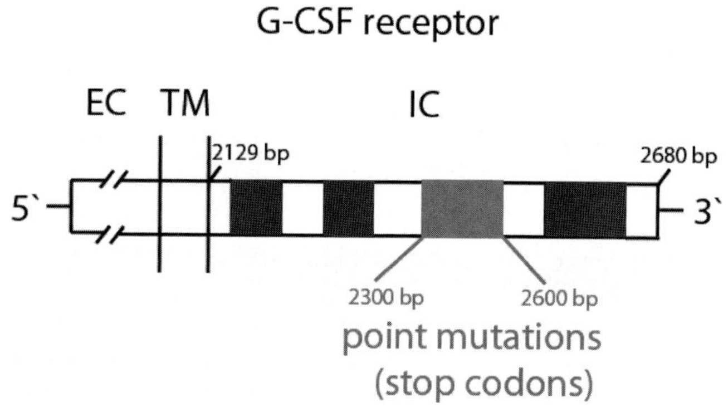

Figure 1 Point mutations within the critical region of the G-CSF receptor gene (2,300 to 2,600 basepairs). EC, extracellular; IC, intracytoplasmic.

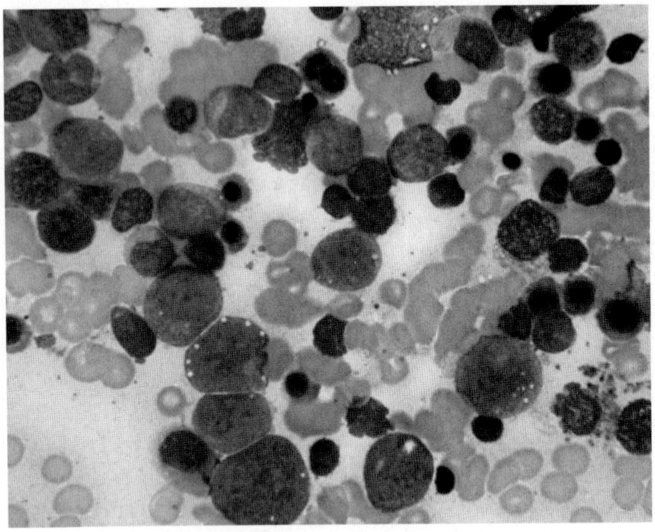

Figure 2 Typical bone marrow morphology in CN.

Studies of the G-CSF receptor gene have shown that mutations occur mainly within a critical region (nucleotide position 2300 to 2600) of the intracellular part of the receptor (Fig 1).[23-29] These mutations are not present at birth, so they are not causative for CN. Analysis of the G-CSF receptor gene to detect acquired mutations can be performed using blood and bone marrow samples.

Onset of Symptoms

Severe bacterial infections frequently occur during the first year of life in children with CN. Omphalitis, beginning directly after birth, may be the first symptom, but otitis media, pneumonitis, and infections of the upper respiratory tract, and abscesses of skin or liver are also common and can lead to the diagnosis of CN. Cultures are mainly positive for staphylococci or streptococci, but other bacteria (*Pseudomonas, Peptostreptococcus*) and, rarely, fungi are detected. In addition, uncommon infections such as clostridial gas gangrene may occur. The outcome of these fulminant infections is often lethal due to the lack of neutrophil defense. Most patients suffer from frequent aphthous stomatitis and gingival hyperplasia, leading to an early loss of permanent teeth.

Differential Diagnosis

The differential diagnosis of congenital neutropenia[10] includes a number of congenital and acquired diseases. The most common difficulty is determining whether the patient has cyclic neutropenia, autoimmune neutropenia of infancy, or idiopathic neutropenia. Cyclic neutropenia is diagnosed by serial measurement of blood neutrophils on at least 3 days per week for at least 6 weeks, graphing the counts and determining if there are regular periods of very severe neutropenia at 3-week intervals. Even with careful serial counts, the diagnosis may be missed because the amplitude of the oscillations may be too small for detection.

An important differential diagnostic evaluation is testing for neutrophilic antibodies.[31] In neutropenic children aged 1 to 3 years, the presence of neutrophil-specific auto-antibodies indicates an increased peripheral destruction of neutrophils in the marrow and blood. Although these infants lack peripheral blood neutrophils, the marrow function is normal; maturation of myeloid precursors to the mature neutrophil stage is usually observed. Patients with autoimmune neutropenia usually do not suffer from severe bacterial infections. Neutrophil or granulocyte-specific antibodies in serum are detectable using immunologic tests.[31]

Treatment

rHuG-CSF has been available for treatment of CN since 1987. Phase I–III studies have demonstrated its efficiency in increasing the number of neutrophils associated with reduction of infections.[6,32] In contrast, GM-CSF treatment does not lead to an increase in blood neutrophils but only in blood eosinophils.[33]

In 1994, the SCNIR was established to collect data on clinical course and outcome of these rare disorders. As of December 2005, 611 patients with CN have been registered, and more than 95% responded to rHuG-CSF treatment with an increase in ANCs to $1.0 \times \geq 10^9$/L (Fig 3). Most CN patients respond to a dose between 3 and 10 μg/kg/d.

After initiation of rHuG-CSF at 5 μg/kg/d, the dose should be escalated to 10 μg/kg/d and then by increments of 10 μg/kg at 14-day intervals if the ANC remains below 1.0×10^9/L. As soon as the ANC can be maintained at 1.0 to 1.5 × 109/L or above, increases of the rHuG-CSF dose can be stopped since the occurrence of bacterial infection is reduced dramatically at this level. The dose of rHuG-CSF can be reduced if the ANC increases to $\geq 5.0 \times 10^9$/L to keep the patient at the lowest dose necessary for maintaining a sufficient neutrophil count to overcome infections.

Nonresponders to rHuG-CSF are defined by failure to benefit at dose levels exceeding 120 μg/kg/d. Partial responders have ANCs increased to 0.5 to 1.0×10^9/L but still have bacterial infections. In some patients, the dose of rHuG-CSF cannot be increased to these levels because of the large volume and frequency of injections required. In research studies, refractory patients received a combination of rHuG-CSF with stem cell factor (SCF), which led to a further increase in ANCs above the levels achieved with G-CSF alone. Because of allergic side effects of SCF, this treatment combination has only been used during severe infections in hospitalized patients receiving concomitant antihistaminic medication.[34]

For patients who do not respond to rHuG-CSF alone or in combination with SCF, HSCT is the only currently available treatment.[11] When successful, after transplantation patients normalize hematopoiesis and do not require cytokine treatment. It remains difficult to recommend transplantation for patients with CN who benefit from rHuG-CSF and show no evidence of impending malignant transformation. For many responding patients, the risks associated with transplant from an HLA-identical sibling may outweigh the risk of leukemic transformation when rHuG-CSF is continued.

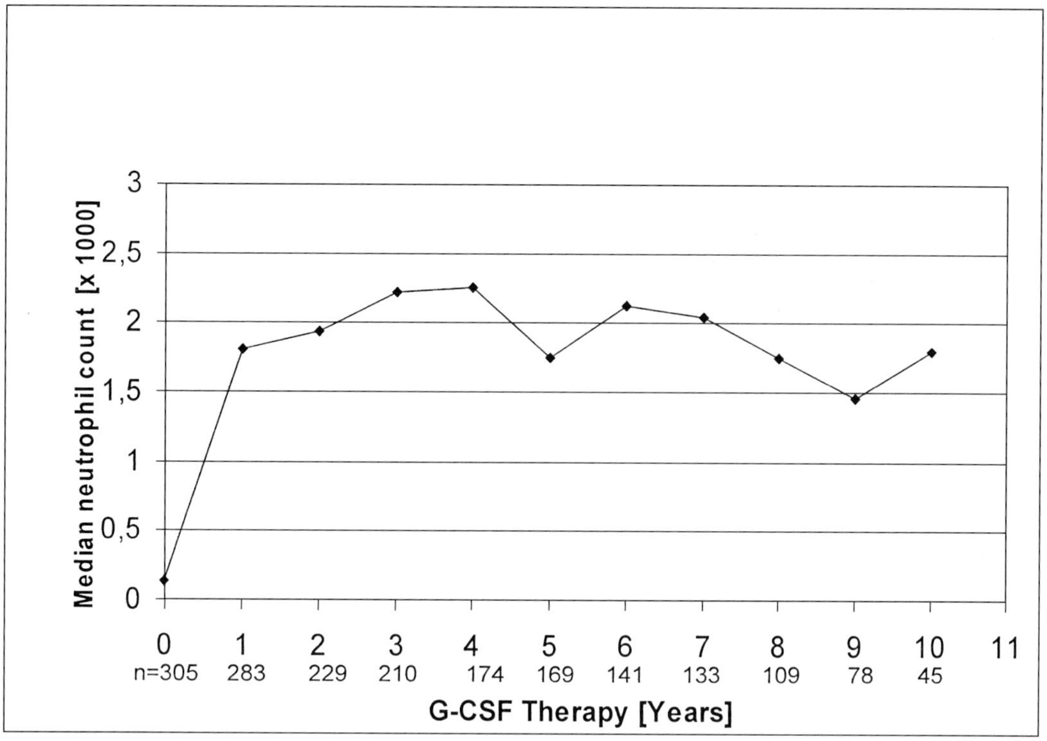

Figure 3 Mean ANC by year of G-CSF treatment in CN.

Long-Term Safety

Prior to the development and availability of G-CSF, complications of severe congenital neutropenia were not well known. There was no organized database for this rare disease. However, a number of reports noting deaths from infections and a few cases evolving to AML are available from the pre–G-CSF era.

Leukemia

Prior to the availability of cytokine therapy, it was already recognized that leukemic transformation occurred in patients with CN.[35,36] However, in the pre-cytokine era, 42% of published cases died in the first 2 years of life, usually from sepsis or pneumonia. Thus, the true risk of CN patients developing MDS/AML was not defined. With G-CSF therapy, most of these patients have survived well beyond 2 years of age. Therefore, it is unknown whether the increased survival allows for a higher risk of the recognized natural expression of leukemogenesis in this population in the absence of G-CSF therapy.

From the initiation of clinical trials with G-CSF in 1987 through December 2005, a total of 70 patients with CN (including five patients with Shwachman-Diamond syndrome) who have developed MDS/AML were reported to the SCNIR. The overall incidence or crude rate of MDS/AML conversion is 11.5% for CN patients (70 cases among 611 exposed cases), with an average follow-up of approximately 5 to 6 years. The leukemias occurred in those CN patients with *ELA 2* mutations, in unclassified CN patients, and in patients with Shwachman-Diamond syndrome but not in the other subgroups listed in Table 1.

The SCNIR recently published a more detailed report on the first 374 patients (1987–2000) with CN on long-term G-CSF enrolled in the registry to identify the risk of leukemic transformation. The hazard of MDS/AML increased significantly during the period of observation on G-CSF, from 2.9% per year after 6 years to 8.0% per year after 12 years. The cumulative incidence of MDS/AML was 21% after 10 years. The risk of MDS/AML increased with the dose of G-CSF. Less responsive patients, defined as those requiring greater than 8 μg/kg/d of G-CSF, had a cumulative incidence of MDS/AML of 40% after 10 years, compared to 11% of more responsive patients.[37] The data were interpreted as indicating that a poor response to G-CSF defines an "at-risk" population and predicts an adverse outcome.

Conversion to MDS/AML in CN patients was associated with one or more cellular genetic abnormalities (such as monosomy 7, ras mutation, or G-CSF receptor mutation), which may be useful for identifying subgroups of patients at high risk. Marrow cells from approximately 75% of the severe CN cases that transformed to MDS/AML also showed point mutations in the gene for the G-CSF receptor, resulting in a truncated C-terminal cytoplasmic region of the receptor that is crucial for maturation signaling.[17,23-25,27-29]

As illustrated by the cases described here, the development of MDS/AML is a multi-step process characterized by a series of cellular genetic changes indicating a genetic predisposition to malignant transformation. If and how G-CSF impacts on this predisposition remains unclear; there are no historical controls for comparison.

To address further the issue of risk-benefit of G-CSF in the CN setting with regard to MDS/AML, all available data were critically reviewed.[37] Although high-level evidence does not exist that would reveal the proper timing of bone marrow surveillance, the SCNIR advisory board recommended annual marrow cytogenetic testing to identify monosomy 7 or other changes indicating transformation; this approach might permit earlier therapeutic interventions such as BMT.

Osteoporosis

Within the SCNIR, bone density measurements have been reported on a total of 121 patients measured by different techniques, including quantitative computer tomography (Q-CT), dual energy x-ray absorptiometry (DEXA), single-photon absorptiometry (SPA), and lumbar x-ray. Of these 121 patients, 66 (54.4%) had varying degrees of abnormal results. These results have not been quantified to interpret the severity of the abnormalities. Most patients did not show clinical symptoms of osteopenia/osteoporosis (bone pain or fractures), which explains why diagnostic procedures for bone density evaluation were not reported in approximately 70% of registry patients. Therefore, the actual incidence continues to be unknown. The pathophysiology of osteopenia/osteoporosis also remains unclear. Serum chemistry did not reveal a typical pattern in patients with osteopenia/osteoporosis. Patients who suffer from osteopenia also did not receive elevated amounts of rHuG-CSF doses compared with all registry patients.[38]

Splenomegaly

The incidence of palpable splenomegaly (2 cm below the costal margin) prior to treatment with rHuG-CSF in CN patients was 21%. During the first year of rHuG-CSF therapy, the incidence increased to 39% and remained approximately at this level of occurrence (34% to 48%) through 10 years of therapy.

Monitoring

The Advisory Board for the SCNIR recommends that all patients should be seen by a physician at least twice per year with assessment for weight and height and documentation of the occurrence of infections. Blood counts (white blood cells, hemoglobin, platelets, and differential blood counts) should be obtained at least every 3 months. Bone marrow examination (morphology plus cytogenetics) is required once per year to search for acquired cytogenetic abnormalities, such as monosomy 7 or trisomy 21. Furthermore, following informed consent, bone marrow samples should be collected for research studies on the molecular analysis of the pathophysiology of CN and risk factors for leukemic evolution.

G-CSF receptor analysis can be performed on heparinized blood or bone marrow samples by laboratories associated with the SCNIR.

Conclusion

In light of the current literature and longitudinal data from the SCNIR, we suggest that the use of rHuG-CSF remain first-line treatment for most CN patients. HSCT from an HLA-identical sibling is beneficial for patients who are refractory to rHuG-CSF. For those patients in whom a G-CSF receptor mutation is identified, HSCT from an HLA-identical sibling is an option. Patients who develop monosomy 7, other significant chromosomal abnormalities, or MDS/leukemia should proceed urgently to HSCT. Data on alternative sources of donor stem cells are insufficient to assess outcome in patients with CN. Other than those patients who fail to respond to rHuG-CSF, the cytokine should be employed to maintain an ANC ranging from 1.0 to 5.0 $\times$ 10^9/L with amelioration of symptoms.

All CN patients, regardless of their treatment or response, are at risk of developing MDS or leukemia at an actual incidence of 11.5% today and a cumulative incidence of 21% after 10 years. With increasing genetic analyses, it may become possible to correlate the leukemic risk with the underlying genetic defect. Careful monitoring for cytogenetic abnormalities and G-CSF receptor mutation is necessary to initiate HSCT as soon as any of these occur. Despite the significant risk of leukemia, HSCT-related morbidity is also significant and, therefore, in patients without signs of leukemia or MDS, HSCT should be restricted to G-CSF nonresponders.

Acknowledgment

The authors thank all colleagues associated with the Data Collection Centers of the Severe Chronic Neutropenia International Registry at the University of Washington, Seattle, WA (Audrey Anna Bolyard and Tammy Cottle), and the Medizinische Hochschule, Hannover, Germany (Beate Schwinzer and Gusal Pracht) for their continued assistance. We are also grateful to the many physicians worldwide who faithfully and generously submitted data on their patients. The authors gratefully acknowledge the important contribution of the Advisory Board and the European Liason Physician Group of the Severe Chronic Neutropenia International Registry and support from the National Institutes of Health (USA), the European Union, and Amgen Inc, Thousand Oaks, CA.

References

1. Kostmann R: Infantile genetic agranulocytosis. Acta Pediatr Scand 45: 1-78, 1956
2. Kostmann R: Infantile genetic agranulocytosis: A review with presentation of ten new cases. Acta Pediatr Scand 64:362-368, 1975
3. Rappeport J, Parkman R, Newburger P, Camitta BM, Chusid MJ: Correction of infantile granulocytosis (Kostmann syndrome) by allogeneic bone marrow transplantation. Am J Med 68:605-609, 1980
4. Souza L, Boone T, Gabrilove J, Lai PH, Zsebo KM, Murdock DC, et al: Recombinant human granulocyte colony-stimulating factor: Effects on normal and leukemic myeloid cells. Science 232:61-65, 1986
5. Bonilla M, Gillio A, Ruggeiro M, Kernan NA, Brochstein JA, Abboud M, et al: Effects of recombinant human granulocyte colony-stimulating factor on neutropenia in patients with congenital agranulocytosis. N Engl J Med 320:1574-1580, 1989
6. Bonilla M, Dale D, Zeidler C, Last L, Reiter A, Ruggeiro M, et al: Long-term safety of treatment with recombinant human granulocyte colony-stimulating factor (r-metHuG-CSF) in patients with severe congenital neutropenias. Br J Hematol 88:723-730, 1994
7. Freedman MH: Safety of long-term administration of granulocyte col-

ony-stimulating factor for severe chronic neutropenia. Curr Opin Hematol 4:217-224, 1997
8. Welte K, Dale D: Pathophysiology and treatment of severe chronic neutropenia. Ann Hematol 72:158-165, 1996
9. Welte K, Boxer L: Severe chronic neutropenia: Pathophysiology and therapy. Semin Hematol 34:267-278, 1997
10. Zeidler C, Boxer L, Dale DC, Freedman MH, Kinsey S, Welte K: Management of Kostmann syndrome in the G-CSF era. Br J Haematol 109: 490-495, 2000
11. Zeidler C, Welte K, Barak Y, Barriga F, Bolyard AA, Boxer L, et al: Stem cell transplantation in patients with severe congenital neutropenia without evidence of leukemic transformation. Blood 95:1195-1198, 2000
12. Mempel K, Pietsch,T, Menzel, Zeidler C, Welte K: Increased serum levels of granulocyte colony-stimulating factor in patients with severe congenital neutropenia. Blood 77:1919-1922, 1991
13. Kyas U, Pietsch T, Welte K: Expression of receptors for granulocyte-colony stimulating factor on neutrtophilsfrom patients with severe congenital neutropenia and cyclic neutropenia. Blood 79:1144-1147, 1992
14. Horwitz, M, Benson KF, Person RE, Aprikyan AG, Dale DC: Mutations in ELA2, encoding neutrophil elastase, define a 21-day biological clock in cyclic haematopoesis. Nat Genet 23:433-436, 1999
15. Ancliff PJ, Gale RE, Watts MJ, Liesner R, Hann IM, Strobel S, Linch DC: Paternal mosaicism proves the pathogenic nature of mutations in neutrophil elastase in severe congenital neutropenia. Blood 100:707-709, 2002
16. Dale DC, Liles WC, Grawicz D, Aprikyan AG: Clinical implications of mutations of neutrophil elastase in congenital and cyclic neutropenia. J Pediatr Hematol Oncol 23:208-210, 2001
17. Donadieu J, Leblanc T, Meunier B, Barkaoui M, Fenneteau O, Bertrand Y, et al: Analysis of risk factors for myelodysplasia/leukemia and infectious death among patients with congenital neutropenia: Experience of the French Severe Chronic Neutropenia Study Group. Haematologica 90:45-53, 2005
18. Dale DC, Person RE, Bolyard AA, Aprikyan AG, Bos C, Bonilla MA, et al: Mutations in the gene encoding neutrophil elastase in congenital and cyclic neutropenia. Blood 96:2317-2322, 2000
19. Massullo P, Druhan LJ, Bunnell BA, Hunter MG, Robinson JM, Marsh CB, et al: Aberrant subcellular targeting of the G185R neutrophil elastase mutant associated with severe congenital neutropenia induces premature apoptosis of differentiating promyelocytes. Blood 105:3397-3404, 2005
20. Germeshausen M, Schulze H, Ballmaier M, Zeidler C, Welte K: Mutations in the gene encoding neutrophil elastase (ELA2) are not sufficient to cause the phenotype of congenital neutropenia. Br J Haematol 115: 1-4, 2001
21. Koellner I, Sodeik B, Schreek S, Heyn H, von Neuhoff N, Germeshausen M, et al.: Mutations in neutrophil elastase causino congenital neutropenia lead to cytoplasmic protein accumulation and induction of the unfolded protein response. Blood March 21, 2006 (Epub ahead of print)
22. Skokowa J, Cario G, Bucan V, Dan L, Wang Z, Scherr M, et al: LEF-1 transcription factor regulates proliferation and differentiation of myeloid progenitors in healthy individuals and in patients with severe congenital neutropenia (CN). Blood 106:390a, 2005 (abstr)
23. Bernard T, Gale R, Evans J, Linch DC: Mutations of the granulocyte-colony stimulating factor receptor in patients with severe congenital neutropenia are not required for transformation to acute myeloid leukaemia and may be a bystander phenomenon. Br J Haematol 101:141-149, 1998
24. Cassinat B, Bellanné-Chantelot C, Notz-Carrère A, Menot ML, Vaury C, Micheau M, et al: Screening for G-CSF receptor mutations in patients with secondary myeloid or lymphoid transformation of severe congenital neutropenia. A report from the French Neutropenia Register. Leukemia 18:1553-1555, 2004
25. Dong F, Russel KB, Tidow N, Freedman M, Fasth A, Neijens HJ, et al: Mutations in the gene for the granulocyte-colony stimulating factor receptor in patients with acute myeloid leukemia preceded by severe congenital neutropenia. N Engl J Med 333:487-493, 1995
26. Germeshausen M, Schulze H, Kratz C, Wilkens L, Repp R, Shannon K, et al: An acquired G-CSF receptor mutation results in increased proliferation of CMML cells from a patient with severe congenital neutropenia. Leukemia 19:611-617, 2005
27. Papadaki HA, Kosteas T, Gemetzi C, Damianaki A, Anagnou NP, Eliopoulos GD: Acute myeloid/NK precursor cell leukemia with trisomy 4 and a novel point mutation in the extracellular domain of the G-CSF receptor in a patient with chronic idiopathic neutropenia. Ann Hematol 83:345-348, 2004
28. Tidow N, Pilz C, Teichmann B, Muller-Brechlin A, Germeshausen M, Kasper B, et al: Clinical relevance of point mutations in the cytoplasmatic domain of the granulocyte-colony stimulating factor gene in patients with severe congenital neutropenia. Blood 88:2369-2375, 1997
29. Tschan CA, Pilz C, Zeidler C, Welte K, Germeshausen M: Time course of increasing numbers of mutations in the granulocyte colony-stimulating factor receptor gene in a patient with congenital neutropenia who developed leukemia. Blood 97:1882-1884, 2001
30. Jeha S, Chan KW, Aprikyan AG, Hoots WK, Culbert S, Zietz H, et al: Spontaneous remission of granulocyte colony-stimulating factor–associated leukemia in a child with severe congenital neutropenia. Blood 96:3647-3649, 2000
31. Bux J, Behrens G, Jaeger G, Welte K: Diagnosis and clinical course of autoimmune neutropenia in infancy: Analysis of 240 cases. Blood 91: 181-186, 1998
32. Dale D, Bonilla M, Davis M, Nakanishi AM, Hammond WP, Kurtzberg J, et al: A randomized controlled phase III trial of recombinant human granulocyte colony-stimulating factor (Filgrastim) for treatment of severe chronic neutropenia. Blood 81:2496-2502, 1993
33. Welte K, Zeidler C, Reiter A, Muller W, Odenwald E, Souza L, Riehm H: Differential effects of granulocyte-macrophage colony-stimulating factor and granulocyte colony-stimulating factor in children with severe congenital neutropenia. Blood 75:1056-1063, 1990
34. Zeidler C, Vogel R, Wyres M, et al: Beneficial effects of stem cell factor (SCF) in children with severe congenital neutropenias refractory to G-CSF. Blood 92:380a, 1998 (abstr)
35. Gilman P, Jackson D, Guild H: Congenital agranulocytosis: Prolonged survival and terminal acute leukemia. Blood 36:576-585, 1971
36. Rosen R, Kang S: Congenital agranulocytosis terminating in acute myelomonocytic leukemia. J Pediatr 94:406-408, 1979
37. Rosenberg PS, Alter BP, Bolyard AA , Bonilla MA, Boxer LA, Cham B, et al: The incidence of leukemia and mortality from sepsis in patients with severe congenital neutropenia receiving long-term G-CSF therapy. Blood, February 23, 2006 (Epub ahead of print)
38. Yakisan E, Schirg E, Zeidler C, Bischop NJ, Reiter A, et al: High incidence of significant bone loss in patients with severe congenital neutropenia (Kostmann's syndrome). J Pediatr 131:592-597, 1997

Seminars in
HEMATOLOGY

Inherited Thrombocytopenia: Congenital Amegakaryocytic Thrombocytopenia and Thrombocytopenia With Absent Radii

Amy E. Geddis

Thrombocytopenia in the newborn period can signify an inherited platelet disorder. Congenital amegakaryocytic thrombocytopenia (CAMT) and thrombocytopenia with absent radii (TAR) share features of isolated thrombocytopenia, reduced or absent marrow megakaryocytes, impaired responsiveness to thrombopoietin (TPO), and high plasma TPO levels. These disorders are most readily distinguished from each other by the finding of radial aplasia in TAR and the presence of *c-MPL* mutations in CAMT. In addition, their long-term outcomes are strikingly different: the development of trilineage marrow failure in CAMT in contrast to the general improvement of thrombocytopenia in TAR. The differential diagnosis for CAMT and TAR also includes other congenital disorders in which thrombocytopenia and radial abnormalities can be seen. In this article we will review our molecular and clinical understanding of these two inherited disorders of amegakaryocytosis.
Semin Hematol 43:196-203

Thrombocytopenia in the neonatal period is a common clinical problem. Although the majority of infants with thrombocytopenia have acquired disorders, it is also important to consider congenital disease in the newborn with low platelet counts as this diagnosis has important consequences for clinical management. At present, mutations in more than 10 different genes have been described in syndromes of inherited thrombocytopenia, including genes involved in the earliest stages of hematopoietic stem cell and megakaryocyte progenitor growth, megakaryocyte maturation, and platelet formation and function.[1,2] Despite advances in our knowledge, the molecular basis of many disorders remains incompletely understood. This chapter will summarize our present understanding of two inherited disorders that present with severe thrombocytopenia at birth: congenital amegakaryocytic thrombocytopenia (CAMT), for which the genetic defect is known, and thrombocytopenia with absent radii (TAR), which despite its distinctive features has eluded genetic explanation.

Department of Pediatrics, Division of Pediatric Hematology-Oncology, University of California San Diego, La Jolla, CA.
The author receives funding from K08 HL04470-06 and Cindy Matters.
Address correspondence to Amy E. Geddis, MD, PhD, 9500 Gilman Dr, Mailcode 0726, La Jolla, CA 92093-0726. E-mail: ageddis@ucsd.edu

Differential Diagnosis of Neonatal Thrombocytopenia: When to Suspect Inherited Disease

Thrombocytopenia in the newborn is a common response to a variety of stressors, as neonates have a limited capacity to increase platelet production when challenged.[3] Placental dysfunction manifest as pre-eclampsia and intrauterine growth retardation, anoxic insult, intrauterine infection with TORCH agents (Toxoplasmosis, Rubella, Cytomegalovirus, Herpes simplex virus, and Other infections including Epstein-Barr virus, hepatitis B, parvovirus, varicella zoster virus, or syphilis), sepsis, disseminated intravascular coagulation, thrombosis, and adverse effects of medications can all contribute to varying degrees of thrombocytopenia. Most of these thrombocytopenic infants are recognizably sick, and most often platelet counts improve with treatment of the underlying disorder and over time. Immune thrombocytopenia, either alloimmune or autoimmune, is an important cause of severe thrombocytopenia in an otherwise well-appearing newborn. In alloimmune thrombocytopenia, the mother's platelets are normal, whereas autoimmune thrombocytopenia can be suspected if the mother's count is low. Antiplatelet antibody detection and platelet antigen typing can be used to confirm the diagnosis of immune thrombocytopenia. Platelet counts may improve in response to the infusion of intrave-

 0037-1963/06/$-see front matter
doi:10.1053/j.seminhematol.2006.04.003

nous immunoglobulin, and in cases of alloimmune thrombocytopenia the symptomatic child should be transfused with washed platelets from the mother or an antigen-negative donor. Platelet counts will increase with time as the maternally derived antibody disappears. Infants of subsequent pregnancies of women who have had children with either form of immune-mediated platelet destruction are at risk for neonatal thrombocytopenia.

It may be difficult to predict which infant with low platelets has an acquired disorder that will improve and which one may have an inherited thrombocytopenia. A family history of thrombocytopenia may suggest an inherited disorder; however, in some cases of recessive inheritance, variable penetrance or sporadic mutation a family history may not be elicited even when a genetic disorder is present. In addition, chronic immune thrombocytopenia in a mother who transmits antibodies to her fetus may create the appearance of an inherited disorder. Physical findings may lead to the suspicion of a congenital disorder; the presence of limb anomalies, cardiac or renal disorders, growth deficiency, or other dysmorphisms suggests genetic disease. However, some genetic disorders are not characterized by physical findings or the signs may not always be present. Laboratory testing can support a diagnosis of inherited disease. A peripheral blood smear should be examined for the confirmation of thrombocytopenia, to assess platelet size and morphology, and to look for associated abnormalities in erythrocytes and neutrophils. Large platelets may be seen in disorders of increased platelet destruction, but they are also characteristic of some inherited disorders of thrombocytopenia, including Bernard Soulier syndrome, MYH9-related disease, and mutations of GATA1, whereas small platelets are associated with Wiskott-Aldrich syndrome. Pale-appearing platelets may indicate a specific granule deficiency. Dysmorphic red blood cells and anemia occur in boys with mutations of GATA1, and neutrophil inclusions are a hallmark of MYH9-related disease. However, in many cases platelet appearance is not remarkable. Determination of megakaryocyte number and morphologic appearance by bone marrow aspiration and biopsy remains important in assessing whether thrombocytopenia is due to impaired production, in which case megakaryocytes are typically absent, reduced, or small, or peripheral platelet destruction, in which megakaryocytes are normal or increased. Cytogenetic testing can be helpful, as an abnormal karyotype suggests a genetic disorder and may even be diagnostic. In some cases, specific genes can be sequenced for mutations known to be associated with inherited thrombocytopenia.

Specialized laboratory assays may provide measures of megakaryopoiesis to distinguish between disorders of platelet production versus platelet destruction. For example, reticulated platelets, similar to erythrocyte reticulocytes, can be used as an indirect measure of platelet production and in neonates correlate with quantitative assays of megakaryocyte progenitors.[4] Measurement of plasma glycocalicin levels also has been used as a marker of platelet turnover.[5] In addition, plasma thrombopoietin (TPO) levels are typically elevated in patients with thrombocytopenia due to absence of megakaryocytes, whereas TPO levels are relatively normal in thrombocytopenia due to peripheral platelet destruction.[6] In vitro colony formation assesses the number of megakaryocyte progenitors in a marrow sample and their responsiveness to TPO. The above assays may be obtained through specialized research laboratories but are not clinically available, and therefore presently are of limited utility for patient management.

Overview of Thrombopoiesis

As with all blood cells, platelets have their ultimate origin in the hematopoietic stem cell. Under the influence of lineage-specific cytokines and transcription factors, hematopoietic stem cells have the potential to survive in a quiescent state, undergo self-renewing divisions, or expand and differentiate to produce the complete spectrum of hematopoiesis, including cells of the myeloid, erythroid, and megakaryocytic lineages. TPO is a critical cytokine for all stages of megakaryocyte development, from hematopoietic stem cell survival and expansion to megakaryocytic progenitor survival, expansion, and differentiation.[7] The receptor for thrombopoietin is c-Mpl, a cytokine receptor without intrinsic kinase activity. Instead, c-Mpl utilizes a cytoplasmic tyrosine kinase, Jak2, to transduce its signals.[8] Consistent with the importance of TPO for both stem cells and megakaryocytes, genetically engineered mice deficient in TPO or c-Mpl demonstrate not only peripheral thrombocytopenia but also reduced numbers of hematopoietic stem cells and progenitors of all lineages.[9,10]

Under normal conditions the liver is the site of production for approximately half of the body's TPO, whereas the remainder is produced by the kidney, muscles and stromal cells of the bone marrow. TPO is removed from the circulation by receptor-bearing cells, primarily megakaryocytes and platelets, creating a feedback mechanism in which increased production of platelets results in the reduction of available TPO.[11] Conversely, circulating TPO levels are elevated when fewer receptor-bearing megakaryocytes and platelets are present. Although production of TPO in the liver is thought to be constitutive, TPO production in the bone marrow can be upregulated in response to thrombocytopenia,[12] and mutations that alter splicing of the TPO transcript can result in significant overproduction of TPO through increased translational efficiency.[13]

We are learning more about the mechanisms by which TPO provides the signals that stimulate stem cells, megakaryocytes, and platelets.[8] Inactive Jak2 normally associates with the unliganded homodimeric c-Mpl receptor. When TPO binds to c-Mpl, a conformational change occurs that brings the two molecules of Jak2 into sufficient proximity that one molecule of Jak2 can phosphorylate and activate the other. In addition, Jak2 phosphorylates the c-Mpl receptor and the transcription factors STAT3 and STAT5 and leads to the activation of the PI3K and Ras/Raf/MAPK pathways. The phosphorylation events that result from the activation of these pathways promote the assembly of signaling complexes, mediate the translocation of molecules to and from the membrane or in and out of the nucleus, and regulate the destruction of proteins within the cell, ultimately controlling cell survival, proliferation, and maturation. Additional cytokines, including stem cell factor, interleukin-3, and interleukin-6, can synergize with TPO in promoting thrombopoiesis, but these cytokines cannot support normal megakaryopoiesis on their own.

In addition to cytokine stimulation described above, megakaryocyte differentiation also requires the concerted action of hematopoietic transcription factors, including members of the Hox family, Runx1, FLI1, GATA1, FOG1, and NF-E2.[1,2,14] Many of these factors also have critical roles in myelopoiesis (Runx1)[15] and erythropoiesis (GATA1, FLI1, and NF-E2),[14,16,17]and mutations involving Runx1 and GATA1 have been implicated in leukemogenesis.[16,18] The discovery of inherited thrombocytopenia syndromes caused by mutations involving these transcription factors contributes enormously to our understanding of the mechanisms by which they direct megakaryopoiesis. Transcription factors may regulate the cell's ability to respond to TPO, for example, by driving expression of c-Mpl,[19] so that cytokine signaling and transcriptional regulation of megakaryocyte maturation are interrelated.

The process of megakaryocyte maturation is complex. As they mature, megakaryocytes become highly polyploid, enlarge, and develop specialized cytoplasmic structures, including alpha and dense granules, a surface-connected canalicular system, and platelet territories. This process culminates in the formation of branching microtubule-based processes, called proplatelets.[20] The microtubules within the shaft of the proplatelets facilitate the transport of granules and mitochondria from the cell body to the ends of the processes where platelets will be released.[21] At the ends of the processes, microtubules form a coiled structure that will support the disc-like shape of the circulating platelet.[20,22] Once released into the circulation, platelets normally survive for approximately 10 days before they senesce and are removed from the blood by the spleen.

Congenital Thrombocytopenia Without Physical Features: CAMT

CAMT is an autosomal recessive disorder that presents at birth with severe thrombocytopenia. Mean platelet counts at diagnosis are 21,000/μL, with platelets of normal size and appearance on peripheral blood smear.[23] Many affected children have cutaneous purpura or hemorrhage within hours of delivery, and they may suffer intracranial bleeding before or after birth.[23] In contrast to neonatal immune thrombocytopenias, at presentation infants with CAMT have normocellular bone marrows with an isolated reduction or absence of megakaryocytes.[24] When they are obtained, plasma TPO levels are high, consistent with the severe deficiency of megakaryocytes and platelets.[6] No specific congenital malformation is characteristic of CAMT. Although physical abnormalities have been described in newborns with hematologic features suggestive of CAMT, these children may have had other syndromes such as Noonan's syndrome (with mutation of PTPN11) or severe X-linked dyskeratosis congenita.[23] However, in large patient series, there is an increased incidence of psychomotor retardation in patients with CAMT, which cannot be fully attributed to the sequelae of intracranial bleeding.[23] In general, strong consideration should be given to diagnoses other than CAMT when a newborn presents with thrombocytopenia and congenital malformations.

Although originally clinically defined as thrombocytopenia with reduced or absent megakaryocytes in the bone marrow and normal radii, CAMT can now be molecularly defined by mutation of the TPO receptor, c-Mpl.[6,25] Prior to 1999,[25] studies of clinically defined CAMT may have included patients that did not have c-Mpl mutations, complicating the interpretation of reports of associated features and outcomes. Today, mutations have been found throughout the *c-MPL* gene, including nonsense, missense, and splicing mutations; in the most severely affected patients, there is a clustering of mutations in exons 2 and 3, encoding the first cytokine receptor homology domain.[23] Some individuals with CAMT have inherited two different mutations of *c-MPL*, resulting in a compound heterozygous state[23,25-27]; in addition, there is a high rate of consanguinity between parents of children with CAMT, leading to the inheritance of homozygous *c-MPL* mutations.[23] Certified mutation analysis of this gene can now be obtained at GeneDx (Gaithersburg, MD), which should facilitate accurate diagnosis of CAMT.

In a child who presents with features of CAMT but does not have a mutation in *c-MPL*, alternative syndromes should be considered. Radial abnormalities suggest the diagnosis of TAR, Fanconi anemia, or ATRUS (discussed below). Platelet size and inheritance pattern can be helpful in formulating the differential diagnosis. Autosomal dominant inheritance of normal sized platelets is seen in familial platelet syndrome with predisposition to acute myeloid leukemia (due to haploinsufficient expression of Runx1)[18] and in families with mutations in the gene for the kinase MASTL.[28] Congenital heart disease and neurologic deficits, with deletion of the terminal position of chromosome 11q, accompany thrombocytopenia in the Paris Trousseau syndrome.[29] Boys with small platelets, with or without eczema, should be evaluated for mutations of WASp.[30] X-linked inheritance of thrombocytopenia with large platelets and dyserythropoiesis or granule deficiency should prompt analysis for mutations of GATA1.[31,32] Autosomal dominant inheritance of macrothrombocytopenia accompanied by leukocyte inclusions suggests MYH9-related disease,[33] and autosomal recessive inheritance of macrothrombocytopenia is seen in Bernard Soulier syndrome.[34] Novel gene mutations are also possible. Curiously, no case of amegakaryocytic thrombocytopenia has been reported that is due to a mutation of TPO, although mouse models would suggest that absence of TPO results in the same phenotype as absence of c-Mpl.[35] Moreover, an acquired case of amegakaryocytic thrombocytopenia with evolution to stem cell failure was described in a patient with anti-TPO antibodies.[36] Similarly, isolated mutations in NF-E2 or FLI1 might be expected to cause amegakaryocytic thrombocytopenia, possibly with anemia, but these mutations have not been described in humans.

Consistent with the importance of TPO for the hematopoietic stem cell, children with CAMT usually progress from isolated thrombocytopenia to aplastic anemia within 5 years of life.[7,23,24] Analysis of large series has defined two groups of patients with CAMT: those with complete loss of functional c-Mpl (type I) and those with a partially functional receptor (type II).[6,23] Children in the latter group frequently showed a transient improvement in their platelet counts to over 50,000/μL during the first year of life, which could persist as long as several years. In addition, these children had a delayed progression to aplastic anemia, with a mean onset of pancytopenia at 5 years of age as compared to almost 2 years in type I patients; one patient was 14 years old and had not yet developed pancytopenia. Thus, a wide range of phenotypes may exist for CAMT, including some children or even young adults with relatively mild thrombocytopenia or trilineage marrow failure in which a thrombocytopenic phase was not recognized. In addition to the development of aplastic anemia, acute myeloid leukemia and myelodysplastic syndrome have been reported to occur in patients with CAMT, although the incidence or underlying mechanism of these complications is unclear.[23,37,38]

Treatment options in CAMT are limited. Bleeding is of primary concern: cutaneous, gastrointestinal, pulmonary, and intracranial hemorrhage.[23,24] Supportive care includes judicious use of unrelated donor platelet transfusions (leukocyte-reduced, and irradiated), avoidance of nonsteroidal anti-inflammatory medications and aspirin, adjunctive therapies such as anti-fibrinolytic agents for minor bleeding, and monitoring for the development of additional cytopenias. Desmopressin acetate (DDAVP) should be avoided in small infants due to the risk of hyponatremia but may be useful in older children and adults. Cytokine therapy with interleukin-3 and granulocyte-macrophage colony-stimulating factor has been attempted but only resulted in transient responses.[39,40] Development of aplastic anemia leads to additional complications including increasing transfusion requirements and risk of infection.

Hematopoietic stem cell transplant remains the only definitive therapy for CAMT. Children and their family members should be human leukocyte antigen (HLA)-typed to identify possible matched related donors. Siblings that are heterozygous for a c-Mpl mutation may have abnormal megakaryopoiesis despite normal peripheral platelet counts,[27] but at least in one case a sibling carrier has been successfully used as a donor.[41] If a matched sibling donor is available, hematopoietic stem cell transplantation is the treatment of choice. If a matched related donor is not available, transplantation may still be necessary, especially when marrow failure ensues, but the reported outcomes using matched unrelated donors have been poor due to regimen-related toxicity and a high rate of engraftment failure.[23,42,43] Stem cell transplantation using low-intensity conditioning, successful in one reported patient with CAMT, may be one approach to lessen transplantation-related mortality if barriers to engraftment can be overcome.[44]

Therapies in development may be beneficial to patients with CAMT. Recent in vitro data suggest that, while patients with CAMT are not sensitive to TPO, patients with type II c-Mpl mutations may respond to engineered c-Mpl agonist antibodies.[45] New TPO-mimetics should be tested as pharmacologic agents for binding and activity towards partially functional c-Mpl receptors.[46] In addition, CAMT is a candidate disease for gene therapy, as restoration of a normal c-Mpl would provide in vivo selection of corrected hematopoietic stem cells.[47]

Congenital Thrombocytopenia With Skeletal Abnormalities: TAR

TAR is a well-defined syndrome characterized by thrombocytopenia of variable severity and bilateral radial aplasia. Importantly, thumbs are present, although they may be hypoplastic or anteriorly placed; this feature can be useful in distinguishing TAR from other congenital disorders in which the radius is abnormal. At birth, platelet counts range from 10,000 to 100,000/μL, and on the peripheral smear platelets are normal in size. Because platelet levels can fluctuate, a normal count in a newborn with the radial features of TAR should be repeated at several intervals prior to excluding the diagnosis. Functional platelet defects have been reported in several patients.[48,49] Eosinophilia and leukemoid reactions also may be seen.[50] As in CAMT, examination of the bone marrow shows a reduction in the number and maturity of megakaryocytes in an otherwise normocellular specimen. Plasma TPO levels are elevated, consistent with decreased megakaryocyte and platelet production.[51] Unlike in CAMT, congenital abnormalities are a prominent characteristic in TAR. Bilateral radial aplasia is the defining skeletal feature of TAR but additional abnormalities are frequent. More extensive upper limb malformations may be present, including hypoplasia of the humerus or even phocomelia. Lower limb malformations occur in approximately 50% of patients, including patellar abnormalities, hip dislocation, bowing of the legs, absence of the tibial/fibular joint, and phocomelia.[24,50,52-54] Nonskeletal abnormalities are also common: gastroenteritis and cow's milk intolerance in 47%, genitourinary tract malformations in 23%, cardiac defects (usually septal defects and tetralogy of Fallot) in 15%, facial dysmorphism in 53%, a tendency to short stature in 95% and macrocephaly in 76%, and capillary hemangiomata in 24%.[52,55] When a child is born with absent radii, consultation from a clinical geneticist and a multisystem evaluation is imperative to evaluate patients for associated congenital malformations and to establish the correct diagnosis.

While seemingly distinctive, TAR must be differentiated from several other genetic syndromes with radial and hematologic abnormalities. Fanconi anemia (FA) is a chromosomal instability syndrome characterized by marrow failure that may present with thrombocytopenia, development of marrow aplasia, predisposition to malignancy, limb malformations, abnormal pigmentation and growth failure[37,56] (reviewed by Bagby and Alter in this volume). Unlike in TAR, in FA thrombocytopenia is usually not present at birth and thumbs may be absent. Alternatively, patients with FA may have no physical findings. FA can be diagnosed by increased chromosomal breakage in the presence of clastogenic agents such as di-epoxybutane. Extensive analysis using cells from patients with FA has identified mutations in at least 12 genes that cooperate in DNA repair. Radial abnormalities are also a characteristic feature of amegakaryocytic thrombocytopenia with radioulnar synostosis (ATRUS), in which thrombocytopenia at birth is associated with bilateral proximal fusion of the radius and ulna. Development of aplastic anemia has been reported in association with radioulnar synostosis.[57,58] In two families with ATRUS, a mutation in the homeobox family member HoxA11 was identified,[59] although additional children with features of ATRUS have been described who may not have HoxA11 mutations; additional genes may be involved.[24,57] The role of the HoxA11 transcription factor in megakaryopoiesis remains unclear. HoxA11 alterations have been described in chromosomal translocations involved in T-cell leukemia and chronic myelogenous leukemia,[60,61] but mouse models of HoxA11 deletion are not reported to have a platelet phenotype.[62] Trisomy involving chromosome 18 can also present with radial hypoplasia and impaired platelet production, accompanied by esophageal atresia.[63] Although esophageal anomalies are not common in TAR, one child with thrombocytopenia and unilateral radial aplasia also had a a tracheo-esophageal fistula.[64]

Several syndromes characterized by radial abnormalities but not associated with thrombocytopenia must be distinguished from TAR. Roberts syndrome is an autosomal recessive disorder of tetraphocomelia and craniofacial anomalies. Recently Roberts syndrome and a milder variant called SC phocomelia were determined to be due to inactivating mutations of ESCO1 (establishment of cohesion homolog 2), a protein important for sister chromatid cohesion in S-phase.[65] Impaired sister chromatid cohesion can be seen microscopically as centromeric "puffing," or splitting. TAR and Roberts syndrome were postulated to be allelic disorders,[66] but no defect in sister chromatid cohesion has been demonstrated in TAR.[52] Several syndromes with overlapping characteristics, including radial aplasia, craniosynostosis, and patellar abnormalities (Baller-Gerold, Rothmund-Thomson, and Rapadilino syndromes), may be due to mutations in RecQ DNA recombinase, which is involved in the initiation of DNA recombination and sister chromatid cohesion.[67] Holt-Oran syndrome, in which radial defects coexist with cardiac malformations, is due to mutations in TBX5, a T-box transcription factor important for patterning of the sternum and forearms and development of the heart.[68,69] The genetic characterization of these phenotypically similar syndromes is helpful in making definitive diagnoses and helps us to understand the molecular mechanisms underlying these fascinating congenital malformations.

Although less common in developed countries today, TAR and other genetic phocomelia syndromes must be distinguished from thalidomide embryopathy.[70]

Despite these advances in phenotypically similar syndromes, the genetic basis of TAR remains unknown. The inheritance pattern of TAR is unclear, and although considered in most cases to be an autosomal recessive disorder, families with a pattern of autosomal dominant inheritance with variable penetrance have been described.[52,66,71-73] Unlike in CAMT, in TAR parental consanguinity is unusual.[74,75] An excess of affected females compared to males (27:7 in one series, 26:14 in another) suggests the possibility of an X-linked dominant trait with lethality in males.[75,76] Karyotypic abnormalities found in a few patients are of unclear significance, and no recurrent chromosomal changes have been seen.[52] Because studies with megakaryocytes and platelets from affected patients indicate that they are insensitive to TPO,[51,77] *TPO* and *c-MPL* were investigated as candidate genes. However, expression of *TPO* and *c-MPL* is normal, and mutations in *c-MPL* have not been identified.[78,79] Mutations have also been sought in Hox family genes in patients with TAR, but none has been identified.[80]

Although both present with isolated thrombocytopenia, the natural history of TAR is distinct from that of CAMT. Hemorrhage in the neonatal period is a problem with both disorders, but in TAR, platelet counts generally improve over the first year of life and may eventually approach normal adult levels. Platelet counts can fluctuate and in particular decrease in response to exacerbations of the gastroenteritis that frequently complicates the course of these patients.[52,55] Unlike CAMT and possibly ATRUS, TAR patients do not develop bone marrow failure; however, like CAMT, the late development of leukemia, including acute myeloid leukemia and acute lymphocytic leukemia, has been reported in TAR.[81-83] Despite one report of nonhematologic malignancy in a patient with the features of TAR whose lymphocytes exhibited radiation hypersensitivity,[84] abnormal chromosomal breakage is not a characteristic of TAR.[52] The basis for a predisposition to leukemia is not understood, and the relative risk of malignancy is not known. It is surprising that despite sharing a resistance to stimulation by TPO, the thrombocytopenia of TAR generally improves and patients do not develop aplastic anemia; in contrast, CAMT patients with defective c- Mpl usually develop pancytopenia.

Treatment

The treatment of TAR is largely supportive, with platelet transfusions in the first year of life as needed to control bleeding symptoms. Adjunctive therapies as described above for CAMT, including fibrinolytic agents and, for older children, DDAVP, can be helpful for minor bleeding. Stem cell transplantation is generally not indicated, as thrombocytopenia is expected to improve and aplastic anemia does not develop, but matched related donor transplantation was successful in a case of persistent thrombocytopenia to facilitate orthopedic surgery.[85] An adult with persistent thrombocytopenia was reported to improve after splenectomy.[86] Although their platelets are insensitive to TPO, administration of interleukin-6 improved platelet counts in a patient with TAR, but use of interleukin-6 causes fevers and chills[87] and its clinical development has been halted. After the first year of life, management of nonhematologic manifestations may dominate the clinical picture. Orthopedic procedures are often necessary, including centralization of the hand to improve function and straightening of the lower extremities to correct varus deformities.[52,54]

Future Directions

Our understanding of the inherited thrombocytopenias including CAMT and TAR is limited by their rarity; much of the published literature consists of case studies and small series, and additional children are likely not diagnosed or reported. The formation of collaborative research efforts to facilitate the collection of data on larger numbers of affected patients will help us to learn more of the incidence, associated complications, and molecular mechanisms of these disorders. Several registries for inherited platelet disorders are seeking to recruit patients, including the Inherited Bone Marrow Failure Registry (National Cancer Institute; http://marrowfailure.cancer.gov), the Study of Megakaryocytes from Patients with Abnormal Platelet Vesicles (National Human Genome Research Institute; http://www.clinicaltrials.gov/ct/show/NCT00086476), and a newly forming Registry and Shared Resource for Inherited Disorders of Platelet Number. In addition, support groups have formed for patients with thrombocytopenia in general (Platelet Disorders Support Association; www.pdsa.org) and for TAR (Thrombocytopenia Absent Radius Syndrome Association, TAR Syndrome Support Group; http://www.ivh.se/TAR). These cooperative efforts are essential to provide access for physicians, researchers and patients to the information and resources necessary to diagnose, manage and understand these rare disorders.

References

1. Geddis AE, Kaushansky K: Inherited thrombocytopenias: Toward a molecular understanding of disorders of platelet production. Curr Opin Pediatr 16:15-22, 2004
2. Balduini CL, Iolascon A, Savoia A: Inherited thrombocytopenias: From genes to therapy. Haematologica 87:860-880, 2002
3. Roberts IA, Murray NA: Thrombocytopenia in the newborn. Curr Opin Pediatr 15:17-23, 2003
4. Saxonhouse MA, Christensen RD, Walker DM, Hutson AD, Sola MC: The concentration of circulating megakaryocyte progenitors in preterm neonates is a function of post-conceptional age. Early Hum Dev 78: 119-124, 2004
5. van den Oudenrijn S, Bruin M, Folman CC, Bussel J, de Haas M, von dem Borne AE: Three parameters, plasma thrombopoietin levels, plasma glycocalicin levels and megakaryocyte culture, distinguish between different causes of congenital thrombocytopenia. Br J Haematol 117:390-398, 2002
6. Ballmaier M, Germeshausen M, Schulze H, Cherkaoui K, Lang S, Gaudig A, et al: c-mpl mutations are the cause of congenital amegakaryocytic thrombocytopenia. Blood 97:139-146, 2001
7. Ballmaier M, Germeshausen M, Krukemeier S, Welte K: Thrombopoietin is essential for the maintenance of normal hematopoiesis in humans: Development of aplastic anemia in patients with congenital amegakaryocytic thrombocytopenia. Ann N Y Acad Sci 996:17-25, 2003
8. Geddis AE, Linden HM, Kaushansky K: Thrombopoietin: A pan-hematopoietic cytokine. Cytokine Growth Factor Rev 13:61-73, 2002
9. Murone M, Carpenter DA, de Sauvage FJ: Hematopoietic deficiencies in c-mpl and TPO knockout mice. Stem Cells 16:1-6, 1998
10. Alexander WS, Roberts AW, Nicola NA, Li R, Metcalf D: Deficiencies in progenitor cells of multiple hematopoietic lineages and defective megakaryocytopoiesis in mice lacking the thrombopoietic receptor c-Mpl. Blood 87:2162-2170, 1996
11. Nagata Y, Shozaki Y, Nagahisa H, Nagasawa T, Abe T, Todokoro K: Serum thrombopoietin level is not regulated by transcription but by the total counts of both megakaryocytes and platelets during thrombocytopenia and thrombocytosis. Thromb Haemost 77:808-814, 1997
12. McCarty JM, Sprugel KH, Fox NE, Sabath DE, Kaushansky K: Murine thrombopoietin mRNA levels are modulated by platelet count. Blood 86:3668-3675, 1995
13. Wiestner A, Schlemper RJ, van der Maas AP, Skoda RC: An activating splice donor mutation in the thrombopoietin gene causes hereditary thrombocythaemia. Nat Genet 18:49-52, 1998
14. Shivdasani RA: Molecular and transcriptional regulation of megakaryocyte differentiation. Stem Cells 19:397-407, 2001
15. Yergeau DA, Hetherington CJ, Wang Q, Zhang P, Sharpe AH, Binder M, et al: Embryonic lethality and impairment of haematopoiesis in mice heterozygous for an AML1-ETO fusion gene. Nat Genet 15:303-306, 1997
16. Crispino JD: GATA1 in normal and malignant hematopoiesis. Semin Cell Dev Biol 16:137-147, 2005
17. Kawada H, Ito T, Pharr PN, Spyropoulos DD, Watson DK, Ogawa M: Defective megakaryopoiesis and abnormal erythroid development in Fli-1 gene-targeted mice. Int J Hematol 73:463-468, 2001
18. Song WJ, Sullivan MG, Legare RD, Hutchings S, Tan X, Kufrin D, et al: Haploinsufficiency of CBFA2 causes familial thrombocytopenia with propensity to develop acute myelogenous leukaemia. Nat Genet 23: 166-175, 1999
19. Deveaux S, Filipe A, Lemarchandel V, Ghysdael J, Romeo PH, Mignotte V: Analysis of the thrombopoietin receptor (MPL) promoter implicates GATA and Ets proteins in the coregulation of megakaryocyte-specific genes. Blood 87:4678-4685, 1996
20. Italiano JE Jr, Lecine P, Shivdasani RA, Hartwig JH: Blood platelets are assembled principally at the ends of proplatelet processes produced by differentiated megakaryocytes. J Cell Biol 47:1299-1312, 1999
21. Richardson JL, Shivdasani RA, Boers C, Hartwig JH, Italiano JE Jr: Mechanisms of organelle transport and capture along proplatelets during platelet production. Blood 106:4066-4075, 2005
22. Italiano JE Jr, Bergmeier W, Tiwari S, Falet H, Hartwig JH, Hoffmeister KM, et al: Mechanisms and implications of platelet discoid shape. Blood 101:4789-4796, 2003
23. King S, Germeshausen M, Strauss G, Welte K, Ballmaier M: Congenital amegakaryocytic thrombocytopenia: A retrospective clinical analysis of 20 patients. Br J Haematol 131:636-644, 2005
24. Cines DB, Bussel JB, McMillan RB, Zehnder JL: Congenital and acquired thrombocytopenia. Hematology (Am Soc Hematol Educ Program) 390-406, 2004
25. Ihara K, Ishii E, Eguchi M, Takada H, Suminoe A, Good RA, et al: Identification of mutations in the c-mpl gene in congenital amegakaryocytic thrombocytopenia. Proc Natl Acad Sci U S A 96: 3132-3136, 1999
26. Gandhi MJ, Pendergrass TW, Cummings CC, Ihara K, Blau CA, Drachman JG: Congenital amegakaryocytic thrombocytopenia in three siblings: Molecular analysis of atypical clinical presentation. Exp Hematol 33:1215-1221, 2005
27. Tonelli R, Scardovi AL, Pession A, Strippoli P, Bonsi L, Vitale L, et al: Compound heterozygosity for two different amino-acid substitution mutations in the thrombopoietin receptor (c-mpl gene) in congenital amegakaryocytic thrombocytopenia (CAMT). Hum Genet 107:225-233, 2000
28. Gandhi MJ, Cummings CL, Drachman JG: FLJ14813 missense mutation: a candidate for autosomal dominant thrombocytopenia on human chromosome 10. Hum Hered 55:66-70, 2003
29. Krishnamurti L, Neglia JP, Nagarajan R, Berry SA, Lohr J, Hirsch B, et al: Paris-Trousseau syndrome platelets in a child with Jacobsen's syndrome. Am J Hematol 66:295-299, 2001
30. Rengan R, Ochs HD: Molecular biology of the Wiskott-Aldrich syndrome. Rev Immunogenet 2:243-255, 2000
31. Nichols KE, Crispino JD, Poncz M, White JG, Orkin SH, Maris JM, et al:

Familial dyserythropoietic anaemia and thrombocytopenia due to an inherited mutation in GATA1. Nat Genet 24:266-270, 2000
32. Balduini CL, Pecci A, Loffredo G, Izzo P, Noris P, Grosso M, et al: Effects of the R216Q mutation of GATA-1 on erythropoiesis and megakaryocytopoiesis. Thromb Haemost 91:129-140, 2004
33. Seri M, Cusano R, Gangarossa S, Caridi G, Bordo D, Lo Nigro C, et al: Mutations in MYH9 result in the May-Hegglin anomaly, and Fechtner and Sebastian syndromes. The May-Heggllin/Fechtner Syndrome Consortium. Nat Genet 26:103-105, 2000
34. Caen JP, Nurden AT, Jeanneau C, Michel H, Tobelem G, Levy-Toledano S, et al: Bernard-Soulier syndrome: A new platelet glycoprotein abnormality. Its relationship with platelet adhesion to subendothelium and with the factor VIII von Willebrand protein. J Lab Clin Med 87: 586-596, 1976
35. Carver-Moore K, Broxmeyer HE, Luoh SM, Cooper S, Peng J, Burstein SA, et al: Low levels of erythroid and myeloid progenitors in thrombopoietin-and c-mpl-deficient mice. Blood 88:803-808, 1996
36. Basser RL, O'Flaherty E, Green M, Edmonds M, Nichol J, Menchaca DM, et al: Development of pancytopenia with neutralizing antibodies to thrombopoietin after multicycle chemotherapy supported by megakaryocyte growth and development factor. Blood 99:2599-2602, 2002
37. Alter BP: Bone marrow failure: A child is not just a small adult (but an adult can have a childhood disease). Hematology (Am Soc Hematol Educ Program) 96-103, 2005
38. Germeshausen M, Ballmaier M, Welte K: Implications of mutations in hematopoietic growth factor receptor genes in congenital cytopenias. Ann N Y Acad Sci 938:305-320, 2001
39. Taylor DS, Lee Y, Sieff CA, Homans A, Garrison L, Guinan EC: Phase I/II trial of PIXY321 (granulocyte-macrophage colony stimulating factor/interleukin-3 fusion protein) for treatment of inherited and acquired marrow failure syndromes. Br J Haematol 103:304-307, 1998
40. Guinan EC, Lee YS, Lopez KD, Kohler S, Oette DH, Bruno E, et al: Effects of interleukin-3 and granulocyte-macrophage colony-stimulating factor on thrombopoiesis in congenital amegakaryocytic thrombocytopenia. Blood 81:1691-1698, 1993
41. Muraoka K, Ishii E, Ihara K, Imayoshi M, Miyazaki S, Hara T, et al: Successful bone marrow transplantation in a patient with c-mpl-mutated congenital amegakaryocytic thrombocytopenia from a carrier donor. Pediatr Transplant 9:101-103, 2005
42. Lackner A, Basu O, Bierings M, Lassay L, Schaefer UW, Revesz T, et al: Haematopoietic stem cell transplantation for amegakaryocytic thrombocytopenia. Br J Haematol 109:773-775, 2000
43. MacMillan ML, Davies SM, Wagner JE, Ramsay NK: Engraftment of unrelated donor stem cells in children with familial amegakaryocytic thrombocytopenia. Bone Marrow Transplant 21:735-737, 1998
44. Steele M, Hitzler J, Doyle JJ, Germeshausen M, Fernandez CV, Yuille K, et al: Reduced intensity hematopoietic stem-cell transplantation across human leukocyte antigen barriers in a patient with congenital amegakaryocytic thrombocytopenia and monosomy 7. Pediatr Blood Cancer 45:212-216, 2005
45. Orita T, Tsunoda H, Yabuta N, Nakano K, Yoshino T, Hirata Y, et al: A novel therapeutic approach for thrombocytopenia by minibody agonist of the thrombopoietin receptor. Blood 105:562-566, 2005
46. Wang B, Nichol JL, Sullivan JT: Pharmacodynamics and pharmacokinetics of AMG 531, a novel thrombopoietin receptor ligand. Clin Pharmacol Ther 76:628-638, 2004
47. Richard RE, Blau CA: Small-molecule-directed mpl signaling can complement growth factors to selectively expand genetically modified cord blood cells. Stem Cells 21:71-78, 2003
48. Zahavi J, Gale R, Kakkar VV: Storage pool disease of platelets in an infant with thrombocytopenic absent radii (TAR) syndrome simulating Fanconi's anaemia. Haemostasis 10:121-133, 1981
49. Day HJ, Holmsen H: Platelet adenine nucleotide "storage pool deficiency" in thrombocytopenic absent radii syndrome. JAMA 221:1053-1054, 1972
50. Hedberg VA, Lipton JM: Thrombocytopenia with absent radii. A review of 100 cases. Am J Pediatr Hematol Oncol 10:51-64, 1988
51. Ballmaier M, Schulze H, Strauss G, Cherkaoui K, Wittner N, Lynen S, et al: Thrombopoietin in patients with congenital thrombocytopenia and absent radii: Elevated serum levels, normal receptor expression, but defective reactivity to thrombopoietin. Blood 90:612-619, 1997
52. Greenhalgh KL, Howell RT, Bottani A, Ancliff PJ, Brunner HG, Verschuuren-Bemelmans CC, et al: Thrombocytopenia-absent radius syndrome: A clinical genetic study. J Med Genet 39:876-881, 2002
53. Ray R, Zorn E, Kelly T, Hall JG, Sommer A: Lower limb anomalies in the thrombocytopenia absent-radius (TAR) syndrome. Am J Med Genet 7:523-528, 1980
54. Schoenecker PL, Cohn AK, Sedgwick WG, Manske PR, Salafsky I, Millar EA: Dysplasia of the knee associated with the syndrome of thrombocytopenia and absent radius. J Bone Joint Surg Am 66:421-427, 1984
55. Whitfield MF, Barr DG: Cows' milk allergy in the syndrome of thrombocytopenia with absent radius. Arch Dis Child 51:337-343, 1976
56. Bagby GC Jr: Genetic basis of Fanconi anemia. Curr Opin Hematol 10:68-76, 2003
57. Sola MC, Slayton WB, Rimsza LM, Perez JA, Fuchs D, Calhoun DA, et al: A neonate with severe thrombocytopenia and radio-ulnar synostosis. J Perinatol 24:528-530, 2004
58. Dokal I, Ganly P, Riebero I, Marsh J, Steed A, Kendra J, et al: Late onset bone marrow failure associated with proximal fusion of radius and ulna: A new syndrome. Br J Haematol 71:277-280, 1989
59. Thompson AA, Nguyen LT: Amegakaryocytic thrombocytopenia and radio-ulnar synostosis are associated with HOXA11 mutation. Nat Genet 26:397-398, 2000
60. Fujino T, Suzuki A, Ito Y, Ohyashiki K, Hatano Y, Miura I, et al: Single-translocation and double-chimeric transcripts: Detection of NUP98-HOXA9 in myeloid leukemias with HOXA11 or HOXA13 breaks of the chromosomal translocation t(7;11)(p15;p15). Blood 99: 1428-1433, 2002
61. Speleman F, Cauwelier B, Dastugue N, Cools J, Verhasselt B, Poppe B, et al: A new recurrent inversion, inv(7)(p15q34), leads to transcriptional activation of HOXA10 and HOXA11 in a subset of T-cell acute lymphoblastic leukemias. Leukemia 19:358-366, 2005
62. Boulet AM, Capecchi MR: Multiple roles of Hoxa11 and Hoxd11 in the formation of the mammalian forelimb zeugopod. Development 131: 299-309, 2004
63. Rabinowitz JG, Moseley JE, Mitty HA, Hirschhorn K: Trisomy 18, esophageal atresia, anomalies of the radius, and congenital hypoplastic thrombocytopenia. Radiology 89:488-491, 1967
64. Bajaj R, Jain M, Kasat L, Naregal A, Borwankar SS: Tar syndrome with unilateral absent radius and associated esophageal atresia: A variant? Indian J Pediatr 66:460-463, 1999
65. Vega H, Waisfisz Q, Gordillo M, Sakai N, Yanagihara I, Yamada M, et al: Roberts syndrome is caused by mutations in ESCO2, a human homolog of yeast ECO1 that is essential for the establishment of sister chromatid cohesion. Nat Genet 37:468-470, 2005
66. Hall JG: Thrombocytopenia and absent radius (TAR) syndrome. J Med Genet 24:79-83, 1987
67. Van Maldergem L, Siitonen HA, Jalkh N, Chouery E, De Roy M, Delague V, et al: Revisiting the craniosynostosis-radial ray hypoplasia association: Baller-Gerold syndrome caused by mutations in RECQL4 gene. J Med Genet 43:148-152, 2005
68. Li QY, Newbury-Ecob RA, Terrett JA, Wilson DI, Curtis AR, Yi CH, et al: Holt-Oram syndrome is caused by mutations in TBX5, a member of the Brachyury (T) gene family. Nat Genet 15:21-29, 1997
69. Basson CT, Bachinsky DR, Lin RC, Levi T, Elkins JA, Soults J, et al: Mutations in human TBX5 [corrected] cause limb and cardiac malformation in Holt-Oram syndrome. Nat Genet 15:30-35, 1997
70. Castilla EE, Ashton-Prolla P, Barreda-Mejia E, Brunoni D, Cavalcanti DP, Correa-Neto J, et al: Thalidomide, a current teratogen in South America. Teratology 54:273-277, 1996
71. Schnur RE, Eunpu DL, Zackai EH: Thrombocytopenia with absent radius in a boy and his uncle. Am J Med Genet 28:117-123, 1987
72. Adeyokunnu AA: Radial aplasia and amegakaryocytic thrombocytopenia (TAR syndrome) among Nigerian children. Am J Dis Child 138: 346-348, 1984
73. Edelberg SB, Cohn J, Brandt NJ: Congenital hypomegakaryocytic

thrombocytopenia associated with bilateral absence of the radius—The TAR syndrome. Hum Hered 27:147-152, 1977

74. Ceballos-Quintal JM, Pinto-Escalante D, Gongora-Biachi RA: TAR-like syndrome in a consanguineous Mayan girl. Am J Med Genet 43:805-807, 1992
75. Teufel M, Enders H, Dopfer R: Consanguinity in a Turkish family with thrombocytopenia with absent radii (TAR) syndrome. Hum Genet 64: 94-96, 1983
76. Hall JG, Levin J, Kuhn JP, Ottenheimer EJ, van Berkum KA, McKusick VA: Thrombocytopenia with absent radius (TAR). Medicine (Baltimore) 48:411-439, 1969
77. Homans AC, Cohen JL, Mazur EM: Defective megakaryocytopoiesis in the syndrome of thrombocytopenia with absent radii. Br J Haematol 70:205-210, 1988
78. Ballmaier M, Schulze H, Cremer M, Folman CC, Strauss G, Weite K: Defective c-Mpl signaling in the syndrome of thrombocytopenia with absent radii. Stem Cells 16:177-184, 1998 (suppl 2)
79. Strippoli P, Savoia A, Iolascon A, Tonelli R, Savino M, Giordano P, et al: Mutational screening of thrombopoietin receptor gene (c-mpl) in patients with congenital thrombocytopenia and absent radii (TAR). Br J Haematol 103:311-314, 1998
80. Fleischman RA, Letestu R, Mi X, Stevens D, Winters J, Debili N, et al: Absence of mutations in the HoxA10, HoxA11 and HoxD11 nucleotide coding sequences in thrombocytopenia with absent radius syndrome. Br J Haematol 116:367-375, 2002
81. Go RS, Johnston KL: Acute myelogenous leukemia in an adult with thrombocytopenia with absent radii syndrome. Eur J Haematol 70: 246-248, 2003
82. Camitta BM, Rock A: Acute lymphoidic leukemia in a patient with thrombocytopenia/absent radii (Tar) syndrome. Am J Pediatr Hematol Oncol 15:335-337, 1993
83. Fadoo Z, Naqvi SM: Acute myeloid leukemia in a patient with thrombocytopenia with absent radii syndrome. J Pediatr Hematol Oncol 24: 134-135, 2002
84. Symonds RP, Clark BJ, George WD, Bryant PE, Liu N, Connor JM: Thrombocytopenia with absent radii (TAR) syndrome: A new increased cellular radiosensitivity syndrome. Clin Oncol (R Coll Radiol) 7:56-58, 1995
85. Brochstein JA, Shank B, Kernan NA, Terwilliger JW, O'Reilly RJ: Marrow transplantation for thrombocytopenia-absent radii syndrome. J Pediatr 121:587-589, 1992
86. Armitage JO, Hoak JC, Elliott TE, Fry GL: Syndrome of thrombocytopenia and absent radii: Qualitatively normal platelets with remission following spenectomy. Scand J Haematol 20:25-28, 1978
87. Aquino VM, Mustafa MM, Vaickus L, Wooley R, Buchanan GR: Recombinant interleukin-6 in the treatment of congenital thrombocytopenia associated with absent radii. J Pediatr Hematol Oncol 20:474-476, 1998

Seminars in
HEMATOLOGY

Erratum

On page ii of the supplement entitled "Current Opinion on Management of Inhibitor Therapy" (Semin Hematol vol 43, no 2, suppl 4, 2006), the first paragraph of the supplement information should read as follows:

The articles in this supplement are based on presentations made during the World Federation of Hemophilia World Congress 2004 in Bangkok, Thailand.

doi:10.1053/j.seminhematol.2006.06.001

Vol 43, No 3, Suppl 5 July 2006

Supplement to

Seminars in HEMATOLOGY

Neal S. Young · Photis Beris
Editors

Review of Therapies for Immune Thrombocytopenic Purpura

James Bussel and Michael Tarantino
Guest Editors

W.B. Saunders

Seminars in HEMATOLOGY

Neal S. Young · Photis Beris
Editors

Peter A. Miescher, *Founding Editor* Ernst R. Jaffé, *Co-Editor Emeritus*

Editorial correspondence should be addressed to Photis Beris, MD, Division d'Hématologie, Hôpital Cantonal Universitaire, 25 rue Micheli-du-Crest, 1211 Geneve 14, Switzerland, or Neal S. Young, MD, 4400 17th Street, NW, Washington, DC 20011.

Business correspondence (subscriptions, change of address) should be addressed to the Publisher, Elsevier, 6277 Sea Harbor Dr, Orlando, FL 32887-4800; Email elspcs@elsevier.com.

Change of address notices, including both the old and new addresses of the subscriber, should be sent at least one month in advance.

Customer Service: 1-800-654-2452; outside the United States and Canada, (407) 345-4000.

Yearly subscription rates: United States and possessions: individual, $169.00; institution, $267.00; single issues, $81.00. All other countries: individual, $239.00; institution, $339.00; single issues, $81.00. Student and resident: United States and possessions, and Canada: $85.00; all other countries: $122.00. To receive student/resident rate, orders must be accompanied by name of affiliated institution, date of term, and the *signature* of program/residency coordinator on institution letterhead. Orders will be billed at individual rate until proof of status is received. Current prices are in effect for back volumes and back issues. Single issues, both current and back, exist in limited quantities and are offered for sale subject to availability. Back issues sold in conjunction with a subscription are on a prorated basis. Prices are subject to change without notice. *Checks* should be made payable to Elsevier and sent to *Seminars in Hematology*, Elsevier, Periodicals Department, PO Box 628239, Orlando, FL 32862-8239.

Other correspondence (copyediting, production) should be addressed to Elsevier, 1600 John F. Kennedy Blvd, Ste 1800, Philadelphia, PA 19103-2899.

Reprints: For 100 or more copies of an article in this publication, please contact the Commercial Reprints Department, Elsevier, 360 Park Ave South, New York, NY 10010-1710. Telephone (212) 633-3813, fax (212) 633-3820; e-mail, reprints@elsevier.com.

Advertising Representative: Cunningham Associates, PO Box 308, Park Ridge, NJ 07656. Telephone (201) 767-4170.

The contents of *Seminars in Hematology* are indexed in *Index Medicus* and *MEDLINE, Current Contents/Clinical Medicine, Current Contents/Life Sciences,* Science Citation Index, and *EMBASE/* Excerpta Medica.

The *Seminars in Hematology* home page is located at *www.seminhematol.org.*

W.B. Saunders **Philadelphia, PA**

Seminars in HEMATOLOGY

Vol 43, No 3, Supplement 5, July 2006

Review of Therapies for Immune Thrombocytopenic Purpura

James Bussel and Michael Tarantino
Guest Editors

Review of Therapies for Immune Thrombocytopenic Purpura S1
James Bussel and Michael Tarantino

Treatment of Immune Thrombocytopenic Purpura in Adults S3
James Bussel

Recent Advances in the Treatment of Childhood Immune Thrombocytopenic Purpura S11
Michael Tarantino

Question and Answer S18

Seminars in
HEMATOLOGY

Review of Therapies for Immune Thrombocytopenic Purpura

James Bussel and Michael Tarantino

Guest Editors

The articles in this supplement are based on presentations made during educational symposia, "International Review of the Therapies for Immune Thrombocytopenic Purpura," held on Thursday, August 11, 2005 during the International Society on Thrombosis and Haemostasis in Sydney, Australia.

This supplement is being supported by an unrestricted educational grant from Baxter BioScience.

The opinions or views expressed in this supplement are those of the authors and do not necessarily reflect the opinions or recommendations of Baxter.

The guest editors, authors, and publisher have tried to ensure that recommended measures and drug dosages discussed in this supplement are accurate and conform to the standards that prevailed at the time of publication. The reader is advised, however, to check the product information available for any product discussed in this supplement to be familiar with any changes in the dosage schedule, techniques of use, or contraindications. Because of the uniqueness of each patient, physicians should use this information only as a general guide in determining the best treatment for each patient. For approved product information, consult the manufacturer's prescribing information.

ELSEVIER

Seminars in HEMATOLOGY

Volume 43, Number 3, Supplement 5 **July 2006**

Review of Therapies for Immune Thrombocytopenic Purpura

Immune thrombocytopenic purpura (ITP) is thought to be caused by autoantibody-mediated platelet destruction with associated thrombocytopenia. In general, the management strategy depends on the clinical course of the disease. Conventional agents, such as corticosteroids or intravenous immune globulin (IVIg), are the initial treatment of choice. However, therapies with different mechanisms of action, such as anti-D globulin, have recently emerged as a promising alternative to, or in combination with some, existing conventional agents. In addition, newer or investigational treatments such as rituximab (anti-CD20 monoclonal antibody) and thrombopoietin (TPO)-like therapies have yielded encouraging results in early clinical trials. Anecdotal evidence suggests that some of these newer agents may be associated with fewer adverse events compared with many conventional agents, while also exhibiting impressive clinical efficacy.

To date, few randomized clinical trials have been conducted to comprehensively evaluate the many available treatments for adult and childhood ITP. Consequently, clear algorithms to treat this disease are not available and the details of management frequently differ among experts.[1] However, with the emerging evidence suggesting that genetics can play a major role in the development and clinical outcome of this disease, and with the progress in designing therapeutics against specific molecular targets that have been implicated, there is now renewed interest and enthusiasm in applying these findings to improve the overall management of ITP.

ITP is often acute and self-limiting in children. Its management is a topic of worldwide debate because of the high percentage of pediatric patients that spontaneously recover in the absence of therapy. In general, the clinical strategy for patients presenting with severe thrombocytopenia and a perceived risk of serious hemorrhage is to increase the platelet count rapidly, while minimizing toxicity from pharmacologic agents. If the risk of severe bleeding is low, management may be limited to close observation and counseling. However, ITP in children may often be treated to reduce the risk of bleeding, especially intracranial bleeding, and to avoid alteration of lifestyle. Corticosteroids might be used for short-term therapy but can lead to significant adverse reactions if too much is given daily for too long. Newer regimens of corticosteroids suggest that a substantial increase in the platelet count can be achieved with short pulses at "high" doses.[2]

Acute ITP in children also responds well to treatment with anti-D globulin or high-dose IVIg. A recent study demonstrated that anti-D globulin therapy compares favorably with IVIg in patients with severe thrombocytopenia.[3] Furthermore, the platelet response to anti-D is dose-dependent.[3–5] A randomized prospective trial of 105 Rh+ children with newly diagnosed ITP, completed in 2004, showed that a 75-μg/kg dose of anti-D globulin raised the platelet count more rapidly than a 50-μg/kg dose of anti-D globulin, and as rapidly as IVIg.[3] The safety profiles of the anti-D globulin and IVIg treatment groups were similar. The use of anti-D globulin has been a safe drug therapy for a majority of patients; however, a very rare, but serious complication, intravascular hemolysis with associated renal compromise, has been reported.[6,7]

In adults (and a minority of children), ITP is often chronic. In these cases, patients may require long-term therapy. Corticosteroids or other immunosuppressive agents are commonly used for initial treatment and in adults splenectomy has been the mainstay after steroid failure. However, splenectomy may lead to serious complications, such as overwhelming bacterial sepsis, and has a long-term success rate of approximately 60% to 70%, factoring in relapse in initially improved patients in the first 5 years after the procedure.[8,9] It remains difficult to gauge outcomes for individual patients and the 20- to 30-year outcome of splenectomy remains unknown.[10–13]

New therapeutic approaches have recently been evaluated in adult patients with ITP. These findings have been particularly important for those patients who would prefer to postpone or avoid splenectomy. Results from one study suggested that 40% to 60% of adults with acute ITP would be able to avoid splenectomy altogether by repeated use of maintenance anti-D globulin,[14] and this was replicated in a second study.[15] In a separate study, approximately 33% of chronic ITP patients achieved durable response with rituximab.[16] Furthermore, in small clinical trials of thrombopoi-

0037-1963/06/$-see front matter
doi:10.1053/j.seminhematol.2006.04.010

etic agents conducted in patients with highly refractory chronic ITP, transient increases in platelet counts sustainable by continued dosing have been observed.[17–19]

The likelihood of a rapid and/or sustained response must be balanced by the likelihood of near- and long-term adverse events when considering drug therapy for ITP. In addition to clinical and laboratory information, social information is important in deciding whether to treat or not treat ITP in a child. As with children, adults should also be evaluated on a case-by-case basis. Patient preferences, tolerance to therapy, age, and lifestyle are important components in treatment decisions.

Although the fundamental pathophysiology of ITP has been known for half a century, important discoveries at the molecular level have been relatively recent. For example, a strong positive correlation was reported of the HH polymorphism of FcRIIa in adult patients receiving anti-D globulin with increases in the proinflammatory cytokines interleukin-6 (IL-6), tumor necrosis factor (TNF), and a chemokine (membrane cofactor protein).[20] Patients receiving IVIg did not demonstrate this same increase. Collectively, these and other recent immunologic findings may herald a new way in designing clinical trials to optimize clinical outcome in ITP patients.

Therapeutic approaches for ITP will continue to evolve with emerging data on the molecular pathogenesis of this disease and outcomes of clinical trials. This supplement will provide a critical review of treatment options for acute and chronic ITP in children and adults. Furthermore, it will examine the differences in the presentation of the disease in children and adults and describe the clinical outcome of treatment strategies, with an emphasis on novel and innovative approaches to treat ITP.

James Bussel, MD
Weill Medical College of Cornell University
New York, NY

Michael Tarantino, MD
University of Illinois College of Medicine at Peoria
Peoria, IL
Guest Editors

References

1. George JN, Woolf SH, Raskob GE, Wasser JS, Aledort LM, Ballem PJ, et al: Idiopathic thrombocytopenic purpura: a practice guideline developed by explicit methods for the American Society of Hematology. Blood 88:3-40, 1996
2. Cines DB, Bussel JB: How I treat idiopathic thrombocytopenic purpura (ITP). Blood 106:2244-2251, 2005
3. Tarantino MD, Young G, Bertolone SJ, Kalinyak KA, Shafer FE, Kulkarni R, et al: for the Acute ITP in Children Study Group: Single dose of anti-D immune globulin at 75 μg/kg is as effective as intravenous immune globulin at rapidly raising the platelet count in newly diagnosed immune thrombocytopenic purpura (ITP) in children. J Pediatr 148:489-494, 2006
4. Bussel JB, Graziano JN, Kimberly RP, Pahwa S, Aledort LM: Intravenous anti-D treatment of immune thrombocytopenic purpura: Analysis of efficacy, toxicity, and mechanism of effect. Blood 77:1884-1893, 1991
5. Newman GC, Novoa MV, Fodero EM, Lesser ML, Woloski BMR, Bussel JB: A dose of 75 μg/kg/d of IV anti-D increases the platelet count more rapidly and for a longer period of time than does 50 μg/kg/d in adults with immune thrombocytopenic purpura (ITP). Br J Haematol 112:1076-1078, 2001
6. Gaines AR: Acute onset hemoglobinemia and/or hemoglobinuria and sequelae following Rh(o)(D) immune globulin intravenous administration in immune thrombocytopenic purpura patients. Blood 95:2523-2529, 2000
7. Gaines AR: Disseminated intravascular coagulation associated with acute hemoglobinemia or hemoglobinuria following Rh(0)(D) immune globulin intravenous administration for immune thrombocytopenic purpura. Blood 106:1532-1537, 2005
8. Schwartz J, Eldor A, Gillis S, Guinta A, Leber M, Bussel JB: Long term follow-up after splenectomy performed for immune thrombocytopenic purpura (ITP). Am J Hematol 72:94-98, 2003
9. Kojouri K, Vesely SK, Terrell DR, George JN: Splenectomy for adult patients with idiopathic thrombocytopenic purpura: A systematic review to assess long-term platelet count responses, prediction of response, and surgical complications. Blood 104:2623-2634, 2004
10. Fabris F, Tassan T, Ramon R, Carraro G, Randi ML, Luzzatto G, et al: Age as the major predictor of long-term response to splenectomy in immune thrombocytopenic purpura. Br J Haematol 112:637-640, 2001
11. Law C, Marcaccio M, Tam P, Heddle N, Kelton JG: High-dose intravenous immune globulin and the response to splenectomy in patients with idiopathic thrombocytopenic purpura. N Engl J Med 336:1494-1498, 1997
12. Holt D, Brown J, Terrill K, Goldsby R, Meyers RL, Heximer J, et al: Response to intravenous immunoglobulin predicts splenectomy response in children with immune thrombocytopenic purpura. Pediatrics 111:87-90, 2003
13. Najean Y, Rain JD, Billotey C: The site of destruction of autologous ^{111}In-labelled platelets and the efficiency of splenectomy in children and adults with idiopathic thrombocytopenic purpura: a study of 578 patients with 268 splenectomies. Br J Haematol 97:547-550, 1997
14. Cooper N, Woloski BM, Fodero EM, Novoa M, Leber M, Beer JH, Bussel JB: Does treatment with intermittent infusions of intravenous anti-D allow a proportion of adults with recently diagnosed immune thrombocytopenic purpura to avoid splenectomy? Blood 99:1922-1927, 2002
15. George JN, Raskob GE, Vesely SK, Moore D Jr, Lyons RM, Cobos E, et al: Initial management of immune thrombocytopenic purpura in adults: A randomized controlled trial comparing intermittent anti-D with routine care. Am J Hematol 74:161-169, 2003
16. Cooper N, Stasi R, Cunningham-Rundles S, Feuerstein MA, Leonard JP, Amadori S, et al: The efficacy and safety of B-cell depletion with anti-CD20 monoclonal antibody in adults with chronic immune thrombocytopenic purpura. Br J Haematol 125:232-239, 2004
17. Kuter D, Bussel JB, Aledort LM, George J, Lyons RM, Conklin GT, et al: A phase 2 placebo controlled study evaluating the platelet response and safety of weekly dosing with a novel thrombopoietic protein (AMG531) in thrombocytopenic adult patients (pts) with immune thrombocytopenic purpura (ITP) [abstract]. Blood 104:148a, 2004 (suppl 1)
18. Newland A, Caulier MT, Schipperus MR, Kappers-Klunne M, Varet BR, Watkins K, et al: An open-label, unit dose-finding study evaluating the safety and platelet response of a novel thrombopoietic protein (AMG531) in thrombocytopenic adult patients (pts) with immune thrombocytopenic purpura (ITP) [abstract]. Blood 104:567a, 2004 (suppl 1)
19. Bussel JB, Kuter DJ, George JN, Aledort LM, Lichtin AE, Lyons RM, et al: Long-term dosing of AMG 531 is effective and well tolerated in thrombocytopenic patients with immune thrombocytopenic purpura. Presented at the 47th ASH Annual Meeting and Exposition, Atlanta, GA, December 10-13, 2005 (abstr 220)
20. Cooper N, Heddle NM, Haas M, Reid ME, Lesser ML, Fleit HB, et al: Intravenous (IV) anti-D and IV immunoglobulin achieve acute platelet increases by different mechanisms: Modulation of cytokine and platelet responses to IV anti-D by FcγRIIa and FcγRIIIa polymorphisms. Br J Haematol 124:511-518, 2004

ELSEVIER

Seminars in
HEMATOLOGY

Treatment of Immune Thrombocytopenic Purpura in Adults

James Bussel

Idiopathic thrombocytopenic purpura (ITP) is a hematologic disorder characterized by the destruction of antibody-coated platelets in the reticuloendothelial system. Whereas 70% to 80% of children experience the acute form of the disease and recover within a few weeks or months after diagnosis, most adults have persistent disease and will require therapy. Principles of management are largely predicated on the extent of thrombocytopenia and symptoms of disease. Minimizing the toxicity associated with treatment while achieving hemostatic platelet counts are essential goals of treatment. Although there are numerous therapeutic options, neither consensus among experts nor clear algorithms to treat this complex disease exist. This article will review appropriate treatment options available for adult patients with ITP prior to splenectomy, at splenectomy, and following splenectomy. In addition to conventional agents such as corticosteroids and intravenous immune globulin (IVIg), the role of newer therapies with diverse mechanisms of action, such as rituximab, anti-D, and thrombopoietin (TPO)-like agents, will be highlighted. When used as either monotherapy or in combination with conventional therapeutics, these treatments may offer a more tolerable side effect profile and improved clinical benefit compared to existing drugs.
Semin Hematol 43(suppl 5):S3-S10

Idiopathic thrombocytopenic purpura (ITP) is a hematologic disorder characterized by platelet antibodies that opsonize the platelet membrane, leading to their destruction by the reticuloendothelial system. Despite the fact that this disease is relatively common and often easily recognizable, the true incidence of adult chronic ITP remains unknown. Estimates of annual incidence range from 55 to 66 new cases per million persons.[1]

Until recently, it was believed that most patients with ITP were primarily women of childbearing age at a ratio of 3:1. Two recent studies conducted in Denmark and the United Kingdom showed more equal female-male ratios of 1.7:1 and 1.2:1, respectively.[2,3] In addition, the age-specific incidence reported in these studies was substantially higher than in previous reports; in the Danish report, the median age at diagnosis was 56 years old, and in the UK study, the age-specific incidence was highest in patients greater than 60 years of age.[2,3] These findings are provocative, but seem consistent with clinical experience elsewhere, with an even female–male ratio in older patients reducing the overall female predominance.

The natural history of ITP in adults is distinct from pediatric ITP, but increasingly some similarities have become apparent. ITP in adults is generally chronic with an insidious onset. A recent study found that approximately 50% of patients with chronic ITP seen at tertiary referral centers have their ITP initially diagnosed on a routine blood count by their internist. In many cases, these counts are initially greater than 50,000/μL and only fall over time to a level requiring treatment. Symptoms often persist for years, however, and many treatment regimens may be required. Spontaneous remissions are rare, but there is a clear pattern of improvement over the first 1 to 2 years after diagnosis in at least 50% of cases. In contrast, childhood ITP is often acute, and in 70% to 80% of affected patients, symptoms resolve within 6 months. Furthermore, childhood ITP may be associated with a preceding viral or other infectious illness, whereas in adult ITP this is not the case.[4]

ITP typically presents with platelet counts of 20,000/μL accompanied with petechiae or purpura that develops over several days; otherwise, most patients are generally healthy.[5] In patients with platelet counts below 10,000/μL, symptoms can be highly variable and may include severe cutaneous

Department of Pediatrics, Division of Hematology and Oncology, and Department of Pediatrics in Medicine and in Obstetrics and Gynecology, Weill Medical College of Cornell University, New York, NY.

Address correspondence to James Bussel, MD, Weil Cornell Medical Center, 525 E 68th St, Payson 695, New York, NY 10021. E-mail: jbussel@med.cornell.edu

0037-1963/06/$-see front matter
doi:10.1053/j.seminhematol.2006.04.009

bleeding, epistaxis, hematuria, gingival or vaginal bleeding, and, rarely, even intracranial hemorrhage.[6] While quite uncommon, the most serious and life-threatening complication associated with ITP is spontaneous intracranial hemorrhage (ICH) with an incidence of up to 3% per year in chronic refractory ITP[7] and 1% in acute disease.[5] The greatest concern for major bleeding that may result in fatal ICH exists in patients with platelet counts less than 20,000/μL but especially less than 10,000/μL.[5,8,9]

The diagnosis of primary ITP remains one of exclusion and therefore it is essential that a careful history be taken and physical examination be performed. It is important that other types of immune-mediated thrombocytopenias, such as drug-induced thrombocytopenia, inherited thrombocytopenia, and post-transfusion purpura, be ruled out.[6] In addition, it has become increasingly obvious that inherited thrombocytopenia is frequently misdiagnosed as ITP.[10] The physical examination should generally be normal except for evidence of bleeding. In addition, laboratory findings should be unremarkable with the exception of isolated thrombocytopenia. Bone marrow examinations are infrequently performed except in patients over 50 to 60 years of age, in cases with atypical features, or where splenectomy is considered. Some experts have stated that the best diagnostic test for ITP is response to specific therapy (eg, intravenous immune globulin [IVIg], anti-D), even if the response is transient.[5]

Many issues regarding the optimal treatment of adult patients with ITP remain unresolved; consequently, principles of management differ among experts and evolve with emerging data. In general, management is predicated primarily on platelet count and symptoms. Four major factors should be considered when evaluating different therapeutic options in addition to the platelet count and comorbid conditions. They include the signs and symptoms of the patient (bleeding diathesis), tolerance to therapy, lifestyle, and patient preferences. Therefore, individualization of approach is a central tenet. It is especially important that a good relationship between the physician and the patient be established because of the potentially long duration of this disease. There also has been recent awareness of substantial quality-of-life issues far exceeding the degree expected in patients with chronic ITP. Attention to these quality-of-life issues will be beneficial with regard to managing important decisions concerning therapy.

With the above background, this article will review treatments for adult ITP with a division into therapeutic options prior to splenectomy, at splenectomy, and after splenectomy. This article will also address secondary ITP, a condition that may be associated with pregnancy, infectious diseases, immunodeficiencies, and lymphoproliferative disorders.

Treatment at Diagnosis in Emergency and Nonemergency Settings: Prior to Splenectomy

Since its introduction in 1950, the standard treatment for adults presenting with moderate or severe thrombocytopenia at diagnosis in a nonemergency setting has been prednisone (1.0 to 2.0 mg/kg).[11] Alternatively, for patients who are intolerant of corticosteroids and are Rh+ and direct antiglobulin–negative, intravenous (IV) anti-D (50 to 75 μg/kg) may be effectively substituted for prednisone.[12,13] Alternatively, if prednisone therapy is initiated but platelet counts remain below 20,000/μL or if there is a need for a rapid response, treatment with prednisone may be supplemented with IV methylprednisolone (5 to 30 mg/kg), IVIg (1 g/kg for 1 to 3 days), and/or IV anti-D (75 μg/kg).[5] Rapid and durable platelet responses have also been reported with high-dose dexamethasone 40 mg/d (400 mg prednisone equivalent) for 4 days, although an optimal repeat schedule has not been established. In patients who fail to demonstrate any acute response to therapy, the diagnosis of ITP should be reevaluated.

In emergency settings, such as hospitalization, urgent treatment is frequently required for acute platelet increases. For patients experiencing profound bleeding, or who present with very low platelet counts (<10,000 to 20,000/μL), therapy is typically initiated with IVIg (1 g/kg for 2 to 3 days) combined with IV methylprednisolone (1 g/d for 1 to 3 days). This may be supplemented with either IV anti-D (75 μg/kg) or with high-dose dexamethasone or prednisone until the platelet count exceeds 50,000/μL.[6] In addition, platelet transfusions may be warranted in patients with ongoing life-threatening hemorrhage, and, in some instances, combination modalities including corticosteroids, IVIg, IV anti-D, and/or vincristine are appropriate.[5]

IV anti-D is increasingly being used in appropriate settings as an alternative to IVIg, or even in combination with IVIg, as experience with this agent confirms its clinical benefit. In early studies, 79% of patients receiving 25 to 50 μg/kg/d anti-D experienced an increased platelet count of greater than 20,000/μL.[14] While encouraging, these findings were less impressive than results with standard IVIg because the platelets did not increase significantly for 72 hours. More recent studies have shown that at higher doses (75 μg/kg), IV anti-D not only increases the platelet count more rapidly, and for a longer duration compared with the standard dose of 50 μg/kg IV anti-D, but platelet responses within 24 hours occur in the majority of patients, faster than those that have been reported with corticosteroids and as fast as those reported with IVIg (Fig 1).[12] To reduce the potential for adverse fever-chill side effects associated with higher-dose IV anti-D, one study administered single doses of prednisone to some patients receiving high-dose (75 μg/kg) IV anti-D.[12] In this trial, six of the seven moderate adverse events were reported in patients who did not receive premedication with prednisone. Overall, 20 adverse events were reported in eight infusions without prednisone compared with seven adverse events in five infusions with prednisone. No serious adverse events were reported.

In an attempt to better understand the biological basis of the increased number of patients experiencing fever and chill reactions on high-dose IV anti-D, levels of specific proinflammatory cytokine levels have been examined and compared with levels in patients receiving IVIg. In a recent study by Cooper et al, dramatic increases in interleukin-6 (IL-6),

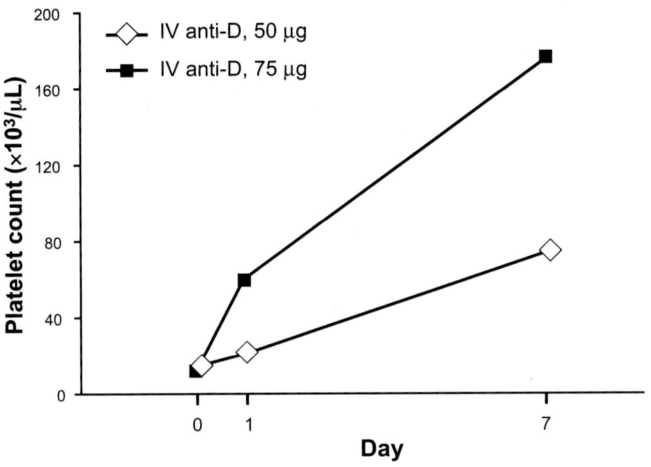

Figure 1 Randomized comparison of two doses of anti-D in adults with acute ITP: 50 versus 75 μg/kg.[12] Platelet count response is plotted for each dosage at day 0 (baseline), day 1 post-infusion, and day 7 post-infusion.

tumor necrosis factor alpha (TNF), and membrane cofactor protein (MCPI) were observed within 1 to 2 hours after a 5-minute infusion of IV anti-D. Higher cytokine levels were seen when higher dose IV anti-D was infused.[15] By contrast, patients receiving IVIg treatment appeared to show a lack of pro-inflammatory responses, possibly due to mediation of the IVIg effect through an inhibitory Fc receptor.[16] Interestingly, adverse events, but not cytokine levels, were significantly reduced by prednisone. Molecular analysis from this study indicated that patients with the HH polymorphism of FcγRIIa had significantly higher IL-6 (P = .001), MCP-1 (P = .002), and TNF (P = .001) levels following infusion than did heterozygotes. This suggests that anti-D interacts with this FcR (FcRIIa) and not solely FcRIIIa.

Maintenance for Persistent ITP: Prior to Splenectomy

More than three quarters of adult patients will fail to achieve a lasting response to an initial short course of prednisone; consequently, thrombocytopenia will recur. The standard of practice for corticosteroid nonresponders and platelet counts below 30,000/μL after 4 to 6 weeks of therapy, either primary nonresponders or relapsers, had been splenectomy.[11] However, many patients wish to avoid the risks associated with surgery and the removal of a "healthy" organ if other alternatives are available. Furthermore, it has become clear that supporting the platelet count for up to 1 to 2 years from diagnosis will allow more than half of the patients to avoid splenectomy. Therapeutic options of the relapsed patient with ITP (platelet count <30,000/μL) are varied and include low-dose prednisone, high-dose dexamethasone, IV anti-D, and rituximab (anti-CD20 monoclonal antibody), and experimental thrombopoietin (TPO)-like agents. Clinical data on the effects of maintenance therapy in persistent ITP have been obtained with three agents: dexamethasone, rituximab, and IV anti-D.

In a small study reported by Andersen, 10 patients with refractory ITP received six cycles of high-dose (40 mg/d) dexamethasone for 4 sequential days.[17] Platelet counts in all patients remained above 100,000/μL for at least 6 months after the last cycle of treatment. These findings were extended in a larger study that assessed the efficacy of a 4-day course of high-dose (40 mg/d) oral dexamethasone. In this study, 53 of 106 (50%) newly diagnosed patients had a sustained response at 6 months, defined as a platelet count greater than 50,000/μL.[18]

The effects of repeated infusions with IV anti-D were examined in a pilot study with 28 patients.[19] All patients had been diagnosed within the last year (median, 3.5 months from diagnosis) and the mean number of prior treatments was two (typically corticosteroids and IVIg). The purpose of the study was to assess whether maintenance IV anti-D therapy could increase platelet counts to sufficient levels (>30,000/μL) for patients to postpone or avoid splenectomy. Patients were randomized to receive initially either 50 or 75 μg/kg IV anti-D and followed for a median of 26 months. The results were promising. At the time of publication, six patients had maintained platelet counts greater than 100,000/μL and six others were maintaining counts for more than 6 months at greater than 30,000/μL without therapy. The remaining 16 patients have continued on with treatment (n = 7), undergone splenectomy (n = 8), or been lost to follow-up (n = 1). After 6 months of treatment, more than 40% of adults in this trial were able to achieve stable platelet counts and avoid splenectomy. Additional patients have come off treatment in the intervening years and one "stable" patient had subsequently undergone splenectomy. These findings were supported by a subsequent study that found that an aggressive regimen of IV anti-D or prednisone could prevent splenectomy in more than 50% of newly diagnosed patients.[13]

Rituximab, an anti-CD20 monoclonal antibody that is indicated for the treatment of patients with relapsed or refractory, low-grade or follicular, $CD20^{+}$, B-cell non-Hodgkin's lymphoma, has recently entered clinical studies in several autoimmune disorders, including chronic ITP. Through several complementary mechanisms including apoptosis, antibody-dependent cell-mediated cytotoxicity (ADCC), and/or complement-dependent cytotoxicity (CDC), rituximab has been demonstrated to effectively cause selective B-cell lysis in vitro and B-cell depletion in vivo.[20] Recovery of B-cell counts in patients receiving this agent generally occurs 6 to 12 months after completion of therapy.

A recent study evaluated the safety and therapeutic benefit of rituximab in 57 splenectomized and nonsplenectomized patients with platelet counts less than 30,000/μL. Eighteen patients receiving the standard dose of 375 mg/m^2 IV every week for 4 weeks achieved a complete response, defined as a platelet count greater than 150,000/μL, and 13 patients had a partial response, defined as a platelet count of 50,000 to 150,000/μL. Overall, 31 patients (55%) responded.[21] Thirty-two splenectomized patients were treated, of whom 16 responded (50%); of these, nine achieved a complete response and seven a partial response. Twenty-five nonsplenectomized patients were treated and 15 responded (60%); of

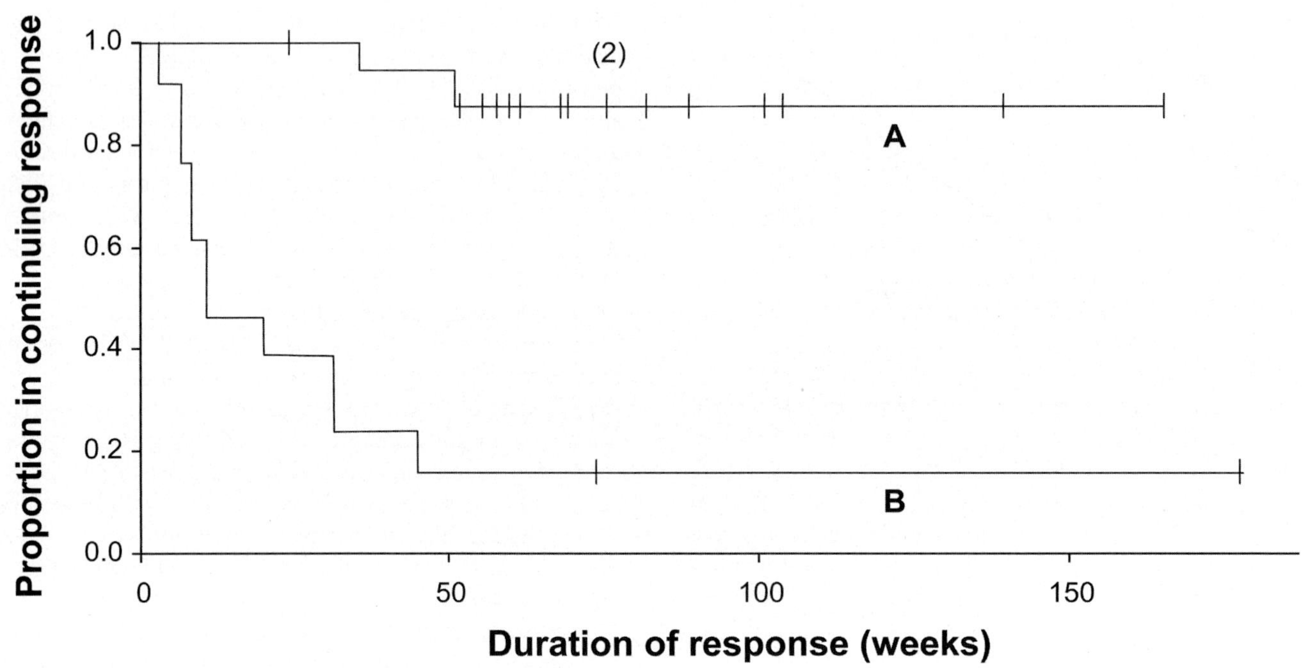

Figure 2 Kaplan-Meier curve for the duration of response for (A) complete responders and (B) partial responders. Duration of response in weeks from initial infusion of rituximab is plotted against proportion of patients in each category that maintained response without additional treatment. Each tick mark represents last follow-up of an ongoing response (one represents two patients). Each vertical line represents the proportion of patients with that amount of follow-up who relapsed at that particular time point. Reprinted with permission from Blackwell Publishing.[21]

these, there were nine complete responses and complete partial responses. The timing of platelet responses was notable. In 29 of the 31 responders to rituximab, the platelet increase (>50,000/μL) occurred by week 9 of the first infusion. Furthermore, in 12 of the 18 complete responses, the platelet increase to greater than 150,000/μL was achieved by week 9. At the time of publication, 16 of 18 patients were still in complete response and 15 of these patients were more than a year past their first infusion. In addition, of the 13 patients who had achieved a partial response, two were still responding at 22 and 36 months. The duration of response in complete and partial responders is illustrated in Fig 2. Interestingly, at week 26, nonresponders had significantly higher numbers of circulating B cells than responders in this study. These findings suggest that the extent of B-cell depletion may be important for response.

None of the patients in this trial experienced a severe adverse event and all patients completed the trial. The most common adverse events were grade 1 or 2 reactions to the first infusion of rituximab. These included transient fever, chills, and rash in 32 of 57 (58%) patients. However, one grade 3 event, a bronchospasm, was reported. Overall, immunoglobulin levels (IgM and IgG) did not change; only one patient had a decrease in IgG levels from normal to just below normal (8.2 g/L to 7.44 g/L). There were no serious infections or serum sickness reported during the study. In contrast, reports of serum sickness have been observed in children receiving rituximab therapy for ITP.[22,23]

Given the promising durability of responses with rituximab in certain refractory patients but the less than 50% response rate and the occurrence of late relapses, new trials are under way that explore whether nonresponders might benefit from rituximab when given at higher doses or in combination with chemotherapeutic agents. Accordingly, an ongoing study is examining augmented rituximab. The two arms are double-dose rituximab versus rituximab with cyclophosphamide, vincristine, and prednisone (R-CVP).[24] Patients with ITP who received standard rituximab 375 mg/m^2 in an earlier trial and either did not respond or responded and relapsed, are being randomized to receive either 4 weekly doses of high-dose rituximab (750 mg/m^2) or standard dose rituximab (375 mg/m^2) combined with standard CVP. Preliminary results suggest that this is not a very promising approach for patients who did not respond to rituximab initially.

Splenectomy

Splenectomy remains the cornerstone of therapy after failure of prednisone or other therapies in chronic ITP.[25] Because splenectomy avoids toxicities associated with persistent application of other therapies and because durable complete responses are achievable in approximately two thirds of adult patients, this therapeutic option is often the most attractive one for patients who desire a lifestyle independent of frequent monitoring.[5,26,27] However, in addition to complications associated with surgery, overwhelming bacterial sepsis currently occurs in a small number of patients (≤1%). In recent years, with marked improvements in perioperative management, including preoperative vaccination and postoperative antibiotics, the estimated risk of fatal bacterial infections has been declining.[11,28] However, preliminary data suggest that certain patients will not respond well to pneumovax, increasing their vulnerability to sepsis.[29]

According to the American Society of Hematology Practice Guidelines, splenectomy is recommended under two hypothetical situations: "(1) patients have had the diagnosis for a minimum of 6 weeks, and still have a platelet count <10,000/μL and (2) patients who have had the diagnosis for 3 months, have experienced a transient or incomplete response to primary treatment, have a platelet count <30,000/μL and who are either bleeding or not bleeding."[11] The benefit of splenectomy may outweigh the risks in certain patients. For example, in individuals who present with significant bleeding and a platelet count of 20,000 to 30,000/μL, and are young and active, splenectomy may indeed be appropriate, and therefore, should not be ruled out.[5] Conversely, in elderly patients, the added risk of the surgery makes splenectomy, even when performed laparoscopically, a less desirable option.

The long-term results and rate of relapse of splenectomy are not well defined.[26,27,30] However, recent studies suggest that the long-term outcome after splenectomy for ITP may be substantially lower than the immediate postoperative complete remission rates. In one report that evaluated 75 patients who underwent splenectomy, the immediate postoperative complete response rate was 77%; however, after 5 years, only 57% of patients remained in complete response.[27] Three patients died of apparently untreated causes prior to the 5-year follow-up. Additional studies in larger numbers of patients are needed to assess the long-term durability of response in patients who choose this approach, especially the adverse events and efficacy more than 5 to 10 years from surgery.

An outstanding issue with regard to splenectomy is predicting response and the optimal timing of this procedure in the treatment algorithm. In most instances, the decision to undergo splenectomy is determined in large part by patient preference. With the advent of other therapeutic modalities that may defer splenectomy, such as rituximab, anti-D, azathioprine–danazol, or TPO-like agents, some patients may decide to wait. In other cases, physicians may treat a relapsed patient with more prednisone. Overall, as suggested by a recent retrospective study as well,[30] Kojouri and colleagues identified younger age as linked to a good response but could not define a specific age in their meta-analysis.[26] Sex, severe hemorrhage, platelet count at diagnosis, duration of thrombocytopenia, and response to medical therapy were not significant risk factors. Thrombocytopenia-free survival among patients less than 40 years of age is illustrated in a Kaplan-Meier curve in Fig 3. An important finding from this study is that response rates appear to decrease over time, although only to 60% to 65%.

An alternative to conventional splenectomy, which has essentially replaced it, is laparoscopic splenectomy.[31] First introduced in 1991, numerous studies have shown reduced blood loss with this procedure and more rapid recovery time[32] and suggested a lower mortality rate compared with open splenectomy (0.2% and 1.0%, respectively).[26,31]

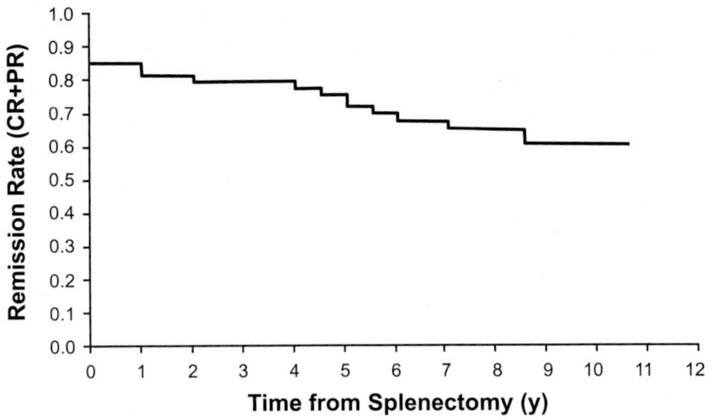

Figure 3 Kaplan-Meier analysis of relapse-free platelet response after splenectomy. The probability of staying in clinical remission (CR+PR) after splenectomy is shown: 73% of the patients were in clinical remission 5 years postoperatively, 62% were in remission 10 years postoperatively. Reprinted with permission.[27]

Currently, less than 50% of US hematologists prefer laparoscopic (or any) splenectomy as their treatment of choice after failure of prednisone, according to informal surveys (J. Bussel, unpublished results). To date, no randomized controlled trials have been conducted comparing the two approaches.

Refractory ITP: Persistent Severe Thrombocytopenia After Splenectomy

Despite a higher "cure" rate than other treatments with ITP, many patients fail to respond to splenectomy. In addition, approximately 15% to 25% of patients will relapse within 10 years of splenectomy.[1,25] These individuals are at increased risk of significant morbidity and mortality. Unfortunately, there are few randomized controlled trials or consensus among experts to guide the optimal management of refractory patients.[5,33]

The objective of treatment for patients with refractory ITP is to achieve stable adequate platelet counts (>20,000 to 30,000/μL) while minimizing the adverse side effects of medication. Deciding on the best treatment can be problematic and should be individualized. Factors such as age of the patient, degree of bleeding, platelet count level, whether the disease is primary refractory or relapsed, and the length of time prior to relapse are considerations.[4] Therapy is generally recommended for patients with platelet counts less than 20,000 to 30,000/μL who have active or intermittent bleeding or are at risk of such.[11]

Therapeutic approaches for patients with refractory ITP include single agents, combination chemotherapy, and experimental therapies. The advantage of single oral agents such as danazol, azathioprine, or cyclophosphamide is their relatively low toxicity. If responses are seen, they may only be apparent in 12 to 16 weeks; rituximab may require 4 to 8 weeks. Corticosteroids are only transiently effective, have low response rates and substantial toxicity with daily use, and may upregulate multidrug resistance genes.[34] Cyclosporine, a powerful immunosuppressant, is effective, but the risk of nephrotoxicity especially, as well as infection and malignancy, limit its long-term use.[35] Another alternative is dapsone. In a study of 66 adults with chronic ITP and platelet counts less than 50,000/μL, response rates in patients receiving 75 to 100 mg/d were 50%.[36] Anti-D is not indicated in patients who have undergone splenectomy.[37] Rituximab may be useful, but increasingly patients have received therapeutic trials of it before splenectomy.

In contrast to single agents, the benefits of multimodal therapy can include a higher response rate and avoidance of multidrug resistance; however, adverse side effects associated with more than one therapy can be more challenging and large clinical trials have not been conducted. Combinations of danazol (10 to 15 mg/kg/d) with either azathioprine (2 mg/kg/d) or mycophenolate mofetil (1.5 to 2.0 g/d) may be useful.[5,38] Other potentially beneficial combinations are oral cyclophosphamide (1 to 2 mg/kg/d) and prednisone combined with vincristine, vincristine and procarbazine, or etoposide; however, results from a small study did not clearly support one form of combination over another,[39] although unmaintained remissions persisted in all but one case.

In recent years, a number of new experimental approaches have been investigated in small pilot studies for patients who are refractory to conventional agents. In some instances, these studies have yielded durable responses with varying toxicity. For example, with a follow-up of 42 months, six of 14 patients treated with high-dose cyclophosphamide with autologous T- and B-lymphocyte–depleted peripheral blood stem cells have achieved durable complete responses, and two patients had partial responses.[40] However, two of the six patients who achieved a complete response died within a year and eight patients experienced gram-positive bacteremia.

One promising therapeutic approach includes the use of thrombopoietic agents to stimulate platelet production. Because TPO levels are inappropriately low (normal) in patients with ITP, this approach may be especially useful in patients who are not responsive to currently available modalities. In recent phase II trials of AMG 531, a protein that binds and activates the TPO receptor, transient but substantial increases in platelet counts were reported at a dose of 3 μg/kg or higher in eight of 12 patients in one study, and 13 of 16 in another study.[41-43] A trend toward a dose-response rate was observed; platelet counts ranging from greater than 100,000 to more than 450,000/μL were observed after a single dose of 3, 6, and 10 μg/kg. The most frequently reported adverse event with this regimen was mild-to-moderate headache. Antibodies to either AMG 531 or TPO antibodies were not observed. Hemoglobin, white blood cell, blood chemistry, and coagulation variables remained stable with no clinically significant changes observed. This agent, and the oral agent eltrombopag developed by GlaxoSmithKline, are likely to be prominent options in the management of ITP prior to splenectomy as well as after. Further trials are ongoing.

A number of other treatment modalities for refractory ITP have been investigated both in vivo and in vitro. However, either because of low response rates or more serious side effects, these therapies are less widely used. These include IL-11,[44] plasmapheresis,[45] accessory splenectomy,[46] dexamethasone,[47] anti-CD40 ligand,[48] and alemtuzumab.[49] Equivocal results have been reported with interferon-α.[11] However, this agent may be useful in patients infected with hepatitis C.

Secondary ITP

In some cases, ITP is a secondary condition—associated with other disorders or with pregnancy. For example, ITP may be initiated or perpetuated by human immunodeficiency virus, hepatitis C, or *Helicobacter pylori* infections. Therefore, testing for these microbes is indicated in at-risk populations.[5] In some studies, platelet recovery has occurred in patients with chronic ITP with *H pylori* infections treated with antibiotics.[50,51] However, other reports found that eradication of *H pylori* did not improve the course of the disease in their patients.[52]

Secondary forms of ITP are also associated with immunodeficiencies (common variable, IgA, and C4); systemic autoimmunity (Evans syndrome) and systemic lupus erythematosus; and lymphoproliferative disorders. Lymphoproliferative disorders include both malignant (chronic lymphocytic leukemia, Hodgkin's disease, and non-Hodgkin's lymphoma) and nonmalignant disorders (autoimmune lymphoproliferative syndrome type 1 or Canale-Smith syndrome).

ITP occurs in approximately one to two of every 1,000 pregnancies and can rarely lead to serious maternal and fetal complications.[32,53] One of the major complications associated with pregnancy is severe neonatal thrombocytopenia (platelet counts <20,000/μL) that carries a 1% risk of intracranial hemorrhage or other serious bleeding.[54,55] Some women present with severe thrombocytopenia for the first time at pregnancy.[4] As with all patients with possible ITP, a differential diagnosis should be performed since platelet counts can fall to 100,000/μL or less in as many as 10% of uncomplicated pregnancies. Special consideration should be given to the etiology of thrombocytopenia that occurs more frequently during pregnancy, such as HELLP syndrome (hemolysis, elevated liver enzyme levels, and low platelet count), microangiopathic hemolytic processes, gestational thrombocytopenia, and obstetrical causes of disseminated intravascular coagulation.[6]

In the absence of therapy or symptoms, platelet counts should be carefully monitored at least monthly through the first 2 trimesters, biweekly in the third, and weekly as term approaches.[5] Most women will tolerate platelet counts of 20,000 to 30,000/μL throughout pregnancy; however, in certain cases (eg, for amniocentesis) IV anti-D or IVIg may be appropriate to increase the count acutely. Prednisone (20 mg/d) may be beneficial to maintain the count.[56]

Unfortunately, no sizeable randomized clinical studies of ITP in pregnant women have been conducted. In addition, expert panels have not reached consensus about appropriate therapy in this population.[11] One of the major difficulties is that performing clinical trials in pregnant women is not feasible and it is difficult to assess differences in low probability outcomes such as neonatal ICH.[53]

Conclusions

Principles of management of adult patients with ITP vary and have evolved with emerging data. In the absence of a consensus among experts as a result of the lack of well-controlled clinical trials, therapeutic strategies are primarily predicated on platelet count and symptoms. Nevertheless, every patient is unique and should be evaluated on a case-by-case basis. In addition to the severity of the disease, factors that help to guide treatment decisions include: the patient's tolerance to specific treatments, his or her lifestyle, and patient preferences. It is hard to disagree forcefully with one of many reasonable choices in the absence of data demonstrating a clear advantage of one option over another.

Many novel therapies are in early stages of investigation or have recently been approved for, or at least tested in, chronic ITP. With a more tolerable side effect profile and potentially improved efficacy, these new therapies—such as rituximab, anti-D, and TPO-like agents—have diverse mechanisms of action and may be used as single agents, in combination with each other, or with conventional therapeutics. While these agents are indeed promising and have changed the landscape of this disease, the prospect of a cure remains elusive. Additional focused therapeutics still need to be invented, which in turn will require a sustained commitment to basic and clinical research committed to a better understanding of the underlying pathophysiology.

References

1. McMillan R: Therapy for adults with refractory chronic immune thrombocytopenic purpura. Ann Intern Med 126:307-314, 1997
2. Frederiksen H, Schmidt K: The incidence of idiopathic thrombocytopenic purpura in adults increases with age. Blood 94:909-913, 1999
3. Neylon AJ, Saunders PWG, Howard MR, Proctor SJ, Taylor PRA, on behalf of the Northern Regional Haematology Group: Clinically significant newly presenting autoimmune thrombocytopenic purpura in adults: A prospective study of a population-based cohort of 245 patients. Br J Haematol 122:966-974, 2003
4. British Committee for Standards in Haematology and General Haematology Task Force: Guidelines for the investigation and management of idiopathic thrombocytopenic purpura in adults, children and in pregnancy. Br J Haematol 120:574-596, 2003
5. Cines DB, Bussel JB: How I treat idiopathic thrombocytopenic purpura (ITP). Blood 106:2244-2251, 2005
6. Cines DB, McMillan R: Management of adult idiopathic thrombocytopenic purpura. Annu Rev Med 56:425-442, 2005
7. Cohen YC, Djulbegovic B, Shamai-Lubovitz O, Mozes B: The bleeding risk and natural history of idiopathic thrombocytopenic purpura in patients with persistent low platelet counts. Arch Intern Med 160: 1630-1638, 2001
8. Cortelazzo S, Finazzi G, Buelli M, Molteni A, Viero P, Barbui T. High risk of severe bleeding in aged patients with chronic idiopathic thrombocytopenic purpura. Blood 77:31-33, 1991
9. Butros LJ, Bussel JB: Intracranial hemorrhage in immune thrombocytopenic purpura: A retrospective analysis. J Pediatr Hematol Oncol 25:660-664, 2003
10. Cines DB, Bussel JB, McMillan RB, Zehnder JL: Congenital and acquired thrombocytopenia. Hematology (Am Soc Hematol Educ Program) 390-406, 2004
11. George JN, Woolf SH, Raskob GE, Wasser JS, Aledort LM, Ballem PJ, et al: Idiopathic thrombocytopenic purpura: A practice guideline developed by explicit methods for the American Society of Hematology. Blood 88:3-40, 1996
12. Newman GC, Novoa MV, Fodero EM, Lesser ML, Woloski BMR, Bussel JB: A dose of 75 μg/kg/d of IV anti-D increases the platelet count more rapidly and for a longer period of time than does 50 g/kg/d in adults with immune thrombocytopenic purpura (ITP). Br J Haematol 112: 1076-1078, 2001
13. George JN, Raskob GE, Vesely SK, Moore D Jr, Lyons RM, Cobos E, et al: Initial management of immune thrombocytopenic purpura in adults: A randomized controlled trial comparing intermittent anti-D with routine care. Am J Hematol 74:161-169, 2003
14. Bussel JB, Graziano JN, Kimberly RP, Pahwa S, Aledort LM: Intravenous anti-D treatment of immune thrombocytopenic purpura: Analysis of efficacy, toxicity, and mechanism of effect. Blood 77:1884-1893, 1991
15. Cooper N, Heddle NM, Haas M, Reid ME, Lesser ML, Fleit HB, et al: Intravenous (IV) anti-D and IV immunoglobulin achieve acute platelet increases by different mechanisms: Modulation of cytokine and platelet responses to IV anti-D by FcγRIIa and FcγRIIIa polymorphisms. Br J Haematol 124:511-518, 2004
16. Samuelsson A, Towers TL, Ravetch JV: Anti-inflammatory activity of IVIg mediated through the inhibitory Fc receptor. Science 291:484-486, 2001
17. Andersen JC: Response of resistant idiopathic thrombocytopenic purpura to pulsed high-dose dexamethasone therapy. N Engl J Med 330: 1560-1564, 1994
18. Cheng Y, Wong RSM, Soo YOY, Chui CH, Lau FY, Chan NP, et al: Initial treatment of immune thrombocytopenic purpura with high-dose dexamethasone. N Engl J Med 349:831-836, 2003
19. Cooper N, Woloski BM, Fodero EM, Novoa M, Leber M, Beer JH, Bussel JB: Does treatment with intermittent infusions of intravenous anti-D allow a proportion of adults with recently diagnosed immune thrombocytopenic purpura to avoid splenectomy? Blood 99:1922-1927, 2002
20. Grillo-López AJ, Hedrick C, Rashford M, Benyunes M: Rituximab: Ongoing and future clinical development. Semin Oncol 29:105-112, 2002
21. Cooper N, Stasi R, Cunningham-Rundles S, Feuerstein MA, Leonard JP, Amadori S, et al: The efficacy and safety of B-cell depletion with anti-CD20 monoclonal antibody in adults with chronic immune thrombocytopenia purpura. Br J Haematol 125:232-239, 2004
22. Bennett CM, Rogers ZR, Kinnamon DD, Bussel JB, Mahoney DH, Abshire TC, et al: Prospective phase I/II study of rituximab in childhood and adolescent chronic immune thrombocytopenic purpura. Blood 107:2639-2642, 2005
23. Wang J, Wiley JM, Luddy R, Greenberg J, Feuerstein MA, Bussel JB: Chronic immune thrombocytopenic purpura in children: assessment of rituximab treatment. J Pediatr 146:217-221, 2005
24. Hasan AN, Bussel JB: Re-treatment with rituximab in ITP: comparison of standard dose with 2 forms of augmented rituximab. Blood 106: 1237, 2005 (abstr)
25. Stasi R, Stipa E, Masi M, Cecconi M, Scimo MT, Oliva F, et al: Long-term observation of 208 adults with chronic idiopathic thrombocytopenic purpura. Am J Med 98:436-442, 1995
26. Kojouri K, Vesely SK, Terrell DR, George JN: Splenectomy for adult patients with idiopathic thrombocytopenic purpura: A systematic review to assess long-term platelet count responses, prediction of response, and surgical complications. Blood 104:2623-2634, 2004
27. Schwartz J, Eldor A, Gillis S, Guinta A, Leber M, Bussel JB: Long term follow-up after splenectomy performed for immune thrombocytopenic purpura (ITP). Am J Hematol 72:94-98, 2003
28. Recommendations of the Advisory Committee on Immunization Practices (ACIP): Use of vaccines and immune globulins in persons with altered immunocompetence. MMWR Morb Mortal Wkly Rep 42:1-11, 1993
29. Wasserstrom HA, Cunningham-Rundles C, Lim LCL, Guerro NT, Wissert MH, Radigan L, et al: Splenectomized patients have reduced $CD27^+$ memory B cells but protective antibody responses to pneumococcal vaccination. Blood 104:3025, 2004 (abstr)

30. Fabris F, Tassan T, Ramon R, Carraro G, Randi ML, Luzzatto G, et al: Age as the major predictor of long-term response to splenectomy in immune thrombocytopenic purpura. Br J Haematol 112:637-640, 2001
31. Marcaccio MJ: Laparoscopic splenectomy in chronic idiopathic thrombocytopenic purpura. Semin Hematol 37:267-274, 2000
32. Cines DB, Blanchette V: Idiopathic thrombocytopenic purpura. N Engl J Med 364:995-1008, 2002
33. Vesely SK, Perdue JJ, Rizvi MA, Terrell DR, George JN: Management of adult patients with persistent idiopathic thrombocytopenic purpura following splenectomy. Ann Intern Med 140:112-120, 2004
34. Levy AS, Cunningham-Rundles S, Mazza B, Simm M, Gorlick R, Bussel J: High P-glycoprotein-mediated export observed in patients with a history of idiopathic thrombocytopenic purpura. Br J Haematol 118: 836-838, 2002
35. Kappers-Klunne MC, van't Veer MB: Cyclosporin A for the treatment of patients with chronic idiopathic thrombocytopenia purpura refractory to corticosteroids or splenectomy. Br J Haematol 114:121-125, 2001
36. Godeau B, Durand J-M, Roudot-Thoraval F, Tenneze A, Oksenhendler E, Kaplanski G, et al: Dapsone for chronic autoimmune thrombocytopenic purpura: A report of 66 cases. Br J Haematol 97:336-339, 1997
37. Scaradavou A, Woo B, Woloski BMR, Cunningham-Rundles S, Ettinger LJ, Aledort LM, et al: Intravenous anti-D treatment of immune thrombocytopenic purpura: Experience in 272 patients. Blood 89:2689-2700, 1997
38. Hou P, Pang J, Shi Y, Zhang C, Qin P, Zhao C, et al: Mycophenolate mofetil (MMF) for the treatment of steroid-resistant idiopathic thrombocytopenic purpura. Eur J Haematol 70:353-357, 2003
39. Figueroa M, Gehlsen J, Hammond D, Ondreyco S, Piro L, Pomeroy T, et al: Combination chemotherapy in refractory immune thrombocytopenic purpura. N Engl J Med 328:1226-1229, 1993
40. Huhn RD, Fogarty PF, Nakamura R, Read EJ, Leitman SF, Rick ME, et al: High-dose cyclophosphamide with autologous lymphocyte-depleted peripheral blood stem cell (PBSC) support for treatment of refractory chronic autoimmune thrombocytopenia. Blood 101:71-77, 2003
41. Kuter D, Bussel JB, Aledort LM, et al: A phase 2 placebo controlled study evaluating the platelet response and safety of weekly dosing with a novel thrombopoietic protein (AMG531) in thrombocytopenic adult patients (pts) with immune thrombocytopenic purpura (ITP). Blood 114:148a, 2004 (suppl 1, abstr)
42. Newland A, Caulier MT, Schipperus MR, et al: An open-label, unit dose-finding study evaluating the safety and platelet response of a novel thrombopoietic protein (AMG531) in thrombocytopenic adult patients (pts) with immune thrombocytopenic purpura (ITP). Blood 104:567a, 2004 (suppl 1, abstr)
43. Bussel JB, George JN, Kuter DJ, Wasser JS, Aledort LM, Chen M-G, Nichol JL: An open-label, dose-finding cohort study evaluating the safety of and platelet response to a novel thrombopoietic protein (AMG531) in thrombocytopenic patients with immune thrombocytopenic purpura (ITP). Blood 102:86a, 2003 (abstr)
44. Bussel JB, Mukherjee R, Stone AJ: A pilot study of rhuIL-11 treatment of refractory ITP. Am J Hematol 66:172-177, 2001
45. Snyder HW Jr, Cochran SK, Balint JP Jr, Bertram JH, Mittelman A, Guthrie TH Jr, et al: Experience with protein A-immunoadsorption in treatment-resistant adult immune thrombocytopenic purpura. Blood 79:2237-2245, 1992
46. Blanchette VS, Price V: Childhood chronic immune thrombocytopenic purpura: Unresolved issues. J Pediatr Hematol Oncol 25:S28-S33, 2003 (suppl 1)
47. Caulier MT, Rose C, Roussel MT, Huart C, Bauters F, Fenaux P: Pulsed high-dose dexamethasone in refractory chronic idiopathic thrombocytopenic purpura: A report on 10 cases. Br J Haematol 91:477-479, 1995
48. Kuwana M, Kawakami Y, Ikeda Y: Suppression of autoreactive T-cell response to glycoprotein IIb/IIIa by blockade of CD40/CD154 interaction: Implications for treatment of immune thrombocytopenic purpura. Blood 101:621-623, 2003
49. Lim SH, Hale G, Marcus RE, Waldmann H, Baglin TP: CAMPATH-1 monoclonal antibody therapy in severe refractory autoimmune thrombocytopenic purpura. Br J Haematol 84:542-544, 1993
50. Emilia G, Longo G, Luppi M, Gandini G, Morselli M, Ferrara L, et al: *Helicobacter pylori* eradication can induce platelet recovery in idiopathic thrombocytopenic purpura. Blood 97:812-814, 2001
51. Kohda K, Kuga T, Kogawa K, Kanisawa Y, Koike K, Kuroiwa G, et al: Effect of *Helicobacter pylori* eradication on platelet recovery in Japanese patients with chronic idiopathic thrombocytopenic purpura and secondary autoimmune thrombocytopenic purpura. Br J Haematol 118: 584-588, 2002
52. Michel M, Cooper N, Jean C, Frissora C, Bussel JB: Does *Helicobacter pylori* initiate or perpetuate immune thrombocytopenic purpura? Blood 103:890-896, 2003
53. Gill KK, Kelton JG: Management of idiopathic thrombocytopenic purpura in pregnancy. Semin Hematol 37:275-289, 2000
54. Fujimura K, Harada Y, Fujimoto T, Kuramoto A, Ikeda Y, Akatsuka J, et al: Nationwide study of idiopathic thrombocytopenic purpura in pregnant women and the clinical influence on neonates. Int J Hematol 75:426-433, 2002
55. Samuels P, Bussel JB, Braitman LE, Tomaski A, Druzin ML, Mennuti MT, et al: Estimation of the risk of thrombocytopenia in the offspring of pregnant women with presumed immune thrombocytopenic purpura. N Engl J Med 323:229-235, 1990
56. Michel M, Novoa MV, Bussel JB: Intravenous anti-D as a treatment for immune thrombocytopenic purpura (ITP) during pregnancy. Br J Haematol 123:142-146, 2003

Seminars in
HEMATOLOGY

Recent Advances in the Treatment of Childhood Immune Thrombocytopenic Purpura

Michael Tarantino

Immune thrombocytopenic purpura (ITP), the most common bleeding disorder in childhood, is a benign condition that typically resolves within 6 months following diagnosis. While all would agree on drug treatment for children with severe hemorrhage, management strategies of the minimally symptomatic child with a very low platelet count can vary widely. The case for treatment is based primarily on the risk for the uncommon complication of intracranial hemorrhage or other serious bleeding. Numerous clinical studies clearly indicate that immune globulins (intravenous immune globulin [IVIg] or anti-D) and corticosteroid therapy (prednisone and megadose methylprednisolone) are effective in rapidly raising platelet counts. However, physicians must ultimately decide whether to use drug therapy for a patient with minimal symptoms and low platelet count or adopt an "observation-only" approach. With this background, three fundamental questions emerge when evaluating different clinical strategies and potential outcomes: (1) Which children with ITP need treatment? (2) Which pharmacologic agent best accomplishes the goals of drug treatment? (3) Can physicians better predict the outcome of treatments?
Semin Hematol 43(suppl 5):S11-S17

Acute immune thrombocytopenic purpura (ITP) in children is widely perceived as an enigmatic, transient autoimmune disorder, frequently associated with a postinfectious illness. An estimated 5,000 cases of childhood ITP are diagnosed annually, with a peak incidence between the ages of 2 and 10 years.[1] Boys and girls are equally affected. Children with newly diagnosed ITP typically present with platelet counts of less than 10,000/μL, and purpura, a condition associated with intradermal and mucous membrane bleeding. In a recent prospective study in children with newly diagnosed ITP, approximately one fourth of patients exhibited oozing of blood from mucous membranes.[2]

It is commonly acknowledged that childhood ITP spontaneously resolves within 6 months, irrespective of drug therapy. However, it is the risk of serious bleeding complications such as gastrointestinal or intracranial hemorrhage (ICH) and the often strikingly low platelet count that compel most clinicians to prescribe drug treatment.

The decision whether to give drug therapy to minimally or moderately symptomatic children with ITP is a topic of lasting controversy. While a number of clinical trials indicate that treatment with corticosteroids or immune globulin induces a rapid increase in platelet count, most clinical trials have been underpowered to demonstrate that pharmacologic intervention can alter the ultimate outcome. Consequently, treatment is frequently based on best clinical judgment, and the need for uniform consensus persists in the therapeutic and diagnostic approaches to this disease.

This review will focus on three unresolved issues with regard to the treatment of childhood ITP. They are:

(1) Which children with ITP need treatment?
(2) Which pharmacologic agent best accomplishes the goals of treatment?
(3) How can physicians better predict the outcome of treatments?

Diagnosis

As is the case with adults, the diagnosis of ITP in children is based primarily on exclusion. Isolated thrombocytopenia is a relatively rare condition. Therefore, it is important that other causes of thrombocytopenia be ruled out through a physical examination and thorough history. In children less than 3 months of age, neonatal alloimmune thrombocytopenia and maternal ITP must be considered.

In approximately 60% of patients, ITP may follow an acute

Comprehensive Bleeding Disorders Center and Department of Pediatrics, University of Illinois College of Medicine at Peoria, Peoria, IL.
M.T. is supported by Baxter and Amgen and serves as a Consultant to Baxter.
Address correspondence to Michael Tarantino, MD, Comprehensive Bleeding Disorders Center, University of Illinois, 5019 N Executive Dr, Peoria, IL 61614. E-mail: mdtara@hemophilia-ctr-peoria.com

0037-1963/06/$-see front matter
doi:10.1053/j.seminhemat.2006.04.008

Table 1 Childhood ITP: Current Initial Therapy Options

Agent	Dose	Schedule	Reference
Prednisone	0.25 mg/kg	Daily × 21	Bellucci, 1988[9]
	2 mg/kg	Daily × 14, then taper	Buchanan, 1984[10]
	60 mg/m²	Daily × 21	Sartorius, 1984[11]
	4 mg/kg	Daily × 7, then taper	Blanchette, 1993[12]; Blanchette, 1994[13]
	4 mg/kg	Daily × 4	Carcao, 1998[14]
Methylprednisolone	30 or 50 mg/kg	Daily × 7	Albayrak, 1994[15]
	20–30 mg/kg	Daily × 2–7	Ancona, 2002[16]
	30 mg/kg	Daily × 3	van Hoff, 1988[17]
IVIg	0.8–1 g/kg	Daily × 1–2	Blanchette, 1993[12]
	0.25 g/kg	Once	Warrier, 1997[18]; Benesch, 2003[19]
Anti-D	25 μg/kg	Daily × 2	Blanchette, 1994[13]
	50–60 μg/kg	Once	Scaradavou, 1997[20]; Tarantino, 1999[21]; Monteleone, 2000[22]
	75 μg/kg	Once	Tarantino, 2003[2]; Newman, 2001[23]

Reprinted with permission.[24]

infection (viral or other) within the preceding 2 months.[3] ITP has also been associated with the measles, mumps, and rubella (MMR) vaccine, with an estimated risk of one in 24,000 doses and occurring within 6 weeks of vaccination.[4]

Children with ITP often present with platelet-type bleeding (purpura, petechiae, conjunctival hemorrhage) that has developed over a 24- to 48-hour period. Otherwise, the physical examination is unremarkable. Inspection of peripheral blood smear reveals thrombocytopenia (<10 to 20×10^9/L), often with normal to large platelets.[5] However, uniformly large platelets may indicate macrothrombocytopenia, such as in Sebastian syndrome, and not ITP. The morphology of red blood cells and white blood cells should be unaffected.

As an initial diagnostic test, bone marrow aspiration is rarely necessary in children; however, it may be useful in more difficult cases with atypical clinical or laboratory features that challenge the diagnosis, or in cases where response to therapy is absent.[6,7] Antiplatelet antibody assays, an additional tool, are usually positive for platelet-associated immune globulin, and are not routinely used because of their limited positive predictive value (80% to 83%); therefore, a negative test cannot exclude the diagnosis.[6,8]

Current Therapy Options

During the last several decades, many therapies have been evaluated in prospective and retrospective clinical trials in children with ITP. The primary outcome measure of these studies has been the rise in platelet count, with the inference that increased platelet counts reduce the risk of serious bleeding, and prevent ICH. The four most commonly used therapeutic agents for childhood ITP include two corticosteroids (prednisone and methylprednisolone) and two immune globulins (intravenous immune globulin [IVIg] and anti-D) (Table 1). Splenectomy is rarely used in children for initial therapy.

Over two decades ago, two randomized, prospective studies independently reported the effectiveness of prednisone in childhood ITP. Both trials demonstrated that prednisone led to a more rapid rise in platelet count in newly diagnosed ITP in children in comparison with no therapy.[10,11] In a randomized cooperative study, Sartorius reported that a moderate dose (60 mg/m²/day orally × 21 days) of prednisolone decreased the duration of severe thrombocytopenia in most patients.[11] In a separate trial, Buchanan and Holtkamp showed that prednisone (2 mg/kg/d × 14 days with subsequent tapering and discontinuation by day 21) resulted in statistically significant differences on day 7 of therapy. Children receiving prednisone had higher platelet counts and lower bleeding scores and bleeding times compared with placebo. Later, Bellucci et al reported that smaller doses of prednisone could avoid some of the adverse events associated with conventional dosing of corticosteroid therapy.[9]

Immune globulin alternatives are widely considered an advance over corticosteroids. In 1984, Imbach et al published a randomized study that demonstrated that pooled immune globulins were at least as effective as corticosteroids at standard doses.[25] Since that time, a variety of corticosteroid regimens, ranging from mid-range doses of prednisone (1 to 2 mg/kg/d) to so-called megadose methylprednisolone (up to 50 mg/kg/d for 2 to 5 days), have been shown to raise the platelet count in 1 to 7 days in the great majority of children with ITP.[15-17,26] The efficacy of corticosteroid and IVIg regimens was recently compared in a meta-analysis.[27] In this study, IVIg regimens yielded a significantly more rapid early rise in the platelet count in children with ITP.

Another immune globulin, anti-D, is available for children with ITP who are Rh D+. An early study suggested that patients receiving a dose of 25 μg/kg/d for 2 consecutive days experienced a slower platelet response compared with either prednisone or IVIg.[13] However, more recent studies have demonstrated that higher, single-day doses of anti-D may increase the platelet count more rapidly and for a longer duration.[21-23] Furthermore, a recently completed randomized clinical trial in newly diagnosed children with ITP confirms that high-dose anti-D (75 μg/kg intravenous once) is more effective than standard-dose anti-D and as effective as IVIg in raising platelet counts rapidly.[2]

Unanswered Questions: Who Really Needs Treatment?

The management of childhood ITP remains controversial because of the low risk of severe hemorrhage and the high likelihood of favorable outcomes in the absence of therapy. Sound clinical judgment supports drug and transfusion treatment of life-threatening bleeding[5]; however, the decision to intervene in the case of a minimally symptomatic child with a very low platelet count is not as clear.

Evidence in support of intervening with drug therapy includes numerous studies that show that patients treated with either corticosteroids or immune globulins experience a more rapid recovery of their platelet count compared with observation alone.[10-12] Furthermore, it has been documented that severe hemorrhage is more likely to occur in patients with platelet counts less than 10 × 10⁹/L.[28] Finally, drug treatment of a minimally symptomatic child may be more cost effective if it prevents high morbidity and mortality associated with intracranial or other severe hemorrhage.[29]

Evidence in support of the observation-only approach to a minimally symptomatic child with ITP is based on low rates of severe hemorrhage (0.1% to 1%), and that one half to one third of pediatric cases recover within 4 weeks in the absence of treatment.[5] In a retrospective assessment of 332 children with ITP over 10 years, a small minority of the 17% with major hemorrhage experienced an immediate rise in platelet count in response to either IVIg, corticosteroid treatment, or both.[30] Furthermore, in a study that specifically examined the "watchful waiting" approach in 55 children with acute ITP (but with no active mucosal bleeding), it was concluded that drug treatment unnecessarily increases the cost of management of this disease.[31] Finally, drug treatment may result in adverse events that outweigh the risk of serious bleeding, including the unlikely complications of thrombosis, overwhelming infection, and renal failure.[24]

Progress in identifying predictors of severe hemorrhage in newly diagnosed patients with low platelet counts who are at increased risk of life-threatening hemorrhage has been slow because of the rarity of this complication. However, a retrospective analysis of 75 children with ITP and ICH has provided preliminary information in identifying causative factors.[28] In 71.4% of patients in this study, the platelet count was less than 10 to 20 × 10⁹/L. Other precipitating events that were identified included head trauma, arteriovenous malformation, and aspirin use. The role of wet purpura or epistaxis as a warning of impending ICH was not specifically investigated because a far larger number of cases of ITP without ICH would have been required. The authors concluded that a low platelet count (<10 × 10⁹/L) constituted a permissive, but not a predictive risk factor.

In an earlier report by Medeiros and Buchanan, the medical records of 332 children diagnosed with ITP were reviewed. In this report, 17% of children had major hemorrhage defined as intracranial bleeding, epistaxis requiring cautery or nasal packing, gross hematuria, or other bleeding causing a decline in hemoglobin concentration.[30] Approximately 75% of bleeding episodes occurred in children with platelet counts less than 10 × 10⁹/L.

To collect data on the rate of severe hemorrhage, natural history, demographics, and management of ITP, an Intercontinental Childhood ITP Study (ICIS) Group was established in 1997. The first registry collected data on 3,000 patients, aged 4 months to 16 years, from 38 countries. Based on the ICIS, intracranial hemorrhage was identified in two of 1,496 children.[32] It is hoped that future studies from this organization will provide additional clinical data on other risk factors for the development of life-threatening hemorrhage.

Therefore, as with any therapy, the pros and cons must be appropriately considered for each patient. In addition, less tangible determinants, such as the likelihood of an accidental injury during times of severe thrombocytopenia or the patient's access (or lack of access) to emergency medical care, should be considered when deciding whether to intervene with drug therapy.

Adverse Events of Drug Therapy

The case for intervening with pharmacologic agents to raise the platelet count would be less controversial if the toxicity of drug therapy were rare. However, because of the risk of adverse events, clinicians must weigh the likelihood of clinical efficacy against the likelihood of clinically relevant adverse events. In most instances, routine monitoring for adverse events is warranted.

The adverse effects of corticosteroid treatment are dose- and duration-dependent and must be carefully monitored. Some of the common adverse events associated with brief courses of corticosteroids include gastritis, weight gain, behavioral changes, osteopenia, and glycosuria.[6] Other adverse events, such as ulcerative esophagitis, aseptic necrosis, and growth-inhibitory effects, may occur with more dose-intensive regimens.

Adverse events of IVIg are common (15% to 75%) and include headache, fever, and chills.[6] Severe headaches are of greatest concern in patients on immune globulin therapy (including anti-D) because when platelet counts fall below 5 × 10⁹/L, the possibility of an ICH as the cause of headache must be considered. Other adverse events associated with high-dose IVIg therapy include aseptic meningitis, intravascular hemolysis, hemolytic anemia, thrombosis, and renal dysfunction.[24,33-36]

Adverse effects associated with anti-D treatment include headache, fever, and chills. An infrequent but serious side effect with anti-D is intravascular hemolysis, which may result in acute renal failure.[1,37-40] The cause of the intravascular hemolysis is not well understood; however, some patients developing this complication have evidence of comorbid immunopathic conditions, including infection with Epstein-Barr virus.[40,41] Therefore, monitoring renal function is strongly recommended when signs of intravascular hemolysis are detected after anti-D infusion. Further, patients at risk for underlying hemolysis should be considered for other agents.

Guidelines for the Treatment of Acute ITP in Children

For a rational approach to the management of adult and pediatric ITP, specific guidelines have been published over the past 10 years. Acknowledging the dearth of randomized clinical trials, these recommendations, based on expert opinion, provide a careful assessment of published evidence. Two of the most widely used sets of recommendations were published by the American Society of Hematology (ASH) in 1996[5] and the British Committee for Standards in Haematology and General Haematology Task Force (BCSH) in 2003.[42] In addition, a set of recommendations was developed in Germany.[43]

Both the UK and ASH guidelines agree with the general principle that therapeutic and diagnostic decisions should be evidence based. However, the ASH task force recommends drug therapy for children with platelet counts of less than 10×10^9/L with little or no purpura.

In contrast to the ASH guidelines, the UK guidelines focus more on the clinical presentation of the patients and recommend that only patients who experience significant mucous membrane bleeding receive treatment. Accordingly, the UK guidelines state that patients with pronounced skin purpura and bruising may not reflect a serious risk of bleeding. Furthermore, the BCSH recommends that IVIg be used only for emergency treatment or for those who do not respond to corticosteroids.

While these different guidelines may reflect diverging philosophies on the likelihood of life-threatening bleeding in newly diagnosed children with ITP who are minimally symptomatic—and therefore, the necessity to initiate treatment—ultimately, a tailored decision is required for each patient. This decision should incorporate not only clinical information but also essential social information, such as the ability of caretakers to prevent a child from engaging in dangerous activities and/or taking medications with antiplatelet activity.

Unanswered Question: Which Agent Best Accomplishes the Treatment Goals?

The goal of ITP treatment must always be clear. While IVIg and megadose methylprednisone are equally effective in raising the mean platelet count after a period of 1 week,[16,44] some studies suggest that megadose methylprednisone is less effective than IVIg after 24 hours.[16] Response rates to higher dose corticosteroids within 24 hours are uniformly less than 50%.[16,26] Hence, the physician must decide whether elevating the platelet count rapidly within 24 hours justifies the higher cost and potential safety risk of IVIg. Corticosteroids (either standard- or high-dose) are inferior to IVIg for rapidly raising the platelet count in children with acute ITP.[27]

Recent studies suggest that platelet response to IVIg therapy is less dose-dependent than was once assumed. In a report by Warrier et al, the safety and efficacy of low-dose IVIg therapy for infants and children was compared with the established higher dose regimen.[18] Results of this study indicated that doses of 250, 400, or 500 mg/kg/d were as well tolerated and as effective in rapidly reversing thrombocytopenia as a dose of 1 g/kg/d. However, in patients with very low platelet counts, high-dose IVIg appears more effective in increasing platelet counts rapidly, within 72 hours.[19]

Reports from the last decade indicate that platelet response to anti-D in acute ITP is dose-dependent.[13,20,21,23] In a randomized trial of IVIg, anti-D, and oral prednisone in newly diagnosed pediatric patients, a 2-day regimen of 25 μg/kg per dose of anti-D resulted in a significantly slower increase in platelet count compared with IVIg.[13] However, in a retrospective analysis, a larger single dose of 45 to 50 μg/kg of anti-D was as effective as IVIg for the treatment of acute ITP in children.[21] These findings were confirmed in a prospective randomized study in adults.[23] A dose of 75 μg/kg/d of anti-D increased the platelet count more rapidly and for a longer period of time than the 50-μg/kg/d regimen.

Until recently, the safety and efficacy of higher-dose anti-D compared with IVIg or standard-dose anti-D have not been prospectively studied in children with ITP. A randomized three-arm trial in 105 children with newly diagnosed ITP and a platelet count less than 20×10^9/L has now been completed (Table 2).[2] Patients received either a single intravenous dose of 50 μg/kg anti-D, 75 μg/kg anti-D, or 0.8 g/kg IVIg. Following initial treatment, at 24 hours, the mean platelet count was greater (but not statistically significant) in the anti-D 75-μg/kg cohort and the IVIg cohort compared to the anti-D 50-μg/kg cohort (45 and 46×10^9/L *v* $33 \pm 5.4 \times 10^9$/L, $P = .12$ and .09, respectively) (Fig 1). By 7 days following initial treatment, the mean platelet counts were significantly greater in the anti-D 75-μg/kg patients compared with the other two cohorts. The most frequently observed adverse events in patients receiving anti-D included fever, headache, and chills (Fig 2). Collectively, these findings indicate that higher dose anti-D increases platelet count more rapidly than standard-dose anti-D and is as effective as IVIg.

Genetics of Childhood ITP

Immune thrombocytopenia is mediated by immune complexes that are formed by autoantibodies (IgG) generated against heterogeneous autoantigens on the platelets. Antibody-coated platelets circulate through the reticular endothelial system until they are recognized nonspecifically by the Fcγ receptors on the splenic or liver tissue macrophages and are subsequently cleared. Because the bone marrow cannot keep up with accelerated destruction of platelets, the result in most patients is thrombocytopenia.

Although the fundamental immune mechanisms of ITP have been known for more than 50 years,[42] some of the major molecular advances have been discovered relatively recently. Indeed, over the past 10 years many isoforms of the Fcγ receptors and their polymorphisms have been identified. These observations have contributed to a greater understanding of the pathogenesis of ITP. For example, it has now been determined that some Fcγ receptors have distinct functional

Table 2 Randomized Trial of Anti-D and IVIg for the Initial Treatment of ITP in Children

Study Patient Demographic Data					
Study group	**No.**	**M:F**	**Age (yrs), mean/median/min-max**	**Purpura***	
				% Dry (n)	**% Wet (n)**
Anti-D 50 μg/kg	35	0.8	4.9/4/1–16	27 (9)	73 (25)
Anti-D 75 μg/kg	35	0.8	4.6/4/1–15	27 (9)	73 (25)
IVIg	35	0.9	5.8/4/1–17	27 (9)	73 (25)

Platelet Response to Immune Globulin Treatment				
Platelet count (× 10⁹/L)	**Anti-D 50 μg/kg**	**Anti-D 75 μg/kg**	**IVIg**	**P**
Day 0				
No.	34	32	35	
Mean	8.5	9.4	9.2	NS
SD	3.1	5.0	5.4	
Day 1				
No.	32	31	35	
Mean	32.7	45.3	46.3	.12†, .09†
SD	5.4	34.6	32.0	
Day 7				
No.	31	29	30	
Mean	175.6	312.5	195.0	.005‡, .03§
SD	79.1	211.8	182.4	

Abbreviation: NS, not significant
Reprinted with permission.[2]
*Wet purpura was defined as one or more of: mucous membrane oozing, epistaxis, hematuria, melana, or hematemesis. Dry purpura was defined as petechiae and/or ecchymoses only.
†Anti-D 50 μg/kg *v* anti-D 75 μg/kg.
‡Anti-D 50 μg/kg *v* IVIg 0.8 g/kg.
§Anti-D 75 μg/kg *v* IVIg 0.8 g/kg.

capacities, such as either inhibiting or stimulating the immune response.

Four recent studies have provided evidence of the important role of particular polymorphisms in the FcγR gene in influencing the clinical outcomes in childhood ITP. In one study, Foster et al studied the FcγR gene in children with chronic ITP and found a greater likelihood of FcγRIIIB NA1 homozygosity than controls.[45] In a study of children with newly diagnosed ITP, however, the FcγRIIB Ile232Thr polymorphism was more prevalent in children with chronic ITP.[46] In a separate study, no association was observed between children with acute and chronic ITP and the occurrence of the polymorphisms FcγRIIIA F158V or FcγRIIA R131H.[47]

From a prospective randomized clinical trial,[48] the FcγRIIIa genotype did not correlate with the degree of purpura or chronicity of ITP in children with acute ITP; however, the VV genotype, which occurs in approximately 15% of the population, correlated with 100% platelet response to initial immunoglobulin treatment in children with acute ITP.[48] These findings are noteworthy because the FF and FV

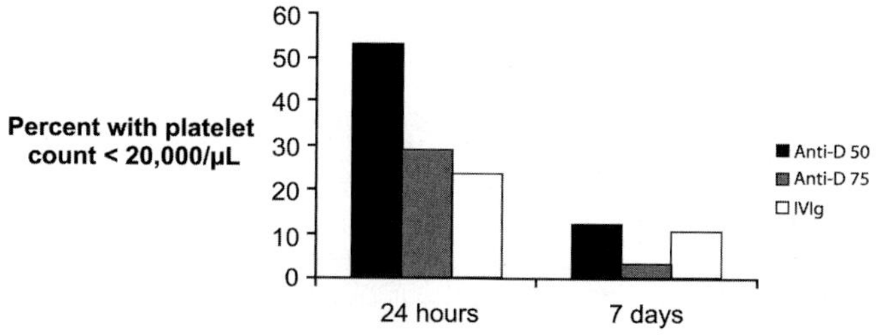

Figure 1 Rate of platelet response post initial treatment. Rate of platelet response at 24 hours and 7 days among patients treated with anti-D 50 μg/kg, anti-D 75 μg/kg, or IVIg 0.8 g/kg. At 24 hours: $P = .09$, anti-D 50 *v* anti-D 75; $P = .02$, anti-D 50 *v* IVIg; $P = .6$, anti-D 75 *v* IVIg. At 7 days, no significant difference was observed in the rate of platelet response among the three groups. Reprinted with permission.[2]

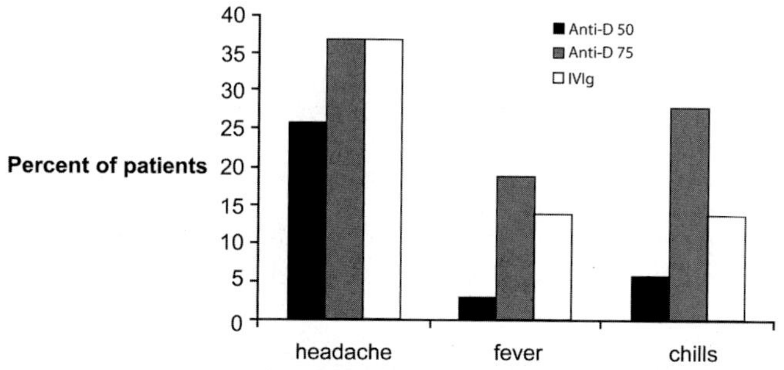

Figure 2 Adverse events. Headache was the most common adverse event, reported with equal frequency in the IVIg and anti-D 75-μg/kg groups. Fever was reported significantly less often in the anti-D 50-μg/kg group compared with the anti-D 75-μg/kg group ($P = .04$) and nearly so compared with the IVIg group ($P = .09$). Chills, during or shortly after the infusion, were reported least often in the anti-D 50-μg/kg group ($P = .015$ *v* the anti-D 75-μg/kg group, and $P = .24$ *v* the IVIg group). Reprinted with permission.[2]

polymorphisms were associated with a significantly lower rate of response.

Conclusions

In managing childhood ITP, physicians should evaluate each patient on an individual basis. The answers to salient clinical questions may be used to determine the optimal management strategy. Does the child have major or minor bleeding manifestations of ITP? Is the platelet count less than $10 \times 10^9/L$? Can the child's physical activity be adequately controlled? Does the child's caregiver have adequate access to emergency care if needed? Does the child have other features that would increase the risk for serious hemorrhage (such as recent head trauma or a family history of other bleeding disorders)? The sanguine, obedient adolescent with only dry purpura and a platelet count of $18 \times 10^9/L$ may do well without drug therapy, whereas the rambunctious toddler with wet purpura and a platelet count of $22 \times 10^9/L$ may be an appropriate candidate for an immune globulin or corticosteroid.

In the future, biological and genetic markers may be useful in predicting which children may develop life-threatening hemorrhage. To date, however, identifying which patients are truly in need of treatment is still unclear.

References

1. Chun NS, Savani B, Seder RH, Taplin ME: Acute renal failure after intravenous anti-D immune globulin in an adult with immune thrombocytopenic purpura. Am J Hematol 74:276-279, 2003
2. Tarantino MD, Young G, Bertolone SJ, Shafer FE, Kulkarni R, Kalinyak K, et al: High-dose anti-D immune globulin is as effective as IVIg in the treatment of newly diagnosed immune thrombocytopenic purpura (ITP) in children. Blood 102:299a-300a, 2003 (suppl 1)
3. Beardsley DS, Nathan DG: Platelet abnormalities in infancy and childhood, in Nathan DG, Orkin SH (eds): Hematology of Infancy and Childhood (ed 5). Philadelphia, PA, Saunders, 1988, pp 1585-1630
4. Farrington P, Pugh S, Colville A, Flower A, Nash J, Morgan-Capner P, et al: A new method for active surveillance of adverse events from diphtheria/tetanus/pertussis and measles/mumps/rubella vaccines. Lancet 345:567-569, 1995
5. George JN, Woolf SH, Raskob GE, Wasser JS, Aledort LM, Ballem PJ, et al: Idiopathic thrombocytopenic purpura: A practice guideline developed by explicit methods for the American Society of Hematology. Blood 88:3-40, 1996
6. Cines DB, Blanchette V: Immune thrombocytopenic purpura. N Engl J Med 346:995-1008, 2002
7. Calpin C, Dick P, Poon A, Feldman W: Is bone marrow aspiration needed in acute childhood idiopathic thrombocytopenic purpura to rule out leukemia? Arch Pediatr Adolesc Med 152:345-347, 1998
8. Warner MN, Moore JC, Warkentin TE, Santos AV, Kelton JG: A prospective study of protein-specific assays used to investigate idiopathic thrombocytopenic purpura. Br J Haematol 104:442-447, 1999
9. Bellucci S, Charpak Y, Chastang C, Tobelem G: Low doses v conventional doses of corticoids in immune thrombocytopenic purpura (ITP): Results of a randomized clinical trial in 160 children, 223 adults. Blood 71:1165-1169, 1988
10. Buchanan GR, Holtkamp CA: Prednisone therapy for children with newly diagnosed idiopathic thrombocytopenic purpura. A randomized clinical trial. Am J Pediatr Hematol Oncol 6:355-361, 1984
11. Sartorius JA: Steroid treatment of idiopathic thrombocytopenic purpura in children. Preliminary results of a randomized cooperative study. Am J Pediatr Hematol Oncol 6:165-169, 1984
12. Blanchette VS, Luke B, Andrew M, Sommerville-Nielsen S, Barnard D, de Veber B, et al: A prospective, randomized trial of high-dose intravenous immune globulin G therapy, oral prednisone therapy, and no therapy in childhood acute immune thrombocytopenic purpura. J Pediatr 123:989-995, 1993
13. Blanchette V, Imbach P, Andrew M, Adams M, McMillan J, Wang E, et al. Randomised trial of intravenous immune globulin G, intravenous anti-D, and oral prednisone in childhood acute immune thrombocytopenic purpura. Lancet 344:703-707, 1994
14. Carcao MD, Zipursky A, Butchart S, Leaker M, Blanchette VS: Short-course oral prednisone therapy in children presenting with acute immune thrombocytopenic purpura (ITP). Acta Pediatr 424:71-74, 1998 (suppl)
15. Albayrak D, Islek I, Kalayci AG, Gurses N: Acute immune thrombocytopenic purpura: A comparative study of very high oral doses of methylprednisolone and intravenously administered immune globulin. J Pediatr 125:1004-1007, 1994
16. Ancona KG, Parker RI, Atlas MP, Prakash D: Randomized trial of high-dose methylprednisolone versus intravenous immune globulin for the treatment of acute idiopathic thrombocytopenic purpura in children. J Pediatr Hematol Oncol 24:540-544, 2002
17. van Hoff J, Ritchey K: Pulse methylprednisolone therapy for acute childhood idiopathic thrombocytopenic purpura. J Pediatr 113:563-566, 1988
18. Warrier I, Bussel JB, Valdez L, Barbosa J, Beardsley DS: Safety and efficacy of low-dose intravenous immune globulin (IVIG) treatment for infants and children with immune thrombocytopenic purpura. Low-Dose IVIG Study Group. J Pediatr Hematol Oncol 19:197-201, 1997
19. Benesch M, Kerbl R, Lackner H, Berghold A, Schwinger W, Triebl-Roth K, et al: Low-dose versus high-dose immune globulin for primary treatment of acute immune thrombocytopenic purpura in children: Results of prospective, randomized single-center trial. J Pediatr Hematol Oncol 25:797-800, 2003
20. Scaradavou A, Woo B, Woloski BM, Cunningham-Rundles S, Ettinger LJ, Aledort LM, et al: Intravenous anti-D treatment of immune thrombocytopenic purpura: Experience in 272 patients. Blood 89:2689-2700, 1997
21. Tarantino MD, Madden RM, Fennewald DL, Patel CC, Bertolone SJ: Treatment of childhood acute immune thrombocytopenic purpura with anti-D immune globulin or pooled immune globulin. J Pediatr 134:21-26, 1999
22. Monteleone PM, Vander Heyden MA, Steele DA, Kelleher JH: Anti-D immunoglobulin in children with newly diagnosed immune thrombocytopenic purpura: A pilot study. Haematologica 85:887-888, 2000
23. Newman GC, Novoa MV, Fodero EM, Lesser ML, Woloski BM, Bussel JB: A dose of 75 microg/kg/d of i.v. anti-D increases the platelet count more rapidly and for a longer period of time than 50 microg/kg/d in adults with immune thrombocytopenic purpura. Br J Haematol 112: 1076-1078, 2001
24. Tarantino MD, Buchanan GR: The pros and cons of drug therapy for immune thrombocytopenic purpura in children. Hematol Oncol Clin North Am 18:1301-1314, 2004
25. Imbach P, Gaedicke G, Joller P: Interim evaluation of two cooperative studies assessing the effects of intravenous immunoglobulin (i.v. IgG) on childhood idiopathic thrombocytopenic purpura (ITP): I. Randomized study comparing i.v. IgG with oral corticosteroids in previously untreated acute ITP. II. Prospective study of i.v. IgG in acute and chronic ITP unresponsive to previous treatment. Blut 48:357-361, 1984
26. Duru F, Fisgin T, Yarali N, Kara A: Clinical course of children with immune thrombocytopenic purpura treated with intravenous immune globulin G or megadose methylprednisolone or observed without therapy. Pediatr Hematol Oncol 19:219-225, 2002
27. Beck CE, Nathan PC, Parkin PC, Blanchette VS, Macarthur C: Corticosteroids versus intravenous immune globulin for the treatment of acute immune thrombocytopenic purpura in children: A systematic review and meta-analysis of randomized controlled trials. J Pediatr 147:521-527, 2005
28. Butros LJ, Bussel JB: Intracranial hemorrhage in immune thrombocytopenic purpura: A retrospective analysis. J Pediatr Hematol Oncol 25:660-664, 2003

29. Adams JR, Nathan DP, Bennett CL: Pharmacoeconomics of therapy for ITP: Steroids, i.v.Ig, anti-D, and splenectomy. Blood Rev 16:65-67, 2002
30. Medeiros D, Buchanan GR: Major hemorrhage in children with idiopathic thrombocytopenic purpura: Immediate response to therapy and long-term outcome. J Pediatr 133:334-339, 1998
31. Dickerhoff R, von Ruecker A: The clinical course of immune thrombocytopenic purpura in children who did not receive intravenous immune globulins or sustained prednisone treatment. J Pediatr 137:629-632, 2000
32. Kuhne T, Imbach P, Bolton-Maggs PH, Berchtold W, Blanchette V, Buchanan GR, Intercontinental Childhood ITP Study Group: Newly diagnosed idiopathic thrombocytopenic purpura in childhood: An observational study. Lancet 358:2122-2125, 2001
33. Centers for Disease Control and Prevention (CDC): Renal insufficiency and failure associated with immune globulin intravenous therapy—United States, 1985-1998. MMWR Morb Mortal Wkly Rep 48:518-521, 1999
34. Schiavotto C, Ruggeri M, Rodeghiero F: Adverse reactions after high-dose intravenous immune globulin: Incidence in 83 patients treated for idiopathic thrombocytopenic purpura (ITP) and review of the literature. Haematologica 78:35-40, 1993 (suppl 2)
35. Zaidan R, Al Moallem M, Wani BA, Shameena AR, Al Tahan AR, Daif AK, et al: Thrombosis complicating high dose intravenous immune globulin: Report of three cases and review of the literature. Eur J Neurol 10:367-372, 2003
36. Gottlieb S: Intravenous immune globulin increases risk of thrombotic events. BMJ 324:1056, 2002
37. Gaines AR: Acute onset hemoglobinemia and/or hemoglobinuria and sequelae following Rh(o)(D) immune globulin intravenous administration in immune thrombocytopenic purpura patients. Blood 95:2523-2529, 2000
38. Gaines AR: Disseminated intravascular coagulation associated with acute hemoglobinemia or hemoglobinuria following Rh(0)(D) immune globulin intravenous administration for immune thrombocytopenic purpura. Blood 106:1532-1537, 2005
39. Roberti I, Bagtas JF, Reisman L, Murphy S: Severe acute renal failure due to hemoglobinuria after use of WinRho for the treatment of idiopathic thrombocytopenic purpura. Clin Pediatr (Phila) 40:61-62, 2001
40. Kees-Folts D, Abt AB, Domen RE, Freiberg AS: Renal failure after anti-D globulin treatment of idiopathic thrombocytopenic purpura. Pediatr Nephrol 17:91-96, 2002
41. Levendoglu-Tugal O, Jayabose S: Intravenous anti-D immune globulin-induced intravascular hemolysis in Epstein-Barr virus-related thrombocytopenia. J Pediatr Hematol Oncol 23:460-463, 2001
42. British Committee for Standards in Haematology and General Haematology Task Force: Guidelines for the investigation and management of idiopathic thrombocytopenic purpura in adults, children and in pregnancy. Br J Haematol 120:574-596, 2003
43. Sutor AH, Dickerhoff R, Gaedicke G, et al: Hămostasiologie: akute postinffektiōse immunthrombozytopenie im kindesalter, in Reinhard D, Cruetzig U, Kiess W, Luthardt T, Michalk D, Schmidt E, et al (eds): Leitlinien Kenderheilkunde und Jugenmedizin. Munich, Germany, Urban & Fischer, 1999, pp 23-27
44. Erduran E, Aslan Y, Gedik Y, Orhan F: A randomized and comparative study of intravenous immune globulin and mega dose methylprednisolone treatments in children with acute idiopathic thrombocytopenic purpura. Turk J Pediatr 45:295-300, 2003
45. Foster CB, Zhu S, Erichsen HC, Lehrnbecher T, Hart ES, Choi E, et al: Early Chronic ITP Study Group: Polymorphisms in inflammatory cytokines and Fcgamma receptors in childhood chronic immune thrombocytopenic purpura: A pilot study. Br J Haematol 113:596-599, 2001
46. Bruin M, Bierings M, Uiterwaal C, Revesz T, Bode L, Wiesman ME, et al: Platelet count, previous infection and FCGR2B genotype predict development of chronic disease in newly diagnosed idiopathic thrombocytopenia in childhood: Results of a prospective study. Br J Haematol 127:561-567, 2004
47. Carcao MD, Blanchette VS, Wakefield CD, Stephens D, Ellis J, Matheson K, et al: Fcgamma receptor IIa and IIIa polymorphisms in childhood immune thrombocytopenic purpura. Br J Haematol 120:135-141, 2003
48. Tarantino MD, Williams SA, Weber LC, Nugent DJ: *FCGR3A* genotype affects the platelet response to immune globulin (Ig) treatment of acute immune thrombocytopenic purpura (ITP) in children. Presented at the XXth Congress of the International Society on Thrombosis and Haemostasis, Sydney, Australia, August 6-12, 2005 (poster P2104)

Seminars in
HEMATOLOGY

Question and Answer

Question 1: Please comment on the use of dexamethasone in immune thrombocytopenic purpura (ITP) compared with methylprednisolone and, also, does the dose of anti-D or intravenous immune globulin (IVIg) have an impact on long-term responses?

Answer (Dr Tarantino): The experience is largely in children, and the long-term response rate in children to 4 days of a maximum of 40 mg/d of dexamethasone, either before or after splenectomy, is around 20%. Although high-dose methylprednisolone has been used as front-line treatment in childhood ITP, dexamethasone has not (at least as reported in the literature). Therefore, a direct comparison cannot be made. Regarding the dose effect of immune globulin treatment on long-term response, no difference was seen in the rate of chronicity among children treated with standard or higher-dose anti-D in our prospective trial. The platelet effect did seem to last longer with the higher dose, similar to the observation of Dr. Bussel as reported in Newman et al, Br J Haematol 2001.

Question 2: What role do you think the thrombopoietic agents and rituximab play in the treatment of ITP? Are they first-line or second-line therapies?

Answer (Dr Bussel): I do not think of those two treatments as first-line therapies. Use of a thrombopoietic agent will not cure somebody, but either taking a pill every day, if using the GSK agent, or getting a once-weekly subcutaneous injection of AMG 531 will commonly elicit a good platelet count. When using rituximab, one is potentially trying to cure people. In the United States, at least so far, where rituximab is available and the thrombopoietic agents are not, an increasing number of hematologists consider rituximab relatively early.

Question 3: Which is the most appropriate drug for chronic infantile ITP if IVIg does not elicit a response? Steroids, cyclosporine. . .?

Answer (Dr Tarantino): Infants with true ITP often are refractory to treatment; however, I think many eventually spontaneously resolve, even if not within 6 months. We are careful about using drugs with no safety data in children under age 3 years. It is a very empirical situation.

(Dr Bussel): The more refractory a patient with ITP is, especially an infant, but even an adult, the more one should consider alternative diagnoses. I believe that, relatively often, especially in infants, refractory ITP may be one of the 21 or more syndromes of inherited thrombocytopenia or perhaps a form of myelodysplasia.

Question 4: What is the appropriate therapy for severe thrombocytopenia associated with antiphospholipid syndrome?

Answer (Dr Bussel): I do not think anybody really knows the answer. When raising the platelet count, one should consider instituting appropriate anticoagulation therapy (eg, in an elderly male) once the platelet count gets over 40,000 or 50,000/μL.

Question 5: What about response rate? Do patients respond similarly?

Answer (Dr Bussel): I would expect that they would not respond very differently from patients without antiphospholipid antibody, but this remains unclear, possibly steroids would be relatively more effective in these patients. Again, if they respond, one runs the risk of a major thrombotic event when the platelets increase, if they have a strong antiphospholipid antibody.

Question 6: Did you evaluate the cost in your trials, eg, for anti-D at high doses compared with IVIg?

Answer (Dr Tarantino): Obviously, there were some major cost considerations between the two groups of patients depending on where they were treated. Between the groups, the re-treatment rate was about the same when the same criteria were used. It appeared, however, that it might have been a bit more cost effective to use anti-D.

Question 7: You mentioned delaying or avoiding splenectomy by using anti-D. Can you elaborate on this? Was this more effective in children or adults?

Answer (Dr Bussel): Specifically, the treatment experience was in adults. If the platelet counts fell to, for example, less than 30,000/μL, treatment was as needed with anti-D, and platelet counts were measured at weekly or biweekly intervals. In one study, six of 28 patients maintained stable platelet counts greater than 100,000/μL after more than 1 year of treatment.

Question 8: At what age do you consider treating the child as an adult?

Answer (Dr Tarantino): The randomized trial did not indicate that older children responded to treatment like adults did. In practice, however, I maintain a watchful eye on patients once they are about 12 years of age. I still treat them with a protocol similar to that for children, but realize that perhaps they are more likely to develop chronic ITP.

Question 9: Is that more related to the likelihood of a spontaneous remission? Is 12 years of age a cutoff for that as well?

Answer (Dr Tarantino): The more recent registry information from the ICIS study challenges that theory. I think we

0037-1963/06/$-see front matter Published by Elsevier Inc.
doi:10.1053/j.seminhematol.2006.04.011

may need different markers than age, or in addition to age, to really set that straight.

Question 10: Did you use IVIg with rituximab to decrease infections? How many times would you repeat the dose of rituximab?

Answer (Dr Bussel): Rituximab, when it is effective as shown by some of the data presented, can take up to 8 weeks to have an effect. Other treatments should be considered for the interim. Unless the patient is a small child under the age of 10 years, one should not have any significant degree of hypogammaglobulinemia with rituximab. As a result, IVIg will not be necessary. Where possible, IVIg should be avoided in favor of anti-D, because IVIg may shorten the half-life of rituximab by saturating FcRn, thereby decreasing the recycling of the antibody.

Question 11: Could you comment on the impact on treatment decisions of identifying the FcγRIIIa receptor phenotype?

Answer (Dr Tarantino): The VV genotype correlates with the best early response. Unfortunately, the VV genotype is the least common in the general population. I do not know whether the technology involved can become sufficiently rapid to affect important treatment decisions. I think, however, that someday we will be able to incorporate such information into our treatment decisions.

Question 12: How do you characterize large platelets and how would you incorporate that into your decision making?

Answer (Dr Bussel): Our experience is largely with the Bayer Advia 120, but the Sysmex XE2100 can automatically give you a reticulated platelet count. I do not know whether the definition of large platelets varies among machines, but I think in the Bayer Advia, they are 20 to 60 μL. Thus, they would not have to be megathrombocytes. These measurements are not included in the regular complete blood cell count and must be selected from the special platelet parameters. We did examine the utility of other variables such as mean platelet mass, platelet crit, and the platelet equivalent of the red blood cell distribution width index, but none were as useful as measuring large platelets for predicting response to treatment as we recently published in *Haematologica*.

ELSEVIER
SAUNDERS
email: reprints@elsevier.com

Vol 43, No 4 October 2006

Seminars in HEMATOLOGY

Neal S. Young · Photis Beris
Editors

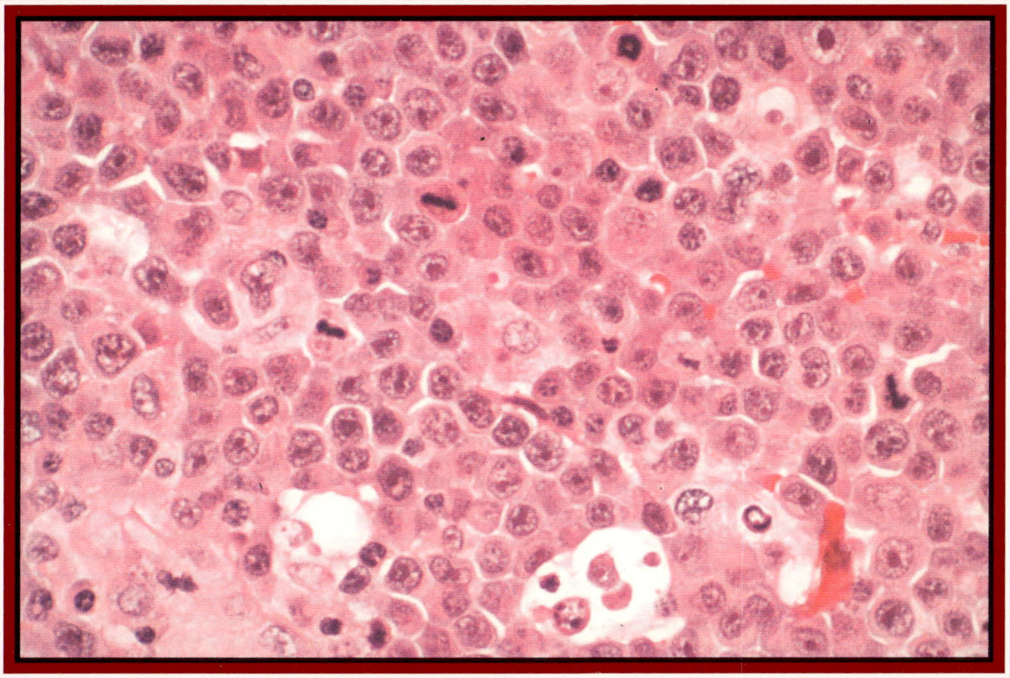

Treatment of Diffuse Large B-Cell Lymphomas

Richard I. Fisher
Guest Editor

W.B. Saunders

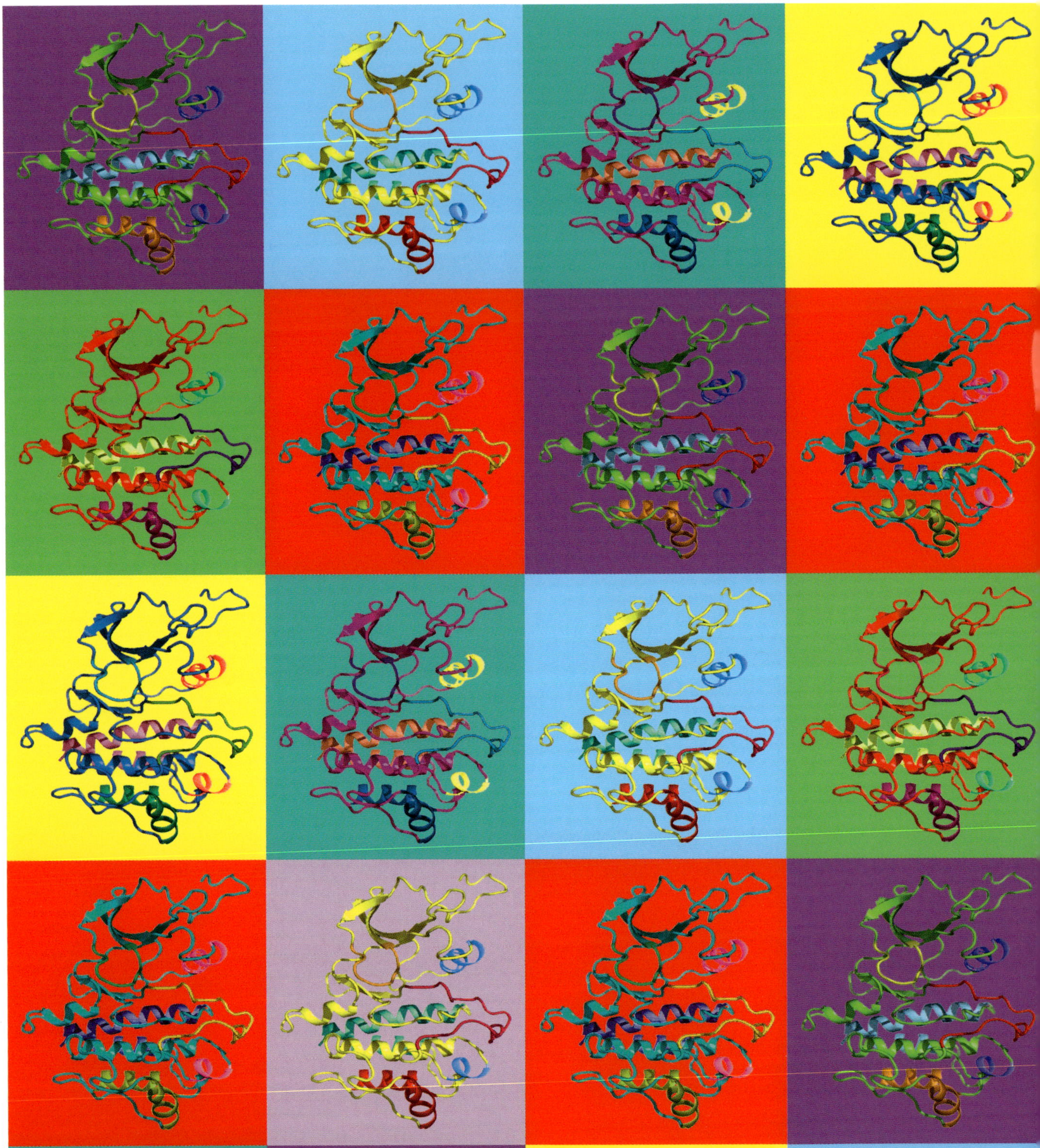

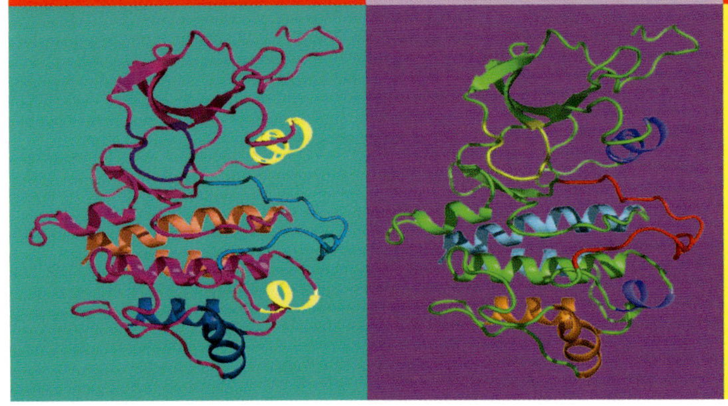

References: 1. Melo JV, Deininger MWN. *Hematol Oncol Clin North Am.* 2004;18:545-568. 2. Deininger MWN, Buchunger E, Druker BJ. *Blood.* 2005;105:2640-2653. 3. Branford S, Rudzki Z, Walsh S, et al. *Blood.* 2003;102:276-283. 4. Hochhaus A, La Rosée P. *Leukemia.* 2004;188:1321-1331. 5. Roche-Lestienne C, Soenen-Cornu V, Grardel-Duflos N, et al. *Blood.* 2002;100:1014-1018. 6. Gorre ME, Skaggs BJ, Sawyers CL. Presented at: Annual Meeting of the American Society of Hematology; December 2-6, 2004; San Diego, Calif. Abstract 556. 7. Donato NJ, Wu JY, Stapley J, et al. *Blood.* 2003;101:690-698. 8. Martinelli G, Soverini S, Rosti G, Cillani D, Baccarani M. *Haematologica.* 2005;90:534-541. 9. Pasquet J-M, Pocaly M, Lagarde V, et al. Presented at: Annual Meeting of the American Society of Hematology; December 2-6, 2004; San Diego, Calif. Abstract 1981. 10. Gorre ME, Ellwood-Yen K, Chiosis G, Rosen N, Sawyers CL. *Blood.* 2002;100:3041-3044. 11. Deininger MWN, Goldman JM, Melo JV. *Blood.* 2000:96:3343-3356.

CML: A Disease of Increasing Molecular Complexity

At present, there is a considerable amount of knowledge on the molecular biology of chronic myeloid leukemia (CML), providing an unparalleled platform for molecularly targeted therapy. While the *BCR-ABL* gene remains the driving force in CML, ongoing research into the inhibition of additional molecular targets, including mutations of the *BCR-ABL* kinase, may lead to new therapies.[1,2]

CML Is a Disease With More Than One Target

BCR-ABL Kinase Mutations within the *ABL* kinase domain are emerging as the most frequent mechanism for the reactivation of *BCR-ABL* activity and, thus, represent important potential targets in CML.[2-5] The development of *BCR-ABL* mutations can occur through either genetic instability or secondary mutational events over the course of the disease and is not limited to late-stage disease.[5]

Recent evidence has also shown that certain mutations may bind and phosphorylate substrates distinct from wild-type *BCR-ABL* and have the potential to activate alternative signaling pathways, providing additional insight into why certain mutations are associated with poor prognosis.[6]

SRC-Family Kinases are independent oncogenic pathways that are believed to be involved in late-stage disease progression. Two members of the *SRC* family in particular, *LYN* and *HCK*, are highly overexpressed and activated in patients with blast crisis and have been implicated in leukemic tumor cell growth, apoptotic protection, and kinase inhibitory activity.[7,8]

Heat-Shock Family Proteins (Hsp) are molecular chaperones capable of maintaining the stability and function of *BCR-ABL*.[9,10]

Downstream BCR-ABL Signal Transduction Pathways are responsible for the development and proliferation of malignant cells through a signaling cascade of multiple oncogenic kinase events.[11] These pathways represent potential new targets for molecular therapy.[1]

BCR-ABL Mitogenic Signaling Pathways*[11]

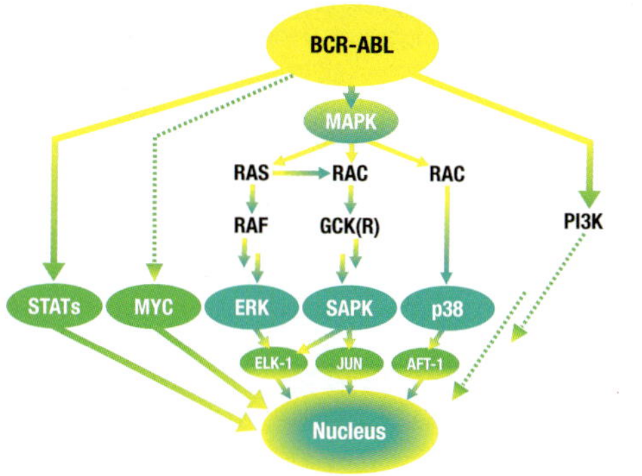

Reprinted with permission from Deininger MWN, et al.

* Note: This is a simplified diagram of the *BCR-ABL* signaling pathways. Numerous additional downstream targets have been reported.

Potential Multi-Targeted Approaches to CML Therapy

Significant progress has been made in the development of therapeutic agents directed against molecular targets specifically expressed or abnormally activated in patients with CML.[1] While *BCR-ABL* remains the primary target for CML therapy, there is hope that new research investigating synergistic approaches, simultaneously addressing multiple targets, may lead to new therapies for patients with CML.

Bristol-Myers Squibb is committed to investigating the molecular causes of cancer and developing potential new treatment alternatives to help address the needs of people living with cancer.

Seminars in HEMATOLOGY

Neal S. Young · Photis Beris
Editors

Peter A. Miescher, *Founding Editor* Ernst R. Jaffé, *Co-Editor Emeritus*

Seminars in Hematology (ISSN 0037-1963) is published quarterly by Elsevier Inc, 360 Park Avenue South, New York, NY 10010-1710. Months of issue are January, April, July and October. Business and Editorial Office: 1600 John F. Kennedy Blvd., Ste. 1800, Philadelphia, PA 19103-2899. Customer Service Office: 6277 Sea Harbor Drive, Orlando, FL 32887-4800. Periodicals postage paid at New York, NY and additional mailing offices.

POSTMASTER: Send address changes to *Seminars in Hematology*, Elsevier Customer Service, 6277 Sea Harbor Drive, Orlando, FL 32887-4800.

Editorial correspondence should be addressed to Photis Beris, MD, Division d'Hématologie, Hôpital Cantonal Universitaire, 25 rue Micheli-du-Crest, 1211 Geneve 14, Switzerland, or Neal S. Young, MD, 4400 17th Street, NW, Washington, DC 20011.

Business correspondence (subscriptions, change of address) should be addressed to the Publisher, Elsevier, 6277 Sea Harbor Dr, Orlando, FL 32887-4800; Email elspcs@elsevier.com.

Change of address notices, including both the old and new addresses of the subscriber, should be sent at least one month in advance.

Customer Service: 1-800-654-2452; outside the United States and Canada, (407) 345-4000.

Yearly subscription rates: United States and possessions: individual, $169.00; institution, $267.00; single issues, $81.00. All other countries: individual, $239.00; institution, $339.00; single issues, $81.00. Student and resident: United States and possessions, and Canada: $85.00; all other countries: $122.00. To receive student/resident rate, orders must be accompanied by name of affiliated institution, date of term, and the *signature* of program/residency coordinator on institution letterhead. Orders will be billed at individual rate until proof of status is received. Current prices are in effect for back volumes and back issues. Single issues, both current and back, exist in limited quantities and are offered for sale subject to availability. Back issues sold in conjunction with a subscription are on a prorated basis. Prices are subject to change without notice. *Checks* should be made payable to Elsevier and sent to *Seminars in Hematology*, Elsevier, Periodicals Department, PO Box 628239, Orlando, FL 32862-8239.

Other correspondence (copyediting, production) should be addressed to Elsevier, 1600 John F. Kennedy Blvd, Ste 1800, Philadelphia, PA 19103-2899.

Reprints: For 100 or more copies of an article in this publication, please contact the Commercial Reprints Department, Elsevier, 360 Park Ave South, New York, NY 10010-1710. Telephone (212) 633-3813, fax (212) 633-3820; e-mail, reprints@elsevier.com.

Advertising Representative: Cunningham Associates, 180 Old Tappan Rd, Old Tappan, NJ 07675. Telephone: (201) 767-4170; fax: (201) 767-8065; email: kdunn@cunnasso.com.

The contents of *Seminars in Hematology* are indexed in *Index Medicus* and *MEDLINE, Current Contents/Clinical Medicine, Current Contents/Life Sciences,* Science Citation Index, and *EMBASE/* Excerpta Medica.

The *Seminars in Hematology* home page is located at *www.seminhematol.org*.

W.B. Saunders **Philadelphia, PA**

Seminars in
HEMATOLOGY

Vol 43, No 4, October 2006

Treatment of Diffuse Large B-Cell Lymphomas

Richard I. Fisher
Guest Editor

Treatment of Diffuse Large B-Cell Lymphomas 205
Richard I. Fisher

Diffuse Agressive Histologies of Non-Hodgkin Lymphoma: Treatment and Biology of Limited Disease 207
Thomas P. Miller, Catherine M. Spier, and Lisa Rimsza

Standard Treatment of Advanced Stage Diffuse Large B-Cell Lymphoma 213
Bertrand Coiffier

Dose-Intensified Treatment of Advanced-Stage Diffuse Large B-Cell Lymphomas 221
Gerhard Held, Joerg Schubert, Marcel Reiser, and Michael Pfreundschuh, for the German High-Grade Non-Hodgkin-Lymphoma Study Group

Drug Resistance in Diffuse Large B-Cell Lymphoma 230
Wyndham H. Wilson

Role of Hematopoietic Stem Cell Transplantation for Advanced-Stage Diffuse Large Cell B-Cell Lymphoma-B 240
Auayporn Nadamanee and Stephen J. Forman

New Drugs for the Treatment of Advanced-Stage Diffuse Large Cell Lymphomas 251
Owen A. O'Connor and Paul Hamlin

Annual Index 262

Cover Illustration: Inguinal lymph node biopsy from a 51-year-old patient showing a homogeneous proliferation of large immunoblastic cells with atypical nuclei, large central nucleoli, and relatively abundant eosinophilic cytoplasm. These B lymphocytes were irf-4–positive and CD10- and bcl-6–negative, suggesting an activated phenotype. Hematoxylin & eosin staining (400×). Courtesy of Thomas McKee, MD, Service de Pathologie Clinique, Hôpital Cantonal, Geneva, Switzerland.

Seminars in HEMATOLOGY

Previous Issues

2005

Vol 42, No 1, January	**von Willebrand Factor in Hemostasis and Thrombosis** *Pier M. Mannucci, Guest Editor*
Vol 42, No 2, April	**Immune Hemolytic Anemia** *George Garratty, Guest Editor*
Vol 42, No 3, July	**Transplant Immunobiology** *Effie W. Petersdorf, Guest Editor*
Vol 42, No 4, October	**Chronic Myeloproliferative Disorders** *Radek Skoda and Josef T. Prchal, Guest Editors*

2004

Vol 41, No 1, January	**Thrombotic Thrombocytopenic Purpura: Advances in Pathophysiology, Diagnosis, and Treatment** *Bernhard Lämmle and James N. George, Guest Editors*
Vol 41, No 2, April	**Erythrocyte Membrane Proteins and Their Diseases** *Narla Mohandas, Guest Editor*
Vol 41, No 3, July	**Chronic Lymphocytic Leukemia** *Kanti R. Rai and Jacques Louis Binet, Guest Editors*
Vol 41, No 4, October	**Gene Therapy in Hematology** *Cynthia E. Dunbar, Guest Editor*

2003

Vol 40, No 1, January	**Management of Chronic Myeloid Leukemia** *John M. Goldman, Guest Editor*
Vol 40, No 2, April	**Herpesvirus in Hematology** *Giovanna Tosato, Guest Editor*
Vol 40, No 3, July	**Hematologic Malignancies of Cytotoxic Cells** *Thomas P. Loughran Jr, Guest Editor*
Vol 40, No 4, October	**Genomics in Hematology** *Louis M. Staudt, Guest Editor*

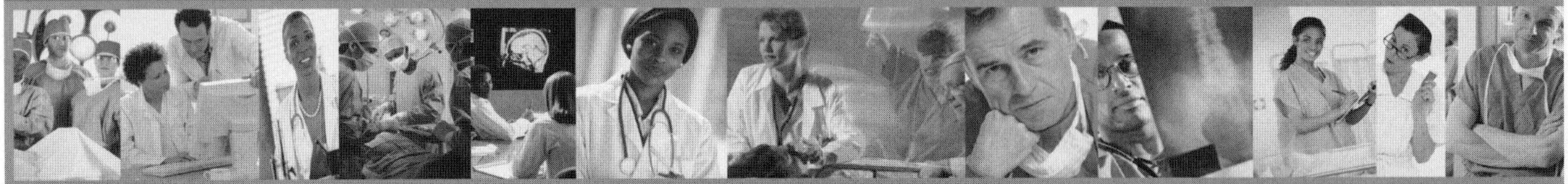

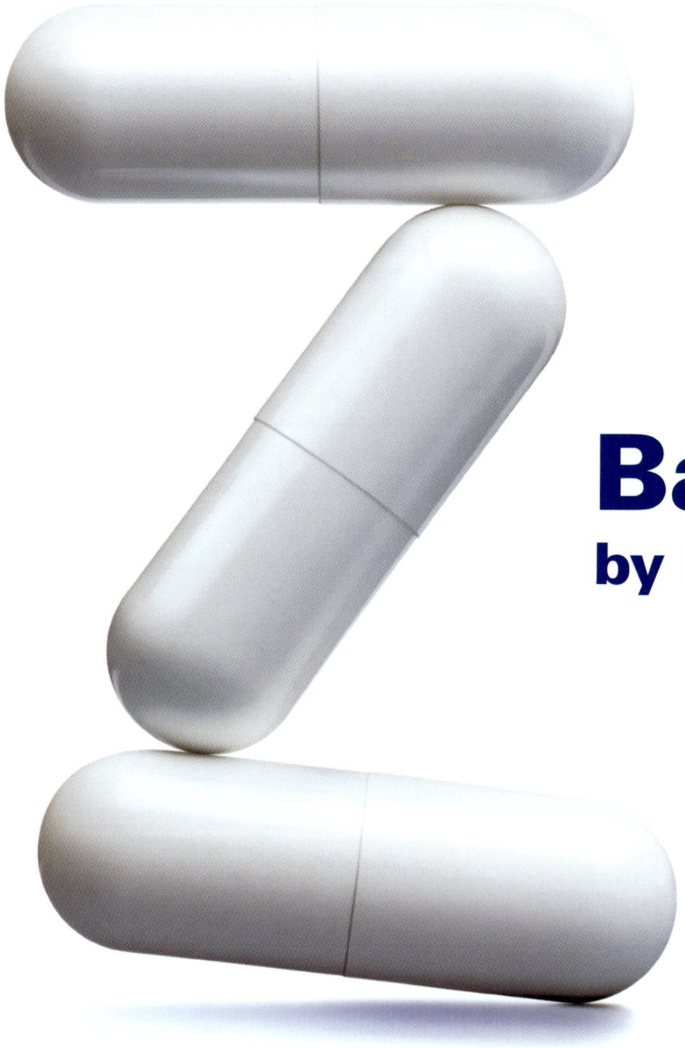

For adults with mild-to-moderate ***type 1 Gaucher disease*** *for whom enzyme replacement therapy is not an option*

Balance
by Substrate Reduction

Substrate Reduction Therapy (SRT) With Zavesca Provides Important Benefits

- Liver and spleen volume reductions seen as early as month 6—continued reductions over 24 months
- Hemoglobin concentration and platelet count improvements seen as early as month 6—significant improvements seen at 24 months

Zavesca Maintained Benefits of Long-Term Enzyme Replacement Therapy (ERT)

- In patients on ERT for a mean of 5.6 years, liver and spleen volume, as well as hemoglobin concentration and platelet count, were maintained after 6 months of Zavesca monotherapy

Important Safety Information

- Peripheral neuropathy has been reported in patients receiving Zavesca
- Zavesca may cause fetal harm if administered to a pregnant woman
- There is a risk of impaired fertility in men

Convenient Oral Dosing

- Recommended at 100 mg tid
- May be taken with or without food

Zavesca may be prescribed only by physicians knowledgeable in the management of Gaucher disease

- **Visit www.ZAVESCA.com or call 1.866.228.3546**

ZAVESCA® 100mg
(miglustat) capsules

Please see brief summary of full prescribing information on following page.

ACTELION

Seminars in
HEMATOLOGY

Future Topics

Vol 44, No 1, January	**Transfusion Medicine in the Early 21st Century** *Harvey Klein, Guest Editor*
Vol 44, No 2, April	**Inherited Thrombophilias** *Michael Greaves, Guest Editor*
Vol 44, No 3, July	**Hematopoietic Growth Factors** *Arnold Ganser, Guest Editor*
Vol 44, No 4, October	**Autologous Stem Cell Transplantation** *Theo De Witte, Guest Editor*

Seminars in
HEMATOLOGY

Forthcoming Issue
January 2007

Transfusion Medicine in the Early 21st Century
Harvey G. Klein, *Guest Editor*

Pulmonary Transfusion Reactions — *David F. Stroncek*

The Structure and Function of the Rh Antigen Complex — *Connie Westhoff*

Emerging Infectious Agents That Threaten the Blood Supply — *Harvey J. Alter, Susan L. Stramer, and Roger Dodd*

Granulocyte Transfusion: Current Status — *Thomas H. Price*

Modifying the Red Blood Cell Surface: Toward An ABO-Universal Blood Supply — *Martin L. Olsson and Henrik Clausen*

Transfusion-Associated Microchimerism: A New Complication of Blood Tranfusions in Severely Injured Patients — *William Reed, Tzong-Hae Lee, Philip J. Norris, Garth H. Utter, and Michael P. Busch*

Red Blood Cell Substitutes — *Robert M. Winslow*

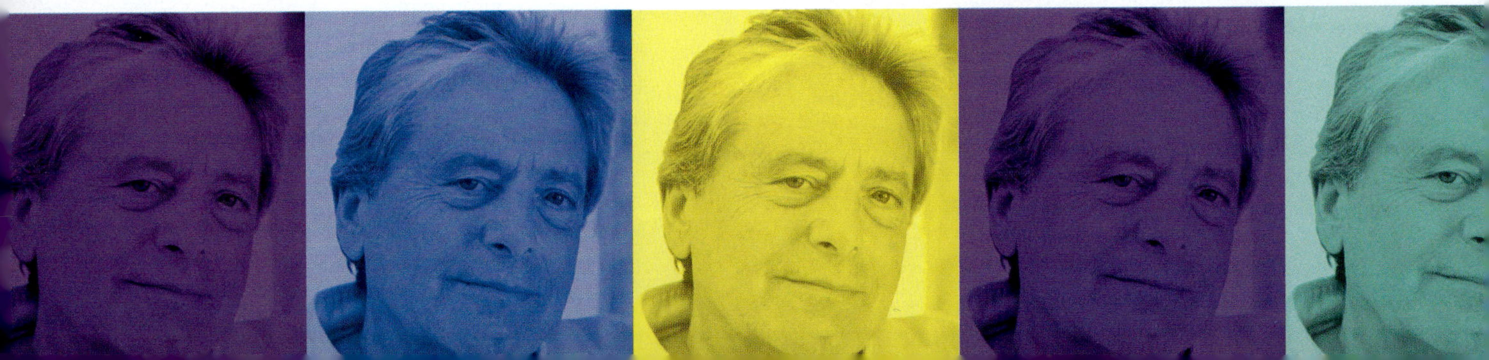

ELSEVIER

Seminars in
HEMATOLOGY

Volume 43, Number 4 **October 2006**

Treatment of Diffuse Large B-Cell Lymphomas

Diffuse large B-cell lymphoma (DLCL-B) is the most common non-Hodgkin's lymphoma throughout the world. An aggressive disease that is uniformly fatal without treatment, DLCL-B represents one of the major successes of combination chemotherapy for the treatment of malignancy. For more than 20 years, combination chemotherapy with CHOP (cyclophosphamide, doxorubicin, vincristine, and prednisone) resulted in cure for over 50% of all DLCL-B patients.[1] However, attempts to improve on those therapeutic results were essentially unsuccessful. Recently, significant improvements in overall survival have been achieved. This issue of *Seminars in Hematology* is dedicated to analyzing, in detail, those current and also future potential therapeutic advances as seen by some of the world's leading DLCL-B investigators. In some sense, this issue is also dedicated to the monoclonal antibody rituximab. Although it had relatively modest single-agent activity in untreated or relapsed patients with DLCL-B,[2] the addition of rituximab to CHOP has resulted in improved complete remission rates, failure-free survival, and even overall survival for these patients.[3]

In the initial article, Miller and colleagues from the University of Arizona and the Southwest Oncology Group (SWOG) discuss the current status of treatment for early stage DLCL-B. Their pioneering studies established three cycles of CHOP plus involved-field radiation as the standard effective treatment for these patients.[4] Whether this therapy should still be the standard is now less clear since late relapses have been observed in patients treated with three cycles of CHOP plus radiation and other investigators have now published data suggesting that radiation may no longer be necessary. In addition, essentially all patients are being treated with CHOP plus rituximab even though currently there is only phase II data in abstract form to support that decision. Miller et al use differences in clinically relevant prognostic factors to try to sort out the different therapeutic results that have been reported recently.

Next, Coiffier describes the pioneering studies from The Groupe d'Etude des Lymphomes de l'Adulte (GELA) that first demonstrated improved survival in elderly patients with advanced-stage DLCL-B receiving CHOP plus rituximab compared to CHOP alone.[3] Coiffier reviews the more recent data from the United States Intergroup study that supports the GELA results,[5] as well as the international trials extending the benefit of CHOP plus rituximab to younger patients.

Pfreundschuh and colleagues from the German High Grade Non-Hodgkin Lymphoma Study Group present the results of their series of studies exploring dose escalation for the treatment of these patients.[6] In Germany, CHOP plus rituximab given on a 14-day schedule (CHOP-14) is now considered the standard for elderly patients as opposed to CHOP given on the historical 21-day schedule (CHOP-21). The debate between the French and German protocols can only be resolved by a prospective phase III comparative study of the two regimens, which is currently being conducted by the GELA group. In addition, these authors postulate that changes in the method of administering rituximab might have important therapeutic consequences.

Wilson from the National Cancer Institute next describes a totally different approach to therapy based on efforts to overcome drug resistance and to administer variable doses of chemotherapy based on the patient's peripheral white blood cell count. This effort has resulted in the EPOCH-R (etoposide, prednisone, vincristine, cyclophosphamide, doxorubicin, and rituximab) series of studies. Currently, EPOCH-R is being compared to CHOP-R in a prospective randomized trial being conducted by the Cancer and Leukemia Group B (CALGB). Wilson also reviews the new and exciting data generated from the gene arrays of patients with DLCL-B. The genetic heterogeneity of DLCL-B can now be documented, rational subgroups can be established, and even targeted therapy may result from an improved understanding of the critical pathways operative in the different subsets of DLCL-B patients.

Nademanee and Forman from the City of Hope and SWOG review the role of stem cell transplantation in these patients. Initially demonstrated to offer curative hope for patients relapsing after initial treatment for DLCL- B, the role of stem cell transplant in the initial treatment of patients presenting with clinical features that predict a poor therapeutic outcome with standard CHOP chemotherapy has been difficult to establish clearly. This issue should be resolved by the results of an ongoing North American Intergroup Study (SWOG-9704) comparing early versus delayed autologous stem cell transplantation in poor-prognosis patients with DLCL-B. These authors also review the most recent data on reduced-intensity allogeneic transplantation for relapsed patients.

doi:10.1053/j.seminhematol.2006.07.007

Finally, O'Connor and Hamlin from Memorial Sloan-Kettering Cancer Center present the hope for future improvements by reviewing the new drugs that are currently in development and likely to impact the treatment of DLCL-B. More targeted therapeutics are clearly on the horizon and may add to or even replace current therapy.

Thus, in less than a decade tremendous progress has been made in the treatment of DLCL-B. All of this progress came from rationally designed, well-conducted clinical trials. The challenge to readers of this issue of *Seminars* is to continue that momentum by ensuring that all of their patients are offered and encouraged to enroll in future clinical studies.

Richard I. Fisher, MD
University of Rochester Medical Center
Rochester, NY
Guest Editor

References

1. Fisher RI, Gaynor ER, Dahlberg S, Oken MM, Grogan TM, Mize EM, et al: Comparison of a standard regimen (CHOP) with three intensive chemotherapy regimens for advanced non-Hodgkin's lymphoma. N Engl J Med 328:1002-10066, 1993
2. Coiffier B, Haioun C, Ketterer N, Engert A, Tilly H, Ma D, et al: Rituximab (anti-CD20 monoclonal antibody) for the treatment of patients with relapsing or refractory aggressive lymphoma: A multicenter phase II study. Blood 92:1927-1932, 1998
3. Coiffier B, Lepage E, Briere J, Herbrecht R, Tilly H, Bouabdallah R, et al: CHOP chemotherapy plus rituximab compared with CHOP alone in elderly patients with diffuse large-B-cell lymphoma. N Engl J Med 346: 235-242, 2002
4. Miller TP, Dahlberg S, Cassady JR, Adelstein DJ, Spier C, Grogan T, et al: Chemotherapy alone compared with chemotherapy plus radiotherapy for localized intermediate- and high-grade non-Hodgkin's lymphoma. N Engl J Med 339:21-26, 1998
5. Haberman TM, Weller EA, Morrison VA, Cassileth PA, Cohn BB, Dakhil SR, et al: Phase III trial of rituximab-CHOP vs. CHOP with a second randomization to maintenance rituximab or observation in patients 60 years of age and older with diffuse large B cell lymphoma. Blood 102:6a, 2003
6. Pfreundschuh M, Trumper L, Kloess M, Schmits R, Feller AC, Rube C, et al: Two-weekly or 3-weekly CHOP chemotherapy with or without etoposide for the treatment of elderly patients with aggressive lymphomas: Results of the NHL-B2 trial of the DSHNHL. Blood 104: 634-641, 2004

ELSEVIER

Seminars in
HEMATOLOGY

Diffuse Aggressive Histologies of Non-Hodgkin Lymphoma: Treatment and Biology of Limited Disease

Thomas P. Miller, Catherine M. Spier, and Lisa Rimsza

A quarter century has passed since the paradigm for treating aggressive histologies of non-Hodgkin lymphoma (NHL) presenting with limited extent of disease (LD) changed from using aggressive surgical staging techniques followed by primary radiotherapy (RT) to clinical staging followed by initial treatment with doxorubicin-containing chemotherapy (CT). This paradigm shift occurred for two reasons. First, unlike the predictable contiguous spread of Hodgkin lymphoma from one lymph node region to the next, the NHLs are largely systemic diseases characterized by early hematogenous spread. Second, the discovery of a potential curative combination of drugs, including cyclophosphamide, doxorubicin, vincristine, and prednisone (CHOP), for use in advanced disease could eradicate micrometastatic disease in patients with LD. The focus of current investigation on controlling the systemic nature of the disease has not changed. In this regard, new effective systemic therapies using combination chemotherapy plus monoclonal antibodies have resulted in improved outcome for patients with advanced disease and those treatment strategies are now under investigation in patients with LD.
Semin Hematol 43:207-212

Prior to 1980 patients with aggressive subtypes of non-Hodgkin lymphoma (NHL) underwent rigorous staging, including laparotomies, to assure that all detectable disease was confined to one or two anatomical sites. These patients then received raditotherapy (RT) using variable doses and fields from involved-field RT to total nodal irradiation. The strategy was successful for the rare patient but the majority of patients relapsed and died within the first 2 years following treatment. In 1979, Miller and Jones proposed an alternative approach using clinical staging followed by initial treatment with cyclophosphamide, doxorubicin, vincristine, and prednisone (CHOP), a regimen that had recently been shown to extend survival for patients with advanced disease.[1] Some patients received consolidative RT. For the 22 study patients, 2-year survival was 100%. For the next 25 years investigators largely focused on optimizing treatment using various drug combinations with or without consolidative RT. During that time more precise definitions of limited disease (LD) emerged, potent risk factors were recognized, new staging technologies were developed, additional effective drugs for treating advanced disease were incorporated into routine use, and insights into relevant biology were discovered. This review addresses some of the issues currently discussed by investigators and questions asked by clinicians pertinent to treating patients with LD lymphoma.

Diagnosis and Histology

Adequate surgical sampling of a tumor mass is a foundation to establish an accurate World Health Organization (WHO) histologic classification of NHL, to recognize potential risk factors, and to gain insight into the nuances of optimal therapy. Fine-needle aspirations (FNA), as practiced in the United States, are inadequate for these purposes.[2] A diagnosis of "NHL," "high-grade lymphoreticular malignancy," or even "follicle center–derived lymphoma" is not adequate to provide optimal care or predict prognosis. However, there is little information relating outcome of patients with LD to histologic subtype.

Prior therapeutic trials of LD have usually included intermediate- and high-grade histologies (except lymphoblastic subtype) using the Working Formulation classification system. Histologies that we now know to have unique biologic and clinical behavior in advanced disease were "lumped" as "aggressive subtypes" in these older studies. Part of the problem has been a change in the classification system used during the period of accrual to some of the larger therapeutic trials for patients with LD. Changes in the classification sys-

Departments of Medicine and Pathology, and Arizona Cancer Center, University of Arizona, Tucson, AZ.

Address correspondence to Thomas P. Miller, MD, Arizona Cancer Center, PO Box 245024, 1515 N Campbell Ave, Tucson, AZ 85724. E-mail: tmiller@azcc.arizona.edu

doi:10.1053/j.seminhematol.2006.07.001

tem based on a better understanding of the biology of lymphoma require immunophenotyping and, on occasion, molecular analysis, techniques that were not routinely performed during the 1980s and early 1990s. Spier et al for the Southwest Oncology Group (SWOG) have attempted to reclassify cases of LD using the SWOG lymphoma tissue bank by applying modern immunohistochemical techniques to the preserved specimens and reclassifying the cases according to WHO criteria.[3] All patients were treated with either eight cycles of CHOP or three cycles of CHOP followed by involved-field RT, a randomized trial previously reported as SWOG 8736.[4] The histologic review of that study resulted in two major unexpected findings. First, there were no perceptible differences in outcome based on histology (Table 1). Overall survival curves for diffuse large cell (DLCL) immunophenotype unknown, diffuse large B-cell (DLBCL), Burkitt-like (BL), follicular grade 3 (FL), and peripheral T-cell not otherwise specified (PTCL) lymphomas had overlapping survival curves ($P = .94$). Five-year estimates of overall survival varied from 78% to 82%. Failure-free survival curves similarly overlapped. Five-year estimates of failure-free survival varied from 70% to 75% except for the nine patients with PTCL, who had a 5-year failure-free survival rate of 56%. Given such small numbers of patients with PTCL, the perceived difference was not statistically significant ($P = .99$). The group from the British Columbia Cancer Agency has reported a similar finding for 21 patients with the T-cell phenotype.[5] The second unexpected finding was that these patients with LD had a relatively constant risk of relapse over a period of 10 years regardless of histology, with survival curves failing to reach a plateau as is seen in advanced disease. These observations taken together suggest either that LD is a product of a unique biology (rather than an early form of advanced disease), or that key molecular events determining outcome are the same for different stages, and LD patients simply require up to 10 years for recurrence to manifest (in this case, one might surmise that the survival curves will plateau, but at the same percent survival as seen in advanced disease). Gene array technology may provide insight into these unexpected observations.

Table 1 Outcome by WHO Histology Subtype of NHL

WHO Histology	No. of Patients	5-yr TTF*	5-yr OS†
DLCL, NOS	104	72%	82%
DLBCL	174	73%	80%
Burkitt-like	27	70%	78%
Follicular, grade 3	37	75%	78%
PTCL, NOS	9	56%	78%

NOTE. There are no significant differences between aggressive histologies.

Abbreviations: WHO, World Health Organization; TTF, time to treatment failure; OS, overall survival; DLCL, diffuse large cell lymphoma; NOS, not otherwise specified; DLBCL, diffuse large B-cell lymphoma; PTCL, peripheral T-cell lymphoma.

*$P = .99$.

†$P = .94$.

Staging

The results of current therapeutic trials for patients with LD were based on history, physical examination, computed tomography (CT) scans of the chest, abdomen, and pelvis, and a bone marrow biopsy to determine the extent of disease. Staging laparotomies were obviated with the development of effective systemic chemotherapy. With the advent of positron emission tomography (PET) and PET-CT fusion scans, the issue of adequate or optimal staging is again relevant.[6] Clearly, PET scans will, on occasion, reveal distant sites of unexpected disease involvement following traditional staging techniques. The issue is what to do with this information, and there are no studies to provide guidance. Should a patient with clinical stage I disease involving the neck be upstaged to stage III disease following a PET scan showing an abnormal area of uptake in the retroperitoneum? Or does such a patient without anatomic evidence of abdominal involvement simply recapitulate the historic information obtained from staging laparotomies? We know that NHL is systemic in nearly all patients from the time of diagnosis. That is why treatment with initial chemotherapy is required for optimal results. The question then is whether the PET scan identifies a critical tumor burden that cannot be eradicated with a brief course of chemotherapy? That question could be answered in a clinical trial wherein PET scans are performed on all patients with LD and then ignored during treatment planning. Outcome could then be correlated with the pretreatment PET scan. Such a trial would determine, in addition, whether PET scans provide any incremental useful information to established staging techniques. In the meantime, investigators using PET imaging will likely see improved results for both patients with LD and for patients with advanced disease, as patients with low tumor burden migrate to higher stages and the costs to treat patients escalate.

Prognostic Factors

The number of statistically significant prognostic factors available to forecast outcome for patients with NHL is seemingly limited only by the number of patients available for study. Most investigators have accepted the International Prognostic Index (IPI) as a standardized means to categorizing advanced disease patients by risk.[7] The IPI works for patients with LD, but does not have much utility because the majority of patients with LD fall into a single low-risk category. LD patients are low risk by definition, having stage I–II disease and one or fewer sites of extranodal disease. In addition, these patients with small tumor volumes seldom have a poor performance status. Thus, they can only have the poor-risk features of older age, elevated serum lactate dehydrogenase (LDH), and rarely, a poor performance status. One might presume then that LD patients are relatively homogeneous with regard to risk (95% fall into the lowest risk factor category using the IPI), but this is not the case.[8] If one modifies the IPI with regard to stage for use in LD patients, and stage II becomes an adverse risk factor, enough variables are created to allow separation of outcome (Table 2). Using this

Table 2 Adverse Risk Factors, as Defined by the International Prognostic Index, Refined for Use in Patients With Limited Disease

Adverse Risk Factor	IPI	Stage-Modified IPI
Stage	III, IV	Non-bulky II
Age	>60	>60
LDH	>normal	>normal
PS	≥2	≥2
"E" sites	≥2	Not applicable

Abbreviations: IPI, International Prognostic Index; LDH, lactate dehydrogenase; PS, performance status; E, extranodal.

simple modification of the IPI we have shown that patients with no adverse risk factors have an outstanding 5-year survival of 94% while patients with 3 or 4 adverse risk factors have a poor 5-year survival of only 50%. The stage-modified IPI appears to be reproducible, as the British Columbia Cancer Agency has retrospectively analyzed their large experience of treating LD using this system and found remarkably similar results (Table 3).[5]

The stage-modified IPI can be used to better select patients for clinical trials. In a recently reported study to test the efficacy of rituximab in LD patients, the stage-modified IPI was used to determine eligibility. Patients with no risk factors were unlikely to relapse in the first 5 years following treatment and, thus, their inclusion in a clinical trial using time to treatment failure as a primary end point would have required a larger study cohort to observe the expected number of failures. In addition, patients with no risk factors would have received additional treatment they did not need. Thus the trial could be directed at those patients with an unacceptable risk for relapse, who could be identified by having at least one adverse risk factor (see "Treatment" below).

The stage-modified IPI for use in LD patients can be used to compare treatment results across trials. In this regard, it is comforting to know that pilot results published by the British Columbia Cancer Agency can be, and were, reproduced by a cooperative group. Virtually all patients in North America with LD seem to carry the same risk for recurrence and the same likelihood of cure when treated with a brief course of CHOP followed by involved-field RT.[5,8] Why then do the results of the Groupe d'Etude des Lymphomes d'Adulte (GELA) differ so dramatically (Table 4)? It would seem that we are either comparing "apples and oranges" or there are significant differences in treatment administration that are not apparent from initial reports.

Table 3 Five-Year Overall Survival Results Compared Between Studies to Test Reproducibility of Stage-Modified IPI in Patients With Limited Disease

Risk Factor	SWOG 5-yr OS	BCCA 5-yr OS
0	94%	97%
1 or 2	74%, 72%	77%
≥1	70%	—
3 or 4	50%	58%

NOTE. SWOG data set combines (averages) the results of patients treated on two different treatment arms (see Table 4).

Abbreviations: SWOG, Southwest Oncology Group; BCCA, British Columbia Cancer Agency; OS, overall survival.

Treatment

The overriding principle of therapy for patients with LD and aggressive-histology NHL is to initiate treatment with systemic chemotherapy of curative potential. At this time, this specifically means using a doxorubicin-containing combination of drugs. Recent data suggest it is prudent to add rituximab to the combination.[9-11] However, there are relatively few combinations of drugs and sequences of therapeutic modalities for which prospective data are available. The following section summarizes completed clinical trials of LD.

As a benchmark for comparison, consider three cycles of CHOP followed by involved-field RT [CHOP(3) plus RT], the most thoroughly tested treatment regimen. CHOP(3) plus RT results in long-term and reproducible disease-free survival for the majority of patients with LD. It outperforms eight cycles of CHOP [CHOP(8)] over the short-term (5 years) but appears to have no advantage by 10 years.[4,8] Progression-free survival and overall survival curves appear to come together between 7 and 9 years. However, long-term follow-up of patients treated on SWOG study 8736 comparing CHOP(3) plus RT to CHOP(8) shows that the area under the survival curves favored CHOP(3) plus RT in patient-years survived and that CHOP(3) plus RT was less toxic.

More recently, investigators from France representing the GELA have reported two large randomized trials challenging the role of RT in the treatment of LD. These trials were designed for specific subsets of patients with LD based on age criteria. In the first trial, Reyes et al compared a dose- and schedule-intense chemotherapy regimen (ACVBP: doxorubicin, cyclophosphamide, vindesine, bleomycin, and prednisone) alone to the CHOP(3) plus RT combination in patients 60 years and younger.[12] Patients treated with ACVBP had considerably more toxicity, but also significantly improved event-free survival and overall survival. These outcome advantages remained after removing from analysis patients with bulky (10 cm) disease, albeit the advantage was diminished. It was important to assess the results after excluding patients with bulky stage II disease since this represents advanced disease and three cycles of CHOP is predictably inadequate for advanced disease. For all patients entered on trial the 5-year survival rates for ACVBP and CHOP(3)

Table 4 Treatment Results Across Studies Compared by Risk Factors

Risk Factor	SWOG CHOP(3) + RT	BCCA CHOP(3) + RT	GELA CHOP(3) + RT	GELA ACVBP
0	95	97	83	91
1	77	77	78	85
2	77	77	—	—

NOTE. Percentage (%) 5-year survival outcome by risk factor.

plus RT were 90% and 81%, respectively (P = .001). After removing patients with bulky disease, the 5-year survival difference between ACVBP and CHOP(3) plus RT was reduced but remained significantly different (P = .01). Toxicity for the ACVBP group was significant and has been reported to include hospitalization for more than 20% of all patients treated with each of three induction cycles of ACVBP. However, there were no treatment-related deaths. Interestingly, and of possible critical importance, 26 patients (8%) did not receive RT on the CHOP(3) plus RT treatment arm and 28% of patients receiving RT relapsed within the planned RT field.

The second randomized trial from the GELA has been reported on several occasions in abstract form and was designed to test whether RT contributes any incremental advantage to CHOP chemotherapy.[13] In this study, 576 older patients (age >60 years) were randomized to receive CHOP(4) plus RT or CHOP(4) alone. Fillet et al demonstrated no detectable difference between treatment regimens. Five-year event-free survival rates were 68% for CHOP(4) and 66% for CHOP(4) plus RT, and overall survival rates were 72% and 68%, respectively. They concluded that four cycles of CHOP alone is as good as four cycles of CHOP plus RT and has less toxicity by virtue of deleting the RT. The results of this study are remarkable, and important, as they indicate that RT adds nothing but toxicity to the treatment of lymphoma in the best possible patient population, those with LD. Why then would RT ever be considered for consolidation in more advanced disease?

Although the GELA investigators have stated that new standards for treating LD have been established, it is probably prudent to look for more details and consider alternative explanations before adopting ACVBP and its remarkable toxicity in young patients and foregoing RT in elderly patients. Consider Table 4, which compares the results of all trials using CHOP(3) plus RT and corrects for risk factors.[5,8,12] For those patients with stage I disease and no other IPI adverse risk factors, the large series from Vancouver and SWOG achieved nearly identical survival results at 5 years of 97% and 95%. The GELA trial by Reyes et al, on the other hand, has a 5-year survival of 83%, an increase in mortality over the first 5 years of follow-up of more than 300%. The question is whether the GELA trial included an adverse group of patients that is not identified using the IPI index, or whether RT as delivered by the GELA is fundamentally different. Many of the details of RT administration in that trial, as well as the trial reported by Fillet et al, are not known. However, the data thus far presented by Reyes et al raise a significant issue regarding RT administration. What is the effect on survival after excluding from analysis 8% of patients not receiving the prescribed treatment (RT), and why are there so many in-field relapses (see above)? Although it is prudent to wait for additional data to judge the effects of RT, the studies by the French GELA raise a fundamental issue in the treatment of LD. Is there a role for RT in the treatment of LD?

Horning et al attempted to determine the utility of RT in an Eastern Cooperative Oncology Group (ECOG) study of patients with somewhat more advanced disease, including bulky stage I and all stage II patients.[14] Patients who achieved a complete remission (CR) after eight cycles of CHOP were randomized to observation or to low-dose (3,000 rad) involved-field RT. Unfortunately, the study was inadequately powered to determine modest or even moderate significant differences in outcome. However, the trends are impressive. For the 172 CR patients randomized, disease-free survival was 73% for the RT group and 56% for the observation group measured at 6 years follow-up (P = .05). No significant survival differences were noted, with 67% of the observation group alive at 6 years compared to 79% for the low-dose RT group (P = .24). It is intriguing to speculate what the outcome of the study might have been had twice the number of patients been randomized. The study does demonstrate excellent disease control within the RT fields, with only three local relapses in the RT group, and a significant difference in disease-free survival (in-field relapses constituted <5% of the treatment failures). These findings are not consistent with the GELA studies and suggest that RT administration differs among treatment sites and that RT planning and administration may be critical to outcome.

The question of RT efficacy in treating LD may never be resolved. The discovery of increased efficacy of the CHOP plus rituximab combination may obviate the need for involved-field RT. Alternatively, the addition of rituximab to CHOP plus RT may allow for additional reductions in total-dose doxorubicin and/or RT, further decreasing the toxicity of the combined treatment regimen. Currently, only pilot trials using rituximab in LD are available for review. Miller et al reported the results of a pilot study in patients with LD who, in addition, had one or more adverse risk factors.[9] Patients received CHOP(3) plus RT plus four infusions of rituximab during the CHOP administration. Rituximab was given on days −7, 1, 22, and 43 with CHOP administered on days 0, 21, and 42. Results were compared to the historic experience of CHOP(3) plus RT using the same selection factors to identify 68 control patients from SWOG 8736.[4] Among 62 patients treated, the results at 2 years demonstrated a 50% reduction in relapses and deaths. It seems unlikely that any group will undertake a randomized trial comparing CHOP alone to CHOP plus rituximab in LD and these pilot results, if still positive with longer follow-up, will likely be the rationale for using CHOP plus rituximab in LD.

Trials underway in the United States and Europe seem to be focusing on the efficacy of radioimmunoconjugates added to CHOP, with or without rituximab. The rationale for testing radioimmunoconjugates derives from the efficacy, ironically, of RT to control NHL. Relapses within the RT fields for patients with LD are uncommon, except as noted above. Consequently, if a radioimmunoconjugate is able to "track" to areas of microscopic disease, the effect of RT may enhance control of distant sites of subclinical disease. Other trials will likely test the efficacy of chemotherapy alone using CHOP plus rituximab.

Biology

Localized DLBCL can occur at any anatomic location with presumed similar biology and outcome. However, in the last few years, several site-specific differences have been described among localized DLBCLs. These differences include (1) altered expression of antigen presentation molecules in the CNS and testicular lymphoma; (2) different histogenesis and outcome in cutaneous DLBCL of the leg versus other cutaneous sites; and (3) different use of the nuclear factor κB (NFκB) and B-cell receptor signaling pathways in mediastinal (thymic) large B-cell lymphoma.

Primary CNS and testicular lymphomas occur in immune-privileged sites and appear to have distinct immunologic properties. In particular, there is reported loss of expression of the major histocompatibility type II antigen (MHC II), HLA-DR, in 61% of testicular cases and 46% of CNS cases as compared to 5% of nodal DLBCLs.[15] This loss of expression is associated with homozygous deletions or hemizygous deletions combined with mutations of the second allele of the involved MHC II gene locus at 6p21.[15-17] How the absence of MHC class II relates to lymphomagenesis or tumor survival mechanisms at these sites is currently unknown. However, the propensity of testicular DLBCL to relapse at CNS sites and vice versa speaks to the predilection of MHC class II–negative DLBCL for immune-privileged locations.[18] It can be speculated that loss of expression of the MHC class II proteins by the tumor cells alters the ability of the lymphoma cells to express tumor-associated antigens, leading to consequent altered immunosurveillance, which may be relevant to immune-privileged sites.[19-22]

Another site-specific difference in localized DLBCL was recently described among primary cutaneous DLBCLs, which have been reclassified into three separate diseases.[23] These diseases include DLBCL-leg type, primary cutaneous follicular center cell lymphoma (PCFCCL), and DLBCL-other. While the DLBCL-other category may represent nodal or extranodal DLBCL disseminated to cutaneous sites, the other two entities are considered primary cutaneous lymphomas. At first glance, distinguishing DLBCL of the leg as different from DLBCL in other locations seems arbitrary. However, DLBCL-leg type has some unique clinical features: presentation in older women, rapid growth of multiple lesions usually below the knee, and a 5-year disease-specific survival of only 55%.[23] Gene expression profiling experiments further demonstrate a pattern of gene usage in DLBCL-leg similar to the activated B-cell type of DLBCL, which is associated with poorer patient survival in noncutaneous DLBCL.[24-26] In contrast, cutaneous DLBCL occurring as part of the spectrum of PCFCCL has a predilection of the head/neck and trunk regions, usually consists of slowly growing single or grouped lesions, and has a disease-specific 5-year survival of 95%.[23] By gene expression profiling, cutaneous DLBCLs that are part of PCFCCL have a gene usage pattern similar to the germinal center subtype of DLBCL, which is associated with good survival in DLBCL from noncutaneous sites.[24-26] The reasons for the differences in gene expression pattern based on cutaneous location are unknown.

Mediastinal (thymic) large B-cell lymphoma (MBCL) is another type of localized DLBCL that has some characteristic clinicopathologic findings: predominant disease initially confined to the mediastinum, locally invasive to other thoracic structures, associated dense fibrosis, predilection for female patients in their third to fourth decades, and fairly good patient survival with combination chemotherapy.[27] Despite these properties, it is unclear whether MBCL is truly a separate entity from other localized DLBCL. Recent gene expression profiling experiments demonstrate a characteristic gene expression pattern in MBCL with high expression levels of genes in the NFκB pathway and low expression levels of genes in the B-cell receptor signaling pathways. Interestingly, these two features are also reported in gene expression profiling of Hodgkin lymphoma, suggesting that at least partially overlapping lymphomagenic mechanisms exist between these two diseases.[28,29] These examples of recently described site-specific differences in the biology of localized DLBCL may have significant clinical and therapeutic implications.

Summary

Substantial progress toward curing patients with aggressive histologies of NHL presenting with LD has been made over the past 25 years. By focusing on the systemic nature of the disease, investigators have improved outcome. These same investigators now challenge the role of RT as they apply new, less toxic, and more effective treatment regimens to patients with early stages of the disease. In addition, surprising discoveries regarding outcome related to histology and site of disease involvement suggest that NHLs may have unique biologies associated with low tumor burdens. The heterogeneity of the disease at the molecular level is recapitulated in the range of outcomes based on clinical features. Understanding these variables will eventually lead to curative therapy for all patients.

References

1. Miller TP, Jones SE: Chemotherapy of localized histiocytic lymphoma. Lancet 8:358-360, 1979
2. Hehn ST, Grogan TM, Miller TP: Utility of fine-needle aspiration as a diagnostic technique in lymphoma. J Clin Oncol 22:3046-3052, 2004
3. Spier CM, LeBlanc M, Chase EM, Fisher RI, Miller TP: Histologic subtypes do not confer unique outcomes in early-stage lymphoma: Long-term followup of SWOG 8736. Blood 104:891a, 2004 (abstr)
4. Miller TP, Dahlberg S, Cassady JR, Adelstein DJ, Spier CM, Grogan TM, et al: Chemotherapy alone compared with chemotherapy plus radiotherapy for localized intermediate and high-grade non-Hodgkin's lymphoma. N Engl J Med 339:21-26, 1989
5. Shenkier TN, Voss N, Fairey R, Gascoyne RD, Hoskins P, Klimo P, et al: Brief chemotherapy and involved-region irradiation for limited-stage diffuse large-cell lymphoma: An 18 year experience from the British Columbia Cancer Agency. J Clin Oncol 20:197-204, 2002
6. Friedberg JW, Chengazi V: PET scans in the staging of lymphoma: Current status. Oncologist 8:438-447, 2003
7. The International Non-Hodgkin's Lymphoma Prognostic Factors Project. A predictive model for aggressive non-Hodgkin's lymphoma. N Engl J Med 329:987-994, 1993
8. Miller TP, LeBlanc M, Spier CM, Chase EM, Fisher RI: CHOP alone compared to CHOP plus radiotherapy for early stage aggressive non-Hodgkin's lymphoma: Update of the Southwest Oncology Group (SWOG) randomized trial. Blood 98:724a, 2001(abstr)
9. Miller TP, Unger JM, Spier C, Stea B, Cantu E, LeBlanc M, Fisher RI: Effect of adding rituximab to three cycles of CHOP, plus involved-field radiotherapy for limited-stage aggressive diffuse B-cell lymphoma (SWOG-0014). Blood 104:48a, 2004 (abstr)

10. Coiffier B, Lepage E, Briere J, Herbrecht R, Tilly H, Bouabdallah R, et al: CHOP chemotherapy plus rituximab compared with CHOP alone in elderly patients with diffuse large B-cell lymphoma. N Engl J Med 346:235-242, 2002
11. Sehn LH, Donaldson J, Chhanabhai M, Fitzgerald C, Gill K, Klasa R, et al: Introduction of combined CHOP-rituximab therapy dramatically improved outcome of diffuse large B-cell lymphoma in British Columbia. Blood 102:29, 2003 (abstr)
12. Reyes F, Lepage E, Ganem G, Molina TJ, Brice P, Coiffier B, et al: ACVBP versus CHOP plus radiotherapy for localized aggressive lymphoma. N Engl J Med 352:1197-1205, 2005
13. Fillet G, Bonnet C, Mounier N, Ganem G, Molina T, Thieblement C, et al: No role for chemoradiotherapy when compared with chemotherapy alone in elderly patients with localized low risk aggressive lymphoma: Final results of the LNH93-4 GELA study. Blood 106:9a, 2005 (abstr)
14. Horning SJ, Weller E, Kim K, Earle JD, O'Connell MJ, Habermann TM, et al: Chemotherapy with or without radiotherapy in limited stage diffuse aggressive non-Hodgkin lymphoma. J Clin Oncol 22:3032-3038, 2004
15. Riemersma SA, Jordanova ES, Schop RF, Phillipo K, Looujenga LH, Schuuring E, et al: Extensive genetic alterations of the HLA region, including homozygous deletions of HLA class II genes in B-cell lymphomas arising in immune-privileged sites. Blood 96:3569-3577, 2000
16. Jordanova ES, Riemersma SA, Philippo K, Giphart-Gassler M, Schuuring E, Kluin PM: Hemizygous deletions in the HLA region account for loss of heterozygosity in the majority of diffuse large B-cell lymphomas of the testis and the central nervous system. Genes Chromosomes Cancer 35:38-48, 2001
17. Jordanova ES, Philippo K, Giphart MJ, Schuuring E, Kluin PM: Mutations in the HLA class II genes leading to loss of expression of HLA-DR and HLA-DQ in diffuse large B-cell lymphoma. Immunogenetics 55: 203-209, 2003
18. Zucca E, Conconi A, Mughal TI, Sarris AH, Seymour JF, Vitolo U, et al: Patterns of outcome and prognostic factors in primary large-cell lymphoma of the testis in a survey by the International Extranodal Lymphoma Study Group. J Clin Oncol 21:20-27, 2003
19. List AF, Spier CM, Miller TP, Grogan TM: Deficient tumor-infiltrating T-lymphocyte response in malignant lymphoma: Relationship to HLA expression and host immunocompetence. Leukemia 7:398-403, 1993
20. Rimsza LM, Roberts RA, Campo E, Grogan TM, Bea S, Salaverria I, et al: Loss of MHC class II gene and protein expression in diffuse large B-cell lymphoma is related to decreased tumor immunosurveillance and poor patient survival regardless of other prognostic factors: A follow-up study from the Leukemia and Lymphoma Molecular Profiling Project. Blood 103:4251-4258, 2004
21. Stopeck AT, Gessner A, Miller TP, Hersh EM, Johnson CS, Cui H, et al: Loss of B7.2 (CD86) and intracellular adhesion molecule 1 (CD54) expression is associated with decreased tumor-infiltrating T lymphocytes in diffuse B-cell large-cell lymphoma. Clin Cancer Res 6:3904-3909, 2000
22. Jacob MC, Piccinni MP, Bonnefoix T, Sotto MF, Couderc P, Bensa JC, et al: T lymphocytes from invaded lymph nodes in patients with B-cell-derived non-Hodgkin's lymphoma: Reactivity toward the malignant clone. Blood 75:1154-1162, 1990
23. Willemze R, Jaffe ES, Burg G, Cerroni L, Berti E, Swerdlow SH, et al: WHO-EORTC classification for cutaneous lymphomas. Blood 105: 3768-3785, 2005
24. Alizadeh AA, Eisen MB, Davis RE, Ma C, Lossos IS, Rosenwald A, et al: Distinct types of diffuse large B-cell lymphoma identified by gene expression profiling. Nature 403:503-511, 2000
25. Hoefnagel JJ, Dijkman R, Basso K, Jansen PM, Hallermann C, Willemze R, et al: Distinct types of primary cutaneous large B-cell lymphoma identified by gene expression profiling. Blood 105:3671-3678, 2005
26. Rosenwald A, Wright G, Chan WC, Connors JM, Campo E, Fisher RI, et al: The use of molecular profiling to predict survival after chemotherapy for diffuse large-B-cell lymphoma. N Engl J Med 346:1937-1947, 2002
27. Jaffe ES: WHO Classification of Tumours, Pathology and Genetics, Tumours of Haematopoietic and Lymphoid Tissues. Lyon, France, IARC, 2001
28. Rosenwald A, Wright G, Leroy K, Yu X, Gaulard P, Gascoyne RD, et al: Molecular diagnosis of primary mediastinal B cell lymphoma identifies a clinically favorable subgroup of diffuse large B cell lymphoma related to Hodgkin lymphoma. J Exp Med 198:851-862, 2003
29. Savage KJ, Monti S, Kutok JL, Cattoretti G, Neuberg D, De Leval L, et al: The molecular signature of mediastinal large B-cell lymphoma differs from that of other diffuse large B-cell lymphomas and shares features with classical Hodgkin lymphoma. Blood 102:3871-3879, 2003

ELSEVIER

Seminars in
HEMATOLOGY

Standard Treatment of Advanced-Stage Diffuse Large B-Cell Lymphoma

Bertrand Coiffier

Diffuse large B-cell lymphoma (DLBCL) is the most frequent lymphoma and is not localized in 70% of the cases. Even if the clinical picture, the morphologic aspect, and the prognostic parameters are different from one patient to another, the standard treatment is the same for all patients. Currently, treatment decision is based on the International Prognostic Index (IPI) and age of the patient. Outcome has been completely modified with the introduction of rituximab in combination with chemotherapy. A review of standard treatment and remaining questions is presented.
Semin Hematol 43:213-220

Diffuse large B-cell lymphoma (DLBCL) is the most frequent non-Hodgkin's lymphoma subtype, accounting for 30% to 35% of all lymphoma cases. It is characterized as an aggressive lymphoma because survival is limited in the absence of effective treatment. Currently, DLBCL may be cured in a significant percentage of patients, depending on the initial characteristics of the tumor and of the host. The treatment of DLBCL has been revolutionized in recent years with the addition of rituximab to combination chemotherapy, resulting in an increased proportion of cured patients. Despite these advances, therapeutic challenges persist, particularly for patients with the highest risk of failure. In this review, new developments will be presented, together with questions to be resolved in the future.

Prognostic Factors and Choice of Treatment

The description of the International Prognostic Index (IPI) for diffuse aggressive lymphoma in 1993 enabled comparisons of published results and the prospective design of studies including patients with similar characteristics.[1] Age, one of the five parameters in the index, is also an important determinant in the choice of treatment because older patients may have comorbid conditions and thus limited therapeutic possibilities. On this basis, the age-adjusted IPI (aa-IPI), which is based on stage, serum lactate dehydrogenase (LDH) level, and performance status (PS), is the most powerful and simplest index to determine the treatment of any patient.[1] Patients with an aa-IPI score of 0 have favorable, localized disease, those with an aa-IPI score of 1 constitute a group with intermediate prognosis, and those with an aa-IPI of 2 or 3 have the worst outcome. Of note, immunophenotype was not considered in the design of the IPI but T-cell lymphomas, which have been associated with a worse outcome in all prospective and retrospective analyses, comprise only a small subset of diffuse aggressive lymphomas.

Prior to the incorporation of rituximab in DLBCL treatment, patients with aggressive B-cell or T-cell lymphoma were treated similarly with doxorubicin-containing combination chemotherapy. Whether a particular presentation or site (mediastinal, gastrointestinal, nodal, or extranodal) would benefit from a specific regimen or strategy was never adequately studied or proven, with the possible exception of primary central nervous system lymphoma.[2] This was also the case for the different histologic entities within the DLBCLs or peripheral T-cell lymphomas.

Although gene expression analyses have defined subtypes of DLBCL based on cell of origin, with different outcomes after treatment with combination chemotherapy,[3] this technology is not widely available or, at this time, practical for routine clinical use. However, molecular profiling allows recognition of important gene signatures involved in the pathobiology of DLBCL and the identification of potential new therapeutic targets. Extrapolation of gene expression results to an immunohistochemistry platform has more immediate potential for clinical application.[3,4]

Development of Dose-Dense and Dose-Intense Regimens

In 1993, the US Intergroup study demonstrated that the CHOP (cyclophosphamide, doxorubicin, vincristine, pred-

Hospices Civils de Lyon and Université Claude Bernard, Lyon, France.
Address correspondence to Professor Bertrand Coiffier, MD, Hematology Department, CH Lyon-Sud, 69495 Pierre Benite, France. E-mail: bertrand.coiffier@chu-lyon.fr

0037-1963/06/$-see front matter
doi:10.1053/j.seminhematol.2006.07.004

Table 1 Number and Type of Events Observed in Both Arms of the LNH-98.5 Study With a Median Follow-up of 5 Years

Event	CHOP N	CHOP %	R-CHOP N	R-CHOP %
PD during treatment	44	22	19	9.5
New treatment	9	4.5	11	5.5
PD after SD	1	1	1	0.5
PD after PR	4	2	6	3
Relapse	67	34	40	20
Death during treatment	12	6	12	6
Death in CR	5	2.5	17	8
All events	**142**	**72**	**106**	**52.5**
No event	55	28	96	47.5
Total patients	**197**	**100**	**202**	**100**

Abbreviations: PD, progressive disease; SD, stable disease; PR, partial response; CR, complete response.

nisone every 3 weeks for eight cycles) regimen was associated with similar complete response (CR) rates, progression-free survival (PFS), and overall survival (OS) to more complicated regimens associated with more toxicity.[5] However, CHOP resulted in only 30% to 40% OS at 5 years and 30% of patients failed to respond or progressed shortly after the completion of treatment. These outcomes prompted the investigation of dose-dense or dose-intense strategies to improve response rates or consolidation with high-dose therapy (HDT) with autologous transplantation to decrease the relapse rates. Even though these therapeutic regimens have not been broadly applied, they have demonstrated significantly better results in many cases.[6] Several phase II studies in the US and randomized phase III studies in Europe have demonstrated superiority of these approaches over the CHOP regimen as described in more detail below.[7-11]

The Rituximab Effect

After the demonstration of the activity of rituximab in aggressive B-cell lymphomas in two phase II studies,[12,13] one with rituximab alone in relapsing patients and the other with rituximab combined with CHOP (R-CHOP) in untreated patients, several groups launched randomized trials in different patient subsets to test the ability of R-CHOP to increase the cure rate over CHOP alone in DLBCL. The first report of a significant benefit for patients treated with R-CHOP came from the study reported by the Groupe d'Etude des Lymphomes de l'Adulte (GELA) in elderly DLBCL patients (Table 1).[14] Since then, the results from three large phase III studies and one population-based study have confirmed the superior efficacy of the combination of rituximab and CHOP in DLCBL patients, setting this as the new standard of care (Table 2).[15-19] Today, the combination of rituximab plus CHOP is the standard care for patients with DLBCL.

The results from the GELA are currently the more mature, with a 5-year median follow-up.[20] Nearly half of R-CHOP patients are event-free at 5 years compared to 28% in the CHOP arm (Table 1). Event-free survival (EFS), PFS, disease-free survival (DFS), and OS remained statistically significant in favor of the combination of R-CHOP with *P* values of .00002, <.00001, .00031, and .0073, respectively (Fig 1). The benefit from R-CHOP was observed in both low-risk and high-risk aa-IPI groups (Fig 2). No additional long-term tox-

Table 2 Results of Different Randomized Studies Comparing Chemotherapy to Rituximab Plus Chemotherapy in Previously Untreated Patients With DLBCL

Study	Setting	CR Rate	Median EFS	Median PFS	Median DFS	Median OS
GELA[14,20]	DLBCL					
R-CHOP	60–80 years, all IPI	75%†	3.8 yr‡	NR‡	NR‡	NR†
CHOP	Intent-to-treat analysis	63%	1.1 yr	1.5 yr	2.45 yr	3.1 yr
Intergroup study[19]	DLBCL	NA	NA	At 3.5 yr	NA	NS
R-CHOP	>60 years			53%*		
CHOP	Not published			46%		
			NA	At 2 yr	NA	NS
R-CHOP + maintenance				79%‡		
R-CHOP w/o maintenance				77%		
CHOP + maintenance				74%		
CHOP w/o maintenance				45%		
MInT[16]	DLBCL		At 3 yr	At 3 yr	NA	At 3 yr
R-chemotherapy	<60 years, IPI score 0–1	86%‡	79%‡	85%‡		93%‡
Chemotherapy	Intent-to-treat analysis	68%	59%	68%		84%
RICOVER[37]	DLBCL	NA	NA	At 2 yr	NA	NS
R-CHOP-14	61–80 years, all IPI			*P* <.001		
CHOP-14	Not published					

Abbreviations: CR, complete remission; EFS, event-free survival; PFS, progression-free survival; DFS, disease-free survival; OS, overall survival; NS, not significantly different; NR, not reached; NA, not available.
$^*P<.05$; $^†P<.01$; $^‡P<.001$.

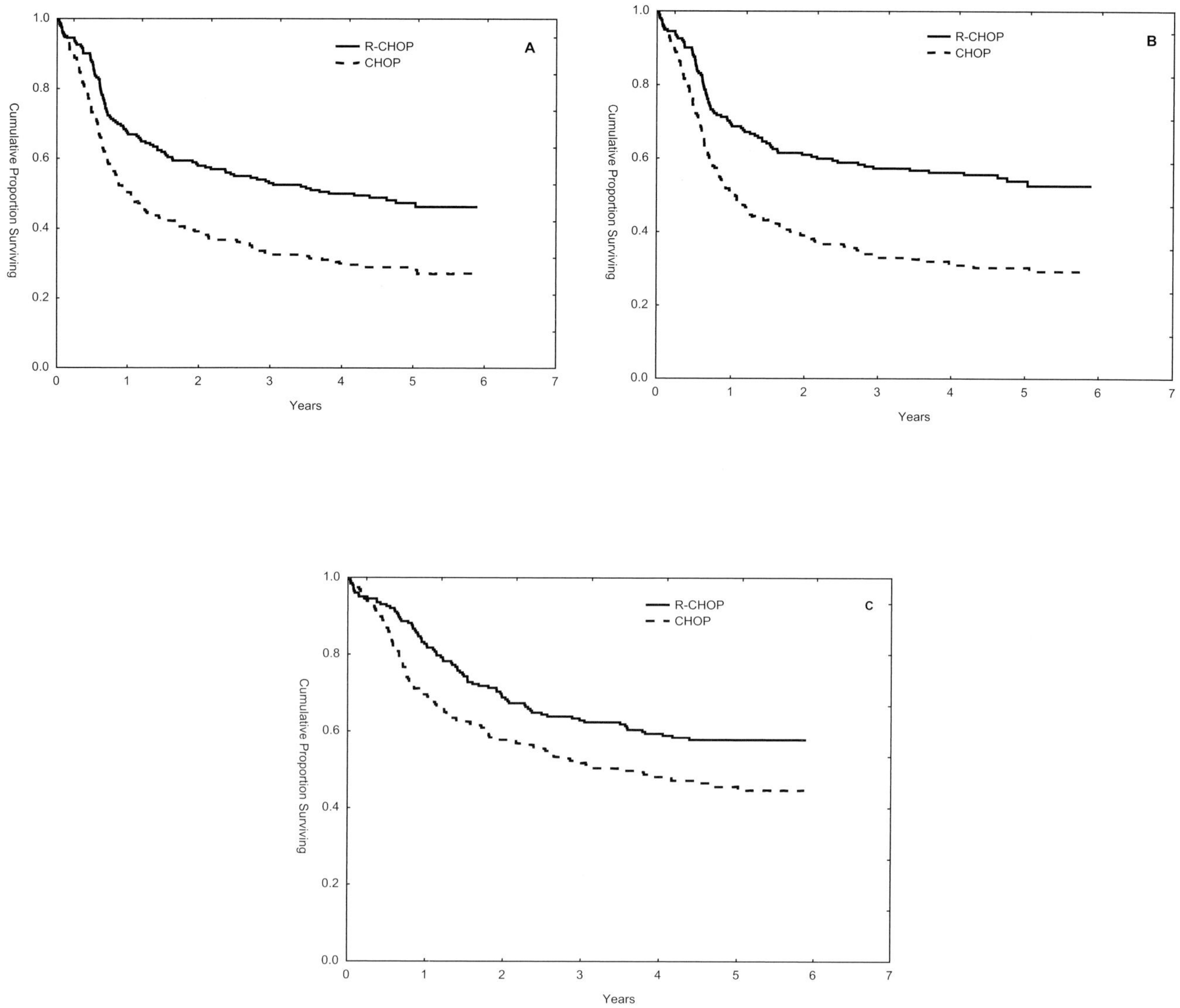

Figure 1 Event-free survival (A), progression-free survival (B), and overall survival (C) with a median follow-up of 5 years in CHOP- and R-CHOP–treated patients in the LNH-98.5 study.[18] Log-rank test *P* values are .00002, <.00001, and .0073, respectively. Reprinted with permission from J Clin Oncol.[18] © 2005 American Society of Clinical Oncology.

icity appeared to be associated with the R-CHOP combination. This study also confirmed that elderly patients must be treated with the aim of cure and that the toxicity of R-CHOP is not greater than that observed in younger patients provided granulocyte colony-stimulating factor (G-CSF) is used in frail patients.

Good-Risk Patients

Patients with an aa-IPI score 0 or 1 have either localized disease or disseminated disease with favorable (normal LDH level and good PS) features. For patients with non-bulky stage I–II diffuse aggressive lymphoma, three cycles of CHOP followed by involved-field radiation therapy became a standard after the study conducted by the Southwest Oncology Group (SWOG).[21] However, the advantage of CHOP–radiotherapy demonstrated in the early publication disappeared with 10-year follow-up.[22] The Eastern Cooperative Oncology Group (ECOG) study evaluated eight cycles of CHOP with or without consolidative radiation therapy in complete responders who presented with unfavorable stage I (bulky or mediastinal or retroperitoneal) or stages IE, II, or IIE disease. In this study, which was underpowered, DFS was greater for radiation therapy patients at 6 years (73% *v* 56%, two-sided *P* = .05) but differences in OS were not statistically significant.[23]

The GELA compared three cycles of CHOP plus involved-field radiotherapy to the ACVBP (doxorubicin, cyclophosphamide, vincristine, bleomycin, prednisone) chemotherapy regimen with sequential consolidation in 747 previously untreated patients younger than 61 years with stage I–II aggressive lymphoma and an aa-IPI of 0.[24] With a median follow-up of 7.7 years, EFS and OS were significantly longer in the chemotherapy-alone group (*P* <.001 and *P* = .001, respec-

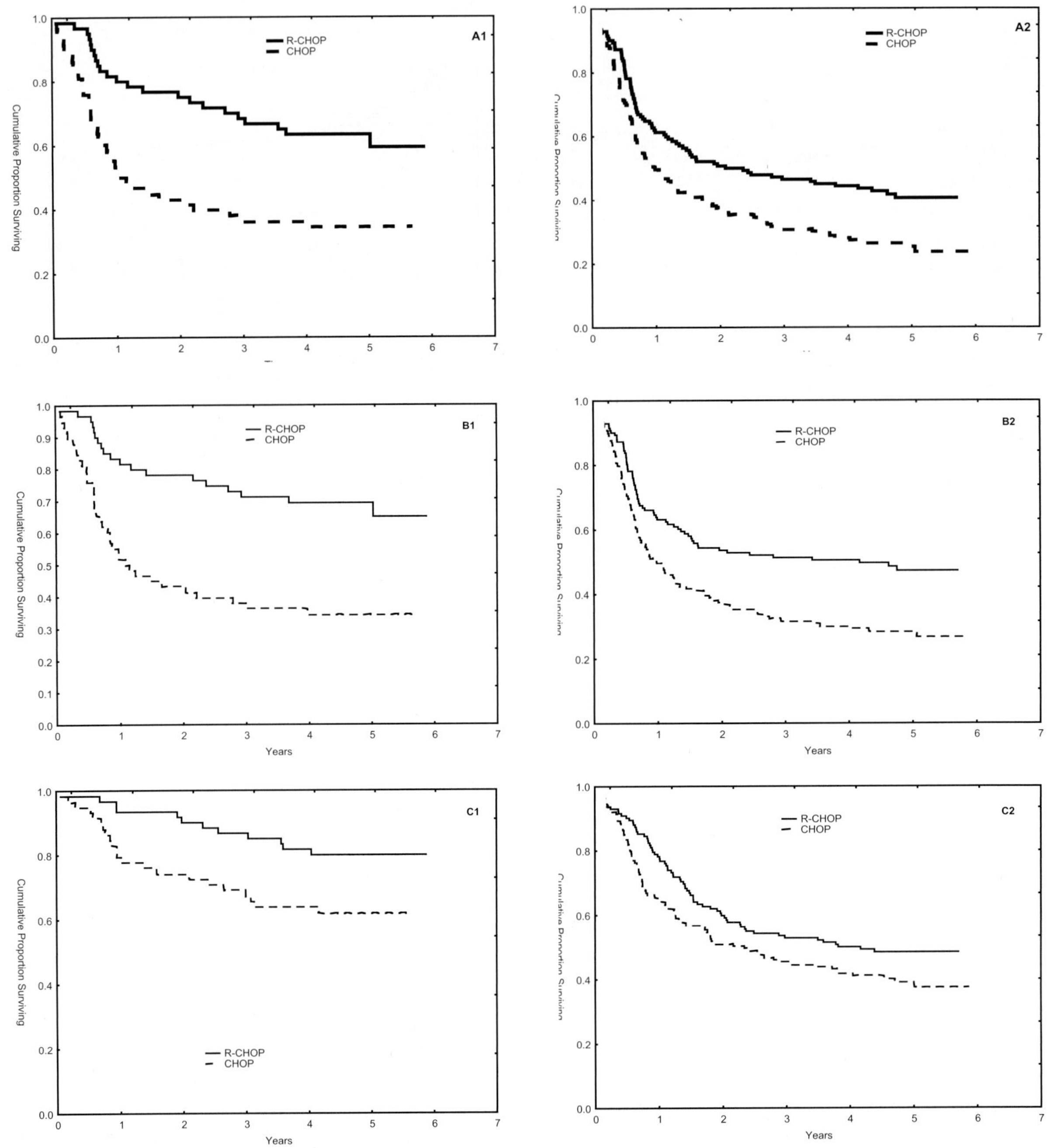

Figure 2 Event-free survival (A), progression-free survival (B), and overall survival (C) with a median follow-up of 5 years of patients treated with R-CHOP and CHOP in the LNH-98.5 study according to the age-adjusted International Prognostic Index score at diagnosis: (1) low-risk patients (scores 0 and 1); (2) high-risk patients (scores 2 and 3). All differences are statistically significant except for overall survival in high-risk patients: *P* values are .00085, .0037, .00013, .00078, .023, and .062, respectively. Reprinted with permission from J Clin Oncol.[18] © 2005 American Society of Clinical Oncology.

tively). The 5-year estimates of EFS were 82% for patients receiving chemotherapy alone and 74% for patients treated with CHOP plus radiotherapy. The 5-year estimates of OS were 90% and 81%, respectively. In a multivariate analysis, EFS and OS were affected by treatment arm, independent of stage and tumor bulk. The GELA has conducted another study in elderly patients that also tests the benefit of the radiotherapy. In the LNH-93.4 study, patients older than 60 years were randomized to either four cycles of CHOP or four cycles of CHOP plus involved-field radiotherapy. In a preliminary analysis, CR rates, EFS, and OS were similar in both groups.[25]

These randomized prospective studies have studied different populations of localized diffuse aggressive lymphoma, leading to variable interpretation. However, none showed a long-term advantage for radiotherapy either with shortened chemotherapy or as consolidation after chemotherapy. In patients with favorable, non-bulky stage I disease, limited chemotherapy plus radiation therapy or a longer course of chemotherapy alone is likely to yield similar long-term results. In localized disease patients with bulky tumor or IPI risk factors, a full course of chemotherapy is indicated and, to date, radiation therapy consolidation has not demonstrated any survival advantage. The most important question currently relates to the added benefit of rituximab for these patients.

Two additional studies are pertinent to the discussion of good-risk patients. The German Non-Hodgkin's Lymphoma Study Group evaluated CHOP given on a 2- or 3-week schedule and the addition of etoposide (CHOEP), also on a 2- or 3-week schedule in younger patients (age 18 to 60 years) with diffuse aggressive lymphoma and a normal LDH.[26] About two thirds of the study group had an aa-IPI of 0. In this study, which also included other histologic subtypes and some T-cell lymphomas, the addition of etoposide resulted in superior response rates and EFS but similar OS at 5 years. Of note, the 2- or 3-week schedule showed similar results, not validating in young patients the alleged superiority of CHOP-14. As noted below, CHOEP and CHOP have also been evaluated in combination with rituximab in the MabThera International Trial (MInT) trial, whereupon the differences in these regimens were no longer apparent.[16]

Elderly Patients With Poor-Risk DLBCL

Classically, elderly patients are defined by an age older than 60 years. They represent 50% of patients with aggressive lymphoma. A subgroup of patients older than 80 years has currently been defined because these patients will be seen more frequently in the future and the strategy in these elderly patients may be different from the standard therapy in patients in the 61 to 79 age group.

Currently, two studies have demonstrated that the combination of rituximab with CHOP is clearly superior to CHOP alone.[14,19,20] The first, reported by the GELA, was described above and in Table 1 and in Figs 1 and 2. The second study is the US Intergroup E4494 study from the ECOG and Cancer and Acute Leukemia Group B (CALGB) with participation from SWOG.[19] The E4494 study compared CHOP versus R-CHOP, and, for responding patients, maintenance with rituximab alone, four infusions every 6 months, for 2 years, versus observation. E4494 differs in several ways from the GELA study: (1) rituximab was given according to the original R-CHOP study of Czuczman et al, resulting in four or five rather than eight rituximab infusions[27]; (2) patients in CR at four cycles received a total of six cycles of CHOP and only 33% of patients received seven or more cycles; (3) half of responding patients received maintenance with rituximab. Patients had nearly the same characteristics as the GELA study: only 50 had aa-IPI score greater than 1 compared to 60% in the GELA study. Median follow-up at time of last presentation of E4494 was 3.5 years. Response rates in this study did not differ by treatment arm; this may have been an artifact of the response definition or related to the schedule of rituximab. Failure-free survival (FFS) at 3 years favored R-CHOP (53%) versus CHOP (46%), $P = .04$. Maintenance rituximab significantly prolonged FFS ($P = .009$). However, the prolongation in FFS with rituximab maintenance was limited to patients treated with CHOP ($P = .0004$) and was not seen after R-CHOP ($P = .81$). No significant differences in OS according to induction therapy or maintenance therapies were observed with current follow-up. However, in an analysis in which patients who received maintenance rituximab were removed, an advantage to R-CHOP was observed for FFS but not for OS.[19]

Other results in the literature may guide the design of future therapeutics in elderly patients. Patients in the 60- to 65-year range may benefit from dose-dense or dose-intense regimens akin to younger patients.[10] In a trial comparing 8× CHOP to ACVBP plus sequential consolidation, the 5-year EFS was 39% in the ACVBP group and 29% in the CHOP group ($P = .005$). The OS at 5 years was also significantly longer for patients treated with ACVBP: 46% compared with 38% for patients treated with CHOP ($P = .036$). However, it appears that ACVBP cannot be used in patients over 65 years because of its toxicity. A German study also has shown improvement over classical CHOP (CHOP given every 3 weeks or CHOP-21) when the CHOP regimen was administered every 2 weeks (CHOP-14) in patients age older than 60 years of age.[11] The conclusions from these studies, employing regimens associated with greater toxicity and expense, must now be reconsidered as their additional benefit over classical CHOP-21 when rituximab is added to standard chemotherapy remains unproven.

Given that current treatment is not satisfactory for poor-risk patients, the GELA is testing whether administering R-CHOP every 2 weeks might increase the response rate and prolong the response duration in these patients. GELA is also testing whether maintaining hemoglobin level at 13 g/dL may render them better able to tolerate the dose-dense regimen.

Young Patients With Intermediate-Risk DLBCL

According to the aa-IPI, these patients have one adverse prognostic factor, usually advanced stage or high LDH. The MInT study led by the German lymphoma group showed that R-CHOP or R-CHOP–like regimens were superior to the same chemotherapy without rituximab in young patients with favorable or intermediate-risk disease.[16] In this trial, 57% patients had an aa-IPI score of 1. After a median follow-up of 34 months, patients receiving the R-CHOP-like regimens had a significantly longer time to treatment failure ($P < .00001$), with estimated 3-year EFS rates of 59% (CHOP-like) versus 79% (R-CHOP–like). Similarly, OS was significantly different ($P < .001$), with 3-year survival rates of 84% (CHOP-like) and 93% (R-CHOP–like), respectively (Fig 3). However, 3-year EFS after R-CHOP–like regimens in patients with bulky disease and/or an aa-IPI score of 1 was

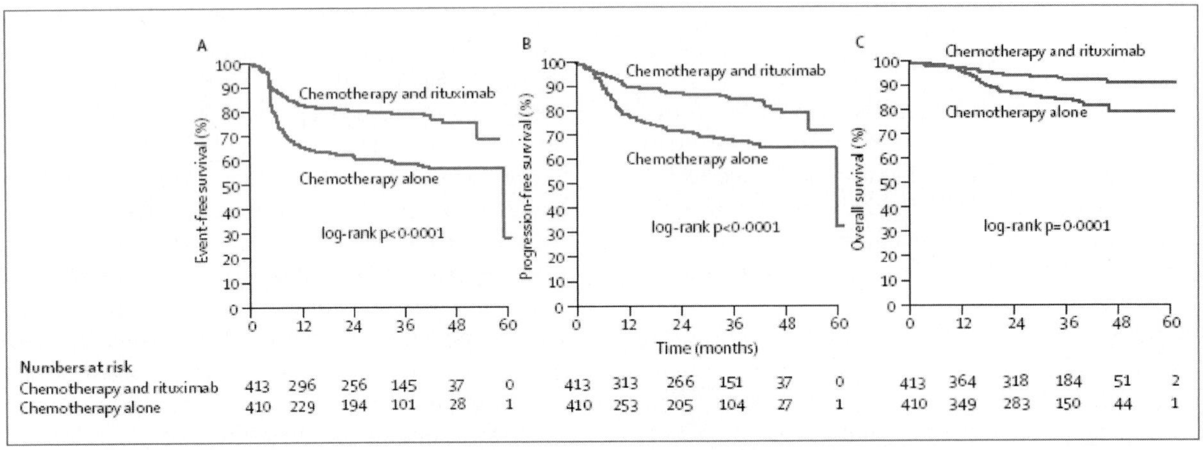

Figure 3 MInT study: (A) event-free survival, (B) progression-free survival, and (C) overall survival of the 823 patients assigned to CHOP-like chemotherapy alone (n = 410) or to CHOP-like chemotherapy and rituximab (n = 413). Reprinted with permission from Lancet Oncol.[16]

significantly worse ($P < .001$) than in patients with an aa-IPI of 0 and no bulk (71% *v* 90%, respectively).

Is it possible to achieve survival greater than 60% to 70% at 10 years? High-dose therapy with autologous transplant (HDT) has not shown any benefit in subgroup analyses of randomized trials in these intermediate-risk patients. To date, no prospective randomized study has concluded that a dose-dense or dose-intense regimen performs better than CHOP or R-CHOP in this group of patients. Currently, the GELA is comparing R-CHOP to R-ACVBP for treating this group of patients with an aa-IPI score of 1. However, the standard regimen remains R-CHOP-21, but a study comparing R-CHOP-14 to R-CHOP-21 would certainly be interesting to test the hypothesis of dose-dense regimen.

Young Patients With Poor-Risk DLBCL

Young patients with poor-risk DLBCL, defined by an aa-IPI score of 2 or 3 and age younger than 60 years, are characterized by truly refractory disease, evidenced by progression during or early after treatment, or later relapse. Attempts to modify treatment to improve the response rate and reduce the proportion of patients with progressive disease have been unsuccessful to date: the best CR rate is currently around 65%. In contrast, some but not all attempts to decrease the relapse rate by consolidation with HDT have succeeded. Two of the positive studies include GELA LNH-87.2 study, which compared the standard consolidation with sequential chemotherapy versus HDT and autologous transplantation after four cycles of ACVBP.[7] With a median follow-up of 8 years, HDT was superior to sequential chemotherapy in the subgroup of poor-risk patients: DFS rates of 55% (95% confidence interval [CI], 46% to 64%) and 39% (95% CI, 30% to 48%), respectively. The 8-year OS rate was significantly superior in the HDT arm (64%) compared with the sequential chemotherapy arm (49%), $P = .04$. Building on prior results, the GELA is currently testing the hypotheses that rituximab added to ACVBP may improve the response rate and the addition of rituximab maintenance after HDT and transplantation may reduce the relapse rate.

A second positive HDT study, in which patients with high-risk disease were excluded, also came from France.[28] Based on these data, HDT with autologous transplantation may be considered for selected patients who achieve CR with a dose-intense and/or dose-dense regimen.[6] However, the role of HDT and transplantation in this setting has been challenged by a recent meta-analysis.[16,29] The current US Intergroup study (S9704), which is assessing the role of HDT and autologous transplantation after five cycles of R-CHOP versus completing eight total cycles in younger patients with high-intermediate or high-risk disease, should further inform this debate.

Very Old Patients With DLBCL

Patients over 80 years old represent a growing group with DLBCL. Most are able to receive life-prolonging treatment, but conventional treatments may not be feasible due to comorbid conditions and inadequate marrow reserve. However, a non-negligible proportion of these patients may be alive in CR 2 years after treatment with an active regimen.[30] Relatively few prospective studies have specifically addressed this group of patients. The addition of rituximab to chemotherapy will certainly increase the response to treatment without additional toxicity as in younger patients, but the nature of the chemotherapy regimen to be used remains unknown. The GELA is currently conducting a study with "adapted" R-CHOP in these patients. "Adapted" means that doses of doxorubicin, cyclophosphamide, and vincristine are reduced for the first cycle (25 mg/m^2, 400 mg/m^2, and 1 mg/m^2, respectively) and may be increased for further cycles if the tolerance is good. In combination with rituximab, it appears feasible to strive for a treatment response that may prolong the survival of these patients without undue toxicity.

Positron Emission Tomography Scan for Evaluation of Response and Prognosis

Positron emission tomography (PET) using ^{18}F-fluorodeoxyglucose (FDG) is a powerful functional imaging tool for staging, restaging, and response assessment in DLBCL patients. The advantage of PET over conventional imaging techniques is its ability to distinguish between viable tumor and fibrosis in residual mass(es) often present following treatment. This information may have important clinical consequences: in a retrospective study of 56 patients with DLBCL, PET not only increased the number of CRs, but unconfirmed CRs were eliminated.[31] Such findings provided rationale for incorporating FDG-PET into revised criteria of the International Working Group on response evaluation.[32]

However, a number of issues with PET need to be considered before applying it to all patients and basing studies on the results obtained. First, the technique for performing and interpreting PET is not yet standardized. There is variability among readers and equipment. PET is also associated with false-positive findings due to nonlymphoma masses such as rebound thymic hyperplasia, infectious or inflammatory changes, or brown fat. Particularly important is false positivity secondary to macrophage activation in large initial tumor mass. So, a histologic confirmation is recommended before intensifying a treatment in case of FDG uptake in the PET examination. False negativity is rare in DLBCL patients.

Currently, PET is strongly recommended prior to treatment for patients with DLBCL to better delineate the extent of disease. PET is essential for the post-treatment assessment of DLBCL, particularly if there are persistent masses on the computed tomography scan. Numerous studies have demonstrated that PET performed after one to four cycles of chemotherapy predicts patient outcome.[33-35] However, there are currently no data demonstrating improvement in patient outcome by altering treatment based on this information. Studies are currently designed with early PET scan evaluation and intensifying treatment in case of FDG uptake confirmed by morphology.

Conclusions

During the last 20 years, the outcome for patients with DLBCL has significantly improved. Major improvements were (1) the addition of rituximab to combination chemotherapy with higher response rates and lower relapse rates; (2) the intensification with high-dose therapy for patients relapsed after conventional treatment and for selected high-risk patients as primary treatment; and (3) the description of benefit associated with dose-dense and dose-intense regimens. There continues to be room for improvement, particularly in patients with higher risk disease, the very elderly, and patients with disease that is initially insensitive to rituximab chemotherapy. However, if rituximab allows a significant improvement when added to CHOP, some preliminary observations showed that it may replace the benefit associated with adding other drugs to CHOP with less toxicity but not increase the benefit observed with these dose-dense or dose-intense regimens. Whether it will be the same observation with dose-dense regimen must be demonstrated.

Advances in these areas and a more individualized approach to therapy will likely emerge from better understanding of the pathogenesis of DLBCL. As a step in that direction, the DA-EPOCH (dose-adjusted, etoposide, prednisone, vincristine, cyclophosphamide, doxorubicin) regimen plus rituximab developed by Wilson and colleagues, is being compared to R-CHOP in a CALGB phase III trial that will also incorporate molecular profiling and pharmacogenomics.[36] Studies such as these with strong biologic underpinnings, together with the discovery of new targets and evaluation of novel therapeutics, will be required to further advance the treatment of DLBCL.

References

1. The International Non-Hodgkin's Lymphoma Prognostic Factors Project. A predictive model for aggressive non-Hodgkin's lymphoma. N Engl J Med 329:987-994, 1993
2. Batchelor T, Loeffler JS: Primary CNS lymphoma. J Clin Oncol 24: 1281-1288, 2006
3. Rosenwald A, Wright G, Chan WC, Connors JM, Campo E, Fisher RI, et al: The use of molecular profiling to predict survival after chemotherapy for diffuse large-B-cell lymphoma. N Engl J Med 346:1937-1947, 2002
4. Hans CP, Weisenburger DD, Greiner TC, Gascoyne RD, Delabie J, Ott G, et al: Confirmation of the molecular classification of diffuse large B-cell lymphoma by immunohistochemistry using a tissue microarray. Blood 103:275-282, 2004
5. Fisher RI, Gaynor ER, Dahlberg S, Oken MM, Grogan TM, Mize EM, et al: Comparison of a standard regimen (CHOP) with three intensive chemotherapy regimens for advanced non-hodgkin's lymphoma. N Engl J Med 328:1002-1006, 1993
6. Coiffier B: Increasing chemotherapy intensity in aggressive lymphomas: A renewal? J Clin Oncol 21:2457-2459, 2003
7. Haioun C, Lepage E, Gisselbrecht C, Salles G, Coiffier B, Brice P, et al: Survival benefit of high-dose therapy in poor-risk aggressive non-Hodgkin's lymphoma: Final analysis of the prospective LNH87-2 protocol—A Groupe d'Etude des Lymphomes de l'Adulte study. J Clin Oncol 18:3025-3030, 2000
8. Blayney DW, LeBlanc ML, Grogan T, Gaynor ER, Chapman RA, Spiridonidis CH, et al: Dose-intense chemotherapy every 2 weeks with dose-intense cyclophosphamide, doxorubicin, vincristine, and prednisone may improve survival in intermediate- and high-grade lymphoma: A phase II study of the Southwest Oncology Group (SWOG 9349). J Clin Oncol 21:2466-2473, 2003
9. Shipp MA, Neuberg D, Janicek M, Canellos GP, Shulman LN: High-dose CHOP as initial therapy for patients with poor-prognosis aggressive non-Hodgkin's lymphoma: A dose-finding pilot study. J Clin Oncol 13:2916-2923, 1995
10. Tilly H, Lepage E, Coiffier B, Blanc M, Herbrecht R, Bosly A, et al: Intensive conventional chemotherapy (ACVBP regimen) compared with standard CHOP for poor-prognosis aggressive non-Hodgkin lymphoma. Blood 102:4284-4289, 2003
11. Pfreundschuh M, Trumper L, Kloess M, Schmits R, Feller AC, Rube C, et al: Two-weekly or 3-weekly CHOP chemotherapy with or without etoposide for the treatment of elderly patients with aggressive lymphomas: Results of the NHL-B2 trial of the DSHNHL. Blood 104:634-641, 2004
12. Vose JM, Link BK, Grossbard ML, Czuczman M, Grillo-Lopez A, Gilman P, et al: Phase II study of rituximab in combination with CHOP chemotherapy in patients with previously untreated, aggressive non-Hodgkin's lymphoma. J Clin Oncol 19:389-397, 2001

13. Coiffier B, Haioun C, Ketterer N, Engert A, Tilly H, Ma D, et al: Rituximab (anti-CD20 monoclonal antibody) for the treatment of patients with relapsing or refractory aggressive lymphoma: A multicenter phase II study. Blood 92:1927-1932, 1998
14. Coiffier B, Lepage E, Briere J, Herbrecht R, Tilly H, Bouabdallah R, et al: CHOP chemotherapy plus rituximab compared with CHOP alone in elderly patients with diffuse large-B-cell lymphoma. N Engl J Med 346:235-242, 2002
15. Sehn LH, Donaldson J, Chhanabhai M, Fitzgerald C, Gill K, Klasa R, et al: Introduction of combined CHOP plus rituximab therapy dramatically improved outcome of diffuse large B-cell lymphoma in British Columbia. J Clin Oncol 23:5027-5033, 2005
16. Pfreundschuh M, Trumper L, Osterborg A, Pettengell R, Trneny M, Imrie K, et al: CHOP-like chemotherapy plus rituximab versus CHOP-like chemotherapy alone in young patients with good-prognosis diffuse large-B-cell lymphoma: A randomised controlled trial by the MabThera International Trial (MInT) Group. Lancet Oncol 7:379-391, 2006
17. Coiffier B: Treatment of diffuse large B-cell lymphoma. Curr Hematol Rep 4:7-14, 2005
18. Coiffier B: Treatment of aggressive lymphomas: Disseminated cases. ASCO 2003 Educational Book 2003, pp 606-611
19. Habermann T, Weller E, Morrison V, Gascoyne R, Cassileth P, Cohn J, et al: Rituximab-CHOP versus CHOP alone or with maintenance rituximab in older patients with diffuse large B-cell lymphoma. J Clin Oncol 2006;24:DOI: 10.1200/JCO.2005.05.1003
20. Feugier P, Van Hoof A, Sebban C, Solal-Celigny P, Bouabdallah R, Ferme C, et al: Long-term results of the R-CHOP study in the treatment of elderly patients with diffuse large B-cell lymphoma: A study by the Groupe d'Etude des Lymphomes de l'Adulte. J Clin Oncol 23:4117-4126, 2005
21. Miller TP, Dahlberg S, Cassady JR, Adelstein DJ, Spier CM, Grogan TM, et al: Chemotherapy alone compared with chemotherapy plus radiotherapy for localized intermediate-and high-grade non-Hodgkin's lymphoma. N Engl J Med 339:21-26, 1998
22. Miller TP, Leblanc M, Spier CM, Chase E, Fischer RI: CHOP alone compared to CHOP plus radiotherapy for early stage aggressive non-Hodgkin's lymphomas: Update of the Southwest Oncology Group (SWOG) randomized trial. Blood 98:742a, 2001 (abstr)
23. Horning SJ, Weller E, Kim K, Earle JD, O'Connell MJ, Habermann TM, et al: Chemotherapy with or without radiotherapy in limited-stage diffuse aggressive non-Hodgkin's lymphoma: Eastern Cooperative Oncology Group study 1484. J Clin Oncol 22:3032-3038, 2004
24. Reyes F, Lepage E, Ganem G, Molina TJ, Brice P, Coiffier B, et al: ACVBP versus CHOP plus radiotherapy for localized aggressive lymphoma. N Engl J Med 352:1197-1205, 2005
25. Fillet G, Bonnet C, Mounier N, et al: Radiotherapy is unnecessary in elderly patients with localized aggressive non-Hodgkin's lymphoma. Results of the GELA LNH 93-4 study. Blood 100:92a, 2002 (abstr)
26. Pfreundschuh M, Trumper L, Kloess M, Schmits R, Feller AC, Rudolph C, et al: Two-weekly or 3-weekly CHOP chemotherapy with or without etoposide for the treatment of young patients with good-prognosis (normal LDH) aggressive lymphomas: Results of the NHL-B1 trial of the DSHNHL. Blood 104:626-633, 2004
27. Czuczman MS, Weaver R, Alkuzweny B, Berlfein J, Grillo-Lopez AJ: Prolonged clinical and molecular remission in patients with low-grade or follicular non-Hodgkin's lymphoma treated with rituximab plus CHOP chemotherapy: 9-year follow-up. J Clin Oncol 22:4711-4716, 2004
28. Milpied N, Deconinck E, Gaillard F, Delwail V, Foussard C, Berthou C, et al: Initial treatment of aggressive lymphoma with high-dose chemotherapy and autologous stem-cell support. N Engl J Med 350:1287-1295, 2004
29. Greb A, Schiefer DH, Bohlius J, et al: High-dose chemotherapy with autologous stem cell support is not superior to conventional-dose chemotherapy in the first-line treatment of aggressive non-Hodgkin lymphoma: Results of a comprehensive meta-analysis. Blood 104:263a, 2004 (abstr)
30. Bairey O, Benjamini O, Blickstein D, Elis A, Ruchlemer R: Non-Hodgkin's lymphoma in patients 80 years of age or older. Ann Oncol 17:928-934, 2006
31. Juweid ME, Wiseman GA, Vose JM, Ritchie JM, Menda Y, Wooldridge JE, et al: Response assessment of aggressive non-Hodgkin's lymphoma by integrated International Workshop Criteria and fluorine-18-fluorodeoxyglucose positron emission tomography. J Clin Oncol 23:4652-4661, 2005
32. Cheson BD, Horning SJ, Coiffier B, Shipp MA, Fisher RI, Connors JM, et al: Report of an international workshop to standardize response criteria for non-Hodgkin's lymphomas. J Clin Oncol 17:1244-1253, 1999
33. Kostakoglu L, Coleman M, Leonard JP, Kuji I, Zoe H, Goldsmith SJ: PET predicts prognosis after 1 cycle of chemotherapy in aggressive lymphoma and Hodgkin's disease. J Nucl Med 43:1018-1027, 2002
34. Spaepen K, Stroobants S, Dupont P, Van Steenweghen S, Thomas J, Vandenberghe P, et al: Prognostic value of positron emission tomography (PET) with fluorine-18 fluorodeoxyglucose. J Clin Oncol 19:414-419, 2001
35. Haioun C, Itti E, Rahmouni A, Brice P, Rain JD, Belhadj K, et al: [18F]fluoro-2-deoxy-D-glucose positron emission tomography (FDG-PET) in aggressive lymphoma: An early prognostic tool for predicting patient outcome. Blood 106:1376-1381, 2005
36. Wilson WH, Gutierrez M, O'Connor P, Frankel S, Jaffe E, Chabner BA, et al: The role of rituximab and chemotherapy in aggressive B-cell lymphoma: A preliminary report of dose-adjusted EPOCH-R. Semin Oncol 29:41-47, 2002
37. Pfreundschuh M, Kloess M, Schmits R, Zeynalova S, Lengfelder E, Franke A, et al: Six, not eight cycles of bi-weekly CHOP with rituximab (R-CHOP-14) is the preferred treatment for elderly patients with diffuse large B-cell lymphoma (DLBCL): Results of the RICOVER-60 Trial of the German High-Grade Non-Hodgkin Lymphoma Study Group (DSHNHL). ASH Annual Meeting Abstracts 106:13, 2005 (abstr)

ELSEVIER

Seminars in
HEMATOLOGY

Dose-Intensified Treatment of Advanced-Stage Diffuse Large B-Cell Lymphomas

Gerhard Held,[a] Joerg Schubert,[a] Marcel Reiser,[b] and Michael Pfreundschuh,[a] for the German High-Grade Non-Hodgkin-Lymphoma Study Group

The introduction of the CHOP (cyclophosphamide, doxorubicin, vincristine, and prednisone) regimen 30 years ago was the great breakthrough in the treatment of advanced-stage aggressive lymphomas. About 50% of all patients treated with CHOP achieved complete remission, and about one third experienced long-term disease-free survival and cure. Attempts to improve results by modifications of CHOP using escalated doses, additional drugs, or the alternative use of putatively non–cross-resistant chemotherapy regimens were not confirmed in randomized trials. With the availability of granulocyte colony-stimulating factor (G-CSF) and the tool of autologous stem cell support in the 1990s, dose escalation, dose densification (by interval reduction), or combinations thereof were pursued to increase dose intensity. While dose-escalation strategies, including high-dose approaches necessitating stem cell support, have not been demonstrated unequivocally yet to be superior to a baseline CHOP-21, dose-dense (biweekly) modifications improved the outcome of young and elderly patients with aggressive lymphomas compared to baseline CHOP-21. The challenges in the era of the monoclonal antibody rituximab are the identification of the ideal chemotherapy partner for rituximab both with respect to potential synergistic effects and to the lack of interference with its effector mechanisms. Finally, the issue of intensifying rituximab within such approaches must be addressed by appropriately designed randomized trials.
Semin Hematol 43:221-229

Risk factor profile and age are the main determinants for the primary therapeutic strategy in aggressive lymphomas. The International Prognostic Index (IPI)[1] sets the cut-off between young and elderly patients at 60 years. According to the number of risk factors present, the IPI distinguishes four prognostic subgroups; however, for practical reasons, low-risk and low-intermediate risk patients are often grouped together as "good-prognosis," and patients with high-intermediate and high risk as "poor-prognosis" patients. In contrast to "good prognosis" as defined here, "limited-stage disease," "early-stage disease," "low-stage disease," and "localized disease" are less well defined. Similarly, the term "advanced stage" is ill-defined and used differently by various cooperative groups.

In the era of chemoimmunotherapy with rituximab, two novel subgroups among the young good-prognosis patients have evolved after a combination of a CHOP (cyclophosphamide, doxorubicin, vincristine, and prednisone)-like chemotherapy regimen and rituximab[2]: a very favorable and a less favorable group. While results of the very favorable subgroup (no age-adjusted IPI [aaIPI] risk factor, no bulky disease) with an estimated 3-year event-free survival rate of 97% and on overall survival rate of 100% after six cycles of CHOP with chemotherapy can hardly be improved, the results in all other subgroups of patients with diffuse large B-cell lymphoma (DLBCL) continue to warrant further improvement. For the purpose of clarity, in this review we include all patients not belonging to the very favorable subgroup under the term "advanced," because outcome of these patients must definitely be improved and approaches aiming at this goal in the different subgroups might be very similar and/or complementary. According to the definition used here, the "advanced disease" group includes all patients with bulky disease, young patients with one or more aaIPI risk factors, and all elderly patients.

The most important development in the treatment of advanced aggressive lymphomas was the demonstration that a combination of cyclophosphamide, doxorubicin, vincristine, and prednisone, known under the acronym of CHOP, was

[a]Innere Medizin I, Saarland University Medical School, Homburg, Germany.
[b]Klinik I für Innere Medizin, Klinikum der Universität zu Köln, Cologne, Germany.
Supported by Deutsche Krebshilfe.
Address correspondence to Michael Pfreundschuh, MD, Klinik für Innere Medizin I, Saarland University Medical School, D-66421 Homburg (Saar), Germany. E-mail: michael.pfreundschuh@uniklinikum-saarland.de

0037-1963/06/$-see front matter © 2006 Elsevier Inc. All rights reserved.
doi:10.1053/j.seminhematol.2006.07.003

demonstrated to induce complete remissions and long-term disease-free survival in a considerable proportion of patients.[3] After its publication in 1976, many attempts were started to improve results further by escalating one or more components of the CHOP combination or by the addition of new drugs. Interpretation of encouraging results in phase II trials evaluating these strategies were difficult, because patient selection was difficult to quantify, because there was no commonly accepted risk factor index according to which the population in the respective trials was characterized. In 1993, the results of the US Southwest Oncology Group (SWOG)/Eastern Cooperative Oncology Group (ECOG) Intergroup trial, which had randomized approximately 1,100 patients to CHOP, m-BACOD, ProMACE-CytaBOM, and MACOP-B, showed a very similar efficacy of these four regimens with a median disease-free survival after 4 years of 40%.[4] At the same time, the IPI was established and allowed for a better characterization of patients and interpretation of treatment results observed in different studies.[1] A subgroup analysis of the Intergroup trial according to the IPI confirmed the equivalent efficacy of the four different regimens in each prognostic subgroup. In contrast to efficacy, the differences between the four regimens with respect to toxicity were considerable: the rates of therapy-associated deaths were 1% after CHOP, 5% after m-BACOD, 4% after ProMACE-CytaBOM, and 6% after MACOP-B.

With the availability of granulocyte colony-stimulating factor (G-CSF) and the tool of autologous stem cell support in the 1990s, different strategies for increasing dose intensity[5] were pursued: dose escalation, dose densification (by interval reduction), or a combination thereof. While numerous phase II studies using either one or both strategies in combination reported encouraging results, only a limited number of randomized trials comparing intensified regimens with baseline CHOP have been reported. Only the latter will be discussed here.

Conventional Dose Escalation Not Necessitating Stem Cell Support

The NHL-B1 trial of the Deutsche Studiengruppe Hochmaligne Non-Hodgkin-Lymphome (DSHNHL) tested in a 2 × 2 factorial design whether the addition of etoposide to the CHOP regimen (CHOEP-21)[6] and/or the reduction of treatment intervals from 3 to 2 weeks (CHOP-14, CHOEP-14) improves the outcome of young good-prognosis patients (defined as those with normal pretreatment serum lactate dehydrogenase [LDH]). CHOEP (CHOP plus etoposide 100 mg/m^2 days 1 to 3) was significantly better than CHOP, suggesting CHOEP as the standard chemotherapy combination for young good-prognosis patients in the pre-rituximab era. The superiority of CHOEP over CHOP in young good-prognosis patients was recently confirmed in the MabThera International Trial Group (MInT) trial.[2]

To improve results further, the DSHNHL compared a maximal dose-escalated version of CHOEP-21 tolerable without stem cell support (Hi-CHOEP-21: cyclophosphamide 1,200 mg/m^2, doxorubicin 65 mg/m^2, vincristine 2 mg, etoposide 175 mg/m^2 × 3, prednisone 100 mg) with baseline CHOEP-21 in a subsequent randomized trial. Despite excellent adherence to the protocol (median relative dose CHOEP-21: 96%; Hi-CHOEP: 93%), there was no difference between Hi-CHOEP-21 and baseline CHOEP-21 after 37 months median observation in low-risk or low-intermediate risk patients.[7] This indicates that the window of opportunity for conventional dose escalation without stem cell support is small, even in young patients. In elderly patients who are more sensitive to the additional toxicities of dose-escalated regimens, this window might be even smaller, as demonstrated by the experience with CHOEP in elderly compared to young patients.[8,9] In contrast to young patients, the addition of etoposide to CHOP was too toxic for elderly patients, and required frequent treatment delays and dose reductions, resulting in a reduced delivered dose intensity and loss of superiority over CHOP.[8]

In summary, the results from randomized trials suggest a small window for conventional dose-escalated modifications of CHOP. This window is smaller in elderly patients due to the higher toxicity of dose-escalated regimens in this population.

High-Dose Chemotherapy With Stem Cell Support

In relapsing aggressive lymphomas, high-dose chemotherapy with stem cell support was superior to conventional chemotherapy[10] and is widely accepted as the standard approach for patients with relapsing aggressive lymphomas, who are fit enough to tolerate the considerable toxicity and morbidity associated with this approach. In contrast, the results of high-dose chemotherapy in the primary treatment of aggressive lymphomas are contradictory. In a small, but pivotal trial, B-cell type aggressive lymphomas were randomly assigned to receive either MACOP-B (50 patients) or a so-called high-dose sequential therapy (48 patients). After a median follow-up of 55 months, the patients given high-dose sequential therapy, as compared with those treated with MACOP-B, had significantly higher rates of complete response, freedom from disease progression, freedom from relapse, and event-free survival. The difference in overall survival at 7 years, which also favored the group assigned to high-dose sequential therapy, was marginally significant (81% *v* 55%, $P = .09$).[11]

Several other randomized trials that evaluated the role of high-dose chemotherapy in the primary treatment of aggressive lymphomas yielded conflicting results.[12-22] As shown in Table 1, most trials did not find differences between the conventionally dosed and high-dosed treatment strategies, some favored the high-dose approach, and some did so only in retrospective subgroup analyses. One randomized trial showed even inferior results for the high-dose approach compared to the conventional chemotherapy.[17]

Several factors might be responsible for the failure of high-dose concepts to improve the outcome of young patients in

Table 1 Randomized Comparisons Between Conventional and High-Dose Chemotherapy With Stem Cell Support in Aggressive Lymphoma

Authors*	Population	Randomized Population	EFS	OS
Haioun et al, 2000[12]	≥1 RF, bulk	CR	NS	NS
	>2 RF	**CR***	**.02***	**.04***
Verdonck et al, 1994[13]	I–IV	<CR	NS	NS
Gianni et al, 1997[11]	**I/II$_{bulky}$, III/IV**	**All**	**.004**	**NS**
Santini et al, 1998[14]	II$_{bulky}$, III/IV	All	NS	NS
		≥2 RF*	.008*	NS
Kluin-Nelemans et al, 2001[15]	All	CR	NS	NS
Kaiser et al, 2002[16]	LDH >ONW	CR, PR	NS	NS
Gisselbrecht et al, 2002[17]	*≥1 RF*	*All*	*.01*	*.009*
Martelli et al, 2003[18]	≥2 RF	CR, PR	NS	NS
Milpied et al, 2004[19]	**1 & 2 RF**	**All**	**.04**	***NS***
		≥1, RF*	**.01***	**.001***
Betticher et al, 2005[20]	>1 RF	All	NS	NS
Olivieri et al, 2005[21]	**II$_{bulky}$, III/IV**	**All**	**NS**	**NS**
Vitolo et al, 2005[22]	**>1 RF**	**All**	**NS**	**NS**

NOTE. Bold studies showed an advantage of high-dose over conventional chemotherapy. In the study in italics (Gisselbrecht et al), high-dose chemotherapy yielded inferior results; all other studies showed no difference between conventional and high-dose chemotherapy.

Abbreviations: RF, risk factor according to aaIPI; CR, complete remission; PR, partial remission; EFS, event-free survival; OS, overall survival; NS, not significant.

*Retrospective subgroup analysis.

these trials. First, the cytotoxic drugs used for the myeloablative therapy are not the most active in aggressive lymphomas; second, in many studies the high-dose chemotherapy was given instead of one to three cycles of conventional chemotherapy but not in addition to a full-cycle conventional chemotherapy, resulting in a compromised total dose. In general, the results of these trials are difficult to interpret because the conventional and high-dose arms differed in more than the dose of chemotherapy. For example, in the trial reported by Gianni et al, their "sequential high-dose chemotherapy" approach[11] used high-dose methotrexate and the repeated application of single maximally dosed cytotoxic drugs. In contrast to the superiority of the high-dose sequential approach observed in the original study,[11] three subsequent trials comparing the high-dose sequential approach with dose-dense Mega-CEOP (dose-escalated cyclophosphamide, epirubicin, vincristine, and prednisone), MACOP-B, and CHOP-21, respectively, observed equal efficacy of the conventionally dosed regimens in young poor-prognosis patients. The Groupe Ouest est d'Etude des Leucemies Aigues et des Maladies du Sang (GOELAMS) trial,[19] which compared eight cycles of CHOP-21 with two cycles of a variant of a biweekly CHOEP (CEEP-15) regimen, followed by high-dose methotrexate plus cytarabine and a myeloablative. BEAM regimen (BCNU, etoposide, cytarabine, and melphalan) with autologous stem cell support in patients with low-intermediate and high-intermediate risk according to the aaIPI, found a significant advantage for the intensified concept with respect to event-free survival for the entire study population and with respect to overall survival after 5 years for the subpopulation with intermediate-high risk only. Despite the suggestive title of the publication in the *New England Journal of Medicine*, it is not clear whether the high-dose component (BEAM) or the dose-dense chemotherapy given early in the experimental arm (two cycles of CEEP-15) was responsible for the superiority of this approach over eight cycles of 3-weekly CHOP (Fig 1). The fact that patients in the experimental arm of the GOELAMS study received all their therapy (including high-dose BEAM) by day 64, while patients in the CHOP-21 arm had received only four of their eight CHOP chemotherapy cycles by day 64, demonstrates that the experimental arm has a much higher dose density than the control arm. Hence, the overall dose-density of the experimental arm in the GOELAMS study rather than its single high-dose component BEAM was likely responsible for its superiority over classical CHOP-21.

Similar to the GOELAMS study, the other randomized trials listed in Table 1 are difficult to interpret with respect to the role of high-dose chemotherapy. All of these studies used different drugs in the conventional and high-dose arms, which makes it impossible to ascribe the results obtained in the high-dose arm to dose escalation or the different combinations of cytotoxic drugs.

In summary, the statement of the Lyon 1997 consensus conference is still valid in 2005: there is no justification of high-dose chemotherapy in the primary treatment of aggressive lymphomas outside clinical trials.[23] Novel approaches to high-dose chemotherapy are evaluating regimens that use the cytotoxic drugs with the highest efficacy in aggressive lymphomas, in particular alkylating agents and anthracyclines, at the maximal tolerated doses and/or try to escalate the total dose of the regimen by applying the high-dose regimen in addition to fully dosed conventional chemotherapy. In the so-called Mega-CHOEP trials of the DSHNHL, patients receive a first cycle of conventionally escalated CHOEP followed by three cycles of high-dose CHOEP, each necessitat-

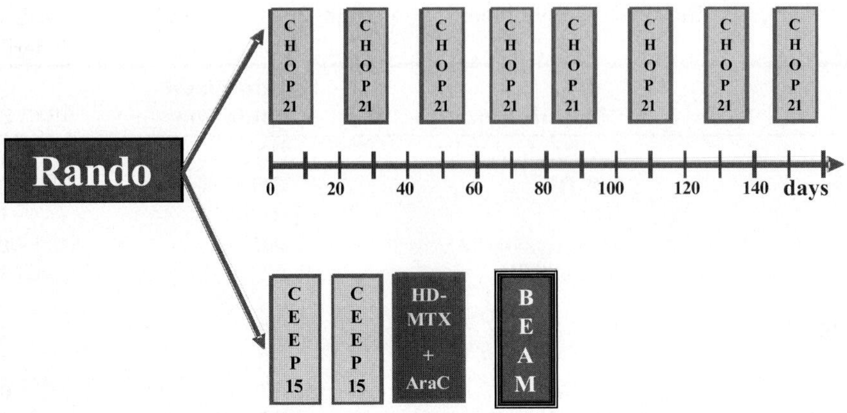

Figure 1 Time scale of the GOELAMS randomized trial comparing CHOP-21 with "high-dose chemotherapy." Patients in the experimental arm received two cycles of dose-dense CEEP (cyclophosphamide, epirubicin, etoposide, and prednisone) followed by high-dose methotrexate/cytarabine and myeloablative BEAM with stem cell support. By the time they had completed their entire chemotherapy (day 64) patients in the control arm had received only four cycles of CHOP-21 or 50% of their planned chemotherapy.

ing stem cell support.[24] The DSHNHL is currently comparing Mega-CHOEP with eight cycles of CHOEP-14 in a randomized fashion, both arms with rituximab.

Dose Densification

As an alternative approach to dose escalation, dose intensity can also be increased by dose densification, ie, reduction of treatment intervals. A reduction of treatment intervals between two cycles of CHOP from 3 to 2 weeks equals an increase of dose intensity, ie, the dose per week[5] by 50%. This compares favorably with strategies that try to increase dose intensity by dose escalation, because increases in excess of 25% compared to classical CHOP-21 cannot be achieved without stem cell support.

Based on these considerations, we designed a dose-dense biweekly version of CHOP plus etoposide (CHOEP-14). After demonstrating its feasibility in a phase II study, the dose-dense biweekly CHOP and CHOEP regimens were compared to their conventional 3-weekly counterparts in two randomized trials in young good-prognosis patients (NHL-B1)[25] and in elderly patients (NHL-B2)[8] in a 2 × 2 factorial design. In the young patients, the addition of etoposide improved the results with respect to the primary end point, event-free survival, while the reduction of treatment intervals from 3 to 2 weeks resulted in a significantly better overall survival.[25] When the three intensified regimens CHOP-14, CHOEP-21, and CHOEP-14 were compared with the standard CHOP-21 regimen, CHOEP-21 improved event-free survival, while CHOEP-14 improved event-free survival, complete remission rates, and overall survival over baseline CHOP-21. The advantage of the 2-weekly over the 3-weekly CHOEP was most pronounced in patients with bulky disease. Therefore, CHOEP-14 appears to be the preferred chemotherapy regimen for young good-prognosis patients, as long as rituximab is not incorporated into the therapeutic strategy.

The results of the elderly patients in the NHL-B2 trial were quite similar to those observed in young patients with the exception that double-intensive CHOEP-14 was too toxic, caused many treatment delays and dose reductions, and was associated with a higher therapy-associated death rate. In contrast, CHOP-14, which was not more toxic than CHOP-21, was significantly better than CHOP-21 with respect to complete remission rate, event-free and overall survival. The advantage of biweekly CHOP-14 over 3-weekly CHOP-21 was most pronounced in patients with elevated LDH and—similar to the situation with younger patients in the NHL-B1 trial (where patients with elevated LDH had been excluded)—in patients with bulky disease.

Another advantage of dose densification is that in contrast to dose escalation, dose densification or interval reduction from 3-weekly to 2-weekly intervals has not only become feasible using G-CSF, but also it shows no or no clinically relevant increase of toxicity,[8,9] allowing for high received relative dose intensities (>90%) even in elderly patients in nationwide trials.

The problem with dose-dense CHOP-14, in particular in the elderly, is that it requires a dedicated therapist who provides all supportive measures necessary to enable strict protocol adherence, which includes, first, a so-called pre-phase treatment consisting of a single shot of 1 mg vincristine and 100 mg prednisone orally per day over 7 days, which results in a significant improvement of patients with poor performance status and ameliorates toxicity of the first chemotherapy cycle; and second, a consequent dose reduction scheme that allows for treatment delay of 3 days increments, but no dose reductions,[8,9] and hydrocortisone substitutions (20 mg in the morning, 10 mg after lunch) after tapering the prednisone. Non-adherence to these recommendations and lack of therapeutic discipline might be responsible for the large differences in outcome after CHOP-14, even in similar patient populations. While the 2.5-year event-free survival after CHOP-14 in elderly patients in the German RICOVER-60 trial (Rituxamab With CHOP Over 60 Years) was greater than 55%,[26] it was only 25% in a Dutch-Scandinavian trial.[27] Unfortunately, there is no standard format for reporting dose

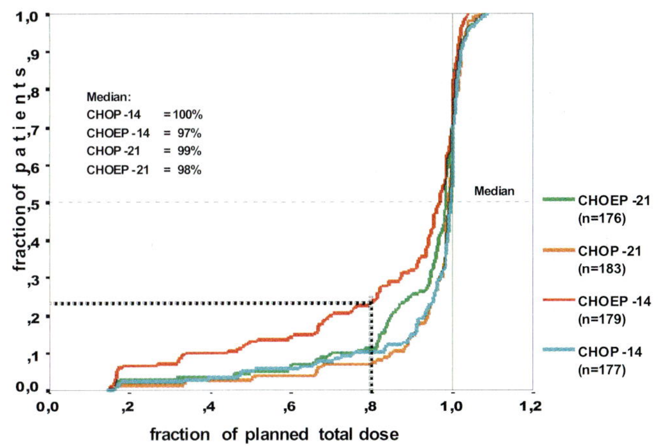

Figure 2 Cumulative dose plot for the description of adherence to planned dose or dose intensity. The cumulative dose plot for cyclophosphamide in the NHL-B2 trial of the DSHNHL[8] shows a rather good median of 97% for the received dose in the CHOEP-14 arm. However, while only 10% or less of the patients in the CHOP-21, CHOEP-21, and CHOP-14 arms, respectively, received less than 80% of the planned dose, the fraction of the patients in the CHOEP-14 regimen who received less than 80% of the planned dose was 23% (dotted line). This demonstrates that reporting median doses or dose intensities is an insufficient format for describing adherence to a protocol.

adherence, and description of the median dose received is not sufficient. Rather, cumulative plots should be used to describe adherence to planned dose and/or dose adherence, because they allow for a better interpretation of the adherence to a given regimen (Fig 2).

Combining Dose Escalation With Dose Densification: Hybrid or Chimeric Approaches

The most prominent example of this hybrid, chimeric or double-intensive strategy, which combines both dose escalation and dose densification, is ACVBP, which was designed by the Groupe d'Etude des Lymphomes des Adultes (GELA). The ACVBP regimen consists of four biweekly courses of doxorubicin (75 mg/m^2), cyclophosphamide (1,200 mg/m^2), vindesine (2 mg/m^2) on days 1 and 5, bleomycin (10 mg) on days 1 and 5, prednisone (60 mg/m^2) orally from day 1 to day 5, and intrathecal methotrexate (15 mg) on day 2. This is followed by a sequential consolidation therapy with high-dose methotrexate (3 g/m^2), etoposide (300 mg/m^2), ifosfamide (1,500 mg/m^2), and cytosine arabinoside (100 mg/m^2). ACVBP achieved a better event-free survival and overall survival rate than CHOP in patients 61 to 69 years of age; however, the therapy-associated death rate was significantly higher (13% *v* 7%), and the authors do not recommend ACVBP in patients older than 65 years.[28]

The already discussed GOELAMS[19] trial, which compared CHOP-21 with an experimental approach consisting of both dose-dense components and a high-dose BEAM regimen in young patients with an aaIPI of 1 or 2, represents another example of a hybrid approach. Recently, the Hemato-Oncologie vor Volwassenen in Nederland (HOVON) presented results with six cycles of dose-escalated I-CHOP-14, which has the same total dose as eight cycles of CHOP-21 but doubles the intensity of cyclophosphamide and doxorubicin. The dose-intense I-CHOP-14 regimen appeared to improve outcome for young patients with low-intermediate risk.[29] Figure 3 compares the dose intensities of cyclophosphamide and doxorubicin in the CHOP-21, CHOP-14, I-CHOP-14, and ACVBP regimens.

Integrating Rituximab Into Dose-Intensified Chemotherapy Regimens

The introduction of rituximab and its combination with standard chemotherapy combination of CHOP represents the major milestone in the treatment of DLBCL for the last 30 years. The toxicity profile of rituximab is excellent and the absence of relevant hematotoxicity allows for its combination with myelosuppressive polychemotherapy regimens without compromising doses and dose intensities of the respective chemotherapy. Combinations of chemotherapy with rituximab are hardly more toxic than the respective chemotherapy alone, except for viral infections, in particular herpes zoster.

The first randomized trial comparing standard eight cycles of 3-weekly CHOP-21 with and without rituximab was performed by the French Cooperative Group, GELA, in previously untreated elderly patients (61 to 80 years) with stages II to IV disease. After a median follow-up of 5 years, event-free survival, progression-free survival, disease-free survival, and overall survival were statistically significantly in favor of the combination of rituximab + CHOP (R-CHOP). Patients with low-risk, but not with high-risk lymphoma according to the IPI had a significantly longer survival if treated with the combination.[30]

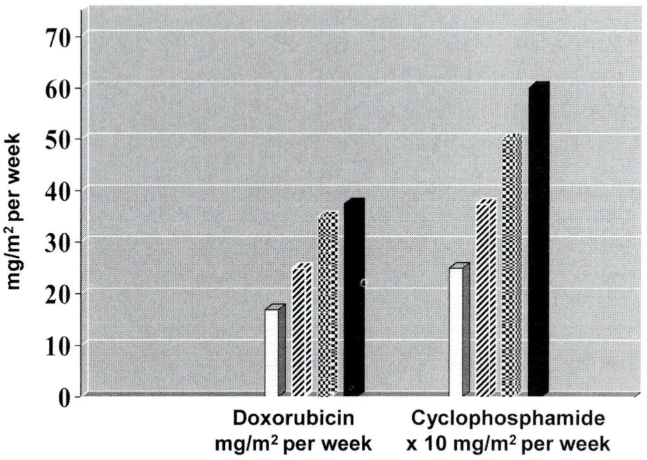

Figure 3 Dose intensities of doxorubicin and cyclophosphamide in dose-dense modifications of CHOP. □, CHOP-21; ▨, CHOP-14[37]; ▩, I-CHOP-14[30]; ■, ACBVP.[12]

A second randomized trial[32] in elderly patients compared CHOP-21 with and without rituximab and yielded similar results. Patients achieving a partial or complete remission had a second randomization into rituximab maintenance or observation. Interestingly, those who received rituximab maintenance had a significantly prolonged event-free survival, but this advantage was only observed in patients who had not received rituximab as part of their induction therapy.

A third randomized trial compared six and eight cycles of dose-dense biweekly CHOP-14 with and without rituximab in elderly patients (61 to 80 years) in a 2 × 2 factorial design. While a planned interim analysis of 828 evaluable patients showed no difference between six and eight cycles, event-free survival after R-CHOP-14 was significantly better than after CHOP-14 alone ($P = .000025$). There was a trend for a better event-free survival after eight cycles of CHOP-14 compared to six cycles, but this trend was neutralized after the addition of rituximab. The advantage of R-CHOP-14 over CHOP-14 with respect to overall survival after 26 months was not yet significant.[26]

Finally, the MInT study showed significantly better 3-year estimates for event-free survival (59% after chemotherapy and 79% after chemotherapy plus rituximab) and overall survival (93% *v* 84%) after chemotherapy plus rituximab compared to rituximab alone in young good-prognosis patients, establishing the combination of CHOP and rituximab as the reference standard also in this population of DLBCL patients.

In contrast, in young high-risk patients, there are no data from randomized trials formally proving the role of rituximab for these patients, even though such a role can be expected from the results of randomized trials in the other therapeutic groups, the young low-risk and elderly patients.

An important issue with respect to integrating rituximab into intensified chemotherapy regimens is the lack of knowledge on the most important effector mechanism of rituximab operative in vivo. If this is indeed antibody-dependent cellular cytotoxicity, then natural killer cells are essential for the efficacy of rituximab and combinations of rituximab with more myelosuppressive chemotherapies would carry an increased risk of compromising its efficacy. In this respect, it is of interest that CHOEP (CHOP + etoposide) was confirmed to be superior to CHOP in the MInT study.[2] However, in combination with rituximab, CHOP was at least as good as CHOEP and there was even a trend that R-CHOP was better than R-CHOEP for some subpopulations of patients. The lack of superiority of R-CHOEP over R-CHOP might be explained by a "chemotherapy regimen–equalizing effect" of rituximab; alternatively, however, this could be due to the more pronounced myelosuppression of CHOEP, which annihilates its greater cytotoxicity in combination with the antibody. The efficacy of rituximab might be even more compromised if rituximab is combined with more myelosuppressive or even myeloablative regimens. Such an interference with rituximab effector mechanisms might explain why the addition of rituximab to the triple high-dose regimen Mega-CHOEP did not improve the results when compared to Mega-CHOEP alone.[32]

In summary, these considerations and the experience with combining rituximab with CHOP or CHOEP in the MInT trial caution against combining rituximab with chemotherapy combinations other than CHOP outside controlled trials.

Intensifying Rituximab

Another key issue with respect to integrating rituximab into dose-intense chemotherapy regimens refers to the lack of pharmacokinetic data available for rituximab in DLBCL, the lack of knowledge of minimal serum levels and areas under the curve necessary to achieve tissue levels that are sufficient to kill the malignant DLBCL clone in situ. The commonly used dosage per application (375 mg/m^2) and the schedule of giving rituximab with each cycle of chemotherapy are mostly based on practicability and economic considerations.

Rituximab has been shown to improve results compared to chemotherapy alone in combination with both CHOP-21[30,31,33] and with dose-dense CHOP-14.[26] However, while the benefit of adding rituximab was much smaller for poor-prognosis patients in the 3-weekly schedule in the French trial (where it even failed to reach significance with respect to survival), poor-prognosis and good-prognosis patients profited from the biweekly application of rituximab to an at least equal extent in the German trial.[34] Pharmacokinetic studies of biweekly rituximab in combination with CHOP-14 showed an increase of pre-infusion rituximab serum concentrations with each additional application for the first four cycles. Rituximab serum levels reached a plateau between cycles 5 and 8 and decreased continuously after the end of treatment with detectable levels even after 9 months. The lower serum levels in the first four cycles are probably due to the destruction of normal B cells together with maximal reduction of tumor load after the first treatment cycle[35] (Fig 4). It must be assumed that rituximab serum levels fall even deeper and possibly below a critical level in a 3-weekly schedule of the drug, in particular in patients with a high tumor load and hence poor prognosis, thus explaining the reduced efficacy of

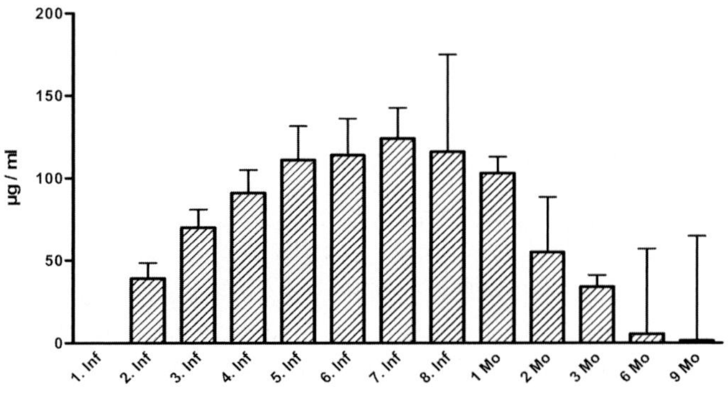

Figure 4 Median (± interquartile range) pre-infusion serum concentrations of biweekly rituximab in combination with CHOP-14 in 10 elderly patients with DLBCL. In a biweekly application schedule of rituximab, trough serum levels increased with each additional cycle, reaching a plateau between cycles 5 and 8 and continuously decreasing after the eighth application with detectable levels as long as 9 months after the last infusion.

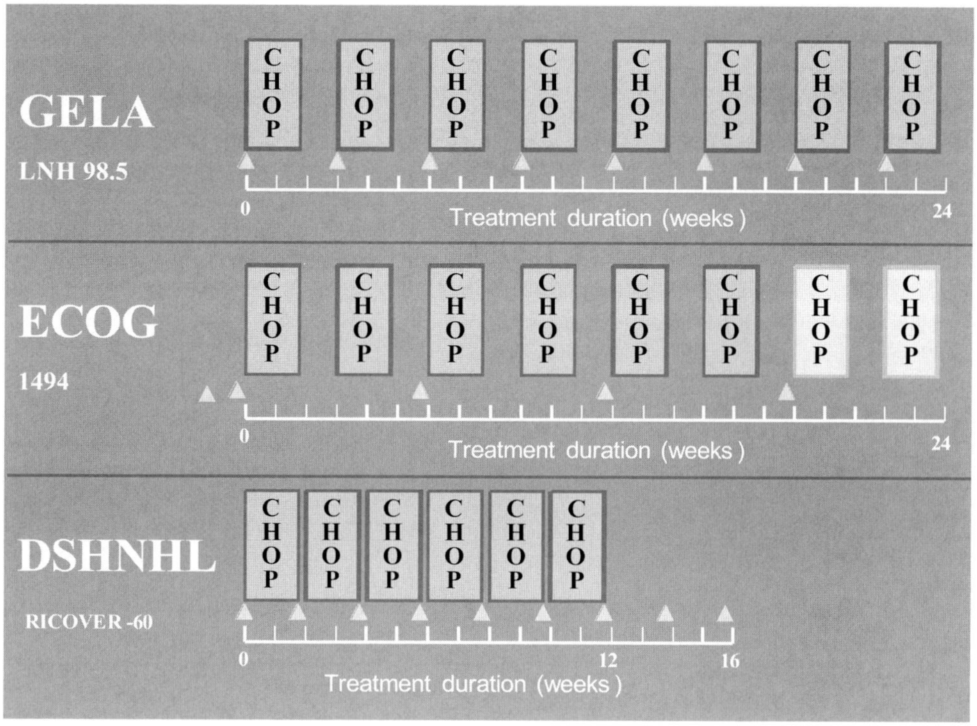

Figure 5 Schedule of rituximab application in combination with CHOP-21 and CHOP-14 in randomized trials all demonstrating superiority of CHOP plus rituximab over CHOP alone. A similar improvement was observed in the GELA[31] and ECOG[32] trials, even though the latter used only five applications of rituximab but had two dose-dense applications before the first chemotherapy cycle. In the DSHNHL trial, biweekly application of rituximab did not prevent a nadir of the serum level after the first application, suggesting that this nadir is more pronounced when the second rituximab is given after 3 weeks only, which was the case in the GELA study.

3-weekly rituximab in high-risk patients in the GELA trial.[30] In this respect, it is noteworthy that the therapeutic gain achieved by the addition of rituximab with eight applications in the GELA LNH 9.5 trial[30,33] was very similar to the one achieved in the ECOG trial,[31] where only five applications (but with a different schedule) were given. Taking into consideration that the first application of rituximab has to eliminate circulating B cells before it can access the tumor site, the rituximab schedule with a loading dose in the ECOG trial, where rituximab was given on days −7 and −3 before the first CHOP cycle, might have been more adequate (Fig 5) than the once-every-3-weeks schedule in the GELA trial.

The pharmacokinetics of biweekly CHOP (Fig 4) also suggest that biweekly rituximab is not dose-dense enough and that smaller intervals are indicated, in particular during the early treatment phase in order to maintain high serum levels. A phase II study evaluating the pharmacokinetics and efficacy of dose-dense rituximab (five applications within the first 2 weeks) in combination with CHOP-14 is currently ongoing in Germany.

Conclusions

Besides the addition of rituximab to standard CHOP chemotherapy, reducing treatment intervals of CHOP from 3 to 2 weeks (CHOP-14) represents a major milestone in the treatment of aggressive lymphomas, where results had stagnated for over 25 years. The recent interim analysis of the RICOVER-60 trial suggests that the combination of both approaches (interval reduction and the addition of rituximab) might be a further step forward, at least in elderly patients with DLBCL. The observation that biweekly rituximab in combination with CHOP-14 in contrast to the 3-weekly application of the antibody in combination with CHOP-21 improves outcome in poor-prognosis as much as in good-prognosis patients suggests that not only densification of the cytotoxic drugs, but also dose-dense application of the antibody contributes to the high efficacy of R-CHOP-14. The key issues with respect to the use of dose-dense chemoimmunotherapy refer to the lack of pharmacokinetic data available for rituximab in DLBCL and the lack of knowledge of minimal serum levels and areas under the curve necessary to achieve tissue levels that are sufficient to kill the malignant DLBCL clone in situ. The chances that current protocols give too much rituximab for DLBCL are as good as the chances that not enough rituximab is given, or that enough rituximab is given but with a suboptimal schedule. Well-designed prospective trials incorporating pharmacokinetic studies are necessary to exploit the full potential of dose-intensified treatment with respect to both its chemotherapy and immunotherapy components in the era of modern chemoimmunotherapy for DLBCL.

References

1. The International Non-Hodgkin's Lymphoma Prognostic Factors Project. A predictive model for aggressive non-Hodgkin's lymphoma. N Engl J Med 329:987-994, 1993
2. Pfreundschuh M, Truemper L, Oesterborg A, Pettengell R, Trneny M, Imrie K, et al: CHOP-like chemotherapy plus rituximab compared with CHOP-like chemotherapy alone in young patients with good-prognosis diffuse large B-cell lymphoma: A randomized trial of the Mabthera International Trial (MInT) Study Group. Lancet Oncol 7:379-391, 2006
3. McKelvey EM, Gottlieb JA, Wilson HE, Haut A, Talley RW, Stephens R, et al: Hydroxyldaunomycin (Adriamycin) combination chemotherapy in malignant lymphoma. Cancer 38:1484-1493, 1976
4. Fisher RI, Gaynor ER, Dahlberg S, Oken MM, Grogan TM, Mize EM, et al: Comparison of a standard regimen (CHOP) with three intensive chemotherapy regimens for advanced non-Hodgkin's lymphoma. N Engl J Med 328:1002-1006, 1993
5. Meyer RM, Hryniuk WM, Goodyear MD: The role of dose intensity in determining outcome in intermediate-grade non-Hodgkin's lymphoma. J Clin Oncol 9:339-347, 1991
6. Koppler H, Pfluger KH, Eschenbach I, Pfab R, Birkmann J, Zeller W, et al: Randomised comparison of CHOEP versus alternating hCHOP/IVEP for high-grade non-Hodgkin's lymphomas: Treatment results and prognostic factor analysis in a multi-centre trial. Ann Oncol 5:49-55, 1994
7. Pfreundschuh M, Zeynalova S, Pflueger K-H, Koch P, Mergenthaler M, Bentz M, et al: Dose-escalated CHOP plus etoposide (Hi-CHOEP) is not superior to base-line CHOEP in young good-prognosis patients with aggressive lymphoma: Results of a randomized DSHNHL trial. J Clin Oncol 24:425s, 2006
8. Pfreundschuh M, Trumper L, Kloess M, Schmits R, Feller AC, Rube C, et al: Two-weekly or 3-weekly CHOP chemotherapy with or without etoposide for the treatment of elderly patients with aggressive lymphomas: Results of the NHL-B2 trial of the DSHNHL. Blood 104:634-641, 2004
9. Pfreundschuh M, Trumper L, Kloess M, Schmits R, Feller AC, Rudolph C, et al: Two-weekly or 3-weekly CHOP chemotherapy with or without etoposide for the treatment of young patients with good-prognosis (normal LDH) aggressive lymphomas: Results of the NHL-B1 trial of the DSHNHL. Blood 104:626-633, 2004
10. Philip T, Guglielmi C, Hagenbeek A, Somers R, Van der Lelie H, Bron D, et al: Autologous bone marrow transplantation as compared with salvage chemotherapy in relapses of chemotherapy-sensitive non-Hodgkin's lymphoma. N Engl J Med 333:1540-1545, 1995
11. Gianni AM, Bregni M, Siena S, Brambilla C, Di Nicola M, Lombardi F, et al: High-dose chemotherapy and autologous bone marrow transplantation compared with MACOP-B in aggressive B-cell lymphoma. N Engl J Med 336:1290-1297, 1997
12. Haioun C, Lepage E, Gisselbrecht C, Salles G, Coiffier B, Brice P, et al: Survival benefit of high-dose therapy in poor-risk aggressive non-Hodgkin's lymphoma: Final analysis of the prospective LNH87-2 protocol—A Groupe d'Etude des Lymphomes de l'Adulte study. J Clin Oncol 18:3025-3030, 2000
13. Verdonck LF, van Putten WL, Hagenbeek A, Schouten HC, Sonneveld P, van Imhoff GW, et al: Comparison of CHOP chemotherapy with autologous bone marrow transplantation for slowly responding patients with aggressive non- Hodgkin's lymphoma. N Engl J Med 332: 1045-1051, 1995
14. Santini G, Salvagno L, Leoni P, Chisesi T, De Souza C, Sertoli MR, et al: VACOP-B versus VACOP-B plus autologous bone marrow transplantation for advanced diffuse non-Hodgkin's lymphoma: Results of a prospective randomized trial by the non-Hodgkin's Lymphoma Cooperative Study Group. J Clin Oncol 16:2796-2802, 1998
15. Kluin-Nelemans HC, Zagonel V, Anastasopoulou A, Bron D, Roozendaal KJ, Noordijk EM, et al: Standard chemotherapy with or without high-dose chemotherapy for aggressive non-Hodgkin's lymphoma: Randomized phase III EORTC study. J Natl Cancer Inst 93:22-30, 2001
16. Kaiser U, Uebelacker I, Abel U, Birkmann J, Trumper L, Schmalenberg H, et al: Randomized study to evaluate the use of high-dose therapy as part of primary treatment for "aggressive" lymphoma. J Clin Oncol 20:4413-4419, 2002
17. Gisselbrecht C, Lepage E, Molina T, Quesnel B, Fillet G, Lederlin P, et al: Shortened first-line high-dose chemotherapy for patients with poor-prognosis aggressive lymphoma. J Clin Oncol 20:2472-2479, 2002
18. Martelli M, Gherlinzoni F, De Renzo A, Zinzani PL, De Vivo A, Cantonetti M, et al: Early autologous stem-cell transplantation versus conventional chemotherapy as front-line therapy in high-risk, aggressive non-Hodgkin's lymphoma: An Italian multicenter randomized trial. J Clin Oncol 21:1255-1262, 2003
19. Milpied N, Deconinck E, Gaillard F, Delwail V, Foussard C, Berthou C, et al: Initial treatment of aggressive lymphoma with high-dose chemotherapy and autologous stem-cell support. N Engl J Med 350:1287-1295, 2004
20. Betticher D, von Rohr A, Kovasovics T, Martinelli G, Cerny TL, Dyer MJS, et al: Sequential high-dose chemotherapy (SHDC) with autologous stem cell transplantation (ASCT) vs standard CHOP regimen for pts with untreated aggressive NHL. Results of the MISTRAL trial from the Swiss Group for Clinical Cancer Research (SAKK). Ann Oncol 16:v101-v102, 2005
21. Olivieri A, Santini G, Patti C, Chisesi T, De Souza C, Rubagotti A, et al: Upfront high-dose sequential therapy (HDS) versus VACOP-B with or without HDS in aggressive non-Hodgkin's lymphoma: long-term results by the NHLCSG. Ann Oncol 16:1941-1948, 2005
22. Vitolo U, Liberati AM, Cabras MG, Federico M, Angelucci E, Baldini L, et al: High dose sequential chemotherapy with autologous transplantation versus dose-dense chemotherapy MegaCEOP as first line treatment in poor-prognosis diffuse large cell lymphoma: An "Intergruppo Italiano Linfomi" randomized trial. Haematologica 90:793-801, 2005
23. Shipp MA, Abeloff MD, Antman KH, Carroll G, Hagenbeek A, Loeffler M, et al: International Consensus Conference on High-Dose Therapy with Hematopoietic Stem Cell Transplantation in Aggressive Non-Hodgkin's Lymphomas: Report of the jury. J Clin Oncol 17:423-429, 1999
24. Glass B, Kloess M, Engert A, Berdel WE, Metzner B, Truemper L, et al: Mega-CHOEP repeated high dose therapy as treatment of aggressive NHL: Critical impact of time scheduling. Blood 100:776a, 2002 (abstr)
25. Pfreundschuh M, Trumper L, Kloess M, Schmits R, Feller AC, Rudolph C, et al: Two-weekly or 3-weekly CHOP chemotherapy with or without etoposide for the treatment of young patients with good-prognosis (normal LDH) aggressive lymphomas: Results of the NHL-B1 trial of the DSHNHL. Blood 104:626-633, 2004
26. Pfreundschuh M, Klöss M, Schmits R, Zeynalova S, Lengfelder E, Franke A, et al: Six, not eight cycles of bi-weekly CHOP with rituximab (R-CHOP-14) is the preferred treatment for elderly patients with diffuse large B-cell lymphoma (DLBCL): Results of the RICOVER-60 trial of the German High-Grade Non-Hodgkin Lymphoma Study Group (DSHNHL). Blood 106:9a, 2005 (abstr)
27. Sonneveld van Putten WL, Holte H, Biesma D, van Marwijk-Kooy M, Kramer M, Wijermans P, et al: Intensified CHOP with rituximab for intermediate or high-risk non-Hodgkin's lymphoma: Interim analysis of a randomized phase III trial in elderly patients by the Dutch HOVON and Nordic Lymphoma groups. Blood 106:10, 2005 (abstr)
28. Tilly H, Lepage E, Coiffier B, Blanc M, Herbrecht R, Bosly A, et al: Intensive conventional chemotherapy (ACVBP regimen) compared with standard CHOP for poor-prognosis aggressive non-Hodgkin lymphoma. Blood 102:4284-4289, 2003
29. Verdonck LF, van Imhoff GW, Raemakers JMM, Verhoef G, Kramer MHH, Ossenkoppele GJ, et al: Six courses of intensified CHOP plus G-CSF compared to eight courses of standard CHOP in patients with intermediate-risk aggressive non-Hodgkin lymphoma. Blood 106:9a, 2005 (abstr)
30. Feugier P, Van Hoof A, Sebban C, Solal-Celigny P, Bouabdallah R, Ferme C, et al: Long-term results of the R-CHOP study in the treatment of elderly patients with diffuse large B-cell lymphoma: A study by the Groupe d'Etude des Lymphomes de l'Adulte. J Clin Oncol 23: 4117-4126, 2005

31. Habermann TM, Weller EA, Morrison VA, Gascoyne RD, Cassileth PA, Cohn JB, et al: Rituximab-CHOP versus CHOP alone or with maintenance rituximab in older patients with diffuse large B-cell lymphoma. J Clin Oncol 24:3121-3127, 2006
32. Glass B, Kloess M, Reiser M, Metzner B, Truemper L, Loeffler M, et al: Dose-escalated CHOP plus etoposide followed by repetitive autologous stem cell transplantation (Mega-CHOEP) with or without rituximab for primary treatment of aggressive NHL. Blood 106:430a, 2005 (abstr)
33. Coiffier B, Lepage E, Briere J, Herbrecht R, Tilly H, Bouabdallah R, et al: CHOP chemotherapy plus rituximab compared with CHOP alone in elderly patients with diffuse large-B-cell lymphoma. N Engl J Med 346:235-242, 2002
34. Schubert J, Pfreundschuh M, Reiser M, Wenger M, Kloess M, Lengenfelder A, et al: Bi-weekly dosing preserves the efficacy of rituximab in elderly patients with poor-prognosis DLBCL: Results from the RICOVER-60 trial of the DSHNHL. J Clin Oncol 24:431s, 2006 (abstr 7536)
35. Reiser M, Wenger M, Nickenig C, Peter N, Metzner B, Pfreundschuh M: Serum levels and pharmacokinetics of rituximab in bi-weekly R-CHOP in elderly patients with DLBCL treated in the RICOVER-60 trial. J Clin Oncol 24:430s, 2006 (abstr)

Seminars in
HEMATOLOGY

Drug Resistance in Diffuse Large B-Cell Lymphoma

Wyndham H. Wilson

Despite significant advances in the treatment of diffuse large B-cell lymphoma (DLBCL), drug resistance remains a major cause of treatment failure. Early strategies to improve outcome were mostly empiric or relied on classical mechanisms of drug resistance and were largely unsuccessful. More recent approaches have been aided by an understanding of the molecular pharmacology of drug action and tumor biology. Microarray profiling in particular has provided important insights into the complex biology of DLBCL and has led to a molecular taxonomy based on cell of origin and pathways of lymphomagenesis. It is now recognized that drug resistance is a complex and dynamic process related to cell cycle and apoptotic pathways, cellular differentiation, and the microenvironment. Drugs that target potential pathways of drug resistance, such as nuclear factor κB (NFκB), cyclin-dependent kinases (CDKs), and BCL-2 have entered clinical trials. However, the complexity of drug resistance requires that future clinical trials incorporate molecular translational endpoints to help identify the biologic basis of treatment failure.
Semin Hematol 43:230-239.

Although diffuse large B-cell lymphoma (DLBCL) is highly curative, treatment failure remains a major therapeutic challenge. Historically, a variety of strategies aimed at overcoming specific drug resistance mechanisms have been attempted but with limited success.[1,2] Their rationale derived from classical concepts of drug resistance, which hypothesize that the acquisition of drug-specific mechanisms, such as overexpression of membrane pumps, increased free radical scavengers, mutation(s) of intracellular targets, and/or increased DNA repair activity, limited cytotoxic damage.[2,3] Much evidence today indicates that the important determinants of chemotherapy sensitivity reside within the apoptotic pathways. Indeed, experimental studies demonstrate apoptosis to be a common final cell death pathway for most drug classes, suggesting its modulation is important for treatment outcome.[4]

The fundamental genetic changes leading to neoplasia involve deregulation of cellular proliferation and death, events that are controlled in large measure by cell cycle checkpoints and the induction and suppression of apoptosis. Evidence also suggests that abnormalities in these pathways may determine the sensitivity of tumor cells, compared with normal cells, to the cytotoxic effects of irradiation and chemotherapy.[5] Clinical strategies that take advantage of the abnormalities that occur in the regulation of the cell cycle and apoptosis are just beginning but have an increasingly important role in the design of therapeutic approaches. However, principles of chemotherapy, including pharmacology, classical drug resistance, and tumor cell kinetics, still comprise the basis for most treatment strategies in DLBCL.

Classical Drug Resistance

Some 25 years ago, Goldie and Coldman proposed the hypothesis that emergence of drug resistance in human tumors correlates with the underlying spontaneous mutation rate of specific drug-resistance genes (Table 1).[6] By extrapolation, they predicted that the emergence of resistant cells would be further hastened by the genomic instability of tumor cells due to mutations in cell cycle regulatory genes such as the p53 tumor suppressor oncogene and by exposure to mutagens such as chemotherapy and irradiation.[7] Resistant clones would eventually predominate as a tumor proliferated and this would increase under the selective pressure of chemotherapy. This hypothesis provided a rational basis for principles already established through empiric observation such as the inverse relationship between tumor bulk and cure and the increased efficacy of combination versus single agent chemotherapy.

The Goldie-Coldman hypothesis provided a rational basis for the "new generation" regimens that began to emerge in the late 1970s. The CHOP regimen (cyclophosphamide, doxorubicin, vincristine, prednisone), the first curative treatment

Center for Cancer Treatment, National Cancer Institute, Bethesda, MD.
Address correspondence to Wyndham H. Wilson, MD, PhD, Center for Cancer Treatment, National Cancer Institute, Bldg 10, Room 4N115, 9000 Rockville Pike, Bethesda, MD 20892. E-mail: wilsonw@mail.nih.gov

 0037-1963/06/$-see front matter.
doi:10.1053/j.seminhematol.2006.07.005

Table 1 Putative "Causes" of Drug Resistance in DLBCL

Drug Resistance "Causes"	Hypothesis/ Mechanism	Detection Method	Therapeutic Strategy	Clinical Outcome
Drug-specific resistance	Goldie-Coldman hypothesis of drug resistance[6]	Target-specific (eg, mutation analysis)	Alternating non–cross-resistant chemotherapy	No difference in phase III trial of CHOP *v* ProMACE-CytoBOM[9]
Multidrug resistance[10]	Cell membrane pumps remove chemotherapy	IHC or PCR of mdr pumps	Pgp inhibitors like (dex)verapamil and quinine; continuous infusion schedules	CVAD + quinine showed no benefit.[2] EPOCH activity modestly increased by dexverapamil[1]
Pharmacokinetic drug resistance	Hryniuk hypothesis of dose-intensity[56]	Dose-intensity calculation	Dose increase and/or dose-dense therapy	Variable benefit of high dose CT and SCT.[17,18] No difference in phase III trial of CHOP and dose dense weekly MACOP-B[9]
	Pharmacodynamic *normalized* PK	PK and biomarker	Dose-adjusted chemotherapy based on neutrophil nadir	DA-EPOCH with variable PK. No association between dose rate and outcome[19]
Tumor proliferation (Ki-67/MIB-I)[24]	Kinetic treatment failures	IHC	Continuous infusion chemotherapy. Dose density	Variable association with outcome[19,24]
NFκB activation and anti-apoptotic pathways	Associated with ABC subtype of DLBCL.[23] ↑ anti-apoptotic proteins (eg, bcl-2)	Microarray; IHC for post-germinal center DLBCL	↓ NFκB by rituximab[44]	Rituximab overcomes bcl-2 and non–GCB-associated resistance[39,40]
			↑ IκB by proteasome inhibition[45]	Bortezomib alone and with chemotherapy not effective in DLBCL[46]
p53 mutation[7,28]	Apoptosis inhibition[7]	Mutation analysis and IHC	None	Rituximab may overcome adverse effects of p53 mutation[57]

Abbreviations: DLBCL, diffuse large B-cell lymphoma; IHC, immunohistochemistry; SCT, stem cell transplant; PK, pharmacokinetics; CT, chemotherapy; PCR, polymerase chain reaction; NFκB, nuclear factor κB; ABC, activated B-cell DLBCL.

for aggressive lymphomas, provided solid evidence for the increased efficacy of combination chemotherapy in aggressive lymphomas. In an effort to improve outcome by overcoming the emergence of drug-resistant cells, new agents were added to later generation regimens, such as m-BACOD (methotrexate, bleomycin, doxorubicin, cyclophosphamide, vincristine, and dexamethasone), and alternated "non–cross-resistant agents, such as in the ProMACE (prednisone, doxorubicin, cyclophosphamide, and etoposide) and CytaBOM (cytarabine, bleomycin, vincristine, and methotrexate) regimens (Table 1).[8] While single-institution studies suggested these regimens were more effective than CHOP, a phase III randomized comparison with CHOP showed no difference in outcome.[9]

Simultaneous resistance to multiple classes of anticancer drugs, known as pleiotropic drug resistance, was another important concept that explained the failure of combination chemotherapy. A major mechanism of pleiotropic drug resistance, associated with resistance to "natural product" based drug classes such as anthracyclines, epipodophyllotoxins, and vinca alkaloids, results from the increased expression of the multidrug resistance gene (*mdr-1*) (Tables 1 and 2).[10] The product of this gene, the P-glycoprotein (Pgp), functions as a membrane efflux pump that decreases intracellular drug levels and confers drug resistance. Increased mdr-1 RNA and Pgp have been found in both untreated and treated lymphomas, suggesting that multidrug resistance plays a role in the development of clinical drug resistance in these tumors.[1,10] Furthermore, the availability of competitive inhibitors, such as verapamil, quinidine, and cyclosporine, led to clinical trials aimed at reversing drug resistance in lymphomas.[1,2] In one trial, 107 patients with relapsed or refractory non-Hodgkin's lymphoma received infusional EPOCH (etoposide, prednisone, vincristine, cyclophosphamide, and doxorubicin) followed by the addition of dex-verapamil, a competitive inhibitor of Pgp, in patients with persistent disease.[1] Of 41 patients treated, 12% each achieved objective and minor responses. Serial analysis of *mdr-1* expression by quantitative polymerase chain reaction (PCR) in 17 patients showed a significant increase, suggesting either induction or

Table 2 Resistance Mechanisms of Major Antineoplastic Agents for DLBCL

Drug Class	Common Agents	Limiting Toxicity*	Resistance Mechanisms
Tubulin binding agents	Vincristine	Neuropathy	Transport (mdr-1) and tubulin mutants
	Vinblastine	Mucositis	
Topoisomerase II inhibitors	Doxorubicin	Cardiomyopathy	Transport (mdr-1) and topo II target modulation
	Etoposide	Mucositis	
Alkylating agents	Cyclophosphamide	Pulmonary	Metabolic detoxification and DNA repair
	Ifosfamide	Nephrotoxicity	
Antimetabolites	Methotrexate	Stomatitis	Polyglutamation; transport and DHFR
	Cytarabine	Neurotoxicity	Activation and transport
Miscellaneous agents	Bleomycin	Pulmonary	Metabolism repair
	Cisplatin	Renal	Transport; detoxification and DNA repair
	Carboplatin		

Abbreviations: mdr, multidrug resistance-1; topo II, topoisomerase II; DHFR, dihydrofolate reductase.
*Nonhematologic toxicity.

selection of *mdr-1* in tumor cells. The Southwest Oncology Group also addressed the role of Pgp resistance in two phase II studies of infusional CVAD (cyclophosphamide, vincristine, doxorubicin, and dexamethasone) alone or with verapamil and quinine (VQ) in untreated aggressive lymphomas.[2] Among 162 assessable patients in the two studies, there was no difference in overall or failure-free survival and the outcomes were similar to historical patients treated with CHOP. While these studies certainly did not support Pgp as a major cause of drug resistance in lymphoma, they could not rule out inadequate Pgp inhibition. However, it is worth noting that infusional chemotherapy schedules may overcome Pgp resistance.[11]

Pharmacokinetics and Drug Resistance

While the dose (concentration)-response relationship is a cornerstone of therapeutics, the complexity of drug action and pharmacokinetics confounds its clinical application. Cell cycle dependent targets like topoisomerase II and p53 may have variable impact depending on drug schedules (Tables 1 and 2). Mechanisms of drug action may also be affected by schedule as observed with doxorubicin where it shifts from free radical formation and alkylation toward topoisomerase II as drug concentrations shift from bolus to continuous infusion schedules.[12] Drugs also have threshold concentrations and this is particularly important for infusion schedules where steady-state concentrations are low.[13] Of course, any practical application of these concepts must also address interpatient drug clearance, which can exceed 10-fold.[14] Such concepts would predict that fixed dose rate/m^2 regimens like R-CHOP will have a lower curative potential in patients with rapid drug clearance and intermediately sensitive tumors.

Dose intensity (DI), defined as the dose per unit time, is generally considered the solution to the dose-response relationship (Table 1). The clinical relevance of DI has been suggested by retrospective studies such as an analysis of 115 untreated diffuse large cell lymphomas where the most important predictor of survival was the relative (R)DI of doxorubicin.[15] However, prospective randomized trials comparing regimens that differ in DI have yielded variable conclusions.[16-18] It is possible that many of these studies failed to show benefit of DI because higher doses only benefit a subset of patients, while unnecessarily increasing toxicity in others, and because DI does not accurately capture dose rate or exposure, which are the relevant indices. It is also important to recall that DI does not distinguish dose rate and dose density, each with a different theoretical benefit. Dose rate is not equivalent to drug exposure because of variable pharmacokinetics, and dose density is more likely to address tumor kinetics. And of course, DI does not capture drug schedule, which is important for some agents.

While the simplicity of DI is appealing, it would be better replaced with measures and strategies that more directly address drug pharmacokinetics and schedule. These principals have been applied in the EPOCH regimen where a dose-adjustment (DA) strategy was employed to "normalize" interpatient drug exposure.[1,19] As an alternative to pharmacokinetic-based dosing, a pharmacodynamic-based approach was adopted whereby dosing is based on the neutrophil nadir. Pharmacodynamic dosing has the advantage that it is practical, and reflects plasma pharmacokinetics and intracellular drug action, which are influenced by genetic polymorphisms. Importantly, a pharmacokinetic analysis showed an inverse correlation between the neutrophil nadir and etoposide and doxorubicin plasma concentrations, providing validation for this pharmacodynamic strategy (unpublished observations, June 2006, W.H. Wilson).[19,20] The study also showed an inverse correlation between patient age and the delivered dose rate and drug clearance, suggesting that younger patients require higher dose rates to achieve equivalent plasma concentrations compared to older patients. Adequate plasma concentrations are particularly important for infusional regimens where the steady-state concentration may fall below the effective threshold concentration in rapid metabolizers.[13] This would be less important with bolus regimens like CHOP where peak concentrations are achieved. Clinically, pharmacodynamic dosing also permits increased DI without excessive toxicity.[19]

Tumor Cell Kinetics

The role of tumor cell kinetics was raised some 30 years ago by Skipper et al who observed that the fraction of cells undergoing DNA replication, termed the "growth fraction," greatly influenced drug sensitivity; a finding that likely reflects the greater sensitivity during S phase to many drug classes.[21] Although a high growth fraction would predict greater drug sensitivity, it could also lead to greater tumor proliferation between cycles. Depending on the relative impact of these two effects, cure could increase due to higher fractional cell kill or decrease if tumor proliferation between cycles lead to a "kinetic" failure. Burkitt lymphoma, where all cells are in cycle, exemplifies these concepts; CHOP has a high failure rate, whereas dose-intense and dose-dense regimens are highly curative.[22]

In aggressive lymphomas, high tumor proliferation determined by Ki-67 or MIB-1 immunohistochemistry has been shown to be an adverse prognostic finding with CHOP chemotherapy, suggesting "kinetic" failure is a problem (Table 1).[23,24] One strategy to overcome "kinetic" failure is to increase dose density through frequent chemotherapy administration. This concept was first addressed by MACOP-B (methotrexate, doxorubicin, cyclophosphamide, vincristine, prednisone, and bleomycin), which was administered weekly for 12 weeks. When compared to CHOP in a randomized study, however, MACOP-B had a similar outcome.[9] More recently, the German High Grade Lymphoma Study Group readdressed this concept in a randomized study of 2-weekly versus 3-weekly CHOP with and without etoposide. In this study of 831 patients older than 60 years with aggressive lymphomas, dose-dense every-14-day CHOP (CHOP-14) was significantly better than every-21-day CHOP (CHOP-21) with overall survival rates of 53.3% and 40.6%, respectively ($P < .001$).[25] When tested in younger patients, dose density was not superior, a finding that lacks an obvious biologic explanation.[26]

An alternative strategy to dose density is to increase the fractional cell kill or efficacy of chemotherapy, thereby reducing the number of tumor cells which can survive and proliferate between cycles. Longer drug exposure may take advantage of the increased sensitivity of cycling cells, and in vitro studies have shown that prolonged low concentration exposure to vincristine and doxorubicin, compared with brief higher-concentration exposure, can increase cytotoxicity by up to 1 log.[11] This approach was incorporated into DA-EPOCH, whereby doxorubicin, vincristine, and etoposide are continuously infused over 96 hours. Interestingly, when DA-EPOCH was tested in untreated DLBCL, high tumor proliferation was associated with a somewhat better outcome.[19] When DA-EPOCH with rituximab was tested in 83 untreated DLBCL patients, it produced both a progression-free survival and overall survival of 82% at 32 months, and a Cancer and Leukemia Group B study in 71 DLBCL patients showed progression-free and overall survivals of 83% and 90%, respectively, at 20 months, suggesting potential improvement over R-CHOP.[19,27]

Cell Cycle Regulation and Apoptosis

Studies now suggest that the clinically important mechanisms of drug resistance in DLBCL are due to alterations in cell cycle and apoptosis pathways. Mutation of the *p53* tumor-suppressor gene, a transcription factor involved in cell cycle arrest and apoptosis, has been associated with treatment failure and poor survival in DLBCL (Table 1).[28,29] P53 controls the cellular responses to DNA damage by arresting cells in G1 of the cell cycle so that repair of DNA damage may occur before the cell proceeds through DNA synthesis and mitosis; if essential repairs are not possible, *p53* may trigger apoptosis.[7] The hypermutable state that may result from inhibition of normal *p53* theoretically could promote the rapid emergence of resistant clones. The importance of *p53* in the development of the malignant phenotype is suggested by the presence of *p53* mutations in most types of cancers, including up to a quarter of DLBCLs.[28]

Increased expression of cyclin D2 and D3 proteins, which regulate the G_1- to S-phase transition, also have been associated with inferior outcome of DLBCL in recent studies.[30,31] On the other hand, the loss of cell cycle–regulatory proteins, p16 (INK4: inhibitor of CDK4) and p14, which inhibit cell cycle progression, are similarly associated with an inferior outcome.[32] Overall, these studies suggest that loss of cell cycle control is associated with a poor outcome in DLBCL and are consistent with studies that show a correlation between high-cycling tumor cells as measured by Ki-67 or microarray and poor outcome.[23,24] Several novel drugs that target the cell cycle and growth pathways are currently under development but have yet to show significant activity in DLBCL. These include inhibitors of cyclin-dependent kinases (CDKs), such as flavopiridol, and the mammalian target of rapamycin (MTOR), such as CCI-779 (Table 3 and Fig 1).[33,34]

Apoptosis is a final common pathway through which many if not most chemotherapy drugs exert their therapeutic effects in DLBCL, thereby providing a biologic explanation for drug cross-resistance. Two main pathways for apoptosis, termed the intrinsic and extrinsic pathways have been identified (Fig 1). The intrinsic pathway is activated by endogenous molecules and is dependent on mitochondrial release of cytochrome c into the cytosol, which in turn activates terminal caspases and cellular death, and is triggered in response to cellular stress. The extrinsic pathway is activated by signals from death receptors such as FAS, which activates caspases and leads to apoptosis. The process of apoptosis can be triggered by multiple events, including cytotoxic cellular stress, loss of essential growth factors, negative regulators such as tumor necrosis factor and transforming growth factor-β, and the loss or induction of specific genes such as *c-myc* and *p53* (Fig 1).[35] As such, drug resistance is a dynamic process that is influenced by multiple cellular pathways, cell cycle state, and the microenvironment.

Multiple genes and proteins regulate the apoptotic response to cellular stress and have been associated with drug

Table 3 Drugs With Novel Mechanisms of Action

Agent	Potential Mechanisms of Action
Flavopiridol	Inhibits cyclin D1, CDK 1, 2, 4; cell cycle arrest in G_1 or G_2 phase of cell cycle; induces apoptosis by caspase 3 activation; ↓ BCL-2 and Mcl-1
CCI-779	mTOR inhibitor
ABT-737	Small molecule inhibitor of BCL-2 and BCL-X_L
Genasense	Reduces BCL-2 and its inhibition on apoptosis
Bortezomib (PS-341)	Inhibits degradation of cell cycle proteins such as cyclin A, B, D, E, and cyclin-dependent kinase inhibitors (CDKI); inhibits NFκB activation
Geldanamycin	HSP 90 inhibitor

Abbreviations: mTOR, mammalian target of rapamycin; HSP 90, heat shock protein 90.

resistance. The anti-apoptotic protein BCL-2 is frequently overexpressed in DLBCL due to a variety of mechanisms, including the t(14;18) translocation, and amplification or nuclear factor κB (NFκB) activation.[23] The apoptosis-repressor activity of BCL-2 affects drug sensitivity, and in vitro, cells with increased levels of BCL-2 are resistant to radiation- and chemotherapy-induced apoptosis.[36] Studies have examined the influence of BCL-2 expression and translocation on clinical outcome in DLBCL. Interestingly, BCL-2 overexpression but not translocation correlates with inferior outcome, suggesting that BCL-2 itself is not a primary cause of drug resistance but a biomarker for other mechanism(s).[23,37] Indeed, agents that putatively targeted BCL-2, such as genasense, and not other anti-apoptotic proteins such as BCL-XL, may not be effective (Fig 1). On the other hand, inhibitors of multiple anti-apoptotic proteins, such as the small molecule inhibitor of BCL-2 and BCL-XL, ABT-737, may be more active and are now entering clinical trial (Table 3).[38]

An important possibility is that BCL-2 is a biomarker for constitutive activation of NFκB, which can increase the ex-

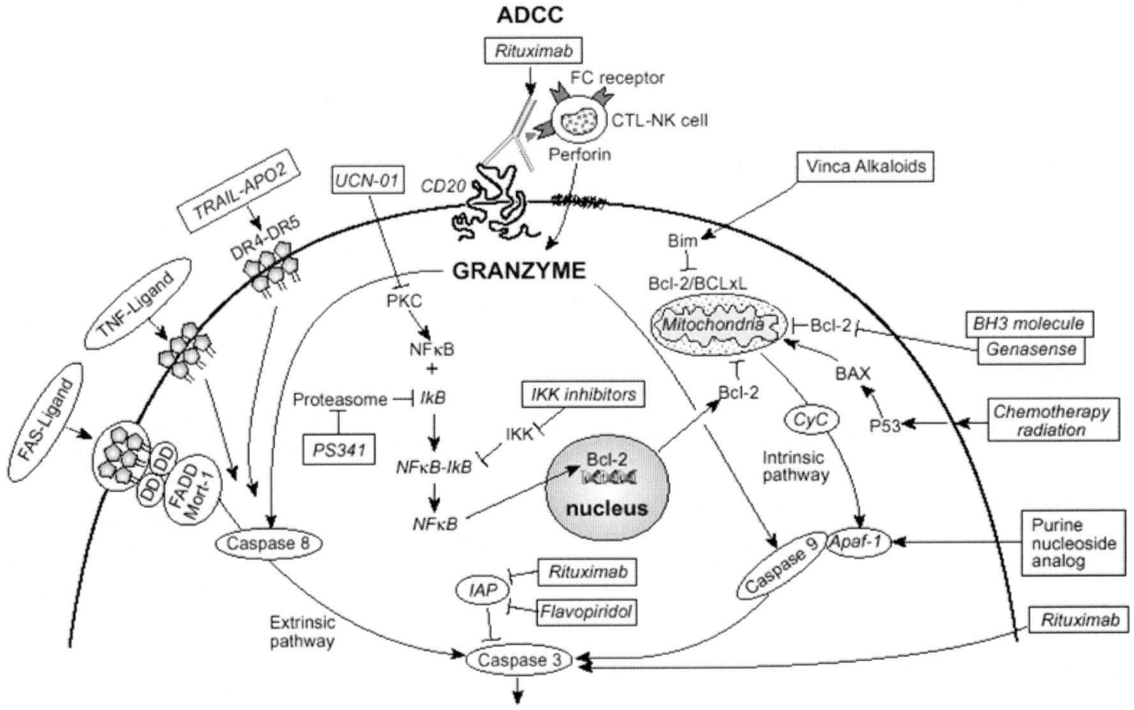

Figure 1 Pathways of apoptosis and novel drug targets (shown in boxes) are shown. The extrinsic and intrinsic apoptosis pathways lead to the activation of effector cysteine proteases (caspases), ultimately leading to apoptosis. The threshold for apoptosis in the intrinsic pathway involves the relative ratios of anti- and pro-apoptotic proteins, including BCL-2, BCL-xL, and BAX. The extrinsic pathway involves the tumor necrosis factor (TNF) family of receptors. Nuclear factor κB (NFκB) is a transcription factor, which activates both pro- and anti-apoptotic genes in response to cellular stress, and is activated by the IκB kinase (IκK). Drugs with putative novel targets include 7-hydroxystaurosporine (UCN-01), a protein kinase inhibitor; flavopiridol, an inhibitor of cyclin D1 and IAP (inhibitor of apoptosis); PS-341 (bortezomib), a proteasome and NFκB inhibitor; and genasense, a BCL-2 inhibitor. Also depicted is the antigen-dependent cellular cytotoxicity (ADCC) pathway for rituximab. Arrows (↓) represent positive regulation and bars (⊥) represent negative regulation.

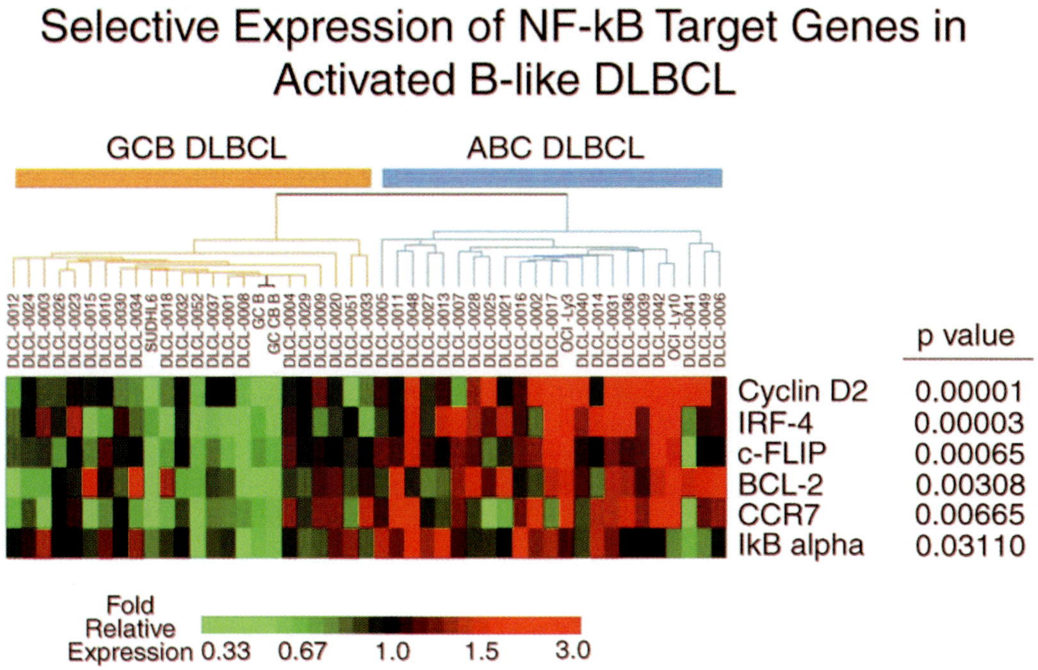

Figure 2 NFκB target genes by c-DNA analysis in germinal center B-like and activate B-like large B-cell lymphomas. Maximum red and green indicate expression threefold above and below baseline, respectively. This array shows a significant ($P_2 = .003$) association between increased BCL-2 expression and the activated B-like genotype, and suggests that BCL-2 protein expression may identify tumors with the activated-B cell genotype. Also shown is increased cyclin D2, which has been associated with a poor prognosis, possibly due to its association with the ABC subtype of DLBCL.[30]

pression of multiple anti-apoptotic proteins, including BCL-2 (Table 1). It is notable that t(14;18)-associated BCL-2 overexpression is found in the germinal center B-cell (GCB) subtype of DLBCL, which has a favorable prognosis, and NFκB-associated BCL-2 overexpression is found in the activated B-cell (ABC) subtype of DLBCL, which has a poor prognosis (Fig 2).[19,23]

Several studies suggest that the adverse prognostic effects of BCL-2 overexpression may be overcome by rituximab.[39,40] The salutary effect of rituximab on BCL-2-associated treatment failure was initially reported in a small study of DA-EPOCH with and without rituximab.[40] A larger study of 292 patients from the pivotal randomized CHOP versus R-CHOP study in elderly patients detected BCL-2 overexpression by immunohistochemistry in 66% of patients and correlated expression with outcome.[39] At a median follow-up of 2 years, R-CHOP was associated with a significantly better overall survival than CHOP in BCL-2–positive patients (67% *v* 48%, respectively, $P = .004$) but not in BCL-2–negative patients. If BCL-2 overexpression is a biomarker for NFκB-positive DLBCL, rituximab should overcome the adverse prognosis associated with the ABC DLBCL subtype where NFκB is expressed. This idea was examined in patients from the US intergroup randomized study of CHOP versus R-CHOP. Using BCL-6 as a marker of GCB DLBCL, the investigators showed that R-CHOP compared to CHOP significantly improved the 2-year failure-free and overall survival (79% *v* 17%, respectively, $P = .0003$) of patients with BCL-6–negative tumors.[41] Perhaps most revealing from this study was the lack of benefit of rituximab in patients with BCL-6–positive tumors, which comprised up to 80% of all cases. When the effects of maintenance rituximab were removed, the 2-year failure-free survival rates for CHOP and R-CHOP were 54% and 58%, respectively, indicating the need for additional therapeutic strategies.

Other clinical studies also suggest that rituximab may benefit NFκB-expressing DLBCL. In a preliminary report, investigators showed that rituximab significantly improves the outcome of primary mediastinal large B-cell lymphomas, which overexpress NFκB.[42,43] In vitro studies also suggest that rituximab can inhibit the NFκB pathway in lymphoma B-cell lines and sensitize them to chemotherapy-induced apoptosis.[44] In one study, rituximab decreased IκB kinase (IκK) activity and phosphorylation of IκB, resulting in reduced NFκB activity (Fig 1). Inhibition of NFκB was associated with downregulation of the Bcl-XL anti-apoptotic protein and chemotherapy sensitization.

Alternative approaches to inhibiting NFκB activity may be important such as blockade of proteasome degradation of IκB, an NFκB inhibitor (Table 3 and Fig 1). In vitro, the proteasome inhibitor bortezomib (PS-341) was shown to be cytotoxic against ABC but not GCB cell lines, suggesting it would be a successful therapeutic agent.[45] However, when tested as a single agent and in combination with DA-EPOCH in relapsed DLBCL, bortezomib did not show significant clinical activity.[46] Drugs that inhibit the IκB kinase (Iκk) are under development and offer a targeted approach to NFκB, while drugs like 7-hydroxystaurosporine (UCN-01) may offer a less targeted approach (Fig 1).[47] Heat shock protein 90 (HSP 90), a molecular chaperone responsible for proper protein folding of client proteins that regulate the cell cycle and apoptosis, is a potential target that leads to NF*κ*B inhibition and cellular dysregulation. Inhibitors of HSP 90 belonging to the geldanamycin drug class are in early clinical development.[48]

Microarray

While mechanisms of lymphomagenesis have important implications for drug resistance, current pathologic classification systems were not designed to take these pathways into account. As a result, treatment strategies have primarily depended on clinical features such as the International Prognostic Index (IPI), which is a surrogate measure.[49] However, large-scale genomic profiling has the potential to classify DLBCLs by molecular subtype and to relate them to treatment outcome.

The initial studies in DLBCL were performed using the specialized lymphochip microarray. Genes associated with cellular proliferation showed a clear distinction, with DLBCL generally showing higher expression than other lymphoma subtypes.[50] The proliferation signature genes were a diverse group and included cell-cycle control and checkpoint genes, and DNA synthesis and replication genes.[19,24] Another prominent feature of DLBCL was the presence of genes that defined a "lymph node" signature, a group including genes associated with infiltrating monocytes and macrophages (CD14, CD105, CSF-1 receptor), genes involved in extracellular matrix remodeling, and T cells. Genes that distinguished germinal center B cells from other stages of B cell differentiation were also differentially expressed in the DLBCL cases.[50] These data suggested that DLBCL can be subdivided into cases derived from a germinal center B-cell (GCB) and an activated post-germinal center B-cell (ABC) DLBCL. Genes associated with GCB DLBCL included known markers of germinal center differentiation such as CD10 and the *BCL-6* gene.[51] In contrast, most genes that defined ABC DLBCL were not expressed by normal germinal center B cells, but instead were induced during in vitro activation of peripheral B cells such as cyclin D2 and CD44. The ABC DLBCL signature also included the *IRF4* (*MUM1*) gene that is transiently induced during normal lymphocyte activation and is necessary for antigen receptor–driven B-cell proliferation.[52] A noteworthy feature of ABC DLBCL was the expression of two anti-apoptotic genes. These included *FLIP* (FLICE-like inhibitory protein), a dominant-negative mimic of caspase 8 that can block Fas-mediated apoptosis, and *BCL-2*, which is induced over 30-fold during peripheral B-cell activation (Fig 2).[23,50] Indeed, most ABC DLBCLs had more than fourfold higher *BCL-2* expression than GCB DLBCLs.[19] Furthermore, two recurrent oncogenic events, the t(14;18) translocation involving the *BCL-2* gene and amplification of c-rel, were ex-

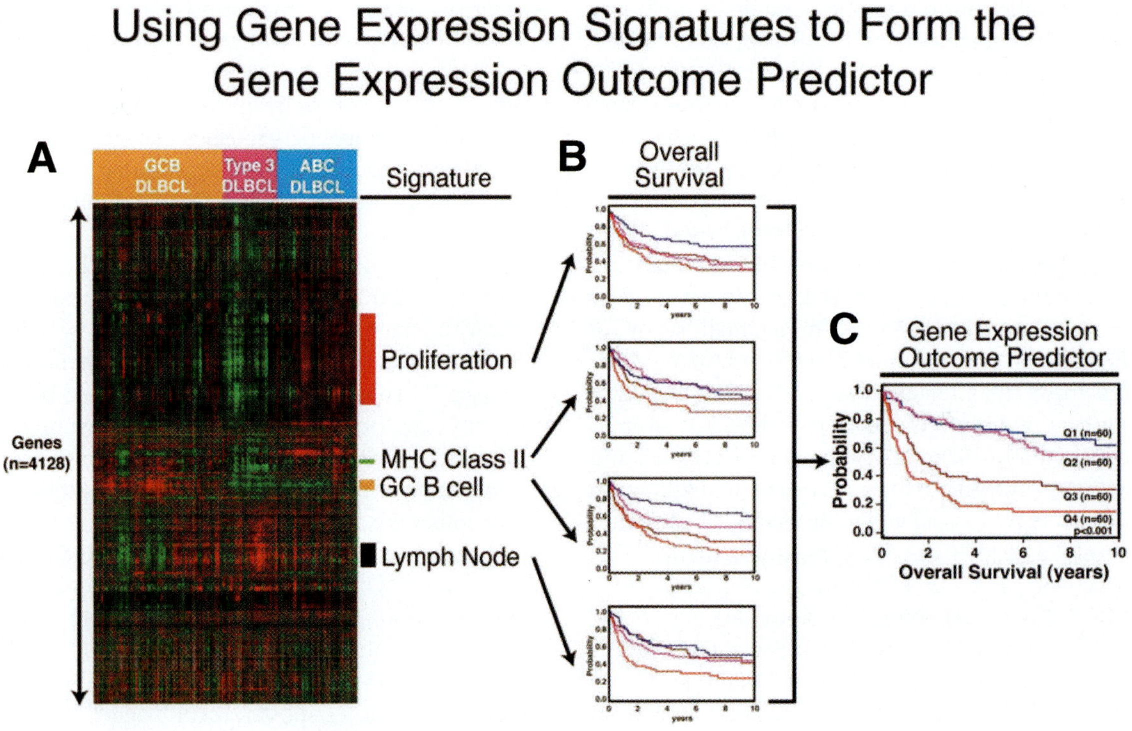

Figure 3 Diagnosis of DLBCL subtypes by gene expression and development of a molecular outcome predictor in previously untreated patients with DLBCL following chemotherapy. (A) The expression levels of 27 genes from the subgroup predictor in 274 DLBCL samples are shown according to the color scale at the left. Six named genes that showed increased expression in either the ABC or GCB subgroups are shown at the right. The likelihood that a DLBCL sample belongs to the ABC or GCB subgroup is shown on top and arranged by probability. (B) Kaplan-Meier estimates of overall survival are shown according to GCB or ABC DLBCL subtype. (C) Kaplan-Meier estimates of overall survival according to the molecular outcome predictor are shown for each quartile.

clusively found in the GCB subgroup, providing further evidence that the GCB and ABC subtypes have distinct mechanisms of lymphomagenesis.

If this new taxonomy defines true DLBCL subtypes, one might predict they would have different clinical outcomes. Because all of the biopsy specimens analyzed in this study were de novo DLBCL and came from untreated patients receiving doxorubicin-based chemotherapy, it was possible to correlate survival and the DLBCL subtype. This analysis revealed a statistically significant difference in overall survival at 5 years of 59% in GCB and 31% in ABC subtypes of DLBCL.[50] Furthermore, these subgroups were also statistically significant within each of the prognostic subgroups identified by the IPI, indicating that molecular profiling identifies different features that influence survival. These results led to a larger study by Rosenwald et al in which samples from 240 patients with DLBCL were analyzed by molecular profiling and for the presence of genomic abnormalities (Fig 3).[23] Using a supervised approach of the gene expression profiles from these cases, a molecular prognostic predictor was developed for DLBCL. The final model combined four expression signatures that were defined by the GCB signature (favorable), major histocompatibility complex (MHC) class II signature (favorable), lymph node signature (favorable) and proliferation signature (unfavorable), and expression of the bone morphogenetic protein 6 (*BMP6*) gene (unfavorable). To estimate survival outcome, each DLBCL case is assigned a score calculated from the weighted sum of these components and ranked in quartiles according to their scores.

This molecular prognostic model provides insight into the complexity of treatment failure and the interplay of multiple biologic factors. The role of lymphomagenesis is illustrated by the ABC subtype whose poor outcome may be related to constitutive expression of NFκB and increased anti-apoptotic proteins (Fig 2). Cell cycle dysregulation, indicated by the tumor proliferation signature, independently influences treatment outcome, as does the microenvironment, which is indicated by the lymph node signature. The biologic role of the MHC class II signature in treatment outcome is uncertain but could be associated with immune surveillance.

Another study by Shipp et al undertook a similar goal to develop an outcome predictor using a different array chip that contained 6,817 genes.[53] Among 58 patients, E2F and vascular endothelial growth factor (VEGF) were highly correlated with cured versus fatal/refractory disease, respectively; findings that are consistent with a previously known association with DLBCL outcome. Using a supervised approach, a highly accurate predictor containing 13 genes was able to discern patients likely to be cured from those who had fatal/refractory disease with a 5-year overall survival of 70% versus 12%, respectively. This predictor, like the one described above, was independent of the IPI. Notably, three of the outcome predictor genes in this model, *NOR1*, *PDE4B* and *PKC-β*, appear to play a role in chemotherapy response and cellular proliferation. The mitogen-inducible nuclear orphan receptor (NOR1) was overexpressed in cured patients, compared to fatal/refractory patients, and may increase the apoptotic response to chemotherapy. In contrast, PDE4B, a cyclic adenosine monophosphate (cAMP)-specific phosphodiesterase, was increased in fatal/refractory patients. The *PDE4B* gene encodes for a protein that limits the inhibitory effects of cAMP protein kinase A (PKA) on cellular proliferation and cytokine release, and may be a useful therapeutic target. *PKC-β* was also overexpressed in fatal/refractory patients and plays a central role in B-cell signaling and survival.[54]

Molecular profiling has also been applied to primary mediastinal B cell lymphoma (PMBL), an important subtype of DLBCL that mostly occurs in young patients. This subtype is defined by a combination of clinical and pathologic features and some cases may have pathologic features reminiscent of Hodgkin's lymphoma, all of which can confound an accurate diagnosis. Two recent studies using molecular profiling have confirmed the unique biological identify of PMBL and have shown a strong relationship between PMBL and Hodgkin's lymphoma.[43,55] Clinically, cases identified as PMBL by gene expression appeared to have a relatively favorable 5-year survival of 64% compared to 59% and 30%, respectively, for the GCB and ABC DLBCL subtypes. These studies, however, have not identified signature associated with an adverse outcome, which may be related to the limited sample size and to the efficacy of involved field radiation.

Conclusions

Understanding the biologic basis of drug resistance is essential for rational treatment design. Molecular techniques like microarray profiling are essential to define the new taxonomy of DLBCL and should be incorporated into future trials to help identify causes of treatment resistance and potential targets. Multiple novel agents are soon to enter or are in clinical development and target important pathways involved in regulation of cell cycle, survival, and death.

References

1. Wilson WH, Bates SE, Fojo A, Bryant G, Zhan Z, Regis J, et al: Controlled trial of dexverapamil, a modulator of multidrug resistance, in lymphomas refractory to EPOCH chemotherapy. J Clin Oncol 13: 1995-2004, 1995
2. Gaynor ER, Unger JM, Miller TP, Grogan TM, White LA Jr, Mills GM, et al: Infusional CHOP chemotherapy (CVAD) with or without chemosensitizers offers no advantage over standard CHOP therapy in the treatment of lymphoma: A Southwest Oncology Group study. J Clin Oncol 19:750-755, 2001
3. Lee WP, Lee CL, Lin HC: Glutathione S-transferase and glutathione peroxidase are essential in the early stage of Adriamycin resistance before P-glycoprotein overexpression in HOB1 lymphoma cells. Cancer Chemother Pharmacol 38:45-51, 1996
4. Alenzi FQ, Wyse RK, Altamimi WG: Apoptosis as a tool for therapeutic agents in haematological diseases. Expert Opin Biol Ther 4:407-420, 2004
5. Lowe SW, Schmitt EM, Smith SW, Osborne BA, Jacks T: p53 is required for radiation-induced apoptosis in mouse thymocytes. Nature 362:847-849, 1993
6. Goldie JH, Coldman AJ: A mathematic model for relating the drug sensitivity of tumors to their spontaneous mutation rate. Cancer Treat Rep 63:1727-1733, 1979
7. Harris CC, Hollstein M: Clinical implications of the p53 tumor-suppressor gene. N Engl J Med 329:1318-1327, 1993
8. Longo DL, DeVita VT Jr, Duffey PL, Wesley MN, Ihde DC, Hubbard S,

et al: Superiority of ProMACE-CytaBOM over ProMACE-MOPP in the treatment of advanced diffuse aggressive lymphoma: Results of a prospective randomized trial. J Clin Oncol 9:25-38, 1991
9. Fisher RI, Gaynor ER, Dahlberg S, Oken MM, Grogan TM, Mize EM, et al: Comparison of a standard regimen (CHOP) with three intensive chemotherapy regimens for advanced non-Hodgkin's lymphoma. N Engl J Med 328:1002-1006, 1993
10. Fojo AT, Ueda K, Slamon DJ, Poplack DG, Gottesman MM, Pastan I: Expression of a multidrug-resistance gene in human tumors and tissues. Proc Natl Acad Sci U S A 84:265-269, 1987
11. Lai GM, Chen YN, Mickley LA, Fojo AT, Bates SE: P-glycoprotein expression and schedule dependence of Adriamycin cytotoxicity in human colon carcinoma cell lines. Int J Cancer 49:696-703, 1991
12. Gewirtz DA: A critical evaluation of the mechanisms of action proposed for the antitumor effects of the anthracycline antibiotics Adriamycin and daunorubicin. Biochem Pharmacol 57:727-741, 1999
13. Lynch A, Harvey J, Aylott M, Nicholas E, Burman M, Siddiqui A, et al: Investigations into the concept of a threshold for topoisomerase inhibitor-induced clastogenicity. Mutagenesis 18:345-353, 2003
14. Cole DE, Balis FM, Lowe ES, et al: Pharmacokinetics (pk) and tolerance of doxorubicin (dox) and etoposide (etop) during treatment of aggressive B-cell lymphomas indicate doses need not be routinely reduced for hepatic dysfunction. Proc Am Soc Clin Oncol 24, 2005 (abstr)
15. Kwak LW, Halpern J, Olshen RA, Horning SJ: Prognostic significance of actual dose intensity in diffuse large-cell lymphoma: Results of a tree-structured survival analysis. J Clin Oncol 8:963-977, 1990
16. Meyer RM, Quirt IC, Skillings JR, Cripps MC, Bramwell VH, Weinerman BH, et al: Escalated as compared with standard doses of doxorubicin in BACOP therapy for patients with non-Hodgkin's lymphoma. N Engl J Med 329:1770-1776, 1993
17. Kaiser U, Uebelacker I, Abel U, Birkmen J, Trumper L, Schmalenberg H, et al: Randomized study to evaluate the use of high-dose therapy as part of primary treatment for "aggressive" lymphoma. J Clin Oncol 20:4413-4419, 2002
18. Haioun C, Lepage E, Gisselbrecht C, Salles G, Coiffier B, Brice P, et al: Survival benefit of high-dose therapy in poor-risk aggressive non-Hodgkin's lymphoma: final analysis of the prospective LNH87-2 protocol—A groupe d'Etude des lymphomes de l'Adulte study. J Clin Oncol 18:3025-3030, 2000
19. Wilson WH, Grossbard ML, Pittaluga S, Cole D, Pearson D, Drbohlav N, et al: Dose-adjusted EPOCH chemotherapy for untreated large B-cell lymphomas: A pharmacodynamic approach with high efficacy. Blood 99:2685-2693, 2002
20. Lowe E, Balis FM, Cole DE, Goodspeed W, Drbohlav N, Wilson WH: Pharmacokinetics of doxorubicin and doxorubicinol in dose-adjusted EPOCH infusional chemotherapy. Am Assoc Cancer Res 2002
21. Skipper HE, Schabel FM Jr, Wilcox WS: Experimental evaluation of potential anticancer agents. Xiii. On the criteria and kinetics associated with "curability" of experimental leukemia. Cancer Chemother Rep 35:1-111, 1964
22. Dave SS, Fu K, Wright G, Lam L, Grenier TC, Weisenberger DD, et al: Gene expression distinguishes Burkitt lymphoma from other aggressive lymphomas and identifies patients who are highly curable with intensive chemotherapeutic regimens. ASH Annual Meeting Abstracts 106: 415, 2000
23. Rosenwald A, Wright G, Chan WC, Connors JM, Campo E, Fisher RI, et al: The use of molecular profiling to predict survival after chemotherapy for diffuse large-B-cell lymphoma. N Engl J Med 346:1937-1947, 2002
24. Miller TP, Grogan TM, Dahlberg S, Spier CM, Braziel RM, Banks PM, et al: Prognostic significance of the Ki-67-associated proliferative antigen in aggressive non-Hodgkin's lymphomas: A prospective Southwest Oncology Group trial. Blood 83:1460-1466, 1994
25. Pfreundschuh M, Trümper L, Kloess M, et al: 2-weekly vs. 3-weekly CHOP with and without etoposide in for patients >60 years of age with aggressive non-Hodgkin's lymphoma (NHL): Results of the completed NHL-B-2 trial of the DSHNHL. Blood 99, 2002 (abstr 3060)
26. Pfreundschuh M, Trümper L, Schmits R, et al: 2-weekly vs. 3-weekly CHOP with and without etoposide in young patients with low-risk (low LDH) aggressive non-Hodgkin's lymphoma: Results of the completed NHL-B-1 trial of the DSHNHL. Blood 99, 2002 (abstr 340)
27. Wilson WH, Porcu P, Hurd D, et al: Phase II study of dose-adjusted EPOCH-R in untreated de novo $CD20^+$ diffuse large B-cell lymphoma (DLBCL)-CALGB 50103. Proc Am Soc Clin Oncol 24, 2005 (abstr)
28. Wilson WH, Teruya-Feldstein J, Fest T, Harris C, Steinberg SM, Jaffe ES, et al: Relationship of p53, bcl-2, and tumor proliferation to clinical drug resistance in non-Hodgkin's lymphomas. Blood 89:601-609, 1997
29. Ichikawa A, Kinoshita T, Watanabe T, Kato H, Nagai H, Tsushita K, et al: Mutations of the p53 gene as a prognostic factor in aggressive B-cell lymphoma. N Engl J Med 337:529-534, 1997
30. Hans CP, Weisenburger DD, Greiner TC, Chan WC, Aoun P, Cochran G, et al: Expression of PKC-beta or cyclin D2 predicts for inferior survival in diffuse large B-cell lymphoma. Mod Pathol 18:1377-1384, 2005
31. Filipits M, Jaeger U, Pohl G, Stranzl T, Simonitsch I, Kaider A, et al: Cyclin D3 is a predictive and prognostic factor in diffuse large B-cell lymphoma. Clin Cancer Res 8:729-733, 2002
32. Paik JH, Jeon YK, Park SS, Kim YA, Kim JE, Huh J, et al: Expression and prognostic implications of cell cycle regulatory molecules, p16, p21, p27, p14 and p53 in germinal centre and non-germinal centre B-like diffuse large B-cell lymphomas. Histopathology 47:281-291, 2005
33. Shapiro GI: Cyclin-dependent kinase pathways as targets for cancer treatment. J Clin Oncol 24:1770-1783, 2006
34. O'Connor OA: Developing new drugs for the treatment of lymphoma. Eur J Haematol 150-158, 2005 (suppl)
35. Sachs L, Lotem J: Control of programmed cell death in normal and leukemic cells: New implications for therapy. Blood 82:15-21, 1993
36. Hockenbery D, Nunez G, Milliman C, Schreiber RD, Korsmeyer SJ: Bcl-2 is an inner mitochondrial membrane protein that blocks programmed cell death. Nature 348:334-336, 1990
37. Gascoyne RD, Adomat SA, Krajewski S, Krajewska M, Horsman DE, Tolcher AW, et al: Prognostic significance of Bcl-2 protein expression and Bcl-2 gene rearrangement in diffuse aggressive non-Hodgkin's lymphoma. Blood 90:244-251, 1997
38. Oltersdorf T, Elmore SW, Shoemaker AR, Armstrong RC, Augeri DJ, Belli BA, et al: An inhibitor of Bcl-2 family proteins induces regression of solid tumours. Nature 435:677-681, 2005
39. Mounier N, Briere J, Gisselbrecht C, Emile JF, Lederlin P, Sebban C, et al: Rituximab plus CHOP (R-CHOP) overcomes bcl-2–associated resistance to chemotherapy in elderly patients with diffuse large B-cell lymphoma (DLBCL). Blood 101:4279-4284, 2003
40. Wilson W, Pittaluga S, O'Connor P, Hegde U, Drbohlav N, Janik J, et al: Rituximab may overcome BCL-2-associated chemotherapy resistance in untreated diffuse large B-cell lymphomas. Proc Am Soc Hematol 99, 2001
41. Winter JN, Weller EA, Horning SJ, Krajewska M, Variakojis D, Habermann TM, et al: Prognostic significance of Bcl-6 protein expression in DLBCL treated with CHOP or R-CHOP: A prospective correlative study. Blood 2005-2010, 2006
42. Dunleavy K, Pittaluga S, Janik J, Grant N, Steinberg S, Staudt L, et al: Primary mediastinal large B-cell lymphoma (PMBL) outcome is significantly improved by the addition of rituximab to dose adjusted (DA)-EPOCH and overcomes the need for radiation. ASH Annual Meeting Abstracts 106:623, 2005 (abstr)
43. Rosenwald A, Wright G, Leroy K, Yu X, Gaulard P, Gascoyne RD, et al: Molecular diagnosis of primary mediastinal B cell lymphoma identifies a clinically favorable subgroup of diffuse large B cell lymphoma related to Hodgkin lymphoma. J Exp Med 198:851-862, 2003
44. Jazirehi AR, Huerta-Yepez S, Cheng G, Bonavida B: Rituximab (chimeric anti-CD20 monoclonal antibody) inhibits the constitutive nuclear factor-{kappa}B signaling pathway in non-Hodgkin's lymphoma B-cell lines: Role in sensitization to chemotherapeutic drug-induced apoptosis. Cancer Res 65:264-276, 2005
45. Davis RE, Brown KD, Siebenlist U, Staudt LM: Constitutive nuclear factor kappaB activity is required for survival of activated B cell-like

diffuse large B cell lymphoma cells. J Exp Med 194:1861-1874, 2001
46. Dunleavy K, Janik J, Gea-Banacloche J, Shovlin M, White T, Goldschmidt N, et al: Phase I/II study of bortezomib alone and bortezomib with dose-adjusted EPOCH chemotherapy in relapsed or refractory aggressive B-cell lymphoma. ASH Annual Meeting Abstracts 104:1385, 2004 (abstr)
47. Wilson WH, Sorbara L, Figg WD, Mont EK, Sausville E, Warren KE, et al: Modulation of clinical drug resistance in a B cell lymphoma patient by the protein kinase inhibitor 7-hydroxystaurosporine: Presentation of a novel therapeutic paradigm. Clin Cancer Res 6:415-421, 2000
48. Georgakis GV, Younes A: Heat-shock protein 90 inhibitors in cancer therapy: 17AAG and beyond. Future Oncol 1:273-281, 2005
49. The International Non-Hodgkin's Lymphoma Prognostic Factors Project. A predictive model for aggressive non-Hodgkin's lymphoma. N Engl J Med 329:987-994, 1993
50. Alizadeh AA, Eisen MB, Davis RE, Ma C, Lossos IS, Rosenwald A, et al: Distinct types of diffuse large B-cell lymphoma identified by gene expression profiling. Nature 403:503-511, 2000
51. Dalla-Favera R, Migliazza A, Chang CC, Niu H, Pasqualucci L, Butler M, et al: Molecular pathogenesis of B cell malignancy: The role of BCL-6. Curr Top Microbiol Immunol 246:257-263, 1999
52. Mittrucker HW, Matsuyama T, Grossman A, Kundig TM, Potter J, Shahinian A, et al: Requirement for the transcription factor LSIRF/IRF4 for mature B and T lymphocyte function. Science 275:540-543, 1997
53. Shipp MA, Ross KN, Tamayo P, Weng AP, Kutok JL, Aguiar RC, et al: Diffuse large B-cell lymphoma outcome prediction by gene-expression profiling and supervised machine learning. Nat Med 8:68-74, 2002
54. Leitges M, Schmedt C, Guinamard R, Davoust J, Schaal S, Stabel S, et al: Immunodeficiency in protein kinase cbeta-deficient mice. Science 273: 788-791, 1996
55. Savage KJ, Monti S, Kutok JL, Cattoretti G, Neuberg D, de Leval L, et al: The molecular signature of mediastinal large B-cell lymphoma differs from that of other diffuse large B-cell lymphomas and shares features with classical Hodgkin's lymphoma. Blood 2003-2006, 2003
56. Hryniuk W, Bush H: The importance of dose intensity in chemotherapy of metastatic breast cancer. J Clin Oncol 2:1281-1288, 1984
57. Wilson WH, et al: Dose-adjusted EPOCH-rituximab in untreated diffuse large B-cell lymphoma: Benefit of rituximab appears restricted to tumors harboring anti-apoptotic mechanisms. ASH Annual Meeting Abstracts 103:356, 2003 (abstr)

Seminars in
HEMATOLOGY

Role of Hematopoietic Stem Cell Transplantation for Advanced-Stage Diffuse Large Cell B-Cell Lymphoma-B

Auayporn Nademanee and Stephen J. Forman

The prognosis of patients with relapsed or refractory diffuse large cell B-cell lymphoma-B (DLCL-B) is poor with conventional salvage chemotherapy; therefore, high-dose therapy (HDT) combined with autologous stem cell transplant (ASCT) has become the treatment of choice for these patients. The outcomes of transplant are better in patients with chemosensitive relapse: those with a longer duration of first remission (>12 month) and those with an age-adjusted low-risk International Prognostic Index (IPI) at relapse. Several high-dose regimens with or without total body irradiation (TBI) have been used with similar outcomes. Relapse remains the most common cause of treatment failure, and thus the use of radioimmunotherapy (RIT) in the high-dose regimens and incorporation of rituximab in the transplant setting have been explored. Several studies have shown that RIT both at conventional dose and at high dose can be given in combination with high-dose chemotherapy regimens without additional toxicity or delay in hematopoietic recovery after ASCT. Additional studies using RIT in combination with high-dose chemotherapy and ASCT are ongoing, and preliminary results suggest that these approaches may be superior to conventional high-dose regimens. Since rituximab is an effective therapy for B-cell non-Hodgkin's lymphoma and given its limited toxicity, rituximab has been incorporated into HDT and ASCT for DLCL-B as in vivo purging, as part of high-dose regimens, and as maintenance therapy to prevent relapse. Preliminary results suggested that rituximab during ASCT and as maintenance therapy post-transplant reduces the risk of relapse and improves survival; however, these results need to be confirmed in phase III randomized trials. The role of ASCT during first remission as consolidative therapy in patients with DLCL-B remains controversial and should not be performed outside of the clinical trial setting. Allogeneic stem cell transplant (allo-SCT) for patients with relapsed DLCL-B is associated with significant toxicity and should be reserved for patients who relapse after ASCT or those with persistent marrow involvement. Innovative approaches are needed for primary refractory and chemoresistant relapsed DLCL-B since these patients have very poor outcomes after ASCT.
Semin Hematol 43:240-250

Despite recent advances in treatment of non-Hodgkin's lymphoma (NHL), most patients with advanced-stage diffuse large cell B-cell lymphoma-B (DLCL-B) are not cured with conventional therapy. High-dose therapy (HDT) followed by autologous stem cell transplant (ASCT) has become the treatment of choice for patients with relapsed or refractory DLCL-B. The benefits of HDT and ASCT in relapsed aggressive lymphoma were clearly shown in the randomized Parma trial,[1] conducted in 215 patients younger than 60 years of age who were in first or second relapse. All patients received two cycles of salvage chemotherapy DHAP (dexamethasone, high-dose cytarabine, and cisplatin). The responders were randomized to receive either four more cycles of DHAP or high-dose carmustine, etoposide, cytarabine, and cyclophosphamide (BEAC) followed by ASCT. The 5-year event-free survival (EFS) was 46% for the ASCT group compared to 12% for the salvage therapy group (P = .001). Overall survival (OS) was also higher in the HDT arm (53% *v* 32%; P = .038). Therefore, two cycles of conventional

Division of Hematology and Hematopoietic Cell Transplantation, City of Hope National Medical Center, Duarte, CA.
Supported in part by United States Public Health Service Grants No. CA30206 and CA33572.
Address correspondence to Auayporn Nademanee, MD, Division of Hematology and Hematopoietic Cell Transplantation, 1500 E Duarte Rd, Duarte, CA 91010. E-mail: anademanee@coh.org

doi:10.1053/j.seminhematol.2006.07.006

salvage chemotherapy followed by HDT and ASCT is considered standard treatment for chemosensitive relapsed aggressive NHL. The value of salvage chemotherapy before transplant has also been confirmed in the LNH-93-RP study,[2] in which patients in first relapse were treated with salvage chemotherapy and randomized to HDT and ASCT on day 30 or to two additional cycles of chemotherapy followed by HDT and ASCT at approximately day 90. The OS was superior in patients receiving two additional cycles (38% *v* 21%, $P < .001$).

Several HDT protocols have been used as preparative regimens for ASCT in patients with NHL. Since NHL is radiosensitive, and based on the experience with acute leukemia, the combination of total body irradiation (TBI) and cyclophosphamide has been widely used as a preparative regimen for patients with NHL. In an attempt to reduce relapse rates, etoposide has been added to the TBI and cyclophosphamide regimen because of its known activity in lymphoma. The results of phase I and II studies of TBI 12.0 Gy, etoposide 60 mg/kg, and cyclophosphamide 100 mg/kg have demonstrated the activity of this regimen in patients with NHL.[3,4] The efficacy of this regimen was tested and confirmed in the Southwestern Oncology Group (SWOG) cooperative trial.[5]

Several high-dose combination chemotherapy regimens have also been developed for patients who were unable to receive TBI due to older age, potential toxicity, prior radiotherapy, and the limited availability of TBI. The two most commonly used regimens are BEAM (carmustine, etoposide, cytarabine, and melphalan) and CBV (cyclophosphamide, carmustine, and etoposide). Thus far, none of these regimens has emerged to be the best combination and randomized trials comparing the efficacy and toxicity between TBI-based and non–TBI-based regimens have not been reported. In a retrospective analysis from Fred Hutchinson Cancer Research Center, the efficacy and toxicity of high-dose TBI, cyclophosphamide, and etoposide was compared to a high-dose regimen of busulfan, melphalan, and thiotepa (Bu/Mel/T) in 451 NHL patients receiving ASCT.[6] No significant differences in toxicities and survival were observed between the two regimens despite the inclusion of patients who had received dose-limiting irradiation in the Bu/Mel/T regimen. Since TBI has been shown to be associated with an increased risk of second malignancies in patients with NHL undergoing ASCT in some studies,[7,8] some centers have stopped using TBI in their high-dose regimens.

Prognostic Factors

Several prognostic factors that predict for outcome of HDT and ASCT in patients with relapsed or refractory NHL have been reported. Chemosensitive disease before transplantation has been identified as the most important prognostic factor predictive of favorable outcome after ASCT. Further analysis of the Parma trial showed that the International Prognostic Index (IPI) at the time of relapse was highly correlated with OS in the conventional chemotherapy DHAP arm but not in the transplant arm.[9] In contrast, time to relapse ($<$12 months *v* $>$12 months) was found to be an independent prognostic factor for both EFS and OS regardless of the treatment arm.[10] Hamlin et al[11] evaluated the age-adjusted IPI at the initiation of second-line chemotherapy (sAAIPI) in 150 patients with DLCL-B who were treated with ICE (ifosfamide, carboplatin, and etoposide) followed by HDT and ASCT for patients with chemosensitive disease. Three risk groups with different progression-free survival (PFS) and OS were identified by sAAIPI: low risk (no factors), 70% and 74%; intermediate (one factor), 39% and 49%; and high-risk (two or three factors), 16% and 18% ($P < .001$ for both PFS and OS). Thus, this prognostic model can be used to evaluate the new treatment approaches and compare results of different regimens. In addition, it can be used to identify poor-risk patients who may benefit from novel treatment approaches designed to improve their curability.

Recently, the prognostic value of pretransplant positron emission tomography using fluorine 18-fluorodeoxyglucose (FDG-PET) in patients with aggressive NHL treated with HDT and ASCT was reported. Spaepen et al[12] retrospectively analyzed the impact of FDG-PET before HDT and ASCT in 60 patients with lymphoma (19 Hodgkin lymphoma, and 41 NHL) who had failed induction chemotherapy or had chemosensitive relapses. Thirty patients had negative FDG-PET before HDT/ASCT; 25 of these remained in remission at median follow-up of 4 years. Two patients died from treatment-related mortality but without evidence of recurrent disease. Only three patients had relapsed. Of the 30 patients with persistent positive FDG-PET, 26 relapsed at a median of 402 days and 16 died of progressive disease. Only four patients remain in remission. For the 41 NHL patients, Cox regression analysis showed a strong prognostic influence of FDG-PET before HDT/ASCT on PFS and OS ($P < .0004$ and $P < .0018$, respectively). Alousi et al[13] evaluated the predictive value of pretransplant PET/gallium in 188 patients with chemosensitive aggressive DLCL-B undergoing HDT and ASCT. Seventy-six percent were PET/gallium-negative whereas 20% were positive. They found that pretransplant PET/gallium-positive status increased the risk of progression after transplant. The PFS at 54 months was 17% for those with positive PET/gallium pretransplant and 55% for the PET/gallium-negative group. Further studies are required to confirm the predictive value of FDG-PET before HDT/ASCT. Furthermore, patients with persistent FDG-PET positivity may require further salvage chemotherapy or novel treatment to achieve a better remission/disease control before proceeding to HDT/ASCT.

High-Dose Sequential Chemotherapy and ASCT

Despite the effectiveness of HDT and ASCT, there is a high rate of relapse (34% to 53%), especially in patients with primary progressive disease. Thus, continued development and evaluation of preparative regimens that will provide a better anti-lymphoma effect is needed. One approach is to deliver sequential high-dose chemotherapy in accordance with the Norton-Simone hypothesis. Following initial cytoreduction, non–cross-resistant agents are given in high doses at short intervals with growth factors support before proceeding to HDT and ASCT. Cortelazzo et al[14] reported the use of high-dose sequential regimen in 103 patients with relapsed (n = 65) or refractory NHL (n = 38). All patients received one or two cycles of APO (doxorubicin, prednisone, and vincristine) for debulking of the disease. The high-dose sequential regimen consisted of high-dose cyclophosphamide 7 g/m^2 on day 0, followed by high-dose methotrexate 8 g/m^2, and vincristine 1.4 mg/m^2 on day +21, and high-dose etoposide 2 g/m^2 on day +28. Bone marrow and stem cells were harvested after high-dose cyclophosphamide and/or etoposide. Patients then underwent ASCT using either high-dose mitoxantrone 60 mg/m^2 in combination with high-dose melphalan 180 mg/m^2 or BEAM regimen. Treatment-related mortality was 4%. After a median follow-up of 24 months, the estimated three-year OS, EFS, and disease-free survival (DFS) were 47%, 44%, and 64%, respectively. Josting et al[15] reported their phase II results of high-dose sequential regimens consisting of two cycles of DHAP; high-dose cyclophosphamide 4 g/m^2 followed by peripheral blood stem cell collection; methotrexate 8 g/m^2 plus vincristine; etoposide 500 g/m^2; then high-dose BEAM and ASCT. The results were encouraging. The toxicity was similar to other high-dose regimens with transplant-related mortality of 1% to 4%. However, further studies are required to confirm the benefit of this approach. In addition, longer follow-up is needed to assess the risk of therapy-induced myelodysplasia/acute leukemia due to repetitive courses of high-dose chemotherapy.

Rituximab and ASCT for B-Cell NHL

Rituximab, a chimeric IgG1 monoclonal antibody that targets CD20, has revolutionized the treatment of B-cell NHL. Two randomized trials have shown that rituximab improves response rate and survival in patients with advanced-stage DLCL-B when administered in combination with standard chemotherapy. The Group d'Etude des lymphomes de l'Adulte (GELA) reported that rituximab in combination with CHOP (cyclophosphamide, doxorubicin, vincristine, and prednisone) produced a higher response rate and survival in older patients (>60 years of age) with advanced-stage DLCL-B when compared to CHOP alone.[16] The MabThera International Trial (MinT) showed that younger patients (<60 years) with DLCL-B who received rituximab in combination with CHOP-like regimen had a significantly better OS and longer time to treatment failure than those receiving chemotherapy alone.[17] The addition of rituximab to salvage chemotherapy regimen has also been shown to improve complete remission (CR) rates. Kewalramini et al[18] showed that CR rates increased from 27% to 53% with the addition of rituximab to ICE in rituximab-naive patients with relapsed or primary refractory DLCL-B. Given its efficacy, its ability to deplete B cells, and its limited toxicity, rituximab has been incorporated into HDT and ASCT for DLCL-B as in vivo purging, as part of high-dose regimen or as maintenance therapy post-transplant to prevent relapse.

Khouri et al[19] evaluated the efficacy and safety of administering high-dose rituximab in combination with high-dose BEAM and ASCT in 67 patients with recurrent aggressive B-cell NHL. Rituximab was administered during stem cell mobilization at 375 mg/m^2 at 1 day before chemotherapy and 1,000 mg/m^2 at 7 days after chemotherapy and on days 1 and 8 after transplant. The results of this treatment were retrospectively compared with a historical control group receiving the same preparative regimen without rituximab. With the median follow-up time for the study group of 20 months, the 2-year OS was 80% for the study group compared to 53% for control group (P = .002). The 2-year DFS rates were 67%, and 43%, respectively, for the study group and the control group (P = .004). The median time to neutrophil recovery of ≥500 cells/μL was 11 days in the rituximab group and 10 days for the matched control group (P = .001). However, there was no increased incidence of infection in the rituximab group. A recent report from the same investigators also showed that the addition of high-dose rituximab decreases the risk of relapse in patients with pretransplant PET/gallium positivity.[13] Even though these results are very encouraging, randomized studies are required, especially considering the cost and potential toxicity of high-dose rituximab.

Horwitz et al[20] evaluated the feasibility and toxicity of rituximab post ASCT in 35 patients with B-cell NHL (25 DLCL-B) who underwent HDT followed by a purged autologous graft. Rituximab schedule was 4 weekly infusions (375 mg/m^2) starting on day 42 and repeated for a second course at 6 months after transplant. With a median follow-up of 30 months, the 2-year EFS rate was 83% and the OS rate was 88%. For 21 patients with relapsed or refractory DLCL-B, the EFS and OS rates were 81% and 85%, respectively. Grade 3 to 4 neutropenia occurred in 54% of patients; however, the incidence of infection was not increased. Delayed B-cell recovery was observed in all patients and suppressed immunoglobulin G level and low pneumococcal titer were observed in a subset of patients. These results are promising and further studies are required to establish whether post-transplant rituximab can improve cure rates in patients with relapsed or refractory DLCL-B, particularly in light of different results from another study reported by Rapaport et al.[21] The role of post-transplant rituximab is being investigated in a US intergroup phase III randomized, controlled trial of patients with relapsed or refractory DLCL-B undergoing HDT/ASCT.

Radioimmunotherapy and ASCT for B-Cell NHL

Recently, the role of radioimmunotherapy (RIT) for the treatment of NHL has emerged. Radioisotope-labeled monoclonal antibodies provide a mechanism by which radioactivity can be directly targeted to tumor sites while sparing normal tissues. B-cell lymphomas are attractive targets for RIT because of their radiosensitivity, their well-defined surface antigens, and the availability of multiple monoclonal antibodies to those antigens. There are two US Food and Drug Administration–approved radioisotope-labeled monoclonal antibod-

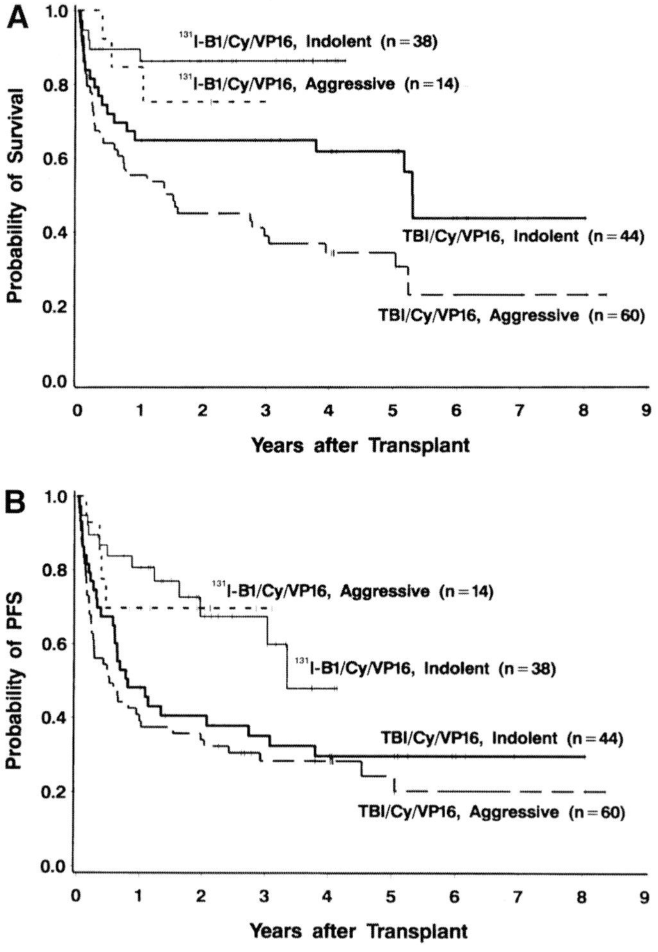

Figure 1 Survival analyses according to type of lymphoma. (A) Overall survival in 38 patients with relapsed indolent lymphomas (thin solid line) and 14 patients with relapsed aggressive lymphomas (short dashes) treated with ^{131}I-tositumomab, etoposide, cyclophosphamide, and ASCT and in 44 patients with relapsed indolent lymphomas (thick solid line) and 60 patients with relapsed aggressive lymphomas (long thick dashes) treated with external-beam TBI (1.5 Gy twice a day for 4 days), etoposide (60 mg/kg), cyclophosphamide (100 mg/kg), and ASCT. (B) Progression-free survival in 38 patients with relapsed indolent lymphomas (thin solid line) and 14 patients with relapsed aggressive lymphomas (short dashes) treated with ^{131}I-tositumomab, etoposide, cyclophosphamide, and ASCT and in 44 patients with relapsed indolent lymphomas (thick solid line) and 60 patients with relapsed aggressive lymphomas (long thick dashes) treated with external-beam TBI (1.5 Gy twice a day for 4 days), etoposide (60 mg/kg), cyclophosphamide (100 mg/kg) and ASCT.

ies for treatment of relapsed or refractory B-cell NHL: the yttrium 90–labeled ibritumomab tiuxetan (^{90}Y-Zevalin, Biogen Idec, San Diego, CA) and the iodine 131–labeled tositumomab (Bexxar, Corixa, Seattle, WA). In an attempt to deliver target radiation to tumor sites, RIT has been evaluated in myeloablative trials with and without high-dose chemotherapy. Press et al[22,23] pioneered the use of high-dose RIT in conjunction with ASCT in two different trials. The first trial used high-dose ^{131}I-tositumomab with autologous bone marrow rescue in 43 patients with B-cell lymphoma in relapse.[22] Nineteen patients received therapeutic infusions of 234 to 777 mCi of ^{131}I-labeled antibodies followed by autologous marrow infusion. Sixteen patients achieved a CR, two a partial response, and one a minor response. Nine of 16 complete responders have remained in CR for 3 to 53 months. Toxicities included myelosuppression, nausea, infection, and two episodes of cardiopulmonary toxicity. The second study was a phase I/II trial of high-dose ^{131}I-tositumomab, etoposide, and cyclophosphamide and ASCT in 52 (38 indolent; 14 aggressive) NHL patients.[23] The maximum tolerated dose of ^{131}I-tositumomab that could be safely combined with high-dose etoposide and cyclophosphamide delivered 25 Gy to critical normal organs. The regimen was well tolerated, with a 15% incidence of grades III and IV toxicity. The estimated OS and PFS at 2 years were 83% and 68%, respectively. The results compared favorably with those in a nonrandomized control group of patients who underwent ASCT using TBI, etoposide, and cyclophosphamide during the same period (53% OS and 36% PFS at 2 years; Fig 1).

Nademanee et al[24] evaluated high-dose ^{90}Y-ibritumomab tiuxetan in combination with high-dose etoposide 40 to 60 mg/kg and cyclophosphamide 100 mg/kg in 31 patients with poor-risk or relapsed B-cell NHL, including 14 patients with DLCL-B. The median number of prior chemotherapy regimens was two (range, one to six). All but two had received rituximab either alone (n = 8) or in combination with chemotherapy (n = 21). The median ^{90}Y-ibritumomab tiuxetan dose delivered was 72 mCi (range, 37 to 105) to deliver a target dose of 1,000 cGy to the highest normal organ. The treatment was well tolerated with mucositis and neutropenic fever being the most common acute toxicities. There was no delay in engraftment. All patients with active disease at transplant achieved remission, although five patients relapsed. At a median follow-up of 22 months, the 2-year estimated OS and DFS were 92%, and 78%, respectively (Fig 2) These results indicate the feasibility of delivering high-dose RIT either ^{90}Y-ibritumomab tiuxetan or ^{131}I-tositumomab in

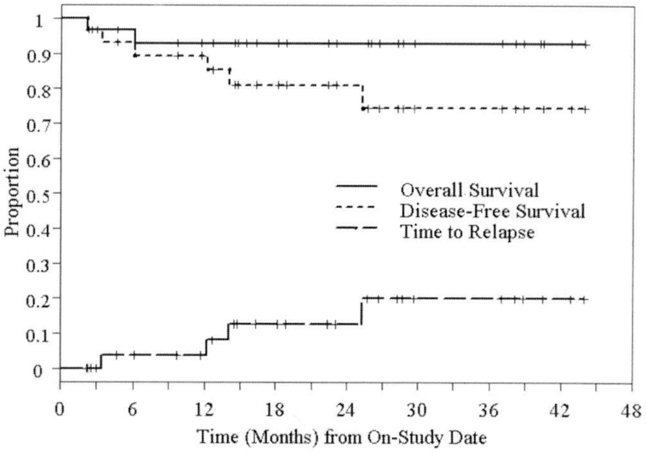

Figure 2 Kaplan-Meier estimated 2-year overall survival, Disease-free survival and relapse for 31 patients who received high-dose ^{90}Y-ibritumomab tiuxetan etoposide and cyclophosphamide plus ASCT in NHL.

combination with high-dose chemotherapy in an ASCT setting for B-cell NHL.

Given the complexity of delivering high-dose RIT, several investigators have chosen to add conventional doses or lower doses of ^{131}I-tositumomab or ^{90}Y-ibritumomab tiuxetan to high-dose BEAM regimen followed by ASCT. Vose et al[25] conducted a phase I/II study evaluating the addition of a standard outpatient dose of ^{131}I-tositumomab in four doses cohorts (30, 45, 60, and 75 cGy) to the BEAM regimen in 23 patients with chemotherapy-refractory or multiply relapsed aggressive B-cell NHL. The treatment was well tolerated without additional toxicity. The CR rate after transplantation was 57% and the overall response rate was 65%. At a median follow-up of 38 months, the 3-year EFS was 39% and OS was 55%. Winter et al[26] evaluated escalating doses of ^{90}Y-ibritumomab tiuxetan to deliver 100, 300, and up to 1,300 cGy to normal organs followed by high-dose BEAM and ASCT. Thirty-five patients with B-cell NHL were treated, including 16 with DLCL-B and seven with transformed NHL. The median number of chemotherapy regimens was three. All patients received individualized RIT doses, which ranged from 100 to 1,300 cGy. Thirteen patients received ^{90}Y-ibritumomab tiuxetan doses of 0.5 mCi/kg or higher. There was no delay in hematopoietic recovery. One patient experienced asymptomatic decreases in diffusion capacity less than 50% and one had grade IV hepatotoxicity. At a median follow-up of 14 months, the median survival had not been reached. Three-year OS and PFS were 65% and 42%, respectively. Krishnan et al[27] evaluated the combination of standard-dose ^{90}Y-ibritumomab tiuxetan 0.4 mCi/kg and high-dose BEAM followed by ASCT in 24 older patients (median age, 60 years) with relapsed aggressive B-cell NHL (10 DLCL, three transformed). Median granulocytes and platelet engraftment occurred at days 11 and 13, respectively. At a median follow-up of 13 months, OS and PFS were 98% and 74%, with a relapse rate of 21%. The regimen was well tolerated even in these older patients and toxicity was similar to high-dose BEAM. These studies suggest that a standard dose of RIT can be added to high-dose chemotherapy in the ASCT setting without additional toxicity. Additional studies with RIT and ASCT are ongoing and preliminary results suggest that these approaches may be superior to conventional high-dose regimens.

Consolidative ASCT for DLCL-B

Several randomized studies have evaluated the role of HDT and ASCT as initial treatment or as consolidative therapy during first remission in patients with poor-risk aggressive NHL. However, these studies have failed to demonstrate conclusively the benefit of HDT and ASCT during first remission and all benefit has been shown only in retrospective subset analyses of larger trials. In addition, there are problems with these trials due to patient selection, variation in the definition of high-risk diseases, a variety of induction chemotherapy regimens, number of cycles given, different high-dose regimens used in ASCT, and timing of ASCT. Moreover, in most studies, one third of the patients who were randomized to receive ASCT never underwent the procedure due to progressive disease or patient choice. There were also significant delays in therapy between the end of chemotherapy and ASCT.

The results of randomized trials of HDT and ASCT as initial therapy or a consolidation therapy are summarized in Table 1. Three studies have shown a benefit for HDT and ASCT during first CR in subsets of patients who were high-intermediate or by age-adjusted IPI (aaIPI). In the LNH87-2 trial reported by the GELA,[2] patients were randomized to treatment with four courses of two anthracycline-containing regimens. Patients who achieved a CR were then randomized to receive additional cycles of sequential chemotherapy or an intensive consolidation with high-dose methotrexate followed by high-dose CBV and ASCT. For the whole group, consolidative CBV followed by ASCT was not superior to sequential chemotherapy. However, a retrospective subset analysis of 451 patients with high or high-intermediate IPI risk group showed that the 8-year OS rate was higher in the ASCT arm than in the sequential chemotherapy arm (64% *v* 49%, P = .04). Santini et al[28] reported the results of the Italian Non-Hodgkin's Lymphoma Cooperative Group in 124 patients with intermediate- and high-grade NHL stage II bulky ($\geq$10 cm), III, and IV. Patients were randomized to receive VACOP-B (etoposide, doxorubicin, cyclophosphamide, vincristine, prednisone, and bleomycin) or VACOP-B plus HDT and ASCT. There was no difference in survival between the two groups. However, in the subset analysis according to aaIPI, the DFS was significantly better for high-intermediate and high-risk group patients who underwent HDT and ASCT (87% *v* 48%, P = .008), with a trend for improved PFS in favor of HDT and ASCT (65% *v* 37%, P = .08).

Recently, the benefit of consolidative ASCT has been confirmed in another randomized trial reported by the Groupe Ouest-Est Leucémies et des Autres Maladies du Sang (GOELAMS).[29] A total of 197 patients (15 to 60 years of age) with aggressive NHL (intermediate or high grade) were randomized to receive either eight cycles of CHOP chemotherapy or CEEP (cyclophosphamide, epirubicin, vindesine, and prednisone) for two cycles followed by consolidation with high-dose methotrexate and cytarabine, then high-dose BEAM and ASCT. Patients with high-risk aaIPI were excluded. Overall, 78% of the patients completed the assigned treatment. The main reasons for not completing the treatment were the lack of an early response or disease progression. After a median follow-up of 4 years, the estimated 5-year EFS was significantly higher for patients who received ASCT than for those who received CHOP (55% *v* 37%, P = .037). Among 105 patients with an aaIPI high-intermediate risk, the 5-year EFS (56% *v* 28%, P = .003) and OS (74% *v* 44%, P = .001) were also significantly better for HDT than CHOP. For patients with low or low-intermediate risk, there was no difference in EFS and OS between the two treatment arms. These three studies support the role of consolidative HDT and ASCT in patients with aaIPI high-intermediate and high-risk aggressive NHL.

However, the outcomes of ASCT were reported to be infe-

Table 1 Results of HDT/ASCT as Part of Initial Treatment or as Consolidation Treatment for Aggressive NHL

Authors	No./Age (yr)	Regimens	Risk Factors	Outcome	Comments
Gianni et al,[51] 1997	90/17–60	MACOP-B × 12 weeks + RT *v* HDS + ASCT + RT	Bulky mass >10cm stage III, IV	Median follow-up 55 months CR rate 70% *v* 96% (*P* = .0001) EFS 49% *v* 76% (*P* = .004) FFP 49% *v* 84% (*P* < .0001)	84% were aaIPI high- and high-intermediate
Haioun et al[2] (GELA), 1997	541/16–55	CR patients ↙ ↘ Sequential Chemotherapy; HDMTX ↓ CBV + ASCT	One of these factors: ECOG 2–4 Tumor bulk ≥10 cm ≥2 extranodal sites BM or CNS+	No difference in DFS or OS between two arms For high-, high-intermediate aaIPI 5-yr DFS 39% *v* 59% (*P* = .01) 5-yr OS 52% *v* 65% (*P* = .06)	Of 125 patients scheduled to receive ABMT, 69% did
Santini et al[28] (NHLCSG), 1998	124/15–60	VACOP-B × 12 weeks *v* VACOP-B × 12wks + HDT + ABMT	Stage II bulky (≥10 cm), III or IV	Median follow-up 42 months 6-yr OS 65% for both 6-yr DFS 60% v 80% (*P* = .1) For aaIPI high-or high-intermediate DFS 48% *v* 87% (*P* = .008)	29% did not undergo HDT + ABMT
Kluin-Nelemans et al[33] (EORTC), 2001	194/15–65	CHVmP/BV × 8 *v* CHVmP/BV × 6 followed by BEAC + ASCT	Stage I bulky, II–IV	Median follow-up 53 months 5-yr OS 77% *v* 88% (*P* = NS) 5-yr TTP 56% *v* 61%, (*P* = NS)	70% low- or low-intermediate IPI
Gisselbrecht et al[30] (GELA), 2002	370/15–60	ACVBP *v* sequential shortened chemotherapy followed by BEAM + ASCT	aaIPI high-, high-intermediate	Median follow-up 60 months 5-yr OS 60% *v* 52 % (*P* = .007) 5-yr EFS 46% *v* 39% (*P* = .01)	74% underwent HDT + ASCT
Kaiser et al[31] (GHNHLSG), 2002	312/18–60	CHOEP × 5 + IFRT *v* CHOEP × 3 + HDT + ASCT + IFRT	↑ LDH level stage II–IV	Median follow-up 45.5 months 3-yr OS 63% *v* 62% (*P* = .68) 3-yr EFS 49% *v* 59% (*P* = .22)	Only 65% randomized to ABMT received transplant
Martelli et al,[32] 2003	150/15–60	MACOP-B × 12 weeks *v* MACOP-B × 8 weeks followed by HDT + ASCT	aaIPI high-, high-intermediate	Median follow-up 24 months 5-yr OS 65% *v* 64% (*P* = .95) 5-yr PFS 49% *v* 61% (*P* = .21)	40% did not undergo ABMT
Milpied et al,[29] 2004	197/15–60	CHOP × 8 v CEEP × 2 + MC Followed by BEAM + ASCT	aaIPI low-, low-intermediate or high-intermediate	Median follow-up 4 years 5-yr EFS 37% *v* 55% (*P* = .037) 5-yr EFS 28% *v* 56% (*P* = .003) For high-intermediate 5-yr OS 44% *v* 74% (*P* = .0001)	78% of patients completed assigned treatment 49% high-intermediate
Olivieri et al,[52] (NHLCSG), 2005	223/15–60	VACOP-B × 12 wks *v* VACOP-B × 8 wks + HDT + ASCT	Advanced stage	Median follow-up 62 months 7-yr DFS 62% *v* 71% (*P* = .2) 7-yr OS 60% *v* 58% (*P* = .5)	Patients with persistent disease after VACOP-B × 12 weeks underwent HDT + ASCT

Abbreviations: GELA, Groupe d' Etude des Lymphomes de l' Adulte; NHLCSG, Non-Hodgkin's Lymphoma Cooperative Study Group; EORTC, European Organization for Research and Treatment of Cancer Lymphoma Group; GHNHLSG, German High-Grade Non-Hodgkin's Lymphoma Study Group; MACOP-B, methotrexate with leucovorin rescue, doxorubicin, cyclophosphamide, vincristine, prednisone, bleomycin; RT, radiotherapy; HDS, high-dose sequential; ASCT, autologous stem cell transplant; EFS, event-free survival; FFP, freedom from progression; OS, overall survival; aaIPI, age-adjusted International Prognostic Index; HDMTX, high-dose methotrexate; CBV, carmustine, cyclophosphamide, etoposide; VACOP-B, etoposide, doxorubicin, cyclophosphamide, vincristine, prednisone, bleomycin; CHVmP/BV, cyclophosphamide, doxorubicin, teniposide, prednisone, bleomycin, vincristine; BEAC, carmustine, etoposide, cytarabine, melphalan; ACVBP, doxorubicin, cyclophosphamide, vindesine, bleomycin, prednisone; BEAM, carmustine, etoposide, cytarabine, melphalan; CHOEP, cyclophosphamide, doxorubicin, oncovin, etoposide, prednisone; IFRT, involved-field radiotherapy; CEEP, cyclophosphamide, epirubicin, vindesine, prednisone.

rior to chemotherapy when an abbreviated course of chemotherapy was used before ASCT or when ASCT was applied as early intensification. Gisselbrecht et al[30] reported the results of randomized trial LNH93-3 in 370 aggressive NHL patients with high or high-intermediate aaIPI. Patients were randomized to receive ACVBP (doxorubicin, cyclophosphamide, vindesine, bleomycin, and prednisone) chemotherapy followed by consolidation chemotherapy or a shortened intensive induction chemotherapy followed by high-dose BEAM and ASCT. After a median follow-up of 60 months, 5-year OS and EFS were significantly superior in the ACVBP arm (OS 60% *v* 46%, $P = .007$; EFS 52% *v* 39%, $P = .01$). The German High-Grade Non-Hodgkin's Lymphoma study group conducted a phase III randomized trial of HDT and ASCT as part of primary treatment for aggressive NHL.[31] Three hundred twelve patients aged ≤60 years with elevated serum lactate dehydrogenase levels (LDH) who had at least a minor response after two cycles of CHOEP (CHOP plus etoposide) were randomized to receive three more cycles of CHOEP followed by involved-field radiotherapy or one more cycle of CHOEP followed by high-dose BEAM and ASCT. When aaIPI was retrospectively applied, 74% of patients were high-intermediate and high risk. At a median follow-up of 45.5 months, the EFS favored the transplant group (59% *v* 49%), but the difference was not statistically significant ($P = .22$). There was also no significant difference in OS between the two groups (63% for CHOEP *v* 62% for HDT/ASCT, $P = .22$). Martelli et al[32] reported similar results from the Italian multi-center randomized trial of early intensification with HDT and ASCT in 150 patients with age-adjusted high-intermediate and high-risk aggressive NHL. Patients were randomized to receive either a conventional chemotherapy regimen of MACOP-B (methotrexate with leucovorin rescue, doxorubicin, cyclophosphamide, vincristine, prednisone, and bleomycin) or an abbreviated regimen of MACOP-B (8 weeks) followed by high-dose BEAC and ASCT. There was no difference in CR rate between the two arms. At a median follow-up of 24 months, there were no differences in OS, PFS, or relapse between the two treatments. The 5-year OS was 65% for MACOP-B alone and 64% for MACOP-B plus HDT/ASCT ($P = .95$). The results from these studies suggest that abbreviated chemotherapy followed by intensification with HDT/ASCT is not superior to conventional chemotherapy. Furthermore, achieving a CR with full courses of induction therapy before transplant is important and HDT should not be performed too early during the course of treatment.

To address the question whether a full course of chemotherapy administration would allow adequate therapy prior to ASCT, the European Organization for Research and Treatment of Cancer (EORTC) Lymphoma Group conducted a phase III randomized trial comparing standard full courses of chemotherapy with or without ASCT.[33] Patients aged 15 to 65 years with aggressive NHL received three cycles of CHVmP/BV (cyclophosphamide, doxorubicin, teniposide, prednisone, bleomycin, and vincristine) and were restaged. Those who achieved a CR or partial remission without bone marrow involvement were randomized to receive five more cycles of CHVmP/BV or three cycles of CHVmP/BV followed by high-dose BEAC and ASCT. After a median follow-up of 53 months, the time to disease progression and OS at 5 years were 61% and 68%, respectively, for the ASCT arm and 56% and 77%, respectively, for the chemotherapy arm. Differences between arms were not statistically significant. Unfortunately, this study was hampered by patient inclusion, 70% of the patients were low or low-intermediate aaIPI, and a significant dropout rate of 39% for patients who were assigned to ASCT arm. Based on the results from this and other studies, conclusion can be made that patients with low- and low-intermediate risk aaIPI do not benefit from ASCT and should not be subjected to toxicity of HDT and ASCT.

Given the improved outcome with CHOP plus rituximab (R-CHOP) in both younger and older patients with DLCL-B, it is possible that the benefit of HDT and ASCT during first CR may be abrogated by the addition of rituximab, as observed when rituximab was added to dose-intensive CHOP-14 or CHOEP chemotherapy. Unfortunately, none of these randomized trials have included rituximab. Therefore, further randomized study comparing R-CHOP to R-CHOP followed by consolidative treatment with HDT and ASCT is needed. Ongoing study comparing R-CHOP for eight cycles to R-CHOP × 6 cycles followed by HDT and ASCT in high or high-intermediate risk DLCL-B patients is being conducted by SWOG in cooperation with the Cancer and Leukemia Group B and the National Cancer Institute of Canada. Until results from this trial are available, ASCT during first CR in poor-risk DLCL-B is not routinely recommended.

ASCT for Elderly Patients (>60 years)

Elderly patients represent a large proportion of patients with NHL. They are less likely to be treated with full-dose chemotherapy and often experience treatment delays due to toxicity, resulting in higher risk of relapse and poorer survival. Most studies of HDT and ASCT have been limited to patients less than 60 years of age; however, a few studies have evaluated the outcome of HDT and ASCT in patients older than 60 years. Gopal et al[34] treated 53 patients older than 60 with HDT and ASCT. Forty-four patients (83%) had aggressive NHL, 75% had chemosensitive disease, and all had failed anthracycline-based chemotherapy. Estimated 4-year survival among 44 patients with aggressive histology and chemosensitive disease was 41%. Interestingly, treatment-related mortality was less in patients who received the TBI-based regimen. Treatment-related mortality was relatively high at 22% for the whole group. Jantunen et al[35] reported a lower early (<100 days) treatment-related mortality of 11% in 88 NHL patients older than 60 years of age who received ASCT in six Finnish transplant centers. Krishnan et al[27] reported that a new regimen of conventional dose ^{90}Y-ibritumomab tiuxetan 0.4 mCi/kg in combination with high-dose BEAM and ASCT was well tolerated in 24 older patients without transplant-related mortality. With a median follow-up of 13 months, OS and PFS were 94% and 74%, respectively. Although treatment-related mortality may be higher than in younger patients,

HDT combined with ASCT is feasible and may result in prolonged survival in selected elderly patients. Patient selection, better supportive therapy, and optimal conditioning regimen to reduce treatment-related mortality may further improve the outcome of ASCT in elderly patients with NHL.

Allogeneic Stem Cell Transplant for DLCL-B

Even though several studies have shown long-term disease control following allogeneic stem cell transplant (allo-SCT) in NHL, the role of allo-SCT in DLCL-B remains limited. Allo-SCT is often reserved for younger patients with bone marrow involvement, chemoresistant patients, or patients who have relapsed after ASCT. In a European Bone Marrow Transplant (EBMT) registry matched-pair analysis, intermediate- (n = 120) and high-grade (n = 255) patients receiving allografts were each matched with three patients receiving autografts.[36] The 4-year PFS rates were 35% and 39% and the treatment-related mortality rates 42% and 33%, respectively, for intermediate- and high-grade NHL patients undergoing allo-SCT. There was no significant difference in PFS between allo-SCT and ASCT in intermediate-grade NHL; however, allo-SCT was associated with a lower relapse rate but a higher treatment-related mortality than ASCT. Freytes et al[37] reported the International Bone Marrow Transplant Registry (IBMTR) results of myeloablative allo-SCT in 114 patients (44 with intermediate-grade NHL) who had relapsed after ASCT. The 100-day mortality rate was 21% and treatment-related mortality was 22% at 1 year. The incidence of disease progression at 3 years was 52%, and with prolonged follow-up nearly all patients experienced disease progression. PFS was 32%, 25%, and 5% at 1, 3, and 5 years after transplantation, respectively. CR at the time of allo-SCT and use of TBI were associated with lower rates of disease progression and higher rates of OS.

To exploit the graft-versus-lymphoma effect while reducing the transplant-related mortality of allo-SCT, reduced-intensity allo-SCTs have been developed. While durable engraftment can be accomplished with low mortality during the first 100 days, graft-versus-host disease (GVHD) and relapse remain significant causes of morbidity and mortality. The EBMT Lymphoma Working Party evaluated the outcome of reduced-intensity allo-SCT in 188 patients with lymphoma.[38] The median age was 40 years, median number of prior treatments was three, and 48% of patients had undergone prior ASCT. Most patients received a fludarabine-based regimen while 10% received BEAM. The 100-day and 1-year treatment-related mortality rates were 12.8% and 25.5%, respectively. For patients with aggressive NHL, the 1-year probability of disease progression and 1-year PFS were 47% and 32%, respectively. Patients with aggressive NHL, mantle cell lymphoma, or chemoresistant disease had a poor outcome. Rodriguez et al[39] retrospectively evaluated the outcome of allo-SCT in 88 patients with NHL; 48 patients received myeloablative regimens and 40 received reduced-intensity allo-SCT. Patients in the reduced-intensity group were older and more had failed autologous transplant. These investigators found that chemosensitive disease at transplant and no prior autologous transplant were associated with improved survival. Reduced-intensity transplant and prior autologous transplant are associated with increased relapse.

In an attempt to reduce the incidence of GVHD, Mackinnon et al[40] incorporated campath-1H (50 to 100 mg/m^2) into a reduced-intensity regimen of fludarabine (150 mg/m^2) and melphalan (140 mg/m^2) in 137 patients (88 NHL, 49 Hodgkin lymphoma). The majority of patients had failed ASCT (51% aggressive NHL) and median number of chemotherapy regimens was more than four. The incidences of grade II to IV acute GVHD and chronic GVHD were less than 20%. When compared to Hodgkin disease and low-grade NHL, the treatment-related mortality was significantly higher in aggressive NHL, 38% ($P < .01$). Despite the high treatment-related mortality, the PFS at 3 to 4 years was 34% for aggressive NHL. These results support the role of reduced-intensity allo-SCT as a potential curative treatment for heavily pretreated lymphoma patients or following autograft failure. A strategy of ASCT for cytoreduction followed by a reduced-intensity allo-SCT could be studied prospectively in selected patients with chemoresistant or primary refractory aggressive DLCL, since these patients do poorly with ASCT. Further investigation with the goals of reduced relapse and treatment-related mortality, as well as development of additional strategies to enhance the graft-versus-leukemia effect, are needed.

In conclusion, HDT and ASCT is the treatment of choice for patients with chemosensitive relapsed DLCL-B. ASCT as consolidation therapy during first CR is not recommended outside the context of a clinical trial. Encouraging results have been reported with incorporation of RIT into high-dose regimens without increased transplant-related toxicity. The role of maintenance rituximab post-transplant is being investigated. Novel strategies are needed for patients with chemoresistant relapse or primary refractory DLCL-B. Allo-SCT for DLCL-B should be reserved for patients with autograft failure or persistent marrow involvement.

Future Considerations

As described earlier, one of the most important determinations of outcome after autologous transplantation is the pretransplant disease status of the patient. Therapies that can improve the response rate and the depth of the response after relapse could be an important contribution to improving outcome. Several trials have been conducted using regimens such as ICE,[41] R-ICE,[18] DHAP,[42] ESHAP,[43] and MIME[44] with varying response rates but rarely higher than 50%. Many patients do not proceed to ASCT because of an inadequate response to chemotherapy and there are increasing data to suggest that the depth of the response (radiologic, molecular quantification of minimal residual disease) prior to transplant correlates with post-transplant outcome. Thus, with the development of new agents focused on epigenetic mechanisms or targeted molecular therapies, there may be further improvement in the response rates and depth of response of regimens used for salvage treatment of relapsed large cell lymphoma and this could improve the patient outcomes.[45,46]

Many studies have been conducted, as discussed here, to determine the clinical and radiographic factors present at diagnosis that would predict a poor outcome from chemotherapy and possibly support the need for transplantation early in the course of disease. Although molecular profiling techniques have been used to refine the classification and diagnosis of lymphoma, they have not been applied to clinical decision-making. Thus, in the same way that newly diagnosed lymphoma can be classified based on the expression profile into the various subtypes of B-cell lymphoma, increasing data suggest that prognosis can also be determined by these profiles. If this can be confirmed in a larger group of patients, it could identify a subset of patients who, at the time of diagnosis and with treatment with the current agents, might benefit from early autologous transplant. Admittedly, a trial would be needed to determine the efficacy of transplant in patients whose initial molecular signature predicts a poor response or early relapse.

In the transplant setting, studies are being conducted to determine molecular predictions of outcome at the time of transplant. One study has been conducted to determine whether there are profiles present at the time of relapse that classify lymphoma into germinal center–like, activated B cell, or type 3 that would predict outcome after ASCT, similar to what has been shown about upfront therapy. Investigators from Memorial Sloan-Kettering sought to determine whether the expression would affect the efficacy of the transplant. They concluded that cells of origin did not influence survival and that molecular markers prognostic in the first-line setting may not be predictive in patients with relapsed disease.[47] Thus, transplant might actually be able to overcome the poor prognosis of certain signatures, but more data are needed to determine if there are other molecular correlates to outcome after transplant.

Although more effective pre-transplant therapy and transplant regimens could improve the overall results, post-transplant therapy is also being recognized as an important component of improving the overall outcome. Post-transplant rituximab appears to have a benefit and clinical trials appear to support this strategy.[19,20] Other investigators are looking at novel ways to augment immune responses against tumor, including the use of immunocytokines (ICK), which fuses an antibody to an immune-enhancing molecule such as the interleukin-2 anti-CD20 ICK.[48] Preclinical data showed that the fusion protein actually is more effective than either compound alone and phase I and II trials will be forthcoming to determine the anti-tumor efficacy of such an approach in patients who have recurrent lymphoma after ASCT. Investigators are also exploring whether an antibody-based cellular immunotherapy approach might be effective by genetically modifying T cells with an immunoreceptor that recognizes the CD19 or CD20 antigen.[49] Cells are then grown to large numbers and infused into patients with recurrent disease, usually after lymphodepletion, to create appropriate space and harness the endogenous homeostatic mechanisms that lead to T-cell expansion.[50] Preclinical work in these models also suggests that T cells can be modified to recognize an antigen on lymphoma cells and could contribute to the post-transplant treatment that is focused on minimal residual disease to reduce the chance of relapse and improve the overall outcome for patients undergoing autologous transplantation for large cell lymphoma.[51,52]

References

1. Philip T, Guglielmi C, Hagenbeek A, Somers R, Van Der Lelie H, Bron D, et al: Autologous Bone marrow transplantation as compared with salvage chemotherapy in relapses of chemotherapy-sensitive non-Hodgkin's lymphoma. N Engl J Med 333:1540-1545, 1995
2. Haioun C, Lepage E, Gisselbrecht C, Bastion Y, Coiffier B, Brice P, et al: Benefit of autologous bone marrow transplantation over sequential chemotherapy in poor-risk aggressive non-Hodgkin's lymphoma: Updated results of the prospective study LNH87-2. J Clin Oncol 15:1131-1137, 1997
3. Weaver CH, Petersen FB, Appelbaum FA, Bensinger WI, Press O, Martin P, et al: High-dose fractionated total-body irradiation, etoposide, and cyclophosphamide followed by autologous stem-cell support in patients with malignant lymphoma. J Clin Oncol 12:2559-2566, 1994
4. Horning SJ, Negrin RS, Chao NJ, Long GD, Hoppe RT, Blume KG: Fractionated total-body irradiation, etoposide, and cyclophosphamide plus autografting in Hodgkin's disease and non-Hodgkin's lymphoma. J Clin Oncol 12:2552-2558, 1994
5. Stiff PJ, Unger JM, Forman SJ, McCall AR, LeBlanc M, Nademanee AP, et al: The value of augmented preparative regimens combined with an autologous bone marrow transplant for the management of relapsed or refractory Hodgkin disease: A Southwest Oncology Group phase II trial. Biol Blood Marrow Transplant 9:529-539, 2003
6. Gutierrez-Delgado F, Maloney DG, Press OW, Golden J, Holmberg LA, Maziarz RT, et al: Autologous stem cell transplantation for non-Hodgkin's lymphoma: Comparison of radiation-based and chemotherapuy-only preparative regimens. Bone Marrow Transplant 28:455-461, 2001
7. Brown JR, Yeckes H, Friedberg JW, Neuberg D, Kim H, Nadler LM, et al: Increasing incidence of late second malignancies after conditioning with cyclophosphamide and total-body irradiation and autologous bone marrow transplantation for non-Hodgkin's lymphoma. J Clin Oncol 23:2208-2214, 2005
8. Darrington DL, Vose JM, Anderson JR, Bierman PJ, Bishop MR, Chan WC, et al: Incidence and characterization of secondary myelodysplastic syndrome and acute myelogeneous leukemia following high-dose chemoradiotherapy and autologous stem-cell transplantation for lymphoid malignancies. J Clin Oncol 12:2527-2534, 1994
9. Blay J, Gomez F, Sebban C, Bachelot T, Biron P, Guglielmi C, et al: The International Prognostic Index correlates to survival in patients with aggressive lymphoma in relapse: Analysis of the PARMA trial. Parma Group. Blood 92:3562-3568, 1998
10. Guglielmi C, Gomez F, Philip T, Hagenbeek A, Martelli M, Sebban C, et al: Time to relapse has prognostic value in patients with aggressive lymphoma enrolled onto the Parma trial. J Clin Oncol 16:3264-3269, 1998
11. Hamlin PA, Zelenetz AD, Kewalramani T, Qin J, Satagopan JM, Verbel D, et al: Age-adjusted International Prognostic Index predicts autologous stem cell transplantation outcome for patients with relapsed or primary refractory diffuse large B-cell lymphoma. Blood 102:1989-1996, 2003
12. Spaepen K, Stroobants S, Dupont P, Vandenberghe P, Maertens J, Bormans G, et al: Prognostic value of pretransplantation positron emission tomography using fluorine 18-fluorodeoxyglucose in patients with aggressive lymphoma treated with high-dose chemotherapy and stem cell transplantation. Blood 102:53-59, 2003
13. Alousi AM, Saliba RM, Okoroji G, Hosing C, Samuels BI, Champlin RE, et al: The influence of PET/gallium (P/G) status and high-dose rituximab (HDR) in patients (pts) with aggressive, large, B-cell lymphoma

(LBCL) receiving autologous stem cell transplants (ASCT). J Clin Oncol (Meeting Abstracts) 24:6518, 2006 (abstr)
14. Cortelazzo S, Rambaldi A, Rossi A, Oldani E, Ghielmini M, Benedetti F, et al: Intensification of salvage treatment with high-dose sequential chemotherapy improves the outcome of patients with refractory or relapsed aggressive non-Hodgkin's lymphoma. Br J Haematol 114:333-341, 2001
15. Josting A, Sieniawski M, Glossmann JP, Staak O, Nogova L, Peters N, et al: High-dose sequential chemotherapy followed by autologous stem cell transplantation in relapsed and refractory aggressive non-Hodgkin's lymphoma: Results of a multicenter phase II study. Ann Oncol 16:1359-1365, 2005
16. Coiffier B, Lepage E, Briere J, Herbrecht R, Tilly H, Bouabdallah R, et al: CHOP chemotherapy plus rituximab compared with CHOP alone in elderly patients with diffuse large-B-cell lymphoma. N Engl J Med 346:235-242, 2002
17. Pfreundschuh M, Trumper L, Osterborg A, Pettengell R, Trneny M, Imrie K, et al: CHOP-like chemotherapy plus rituximab versus CHOP-like chemotherapy alone in young patients with good prognosis diffuse large B-cell lymphoma: A randomised controlled trial by the MabThera International Trial (MInT) Group. Lancet Oncol 7:379-391, 2006
18. Kewalramani T, Zelenetz AD, Nimer SD, Portlock C, Straus D, Noy A, et al: Rituximab and ICE as second-line therapy before autologous stem cell transplantation for relapsed or primary refractory diffuse large B-cell lymphoma. Blood 103:3684-3688, 2004
19. Khouri IF, Saliba RM, Hosing C, Okoroji GJ, Acholonu S, Anderlini P, et al: Concurrent administration of high-dose rituximab before and after autologous stem-cell transplantation for relapsed aggressive B-cell non-Hodgkin's lymphomas. J Clin Oncol 23:2240-2247, 2005
20. Horwitz SM, Negrin RS, Blume KG, Breslin S, Stuart MJ, Stockerl-Goldstein KE, et al: Rituximab as adjuvant to high-dose therapy and autologous hematopoietic cell transplantation for aggressive non-Hodgkin lymphoma. Blood 103:777-783, 2004
21. Rapoport AP, Meisenberg B, Sarkodee-Adoo C, Fassas A, Frankel SR, Mookerjee B, et al: Autotransplantation for advanced lymphoma and Hodgkin's disease followed by post-transplant rituxan/GM-CSF or radiotherapy and consolidation chemotherapy. Bone Marrow Transplant 29:303-312, 2002
22. Press OW, Eary JF, Appelbaum FR, Martin PJ, Badger CC, Nelp WB, et al: Radiolabeled-antibody therapy of B-cell lymphoma with autologous bone marrow support. N Engl J Med 329:1219-1224, 1993
23. Press OW, Eary JF, Gooley T, Gopal AK, Liu S, Rajendran JG, et al: A phase I/II trial of iodine-131-tositumomab (anti-CD20), etoposide, cyclophosphamide, and autologous stem cell transplantation for relapsed B-cell lymphomas. Blood 96:2934-2942, 2000
24. Nademanee A, Forman S, Molina A, Fung H, Smith D, Dagis A, et al: A phase 1/2 trial of high-dose yttrium-90-ibritumomab tiuxetan in combination with high-dose etoposide and cyclophosphamide followed by autologous stem cell transplantation in patients with poor-risk or relapsed non-Hodgkin lymphoma. Blood 106:2896-2902, 2005
25. Vose JM, Bierman PJ, Enke C, Hankins J, Bociek G, Lynch JC, et al: Phase I trial of iodine-131 tositumomab with high-dose chemotherapy and autologous stem-cell transplantation for relapsed non-Hodgkin's lymphoma. J Clin Oncol 23:461-467, 2005
26. Winter JN, Inwards D, Erwin W, Wiseman G, Rademaker A, Patton DR, et al: Zevalin dose-escalation foolowed by high-dose BEAM and autologous peripheral blood progenitor cell (PBPC) transplant in non-Hodgkin's lymphoma: Early outcome results. Blood 100:411a, 2002 (abstr)
27. Krishnan AY, Nademanee A, Forman SJ, Fung H, Molina A, Yamauchi D, et al: The outcome of ZBEAM, a regimen combining 90Y ibritumomab tiuxetan with high dose chemotherapy in elderly patients with non-Hodgkin's lymphoma (NHL). J Clin Oncol (Meeting Abstracts) 23:6566, 2005 (abstr)
28. Santini G, Salvagno L, Leoni P, Chisesi T, De Souza C, Sertoli MR, et al: VACOP-B versus VACOP-B plus autologous bone marrow transplantation for advanced diffuse non-Hodgkin's lymphoma: Results of a prospective randomized trial by the non-Hodgkin's Lymphoma Cooperative Study Group. J Clin Oncol 16:2796-2802, 1998
29. Milpied N, Deconinck E, Gaillard F, Delwail V, Foussard C, Berthou C, et al: Initial treatment of aggressive lymphoma with high-dose chemotherapy and autologous stem-cell support. N Engl J Med 350:1287-1295, 2004
30. Gisselbrecht C, Lepage E, Molina T, Quesnel B, Fillet G, Lederlin P, et al: Shortened first-line high-dose chemotherapy for patients with poor-prognosis aggressive lymphoma. J Clin Oncol 20:2472-2479, 2002
31. Kaiser U, Uebelacker L, Abel U, Birkmann J, Trümper L, Schmalenberg H, et al: Randomized study to evaluate the use of high-dose therapy as part of primary treatment for "aggressive" lymphoma. J Clin Oncol 20:4413-4419, 2002
32. Martelli M, Gherlinzoni F, De Renzo A, Zinzani PL, de Vivo A, Cantonetti M, et al: Early autologous stem-cell transplantation versus conventional chemotherapy as front-line therapy in high-risk, aggressive non-Hodgkin's lymphoma: An Italian multicenter randomized trial. J Clin Oncol 21:1255-1262, 2003
33. Kluin-Nelemans HC, Zagonel V, Anastasopoulou A, Bron D, Roozendaal KJ, Noordijk EM, et al: Standard chemotherapy with or without high-dose chemotherapy for aggressive non-Hodgkin's lymphoma: Randomized phase III EORTC study. J Natl Cancer Inst 93:22-30, 2001
34. Gopal AK, Gooley TA, Golden JB, Maloney DG, Bensinger WI, Petersdorf SH: Efficacy of high-dose therapy and autologous hematopoietic stem cell transplantation for non-Hodgkin's lymphoma in adults 60 years of age and older. Bone Marrow Transplant 27:593-599, 2001
35. Jantunen E, Itala M, Juvonen E, Leppa S, Keskinen L, Vasala K, et al: Autologous stem cell transplantation in elderly (>60 years) patients with non-Hodgkin's lymphoma: A nation-wide analysis. Bone Marrow Transplant 37:367-372, 2006
36. Peniket AJ, De Elvira MCR, Taghipour G, Cordonnier C, Gluckman E, De Witte T, et al: An EBMT registry matched study of allogeneic stem cell transplants for lymphoma: Allogeneic transplantation is associated with a lower relapse rate but a higher procedure-related mortality rate than autologous transplantation. Bone Marrow Transplant 31: 667-678, 2003
37. Freytes CO, Loberiza FR, Rizzo JD, Bashey A, Bredeson CN, Cairo MS, et al: Myeloablative allogeneic hematopoietic stem cell transplantation in patients who experience relapse after autologous stem cell transplantation for lymphoma: A report of the International Bone Marrow Transplant Registry. Blood 104:3797-3803, 2004
38. Robinson SP, Goldstone AH, Mackinnon S, Carella A, Russell N, de Elvira CR, et al: Chemoresistant or aggressive lymphoma predicts for a poor outcome following reduced-intensity allogeneic progenitor cell transplantation: An analysis from the Lymphoma Working Party of the European Group for Blood and Bone Marrow Transplantation. Blood 100:4310-4316, 2002
39. Rodriguez R, Nademanee A, Carter N, Smith E, Krishnan A, Popplewell L, et al: Comparison of reduced intensity with conventional myeloablative regimens for allogeneic transplant of non-Hodgkin lymphoma. (submitted for publication)
40. Mackinnon S: Reduced intensity allogeneic stem cell transplantation for relapsed Hodgkin and non-Hodgkin's lymphoma lowers regimen toxicity and facilitates a graft-versus-lymphoma effect. Ann Oncol 16: v34, 2005 (abstr)
41. Moskowitz CH, Bertino JR, Glassman JR, Hedrick EE, Hunte S, Coady-Lyons N, et al: Ifosfamide, carboplatin, and etoposide: a highly effective cytoreduction and peripheral-blood progenitor-cell mobilization regimen for transplant-eligible patients with non-Hodgkin's lymphoma. J Clin Oncol 17:3776-3785, 1999
42. Velasquez WS, Cabanillas F, Salvador P, McLaughlin P, Fridrik M, Tucker S. Effective salvage therapy for lymphoma with cisplatin in combination with high-dose Ara-C and dexamethasone (DHAP). Blood 71:117-122, 1988
43. Velasquez WS, McLaughlin P, Tucker S, Hagemeister FB, Swan F, Rodriguez MA, et al: ESHAP—An effective chemotherapy regimen in refractory and relapsing lymphoma: A 4 year follow-up study. J Clin Oncol 12:1169-1176, 1994
44. Cabanillas F, Hagemeister FB, McLaughlin P, Velasquez WS, Riggs S,

Fuller L, et al: Results of MIME salvage regimen for recurrent or refractory lymphoma. J Clin Oncol 5:407-412, 1987
45. Johnstone RW: Histone-deacetylase inhibitors: Novel drugs for the treatment of cancer. Nat Rev Drug Discov 1:287-299, 2002
46. O'Connor OA, Heaney ML, Schwartz L, Richardson S, William R, MacGregor-Cortelli B, et al: Clinical experience with intravenous and oral formulations of the novel histone deacetylase inhibitor suberoylanilide hydroxamic acid in patients with advanced hematologic malignancies. J Clin Oncol 24:166-173, 2006
47. Moskowitz CH: Pretreatment prognostic factors and outcome in patients with relapsed or primary-refractory diffuse large B-cell lymphoma treated with second-line chemotherapy and autologous stem cell transplantation. Ann Oncol 17:iv37-iv39, 2006
48. Gillies SD, Lan Y, Williams S, Carr F, Forman S, Raubitschek A, et al: An anti-CD20-IL-2 immunocytokine is highly efficacious in a SCID mouse model of established human B lymphoma. Blood 105:3972-3978, 2005
49. Cooper LJ, Kalos M, DiGiusto D, Brown C, Forman SJ, Raubitschek A, et al: T-cell genetic modification for re-directed tumor recognition. Cancer Chemother Biol Response Modif 22:293-324, 2005
50. Jensen M: Strategies to enhance the therapeutic efficacy of autologous hematopoietic stem cell transplantation by posttransplantation adoptive transfer of T cells with engineered graft-versus-tumor activity. Biol Blood Marrow Transplant 11:34-39, 2005
51. Gianni AM, Bregni M, Siena S, Brambilla C, Nicola MD, Lombardi F, et al: High-dose chemotherapy and autologous bone marrow transplantation compared with MACOP-B in aggressive B-cell lymphoma. N Engl J Med 336:1290-1297, 1997
52. Olivieri A, Santini G, Patti C, Chisesi T, De Souza C, Rubagotti A, et al: Upfront high-dose sequential therapy (HDS) versus VACOP-B with or without HDS in aggressive non-Hodgkin's lymphoma: Long-term results by the NHLCSG. Ann Oncol 16:1941-1948, 2005

Seminars in
HEMATOLOGY

New Drugs for the Treatment of Advanced-Stage Diffuse Large Cell Lymphomas

Owen A. O'Connor[a,b] and Paul Hamlin[b]

The rapid pace of discovering new signaling pathways that influence the growth and survival of different types of cancer cells has produced a daunting array of potentially new, "drugable" targets for the treatment of cancer. This has been particularly true for the lymphomas. The empiric observation that many kinds of "novel targeted" drugs appear to exhibit relatively selective patterns of activity is testament to the concept that the lymphomas represent an incredibly diverse group of human cancers. Targeting one pathway in a subtype of lymphoma may not be universally effective against all subtypes of lymphoma, even closely related ones. These observations suggest that pharmacologically driven "target identification" plays an important role in the continued development of new therapeutic agents, and underscores the need for more research into the biologic basis for different subtypes of lymphoma. Over the past 10 years, there has been an explosion of new drugs making their way through preclinical laboratories and early clinical studies. These experiences have taught us some frustrating lessons. Sometimes, the strongest biologic rationale is associated with the poorest clinical results. Sometimes, where no rationale exists, golden therapeutic opportunities emerge. In either case, both experiences typically end up teaching us something about the disease we didn't historically appreciate. In this review, we will take a close look at some of the more intriguing targets in aggressive large B-cell lymphomas, all of which now have small molecules that can profoundly affect their activity, activity we hope will lead to new treatment opportunities. We will focus on the biologic rationale for targeting novel pathways regulated by Bcl-6, Bcl-2, BLysS, and APRIL for example. In addition, we will review how new concepts in structural biology and chemical design can help produce new generation compounds with novel activity, as is the case for pralatrexate and targeting the reduced folate carrier-type-1. Clearly, given the breadth and depth of information emerging on these and other relevant biologic pathways, we are limited to discussing only a few illustrative examples, which should in no way detract from the importance of other critical signaling and survival pathways now being exploited in the treatment of lymphoma.
Semin Hematol 43:251-261

The intrinsic biological heterogeneity of the lymphomas continues to provide a unique platform for thinking about the molecular events that drive both normal lymphocyte development, as well as the complex pathways leading to malignant transformation. At the heart of understanding the critical growth and survival pathways contributing to lymphomagenesis, is the need to try and understand the cell of origin of these discrete diseases, as well as the particular molecular features that distinguish the diverse array of lymphoma subtypes. What remains unclear at the moment however, is precisely how we should be selecting which targets to modulate in order to find the most effective therapeutic agents. Will the world's best inhibitor of bcl-2 become the most effective drug for a disease like follicular lymphoma, which is essentially defined by constitutive Bcl-2 expression? Will the world's best inhibitor of cyclin D1 be the answer for a disease like mantle cell lymphoma, which is essentially defined by translocations leading to overexpression of cyclin D1? The answer, of course, is probably not. Rather, it will

[a]Laboratory of Experimental Therapeutics for the Lymphoproliferative Malignancies, Memorial Sloan-Kettering Cancer Center, New York, NY.
[b]Department of Medicine, Lymphoma Service, Memorial Sloan-Kettering Cancer Center, New York, NY.
O.A.O. is the recipient of the Leukemia and Lymphoma Society Scholar in Research Award. O.A.O. is supported by the The Werner and Elaine Dannheisser Fund for Research on the Biology of Aging of the Lymphoma Foundation.
Address correspondence to Owen A. O'Connor, MD, PhD, Department of Medicine, Lymphoma and Developmental Chemotherapy Services, Box 329, 1275 York Ave, New York, NY 10021. E-mail: oconnoro@mskcc.org

0037-1963/06/$-see front matter
doi:10.1053/j.seminhematol.2006.07.002

Table 1 Emerging Novel Targets in the Treatment of Lymphoma

Target	Biologic Responsibilities	Potential Drugs
BLys ± APRIL		• TACI-Ig • Belimumab • BAFF-R-Ig • AMG-623
cMyc	Affect the proliferative states of cycling cells	• HMG-Co A-reductase inhibitors
PKC-β		• Enzastaurin
Constitutive 26S proteaseome and immunoproteasome	Affect a variety of intracellular signaling pathways influencing growth and survival	• Bortezomib • PR-171 • IPSI - 001
Microtubule assembly and function	Impair mitosis and the dynamics of intracellular organelle movement	• Kinesin spindle protein inhibitors • Ixabepilone • Epothilone B
Reduced folate carrier and thymidylate cycle	Affect the proliferative states of cycling cells	• Pralatrexate (PDX) • Premetrexed
Histone deacetylases	Modulate chromatin remodeling and activation of transcriptional states	• SAHA • MS-275 • Depsipeptide
BCL-2 family members	Affect survival pathways	• AT-101 • ABT-737 • GX15-070 • TRAIL antibodies
BCL-6	Cell growth and survival pathways	• SAHA • BCL6 BTB peptides

likely be the combination of new and old agents that can simultaneously affect a multitude of critical biologic pathways important in growth dysregulation and survival of that particular disease. And, in all likelihood, it will be the integration of novel agents into the conventional standards of care that now have become the backbone of lymphoma management that will ultimately lead to the most significant breakthroughs in treating these diseases. In this review, we will discuss some of the latest, and potentially most promising, new targets and agents that may soon become part of the lymphoma treatment landscape (Table 1). Not all of these agents or targets belong under the category of absolutely novel—some are twists on past themes that appear to offer an incremental improvement over other structural analogs in the same class.

Targeting Bcl-6 and Gene Transcription

Biological Significance of Bcl-6 in Lymphoma

Over the past several years, the role of Bcl-6 in the molecular pathogenesis of lymphoma has become well established. Dysregulation of Bcl-6, like so many other molecular derangements in lymphoma, is mediated by reciprocal and balanced chromosomal translocations between two specific chromosomal sites.[1-4] BCL6 is actually a nuclear phosphoprotein belonging to the BTB/POZ zinc finger family of transcription factors that bind DNA as a transcriptional repressor.[5] Translocations involving the Bcl-6 locus at 3q27 are seen in about 35% of diffuse large B-cell lymphomas, and can typically be found using routine karyotypic analyses.

Interestingly, the chromosomal translocation affecting the 3q27 band is now widely considered to be one of the most common genetic abnormalities in non-Hodgkin's lymphoma (NHL). Bcl-6, which is expressed predominantly by mature B-cells within the germinal center, plays an essential role in germinal center development.[6] As a result, dysregulation of Bcl-6 is commonly seen in follicular and diffuse large B-cell lymphomas.[7] In addition, Bcl-6 has been shown to be important in T-cell–dependent humoral responses, where it functions as a transcriptional repressor to suppress an array of genes involved in differentiation, lymphocyte activation, and apoptosis in the germinal center.

Bcl-6 itself is typically regulated by a number of factors that includes, for example, activation of the B-cell receptors by antigen, which appears to induce mitogen-activated protein (MAP) kinase–mediated phosphorylation, leading to Bcl-6 proteolysis via the ubiquitin proteasome pathway. Another surprising mechanism revolves around the fact that Bcl-6 appears to be subject to the same set of enzymatic reactions that control chromatin remodeling, namely, the histone acetyltransferases (HAT) and the histone deacetyltransferases (HDAC).[8]

Normally, in quiescent cells, DNA exists in a supercoiled condensed state tightly wrapped around basic proteins called histones. Such tightly coiled DNA preempts access by transcription factors, leading to a transcriptionally silent state. This state of chromatin folding is facilitated by HDAC, which remove acetyl-groups from the lysine tails of histone, leading to condensation of the chromatin structure. In contrast, acetylation of the lysine tails facilitates an unraveling of the DNA from the histones, leading to a more open chromatin structure, which allows access by transcription factors, leading to a more active state of gene transcription. This state is achieved by enzymes called HATs, which add the acetyl-groups to the lysine tails. Hence, the balance between condensed and open chromatin is tightly managed by the relative activity of HATs and HDACs. Drugs that inhibit histone deacetylase (HDAC inhibitors or HDACI) would be expected to inhibit the removal of acetyl-groups from the lysine tails of the histone, facilitating a more transcriptionally active open chromatin state. While only a very small percentage of the genome appears to be affected by these drugs, that is, they do not result in global chromatin changes, it is interesting to note that tumor cell lines treated with HDAC inhibitors undergo cytodifferentiation, cell cycle arrest, and apoptosis.

Interestingly, as alluded to earlier, these very same reactions can influence the activation and deactivation of Bcl-6 (Fig 1). Bcl-6 is subject to acetylation by the p300 acetylase (aHAT), which completely abrogates its transcriptional repressor function, allowing a number of Bcl-6–dependent genes to be transcribed.[8] Alternatively, deacetylation of Bcl-6 by HDACs leads to protein that can now bind to DNA, allowing the transcriptional factor to repress BCL6-dependent genes.

These two pathways converged recently when it was demonstrated that HDACIs can influence gene expression in lymphoma in one of two ways: (1) by modulating the balance of open and closed chromatin available for transcription, or (2) by influencing the acetylation state of BCL6. For example, trichostatin A (TSA), a potent and specific HDAC inhibitor, results in a dose-dependent inhibition of Bcl6-mediated repression. Furthermore, treatment with TSA leads to the accumulation of acetylated Bcl-6 in the RAMOS B-cell lymphoma cell line. In addition to HDACs, it turns out Bcl-6 can undergo deacetylation through a second independent pathway known as the SIR-2 pathway, which happens to be potently inhibited by niacinamide (NIA). Treatment of cells with NIA results in accumulation of acetylated BCL6, while combined treatment with NIA and TSA is additive.[9-11]

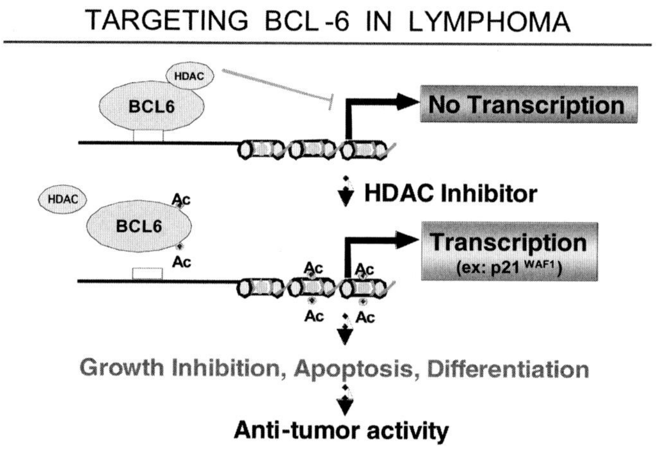

Figure 1 BCL-6 is constitutively expressed in a large proportion of B-cell lymphomas and is involved in the suppression of genes involved in the control of lymphocyte activation, differentiation, and apoptosis. In the acetylated state, BCL-6 is inactive and loses its ability to repress transcription and to induce cell transformation. Pharmacologic inhibition of HDAC with agents such as vorinostat may result in the accumulation of acetylated BCL-6, expression of the cell-cycle regulator p21^{WAF1}, and ultimately growth inhibition, apoptosis, and differentiation of B-cell lymphoma cells.

Therapeutic Prospects of HDAC Inhibitors

To date, at least four major classes of HDACIs have been identified,[12] including: (1) short chain fatty acids (such as 4-phenylbuterate and valproic acid), (2) hydroxamic acids (such as trichostatin [TSA] and SAHA), (3) cyclic tetrapeptides (like depsipeptide [FR901228]), and (4) benzamides (for example, MS-275).

Of these classes of HDACIs, significant experience has emerged with the hydroxamic acid SAHA (suberoylanilde hydroxamic acid) and the cyclic tetrapeptide depsipeptide. SAHA has been studied in phase I trials of patients with advanced cancers, including lymphoma, as both an intravenous infusion[13,14] and as an oral formulation.[15] Interestingly, there may be class effects for these drugs that include transient thrombocytopenia, dehydration, anorexia, diarrhea, and fatigue. Among the patients with lymphoma treated on the phase I studies with SAHA, major responses were seen in two patients with aggressive transformed B-cell lymphoma who attained a complete remission (CR) and partial remission (PR) on study, both of which were very durable (18 and 6 months, respectively). In addition, other responses in patients with Hodgkin's disease and T-cell lymphoma were noted. The activity in T-cell lymphoma has also emerged as an area with great promise. Both SAHA and depsipeptide have demonstrated marked activity in cutaneous T-cell lymphomas.[16-18] In addition, and though still early, another HDACI, MS-275, has completed phase I studies, where an oral formulation was found to be best tolerated when given on a daily for 14 day basis, where the dose-limiting toxicities included nausea, vomiting, and fatigue.[19] Ongoing studies are beginning to clarify the role of SAHA in relapsed de novo large B-cell lymphoma, follicular lymphoma, and Hodgkin's disease. Future studies are planned to explore the potential complementary effects of HDACI with other active drugs in lymphoma like rituximab.

Recently, new biologic approaches to selectively inhibiting Bcl-6 have emerged that do not appear to affect global chromatin remodeling. Based on a detailed understanding of the protein–protein interactions between Bcl-6 and other corepressors that bind Bcl-6 on DNA, small interfering peptides have been synthesized that seem to impair co-repressor binding, and essentially abrogate the transcriptional repressor capabilities of Bcl-6. As discussed above, Bcl-6 contains an N-terminal BTB/POZ (Bric-a-brac, Tramtrack, Broad complex/Poxvirus zinc finger) domain, which is a highly conserved motif found in more than 200 intracellular proteins.[20,21] A subset of BTB proteins are also known to act as transcriptional repressors, including important proteins like PLZF (promyelocytic leukemia zinc finger) and HIC-1 (hypermethylated in cancer-1). The BTB domain on Bcl-6 is a critical site of interaction for a number of co-repressors like SMRT (silencing mediator of retinoid and thyroid receptors), NCoR (nuclear receptor co-repressor), and BCoR (Bcl-6 co-repressor). Polo et al[21] have successfully designed peptides that specifically bind to Bcl-6 and interrupt the recruitment of co-repressors. The peptide inhibitor disrupts Bcl-6–mediated repression, leading to the reactivation of natural Bcl-6 target genes, abrogating Bcl-6 biologic function in B cells, which leads to apoptosis and cell cycle arrest. This type of strategy, while clearly requiring a sophisticated understanding of very detailed protein–protein interactions, may be able to create novel therapeutic venues for very selectively inhibiting discrete signaling pathways involved in lymphomagenesis.

Targeting HDAC with any inhibitor is going to be associated with a remarkable number of different biologic sequelae. These agents, at least in lymphoma, may have effects on chromatin remodeling and important disease-specific pathways like the one discussed above with Bcl-6. Certainly, they appear to have a class effect in cutaneous T-cell lymphoma, and possibly some effects in other subtypes of lymphoma like Hodgkin's disease and transformed large cell lymphoma, although this experience is limited. Clearly, after defining the single-agent activity of these drugs in lymphoma, future studies will need to focus on combining these agents with other active drugs in lymphoma. The simple oral administration of SAHA and MS-275 makes them good candidates to combine with a host of drugs. One looming question with the HDACIs revolves around the best pharmacokinetic profile to use in the clinical setting. Daily oral dosing will likely provide high area under the curve (AUC) exposure, with a relatively low maximum concentration (C_{max}), which would be considerably higher in intravenous bolus dosing schedules. Future studies will need to identify the efficacy and toxicity in terms of these basic pharmacokinetic parameters to be sure that only the best dosing schedules are moved forward in clinical trials.

In addition, understanding the differences in gene expression influenced by different HDACIs in different NHL subtypes will create more rationale approaches for the use of these compounds across many different types of lymphoma. While targeting chromatin remodeling and or Bcl-6 represent novel therapeutic approaches for treating lymphoma, it is certain that these drugs are going to have a very pleiotropic set of effects on malignant cells, effects we will need to understand better with time.

Targeting Survival Pathways: Modulating the Anti-apoptotic Influence of BCL-2 Family Members

Biologic Significance of Bcl-2 Family Members

BCL-2 and related proteins are key regulators of programmed cell death and have been implicated in a variety of human diseases, including cancer.[22,23] Bcl-2 protein can be differentially expressed in different malignancies. For example, Bcl-2 is constitutively overexpressed in follicular lymphoma. Follicular lymphomas are well characterized by the translocation of the bcl-2 proto-oncogene from chromosome 18q21 to the immunoglobulin heavy chain locus (IgH) at chromosome 14q32.[24-26] The resulting translocation, t(14:18), is the hallmark lesion seen in follicular lymphoma, and leads to the overexpression of the anti-apoptotic bcl-2 protein, protecting cells from programmed cell death. In addition, overexpression of Bcl-2 family members is, not surprisingly, seen as a

Table 2 Emerging Drugs Affecting Apoptosis

Drug	BCL-2 Family Members Affected	Status of Clinical Development
Oblimersen (BCL-2 antisense molecule)	BCL-2 mRNA	Completion of phase III in CLL, ongoing phase II studies in combination with chemotherapy in aggressive NHL
AT-101 (gossypol enantiomer)	BCL-2 $BCL\text{-}_{XL}$ MCL-1	Single-agent phase I ongoing in CLL and solid tumors
ABT-737	$BCL\text{-}_{XL}$	Single-agent phase I (to begin summer 2006)
GX15-070	Broad pro-survival Bcl-2 family members	Completed phase I
HGS-ETR1/2	Agonist human monoclonal antibody to TRAIL receptor-1	Completed phase I

Abbreviations: CLL, chronic lymphocytic leukemia; NHL, non-Hodgkin's lymphoma.

major mechanism of chemotherapy resistance. Bcl-2 protein typically functions by inhibiting cytochrome c translocation, preempting caspase activation and the induction of the apoptotic cascade.[27,28] Clinically, the prevalence of Bcl-2 overexpression in NHL is high, being found in approximately 90% of follicular and mantle cell histologies and approximately 50% of diffuse large cell lymphomas.[24-26] Clearly, modulating this pathway through the use of drugs that can lower the threshold for apoptosis represents an important therapeutic advance, especially in diseases where Bcl-2 plays a pivotal role in lymphocyte ontogeny.

Clinical and Preclinical Experiences With Bcl-2–Targeted Drugs

To date, there are a large number of agents available that appear to modulate the various aspects of this all important biology. Table 2 lists some of these agents, and approximately where they are in clinical development. Perhaps the most matured of this class of drugs is the Bcl-2 antisense molecule oblimersen. While a number of studies have been published with this agent in melanoma and other diseases, a recent randomized phase III trial was reported which compared fludarabine and cyclophosphamide with the combination of fludarabine, cyclophosphamide, and oblimerson in patients with intermediate- or high-risk relapsed/refractory chronic lymphocytic leukemia.[29,30] The concept behind these sorts of combination studies with conventional chemotherapy focuses on the idea that drugs targeting these particular pathways will lower the threshold for inducing apoptosis with conventional agents. Of 241 patients treated on study, there were more than twice as many major responses when oblimersen was added to the chemotherapy arm (16% *v* 7%, $P = .039$). Hematopoietic toxicities were similar in the two groups, with the exception of more grade 3–4 thrombocytopenia in the oblimersen-containing arm (55% *v* 32%). Recently, preclinical data have demonstrated that the combination of the proteasome inhibitor bortezomib with oblimersen can potentially increase the sensitivity of aggressive diffuse large B-cell lymphoma to cyclophosphamide, leading to marked improvements in overall response and duration of chemotherapy benefit from the three-drug combination compared to the single- or any two-drug combination.[31]

Another very promising drug that can nullify the anti-apoptotic influence of Bcl-2 family members is the orally available gossypol derivative AT-101. Gossypol is a natural polyphenolic compound extracted from cottonseeds that was initially investigated as an antifertility agent.[32-36] In the 1980s and 1990s, when preclinical studies determined that racemic gossypol exhibited cytotoxic effects in human breast, prostate, colon, melanoma, and adrenal carcinoma cell lines,[32-36] orally administered racemic gossypol was evaluated in more than 100 cancer patients in four clinical trials conducted in the United Kingdom and the United States. While tumor responses and disease stabilization were reported in these preliminary studies, overall the drug was considered to be only marginally active.[37-39] In the late 1980s, it was discovered that the effects of gossypol were stereoselective, in that only the R-(−)-gossypol exhibited potent anticancer activity in comparison to the racemic mixture or the S-(+)-gossypol enantiomer. In the National Cancer Institute (NCI) in vitro screen of 60 cancer cell lines, the average growth inhibition (GI_{50}) for R-(−)-gossypol was 0.57 μmol/L, whereas the GI_{50} for racemic and S-(+)-gossypol was 2.1 μmol/L and 14.5 μmol/L, respectively. Through determination of nuclear magnetic resonance (NMR) experimental three-dimensional solution structure of R-(−)-gossypol in complex with bcl-X_L, several crucial interactions were identified, which accounted for the anti-apoptotic function of R-(−)-gossypol.[40,41]

The (−)-enantiomer of gossypol (AT-101) is a potent small-molecule inhibitor of Bcl-2 and Bcl-X_L. Preclinical studies to date have demonstrated that AT-101 exhibits marked in vitro and in vivo anti-tumor activity in combination with rituximab and cyclophosphamide in a SCID mouse xenograft model bearing a diffuse large B-cell lymphoma (DLBCL) cell line (RL) that carries the t(14:18) translocation.[42] Early single-agent phase I studies have established that this drug is safe, producing modest elevations in liver function tests at higher doses. Ongoing studies in a number of lymphoproliferative malignancies also have begun to suggest some interesting single-agent activity in chronic lymphocytic leukemia, as many future studies begin to explore the best approach for integrating AT-101 into conventional chemotherapy regimens.

In addition to AT-101, Fesik et al reported on the development of another Bcl-2–targeted compound, ABT-737, which appears to target Bcl-X_L.[43,44] In an effort to rationally optimize the design and efficacy of their drug, the group from Abbott Laboratories used NMR-based screening, parallel synthesis, and structure-based design to synthesize and purify a protein that was able to bind and interfere with the function of Bcl-2 without significant albumin binding. Sixty-seven cell lines were then screened for cytotoxicity with ABT-737, with cell lines derived from lymphoid malignancies and small cell lung cancer lines showing the most sensitivity to the compound. As expected from drugs that target Bcl-2, ABT-737 was also found to sensitize cell lines to the cytotoxic effects of several different chemotherapeutic agents and radiation.[43,44] Phase I studies with a derivative of ABT-737, ABT-263, are scheduled to begin in early summer.

While admittedly very early in development, there are now a host of new agents and strategies for targeting survival pathways in cancer. While some of these agents are expected to have some, perhaps even modest single-agent activity, it will be their integration into conventional chemotherapy regimens that will establish the proof of principle, "can targeting Bcl-2 family members lower the threshold to induce apoptosis in lymphoma?" These strategies could prove to be a novel approach to overcoming both intrinsic and acquired drug resistance across many subtypes of cancer.

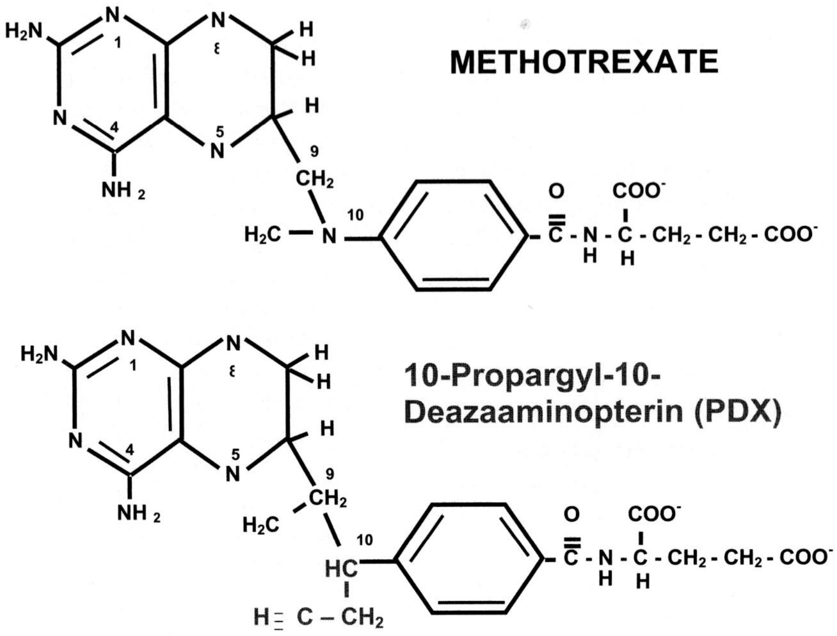

Figure 2 Comparison of methotrexate and pralatrexate (PDX).

New Classes of Familiar Agents Affecting Historically Important Growth and Survival Pathways: Targeting the Reduced Folate Carrier With New Generation Antifols

The Biologic Significance of Targeting the Reduced Folate Carrier and Inhibiting DNA Synthesis

The 10-deazaaminopterins (Fig 2) are a class of folate analogues that demonstrate greater anti-tumor effects than methotrexate against murine tumor models and human tumor xenografts in nude mice.[45-47] The improved activity is due to the more effective internalization by the 1-carbon, reduced folate transporter (RFC-1) and the subsequent accumulation in tumor cells through the formation of polyglutamylated metabolites.

RFC-1 is a fetal oncoprotein that is almost exclusively expressed on fetal and malignant tissue, and is felt to be the principal means through which natural folates and select antifols enter the cell.[48] This carrier protein has evolved to efficiently transport reduced natural folates into highly proliferative cells, in order to meet the demands for purine and pyrimidine nucleotides during DNA synthesis. Interestingly, RFC-1 expression has recently been found to be significantly influenced by a variety of oncogenes, including Hras and c-myc.[48,49] Transfection of wild-type cells lines with either of these oncogenes leads to a marked increase in the surface expression of RFC-1, which has been shown to more rapidly facilitate the internalization of folate analogs in the oncogene transfected cells. Table 3 presents some of the essential pharmacokinetic properties of pralatrexate compared to a number of other well known antifolates, including methotrexate. As can be seen from the influx V_{max}/K_m data, pralatrexate is far more efficiently transported, being incorporated at a rate nearly 14 times greater than that appreciated for methotrexate. Similarly, the V_{max}/K_m for the folylpolyglutamyl synthetase (FPGS)-mediated glutamylation reactions suggest that pralatrexate is also 10 times more efficiently polyglutamylated compared to methotrexate. These biochemical features suggest that pralatrexate should be a more potent antineoplastic

Table 3 Biochemical Properties of Aminopterin, Methotrexate, Edatrexate, and Pralatrexate in CCRF-CEM Cells

Treatment	DHFR Inhibition K_i (pmol/L)	Influx K_m (μmol/L)	Influx V_{max} (pmol/min/mg protein)	Influx V_{max}/K_m	FPGS Activity K_m (μmol/L)	FPGS Activity V_{max} (pmol/min/mg protein)	FPGS Activity V_{max}/K_m
Aminopterin	4.9 ± 1	1.2 ± 0.2	3.6 ± 1.0	3.0	5.8 ± 1	117 ± 18	20.2
Methotrexate	5.4 ± 2	4.8 ± 1.0	4.1 ± 1.2	0.9	32.2 ± 5	70 ± 10	2.2
Edatrexate	5.8 ± 1	1.1 ± 0.1	3.9 ± 0.9	3.5	6.3 ± 1	65 ± 9	10.3
Pralatrexate	13.4 ± 3	0.3 ± 0.1	3.8 ± 1.3	12.6	5.9 ± 1	137 ± 26	23.2

Abbreviations: K_i, inhibitory constant; K_m, binding constant; V_{max}, maximum rate constant.

agent in comparison to methotrexate, and could overcome known mechanisms of methotrexate resistance where downregulation of RFC-1 and/or FPGS leads to frank resistance. One folate analogue in this class, edatrexate (10-ethyl-10-deazaaminopterin), has undergone extensive clinical testing and has been shown in phase II trials to have significant activity in non-small cell lung cancer (NSCLC), breast cancer, and malignant fibrous histiocytoma.

Preclinical Experience in Models of Aggressive Lymphoma

Pralatrexate is structurally similar to edatrexate except for a propargyl-group substitution at the 10-carbon position.[50] Pralatrexate was initially developed by Sirotnak and colleagues at Memorial Sloan-Kettering Cancer Center (MSKCC) in collaboration with Southern Research Institute (SRI). In lymphoma, pralatrexate was consistently more potent than methotrexate in a panel of cell lines representing a variety of lymphproliferative malignancies (one transformed follicular lymphoma, two DLBCL, one Burkitt's, and one Hodgkin's disease). The in vitro experiments demonstrated that pralatrexate was found to produce IC_{50}s consistently 1 log below that typically seen for methotrexate in a library of lymphoma cell lines representing a number of different diseases including DLBCL, T-cell lymphoma, mantle cell lymphoma, and even a very chemotherapy-refractory transformed lymphoma carrying the 14:18 translocation.

In vivo, pralatrexate was consistently found to be superior to methotrexate as well. In a NOD-SCID xenograft model of these lymphomas, complete regression of disease was observed in mice bearing the HT lymphoma (a de novo diffuse large B-cell lymphoma) following treatment with pralatrexate, while methotrexate-treated mice experienced only a 17% reduction in tumor growth. In the RL lymphoma (a transformed large B-cell lymphoma) xenograft model, mice treated with pralatrexate exhibited significant tumor regression, with two thirds of the mice in the pralatrexate-treated cohort experiencing a complete regression of their disease, while mice treated with methotrexate experienced only a modest growth delay compared to the control cohort. These data established the superior therapeutic activity of pralatrexate against human NHL in both in vitro and in vivo models of these diseases. Interestingly, characterization of these cell lines by reverse transcription polymerase chain reaction (RT-PCR) for a number of the determinants of antifolate activity (RFC-1, FPGS, gamma-glutamyl hydrolase [GGH]) revealed a striking correlation between the level of RFC-1 expression and the incidence of complete remission in the NOD-SCID mouse models, with no CRs ever being appreciated in any methotrexate treated mouse cohort. For example, the CR rates for pralatrexate in the in vivo mouse models were approximately 90%, 55%, and 30% for the HT, RL, and SKI-DLCL-1 cell lines, respectively. There was a statistically significant correlation between these CR rates in mice and the total reduced folate carrier expression (RFC-1) by RT-PCR, with the HT, RL, and SKI-DLCL-1 lines having RFC-1 expression levels of 0.96, 0.41, and 0.30. These data provided a strong rationale for conducting a presently ongoing single-agent phase I/II study (MSKCC study 02-078) of pralatrexate in patients with multiply relapsed and refractory aggressive NHL and Hodgkin's disease.

Clinical Experience With Pralatrexate in Lymphoma

Early phase I studies of pralatrexate demonstrated that the dose-limiting toxicity on an every-other-week schedule was stomatitis. In patients with advanced NSCLC, the maximum tolerated dose was considered to be approximately 150 mg/m^2. In a pilot phase II experience in patients with advanced drug-resistant Hodgkin's disease and NHL, the incidence of stomatitis was found to be significantly higher than was appreciated in patients with NSCLC.[51] In fact, there was a statistically significant correlation between the mean total homocysteine (Hcy), methylmalonic acid (MMA) level pretreatment, and the post-treatment AUC exposure, and the relative risk of developing stomatitis. For example, the mean total Hcy and MMA in patients who experienced grade 0 or 1 stomatitis were 7.8 (upper limit of normal, 10) and 118 (upper limit of normal, 200), respectively. In contrast, the mean total Hcy and MMA in patients experiencing grade 3 or 4 stomatitis were 10 and 250, respectively. Interestingly, those patients who presented with the lowest total Hcy and MMA were those who tolerated the greatest dose escalations, which for two patients, both of whom underwent tandem peripheral blood stem cell transplants, was a dose of 240 mg/m^2 administered on an every-other-week basis. For those patients who developed stomatitis after the first cycle, institution of folic acid and vitamin B_{12} resulted in a marked lowering of the Hcy and MMA, and no recurrent stomatitis on rechallenge. These data established the importance of these nutritional covariates in predicting the risk of stomatitis with pralatrexate, allowing subsequent studies to explore further dose escalation in the setting of vitamin repletion.[51]

Based on these data, and the experience that patients on the every-other-week pralatrexate schedule appeared to experience cytokinetic failures, a revised weekly schedule phase I was performed, revealing a maximum tolerated dose of 30 mg/m^2 weekly for 6 of 7 consecutive weeks. To date, of 20 patients treated with pralatrexate, four CRs have been seen. All CRs were in patients with T-cell lymphoma, with no responses yet in B-cell lymphoma. These remissions have proved durable, with some patients sustaining a response for nearly 18 months.[51] These results are even more provocative when one considers the subtypes of T-cell lymphoma that have responded, including patients with $\gamma\,\delta$-panniculitic T-cell lymphoma, human T-lymphotropic virus type 1 (HTLV-1)–associated ATLL, peripheral T-cell lymphoma not otherwise specified, and T-cell lymphoblastic lymphoma. Both the patients with T-cell lymphomablastic lymphoma and $\gamma\,\delta$-panniculitic T-cell lymphoma developed progressive disease either on, or shortly after, a course of methotrexate,

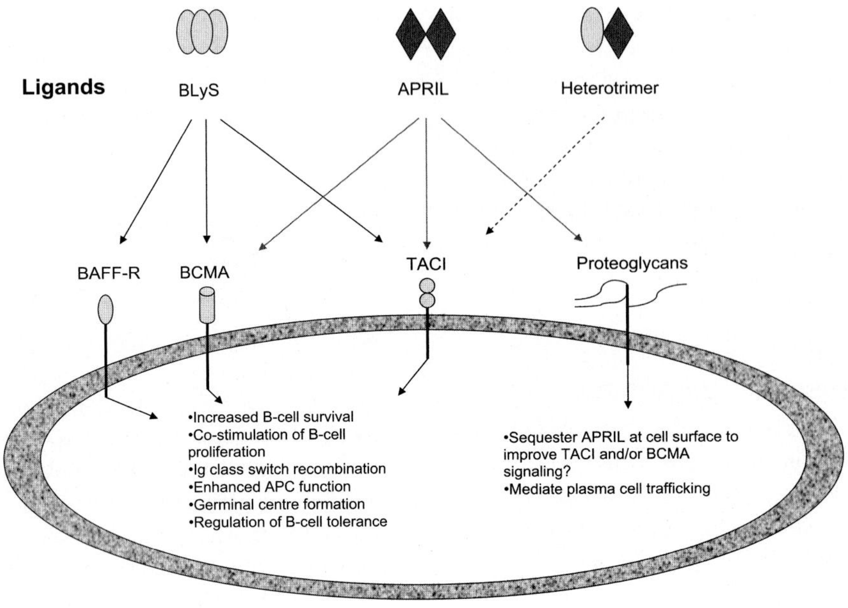

Figure 3 Schematic of BLyS and APRIL and their interactions with TNF family.

suggesting some non–cross-resistant mechanisms of action with pralatrexate.

While admittedly early, these data suggest that pralatrexate exhibits an unusually restricted spectrum of activity against T-cell lymphomas. If pralatrexate was functioning merely as a more potent form of methotrexate, one would reasonably expect some demonstration of activity in B-cell lymphomas. These findings are now giving rise to speculation that there may be alternative pathways in T-cell diseases that may account for some of this differential activity. Additional preclinical and clinical studies are now focusing on the mechanistic basis for this dramatic and unusual spectrum of activity.

Targeting Unique Survival Pathways in B-Cell Survival: Inhibiting the B-Cell Lymphocyte Stimulator and APRIL Pathways

Targeting Unique Survival Pathways Exclusive to B-Cell Lymphomas

One recently novel target that has emerged as a potentially important therapeutic avenue in the treatment of B-cell lymphomas revolves around the role the tumor necrosis factor (TNF) family members play in B-cell development and homeostasis. The TNF family consists of 19 different ligands and 29 different receptors that modulate a panoply of biologic functions, ranging from regulation of cell activation to apoptosis. Recently, two new ligands have been described, including B-lymphocyte stimulator (BLyS; also known as B-cell activating factor of the TNF family [BAFF]) and a proliferation-inducing ligand (APRIL). These ligands are TNF family members that appear to be critical for the maintenance of normal B-cell development and homeostasis. Interestingly, overexpression of BLyS in transgenic mice results in the development of autoimmune-like syndromes resembling systemic lupus erythematosus and Sjögren's syndrome. These mice also develop elevated numbers of circulating B lymphocytes, although they do not appear to be clonal.[52-54] However, BLyS does appear to be important in the growth and survival of malignant B cells and can be elaborated by both normal (different leukocytes, including monocytes, macrophages, dendritic cells, and neutrophils) and malignant cells in an autocrine type fashion. BLyS has been shown to bind to the surface of malignant B cells from patients with chronic lymphocytic leukemia, various forms of NHL, and cells from patients with multiple myeloma.[55,56]

BLyS is thought to bind to three separate receptors, including the B-cell maturation antigen (BCMA), the transmembrane activator and CAML interactor (TACI), and the BAFF-receptor (BAFF-R).[57] BCMA and BAFF-R are usually found on B lymphocytes, while TACI is found on both B and activated T cells as well. The binding of BLyS to TACI has been shown to activate the nuclear factor-κB (NFκB), which in and of itself can contribute to the malignant phenotype by augmenting cellular growth and inhibiting apoptosis. In addition to the ability of the BLyS and APRIL homodimers to bind various ligands, it is now clear that these two ligands can form heterodimers, which appear to only bind TACI as shown in Fig 3.

To date, several biotechnology companies have begun to focus their efforts on designing and developing strategies to neutralize the biological activity of APRIL and/or BLyS. For example, Belimumab (LymphoStat-B) is a human anti-BLyS monoclonal antibody developed collaboratively between GlaxoSmithKline (GSK) and Human Genome Sciences (HGS). This antibody has been tested in phase II trials in a number of autoimmune disorders, including systemic lupus erythematosus and rheumatoid arthritis. The observation that TACI-immunoglobulin (TACI-Ig), and not BCMA-Ig or BAFF-Ig, can neutralize the biologic activity of the BLyS–APRIL heterodimers has raised the interesting prospect that this antibody could be used as a potential therapeutic agent in B-cell lymphomas. TACI-Ig binds to APRIL with a K_D of 0.45 to 1.5 nmol/L, while the K_D for BLyS has been shown to be in the range of 0.16 to 0.79 nmol/L. Currently, TACI-Ig is in phase I trials in systemic lupus erythematosus, multiple myeloma, chronic lymphocytic leukemia, and other subtypes of NHL. Phase Ib trials are underway in rheumatoid arthritis.

While only in its infancy, it is clear that our ever-expanding understanding of the complex biology that governs lymphocyte ontogeny is paving the way for more innovative strategies to assault the fundamental biology of malignant lymphoma. While it is too early to comment on whether these agents will be integrated into future standards of care, it is likely that future approaches to the treatment of aggressive lymphomas will involve a rationally orchestrated combination of agents that will adversely affect very specific growth and survival pathways in discrete subtypes of lymphoma.

New Developments in Arming CD20 Targeted Monoclonal Antibodies With Radioisotopes for the Treatment of Aggressive Large B-Cell Lymphoma

The CD20 B-cell antigen represents an ideal target for immunotherapy. It is present on more than 90% of B-cell malignancies, it is not shed into the cytoplasm or internalized, and it does not appear to undergo significant modulation. Initially approved for use in indolent lymphomas, rituximab (Rituxan, Genentech/Biogen-IDEC) received US Food and Drug Administration (FDA) approval for use in combination with anthracycline containing chemotherapy for the upfront treatment of DLBCL in 2006 (Rituximab PI, 2006). This approval was based on demonstrated improvements in outcome measures in DLBCL for both elderly (≥60 years)[58-60] and low risk (International Prognostic Index [IPI] = 0 or 1) younger patients (age 18 to 59 years).[61] Efforts to build upon this successful strategy have sought to exploit the benefits of targeted immunotherapy with continuous low-dose-rate irradiation in the form of the therapeutic radioimmunoconjugates, called radioimmunotherapy (RIT).

Currently available radioimmunoconjugates use the tumor-targeting capabilities of murine anti-CD20 monoclonal antibodies to deliver cytotoxic radiation via some radionuclide to targeted B cells, ultimately exploiting both the immune-mediated cell killing (antibody-dependent cellular cytoxicity [ADCC]) of the naked antibody and the cytotoxic effects of the radiotherapy . There is also evidence that antibody binding to the CD20 antigen may augment the pro-apoptotic effects of radiation.[62] Additionally, radionuclides exert their cytotoxic effects via the emission of ionizing radiation, which occurs in a sphere whose volume is determined by the path length of the relevant isotope. In this manner, RIT has the advantage of targeting not only the cell to which the antibody is bound, but also the neighboring cells and tumor microenvironment. The two FDA-approved agents are yttrium-90–labeled ibritumomab tiuxetan (Zevalin, Biogen-IDEC) and iodine-131 tositumomab (^{131}I-tositumomab, Bexxar, GSK), indicated for the treatment of relapsed and transformed indolent lymphoma. Based on a clear biologic rationale and evidence of activity in DLBCL and transformed indolent lymphoma, the integration of these agents into the DLBCL treatment paradigm is currently being explored.

In the initial phase I/II trial of ^{90}Y ibritumomab tiuxetan, the reported response rate for the subset with relapsed DLBCL was 43%.[63] Zelenetz reviewed the experience with ^{131}I-tositumomab in patients with transformed NHL not eligible for stem cell transplantation.[64] In this setting, 71 patients across five reported trials were identified, with single-agent activity demonstrating an overall response rate of 39% and a CR rate of 25% at 19.4 months median follow-up. For responding patients, the median time to progression was 20.2 months (12.4 months to not reported). This initial experience formed the basis for a dedicated single agent ^{90}Y ibritumomab tiuxetan study in relapsed and refractory elderly DLBCL patients not eligible for stem cell transplantation.[65] The preliminary report demonstrated a response in 44% of 104 patients. Progression-free survival differed based on prior rituximab exposure, with rituximab-naive patients having progression-free survival of 5.9 months, compared with only 1.6 months for rituximab-exposed patients.

Given the modest activity as a single agent in the relapsed and refractory setting, and the current ubiquitous use of rituximab in the upfront treatment program, new strategies in DLBCL are focusing on the integration of RIT into sequential programs with chemotherapy as part of the conditioning regimens for autologous stem cell transplant (ASCT). Hamlin et al reported early efficacy and safety results of a phase II study evaluating the sequential application of RCHOP (rituxamab, cyclophosphamide, doxorubicin, vincristine, prednisone) for six cycles followed by ^{90}Y ibritumomab tiuxetan 6 to 9 weeks later in high-risk (age-adjusted [aa]IPI = 2 and 3) elderly patients not eligible for ASCT.[66] This strategy is designed to utilize the RIT as a means to eradicate minimal residual disease post chemotherapy. The median age of the 26 evaluable patients was 75 years (range, 65 to 85), with aaIPI high-intermediate risk disease present in 46% and high-risk disease present in 54%; stage IV disease was present in 88.5% and more than half of the patients had a Karnofsky performance status score below 80% (median, 70%; range, 60% to 90%). At a median follow-up of 19 months, the overall survival for all patients by intent to treat was 63%, with an event-free survival of 59%. All patients who received RIT remained relapse free at a median follow-up of 21 months; one patient died of suspected CNS hemorrhage at week 7 post RIT. This strategy appears feasible and relatively safe, and is currently being evaluated in an international randomized phase III study for all risk levels of elderly DLBCL. In a phase II study, Gopal et al used myeloablative doses of ^{131}I tositumomab tiuxetan (25 to 27 Gy to critical normal organs) as the conditioning regimen of a HDT/ASCT program for elderly (age ≥60 years) B-cell lymphoma patients with high-risk relapsed or refractory disease.[67] In an early report on 24 patients, they have demonstrated the feasibility of this approach, with a median time to platelet (defined as >20,000/μL) and neutrophil (absolute neutophil count >500/μL) engraftment of 10 and 15 days, respectively. With a median follow-up of 2.2 years, 42% are alive and progression-free; 38% of patients had DLBCL in this study.

These initial reports are encouraging, in that the integration of RIT into existing treatment schemas appears feasible and potentially efficacious, likely offering greater therapeutic benefit than single-agent drugs in these diseases. As more definitive studies in DLBCL are presently underway, attempts to augment the cytotoxic effects of RIT further by combining it with radiosensitizers are now being explored. For example, mouse models of DLBCL suggest potential benefit for use of the proteasome inhibitor bortezomib in conjunction with ^{90}Y ibritumomab tiuxetan,[68] which is now being studied in phase I clinical trials. Likewise, motexafin gadolinium (MGd), a radiosensitizer known to modulate intracellular redox potentials, appears to be complementary with radiotherapy, which has led to early phase dose-finding trials.

Collectively, these data are encouraging in that they provide a variety of new strategies by which we can modulate important intracellular growth and survival pathways in a fashion that should improve our ability to cure more patients with these diseases.

Summary

There has probably never been a more exciting time to work in the field of cancer drug discovery and development. As we develop an ever-increasing appreciation of the fundamental biology of these complex lymphoproliferative diseases, it is certain we will discover new avenues and opportunities to perturb and inhibit those essential pathways that render malignant cells malignant. The challenge, of course, will be to try to optimize the use of our new agents as best as possible, in realistic preclinical models, where an emphasis on the general principles of pharmacology will guide successful clinical development. Understanding the often subtle and intimate relationships that exist between pharmacokinetic and pharmacodynamic factors and optimal antineoplastic activity will advance our ability to translate sound preclinical observations into sound clinical practice. However, what remains rate limiting in this remarkable process is clearly not our ability to discover new and interesting biology, or even our ability to identify new agents, it is our ability to accrue patients to important clinical trials in a timely fashion.

References

1. Ye BH, Lista F, Lo Coco F, et al: Alterations of a zinc finger-encoding gene, BCL-6, in diffuse large-cell lymphoma. Science 262:747-750, 1993
2. Ye BH, Rao PH, Chaganti RS, et al: Cloning of bcl-6, the locus involved in chromosome translocations affecting band 3q27 in B-cell lymphoma. Cancer Res 53:2732-2735, 1993
3. Ye BH, Chaganti S, Chang CC, et al: Chromosomal translocations cause deregulated BCL6 expression by promoter substitution in B cell lymphoma. EMBO J 14:6209-62017, 1995
4. Dent AL, Shaffer AL, Yu X, et al: Control of inflammation, cytokine expression, and germinal center formation by BCL-6. Science 276:589-592, 1997
5. Shaffer AL, Yu X, He Y, et al: BCL-6 represses genes that function in lymphocyte differentiation, inflammation, and cell cycle control. Immunity 13:199-212, 2000
6. Pasqualucci L, Bereschenko O, Niu H, et al: Molecular pathogenesis of non-Hodgkin's lymphoma: The role of Bcl-6. Leuk Lymphoma 44:S5-S12, 2003 (suppl 3)
7. Capello D, Vitolo U, Pasqualucci L, et al: Distribution and pattern of BCL-6 mutations throughout the spectrum of B-cell neoplasia. Blood 95:651-659, 2000
8. Bereshchenko OR, Gu W, Dalla-Favera R: Acetylation inactivates the transcriptional repressor BCL6. Nat Genet 32:606-613, 2002
9. Luo J, Nikolaev AY, Imai S, et al: Negative control of p53 by Sir2alpha promotes cell survival under stress. Cell 107:137-148, 2001
10. Vaziri H, Dessain SK, Ng Eaton E, et al: hSIR2(SIRT1) functions as an NAD-dependent p53 deacetylase. Cell 107:149-159, 2001
11. Imai S, Armstrong CM, Kaeberlein M, et al: Transcriptional silencing and longevity protein Sir2 is an NAD-dependent histone deacetylase. Nature 403:795-800, 2000
12. Kelly WK, O'Connor OA, Marks PA: Histone deacetylase inhibitors: from target to clinical trials. Expert Opin Investig Drugs 11:1695-1713, 2002
13. Kelly WK, Richon VM, O'Connor O, et al: Phase I clinical trial of histone deacetylase inhibitor: Suberoylanilide hydroxamic acid administered intravenously. Clin Cancer Res 9:3578-3588, 2003
14. O'Connor OA, Heaney ML, Schwartz L, et al: Clinical experience with intravenous and oral formulations of the novel histone deacetylase inhibitor suberoylanilide hydroxamic acid in patients with advanced hematologic malignancies. J Clin Oncol 24:166-173, 2006
15. Kelly WK, O'Connor OA, Krug LM, et al: Phase I study of an oral histone deacetylase inhibitor, suberoylanilide hydroxamic acid, in patients with advanced cancer. J Clin Oncol 23:3923-3931, 2005
16. Piekarz RL, Robey RW, Zhan Z, et al: T-cell lymphoma as a model for the use of histone deacetylase inhibitors in cancer therapy: impact of depsipeptide on molecular markers, therapeutic targets, and mechanisms of resistance. Blood 103:4636-4643, 2004
17. Piekarz RL, Robey R, Sandor V, et al: Inhibitor of histone deacetylation, depsipeptide (FR901228), in the treatment of peripheral and cutaneous T-cell lymphoma: A case report. Blood 98:2865-2868, 2001
18. Duvic MTR, Zhang C, Goy A, Richon V, Frankel S: Phase II trial of oral suberoylanilide hydroxamic acid (SAHA) for cutaneous T-cell lymphoma (CTCL) unresponsive to conventional therapy. J Clin Oncol 23, 16S, 2005 (abstr 6571)
19. Ryan QC, Headlee D, Acharya M, et al: Phase I and pharmacokinetic study of MS-275, a histone deacetylase inhibitor, in patients with advanced and refractory solid tumors or lymphoma. J Clin Oncol 23: 3912-3922, 2005
20. Prive GG, Melnick A, Ahmad KF, Licht JD: The BTB domain zinc finger proteins, in Iuchi S, Kuldell N (eds): Zinc Finger Proteins: From Atomic Contact to Cellular Function. Austin, TX, Landes Bioscience, 2005.
21. Polo JM, Dell'Oso T, Ranuncolo SM, et al: Specific peptide interference reveals BCL6 transcriptional and oncogenic mechanisms in B-cell lymphoma cells. Nat Med 10:1329-1335, 2004
22. Reed JC: Dysregulation of apoptosis in cancer. J Clin Oncol 17:2941-2953, 1999
23. Reed JC: Bcl-2 and the regulation of programmed cell death. J Cell Biol 124:1-6, 1994
24. Cleary ML, Smith SD, Sklar J: Cloning and structural analysis of cDNAs for bcl-2 and a hybrid bcl-2/immunoglobulin transcript resulting from the t(14;18) translocation. Cell 47:19-28, 1986
25. Tsujimoto Y, Gorham J, Cossman J, et al: The t(14;18) chromosome translocations involved in B-cell neoplasms result from mistakes in VDJ joining. Science 229:1390-1393, 1985
26. Tsujimoto Y, Croce CM: Analysis of the structure, transcripts, and protein products of bcl-2, the gene involved in human follicular lymphoma. Proc Natl Acad Sci U S A 83:5214-5218, 1986
27. Yang J, Liu X, Bhalla K, et al: Prevention of apoptosis by Bcl-2: Release of cytochrome c from mitochondria blocked. Science 275:1129-1132, 1997
28. Kluck RM, Bossy-Wetzel E, Green DR, et al: The release of cytochrome

c from mitochondria: A primary site for Bcl-2 regulation of apoptosis. Science 275:1132-1136, 1997
29. Rai K, Wallace P, Soho C, Landrigan B, Meyn P, Wei T, et al: Efficacy and safety of the combination of genasense fludarabine and rituximab in previously treated and untreated subjects with chronic lymphocytic leukemia. Blood 106, 2005 (abstr 2129)
30. O'Brien SM, Cunningham CC, Golenkov AK, et al: Phase I to II multicenter study of oblimersen sodium, a Bcl-2 antisense oligonucleotide, in patients with advanced chronic lymphocytic leukemia. J Clin Oncol 23:7697-7702, 2005
31. O'Connor OA, Smith EA, Toner LE, et al: The combination of the proteasome inhibitor bortezomib and the bcl-2 antisense molecule oblimersen sensitizes human B-cell lymphomas to cyclophosphamide. Clin Cancer Res 12:2902-2911, 2006
32. Wu D: An overview of the clinical pharmacology and therapeutic potential of gossypol as a male contraceptive agent and in gynaecological disease. Drugs 38:333-341, 1989
33. Tuszynski GP, Cossu G: Differential cytotoxic effect of gossypol on human melanoma, colon carcinoma, and other tissue culture cell lines. Cancer Res 44:768-771, 1984
34. Coyle T, Levante S, Shetler M, et al: In vitro and in vivo cytotoxicity of gossypol against central nervous system tumor cell lines. J Neurooncol 19:25-35, 1994
35. Gilbert NE, O'Reilly JE, Chang CJ, et al: Antiproliferative activity of gossypol and gossypolone on human breast cancer cells. Life Sci 57: 61-67, 1995
36. Wang X, Wang J, Wong SC, et al: Cytotoxic effect of gossypol on colon carcinoma cells. Life Sci 67:2663-2671, 2000
37. Flack MR, Pyle RG, Mullen NM, et al: Oral gossypol in the treatment of metastatic adrenal cancer. J Clin Endocrinol Metab 76:1019-1024, 1993
38. Van Poznak C, Seidman AD, Reidenberg MM, et al: Oral gossypol in the treatment of patients with refractory metastatic breast cancer: A phase I/II clinical trial. Breast Cancer Res Treat 66:239-248, 2001
39. Bushunow P, Reidenberg MM, Wasenko J, et al: Gossypol treatment of recurrent adult malignant gliomas. J Neurooncol 43:79-86, 1999
40. Liu S, Kulp SK, Sugimoto Y, et al: The (−)-enantiomer of gossypol possesses higher anticancer potency than racemic gossypol in human breast cancer. Anticancer Res 22:33-38, 2002
41. Oliver CL, Bauer JA, Wolter KG, et al: In vitro effects of the BH3 mimetic, (−)-gossypol, on head and neck squamous cell carcinoma cells. Clin Cancer Res 10:7757-7763, 2004
42. Paoluzzi L, Gonen M, Toner L, Smith E, Yang D, Holmund J, et al: Targeting antiapoptotic BcL-2 family members with AT-101 in preclinical models of aggressive lymphoma in combination with cyclophosphamide (C) and rituximab (R) produces a marked improvement in therapeutic efficacy. Blood 106, 2005 (abstr 926)
43. Oltersdorf T, Elmore SW, Shoemaker AR, et al: An inhibitor of Bcl-2 family proteins induces regression of solid tumours. Nature 435:677-681, 2005
44. Petros AM, Dinges J, Augeri DJ, et al: Discovery of a potent inhibitor of the antiapoptotic protein Bcl-xL from NMR and parallel synthesis. J Med Chem 49:656-663, 2006
45. Sirotnak FM, DeGraw JI, Moccio DM, et al: New folate analogs of the 10-deaza-aminopterin series. Basis for structural design and biochemical and pharmacologic properties. Cancer Chemother Pharmacol 12: 18-25, 1984
46. Wang ES, O'Connor O, She Y, et al: Activity of a novel anti-folate (PDX, 10-propargyl 10-deazaaminopterin) against human lymphoma is superior to methotrexate and correlates with tumor RFC-1 gene expression. Leuk Lymphoma 44:1027-1035, 2003
47. Sirotnak FM, DeGraw JI, Chello PL, et al: Biochemical and pharmacologic properties of a new folate analog, 10-deaza-aminopterin, in mice. Cancer Treat Rep 66:351-358, 1982
48. Sirotnak FM: Obligate genetic expression in tumor cells of a fetal membrane property mediating "folate" transport: Biological significance and implications for improved therapy of human cancer. Cancer Res 45: 3992-4000, 1985
49. Chiao JH, Roy K, Tolner B, et al: RFC-1 gene expression regulates folate absorption in mouse small intestine. J Biol Chem 272:11165-11170, 1997
50. DeGraw JI, Colwell WT, Piper JR, et al: Synthesis and antitumor activity of 10-propargyl-10-deazaaminopterin. J Med Chem 36:2228-2231, 1993
51. O'Connor OA, Hamlin P, Neylon E, Moskowitz C, Portlock C, Straus D, et al: Pralatrexate (10-Propargyl-10-Deazaaminopterin(PRX)), a novel antifolate, effects durable complete remissions (CR) in patients with a diversity of drug resistant T-cell lymphomas with minimal toxicity. Blood 106, 2005 (abstr 2678)
52. Mackay F, Woodcock SA, Lawton P, et al: Mice transgenic for BAFF develop lymphocytic disorders along with autoimmune manifestations. J Exp Med 190:1697-1710, 1999
53. Do RK, Hatada E, Lee H, et al: Attenuation of apoptosis underlies B lymphocyte stimulator enhancement of humoral immune response. J Exp Med 192:953-964, 2000
54. Khare SD, Sarosi I, Xia XZ, et al: Severe B cell hyperplasia and autoimmune disease in TALL-1 transgenic mice. Proc Natl Acad Sci U S A 97:3370-3375, 2000
55. Novak AJ, Grote DM, Ziesmer SC, et al: Elevated serum B-lymphocyte stimulator levels in patients with familial lymphoproliferative disorders. J Clin Oncol 24:983-987, 2006
56. Elsawa SF, Novak AJ, Grote DM, et al: B-lymphocyte stimulator (BLyS) stimulates immunoglobulin production and malignant B-cell growth in Waldenstrom macroglobulinemia. Blood 107:2882-2888, 2006
57. Dillon SR, Gross JA, Ansell SM, et al: An APRIL to remember: Novel TNF ligands as therapeutic targets. Nat Rev Drug Discov 5:235-246, 2006
58. Coiffier B, Lepage E, Briere J, et al: CHOP chemotherapy plus rituximab compared with CHOP alone in elderly patients with diffuse large-B-cell lymphoma. N Engl J Med 346:235-242, 2002
59. Feugier P, Van Hoof A, Sebban C, et al: Long-term results of the R-CHOP study in the treatment of elderly patients with diffuse large B-cell lymphoma: A study by the Groupe d'Etude des Lymphomes de l'Adulte. J Clin Oncol 23:4117-4126, 2005
60. Habermann TWE, Morrison VA, Cassileth PA, Cohn J, Dakhil S, Gascoyne RD, et al: Rituximab-CHOP versus CHOP with or without maintenance rituximab in patients 60 years of age or older with diffuse large B-cell lymphoma (DLBCL). Blood 104:40a, 2004 (abstr)
61. Pfreundschuh M, Trumper L, Osterborg A, et al: CHOP-like chemotherapy plus rituximab versus CHOP-like chemotherapy alone in young patients with good-prognosis diffuse large-B-cell lymphoma: A randomised controlled trial by the MabThera International Trial (MInT) Group. Lancet Oncol 7:379-391, 2006
62. Skvortsova I, Popper BA, Skvortsov S, et al: Pretreatment with rituximab enhances radiosensitivity of non-Hodgkin's lymphoma cells. J Radiat Res (Tokyo) 46:241-248, 2005
63. Witzig TE, White CA, Wiseman GA, et al: Phase I/II trial of IDEC-Y2B8 radioimmunotherapy for treatment of relapsed or refractory CD20(+) B-cell non-Hodgkin's lymphoma. J Clin Oncol 17:3793-3803, 1999
64. Zelenetz A, Salen M, Vose J, Younes A, Kaminski M: Patients with transformed low grade lymphoma attain durable responses following out-patient radioimmunotherapy with tositumomab and iodine I 131 tositumomab. Blood 100:357, 2002 (abstr 1384)
65. Morschhauser F, Huglo D, Martinelli G: Yttrium-90 ibrituomomab tiuxetan (Zevalin) for patients with relapsed/refractory diffuse large b-cell lymphoma not appropriate for autologous stem cell transplantation: results of an open-label phase II trial. Blood 104:41a, 2004 (abstr)
66. Hamlin P, Moskowitz CH, Wegner B: Early safety and efficacy analysis of a phase II study of sequential R-CHOP and yttrium-90 ibritumomab tiuxetan (Zevalin) for elderly high risk patients with untreated DLBCL. Blood 106, 2005 (abstr 926)
67. Gopal A, Rajendran J, Gooley TA, Pagel J, Fisher D, Petersdorf S, et al: A phase II study of myeloablative I-131-anti-CD20 (tositumomab) radioimmunotherapy (RIT) and autologous hematopoietic stem cell transplantation (ASCT) for adults ≥ 60 years of age with high-risk, relapsed, or refractory B-cell lymphoma. Blood 106, 2005 (abstr 487)
68. Pervan Milena JC, Matso D, et al: Active combination therapy of bortezomib (Velcade) and ibritumomab tiuxetan (Zevalin) in an in vivo diffuse large B-cell lymphoma model. Blood 2005

ELSEVIER

Seminars in HEMATOLOGY

AUTHOR INDEX

Alter, B.P., 147
Antin, J.H., 24

Bagby, G.C., 145, 147
Bow, E.J., 134
Bowen, D.T., 82
Burnett, A.K., 96

Caligiuri, M.A., 118
Chao, N.J., 32
Chen, B.J., 32
Coiffier, B., 213
Cooke, K.R., 42

Dale, D.C., 189
de Lima, M., 107
Deeg, H.J., 24
Dokal, I., 157

Edinger, M., 62
Estey, E.H., 89

Farag, S.S., 118

Ferrara, J.L.M., 1, 3
Fisher, R.I., 205
Forman, S.J., 240

Geddis, A.E., 196
Gilman, A.L., 70
Gingerich, J., 134
Giralt, S., 107

Hamlin, P., 251
Held, G., 221
Hoffmann, P., 62

Larson, R.A., 126
Levine, J.E., 1, 53
Lipton, J.M., 167

Malkki, M., 11
Miller, T.P., 207
Mohite, U., 96

Nadamanee, A., 240

O'Connor, O.A., 251

Petersdorf, E.W., 11
Pfreundschuh, M., 221
Porter, D., 53

Reddy, P., 3
Rimsza, L., 207
Reiser, M., 221

Schubert, J., 221
Serody, J., 70
Shimamura, A., 178
Spier, M.C., 207

Vulliamy, T., 157

Welte, K., 189
Wilson, W.H., 230

Yanik, G., 42

Zeidler, C., 189

SUBJECT INDEX

ABT-737, for advanced-stage DLBCL, 255
Acute leukemia. *See* Leukemia, acute
Acute lung injury. *See* Idiopathic pneumonia syndrome
Acute lymphoblastic leukemia (ALL), in the elderly
  age-related differences
    clinical and biologic, 126-128
    cytogenetic, 128
  challenge of Ph^+ ALL, 130-131
  newer drugs, 131-132
  patient management, 129-130
  prospective clinical trials, 128-129
Acute myelogenous leukemia. *See* Acute myeloid leukemia
Acute myeloid leukemia (AML), in the elderly
  etiology
    biology, 82-83
    demographics, 82
    environmental and occupational exposures, 83-84
    inflammatory/infectious disorders, 84
    lifestyle factors, 84
    and MDS, therapy-related, 84-86
    molecular epidemiology, 84
  immunotherapy for, 118-125
    ADCC, 122
    biology of NK cells, 119-120

Acute myeloid leukemia (AML), in the elderly (*Continued*)
      blockade of inhibitory interactions between NK cells and leukemia cells, 122
      cytokine therapy, 120-121
      novel approaches to improve, 121-122
    KIR mismatched allogeneic NK cells, 122-123
  introduction, 81
  investigational therapy for newly-diagnosed disease
    delaying the start of therapy, 93
    new response criteria, 93-94
    perspectives on clinical trial methodology, 94
    rationale, 89-91
    role of allogeneic SCT, 91
    types of, 92
  or MDS, allogeneic transplantation for
    immunologic senescence, 109
    impact of aging on incidence and biology of, 107-108
    impact of comorbidities, 109-110
    nonmyeloablative and reduced-intensity regimens, 108-109
    preparative regimen intensity, 110-112
    therapy results, 108
    timing of, and effect of selection bias, 112-114
    unsolved controversies, 114-115
  new drugs
    antibody-directed treatment, 99-100

Acute myeloid leukemia (AML), in the elderly (*Continued*)
clofarabine, 100
in combination, 101
cloretazine, 101
farnesyl transferase inhibitors, 102-103
FLT-3 inhibitors, 101-102
low-dose Ara-C, 96-98
MLN518, 102
for modulating drug resistance
cyclosporine, 98
PSC-833, 98-99
new approaches to trial design, 103
PKC412, 102
SU5416, 102
SU11248, 102
ACVBP therapy
for advanced-stage DLBCL, 225
for aggressive NHL with limited disease, 209-210
ADCC. *See* Antibody-dependent cellular cytotoxicity
Aging, impact on incidence and biology of AML and MDS, 107-108
Alemtuzumab, for ALL in the elderly, 131-132
ALL. *See* Acute lymphoblastic leukemia
Allogeneic stem cell transplantation
for advanced-stage DLBCL-B, 247
investigational, for newly-diagnosed AML in the elderly, 91
Allogeneic transplantation, for AML or MDS in the elderly
immunologic senescence, 109
impact of aging on incidence and biology of, 107-108
impact of comorbidities, 109-110
nonmyeloablative and reduced-intensity regimens, 108-109
preparative regimen intensity, 110-112
therapy results, 108
timing of, and effect of selection bias, 112-114
unsolved controversies, 114-115
AML. *See* Acute myeloid leukemia
AMN107, for ALL in the elderly, 131-132
Androgen therapy, for FA, 153
Anthracycline, plus cytarabine, for newly-diagnosed AML in the elderly, inadequacy of, 89-91
Antibody-dependent cellular cytotoxicity (ADCC), for AML in the elderly, 122
Antibody-directed therapy, for AML in the elderly, 99-100
Anti-CD20 monoclonal antibodies, with radioisotopes for advanced-stage DLBCL, 259-260
Aplastic anemia, and DC, TERT mutations in, 162-163
Apoptosis, role in drug resistance in DLBCL, 233-235
Ara-C. *See* Cytarabine
ASCT. *See* Autologous stem cell transplantation
AT-101, for advanced-stage DLBCL, 255
Autologous stem cell transplantation (ASCT)
for advanced-stage DLBCL, with high-dose chemotherapy, 222-223
for advanced-stage DLBCL-B
consolidative transplantation, 244-246
in elderly patients, 246-247
with high-dose chemotherapy, 241-242
with radioimmunotherapy, 242-244
with rituximab, 242
Autologous transplantation, acute GVHD after, 28
Autosomal recessive dyskeratosis congenita, 163
Bcl-2, in advanced-stage DLBCL
biologic significance of, 254
targeted drugs, 254-255
Bcl-2, in advanced-stage DLBCL (*Continued*)
Bcl-6, in advanced-stage DLBCL
biologic significance of, 252-253
inhibition with HDAC inhibitors, 253-254
Belimumab (LymphoStat-B), for advanced-stage DLBCL, 258-259
Benzene exposure, as risk factor of AML in the elderly, 83
Blood counts, in severe CN diagnosis, 191
B-lymphocyte stimulator, targeting of, in advanced-stage DLBCL, 258-259
BMS354825. *See* Dasatinib
Bone marrow, morphology in severe CN diagnosis, 191
Bone marrow diseases. *See also specific diseases*
introduction, 145-146

CAMT. *See* Congenital amegakaryocytic thrombocytopenia
Cancer, and DBA, 172
$CD4^+CD25^+$ regulatory T cells, and GVHD, 62-69
in clinical HSCT, 66-67
in murine models, 64-66
Cell cycle regulation, role in drug resistance in DLBCL, 233-235
Chemotherapy, high-dose, with ASCT
for advanced-stage DLBCL, 222-223
for advanced-stage DLBCL-B, 241-242
Chronic myelogenous leukemia (CML), GVL and GVHD after DLI for, 53-54
Chronic obstructive lung disease, after HSCT
definition, clinical course and risk factors, 47-48
pathogenesis, 48
treatment, 49
Clofarabine, for elderly patients
with ALL, 131-132
with AML, 100-101
Cloretazine, for AML in the elderly, 101
CMA-676. *See* Gemtuzumab ozogamicin
CML. *See* Chronic myelogenous leukemia
CN. *See* Congenital neutropenia
Compound 506U78. *See* Nelarabine
Congenital amegakaryocytic thrombocytopenia (CAMT), 198-199
treatment, 200-201
Congenital anomalies, in DBA, 171
Congenital neutropenia (CN), severe, 189-195
complications
leukemia, 193-194
osteoporosis, 194
splenomegaly, 194
diagnosis
blood counts, 191
bone marrow, 191
cytogenetic evaluation and molecular testing, 191-192
differential, 192
onset of symptoms, 192
pathophysiology, 190-191
patient monitoring, 194
treatment, 192
Congenital thrombocytopenia. *See* Inherited thrombocytopenia
Cord blood stem cell transplantation, role of HLA in risk of GVHD, 14-15
Corticosteroids
for acute GVHD, 37-38
for DBA, 172-173
outcomes, 173-174
Cyclophosphamide, with doxorubicin, vincristine and prednisone
for advanced-stage DLBCL
plus etoposide, 222

Cyclophosphamide, with doxorubicin, vincristine and prednisone (*Continued*)
dose densification, 224
plus rituximab, 225-227
for aggressive NHL with limited disease, 209-210
Cyclosporine
for chronic GVHD, 76
for modulating drug resistance in AML in the elderly, 98
Cytarabine (Ara-C), for AML in the elderly
low-dose, 96-98
plus anthracycline, inadequacy for newly-diagnosed disease, 89-91
Cytokines
for AML in the elderly, 120-121
novel approaches to improve immunotherapy, 121-122
axis, in pathophysiology of experimental IPS following allogeneic HSCT, 45-46
in GVHD
pathophysiology of, 5
risk of
genetic diversity, 16-17
IL-10, 17-19
sequence polymorphism of genes, 17
TNF-α, 17
Dasatinib (BMS354825), for ALL in the elderly, 131-132
Daunorubicin, liposomal, for ALL in the elderly, 132
DBA. *See* Diamond Blackfan anemia
DC. *See* Dyskeratosis congenita
Diamond Blackfan anemia (DBA), 167-177
cancer and, 172
congenital anomalies in, 171
diagnosis, 170
pathophysiology and genetics, 168-169
treatment
corticosteroids, 172-173
outcomes and, 173-174
red cell transfusion, 172-173
SCT, 173
Diet, as risk factor of AML in the elderly, 84
Diffuse large B-cell lymphoma (DLBCL)
advanced-stage
development of dose-dense and dose-intense regimens, 213-214
DLBCL-B. *See* Diffuse large B-cell lymphoma-B
dose-intensified treatment, 221-229
dose densification, 224
dose escalation with dose densification, 225
dose escalation without stem cell support, 222
high-dose chemotherapy with ASCT, 222-223
rituximab, 225-227
good-risk patients, 215-217
intermediate-risk young patients, 217-218
new drugs for, 251-261
CD20 targeted monoclonal antibodies with radioisotopes, 259-260
targeting of Bcl-2, 254-255
targeting of Bcl-6, 252-254
targeting of reduced folate carrier and inhibiting DNA synthesis, 255-257
targeting of unique survival pathways, 258-259
PET for evaluation of response and prognosis, 219
poor-risk patients
elderly, 217
youth, 218
prognostic factors and treatment choice, 213
Diffuse large B-cell lymphoma (DLBCL) (*Continued*)
rituximab, 214-215
very old patients, 218
aggressive NHL with limited disease
biology, 210-211
diagnosis and histology, 207-208
prognostic factors, 208-209
staging, 208
treatment, 209-210
drug resistance in
apoptosis and, 233-235
cell cycle regulation and, 233-235
classical form of, 230-232
microarray analysis, 235-237
pharmacokinetics and, 232
tumor cell kinetics and, 232-233
introduction, 205-206
Diffuse large B-cell lymphoma-B (DLBCL-B), advanced-stage, 240-250
allogeneic stem cell transplantation for, 247
ASCT for
consolidative transplantation, 244-246
elderly patients, 246-247
with high-dose sequential chemotherapy, 241-242
with radioimmunotherapy, 242-244
with rituximab, 242
prognostic factors, 241
DLBCL. *See* Diffuse large B-cell lymphoma
DLBCL-B. *See* Diffuse large B-cell lymphoma-B
DLI. *See* Donor leukocyte infusion
Donor leukocyte infusion (DLI), GVL and GVHD after, 53-61
after reduced intensity transplantation, 56-58
for acute leukemia, 54-55
for CML, 53-54
for Hodgkin's disease, 55
for myeloma, 55
for NHL, 55
tumor-specific DLI, 58
unrelated, 55-56
Doxorubicin, with cyclophosphamide, vincristine and prednisone
for advanced-stage DLBCL
plus etoposide, 222
dose densification, 224
plus rituximab, 225-227
for aggressive NHL with limited disease, 209-210
Dyskeratosis congenita (DC), 157-166
and aplastic anemia, TERT mutations in, 162-163
autosomal recessive form, 163
dyskerin mutations, 159-160
genetics, 158-159
telomerase and, 160
mutations in RNA component of, 160-162

Elderly
ALL in
age-related differences
clinical and biologic, 126-128
cytogenetic, 128
challenge of Ph^+ ALL, 130-131
newer drugs, 131-132
patient management, 129-130
prospective clinical trials, 128-129

Elderly (*Continued*)
AML in
etiology
biology, 82-83
demographics, 82
environmental and occupational exposures, 83-84
inflammatory/infectious disorders, 84
lifestyle factors, 84
and MDS, therapy-related, 84-86
molecular epidemiology, 84
immunotherapy for, 118-125
ADCC, 122
biology of NK cells, 119-120
blockade of inhibitory interactions between NK cells and leukemia cells, 122
cytokine therapy, 120-122
KIR mismatched allogeneic NK cells, 122-123
introduction, 81
investigational therapy for newly-diagnosed disease
delaying the start of therapy, 93
new response criteria, 93-94
perspectives on clinical trial methodology, 94
rationale, 89-91
role of allogeneic SCT, 91
types of, 92
or MDS, allogeneic transplantation for
immunologic senescence, 109
impact of aging on incidence and biology of, 107-108
impact of comorbidities, 109-110
nonmyeloablative and reduced-intensity regimens, 108-109
preparative regimen intensity, 110-112
therapy results, 108
timing of, and effect of selection bias, 112-114
unsolved controversies, 114-115
new drugs
antibody-directed treatment, 99-100
clofarabine, 100-101
cloretazine, 101
farnesyl transferase inhibitors, 102-103
FLT-3 inhibitors, 101-102
low-dose Ara-C, 96-98
MLN518, 102
for modulating drug resistance, 98-99
new approaches to trial design, 103
PKC412, 102
SU5416, 102
SU11248, 102
ASCT for advanced-stage DLBCL-B, 246-247
with poor-risk advanced-stage DLBCL, 217
therapy-related complications of acute leukemia in
defining patient population, 134-135
defining patients for treatment, 137
identifying important age-related physiologic differences, 135-137
treatment
fever, 138-139
infection, 138-139
neutropenia, 138-139
oral and gastrointestinal mucositis, 137-138
pain, 138
role of myeloid growth factors, 137

Elderly (*Continued*)
Engraftment syndrome, in acute GVHD, 27
Environmental exposure, as risk factor of AML in the elderly, 83-84
Etoposide, with vincristine, doxorubicin, cyclophosphamide and prednisone for advanced-stage DLBCL, 222
dose densification, 224
Exocrine pancreatic insufficiency, in SDS, 179
clinical management and treatment, 185
FA. *See* Fanconi anemia
Fanconi anemia (FA)
clinical management, 153
malignancy in, 153-154
diagnosis
clinical, 151
FA without MMC hypersensitivity, 152-153
laboratory, 152
genetic heterogeneity, 147-148
molecular pathogenesis of clonal evolution, 154
non-FA binding partners
GSTP1, 150
heat shock proteins, 149
STAT proteins, 149
prevention, 154
protein complex, 148
structural evidence of molecular multifunctionality, 151
Farnesyl transferase inhibitors, for AML in the elderly, 102-103
Fever, as therapy-related complication of acute leukemia in the elderly, treatment of, 138-139
FLT-3 inhibitors, for AML in the elderly, 101-102
Gastrointestinal mucositis, as therapy-related complication of acute leukemia in the elderly, treatment of, 137-138
Gemtuzumab ozogamicin (CMA-676; Mylotarg), for AML in the elderly, 99-100
Gene therapy, for FA, 153
Gene transfer, retroviral-mediated, for FA diagnosis, 152
Genetic heterogeneity, of FA, 147-148
Graft-versus-host disease (GVHD)
acute
corticosteroid-resistant, treatment of, 38
description and diagnosis, 24-25
intestinal involvement, 26
liver involvement, 25-26
other organ involvement, 26
skin manifestations, 25
time of onset, 25
differential diagnosis, 27
engraftment syndrome in, 27
histopathology, 26-27
new perspectives in the 21st century, 1-2
prophylaxis and treatment, 32-41
allogeneic NK cells, 37
corticosteroids, 37-38
effector phase, 35
insertion of suicide genes, 36
minor histocompatibility antigen-specific T cells, 36
NK T-cells, 37
other supportive approaches, 38
pan T-cell depletion, 35
pretransplant phase, 32-33
removal of alloreactive T cells, 35-36
removal of naive T cells, 36

Graft-versus-host disease (GVHD) (*Continued*)
T cell activation phase, 33-35
risk factors, 27
staging and grading, 27-28
syngeneic and autologous, 28
transfusion-associated, 28-29
$CD4^+CD25^+$ regulatory T cells and, 62-69
in clinical HSCT, 66-67
in murine models, 64-66
chronic
clinical manifestations
eyes, 71
gastrointestinal tract, 72-73
heart, 74
hematologic system, 74
immune system, 74
kidneys, 74
liver, 72
lungs, 73-74
mouth, 71-72
musculoskeletal system, 74
nervous system, 74
skin/hair/nails, 71
vulva/vagina, 74
diagnosis, 70-71
pathophysiology, 74-75
supportive care, 78
treatment, 75-76
cyclosporine, 76
high-dose methylprednisolone, 77
hydroxychloroquine, 77
local, 78
multi-agent approach, 78
mycophenolate mofetil, 76-77
pentostatin, 77
photopheresis, 78
prednisone, 76
recommendations, 78
rituximab, 77
sirolimus, 77
thalidomide, 76
after DLI, 53-61
for acute leukemia, 54-55
approaches to minimize, 58
for CML, 53-54
for Hodgkin's disease, 55
for myeloma, 55
for NHL, 55
in reduced intensity transplantation, 56-58
unrelated, 55-56
pathophysiology, 3-10
cellular and inflammatory effectors, 5-6
donor T-cell activation and cytokine secretion, 5
role of HSCT conditioning, 4-5
risk factors
genetics of, 11-23
in cord blood transplantation, 14-15
cytokine genes, 16-17
cytokines, 16-20
HLA barrier, 11-12

Graft-versus-host disease (GVHD) (*Continued*)
role of NK inhibitory receptors and their ligands, 15-16
translating genomic data to clinical practice, 20
and prevention
blockade of inflammatory stimuli and effectors, 7-8
modulation of donor T cells, 7
reduced intensity conditioning regimens, 6-7
Graft-versus-leukemia effect (GVL)
$CD4^+CD25^+$ regulatory T cells
in murine models, 64-66
after DLI, 53-61
for acute leukemia, 54-55
for CML, 53-54
for Hodgkin's disease, 55
for myeloma, 55
for NHL, 55
in reduced intensity transplantation, 56-58
unrelated, 55-56
Granulocyte-colony stimulating factor, recombinant human, for severe CN, 192
Growth disorders, in SDS, 182
GSTP1, as non-FA binding partners of FA proteins, 150
GVHD. *See* Graft-versus-host disease
GVL. *See* Graft-versus-leukemia effect

HDAC inhibitors. *See* Histone deacetyltransferase (HDAC) inhibitors
Heat shock proteins, as non-FA binding partners of FA proteins, 149
Hematologic diseases, in SDS, 179-182
management and treatment, 185
Hematopoietic stem cell transplantation (HSCT)
chronic obstructive and restrictive lung diseases after
definition, clinical course and risk factors, 47-48
pathogenesis, 48
treatment, 49
clinical, $CD4^+CD25^+$ regulatory T cells in GVHD, 66-67
conditioning, role in GVHD pathophysiology, 4-5
IPS after, 42-52
animal models, 44
definition, clinical course and spectrum, 42-43
etiology, 44
pathophysiology
inflammatory cytokine axis, 45-46
T lymphocyte axis, 44-45
risk factors, 44
treatment strategies, 46-47
reduced intensity, GVHD and GVL after DLI in, 56-58
risk of GVHD in
nonmyeloablative, HLA mismatching in, 14
role of NK inhibitory receptors and their ligands, 15-16
for SDS, 186
for severe CN, 192
unrelated, large-scale analyses of high-resolution donor matching in, 12-13
Histone deacetyltransferase (HDAC) inhibitors, for advanced-stage DLBCL, 253-254
HLA. *See* Human leukocyte antigens
Hodgkin's disease, GVL and GVHD after DLI for, 55
HSCT. *See* Hematopoietic stem cell transplantation
Human leukocyte antigens (HLA), role in risk of GVHD
barrier, 11-12
in cord blood transplantation, 14-15
and KIR, 15-16
mismatches

Human leukocyte antigens (HLA), role in risk of GVHD (*Continued*)
factors that govern permissibility of, 13-14
multiple, additive effects of, 13
in nonmyeloablative HSCT, 14
Hydroxychloroquine, for chronic GVHD, 77
Idiopathic pneumonia syndrome (IPS), after HSCT, 42-52
animal models, 44
definition, clinical course and spectrum, 42-43
etiology, 44
pathophysiology
inflammatory cytokine axis, 45-46
T lymphocyte axis, 44-45
risk factors, 44
treatment strategies, 46-47
Imatinib mesylate, for ALL in the elderly, 131-132
Immune disorders, in SDS, 183
Immunoblotting, for FA diagnosis, 152
Immunotherapy, for AML in the elderly, 118-125
ADCC, 122
biology of NK cells, 119-120
blockade of inhibitory interactions between NK cells and leukemia cells, 122
cytokine therapy, 120-121
novel approaches to improve, 121-122
KIR mismatched allogeneic NK cells, 122-123
Infections
in chronic GVHD, supportive care for, 78
in SDS, 183
as therapy-related complications of acute leukemia in the elderly, treatment of, 138-139
Infectious disorders, as risk factor of AML in the elderly, 84
Inflammatory disorders, as risk factor of AML in the elderly, 84
Inherited thrombocytopenia
CAMT, 198-199
differential diagnosis, 196-197
overview of thrombopoiesis, 197-198
TAR, 199-200
treatment, 200-201
Interleukin-2, recombinant human
for AML in the elderly, 120-121
novel approaches to improve immunotherapy, 121-122
Interleukin-10, role in risk of GVHD, 17-19
Investigational therapy, for newly-diagnosed AML in the elderly
delaying the start of therapy, 93
new response criteria, 93-94
perspectives on clinical trial methodology, 94
rationale, 89-91
role of allogeneic SCT, 91
types of, 92
Iodine-131 tositumomab, for advanced-stage DLBCL, 259-260
IPS. *See* Idiopathic pneumonia syndrome
Killer immunoglobulin-like receptors (KIR)
ligand mismatched allogeneic NK cells, for AML in the elderly, 122-123
role in risk of GVHD in HSCT, 15-16
KIR. *See* Killer immunoglobulin-like receptors
Leukemia
acute
in the elderly, therapy-related complications of
defining patient population, 134-135
defining patients for treatment, 137
identifying important age-related physiologic differences, 135-137
Leukemia (*Continued*)
treatment, 137-139
GVL and GVHD after DLI for, 54-55
as complication of severe CN, 193-194
in SDS, clinical management and treatment of, 185-186
Liver diseases, in SDS, 179
LymphoStat-B. *See* Belimumab
Malignancy
in FA, development and treatment of, 153-154
in SDS, 182
MDS. *See* Myelodysplastic syndrome
Methotrexate, for advanced-stage DLBCL, 256-257
Methylprednisolone, high-dose, for chronic GVHD, 77
Microarray analysis, of DLBCL, 235-237
Mitomycin C (MMC), diagnosis of FA without hypersensitivity to, 152-153
MLN518, for AML in the elderly, 102
MMC. *See* Mitomycin C
Monoclonal antibodies, anti-CD20, with radioisotopes for advanced-stage DLBCL, 259-260
Mutations
in DC
and aplastic anemia, of TERT, 162-163
of dyskerin, 159-160
of RNA component of telomerase, 160-162
of *RPS19* in DBA, 168-169
Mycophenolate mofetil, for chronic GVHD, 76-77
Myelodysplastic syndrome (MDS), in the elderly
or AML, allogeneic transplantation for
immunologic senescence, 109
impact of aging on incidence and biology of, 107-108
impact of comorbidities, 109-110
nonmyeloablative and reduced-intensity regimens, 108-109
preparative regimen intensity, 110-112
therapy results, 108
timing of, and effect of selection bias, 112-114
unsolved controversies, 114-115
therapy-related, 84-86
Myeloid growth factors, role in treatment of therapy-related complications of acute leukemia in the elderly, 137
Myeloma, GVL and GVHD after DLI for, 55
Mylotarg. *See* Gemtuzumab ozogamicin
Natural killer (NK) cells
and AML cells, blockade of inhibitory interactions, 122
biology of, 119-120
in GVHD
acute disease, prophylaxis and treatment, 37
inhibitory receptors and their ligands, 15-16
KIR ligand mismatched allogeneic, for AML in the elderly, 122-123
Nelarabine (compound 506U78), for ALL in the elderly, 131-132
Neonatal thrombocytopenia. *See* Inherited thrombocytopenia
Neutropenia, as therapy-related complication of acute leukemia in the elderly, treatment of, 138-139
NHL. *See* Non-Hodgkin's lymphoma
Non-Hodgkin's lymphoma (NHL)
diffuse aggressive, with limited disease
biology, 210-211
diagnosis and histology, 207-208
prognostic factors, 208-209
staging, 208
treatment, 209-210
GVL and GVHD after DLI for, 55

Non-Hodgkin's lymphoma (NHL) (*Continued*)
Nutrition, supportive care in chronic GVHD, 78
Oblimersen, for advanced-stage DLBCL, 255
Occupational exposure, as risk factor of AML in the elderly, 83-84
Oral mucositis, as therapy-related complication of acute leukemia in the elderly, treatment of, 137-138
Osteoporosis, as complication of severe CN, 194
Pain, as therapy-related complication of acute leukemia in the elderly, treatment of, 138
Pentostatin, for chronic GVHD, 77
PET. *See* Positron emission tomography
Ph^+ ALL. *See* Philadelphia chromosome-positive acute lymphoblastic leukemia
Philadelphia chromosome–positive acute lymphoblastic leukemia (Ph^+ ALL), in the elderly, challenge of, 130-131
Photopheresis, for chronic GVHD, 78
PKC412, for AML in the elderly, 102
Positron emission tomography (PET), for evaluation of response and prognosis of advanced-stage DLBCL, 219
Pralatrexate, for advanced-stage DLBCL, 255-256
  clinical experience, 257
  preclinical experience, 256-257
Prednisone
  for chronic GVHD, 76
  with vincristine, doxorubicin and cyclophosphamide
    for advanced-stage DLBCL
      plus etoposide, 222, 224
      plus rituximab, 225-227
    for aggressive NHL with limited disease, 209-210
PSC-833 (valspodar), for modulating drug resistance in AML in the elderly, 98-99
Radiation exposure, as risk factor of AML in the elderly, 83
Radioimmunotherapy
  for advanced-stage DLBCL, 259-260
  with ASCT for advanced-stage DLBCL-B, 242-244
Radiotherapy, for aggressive NHL with limited disease, 209-210
Recombinant human granulocyte-colony stimulating factor, for severe CN, 192
Recombinant human interleukin-2, for AML in the elderly, 120-121
  novel approaches to improve immunotherapy, 121-122
Red cell transfusion, for DBA, 172-173
  outcomes, 173-174
Reduced folate carrier, targeting of, in advanced-stage DLBCL, 255-257
Restrictive lung disease, after HSCT
  definition, clinical course and risk factors, 47-48
  pathogenesis, 48
  treatment, 49
Retroviral-mediated gene transfer, for FA diagnosis, 152
Rituximab
  for advanced-stage DLBCL, 214-215
    in dose-intensified chemotherapy regimens, 225-227
  for ALL in the elderly, 131-132
  with ASCT, for advanced-stage DLBCL-B, 242
  for chronic GVHD, 77
RPS19 mutations, in DBA, 168-169
SCT. *See* Stem cell transplantation
SDS. *See* Shwachman-Diamond syndrome
Selection bias, effect on results of allogeneic transplantation for MDS and AML, 112-114
Severe congenital neutropenia. *See* Congenital neutropenia (CN), severe
Shwachman-Diamond syndrome (SDS)
  additional medical issues, 186-187
  clinical presentation, 178
    additional features, 183
    exocrine pancreatic insufficiency, 179
      management and treatment, 185
    growth, 182
    hematologic features, 179-182
      management and treatment, 185
    immune abnormalities, 183
    infection, 183
    liver, 179
    malignancy, 182
      management and treatment, 185-186
    skeletal abnormalities, 182-183
  diagnosis, 184-185
  genetics, 178
  HSCT for, 186
  molecular pathogenesis, 183-184
Sirolimus, for chronic GVHD, 77
Skeletal abnormalities, in SDS, 182-183
Splenomegaly, as complication of severe CN, 194
STAT proteins, as non-FA binding partners of FA proteins, 149
Stem cell transplantation (SCT)
  allogeneic. *See* Allogeneic stem cell transplantation
  autologous. *See* Autologous stem cell transplantation
  for DBA, 173
    outcomes, 173-174
  for FA, 153
SU5416, for AML in the elderly, 102
SU11248, for AML in the elderly, 102
Sun block, for chronic GVHD, 78
Syngeneic transplantation, acute GVHD after, 28
T cells
  in acute GVHD prophylaxis and treatment
    activation phase, 33-35
    effector phase, 35
    modulation of response
      alloreactive, removal of, 35-36
      insertion of suicide genes, 36
      minor histocompatibility antigen-specific, 36
      naive, removal of, 36
      NK cells, 37
      pan T-cell depletion, 35
  axis, in pathophysiology of experimental IPS following allogeneic HSCT, 44-45
  $CD4^+CD25^+$ regulatory. *See* $CD4^+CD25^+$ regulatory T cells
  donor
    activation of, role in GVHD pathophysiology, 5
    genetic modification to minimize GVHD after DLI, 58
    modulation of, in GVHD prevention, 7
  tolerance, 62-63
T lymphocytes. *See* T cells
Telomerase, and DC, 160
  mutations in RNA component of, 160-162
Telomerase reverse transcriptase (TERT), mutations, in aplastic anemia and DC, 162-163
TERT. *See* Telomerase reverse transcriptase
Thalidomide, for chronic GVHD, 76
Thrombocytopenia with absent radii (TAR), 199-200
  treatment, 200-201

Thrombocytopenia with absent radii (TAR), 199-200 (*Continued*)
Thrombopoiesis, overview of, 197-198
TNF-α. *See* Tumor necrosis factor-α
Tobacco smoking, as risk factor of AML in the elderly, 84
Transfusion-associated acute graft-versus-host disease (GVHD), 28-29
Transplantation conditioning, reduced-intensity
  GVHD and GVL after DLI in HSCT, 56-58
  for GVHD prevention, 6-7
  and nonmyeloablative, for AML or MDS in the elderly, 108-109
Tumor cell, kinetics of, role in drug resistance in DLBCL, 232-233
Tumor necrosis factor-α (TNF-α), role in risk of GVHD, 17
Valspodar. *See* PSC-833
Vincristine
  with doxorubicin, cyclophosphamide and prednisone
    for advanced-stage DLBCL
      plus etoposide, 222, 224
      plus rituximab, 225-227
    for aggressive NHL with limited disease, 209-210
  liposomal, for ALL in the elderly, 132
X-linked dyskeratosis congenita. *See* Dyskeratosis congenita
Yttrium-90–labeled ibritumomab tiuxetan, for advanced-stage DLBCL, 259-260

United States Postal Service

Statement of Ownership, Management, and Circulation

1. Publication Title	2. Publication Number	3. Filing Date
Seminars in Hematology	4 8 9 - 2 4 0	9/15/06
4. Issue Frequency	5. Number of Issues Published Annually	6. Annual Subscription Price
Jan, Apr, Jul, Oct	4	$169.00

7. Complete Mailing Address of Known Office of Publication (*Not printer*) (*Street, city, county, state, and ZIP+4*)

Elsevier Inc.
360 Park Avenue South
New York, NY 10010-1710

Contact Person: Stephen Bushing
Telephone: 215-239-3688

8. Complete Mailing Address of Headquarters or General Business Office of Publisher (*Not printer*)

Elsevier Inc., 360 Park Avenue South, New York, NY 10010-1710

9. Full Names and Complete Mailing Addresses of Publisher, Editor, and Managing Editor (*Do not leave blank*)

Publisher (*Name and complete mailing address*)

Livia Berardi, Elsevier Inc., 1600 John F. Kennedy Blvd., Ste. 1800, Philadelphia, PA 19103-2899

Editor (*Name and complete mailing address*)

Photis Beris, MD, Division d'hematologie, Hopital Cantonal Universitaire de Geneve, 25 rue Micheli-du-Crest, 1211 Geneve 14, Switzerland or Neal S. Young, MD, 4400 17th St., NW, Washington, DC 20011

Managing Editor (*Name and complete mailing address*)

Phil Schafer, Elsevier Inc., 360 Park Avenue South, New York, NY 10010-1710

10. Owner (*Do not leave blank. If the publication is owned by a corporation, give the name and address of the corporation immediately followed by the names and addresses of all stockholders owning or holding 1 percent or more of the total amount of stock. If not owned by a corporation, give the names and addresses of the individual owners. If owned by a partnership or other unincorporated firm, give its name and address as well as those of each individual owner. If the publication is published by a nonprofit organization, give its name and address.*)

Full Name	Complete Mailing Address
Wholly owned subsidiary of	4520 East-West Highway
Reed/Elsevier Inc., US holdings	Bethesda, MD 20814

11. Known Bondholders, Mortgagees, and Other Security Holders Owning or Holding 1 Percent or More of Total Amount of Bonds, Mortgages, or Other Securities. If none, check box → None

Full Name	Complete Mailing Address
N/A	

12. Tax Status (*For completion by nonprofit organizations authorized to mail at nonprofit rates*) (*Check one*)
The purpose, function, and nonprofit status of this organization and the exempt status for federal income tax purposes:
Has Not Changed During Preceding 12 Months
Has Changed During Preceding 12 Months (*Publisher must submit explanation of change with this statement*)

(*See Instructions on Reverse*)

PS Form **3526**, October 1999

13. Publication Title: Seminars in Hematology

14. Issue Date for Circulation Data Below: July 2006

15. Extent and Nature of Circulation			Average No. Copies Each Issue During Preceding 12 Months	No. Copies of Single Issue Published Nearest to Filing D
a. Total Number of Copies (*Net press run*)			3825	30
b. Paid and/or Requested Circulation	(1)	Paid/Requested Outside-County Mail Subscriptions Stated on Form 3541. (*Include advertiser's proof and exchange copies*)	1470	13
	(2)	Paid In-County Subscriptions Stated on Form 3541 (*Include advertiser's proof and exchange copies*)		
	(3)	Sales Through Dealers and Carriers, Street Vendors, Counter Sales, and Other Non-USPS Paid Distribution	859	9
	(4)	2816		
c. Total Paid and/or Requested Circulation [*Sum of 15b. (1), (2), (3), and (4)*] →			2329	22
d. Free Distribution by Mail (*Samples, compliment-ary, and other free*)	(1)	Outside-County as Stated on Form 3541	667	2
	(2)	In-County as Stated on Form 3541		
	(3)	Other Classes Mailed Through the USPS		
e. Free Distribution Outside the Mail (*Carriers or other means*)				
f. Total Free Distribution (*Sum of 15d. and 15e.*) →			667	2
g. Total Distribution (*Sum of 15c. and 15f.*) →			2996	24
h. Copies not Distributed			829	5
i. Total (*Sum of 15g. and h.*) →			3825	30
j. Percent Paid and/or Requested Circulation (*15c. divided by 15g. times 100*)			77.74%	90.

16. Publication of Statement of Ownership
Publication required. Will be printed in the **October 2006** issue of this publication. Publication not required

17. Signature and Title of Editor, Publisher, Business Manager, or Owner

Jean Fanucci, Executive Director of Subscription Services — Date: 9/15/06

I certify that all information furnished on this form is true and complete. I understand that anyone who furnishes false or misleading information on this form or who omits material or information requested on the form may be subject to criminal sanctions (including fines and imprisonment) and/or civil sanctions (including civil penalties).

Vol 43, No 4, Suppl 6 October 2006

Supplement to

Seminars in HEMATOLOGY

Neal S. Young · Photis Beris
Editors

Role of Intravenous Iron Therapy in Anemia Management

Alice Maniatis and Photis Beris
Guest Editors

W.B. Saunders

Seminars in HEMATOLOGY

Neal S. Young · Photis Beris
Editors

Peter A. Miescher, *Founding Editor* Ernst R. Jaffé, *Co-Editor Emeritus*

Editorial correspondence should be addressed to Photis Beris, MD, Division d'Hématologie, Hôpital Cantonal Universitaire, 25 rue Micheli-du-Crest, 1211 Geneve 14, Switzerland, or Neal S. Young, MD, 4400 17th Street, NW, Washington, DC 20011.

Business correspondence (subscriptions, change of address) should be addressed to the Publisher, Elsevier, 6277 Sea Harbor Dr, Orlando, FL 32887-4800; Email elspcs@elsevier.com.

Change of address notices, including both the old and new addresses of the subscriber, should be sent at least one month in advance.

Customer Service: 1-800-654-2452; outside the United States and Canada, (407) 345-4000.

Yearly subscription rates: United States and possessions: individual, $169.00; institution, $267.00; single issues, $81.00. All other countries: individual, $239.00; institution, $339.00; single issues, $81.00. Student and resident: United States and possessions, and Canada: $85.00; all other countries: $122.00. To receive student/resident rate, orders must be accompanied by name of affiliated institution, date of term, and the *signature* of program/residency coordinator on institution letterhead. Orders will be billed at individual rate until proof of status is received. Current prices are in effect for back volumes and back issues. Single issues, both current and back, exist in limited quantities and are offered for sale subject to availability. Back issues sold in conjunction with a subscription are on a prorated basis. Prices are subject to change without notice. *Checks* should be made payable to Elsevier and sent to *Seminars in Hematology,* Elsevier, Periodicals Department, PO Box 628239, Orlando, FL 32862-8239.

Other correspondence (copyediting, production) should be addressed to Elsevier, 1600 John F. Kennedy Blvd, Ste 1800, Philadelphia, PA 19103-2899.

The contents of *Seminars in Hematology* are indexed in *Index Medicus* and *MEDLINE, Current Contents/Clinical Medicine, Current Contents/Life Sciences,* Science Citation Index, and *EMBASE/* Excerpta Medica.

The *Seminars in Hematology* home page is located at *www.seminhematol.org.*

W.B. Saunders **Philadelphia, PA**

Seminars in HEMATOLOGY

Vol 43, No 4, Supplement 6, October 2006

Role of Intravenous Iron Therapy in Anemia Management

Alice Maniatis and Photis Beris
Guest Editors

Role of Intravenous Iron Therapy in Anemia Management: State of the Art S1
Photis Beris and Alice Maniatis

The Relevance of Iron in Erythropoietin-Stimulated Erythropoiesis S3
Lawrence Tim Goodnough

Experience With Intravenous Iron in Nephrology S9
Iain C. Macdougall

Iron Metabolism and Iron Supplementation in Anemia of Cancer S13
Heinz Ludwig

Intravenous Iron in Inflammatory Bowel Disease S18
Christoph Gasche and Stefanie Kulnigg

Iron Administration in the Critically Ill S23
Michael Piagnerelli, Alessandro Rapotec, Frédéric Cotton, and Jean-Louis Vincent

The Use of Iron Sucrose Complex for Anemia in Pregnancy and the Postpartum Period S28
Christian Breymann

Role of Intravenous Iron in Elective and Non-elective Orthopedic Surgery S32
José Antonio García-Erce, Jorge Cuenca, and Manuel Muñoz

Intravenous Iron in Colorectal Cancer Surgery S36
Manuel Muñoz, Arturo Campos, and José Antonio García-Erce

Intravenous Iron in Cardiac Surgery S39
Manuel Muñoz, Ramón Leal-Noval, and José Antonio García-Erce

Seminars in HEMATOLOGY

Role of Intravenous Iron Therapy in Anemia Management

Alice Maniatis and Photis Beris
Guest Editors

Proceedings of a Network for Advancement of Transfusion Alternatives (NATA) expert meeting held in Paris, France, on November 28, 2005.

This supplement was made possible by an unrestricted educational grant from Vifor (International) Inc., St. Gallen, Switzerland.

ELSEVIER

Seminars in
HEMATOLOGY

Volume 43, Number 4, Supplement 6 October 2006

Role of Intravenous Iron Therapy in Anemia Management: State of the Art

Iron-deficiency anemia may have been first described in about 1500 BC in the Egyptian Ebers Papyrus, and treatment of the anemia with iron salts was instituted already by the mid 17th century in France. Despite its long history, iron-deficiency anemia continues to occupy center stage (30 publications in the first month of 2006), especially in developing countries, and new iron formulations continue to evolve in order to improve their tolerance and efficacy.

Anemia can result from absolute iron deficiency but also from "functional iron deficiency" as is the case in chronic diseases. Both are characterized by reduced serum iron and transferrin saturation, but ferritin is usually high in the anemia of chronic disease. In the latter, iron is sequestered in the reticuloendothelial system and is not available for erythropoiesis, resulting in "iron-restricted erythropoiesis."

In absolute iron deficiency, iron absorption is increased and, provided there is no pathology of the gastrointestinal tract, oral iron administration usually leads to correction of the anemia, whereas in anemia of chronic disease absorption is downregulated, possibly through increased hepcidin production,[1] and the small amount of iron absorbed is directed into the reticuloendothelial system.[2] Parenteral iron would be a more effective mode of administration in this case, but with older formulations of intravenous iron serious adverse events were not rare. More recent formulations, however, such as iron sucrose, are better tolerated and intravenous iron administration has gained ground in Europe.[3] That does not mean there are no concerns; if parenteral iron is given to patients with transferrin saturation greater than 20%, it may increase the risk of bacteremia and, in the setting of immune activation, may cause tissue damage. In anemia of chronic disease, evidence of the beneficial effect of intravenous iron in correcting the anemia is accumulating; in addition, iron, by inhibiting tumor necrosis factor-alpha (TNF-α), reduces disease activity.

In order to further clarify the indications for iron therapy in a number of settings, with the ultimate goal of developing practice guidelines, the Network for Advancement of Transfusion Alternatives (NATA; *www.nataonline.com*) convened a panel of experts in November 2005. Areas explored were:

- Chronic renal disease
- Oncology
- Inflammatory bowel diseases
- Critical care
- Pregnancy and obstetrics
- Surgery (orthopedic/trauma, cardiac, malignancy)

Information on the relationship between erythropoietin (EPO), iron, and erythropoiesis obtained from experience with autologous blood donation was reviewed by Professor Lawrence Tim Goodnough.[4] Under standard conditions of phlebotomy (one unit per week), without exogenous EPO administration there is a net red blood cell (RBC) volume expansion of 19%. With aggressive phlebotomy plus EPO and oral iron, RBC expansion was 40% to 50%; even patients with rheumatoid arthritis, a chronic inflammatory disease, had a similar RBC expansion. Professor Goodnough concluded that when erythropoiesis is vigorous, functional iron deficiency does occur and novel approaches to iron supplementation in these circumstances are needed.

The experience of renal anemia patients treated with EPO and iron is already substantial and, as a result, transfusion-dependent patients are few.[5,6] Regarding intravenous iron administration, despite lingering concerns for predisposing patients to infection and oxidative stress, Professor Iain Macdougall concluded that intravenous iron both improves the anemia of renal failure even in the absence of EPO therapy and enhances patients' response to EPO administration, and that benefits outweigh these potential concerns.[7]

In oncology, the advantage of intravenous versus oral iron administration was shown in a randomized trial comparing EPO plus oral iron versus EPO plus intravenous iron in patients with chemotherapy-related anemia.[8] Professor Heinz

0037-1963/06/$-see front matter
doi:10.1053/j.seminhematol.2006.08.001

Ludwig suggested, as target values for iron substitution in oncology patients, the following levels:

Ferritin levels in the 300–500 μg/L range
Transferrin saturation >20%, close to 30%–40%
Withhold parenteral iron when ferritin >1,000 μg/L, or transferrin saturation >50%

In inflammatory bowel disease, Dr Christoph Gashe presented data from a multicenter trial comparing oral and intravenous iron.[9] In both groups, results regarding anemia correction were significant, but ferritin levels at the end of the study were significantly higher only in the intravenous group. Furthermore, in colitis patients oral iron induces oxidative stress and increases inflammation, complications that are avoided with parenteral iron.

Anemia in patients admitted to the intensive care unit was discussed by Professor Jean-Louis Vincent. An ongoing observational study of patients in hospital for less than 2 days shows an early reduction in blood iron levels, a substantial increase in ferritin levels, and a reduction in transferrin levels. Professor Vincent suggested that studies of iron metabolism are needed to identify those patients that would benefit from intravenous iron supplementation, with or without EPO administration.[10]

Dr Christian Breymann, discussing the anemia of pregnancy, stressed the need for aggressive intravenous iron therapy. He pointed out that the World Health Organization's efforts with regard to oral iron supplementation have failed in that the number of cases of anemia has not decreased between 1996 and 2003. In women who did not respond to oral iron, administration of intravenous iron sucrose led to a 2-g/dL increase in hemoglobin in 25 days. Experience over 14 years at the University hospital in Zurich, treating 2,000 patients using 2,500 ampoules per year, demonstrates the safety of iron sucrose in obstetrics (0.012% adverse events) as well as its efficacy. Both the number of patients and the number of blood units transfused were significantly reduced, as was the rate of postoperative infections.[11,12]

Perioperative anemia is quite frequent, with 30% to 50% of patients anemic preoperatively and 90% postoperatively. Dr. José Garcia-Erce and Professor Manuel Muñoz commented on their experience with intravenous iron in surgery. In surgery for oncology patients, particularly those with colon cancer, preoperative administration of EPO with intravenous iron reduces the number of transfused patients. In hip replacement surgery, preliminary results of the administration of 300 mg of iron sucrose showed a reduction in the amount of blood transfused and the rate of infection, and a trend toward reduction of length of hospital stay.[13,14] All participants agreed that, although the use of intravenous iron is increasing, further research in all areas discussed is necessary.

Although this supplement does not pretend to express a statement of a group of experts, concerning intravenous iron use in clinical practice, it does, however, give a complete picture of the state of the art of intravenous iron therapy in different settings of anemia. We hope that this special issue of *Seminars in Hematology* will greatly help clinicians in their daily confrontation with anemia.

Photis Beris, MD
Professor of Clinical Hematology
Geneva University Hospital
Geneva, Switzerland
Photis.beris@hcuge.ch
and

Alice Maniatis, MD
NATA Chair
Professor Emeritus, University of Patras
Director, Hematology Division
Henry Dunant Hospital
Athens, Greece
alicemaniatis@yahoo.com
Guest Editors

References

1. Ganz T, Nemeth E: Iron imports. IV. Hepcidin and regulation of body iron metabolism. Am J Physiol Gastrointest Liver Physiol 290:G199-G203, 2006
2. Weiss G, Goodnough LT: Anemia of chronic disease. N Engl J Med 352:1011-1023, 2005
3. Beris P: The use of iron to increase red cell mass. Can J Anaesth 50:S3-S9, 2003 (suppl)
4. Goodnough LT, Skikne B, Brugnara C: Erythropoietin, iron, and erythropoiesis. Blood 96:823-833, 2000
5. National Kidney Foundation Kidney Disease Outcomes Quality Initiative: KDOQI clinical practice guidelines and clinical practice recommendations for anemia in chronic kidney disease. Am J Kidney Dis 47:S1-S145, 2006 (suppl 3)
6. Locatelli F, Aljama P, Barany P, Canaud B, Carrera F, Eckardt KU, et al: Revised European best practice guidelines for the management of anaemia in patients with chronic renal failure. Nephrol Dial Transplant 19:ii1-ii47, 2004 (suppl 2)
7. Macdougall IC, Roche A: Administration of intravenous iron sucrose as a 2-minute push to CKD patients: A prospective evaluation of 2,297 injections. Am J Kidney Dis 46:283-289, 2005
8. Auerbach M, Ballard H, Trout JR, McIlwain M, Ackerman A, Bahrain H, et al: Intravenous iron optimizes the response to recombinant human erythropoietin in cancer patients with chemotherapy-related anemia: a multicenter, open-label, randomized trial. J Clin Oncol 22:1301-1307, 2004
9. Schröder O, Mickisch O, Seidler U, de Weerth A, Dignass AU, Herfarth H, et al: Intravenous iron sucrose versus oral iron supplementation for the treatment of iron deficiency anemia in patients with inflammatory bowel disease—A randomized, controlled, open-label, multicenter study. Am J Gastroenterol 100:2503-2509, 2005
10. Piagnerelli M, Vincent JL: Role of iron in anaemic critically ill patients: It's time to investigate! Crit Care 8:306-307, 2004
11. Breymann C, Richter C, Huttner C, Huch R, Huch A: Effectiveness of recombinant erythropoietin and iron sucrose vs. iron therapy only, in patients with postpartum anaemia and blunted erythropoiesis. Eur J Clin Invest 30:154-161, 2000
12. Breymann C, Visca E, Huch R, Huch A: Efficacy and safety of intravenously administered iron sucrose with and without adjuvant recombinant human erythropoietin for the treatment of resistant iron-deficiency anemia during pregnancy. Am J Obstet Gynecol 184:662-667, 2001
13. Cuenca J, Garcia-Erce JA, Martinez AA, Solano VM, Molina J, Munoz M: Role of parenteral iron in the management of anaemia in the elderly patient undergoing displaced subcapital hip fracture repair: Preliminary data. Arch Orthop Trauma Surg 125:342-347, 2005
14. Garcia-Erce JA, Cuenca J, Munoz M, Izuel M, Martinez AA, Herrera A, et al: Perioperative stimulation of erythropoiesis with intravenous iron and erythropoietin reduces transfusion requirements in patients with hip fracture. A prospective observational study. Vox Sang 88:235-243, 2005

Seminars in
HEMATOLOGY

The Relevance of Iron in Erythropoietin-Stimulated Erythropoiesis

Lawrence Tim Goodnough

Several clinical models have generated insight into the relationship between erythropoietin (EPO), iron, and erythropoiesis. Patients with chronic hemolytic anemias or hemochromatosis can increase erythropoiesis six- to eightfold over basal rates, whereas patients with blood loss, such as those donating autologous blood, can increase erythropoiesis only two- to fourfold over basal levels, even with pharmacologic doses of recombinant human EPO. A substantial limitation to the dose/response relationship between EPO therapy and the erythropoietic response is iron-restricted erythropoiesis, even in the presence of storage iron. Novel approaches to iron supplementation therapy when erythropoietic agents are used are indicated.

Semin Hematol 43(suppl 6):S3-S8

Twenty years ago, Finch summarized knowledge gained primarily from studies of normal individuals, patients with hereditary hemolytic anemias, and patients with hemochromatosis.[1] Under conditions of basal erythropoiesis in normal subjects, plasma iron turnover (as an index of marrow erythropoietic response) is little affected, whether transferrin saturation ranges from very low to very high levels. In contrast, the erythropoietic response in individuals with congenital hemolytic anemia, in whom erythropoiesis is chronically elevated up to sixfold over basal levels,[2] is affected (and limited) by serum iron levels and by transferrin saturation.[3] Patients with hemochromatosis who underwent serial phlebotomy were observed to mount erythropoietic responses of up to eightfold over basal rates, attributed to the maintenance of very high serum iron and transferrin saturation levels in these patients,[4] whereas normal individuals were shown to have difficulty providing sufficient iron to support rates of erythropoiesis greater than three times basal rates.[5] These observations led Finch to identify a "relative iron deficiency" state, also known as "functional iron deficiency," which he defined as circumstances in which increased erythron iron requirements exceed the available supply of iron.[6] In another clinical setting, patients undergoing autologous blood donation can serve as a model for perioperative blood loss; insights gained regarding the relationship between erythropoietin (EPO), iron, and erythropoiesis were summarized,[7] and will be reviewed here.

Departments of Pathology and Medicine, Stanford University, Stanford, CA.
Address correspondence to Lawrence T. Goodnough, MD, Professor, Pathology and Medicine, Stanford University Medical Center, 300 Pasteur Dr, H-1402, Stanford, CA 94305-5626. E-mail: ltgoodno@stanford.edu

Autologous blood donation in patients scheduled for elective surgery results in blood-loss anemia. Patients undergoing autologous blood phlebotomy may donate a unit (450 ± 45 mL) of blood as often as twice weekly, until 72 hours before surgery.[8] Under routine conditions, patients usually donate once weekly.[9] Oral iron supplements are routinely prescribed. This iatrogenic blood loss is accompanied by a response in endogenous EPO levels that, while increased significantly over basal levels, remain within the normal range (4 to 26 IU/L).[10] The erythropoietic response that occurs under these conditions is modest.[7,8] A summary of selected prospective, controlled trials[11-16] of patients undergoing phlebotomy is presented in Table 1. Calculated estimates of red blood cell (RBC) volume expansion (erythropoiesis in excess of basal rates) were determined.[17] Two hundred twenty to 351 mL (11% to 19% RBC expansion[11,12] or the equivalent of 1 to 1.75 blood units[18]) are produced in excess of basal erythropoiesis, defining the efficacy of this blood-conservation practice.

For patients subjected to more aggressive phlebotomy (up to two units weekly), the endogenous EPO response is more substantial.[13-16] In one clinical trial,[14] a linear-logarithmic relationship was demonstrated between change in hemoglobin level and EPO response,[19] predicted previously by phlebotomy experiments in normal subjects.[20] EPO-mediated erythropoiesis in this setting is 397 to 568 mL (19% to 26% RBC expansion,[13-16] or the equivalent of two to three blood units[18]).

Clinical trials have demonstrated a dose-response relationship between exogenous EPO therapy and RBC expansion.[16] A study of EPO therapy in autologous blood donors found

0037-1963/06/$-see front matter
doi:10.1053/j.seminhematol.2006.08.003

Table 1 Endogenous Erythropoietin-Mediated Erythropoiesis

Patients (n)	Baseline RBC (mL)	Requested/ Donated Units (U)		RBC Donated (mL)	RBC Produced (mL)	RBC Expansion (%)	Iron Therapy	References
Standard phlebotomy								
108	1,884	3	2.7	522	351	19	PO	11
22	1,936	3	2.8	590	220	11	None	12
45	1,991	3	2.9	621	331	17	PO	12
41	1,918	3	2.9	603	315	16	PO + IV	12
Aggressive phlebotomy								
30	2,075	>3	3.0	540	397	19	None	13
30	2,024	>3	3.1	558	473	23	PO	13
30	2,057	>3	2.9	522	436	21	IV	13
24	2,157	6	4.1	683	568	26	PO	14, 15
23	2,257	6	4.6	757	440	19	PO	16

NOTE. Data are expressed as means.
Abbreviations: IV, intravenous; PO, (oral); RBC, red blood cell.
Modified from *Blood.* Goodnough et al.[7]

that 400 IU/kg administered over a 2-week interval resulted in clinically significant erythropoiesis.[21] Table 2 details RBC volume expansion in 134 patients treated with EPO therapy during aggressive blood phlebotomy,[14-16,22,23] ranging from 358 to 1,764 mL (28% to 79% RBC expansion) over 25 to 35 days, or the equivalent of two to nine blood units.[18] The range in response (erythropoiesis) to dose (EPO) is not related to patient gender or age,[24,25] suggesting that iron-restricted erythropoiesis may account for the variability in erythropoietic response to EPO.

Iron-Restricted Erythropoiesis

Erythropoiesis in response to aggressive autologous phlebotomy via endogenous EPO has been estimated to increase up to threefold.[16,26] No apparent relationship exists between basal iron stores and this magnitude of erythropoiesis, suggesting that under conditions of moderate erythropoiesis, serum iron and transferrin saturation for erythron requirements are adequately maintained by storage iron.[13-16] Oral iron supplementation was found to be of benefit,[12,13,27] whereas intravenous iron supplementation was not found to be of value in enhancing erythropoiesis under these conditions of moderate blood loss.[12,13]

With enhanced erythropoiesis during EPO therapy, iron-restricted erythropoiesis occurs even in patients with measurable storage iron. Despite an eightfold increase in gastrointestinal iron absorption,[28] serum ferritin and transferrin saturation levels decline up to 50% with EPO therapy.[29] A fourfold increase in erythropoietic activity is accompanied by declining reticulocyte counts and the appearance of hypochromic RBCs by the second week of EPO therapy.[23,30] In a study of escalating (fourfold) increase in EPO dose administered to patients undergoing aggressive phlebotomy, the marrow erythropoietic index increased from 2.9-fold (with endogenous erythropoietin stimulation) to 3.6-fold over basal rates of erythropoiesis, representing only a 58% increase in erythropoiesis (Figure 1). The superior erythropoietic response in a patient with hemochromatosis further suggests iron-restricted erythropoiesis in patients treated with EPO (Table 2).[23]

Table 2 Erythropoiesis During Blood Loss and Erythropoietin Therapy

Patients (n/sex)	Baseline RBC Volume (mL)	Total EPO Dose (IU/kg)	Units Donated (U)	RBC Volume Donated (mL)	RBC Volume Produced (mL)	RBC Volume Expansion (%)	Iron Therapy	References
10/F	1,285	900 SC	3.4	435	358	28	IV	22
24	1,949	900 IV	5.2	864	621	32	PO	16
10/F	1,293	1,800 SC	4.3	526	474	37	IV	22
26	2,032	1,800 IV	5.5	917	644	32	PO	16
11/F	1,796	3,600 IV	4.9	809	701	39	PO	14, 15
12/M	2,296	3,600 IV	5.9	1097	1102	48	PO	14, 15
23	2,049	3,600 IV	5.4	970	911	45	PO	14, 15
18	2,019	3,600 IV	5.6	972	856	42	PO	16
1/M	2,241	4,200 IV	8	1600	1764	79	Hemochromatosis	23

NOTE. Data expressed as means.
Abbreviations: IV, intravenous; PO, per os (oral); RBC, red blood cell; SC, subcutaneous; EPO, erythropoietin.
Modified from *Blood.* Goodnough et al.[7]

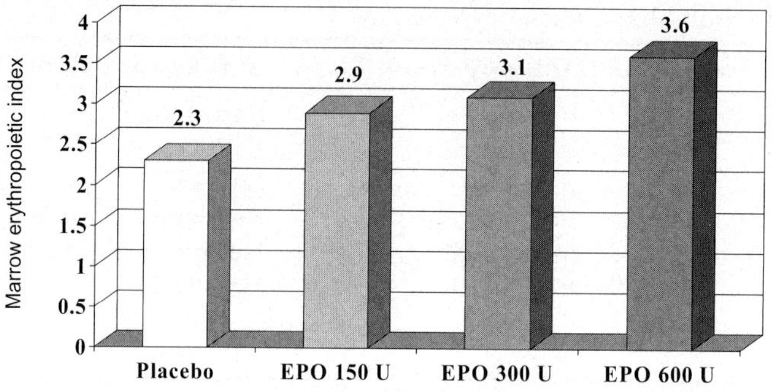

Figure 1 Erythropoietic response, as reflected in the bone marrow erythropoietic index, in four cohorts of autologous donors treated with placebo or escalating doses of EPO therapy. The erythropoietic response (mL/kg/d) was estimated for each treatment group, according to the formula: bone marrow erythropoietic index = [(RBC volume expansion) + (baseline RBC volume production)]/(baseline RBC volume production). Originally published in *Blood*. Goodnough et al. Erythropoietin, iron, and erythropoiesis. Blood. 2000; 96:823-833.

Iron Therapy

The success of EPO therapy in correcting the anemia of chronic renal failure has led to substantial clinical experience in iron therapy and erythropoiesis in this setting.[31,32] Hyporesponsiveness to EPO therapy is a common phenomenon[33,34] due to a variety of comorbid conditions, particularly aluminum toxicity and iron deficiency.

Anemic patients undergoing dialysis may show suboptimal response to oral iron therapy for several reasons. During EPO therapy, absorption of iron increases up to fivefold.[28] However, external iron losses, including hemodialysis and blood testing, exceed gastrointestinal iron absorption.[32] Poor compliance due to gastrointestinal symptoms is problematic, and significantly reduced iron absorption may occur with some newer iron formulations.[35] Iron-restricted erythropoiesis is evident by clinical responses to ascorbate supplementation, thought to facilitate the release of iron from reticuloendothelial stores and increased iron utilization by erythrons,[34] as well as the success of intravenous iron therapy in reducing EPO dose requirements.[32]

Intravenous iron administration has become standard therapy in renal dialysis patients undergoing EPO therapy.[36] Patients treated with intravenous iron (100 mg twice weekly) achieved a 46% reduction in EPO dosage required to maintain hematocrit levels between 30% and 34%, compared to patients supplemented with oral iron.[37] In a study of chronic renal failure (nondialysis) patients, two thirds of patients who were unresponsive to oral iron responded to weekly intravenous iron therapy.[37] Improved erythropoiesis occurred despite initial serum ferritin levels as high as 400 μg/L,[38] indicating that biochemical markers of storage iron in these patients are not helpful in evaluating iron-restricted erythropoiesis.

Intravenous iron therapy in iron-deficient patients with inflammatory bowel disease also result in improved responses to EPO therapy,[39] compared to a similar patient group who received oral iron supplementation.[40] The clinical response to intravenous iron may be attributed to the effect of EPO therapy on iron mobilization from the reticuloendothelial system into RBC precursors.[41] The risk/benefit profile of intravenous iron is controversial in anemic renal dialysis patients,[42,43] as well as in patients with anemia of chronic disease.[44]

Intravenous iron can allow up to a fivefold erythropoietic response to significant blood-loss anemia in normal individuals.[3,45] A greater rate of hemoglobin production is probably not possible unless red marrow expands into yellow marrow space, as is seen in hereditary anemias.[2,45] One limitation to intravenous iron therapy in patients not undergoing EPO therapy may be that much of the administered iron is transported into the reticuloendothelial system as storage iron, where it is less readily available for erythropoiesis.[46] For iron-deficient patients, 50% of intravenous iron is incorporated into hemoglobin within 3 to 4 weeks,[47] whereas for patients with anemia of chronic disease or renal failure, intravenous iron is less rapidly mobilized from the reticuloendothelial system.[48]

Laboratory Evaluation

The diagnosis of iron deficiency is traditionally based on a combination of parameters, including iron metabolism and hematological indices. Technical and biologic issues limit the usefulness of these assays in the clinical setting,[49-51] and the value of iron, transferrin, and transferrin saturation is limited to uncomplicated iron deficiency. Transferrin saturation falls below 16% only when iron stores are exhausted, in contrast to EPO therapy-induced erythropoiesis, in which iron saturation falls even in the presence of storage iron.[52] Detection of iron-restricted erythropoiesis during EPO therapy[52-54] therefore poses additional challenges.

Ferritin is widely used as a marker of iron storage,[55,56] with a cutoff of 15 μg/L indicating absent iron stores in normal individuals.[57] However, one study found that 25% of women with no stainable bone marrow iron had serum ferritin levels above the 15-μg/L cutoff.[58] A level of 30 μg/L[59] to 40 μg/L[60] for anemic patients is therefore desirable in order to provide optimal diagnostic efficiency (positive predictive values of 92% to 98%, respectively), even without clinical evidence of infection or inflammation. For patients with anemia of chronic disease; however, ferritin levels are normal or increased (Table 3).[44] Subjects treated with EPO exhibit a rapid decrease in ferritin to levels 50% to 75% below baseline.[61] Under these conditions, ferritin most likely reflects the iron content of a smaller, more labile pool in equilibrium with both the erythropoietic compartment and storage iron.

Many patients have underlying disorders with "inappropriately high" serum ferritin levels. Ferritin levels are elevated in conditions such as hyperthyroidism, inflammation/infection, hepatocellular disease, malignancies, alcohol consumption, and oral contraceptives.[62] Two thirds of renal dialysis patients respond to intravenous iron therapy, with mean ferritins of 94 μg/L and mean transferrin saturations of 22% that are no different from patients who are not responsive to in-

Table 3 Serum Levels That Differentiate Anemia of Chronic Disease From Iron-Deficiency Anemia

Variable	Anemia of Chronic Disease	Iron-Deficiency Anemia	Both Conditions*
Iron	Reduced	Reduced	Reduced
Transferrin	Reduced to normal	Increased	Reduced
Transferrin saturation	Reduced	Reduced	Reduced
Ferritin	Normal to increased	Reduced	Reduced to normal
Soluble transferrin receptor	Normal	Increased	Normal to increased
Ratio of soluble transferrin receptor to log ferritin	Low (<1)	High (>2)	High (>2)
Cytokine levels	Increased	Normal	Increased

NOTE. Relative changes are given in relation to the respective normal values.
*Patients with both conditions include those with anemia of chronic disease and true iron deficiency.
Reproduced with permission from Weiss et al.[44]

travenous iron.[38] This has led to suggested guidelines[43] for renal dialysis patients, in which a ferritin level of less than 200 μg/L alone, or less than 400 μg/L with a transferrin saturation less than 20%, are used to determine the need for intravenous iron therapy; only at transferrin saturations greater than 50%, or ferritin levels in excess of 800 μg/L, are these patients considered unlikely to benefit from iron therapy.

In patients with the anemia of cancer, up to 50% are unresponsive to EPO therapy.[63] After 2 weeks of EPO therapy, ferritin levels greater than 400 μg/L correctly predicted lack of response in 88% of the cases, while levels less than 400 νg/L correctly predicted response in 75% of cases.[63] However, several studies have failed to show a role for ferritin in either predicting response to EPO therapy or in identifying functional iron deficiency in patients with cancer-related anemia.[64-66] Parenteral iron has been demonstrated to enhance rates of response (compared to a placebo or oral iron supplementation) to therapy with erythropoietic agents in cancer patients who are undergoing chemotherapy.[67] Further clinical studies to determine the level of ferritin that would predict response to intravenous iron in oncology patients undergoing EPO therapy are needed.

A classification of anemias has been proposed around the concept of an adequate or an inadequate EPO response to the degree of anemia, using patients with iron deficiency or chronic hemolytic anemia as reference populations.[68] The correlation between the percentage of patients showing an "inadequate" EPO response to anemia and the percentage of patients responding to EPO therapy (according to the author's criteria) can be illustrated for several diseases, with a wide range in response in myelodysplastic syndromes,[69] multiple myeloma,[70] and rheumatoid arthritis.[71]

There are several problems with the use of EPO levels in the management of individual patients. The interpretation of an EPO level must take into account the degree of anemia at the time of measurement; commercial assay results do not take this into consideration, so that clinicians need to be familiar with mathematical corrections such as observed/predicted ratios.[68] A retrospective analysis of EPO therapy in anemic cancer patients not receiving chemotherapy[72] found that pretreatment EPO levels of less than 200 IU/L were correlated with RBC response to EPO therapy; however, subsequent analyses have found that EPO levels are not predictive for response in cancer patients receiving chemotherapy.[73,74] Since almost all anemic cancer patients and renal dialysis patients have EPO levels that are inadequate for the degree of anemia,[68] measuring EPO levels is not useful in these settings. Furthermore, guidelines recommend that EPO therapy be instituted before hemoglobin levels fall below 10 g/dL, a level at which interpretation of EPO level is not valid.[68] The EPO assay may be most useful as a determinant of response to therapy in certain settings such as patients with multiple myeloma, malignant lymphoma, or myelodysplasia.[64,69,75]

Conclusion

Under conditions of normal iron stores, the maximal erythropoietic response to anemia, with or without pharmacologic doses of erythropoietic agents, is a 350% or 200% increase, respectively, over basal erythropoiesis.

This two- to fourfold increase is limited by functional iron deficiency. The availability of safer intravenous iron preparations allows an opportunity to study their value in optimizing the erythropoietic response to anemia.

References

1. Finch CA: Erythropoiesis, erythropoietin, and iron. Blood 60:1241-1246, 1982
2. Crosby WH: The metabolism of hemoglobin and bile pigment in hemolytic disease. Am J Med 18:112-122, 1955
3. Hillman RS, Henderson PA: Control of marrow production by the level of iron supply. J Clin Invest 48:454-460, 1969
4. Crosby WH: Treatment of haemochromatosis by energetic phlebotomy; one patient's response to the letting of 55 litres of blood in 11 months. Br J Haematol 4:82-88, 1958
5. Coleman DH, Stevens AR, Dodge HT, Finch CA: Rate of regeneration after blood loss. AMA Arch Intern Med 92:341-349, 1953
6. Finch CA: Perspectives in iron metabolism. N Engl J Med 306:1520-1528, 1982
7. Goodnough LT, Skikne B, Brugnara C: Erythropoietin, iron, and erythropoiesis. Blood 96:823-833, 2000
8. Menitove J (ed): Standards for Blood Banks and Transfusion Services (ed 19). Bethesda, MD, American Association of Blood Banks, 1999, p 76
9. Goodnough LT, Brittenham G: Limitations of the erythropoietic response to serial phlebotomy: Implications for autologous blood donor programs. J Lab Clin Med 115:28-35, 1990

10. Kickler TS, Spivak JL: Effect of repeated whole blood donations on serum immunoreactive erythropoietin levels in autologous donors. JAMA 260:65-67, 1988
11. Kasper SM, Gerlich W, Buzello W: Preoperative red cell production in patients undergoing weekly autologous blood donation. Transfusion 37:1058-1062, 1997
12. Kasper SM, Lazansky H, Stark C, Klimek M, Laubinger R, Börner Y: Efficacy of oral iron supplementation is not enhanced by additional intravenous iron during autologous blood donation. Transfusion 38: 764-770, 1998
13. Weisbach V, Skoda P, Rippel R, Lauer G, Glaser A, Zingsem J, et al: Oral or intravenous iron as an adjunct to autologous blood donation in elective surgery: A randomized, controlled study. Transfusion 39:465-472, 1999
14. Goodnough LT, Rudnick S, Price TH, Ballas SK, Collins ML, Crowley JP, et al: Increased preoperative collection of autologous blood with recombinant human erythropoietin therapy. N Engl J Med 321:1163-1168, 1989
15. Goodnough LT, Price TH, Rudnick S, Soegiarso RW: Preoperative red blood cell production in patients undergoing aggressive autologous blood phlebotomy with and without erythropoietin therapy. Transfusion 32:441-445, 1992
16. Goodnough LT, Price TH, Friedman KD, Johnston M, Ciavarella D, Khan N, et al: A phase III trial of recombinant human erythropoietin therapy in nonanemic orthopedic patients subjected to aggressive removal of blood for autologous use: dose, response, toxicity, efficacy. Transfusion 34:66-71, 1994
17. Brecher ME, Monk T, Goodnough LT: A standardized method for calculating blood loss. Transfusion 37:1070-1074, 1997
18. Goodnough LT, Bravo JR, Hsueh YS, Keating LJ, Brittenham GM: Red blood cell mass in autologous and homologous blood units. Implications for risk/benefit assessment for autologous blood crossover and directed blood transfusion. Transfusion 29:821-822, 1989
19. Goodnough LT, Price TH, Parvin CA, Friedman KD, Vogler WR, Khan N, et al: Erythropoietin response to anaemia is not altered by surgery or recombinant human erythropoietin therapy. Br J Haematol 87:695-699, 1994
20. Adamson JW: The erythropoietin-hematocrit relationship in normal and polycythemic man: Implications of marrow regulation. Blood 32: 597-609, 1968
21. Sans T, Bofil C, Joven J, Cliville X, Simo JM, Llobet X, et al: Effectiveness of very low doses of subcutaneous recombinant human erythropoietin in facilitating autologous blood donation before orthopedic surgery. Transfusion 36:822-826, 1996
22. Mercuriali F, Inghilleri G, Biffi E, Colotti MT, Vinci A, Oriani G: Epoetin alfa in low hematocrit patients to facilitate autologous blood donation in total hip replacement: A randomized, double-blind, placebo-controlled, dose-ranging study. Acta Haematol 100:69-76, 1998
23. Brugnara C, Chambers LA, Malynn E, Goldberg MA, Kruskall MS: Red blood cell regeneration induced by subcutaneous recombinant erythropoietin: Iron-deficient erythropoiesis in iron-replete subjects. Blood 81:956-964, 1993
24. Goodnough LT, Verbrugge D, Marcus RE, Goldberg V: The effect of patient size and dose of recombinant human erythropoietin therapy on red blood cell volume expansion in autologous donors for elective orthopedic operation. J Am Coll Surg 179:171-176, 1994
25. Goodnough LT, Price TH, Parvin CA: The endogenous erythropoietin response and the erythropoietic response to blood loss anemia: the effects of age and gender. J Lab Clin Med 126:57-64, 1995
26. Goodnough LT, Marcus RE: Erythropoiesis in patients stimulated with erythropoietin: The relevance of storage iron. Vox Sang 75:128-133, 1998
27. Biesma DH, Kraaijenhagen RJ, Poortman J, Marx JJ, van de Wiel A: The effect of oral iron supplementation on erythropoiesis in autologous blood donors. Transfusion 32:162-165, 1992
28. Skikne BS, Cook JD: Effect of enhanced erythropoiesis on iron absorption. J Lab Clin Med 120:746-751, 1992
29. Heiss MM, Tarabichi A, Delanoff C, Allgayer H, Jauch KW, Hernandez-Richter T, et al: Perisurgical erythropoietin application in anemic patients with colorectal cancer: A double-blind randomized study. Surgery 119:523-527, 1996
30. Biesma DH, Van de Wiel A, Beguin Y, Kraaijenhagen RJ, Marx JJ: Erythropoietic activity and iron metabolism in autologous blood donors during recombinant human erythropoietin therapy. Eur J Clin Invest 24:426-432, 1994
31. Eschbach JW, Egrie JC, Downing MR, Browne JK, Adamson JW: Correction of the anemia of end-stage renal disease with recombinant human erythropoietin. Results of a combined phase I and II clinical trial. N Engl J Med 316:73-78, 1987
32. Fishbane S, Frei GL, Maesaka J: Reduction in recombinant human erythropoietin doses by the use of chronic intravenous iron supplementation. Am J Kidney Dis 26:41-46, 1995
33. Means RT Jr: Commentary: An anemia of chronic disease, after all? J Investig Med 47:203, 1999
34. Tarng DC, Huang TP, Chen TW, Yang WC: Erythropoietin hyporesponsiveness: From iron deficiency to iron overload. Kidney Int 69: S107-S118, 1999 (suppl)
35. Wingard RL, Parker RA, Ismail N, Hakim RM: Efficacy of oral iron therapy in patients receiving recombinant human erythropoietin. Am J Kidney Dis 25:433-439, 1995
36. Adamson JW, Eschbach JW: Erythropoietin for end-stage renal disease. N Engl J Med 339:625-627, 1998
37. Silverberg DS, Iaina A, Peer G, Kaplan E, Levi BA, Frank N, et al: Intravenous iron supplementation for the treatment of the anemia of moderate to severe chronic renal failure patients not receiving dialysis. Am J Kidney Dis 27:234-238, 1996
38. Taylor JE, Peat N, Porter C, Morgan AG: Regular low-dose intravenous iron therapy improves response to erythropoietin in haemodialysis patients. Nephrol Dial Transplant 11:1079-1083, 1996
39. Gasche C, Dejaco C, Waldhoer T, Tillinger W, Reinisch W, Fueger GF, et al: Intravenous iron and erythropoietin for anemia associated with Crohn disease. A randomized, controlled trial. Ann Intern Med 126: 782-787, 1997
40. Schreiber S, Howaldt S, Schnoor M, Nikolaus S, Bauditz J, Gasche G, et al: Recombinant erythropoietin for the treatment of anemia in inflammatory bowel disease. N Eng J Med 334:619-623, 1996
41. Weiss G, Houston T, Kastner S, Johrer K, Grunewald K, Brock JH: Regulation of cellular iron metabolism by erythropoietin: Activation of iron-regulatory protein and upregulation of transferrin receptor expression in erythroid cells. Blood 89:680-687, 1997
42. Eschbach JW, Adamson JW: Iron overload in renal failure patients: Changes since the introduction of erythropoietin therapy. Kidney Int 69:S35-S43, 1999 (suppl)
43. NFK-DOQI clinical practice guidelines for the treatment of anemia of chronic renal failure. National Kidney Foundation-Dialysis Outcomes Quality Initiative. Am J Kidney Dis 30:S192-S240, 1997 (suppl 3)
44. Weiss G, Goodnough LT: Anemia of chronic disease. N Engl J Med 352:1011-1023, 2005
45. Hamstra RD, Block MH: Erythropoiesis in response to blood loss in man. J Appl Physiol 27:503-507, 1969
46. Beutler E: The utilization of saccharated Fe^{59} oxide in red cell formation. J Lab Clin Med 51:415-419, 1958
47. Wood JK, Milner PF, Pathak UN: The metabolism of iron-dextran given as a total-dose infusion to iron deficient Jamaican subjects. Br J Haematol 14:119-129, 1968
48. Beamish MR, Davies AG, Eakins JD, Jacobs A, Trevett D: The measurement of reticuloendothelial iron release using iron-dextran. Br J Haematol 21:617-622, 1971
49. Cavill I: Disorders of iron metabolism. Diagnostic methods. Clin Haematol 11:259-273, 1982
50. Eckfeldt JH, Witte DL: Serum iron: Would analytical improvement enhance patient outcome? Clin Chem 40:505-507, 1994
51. Tietz NW, Rinker AD, Morrison SR: When is a serum iron really a serum iron? The status of serum iron measurements. Clin Chem 40: 546-551, 1994
52. Cazzola M, Pootrakul P, Bergamaschi G, Huebers HA, Eng M, Finch CA: Adequacy of iron supply for erythropoiesis: In vivo observations in humans. J Lab Clin Med 110:734-739, 1987

53. Goodnough LT, Price TH, Rudnick S: Iron-restricted erythropoiesis as a limitation to autologous blood donation in the erythropoietin-stimulated bone marrow. J Lab Clin Med 118:289-296, 1991
54. Hastka J, Lasserre JJ, Schwarzbeck A, Reiter A, Hehlmann R: Laboratory tests of iron status: Correlation or common sense? Clin Chem 42:718-724, 1996
55. Cook JD, Lipschitz DA, Miles LE, Finch CA: Serum ferritin as a measure of iron stores in normal subjects. Am J Clin Nutr 27:681-687, 1974
56. Lipschitz DA, Cook JD, Finch CA: A clinical evaluation of serum ferritin as an index of iron stores. N Engl J Med 290:1213-1216, 1974
57. Olivieri NF, Brittenham GM, Matsui D, Berkovitch M, Blendis LM, Cameron RG, et al: Iron-chelation therapy with oral deferiprone in patients with thalassemia major. N Engl J Med 332:918-922, 1995
58. Hallberg L, Bengtsson C, Lapidus L, Lindstedt G, Lundberg PA, Hulten L: Screening for iron deficiency: An analysis based on bone-marrow examinations and serum ferritin determinations in a population sample of women. Br J Haematol 85:787-798, 1993
59. Punnonen K, Irjala K, Rajamaki A: Serum transferrin receptor and its ratio to serum ferritin in the diagnosis of iron deficiency. Blood 89: 1052-1057, 1997
60. Mast AE, Blinder MA, Gronowski AM, Chumley C, Scott MG: Clinical utility of the soluble transferrin receptor and comparison with serum ferritin in several populations. Clin Chem 44:45-51, 1998
61. Brugnara C, Colella GM, Cremins J, Langley RC Jr, Schneider TJ, Rutherford CJ, et al: Effects of subcutaneous recombinant human erythropoietin in normal subjects: development of decreased reticulocyte hemoglobin content and iron-deficient erythropoiesis. J Lab Clin Med 123:660-667, 1994
62. Leggett BA, Brown NN, Bryant SJ, Duplock L, Powell LW, Halliday JW: Factors affecting the concentrations of ferritin in serum in a healthy Australian population. Clin Chem 36:1350-1355, 1990
63. Ludwig H, Fritz E, Leitgeb C, Pecherstorfer M, Samonigg H, Schuster J: Prediction of response to erythropoietin treatment in chronic anemia of cancer. Blood 84:1056-1063, 1994
64. Cazzola M, Messinger D, Battistel V, Bron D, Cimino R, Enller-Ziegler L, et al: Recombinant human erythropoietin in the anemia associated with multiple myeloma or non-Hodgkin's lymphoma: Dose finding and identification of predictors of response. Blood 86:4446-4453, 1995
65. Henry D, Abels R, Larholt K: Prediction of response to recombinant human erythropoietin (r-HuEPO/epoetin-alpha) therapy in cancer patients. Blood 85:1676-1678, 1995
66. Kasper C, Terhaar A, Fossa A, Welt A, Seeber S, Nowrousian MR: Recombinant human erythropoietin in the treatment of cancer-related anaemia. Eur J Haematol 58:251-256, 1997
67. Auerbach M, Ballard H, Trout JR, McIlwain M, Ackerman A, Bahrain H, et al: Intravenous iron optimizes the response to recombinant human erythropoietin in cancer patients with chemotherapy-related anemia: A multicenter, open-label, randomized trial. J Clin Oncol 22:1301-1307, 2004
68. Barosi G: Inadequate erythropoietin response to anemia: Definition and clinical relevance. Ann Hematol 68:215-223, 1994
69. Thompson JA, Gilliland DG, Prchal J, Bennett JM, Larholt K, Nelson RA, et al: Effects of recombinant human erythropoietin combined with granulocyte/macrophage colony-stimulating factor in the treatment of patients with myelodysplastic syndrome. GM/EPO MDS Study Group. Blood 95:1175-1179, 2000
70. Ludwig H, Fritz E, Kotzmann H, Hocker P, Gisslinger H, Barnas U: Erythropoietin treatment of anemia associated with multiple myeloma. N Engl J Med 322:1693-1699, 1990
71. Pincus T, Olson NJ, Russel IJ, Wolfe F, Harris ER, Schnitzer TJ, et al: Multicenter study of recombinant human erythropoietin in correction of anemia in patients with rheumatoid arthritis. Am J Med 89:161-168, 1990
72. Abels R, Larholt K, Krantz K, Bryant E: Recombinant human erythropoietin for the treatment of the anemia of cancer, in Murphy MJ Jr (ed): Blood Cell Growth Factors: Their Present and Future Use in Hematology and Oncology. Dayton, OH, Alpha Med, 1991, pp 121-141
73. Glaspy J, Bukowski R, Steinberg D, Taylor C, Tchekmedyian S, Vadhan-Raj S: Impact of therapy with epoetin alfa on clinical outcomes in patients with nonmyeloid malignancies during cancer chemotherapy in community oncology practice. J Clin Oncol 15:1218-1234, 1997
74. Glaspy J, Demetri G, Cremieux P: Does baseline endogenous erythropoietin level impact hemoglobin (Hb) response to rHuEPO in cancer patients? Blood 94:15B, 1999
75. Osterborg A, Boogaerts MA, Cimino R, Essers U, Holowiecki J, Juliusson G, et al: Recombinant human erythropoietin in transfusion-dependent anemic patients with multiple myeloma and non-Hodgkin's lymphoma—A randomized multicenter study. The European Study Group of Erythropoietin (Epoetin Beta) Treatment in Multiple Myeloma and Non-Hodgkin's Lymphoma. Blood 87:2675-2682, 1996

ELSEVIER

Seminars in
HEMATOLOGY

Experience With Intravenous Iron in Nephrology

Iain C. Macdougall

Over the last two decades, the use of intravenous iron in nephrology practice has increased considerably. This is due to several factors: first, there has been increased recognition of the benefits of intravenous iron in the management of renal anemia; second, the advent of erythropoiesis-stimulating agent (ESA) therapy has increased the demand for intravenous iron supplementation; and third, the older dextran-containing iron preparations have been replaced by newer intravenous iron compounds that are safer and not associated with life-threatening anaphylaxis. Intravenous iron can potentiate the response to ESA therapy and allow a reduction in ESA dose requirements, and in some patients it may improve hemoglobin levels when administered alone. Safety concerns such as increased risk of exacerbating infections or oxidative stress are largely based on in vitro data, and clinical data to support these concerns are sparse. Intravenous iron may be administered as a slow bolus injection or as an infusion, and there is a need for further studies to elucidate which, if any, of these regimens should be recommended.
Semin Hematol 43(suppl 6):S9-S12

Patients with chronic kidney disease (CKD) show a tendency to be in negative iron balance. This is due to several factors. First, on the intake side, many CKD patients have a reduced appetite, with an associated low intake of iron in their diet. Furthermore, their uremic state also results in impaired iron absorption from the gastrointestinal tract, and this is probably mediated by hepcidin. Second, iron losses in CKD patients are greater than in healthy individuals. The latter lose approximately 1 mg of iron per day in the feces, whereas some patients on dialysis may have iron losses of 5 to 6 mg or more daily. This is due to uremic gastroenteropathy, with an increased risk of esophagitis, gastritis, duodenitis, and even frank peptic ulceration. Bleeding (and hence iron loss) may be further exacerbated by aspirin (which many patients are prescribed), heparin administration on dialysis, and uremic platelet dysfunction. The advent of erythropoiesis-stimulating agents (ESAs) also produced an increase in iron requirements due to the need to support greater red blood cell production in the bone marrow. As a result, many CKD patients require iron supplementation. Although simple and cheap, oral iron is unfortunately not well absorbed in uremia, and thus parenteral iron is required. Intramuscular injections are painful, and result in brownish discoloration of the skin and increased risk of intramuscular hemorrhage. Thus, intravenous iron has become the favored route of administration in the majority of CKD patients, particularly those receiving regular hemodialysis. This review will discuss, in turn, the benefits of intravenous iron supplementation, followed by concerns regarding the safety of intravenous iron and, finally, regimens for administering intravenous iron.

Benefits

The proven benefits of intravenous iron in CKD patients can be considered in two distinct clinical settings.

Intravenous Iron Can Improve the Anemia Associated With CKD Even in the Absence of ESA Therapy

Even before the days when ESA therapy became available, the effects of intravenous iron in partially correcting the anemia of CKD was demonstrated.[1] More recently, Sargent and Acchiardo[2] preloaded a cohort of candidate patients for erythropoietin (EPO) therapy with intravenous iron (900 to 1,525 mg). Seventy percent of patients demonstrated an increase in hematocrit without EPO, and 40% of patients achieved hematocrits greater than 30%. Similarly, in a cohort of 60 anemic nondialyzed CKD patients without overt iron deficiency, Mircescu et al[3] administered 200 mg of intravenous iron sucrose every month for 12 months and observed a significant increase in hemoglobin (9.7 ± 1.1 g/dL at baseline to 11.3 ± 2.5 g/dL after 12 months); 36% of patients reached the study target hemoglobin of 10 g/dL, and no adverse ef-

Department of Renal Medicine, King's College Hospital, London, United Kingdom.
Address correspondence to Iain C. Macdougall, MD, Consultant Nephrologist, Renal Unit, King's College Hospital, London SE5 9RS, UK. E-mail: Iain.macdougall@kingsch.nhs.uk

0037-1963/06/$-see front matter
doi:10.1053/j.seminhematol.2006.08.004

fects were observed. Silverberg et al[4] examined the effect of intravenous iron alone or in combination with low-dose EPO in the correction of anemia in nondialysis CKD patients, and although the hemoglobin response was more rapid in the group supplemented with EPO and intravenous iron, nearly 50% of patients given intravenous iron alone showed an increase in hematocrit greater than 3%; 28.9% of such patients reached the target hematocrit of 35% compared with 40% of those given both EPO and intravenous iron. Thus, it is clear that intravenous iron alone can achieve some correction of anemia in CKD, but many patients will also require EPO supplementation.

Intravenous Iron Can Significantly Enhance the Response to ESAs, Even in Iron-Replete Patients

Several studies have demonstrated potentiation of the response to ESA therapy even in patients who were iron-replete at baseline. Two of the earlier randomized controlled trials compared the effect of intravenous iron administration with oral iron supplementation in CKD patients, one in the correction phase of ESA therapy and one in the maintenance phase. In the correction phase study, Macdougall et al[5] randomized 37 patients to receive intravenous (n = 12), oral (n = 13), or no iron (n = 12) supplementation. The hemoglobin response in the group receiving intravenous iron was significantly greater than that in the other two groups, and there was no difference between the groups supplemented with oral and no iron. EPO dose requirements were significantly less in the intravenous iron group compared with the other two groups.

In the maintenance phase study, Fishbane et al[6] compared the efficacy of oral and intravenous iron for the chronic maintenance of iron stores in a cohort of 52 hemodialysis patients. The 20 patients randomized to intravenous iron supplementation (100 mg twice weekly) had a significantly greater hematocrit increase compared with the group of 32 patients supplemented with oral iron therapy, and the final mean EPO dose was 46% lower in the intravenous iron group compared with the oral iron group (4050 ± 634 units per treatment *v* 7563 ± 378 units per treatment). More recently, Van Wyck et al[7] performed a similar randomized controlled trial comparing intravenous iron sucrose to oral iron in nondialysis CKD patients. The proportion of patients achieving the primary outcome of a hemoglobin increase ≥1 g/dL was greater in the intravenous iron-supplemented group compared with the oral iron-supplemented group (44.3% *v* 28.0%, $P = .0344$), as was the mean increase in hemoglobin by day 42 (0.7 *v* 0.4 g/dL, $P = .0298$).

Thus, the contribution of intravenous iron to the management of anemia in CKD patients is well established, both with and without concomitant ESA therapy.

Concerns Regarding Safety and Adverse Effects

Concerns about the safety of intravenous iron can be considered under short-lived acute reactions and potential long-term detrimental effects (Fig 1).

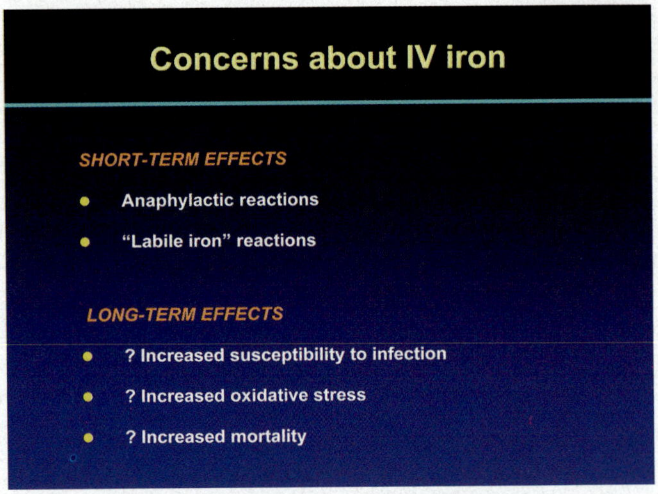

Figure 1 Short-term acute reactions and potential long-term effects of intravenous iron.

Reactions to Intravenous Iron

The administration of intravenous iron is usually not associated with any immediate adverse effects. However, some patients will experience an acute reaction either during or immediately following the administration of iron. Typical reactions are characterized by sudden-onset hypotension, breathlessness, abdominal or back pain, and flushing.

Anaphylaxis may occur with iron dextran, probably mediated immunologically via preformed dextran antibodies.[8] However, the cause of the milder anaphylactoid reactions, which are a characteristic of all intravenous iron preparations is not clear, but it seems apparent that the latter reactions are generally encountered when too much iron is administered too rapidly. Many patients not receiving dextran-containing intravenous iron can be rechallenged with a lower dose administered more slowly. The incidence of severe anaphylactic reactions to iron dextran has been estimated to occur in approximately 0.7% of patients treated with this preparation, and although this catastrophic reaction is rare, hospitalization and death may occur.[9] It seems apparent that the nondextran iron preparations (iron sucrose and ferric gluconate) have a lower risk for severe life-threatening reactions than iron dextran. However, it is very difficult to define the relative rates of reactions with the different iron preparations, and there have been no well-designed, adequately powered comparative studies examining this issue, most of the evidence coming from retrospective analyses of clinical databases.

Risk of Infection

Another safety concern with intravenous iron supplementation relates to the risk of infection. Since iron is an important growth factor for bacteria and other infectious microorganisms, supplemental iron can exacerbate bacterial proliferation.[10] In animal studies, administration of iron has been shown to promote infection.[11] Furthermore, iron supplementation may inhibit important defense mechanisms, such as polymorphonuclear leukocyte function.[12] In short, intravenous iron can potentially enhance bacterial proliferation while reducing the body's ability to fight infection. The supportive evidence for this, however, originates from in vitro studies, and a large multicenter prospective European study did not find any relationship between serum ferritin or iron treatment and risk for infection.[13] Nevertheless, despite this absence of definitive clinical data, it seems sensible to avoid intravenous iron administration in the setting of acute infection.

Risk of Oxidative Stress

Another safety concern with intravenous iron therapy is the potential to induce oxidative tissue injury. Although it is recognized that iron may indeed cause oxidative changes in DNA, protein, or lipids, this should only occur in direct contact between iron and the tissues, and not in iron safely bound in biological complexes such as ferritin, transferrin, and hemosiderin, or when tightly bound in a carbohydrate shell, as occurs with the parenteral iron preparations. Following injection of intravenous iron, however, there may be some release of iron into the circulation, and this free iron may cause a significant increase in oxidative stress.[14,15] Again, the in vitro studies of Zager et al[16] found that iron dextran, iron sucrose, and ferric gluconate all led to some degree of lipid peroxidation, and more recently Leehey et al[17] found evidence of increased oxidative stress following administration of ferric gluconate to CKD patients. These and other studies, therefore, suggest that there is probably some release of free iron into the circulation after injection of intravenous iron and that some degree of oxidative stress occurs. What is not clear is whether this oxidative stress leads to any harmful effects, either tissue injury or worse outcomes. CKD patients are exposed to frequent events causing oxidative stress, including hemodialysis itself. Indeed, in a randomized controlled study, Scheiber-Mojdehkar et al[18] compared the levels of lipid peroxidation in hemodialysis patients who received and who did not receive intravenous iron across the hemodialysis session. There was a transient increase in peroxide generation in both groups of patients, but the addition of intravenous iron did not enhance this. Regarding mortality, Feldman et al[19] examined the incidence of all-cause mortality in a large cohort study involving 32,566 hemodialysis patients from Fresenius dialysis centers, using a multivariate model to account for the timing of intravenous iron. There was absolutely no relationship between the accumulative 6-month iron dose and the probability of mortality in this study. In summary, although nephrologists should be cautious about the potential effects of intravenous iron in increasing oxidative stress, it is not clear just how much additional oxidative stress is achieved by administration of intravenous iron and whether this has any adverse implications. Further research is needed with regard to this important issue.

How to Administer Intravenous Iron

Given the frequent need for iron supplementation in CKD patients, nephrologists have to decide whether to adopt a preemptive or a reactive approach to administration of intravenous iron. Thus, should the nephrologist simply monitor the laboratory parameters of iron status and prescribe intravenous iron supplementation only when iron deficiency becomes evident? Or does the nephrologist administer intravenous iron routinely in order to prevent iron deficiency developing?

The main determinant of which regimen is adopted is the patient population. Hemodialysis patients attend hospital regularly, usually 3 days per week, and have ready vascular access. Thus, in many dialysis units worldwide, intravenous iron is prescribed on a regular basis in order to maintain a background iron supply. This may be intensified as required, depending on the laboratory iron parameters. The exact iron dosing regimen depends on the individual unit. Some units will administer low-dose intravenous iron (20 to 60 mg) every dialysis, while others will give 100 mg every week, reducing to 100 mg every month if the ferritin becomes greater than 400 μg/L. Both the US[20] and European[21] anemia guidelines recommend that intravenous iron should be stopped completely if the ferritin becomes greater than 800 μg/L since, first, there is less evidence that going above this threshold results in significant benefits and, second, this may potentially cause increased harm.

In nonhemodialysis patients such as those receiving peritoneal dialysis or those not yet requiring dialysis, it is clearly less practical to adopt a preemptive approach. Thus, many of these patients have their iron status monitored regularly and intravenous iron administered as required. Since these patients are not attending hospital as regularly, larger doses of intravenous iron are usually given. This may be administered either as a slow bolus injection or as an intravenous iron infusion, depending on the dosage required. Chandler et al,[22] for example, showed that with iron sucrose the risk of acute anaphylactoid reactions increased when more than 400 mg was administered as a 2-hour infusion. Macdougall and Roche[23] investigated the safety of administering 200 mg of

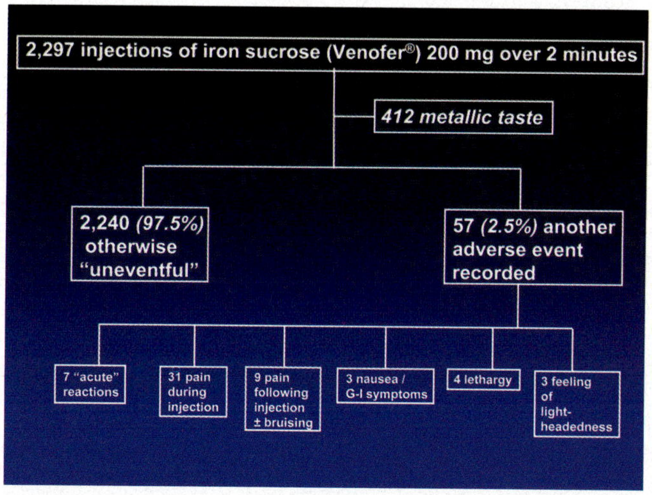

Figure 2 Safety of intravenous iron administration (200 mg of iron sucrose) in 2,297 injections. Prospective data collected by Macdougall and Roche.[23]

iron sucrose as a 2-minute bolus injection, and prospective data were collected for 2,297 injections (Fig 2). During 412 of the injections, patients experienced a transient metallic taste in their mouth. Excluding this, 2,240 of the injections proceeded uneventfully, and in the other 57 injections, an adverse event was recorded. Most of these adverse events were trivial, and of the seven immediate reactions, all were short-lived, usually characterized by hypotension and dizziness, and none required hospitalization. The cost and time savings of adopting this regimen in the study were substantial.

Conclusions

Intravenous iron supplementation has become a mainstay of therapy in the management of CKD-associated anemia. It can potentiate the response to ESAs and may even improve hemoglobin levels when administered alone. There is in vitro evidence that intravenous iron may exacerbate the risk of infection or oxidative stress, although there is no clinical evidence that this is the case. Generally, the benefits of intravenous iron outweigh these potential concerns. Nevertheless, it seems sensible to avoid giving intravenous iron to patients with acute infection or sepsis, since not only might this be hazardous but there is no evidence that intravenous iron is efficacious in this clinical setting.[8]

References

1. Strickland ID, Chaput de Saintonge DM, et al: The therapeutic equivalence of oral and intravenous iron in renal dialysis patients. Clin Nephrol 7:55-57, 1977
2. Sargent JA, Acchiardo SR: Iron requirements in hemodialysis. Blood Purif 22:112-123, 2004
3. Mircescu G, Garneata L, Capusa C, Ursea N: Intravenous iron supplementation for the treatment of anaemia in pre-dialyzed chronic renal failure patients. Nephrol Dial Transplant 21:120-124, 2006
4. Silverberg DS, Blum M, Agbaria Z, et al: The effect of i.v. iron alone or in combination with low-dose erythropoietin in the rapid correction of anemia of chronic renal failure in the predialysis period. Clin Nephrol 55:212-219, 2001
5. Macdougall IC, Tucker B, Thompson J, Tomson CR, Baker LR, Raine AE: A randomized controlled study of iron supplementation in patients treated with erythropoietin. Kidney Int 50:1694-1699, 1996
6. Fishbane S, Frei GL, Maesaka J: Reduction in recombinant human erythropoietin doses by the use of chronic intravenous iron supplementation. Am J Kidney Dis 26:41-46, 1995
7. Van Wyck DB, Roppolo M, Martinez CO, Mazey RM, McMurray S, United States Iron Sucrose (Venofer) Clinical Trials Group: A randomized, controlled trial comparing IV iron sucrose to oral iron in anemic patients with nondialysis-dependent CKD. Kidney Int 68:2846-2856, 2005
8. Fishbane S, Ungureanu VD, Maesaka JK, Kaupke CJ, Lim V, Wish J: The safety of intravenous iron dextran in hemodialysis patients. Am J Kidney Dis 28:529-534, 1996
9. Faich G, Strobos J: Sodium ferric gluconate complex in sucrose: Safer intravenous iron therapy than iron dextrans. Am J Kidney Dis 33:464-470, 1999
10. Bullen JJ, Ward CG, Wallis SN: Virulence and the role of iron in Pseudomonas aeruginosa infection. Infect Immun 10:443-450, 1974
11. Rogers HJ, Bullen JJ, Cushnie GH: Iron compounds and resistance to infection. Further experiments with Clostridium welchii type A in vivo and in vitro. Immunology 19:521-538, 1970
12. Deicher R, Ziai F, Cohen G, Mullner M, Horl WH: High-dose parenteral iron sucrose depresses neutrophil intracellular killing capacity. Kidney Int 64:728-736, 2003
13. Hoen B, Paul-Dauphin A, Hestin D, Kessler M: EPIBACDIAL: A multicenter prospective study of risk factors for bacteremia in chronic hemodialysis patients. J Am Soc Nephrol 9:869-876, 1998
14. Agarwal R, Vasavada N, Sachs NG, Chase S: Oxidative stress and renal injury with intravenous iron in patients with chronic kidney disease. Kidney Int 65:2279-2289, 2004
15. Rooyakkers TM, Stroes ES, Kooistra MP, et al: Ferric saccharate induces oxygen radical stress and endothelial dysfunction in vivo. Eur J Clin Invest 32:9-16, 2002 (suppl 1)
16. Zager RA, Johnson AC, Hanson SY, Wasse H: Parenteral iron formulations: A comparative toxicologic analysis and mechanisms of cell injury. Am J Kidney Dis 40:90-103, 2002
17. Leehey DJ, Palubiak DJ, Chebrolu S, Agarwal R: Sodium ferric gluconate causes oxidative stress but not acute renal injury in patients with chronic kidney disease: A pilot study. Nephrol Dial Transplant 20:135-140, 2005
18. Scheiber-Mojdehkar B, Lutzky B, Schaufler R, Sturm B, Goldenberg H: Non-transferrin-bound iron in the serum of hemodialysis patients who receive ferric saccharate: No correlation to peroxide generation. J Am Soc Nephrol 15:1648-1655, 2004
19. Feldman HI, Joffe M, Robinson B, et al: Administration of parenteral iron and mortality among hemodialysis patients. J Am Soc Nephrol 15:1623-1632, 2004
20. National Kidney Foundation Kidney Disease Outcomes Quality Initiative: KDOQI clinical practice guidelines and clinical practice recommendations for anemia in chronic kidney disease. Am J Kidney Dis 47:S1-S145, 2006 (suppl 3)
21. Locatelli F, Aljama P, Barany P, Canaud B, Carrera F, Eckardt KU, et al: Revised European best practice guidelines for the management of anaemia in patients with chronic renal failure. Nephrol Dial Transplant 19:ii1-ii47, 2004 (suppl 2)
22. Chandler G, Harchowal J, Macdougall IC: Intravenous iron sucrose: Establishing a safe dose. Am J Kidney Dis 38:988-91, 2001
23. Macdougall IC, Roche A: Administration of intravenous iron sucrose as a 2-minute push to CKD patients: A prospective evaluation of 2,297 injections. Am J Kidney Dis 46:283-289, 2005

ELSEVIER

Seminars in
HEMATOLOGY

Iron Metabolism and Iron Supplementation in Anemia of Cancer

Heinz Ludwig

Iron is an essential trace element important for hematopoiesis, oxygen transport and delivery, and other biologic functions. Iron uptake and utilization are strictly regulated but severely altered in anemia of chronic disease. In this condition, availability of iron for erythropoiesis is insufficient and a limiting factor for red blood cell production, in spite of normal or increased storage iron. Although concomitant oral iron supplementation is recommended in guidelines for treatment of cancer-associated anemia with erythropoietic agents, its efficacy is not documented. Recent studies evaluated the impact of parenteral iron supplementation in comparison with oral iron therapy and with control in anemic cancer patients treated with epoetin alfa or beta, or with darbepoetin. Concomitant treatment with parenteral iron proved superior to oral iron or no treatment. Hematologic response rates were higher, time to increase of hemoglobin was shorter, the need for red blood cell transfusions lower, and the quality of life better than in patients treated with oral or no iron at all. Severe side effects were rare and tolerance was remarkably good in most patients. However, information on long-term safety is not available as yet. Taken together, parenteral iron administration seems likely to evolve as an important adjunct to treatment with erythropoietic agents in patients with treatment-induced or chronic anemia of cancer.
Semin Hematol 43(suppl 6):S13-S17

The human body contains 30 to 40 mg/kg iron, adding up to approximately 3 to 4 g iron per individual. Body iron is mostly contained in hemoglobin (~2.5 g), ferritin (1 g), myoglobin, and other heme proteins (~0.5 g). Only 3 mg is transported in plasma. Intestinal iron absorption is tightly regulated by four important proteins. The divalent iron transporter binds intestinal iron and incorporates it into the enterocytes. Ferroportin binds to and exports divalent iron into the circulation where it is taken up by the main iron transporter, transferrin. Finally, hepcidin, a recently described acute-phase protein, is the major regulator of iron absorption. Hepcidin is mainly synthesized in the liver and its production increases significantly during inflammation. Hepcidin interacts with membrane-bound ferroportin and leads to its internalization and degradation, thereby limiting the transport of iron into the circulation. Increased hepcidin levels result in significant reduction of iron absorption, decreased iron release from cells of the reticuloendothelial system, and an increase in storage iron. The normal daily dietary iron supply amounts to 10 to 15 mg, but only 1 to 2 mg are actually absorbed and the same amount is lost by cells sequestered from the gastrointestinal tract and skin.

Formation of red blood cells depends on adequate formation of hemoglobin, which consists of two alpha and two beta globin subunits and four heme groups, each of which contains one atom of iron bound to protoporphyrin. Adequate iron supply, hence, is an important rate-limiting factor of erythropoiesis. Iron is mainly supplied via transferrin, which normally contains two atoms of trivalent iron. Transferrin saturation is significantly decreased (<20%) in iron deficiency and in functional iron deficiency, defined as a state with suboptimal iron supply to the erythron in spite of adequate body iron stores. Functional iron deficiency ensues in inflammatory diseases, infections, and chronic anemia of cancer when a cascade of inflammatory cytokines, as well as hepcidin, induces a major shift of circulating iron into the reticuloendothelial system and almost abolishes intestinal iron absorption, resulting in an inadequate iron supply to the proliferating erythroid compartment that finally results in anemia.

Iron Status in Patients With Anemia of Cancer

Patients with anemia of cancer usually present with normocytic, normochromic red blood cells with reduced serum iron (<60 μg/mL) and normal or increased serum ferritin

Department of Medicine I, Center for Oncology and Hematology, Wilhelminenspital, Vienna, Austria.
Supported by the Austrian Forum Against Cancer.
Address correspondence to Heinz Ludwig, MD, Department of Medicine I, Center for Oncology and Hematology, Montleartstrasse 37, 1171 Vienna, Austria. E-mail: heinz.ludwig@wienkav.at

0037-1963/06/$-see front matter © 2006 Elsevier Inc. All rights reserved.
doi:10.1053/j.seminhematol.2006.08.008

Table 1 Main Features of Functional Iron Deficiency

Serum ferritin	>20 μg/L
Serum iron	<60 μg/dL
Transferrin saturation	<20%
Percentage of hypochromic red blood cells	>5%
Reticulocyte hemoglobin content	<26 pg
Soluble transferrin receptor	Normal
Erythrocyte protoporhyrin	>70 μg/dL

NOTE. Cutoff values may vary slightly depending on the test system used.

levels, reduced transferrin saturation (<20%), but normal or increased iron stores, and normal levels of circulating transferrin receptors. Other, usually not generally available, parameters include increased percentage of hypochromic red blood cells (>5%), increased erythrocyte protoporphyrin levels (>70 μg/dL), and decreased reticulocyte hemoglobin content (<26 pg) (Table 1). In these patients, inflammatory cytokines usually inhibit iron release from storage pools, leading to rapid depletion of the labile serum iron pool and hence to insufficient iron supply to proliferating red blood cell precursors. However, some cancer patients, particularly those with gastrointestinal blood loss, may present with true iron deficiency (serum iron <20 μg/dL, serum ferritin <15 μg/L, transferrin saturation <20%, empty iron stores, and increased circulating transferrin receptors >7 mg/L).[1] In patients with chronic inflammation, absolute iron deficiency may be associated with impaired iron utilization. Information on iron stores and parameters of iron metabolism in different types of anemia is given in Figure 1.

Iron Supplementation in Non-cancer Anemia

Iron supplementation is standard treatment in patients with absolute iron deficiency, and parenteral application results in faster replenishment of iron stores and increased erythropoiesis in patients with absolute or functional iron deficiency. The efficacy of this approach has been documented in patients with increased iron needs due to increased erythropoiesis[2,3] and in patients with functional iron deficiency due to chronic inflammatory diseases such as rheumatoid arthritis[4] and chronic inflammatory bowel disease.[3,5] Besides the increase in circulating iron, inhibition of tumor necrosis factor (TNF) production by intravenous iron has been postulated as an important contributory factor.[6]

In renal anemia, parenteral iron therapy resulted in a rapid increase in hemoglobin levels, whereas oral iron supplementation remained without significant effect.[7] These observations led to the incorporation of intravenous iron supplementation into the guidelines for treating anemia in renal diseases.[8] Additional studies revealed a 40% reduction in erythropoietin doses in iron-supplemented patients compared to patients without iron therapy during maintenance therapy.[7]

Oral Iron Supplementation

Although supplementation with oral iron is recommended for patients with anemia of cancer and concomitant erythropoietin treatment in the guidelines issued by the American Society of Clinical Oncology (ASCO), the American Society of Hematology (ASH),[9] the National Comprehensive Cancer Network (NCCN),[10] and the European Organisation for Research and Treatment of Cancer (EORTC),[11] evidence supporting the efficacy of such supplementation is scarce. The only published prospective randomized trial was a study that also evaluated the efficacy of parenteral iron substitution. The four-arm study showed no significant improvement with twice-daily 325 mg oral iron (ferrous sulfate) over no iron administration in erythropoietin-treated patients with chemotherapy-induced anemia.[12] However, the treatment duration was rather short for a meaningful comparison. Interestingly, the deterioration in certain parameters of quality of life and general activity observed in patients receiving no iron was not seen in patients receiving oral iron supplementation.

Parenteral Iron Supplementation

The hypothesis that unresponsiveness to initial erythropoietin treatment can be overcome by concomitant treatment with intravenous iron was recently tested by Katodritou et al[13] in a small phase II study. The investigators treated 27 anemic patients with myeloma or lymphoma with erythropoietin (30,000 IU once weekly) and observed a hematologic response in 19 patients (70%). Subsequently, intravenous iron (iron sucrose 200 mg once weekly over 6 weeks) was given to the eight patients who did not respond to erythropoietin treatment alone. Six of the eight patients finally responded to combined therapy with erythropoietin and intravenous iron.

Henry et al[14] conducted a larger prospective randomized trial in 187 patients with chemotherapy-induced anemia

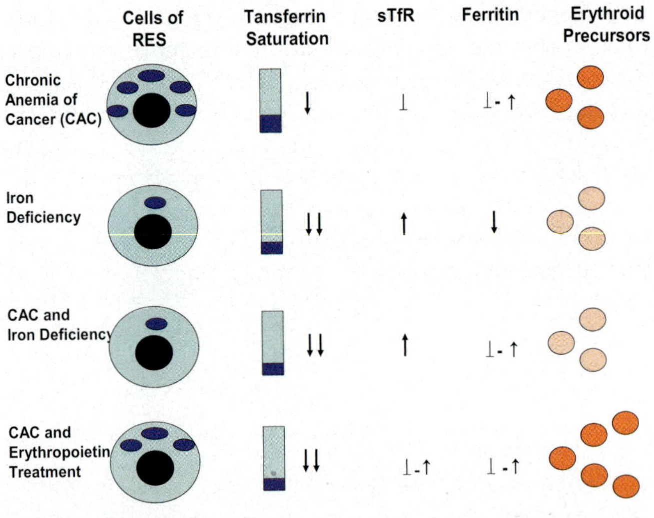

Figure 1 Parameters of iron metabolism and erythropoiesis in different types of anemia. Blue granula in RES cells denote iron deposits. RES, reticuloendothelial system; sTfR, soluble transferrin receptor.

treated with erythropoietin. Patients were randomized to either oral iron supplementation (ferrous sulfate 325 mg, twice daily), parenteral iron therapy (ferric gluconate, 125 mg/wk), or to an untreated control group. Intravenous iron in addition to erythropoietin led to a significantly higher response rate (73%) compared to oral iron (45%) or no iron at all (41%). Median increases in hemoglobin were 2.4 g/dL, 1.6 g/dL, and 1.5 g/dL in patients receiving intravenous, oral, or no iron supplementation, respectively. Furthermore, transferrin saturation fell by 13.7% in patients without iron supplementation but only by 2.7% and 1.8%, respectively, in those with oral or intravenous iron therapy.

The only hitherto fully published prospective randomized trial comparing intravenous iron with oral iron or no iron at all has been published by Auerbach et al.[12] The authors treated 157 anemic patients (hemoglobin <10.5 g/dL, serum ferritin ≤450 nmol/mL, or ≤675 nmol/mL and transferrin saturation ≤19%) with solid tumors receiving erythropoietin therapy (40,000 IU/wk) concomitantly to standard chemotherapy. Patients were randomized to no additional iron, oral iron (iron sulfate 325 mg, twice daily), weekly parenteral iron (iron dextran 100 mg weekly), or single iron-dextran infusion with the calculated total iron demand according to the formula: 0.0442 × (target hemoglobin [14 g/dL] − observed hemoglobin) × body weight + (0.26 × body weight).[15] After 6 weeks of treatment, hematologic responses were observed in 25%, 36%, 68%, and 68% of patients, respectively (Table 2). Mean increases in hemoglobin levels from baseline were 0.9 g/dL, 1.5 g/dL, 2.5 g/dL, and 2.4 g/dL for the non-iron, oral, intravenous bolus, and total-dose iron groups, respectively. Importantly, the hemoglobin response was found to be independent of the baseline transferrin saturation: no difference was seen between patients who had very low or only low (<15% or >15%) transferrin saturation, which indicates a benefit of iron supplementation even in patients with less pronounced functional iron deficiency. In addition, a significant improvement in several parameters of quality of life (especially energy, activity and general quality of life) was observed in the latter two groups. Quality of life deteriorated in patients without any iron therapy and remained unchanged—with the exception of a minor increase in energy—in patients on oral iron.

Two other randomized studies comparing parenteral iron substitution with standard treatment in anemic patients treated with erythropoietic agents have only been presented at meetings as yet.[16,17] Vandebroek et al[16] randomized 198 patients with non-myeloid cancers and treated with darbepoetin alfa every 3 weeks into a group treated with intravenous iron sucrose and a control group treated according to standard practice including oral iron substitution. The full analysis data set was available for 196 patients. Seventy-nine percent of the patients receiving intravenous iron achieved a hemoglobin level of ≥11 g/dL, compared to 70.8% in the standard practice group. The median time to target hemoglobin (≥11 g/dL) was 34 days in the former and 43 days in the latter group. The higher response rate in the intravenous iron group was also reflected by the percentage of patients achieving a hemoglobin level of ≥11g/dL between week 5 and the end of treatment: 79.8% of patients treated with intravenous iron achieved the target level compared to 65.3% on standard therapy. The requirement for transfusion until week 5 was almost halved in patients on intravenous iron (10.6% *v* 22.8%). Quality of life measured by a FACT-F (Functional Assessment of Cancer Therapy: Fatigue) score and by a FACT-G (Functional Assessment of Cancer Therapy: General) score was significantly better in the first 5 treatment weeks in the group receiving parenteral iron. The increases in the mean FACT-F and FACT-G scores were 3.1 versus 1.6 and 2.4 versus 0.94, respectively. Side effects were similar in

Table 2 Hematologic Response (increase of Hb ≥2 g/dL, or achievement of Hb ≥12 g/dL) in Erythropoietin-Treated Anemic Cancer Patients Randomized to Either Oral or Intravenous Iron Supplementation or to an Untreated Group

Authors	Erythropoietic Agent Dose	Untreated Control	Oral Iron Sulfate	Intravenous Iron, Once Weekly	Intravenous Iron, Total Dose Infusion
Henry et al (2004)[1]	Epoetin alfa 40,000 IU once weekly	41%	45%	73%*	
Auerbach et al (2004)[12]	Epoetin alfa 40,000 IU once weekly	25%	36%	68%†	68%‡
Vandebroek et al (2006)[16]	Darbepoetin alpha 500 μg, every 3 weeks	70.8%§		79%‖	
Hedenus et al (2006)[17]	Epoetin beta 30,000 IU once weekly	50%¶		79%¶	

Abbreviation: Hb, hemoglobin.
*Ferric gluconate 125 mg weekly over 8 weeks.
†Iron dextran 100 mg weekly over 6 weeks.
‡Calculated total dose of iron needed given as iron dextran in one infusion.
§Control group included patients with oral iron substitution.
‖Hematologic response defined as achievment of Hb ≥11 g/dL, 200 mg iron sucrose every 3 weeks or two doses (2 × 100 mg) over a 3- week period.
¶Hematologic response defined as increase in Hb ≥2 g/dL, iron sucrose 100 mg once weekly over 6 weeks.

the two groups and no specific adverse events related to parenteral iron substitution were noted.

Hedenus et al[17] randomized 67 patients with indolent lymphoproliferative disease (non-Hodgkin's lymphoma: 19, chronic lymphocytic leukemia: 23, and multiple myeloma: 25) treated with epoetin beta 30,000 IU once weekly to a group receiving 100 mg iron sucrose once weekly (for 6 weeks) or to a control arm. Sixty patients remained on erythropoietin treatment for 16 weeks and, hence, completed the study. Three of them needed red blood cell transfusion during the study and were considered as failures but had been included in the intention-to-treat analysis. The patient group treated with epoetin plus intravenous iron achieved a significantly higher mean change in hemoglobin levels from baseline to the end of the study (2.76 *v* 1.56 g/dL, $P < .0002$). Significantly more patients achieved a hemoglobin response (increase in hemoglobin >2 g/dL) in a shorter time (79% *v* 50%, $P < .02$). Furthermore, a lower dose of erythropoietin was required in the group receiving intravenous iron ($P = .051$).

The side effects of parenteral iron therapy depend largely on the iron preparation used as well as on the dose and velocity of the injection or infusion but are usually less frequently observed with iron sucrose and ferric gluconate than with iron dextran. In the Auerbach study, side effects were noted in 7% of the 41 patients with single infusion of the total iron dose, and in 8% of the 37 patients with weekly infusions of iron dextran.[12] A significant side effect in terms of an anaphylactic reaction with flush, hypotension, emesis, and vomiting was noted in one patient after a test dose of iron dextran. Common side effects of intravenous iron reported in other studies included arthralgias, exanthemas, and increased body temperature. Oral iron supplementation is usually well tolerated but gastrointestinal side effects such as nausea, abdominal discomfort, and constipation are not uncommon and may necessitate discontinuation of treatment in some patients.

Treatment Considerations

Patients with anemia of cancer and absolute iron deficiency are candidates for intravenous iron therapy, particularly if severe symptoms of anemia demand for fast improvement. In anemic cancer patients with functional iron deficiency, there is increasing evidence for the benefits of intravenous iron substitution. In all studies in anemic cancer patients conducted so far, iron was given concomitantly to erythropoietin therapy, indicating the need for data on the efficacy of iron as sole therapy in this situation. Importantly, in the presently available studies, iron was given for very short periods only and information on long-term use is lacking. It is, however, questionable whether iron should be given over prolonged periods to patients with cancer. Iron has been identified as an important growth factor for microorganisms and tumor cells, and some authors consider the shift of circulating iron into iron stores as an important defense mechanism of the body against the aforementioned threats.[18] In addition, free circulating iron results in the formation of hydroxyl radicals that are toxic to various tissues. An increase in cancer incidence has been noted in patients with elevated serum or body iron,[19] while no increase in cancer incidence has been reported in patients with continuous parenteral iron supplementation due to renal anemia.[20] In contrast, in patients on hemodialysis, treatment with iron sucrose resulted in reduced hospitalization and mortality.[20] Treating anemic patients with red blood cell transfusions is always associated with substantial iron supply, and perioperative use of allogeneic blood transfusions has been associated with increased risk of infections.[21] One unit of red blood cells usually confers 200 mg of iron to the recipient. Nevertheless, the unresolved questions regarding the safety of long-term parenteral iron supplementation in patients with anemia of cancer illustrate the need for further studies evaluating the true benefit of long-term iron supplementation. However, short-term use of intravenous iron seems to be relatively safe, efficient, and cost-effective, and represents the only option in patients who do not tolerate oral iron therapy and in those with gastrointestinal deficiency in iron absorption. Intravenous iron in conjunction with erythropoietin should shorten the time to hematologic response, enhance response rate, spare doses of erythropoietin, and help to distinguish responders to erythropoietin from nonresponders.

Practical Considerations

Although formulas to calculate total body iron needs are available,[15] it is still unclear whether the administration of the calculated total body iron need (2 to 3 g) in one infusion is really safe and represents the optimal approach for iron administration, particularly for the treatment of functional iron deficiency. For the time being, there are more arguments in favor of administrating parenteral iron in weekly or at least adequately timed treatment intervals.

The major goal of treatment is of course to rapidly increase the hemoglobin concentration to the recommended target level of 12 to 13 g/dL,[11] and thereby to improve quality of life and reduce transfusion needs. In renal anemia the target levels of important parameters of iron metabolism have been defined as 25% to 40% for transferrin saturation, 200 to 500 μg/L for serum ferritin and <2.5% for hypochromic red cells. High levels of circulating iron expressed by high transferrin saturation (>50%) and high serum ferritin levels (>1,000 μg/L) are considered toxic and should therefore be avoided.[22]

In anemia of cancer, adaptation of these practices seems plausible with the exception of the recommended target level of serum ferritin, which is often increased in patients with cancer without any correlation with body iron store because of its nature as an acute phase protein and nonspecific tumor marker as well.

The selection of the appropriate drug depends on local conditions. Presently, three major iron formulations, namely, iron sucrose, iron gluconate, and iron dextran, are available, both in the United States and in Europe, for intravenous supplementation therapy. The maximal dose for one infusion is ≤500 mg for iron sucrose, ≤125 mg for ferric gluconate, and less than 3,000 mg for iron dextran. The former two formulations may even be administered by slow injection, but intravenous infusion may be preferable. Before administration of the planned dose of iron sucrose or iron dextran, a test dose should be given in order to assure adequate tolerance.

Conclusion

Evidence for the advantages of intravenous iron therapy concomitantly with erythropoietin treatment in patients with anemia of cancer is increasing. Although still not accepted as standard therapy, parenteral iron supplementation seems to shorten the time to hematologic response (hemoglobin ~12 g/dL), increase response rate, convert erythropoietin nonresponder to erythropoietin responder, and to reduce costs by limiting expensive erythropoietin therapy only to those patients who respond within few weeks to combined intravenous iron–erythropoietin therapy. It benefits not only patients with true iron deficiency but, importantly, also those with functional iron impairment induced either by chronic inflammation or by a highly increased demand for iron supply in patients with erythropoietin-stimulated erythropoiesis. However, the optimal use of intravenous iron preparations, the best treatment regimen, and treatment duration remain to be defined. Moreover, additional data on the safety of intravenous iron administration, particularly in patients with cancer, is needed.

Acknowledgment

Silvia Bakos carefully typed and proofread the manuscript.

References

1. Henry DH, Dahl NV, Ferrlecit Cancer Study Group: Iron and B12 parameters in anemic cancer patients on chemotherapy presenting for epoetin alpha (EPO) therapy. J Clin Oncol 22:8091, 2004 (suppl, abstr)
2. Goodnough LT, Skikne B, Brugnara C: Erythropoietin, iron, and erythropoiesis. Blood 96:823-833, 2000
3. Brugnara C: Iron deficiency and erythropoiesis: New diagnostic approaches. Clin Chem 49:1573-1578, 2003
4. Kaltwasser JP, Kessler U, Gottschalk R, Stucki G, Moller B: Effect of recombinant human erythropoietin and intravenous iron on anemia and disease activity in rheumatoid arthritis. J Rheumatol 28:2430-2436, 2001
5. Gasche C, Waldhoer T, Feichtenschlager T, Maie C, Mayer A, Mittermaier C, et al: Prediction of response to iron sucrose in inflammatory bowel disease-associated anemia. Am J Gastroenterol 96:2382-2387, 2001
6. Weiss G, Meusburger E, Radacher G, Garimorth K, Neyer U, Mayer G: Effect of iron treatment on circulating cytokine levels in ESRD patients receiving recombinant human erythropoietin. Kidney Int 64:572-578, 2003
7. Macdougall IC, Tucker B, Thompson J, Tomson CR, Baker LR, Raine AE: A randomized controlled study of iron supplementation in patients treated with erythropoietin. Kidney Int 50:1694-1699, 1996
8. NKF-DOQI clinical practice guidelines for vascular access. National Kidney Foundation-Dialysis Outcomes Quality Initiative. Am J Kidney Dis 30:S150-191, 1997 (suppl 3)
9. Rizzo JD, Lichtin AE, Woolf SH, Seidenfeld J, Bennett CL, Cella D, et al: Use of epoetin in patients with cancer: Evidence-based clinical practice guidelines of the American Society of Clinical Oncology and the American Society of Hematology. J Clin Oncol 20:4083-4107, 2002
10. NCCN 2005. http://professional.cancerconsultants.com/conference_nccn_2005.aspx?id=33902
11. Bokemeyer C, Aapro MS, Courdi A, Foubert J, Link H, Osterborg A, et al: EORTC guidelines for the use of erythropoietic proteins in anaemic patients with cancer. Eur J Cancer 40:2201-2216, 2004
12. Auerbach M, Ballard H, Trout JR, Mcllwain M, Ackerman A, Bahrain H, et al: Intravenous iron optimizes the response to recombinant human erythropoietin in cancer patients with chemotherapy-related anemia: a multicenter, open-label, randomized trial. J Clin Oncol 22:1301-1307, 2004
13. Katodritou E, Speletas M, Kapetanos D, Zervas K, Pavlitou A, Georgiou E, et al: Evaluation of traditional and novel predictive markers of anemia response to recombinant human erythropoietin (rh-Epo) in patients with multiple myeloma and lymphoma: emerging role of functional iron deficiency. Blood 104:3690, 2004 (abstr)
14. Henry DH, Dahl NV, Auerbach M, Aauerbach M, Tchekmedyian S, Laufman LR, Ferrlecit Cancer Study Group: Intravenous ferric gluconate (FG) for increasing response to epoetin (EPO) in patients with anemia of cancer chemotherapy—Results of a multicenter, randomized trial. Blood 104:3696, 2004 (abstr)
15. Auerbach M, Witt D, Toler W, Fierstein M, Lerner RG, Ballard H: Clinical use of the total dose intravenous infusion of iron dextran. J Lab Clin Med 111:566-70, 1988
16. Vandebroek A, Gaede B, Altintas S, Smith K, Yao B, Schupp M, et al: ASCO Poster Session, Atlanta, GA, June 2-6, 2006 (abstr 8612)
17. Hedenus M, Birgegard G, Näsman P, Ahlberg L, Karlsson T, Lauri B, et al: Adjuvant intravenous iron therapy potentiates epoetin b treatment in anemic, non iron-depleted patients with lymphoproliferative disorders: Results of the NIFe Study. EHA Meeting, Amsterdam, the Netherlands, June 15-18, 2006 (abstr 0996)
18. Weiss G, Goodnough LT: Anemia of chronic disease. N Engl J Med 352:1011-1023, 2005
19. Stevens RG, Jones DY, Micozzi MS, Taylor PR: Body iron stores and the risk of cancer. N Engl J Med 319:1047-1052, 1988
20. Aronoff GR, Bennett WM, Blumenthal S, Charytan C, Pennell JP, Reed J, et al: Iron sucrose in hemodialysis patients: Safety of replacement and maintenance regimens. Kidney Int 66:1193-1198, 2004
21. Innerhofer P, Klingler A, Klimmer C, Fries D, Nussbaumer W: Risk for postoperative infection after transfusion of white blood cell-filtered allogeneic or autologous blood components in orthopedic patients undergoing primary arthroplasty. Transfusion 45:103-110, 2005
22. Beguin Y: Erythropoietic Agents and Iron. ESO Scientific Updates, vol. 6: Anemia in Cancer. 2005

ELSEVIER

Seminars in
HEMATOLOGY

Intravenous Iron in Inflammatory Bowel Disease

Christoph Gasche and Stefanie Kulnigg

One of the key symptoms of inflammatory bowel diseases (IBD) is anemia. The reported prevalence of IBD-associated anemia varies between 6% and 74%. Although the therapy of the underlying disease has improved during the past decade, significant anemia continues to be a relevant burden. Iron deficiency and anemia of chronic disease are frequently combined in these patients. Oral iron therapy has been associated with flares in ulcerative colitis, similar to what has been observed in animal models of colitis. Parenteral iron supplementation has become the preferred route as the safety and efficacy of iron sucrose has been demonstrated in several trials. Open questions relate to the use of iron sucrose for prevention of anemia, the target hemoglobin levels, and the immunologic role of iron in the setting of chronic bowel inflammation.
Semin Hematol 43(suppl 6):S18-S22

Inflammatory bowel diseases (IBD) are a group of intestinal diseases that share a variety of symptoms such as chronic or recurrent diarrhea, abdominal pain, fever, thrombocytosis, and anemia. Two major forms of IBD are typically recognized: Crohn's disease and ulcerative colitis. Further subforms involve indeterminate colitis and microscopic (collagenous) colitis. Besides intestinal inflammation, this syndrome is associated with extra-intestinal manifestations of the skin (pyoderma gangrenosum, erythema nodosum), joints (althralgia, peripheral arthritis, or spondylarthritis), or eyes (uveitis or conjunctivitis). Furthermore, IBD runs together with chronic inflammatory diseases of other tissues such as psoriasis, primary sclerosing cholangitis, and ankylosing spondylitis.

The cause of IBD has not been identified yet. Several genetic loci have been linked to IBD at various chromosomes (IBD1 to IBD8).[1] At some of these loci the responsible gene with its variants has been identified (eg, IBD1 locus: CARD15 or Nod2).[2] However, the genetic mutations explain only part of the general disease susceptibility.[3] Environmental factors that have changed over the past 100 years are significantly more important. In this respect, Crohn's disease has been first described in the early 1900s.[4] Epidemiologic data demonstrate a significant increase in both Crohn's disease and ulcerative colitis in Western Europe during the 1960s and 1970s, while these diseases were significantly less common in populations of Eastern or Central Europe, which had been separated from Western life style (by the Iron Curtain).[5] Incidence numbers are still picking up to almost 15/100,000 in Canada for Crohn's disease.[6] Prevalence ranges between 200 and 400/100,000. The best understood environmental factor is cigarette smoking.[7] It has an aggravating effect on Crohn's disease and is associated with a higher number of flares, more steroid intake, and frequent operations. In contrast, smoking and nicotine therapy protect from ulcerative colitis.[8] It is not uncommon that patients develop their first flare when they quit smoking. This just points to the fact that we are dealing with two distinct phenotypes that share symptoms and genetic predisposition but are triggered by different environmental factors and display different types of intestinal inflammation.

IBD-Associated Anemia

Hematologic changes such as anemia and thrombocytosis are among the most common symptoms of these diseases with a prevalence between 6% and 74% (Table 1). Anemia has long been regarded as a marker of inflammation. This is well established since hematocrit or hemoglobin are the only laboratory parameters that are included in disease activity scores such as Crohn's disease activity index or the colitis activity index.[9,10] However, the underlying cause of anemia is considered to be primarily due to chronic intestinal blood loss through ulcerations, which leads to a negative iron balance and thereby to the development of iron-deficiency anemia. Mediators of intestinal inflammation such as tumor necrosis factor (TNF)-α or interferon (INF)-γ, however, may also af-

Medical University of Vienna, Department of Internal Medicine IV, Division of Gastroenterology and Hepatology, Vienna, Austria.
Address correspondence to Christoph Gasche, MD, Medical University of Vienna, Department of Internal Medicine IV, Division of Gastroenterology and Hepatology, Währinger Gürtel 18-20, A-1090 Vienna, Austria. E-mail: christoph.gasche@meduniwien.ac.at

 0037-1963/06/$-see front matter © 2006 Elsevier Inc. All rights reserved.
doi:10.1053/j.seminhematol.2006.08.010

Table 1 Prevalence of Anemia in Inflammatory Bowel Disease

Study	Year of Publication	Country	n	Phenotype	Prevalence (%)
Vijverman et al[36]	2006	Belgium	80 (1993) 90 (2003)	IBD	34 (1993) 17 (2003)
Ershler et al[37]	2005	USA	7,200	IBD	12.9
Ebinger et al[38]	2004	Germany	390	Crohn's disease	6.2
Lakatos et al[39]	2003	Hungary	254	Crohn's disease	57.8
Oldenburg et al[40]	2001	Netherlands	?	Crohn's disease	29.0
Revel-Vilke et al[41]	2000	Israel	63	IBD	41.3
Schreiber et al[42]	1996	Germany	334	Crohn's disease	26.3
Gasche et al[15]	1994	Austria	49	Crohn's disease	32.7
Horina et al[43]	1993	Austria	85	IBD	32.9
Harries et al[44]	1984	England	55	Crohn's disease	43.6
Bambach and Hill[45]	1982	Australia	36	Crohn's disease	16.7
Werlin and Grand[46]	1977	USA	19	Severe Colitis	73.7
Reilly et al[47]	1976	USA	9	Small bowel Crohn's disease	33.3
Reilly et al[48]	1976	USA	14	Large bowel Crohn's disease	71.4
Greenstein et al[49]	1975	USA	160	Crohn's disease	71.3
Burbige et al[50]	1975	USA	58	Crohn's disease	51.7
Beeken[51]	1975	USA	63	Crohn's disease	69.8
Beeken[52]	1973	USA	11	Crohn's disease	72.7
Dyer et al[53]	1972	England	63	Crohn's disease	63.5
Hoffbrand et al[54]	1968	England	64	Crohn's disease	43.8

fect erythropoiesis and iron metabolism, which reflects the presence of anemia of chronic disease (ACD). Iron deficiency and ACD are frequently combined in this type of patient.[11] Besides, various pharmacologic drugs that are used for treatment of IBD, eg, sulfasalazine, mesalazine, azathioprine, and 6-mercaptopyrin, may interfere with erythropoiesis. Extensive ileal resection in Crohn's disease may be associated with vitamin B_{12} deficiency. A series of case reports on hemolytic anemias mainly associated with ulcerative colitis has highlighted a possible shared autoimmune mechanism.[12] Also, myelodysplastic syndrome, aplasia, and inborn disorders of erythropoiesis have been reported.

The diagnosis of iron deficiency in the setting of ACD may be difficult. Bone marrow studies in patients with rheumatoid arthritis have shown that even ferritin levels above 55 μg/L do not necessarily mean that iron is present.[13] Therefore, in the recent literature a ferritin cutoff level of 100 μg/L is recommended when ACD is also present.[14] However, in a series of 49 Crohn's patients, the average ferritin level was 28.7 μg/L in anemic cases and 63.2 μg/L in non-anemic cases, pointing to the importance of iron deficiency.[15] As indicated above, ACD alters the body's iron metabolism possibly through the expression of hepcidin.[16] Hepcidin blocks iron release from the macrophages and therefore reduces the availability of iron in the bone marrow. In our set of Crohn's patients, the average transferrin saturation was 6.2% in anemic cases and 11.5% in non-anemic cases, which is quite low and fits with the iron-withholding model in ACD. Last but not least, erythropoietin levels may be inappropriately low when compared to the corresponding hemoglobin level. Indeed, several patients with hemoglobin levels as low as 8 g/dL did not display a corresponding elevation of the erythropoietin concentration.[15]

Oral or Parenteral Iron Therapy

Under physiologic conditions, about 1 mg of iron is absorbed every day. Studies have shown that, in the setting of iron deficiency, iron absorption may increase. To prevent iron overload, however, iron absorption is tightly regulated. In ACD increased hepcidin may inhibit iron absorption.[17] When considering oral iron therapy, more than 90% of a given dose is not absorbed and passes with stool. However, when this non-absorbed iron is in contact with mucosal ulcerations in IBD it may induce oxidative stress (through the Fenton reaction) and trigger local inflammation.[18] In fact, reported side effects in Crohn's patients differ from controls.[19] It was observed that IBD patients mostly complain about an increase in stool frequency while control individuals typically report constipation upon oral iron therapy. Studies from Norway also showed a reduction of oxygen scavengers upon oral iron therapy, which is indicative of oxidative stress at the mucosal surface.[19] A recent study from England demonstrated a worsening of clinical and mucosal disease activity in patients with ulcerative colitis treated with ferrous sulfate for four weeks.[20] This is in line with several animal models of colitis that showed an increase in oxidative stress, proinflammatory cytokine production or mucosal inflammation when treated with iron-enriched drinking water.[21-25] Because of these limitations, parenteral iron therapy should be considered in IBD.[26]

Most of the available data on parenteral iron replacement therapy concern iron sucrose. Iron sucrose is a semi-stable iron–sugar complex with a molecular weight between 34 and 60 kd. When applied intravenously, the complexed iron is taken up by macrophages and iron is released secondarily to transferrin. However, parts of the sugar-bound ferric iron are directly released to transferrin or other negatively charged serum proteins, such as albumin. Single doses up to 7 mg/kg body weight can be given in IBD and are well tolerated.[27] In controlled trials, short infusions of 200 to 300 mg iron sucrose diluted in sodium chloride were typically applied once or twice per week. In a controlled randomized trial for treatment of anemia in Crohn's disease 2,000 mg of iron sucrose was infused over an 8-week period.[28] The iron sucrose group showed a significant increase in hemoglobin levels from 8.5 g/dL to almost 12 g/dL. When iron sucrose was combined with erythropoietin, the increase was even faster and higher, with hemoglobin levels reaching about 13.5 g/dL at 8 weeks. During a second, open phase, an additional 1,600 mg of iron sucrose was applied. On this regimen and in combination with erythropoietin, anemia was successfully managed in all patients and led to an improvement in quality of life.

Another prospective trial tested the same regimen for ulcerative colitis-associated anemia. Response rates to iron sucrose were comparable to Crohn's disease (65% in 4 weeks, 85% in 8 weeks) and again the drug was well tolerated.[29] Side effects were limited to pain at the infusion site, bitter taste, temporary hypotension, fever, or an increase in diarrhea. No anaphylactic reactions or severe side effects were observed. In a retrospective analysis of 61 anemic IBD patients with a mean hemoglobin of 9.7 g/dL, Bodemar and colleagues reported a 60% response rate within 8 weeks and 91% within 12 weeks.[30] The total iron sucrose dose was 1.4 g on average and 32% of patients needed a second treatment series. This study best reflects the use of iron sucrose in clinical practice.

In a German multicenter trial, iron sucrose was compared to oral iron over a 6-week period.[31] In this trial the head to head comparison between oral and intravenous iron led to a comparable increase in hemoglobin levels; however, only the intravenous group showed a gain in serum ferritin concentrations indicative of building up iron stores (the ferritin was approximately 200 μg/L at week 6). In contrast, the oral iron group did not build up any iron reserve. In another comparative, crossover trial, the clinical disease activity increased in the oral iron group while it was unchanged in the intravenous iron group, again questioning the safety of oral iron therapy in IBD.[32]

To answer the question whether patients will respond to iron sucrose or would need additional erythropoietin therapy, a large Austrian multicenter study was performed.[33] Of eight variables that had been tested as predictive parameters, serum erythropoietin, transferrin, and the soluble transferrin receptor concentrations proved to be of good predictive value. The quality of these parameters was similar; the clinical availability of transferrin, however, is best. Individuals with high pretreatment transferrin values are likely to respond to iron sucrose. As soon as the transferrin level is below 3 g/L this likelihood drops below 50%. In such individuals, it is recommended to start with a combination therapy of iron sucrose and erythropoietin.[26] In this regard, it is interesting to note that the endogenous erythropoietin level drops rapidly upon iron sucrose therapy (Fig 1). The mechanism behind this observation is unknown; however, we believe that it is rapid erythropoietin utilization by the bone marrow rather than lack of erythropoietin production.

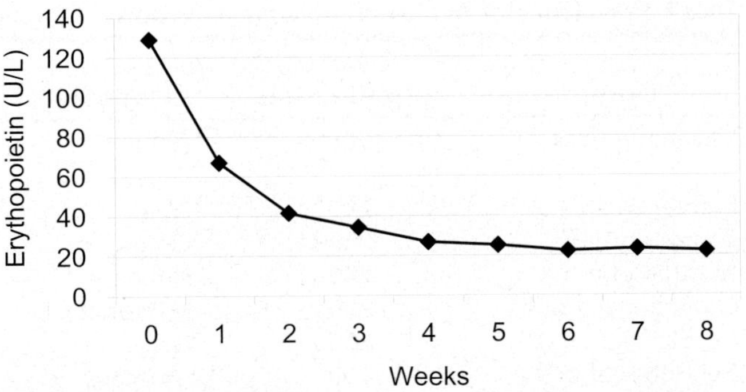

Figure 1 Serum erythropoietin levels were measured in 20 Crohn's patients that had been treated with iron sucrose (2000 mg) as part of a randomized controlled trial.[28] The mean erythropoietin levels dropped within 2 weeks of therapy before an increase in hemoglobin was seen. The mechanism behind this observation is unknown. However, the kinetic is suggestive of fast erythropoietin utilization that is caused by stimulation of erythropoiesis (through iron sucrose) rather than suppression of erythropoietin production.

The Future

Data are accumulating indicating that in the setting of IBD-associated anemia appropriate interventions increase the quality of life[28] and possibly also the cognitive functions.[34] In some studies, the disease-specific quality-of-life scores, such as the Inflammatory Bowel Disease Questionnaire (IBDQ) scores, also improve without any change in concomitant IBD-specific therapy.[20] A number of questions remain: What is the appropriate timing to start intravenous iron therapy? Do we need to wait for the hemoglobin level to drop below a certain trigger, or should we already prevent anemia by ensuring high iron stores? What is the appropriate hemoglobin target level? In the oncology setting, improvements in quality of life paralleled hemoglobin increases up to 14 g/dL.[35] Also, what is the appropriate ferritin target level that reflects adequate amounts of iron stores? Lastly, how does iron therapy affect the underlying inflammatory disease? Data from animal models and colitis patients are provoking the notion that oral iron therapy should be avoided in the IBD setting. Further studies are needed that investigate the immunological consequences of iron in the pathophysiology of chronic intestinal inflammation.

Acknowledgment

The authors are grateful to Alexandra Weisgram for her assistance in the preparation of this manuscript.

References

1. Cho JH, Nicolae DL, Gold LH, Fields CT, LaBuda MC, Rohal PM, et al: Identification of novel susceptibility loci for inflammatory bowel disease on chromosomes 1p, 3q, and 4q: Evidence for epistasis between 1p and IBD1. Proc Natl Acad Sci U S A 95:7502-7507, 1998

2. Hugot JP, Chamaillard M, Zouali H, Lesage S, Cezard JP, Belaiche J, et al: Association of NOD2 leucine-rich repeat variants with susceptibility to Crohn's disease. Nature 411:599-603, 2001
3. Gasche C, Grundtner P: Genotypes and phenotypes in Crohn's disease: Do they help in clinical management? Gut 54:162-167, 2005
4. Dalziel TK: Chronic interstitial enteritis. Br Med J 2:1068, 1913
5. Moum B, Ekbom A: Epidemiology of inflammatory bowel disease—Methodological considerations. Dig Liver Dis 34:364-369, 2002
6. Blanchard JF, Bernstein CN, Wajda A, Rawsthorne P: Small-area variations and sociodemographic correlates for the incidence of Crohn's disease and ulcerative colitis. Am J Epidemiol 154:328-335, 2001
7. Cosnes J, Carbonnel F, Beaugerie L, Le Quintrec Y, Gendre JP: Effects of cigarette smoking on the long-term course of Crohn's disease. Gastroenterology 110:424-431, 1996
8. Sandborn WJ, Tremaine WJ, Offord KP, Lawson GM, Petersen BT, Batts KP, et al: Transdermal nicotine for mildly to moderately active ulcerative colitis. A randomized, double-blind, placebo-controlled trial. Ann Intern Med 126:364-371, 1997
9. Best WR, Becktel JM, Singleton JW, Kern FJ: Development of a Crohn's disease activity index. National Cooperative Crohn's Disease Study. Gastroenterology 70:439-444, 1976
10. Truelove SC, Witts LJ: Cortisone in ulcerative colitis: Final report on a therapeutic trial. Br Med J 4947:1041-1048, 1955
11. Gasche C: Anemia in IBD: The overlooked villain. Inflamm Bowel Dis 6:142-150, 2000
12. Yates P, Macht LM, Williams NA, Elson CJ: Red cell autoantibody production by colonic mononuclear cells from a patient with ulcerative colitis and autoimmune haemolytic anaemia. Br J Haematol 82:753-756, 1992
13. Hansen TM, Hansen NE, Birgens HS, Holund B, Lorenzen I: Serum ferritin and the assessment of iron deficiency in rheumatoid arthritis. Scand J Rheumatol 12:353-359, 1983
14. Weiss G, Goodnough LT: Anemia of chronic disease. N Engl J Med 352:1011-1023, 2005
15. Gasche C, Reinisch W, Lochs H, Parsaei B, Bakos S, Wyatt J, et al: Anemia in Crohn's disease. Importance of inadequate erythropoietin production and iron deficiency. Dig Dis Sci 39:1930-1934, 1994
16. Ganz T: Hepcidin, a key regulator of iron metabolism and mediator of anemia of inflammation. Blood 102:783-788, 2003
17. Nemeth E, Tuttle MS, Powelson J, Vaughn MB, Donovan A, Ward DM, et al: Hepcidin regulates cellular iron efflux by binding to ferroportin and inducing its internalization. Science 306:2090-2093, 2004
18. Babbs CF: Oxygen radicals in ulcerative colitis. Free Radic Biol Med 13:169-181, 1992
19. Erichsen K, Hausken T, Ulvik RJ, Svardal A, Berstad A, Berge RK: Ferrous fumarate deteriorated plasma antioxidant status in patients with Crohn disease. Scand J Gastroenterol 38:543-548, 2003
20. De Silva AD, Tsironi E, Feakins RM, Rampton DS: Efficacy and tolerability of oral iron therapy in inflammatory bowel disease: A prospective, comparative trial. Aliment Pharmacol Ther 22:1097-1105, 2005
21. Erichsen K, Milde AM, Arslan G, Helgeland L, Gudbrandsen OA, Ulvik RJ, et al: Low-dose oral ferrous fumarate aggravated intestinal inflammation in rats with DSS-induced colitis. Inflamm Bowel Dis 11:744-748, 2005
22. Oldenburg B, Berge Henegouwen GP, Rennick D, Van Asbeck BS, Koningsberger JC: Iron supplementation affects the production of pro-inflammatory cytokines in IL-10 deficient mice. Eur J Clin Invest 30: 505-510, 2000
23. Carrier J, Aghdassi E, Platt I, Cullen J, Allard JP: Effect of oral iron supplementation on oxidative stress and colonic inflammation in rats with induced colitis. Aliment Pharmacol Ther 15:1989-1999, 2001
24. Carrier J, Aghdassi E, Cullen J, Allard JP: Iron supplementation increases disease activity and vitamin E ameliorates the effect in rats with dextran sulfate sodium-induced colitis. J Nutr 132:3146-3150, 2002
25. Carrier JC, Aghdassi E, Jeejeebhoy K, Allard JP: Exacerbation of dextran sulfate sodium-induced colitis by dietary iron supplementation: role of NF-kappaB. Int J Colorectal Dis 21:381-387, 2006
26. Gasche C, Lomer MC, Cavill I, Weiss G: Iron, anaemia, and inflammatory bowel diseases. Gut 53:1190-1197, 2004
27. Schroder O, Schrott M, Blumenstein I, Jahnel J, Dignass AU, Stein J: A study for the evaluation of safety and tolerability of intravenous high-dose iron sucrose in patients with iron deficiency anemia due to gastrointestinal bleeding. Z Gastroenterol 42:663-667, 2004
28. Gasche C, Dejaco C, Waldhoer T, Tillinger W, Reinisch W, Fueger GF, et al: Intravenous iron and erythropoietin for anemia associated with Crohn disease. A randomized, controlled trial. Ann Intern Med 126: 782-787, 1997
29. Gasche C, Dejaco C, Reinisch W, Tillinger W, Waldhoer T, Fueger GF, et al: Sequential treatment of anemia in ulcerative colitis with intravenous iron and erythropoietin. Digestion 60:262-267, 1999
30. Bodemar G, Kechagias S, Almer S, Danielson BG: Treatment of anaemia in inflammatory bowel disease with iron sucrose. Scand J Gastroenterol 39:454-458, 2004
31. Schroder O, Mickisch O, Seidler U, de Weerth A, Dignass AU, Herfarth H, et al: Intravenous iron sucrose versus oral iron supplementation for the treatment of iron deficiency anemia in patients with inflammatory bowel disease—A randomized, controlled, open-label, multicenter study. Am J Gastroenterol 100:2503-2509, 2005
32. Erichsen K, Ulvik RJ, Nysaeter G, Johansen J, Ostborg J, Berstad A, et al: Oral ferrous fumarate or intravenous iron sucrose for patients with inflammatory bowel disease. Scand J Gastroenterol 40:1058-1065, 2005
33. Gasche C, Waldhoer T, Feichtenschlager T, Male C, Mayer A, Mittermaier C, Petritsch W: Prediction of response to iron sucrose in inflammatory bowel disease-associated anemia. Am J Gastroenterol 96:2382-2387, 2001
34. Wells CW, Lewis S, Barton JR, Corbett S: Effects of changes in hemoglobin level on quality of life and cognitive function in inflammatory bowel disease patients. Inflamm Bowel Dis 12:123-130, 2006
35. Crawford J, Cella D, Cleeland CS, Cremieux PY, Demetri GD, Sarokhan BJ, et al: Relationship between changes in hemoglobin level and quality of life during chemotherapy in anemic cancer patients receiving epoetin alfa therapy. Cancer 95:888-895, 2002
36. Vijverman A, Piront P, Belaiche J, Louis E: Evolution of the prevalence and characteristics of anemia in inflammatory bowel diseases between 1993 nd 2003. Acta Gastroenterol Belg 69:1-4, 2006
37. Ershler WB, Chen K, Reyes EB, Dubois R: Economic burden of patients with anemia in selected diseases. Value Health 8:629-638, 2005
38. Ebinger M, Leidl R, Thomas S, Von Tirpitz C, Reinshagen M, Adler G, et al: Cost of outpatient care in patients with inflammatory bowel disease in a German University Hospital. J Gastroenterol Hepatol 19:192-199, 2004
39. Lakatos L, Pandur T, David G, Balogh Z, Kuronya P, Tollas A, et al: Association of extraintestinal manifestations of inflammatory bowel disease in a province of western Hungary with disease phenotype: Results of a 25-year follow-up study. World J Gastroenterol 9:2300-2307, 2003
40. Oldenburg B, Koningsberger JC, Berge Henegouwen GP, Van Asbeck BS, Marx JJ: Iron and inflammatory bowel disease. Aliment Pharmacol Ther 15:429-438, 2001
41. Revel-Vilk S, Tamary H, Broide E, Zoldan M, Dinari G, Zahavi I, et al: Serum transferrin receptor in children and adolescents with inflammatory bowel disease. Eur J Pediatr 159:585-589, 2000
42. Schreiber S, Howaldt S, Schnoor M, Nikolaus S, Bauditz J, Gasche C, et al: Recombinant erythropoietin for the treatment of anemia in inflammatory bowel disease. N Engl J Med 334:619-623, 1996
43. Horina JH, Petritsch W, Schmid CR, Reicht G, Wenzl H, Silly H, et al: Treatment of anemia in inflammatory bowel disease with recombinant human erythropoietin: Results in three patients. Gastroenterology 104: 1828-1831, 1993
44. Harries AD, Fitzsimons E, Dew MJ, Heatley RV, Rhodes J: Association between iron deficiency anaemia and mid-arm circumference in Crohn's disease. Hum Nutr Clin Nutr 38:47-53, 1984
45. Bambach CP, Hill GL: Long term nutritional effects of extensive resection of the small intestine. Aust N Z J Surg 52:500-506, 1982
46. Werlin SL, Grand RJ: Severe colitis in children and adolescents: diagnosis. Course, and treatment. Gastroenterology 73:828-832, 1977

47. Reilly J, Ryan JA, Strole W, Fischer JE: Hyperalimentation in inflammatory bowel disease. Am J Surg 131:192-200, 1976
48. Reilly J, Ryan JA, Strole W, Fischer JE: Hyperalimentation in inflammatory bowel disease. Am J Surg 131:192-200, 1976
49. Greenstein AJ, Kark AE, Dreiling DA: Crohn's disease of the colon. II. Controversial aspects of hemorrhage, anemia and rectal involvement in granulomatous disease involving the colon. Am J Gastroenterol 63:40-48, 1975
50. Burbige EJ, Huang SH, Bayless TM: Clinical manifestations of Crohn's disease in children and adolescents. Pediatrics 55:866-871, 1975
51. Beeken WL: Remediable defects in Crohn disease: A prospective study of 63 patients. Arch Intern Med 135:686-690, 1975
52. Beeken WL: Absorptive defects in young people with regional enteritis. Pediatrics 52:69-74, 1973
53. Dyer NH, Child JA, Mollin DL, Dawson AM: Anaemia in Crohn's disease. Q J Med 41:419-436, 1972
54. Hoffbrand AV, Stewart JS, Booth CC, Mollin DL: Folate deficiency in Crohn's disease: Incidence, pathogenesis, and treatment. Br Med J 597:71-75, 1968

ELSEVIER

Seminars in
HEMATOLOGY

Iron Administration in the Critically Ill

Michael Piagnerelli,[a] Alessandro Rapotec,[a] Frédéric Cotton,[b] and Jean-Louis Vincent[a]

Anemia is a common pathology in intensive care unit (ICU) patients. The pathophysiology of anemia includes altered iron metabolism with decreased erythropoiesis. Under normal conditions, there is a balance between iron transport by transferrin, making iron available for incorporation in hemoglobin, and iron storage as ferritin. In inflammatory processes, this balance is disturbed and plays a central role in the development of anemia. Typically, the inflammatory process is associated with a low concentration of serum iron, high ferritin and low transferrin. Effective erythropoiesis requires both erythropoietin (EPO) and iron. Critically ill patients have inappropriately low EPO levels, and several studies have been conducted to assess the potential benefits of exogenous EPO supplementation. EPO treatment plus iron administration reduced the number of red blood cell (RBC) transfusions needed but had no effects on outcome in terms of ICU infection rates or mortality. Iron can have adverse effects, including inhibition of phagocytosis, inhibition of intracellular killing of bacteria, and altered polymorphonuclear cell function. Iron overload has also been shown to cause increased apoptosis in patients with hemochromatosis. Further study is needed to accurately define the precise role of iron in the development of anemia in critically ill patients, and to determine the potential benefits and risks of iron supplementation.
Semin Hematol 43(suppl 6):S23-S27

Iron is essential for oxygen transport by hemoglobin and myoglobin; hemoglobin contains 80% of the total body iron stores.[1] Under physiologic conditions, there is a balance between iron transport and iron storage. Iron transport is provided by transferrin, which makes iron available for incorporation into hemoglobin. Iron storage is in the form of ferritin.[1] This transport/storage balance is disturbed in inflammatory processes, both acute—as often seen in acutely ill patients in the intensive care unit (ICU)—and chronic. These disturbances play a central role in the development of anemia in these patients.[2]

Typically, the inflammatory process is associated with decreased concentrations of serum iron, increased ferritin, and decreased transferrin concentrations.[3] The underlying mechanisms are very complex and not entirely understood, although the final teleologic aim is primarily to deprive bacteria of their nutritionally required iron.[4] In fact, already within a few hours following exposure to an inflammatory stimulus, pro- and anti-inflammatory cytokines can decrease blood iron levels. Pro-inflammatory cytokines, such as tumor necrosis factor (TNF)-α, interleukin (IL)-1β, and IL-6 induce the transcription and the translation of ferritin, modulate the binding affinity of cytoplasmic iron regulatory proteins (IRP)-1 and -2 with iron-responsive elements, and rapidly decrease the mRNA expression of transferrin receptors.[5] Interferon (INF)-γ stimulates iron absorption by enterocytes via the divalent metal transporter-1 (DMT-1) but has an inhibitory effect on ferroportin internalization into these cells. These alterations result in iron storage in enterocytes.[6] Anti-inflammatory cytokines like IL-4, IL-10, and IL-13 induce the expression of heme-oxygenase-1 to favor heme degradation and iron storage in monocytes and in the reticuloendothelial system.[7,8]

Nitric oxide (NO) reduces red blood cell (RBC) production by stimulating IRP and by reducing ferrochelatase activity, which inhibits the final step of heme synthesis.[9] Recent studies have highlighted the fundamental role of hepcidin, a 25–amino acid protein that is produced by the liver in response to inflammation. This production occurs very rapidly, even before acute-phase reactants like C-reactive protein (CRP).[10-12] Hepcidin decreases iron absorption in the gut and downregulates the iron exporter ferroportin at the plasma membrane of macrophages and enterocytes.[11]

This review will focus on some of the key studies on iron metabolism in the critically ill patient and the effects of iron administration in animals and critically ill patients, especially in septic conditions.

[a]Department of Intensive Care, Erasme University Hospital, Free University of Brussels, Brussels, Belgium.
[b]Clinical Chemistry, Erasme University Hospital, Free University of Brussels, Brussels, Belgium.
Address correspondence to Jean-Louis Vincent, MD, PhD, Department of Intensive Care, Erasme Hospital, Free University of Brussels, Brussels, Belgium. E-mail: jlvincen@ulb.ac.be

0037-1963/06/$-see front matter
doi:10.1053/j.seminhematol.2006.08.007

Alterations of Iron Metabolism in Critically Ill Patients

A number of studies have reported alterations of iron metabolism in nonbleeding ICU patients (postsurgery, trauma or medical, septic or nonseptic patients). These studies were recently reviewed by Darveau et al[13] and are summarized in Table 1. Four studies evaluated the prognostic value of ferritin concentration on the risk of development of acute respiratory distress syndrome (ARDS) in ICU patients.[14-17] In these studies, ferritin concentration was significantly increased at the time of ICU admission in patients who developed ARDS. There are two possible explanations for this finding. One is that pro-inflammatory cytokines, which are implicated in the development of ARDS, do increase ferritin synthesis. A second is that the oxidative stress present in patients at risk of developing ARDS might liberate iron from ferritin, accelerating the formation of toxic hydroxyl radicals.[16]

The time course of these measurements is of great importance. This was recently demonstrated by Kemna et al,[12] who observed a significant decrease in blood iron concentrations as early as 22 hours after administration of a small dose of endotoxin in human healthy volunteers. Only a few of the studies listed in Table 1 included blood iron measurements

Table 1 Studies Describing Iron Metabolism in ICU Patients

Study	Type of Patients (no.)	Time of Measurement	Iron (μmol/L)	Ferritin (μg/L)	Transferrin (g/L)	Transferrin Saturation (%)
Risk of ARDS						
Gutteridge[14]	ARDS (10)	ND	2.7	ND	3.06 ± 0.41	26 ± 9
	ARDS retrospective (5)	ND	3.3	ND	0.82 ± 0.13	71 ± 7
Gutteridge[15]	ARDS proven (10)	When ARDS developed	2.7 ± 0.4	ND	1.76 ± 0.13	34 ± 4
	At risk of ARDS (10)	Before surgery	3.7 ± 0.4	ND	1.98 ± 0.14	41 ± 5
Connelly[16]	Medicosurgical (83)					
	At risk of ARDS (75)	ND	ND	280 [230–500] females	ND	ND
				480 [270–738] males	ND	ND
	With ARDS (8)	ND	ND	293 [180–758] females	ND	ND
				1,450 [928–3,750] males	ND	ND
Sharkey[17]	Trauma plus ARDS (42)	At admission	ND	240 [12–4,500]	ND	ND
Medical and/or surgical						
Bobbio-Pallavicini[30]	Surgical (51)	Week 1	4.1	652	1.7	12.8
von Ahsen[31]	Medical (71)	Day 1–2	4.8	471	1.4	16
Rodriguez[32]	Medicosurgical (160)	Day 2 to 3	4.9	727	ND	16
Patteril[33]	Medicosurgical (51)					
	Functional iron deficiency	Day 1	ND	342	ND	ND
	No functional iron deficiency	Day 1	ND	292	ND	ND
Piagnerelli[19]	Medicosurgical (29)	Day 1				
	Septic		ND	ND	1.2 [1.1–1.7]	ND
	Nonseptic		ND	ND	2.2 [2.0–2.6]	ND
Muñoz[22]	Medicosurgical (131)	Day 0 to 6	7.5 ± 6.8	387 ± 462	1.9 ± 0.7	28 ± 25
Piagnerelli[20]	Medicosurgical (51)	Day 1				
	Nonseptic		7.2 [5.0–14.0]	461 [215–973]	2.2 ± 0.6	14 [9–39]
	Septic		3.6 [2.9–5.7]	204 [69–404]	1.7 ± 0.5	11 [7–13]
Septic shock						
Mumby[34]	Septic shock (15)	At diagnosis of infection	7.8 ± 1.8	ND	0.87 ± 0.01	35 ± 7
Trauma						
Hobish-Hagen[18]	Trauma (23)	At admission	9.5	832	1.7	ND
Erythropoietin studies						
van Iperen[21]	Medicosurgical (36)	At admission				
	Control group		2.05 ± 0.8	891 ± 469	1.4 ± 0.4	12 ± 6
	Iron group		2.7 ± 1.3	900 ± 909	1.5 ± 0.4	15 ± 12
	EPO group		3.4 ± 1.9	1042 ± 487	1.5 ± 0.3	16 ± 9
Corwin[25]	Medicosurgical					
	Placebo group (652)	Day 1 to 3	5.03 ± 6.1	562 ± 1,169	ND	17 ± 19
	EPO group (650)	Day 1 to 3	6.5 ± 8.8	684 ± 1,385	ND	20 ± 21
Vincent[26]	Medicosurgical (73)					
	Placebo group (25)	Day 1 to 3	6.9 ± 7.6	642 ± 781	ND	26 ± 26
	EPO group (48)	Day 1 to 3	4.4 ± 3.7	435 ± 299	ND	15 ± 14

on ICU admission,[14,15,17-21] and, unfortunately, the time delay between hospital and ICU admission was usually not defined. Yet, this information is important in order to exclude patients with alterations in iron metabolism due to an inflammatory syndrome that was present prior to ICU admission.

We recently studied iron metabolism in patients admitted to the ICU with a previous hospital length of stay of 2 days or less.[20] Despite identical hemograms at ICU admission, septic patients had more severe alterations in iron metabolism, characterized by decreased iron and transferrin concentrations and increased ferritin concentration. No difference was observed for the transferrin saturation and the concentration of soluble transferrin receptor. Interestingly, for all patients at admission, CRP concentration was directly correlated with ferritin and inversely correlated with transferrin concentration.[20] Muñoz et al[22] also observed a correlation between CRP, iron and transferrin concentration but blood sampling was performed just 1 day per week, and in addition some patients had abnormal RBC mean corpuscular volume (range, 78.4 to 109.7 fL), suggesting prior hematologic disease.

All studies except two[19,20] excluded patients who had received a RBC transfusion prior to ICU admission or during the ICU stay. Indeed, these patients should be excluded from studies on iron metabolism due to the large quantity of iron provided with RBC transfusions.

In summary, alterations in iron metabolism are frequent in ICU patients, but studies evaluating this phenomenon are limited. To understand the primordial role of iron in the development of anemia, we need more studies exploring the time course of events and, particularly, the role of other major regulators of iron metabolism, such as hepcidin or soluble transferrin receptor.[23]

Iron Administration in the Critically Ill

The effects of iron administration in ICU patients have not been well studied. The only available data concern subgroups of patients in studies comparing the effects of iron alone or with erythropoietin (EPO) administration in ICU patients.[21,24-26] In vitro studies have shown that iron can have adverse effects on polymorphonuclear cell functions, including inhibition of phagocytosis and intracellular killing of bacteria.[27] Mice without the *hfe* gene (*hfe*$^{-/-}$) represent a clinically relevant model of hemochromatosis. When these mice were submitted to cecal ligation and puncture (CLP), Wizorek et al[28] observed a higher mortality rate after a high than after a low iron diet (75% *v* 45% at day 7; $P<.001$). Also after CLP, Javadi et al[29] observed a higher mortality rate in mice who received high-dose exogenous iron (daily subcutaneous injection of 5 mg of iron dextran). Interestingly, these authors observed increased apoptosis in the intestinal epithelium and in the spleen in the 24 hours following the onset of infection but no difference in bacteremia, suggesting that causes other than bacterial overgrowth may explain these higher mortality rates.

Four studies in adult ICU patients compared the effects of iron administration alone or with EPO.[21,24-26] These studies actually focused on the potential benefit of EPO rather than the effect of iron administration. Van Iperen et al[21] studied the effects of intravenous administration of 20 mg of iron sucrose daily for 14 days in 12 ICU patients. These authors observed an insignificant increase in reticulocyte count compared to 12 patients treated with 1 mg of folic acid. Iron administration had no effect on EPO or ferritin concentrations, or on transferrin saturation (remaining below 20%). Serum transferrin and iron concentrations increased significantly only after 10 and 21 days, respectively. These modifications could be due to a significant decrease in the inflammatory syndrome (CRP concentrations decreased from 150 ± 71 to 48 ± 53 mg/L; $P<.05$ at day 10) rather than to an effect of the iron administration. This suggestion was confirmed by the absence of change in serum transferrin receptor concentration during iron therapy, indicating the lack of resumption of erythropoiesis. The limit of this study was the small number of patients studied in each group, the very low dose of iron administered, and the non-exclusion of patients who had received a blood transfusion during the study period. This latter factor could modify iron metabolism quite substantially, as this group received a total of 63 units of RBCs (5 ± 7 U per patient).[21]

In 1999, Corwin et al[24] studied the efficacy of 300 U/kg of EPO started 3 days after ICU admission and continued daily for a total of 5 days, versus placebo in a series of 160 ICU patients. Both groups received oral iron (liquid preparation), at a dose of at least 150 mg of elemental iron, either orally or via a nasogastric tube, starting on ICU day 3 or whenever bowel sounds were present. Parenteral iron was given to patients who were either unable to take oral iron or who demonstrated an inadequate response to oral iron, as reflected by a transferrin saturation below 20% and a decrease in serum ferritin to less than 100 μg/L. For the same hematocrit value (around 30%) in both groups before treatment, the increase in reticulocyte count was more pronounced in the EPO group than in the iron group (2.5% *v* 0.8 %). There were fewer RBC transfusions in the EPO than in the iron groups (166 *v* 305). No differences were observed in adverse events, including mortality, but the incidence of new infections was not specified. A limitation of this study is the lack of information about the iron metabolism parameters at baseline and during treatment.

In a larger prospective, randomized, double-bind, placebo-controlled, multicenter trial, Corwin et al[25] compared the effect of EPO to a placebo in patients who received the same dosage of iron as in the first study. They also observed fewer RBC transfusions in patients who received 40,000 units of EPO weekly (50.5% *v* 60.4%; $P<.001$) but no difference in mortality (14% in the EPO and 15% in the placebo group). No data were provided about the time course of iron metabolism during treatment but the alterations in iron metabolism were more marked at baseline in the placebo than in the EPO group. Indeed, iron concentration and transferrin saturation were significantly lower (28.1 ± 34.3 *v* 36.2 ± 48.9 μg/dL, $P<.001$, and 17.2 ± 18.5 *v* 20.3 ± 21.2%, $P=.006$, respectively). Moreover, ferritin concentration was also somewhat lower in the placebo than in the EPO group (562 ± 1,169 *v* 684 ± 1,385 μg/L, $P = .09$). More pronounced alterations in iron metabolism in the placebo group at baseline may perhaps explain the limited erythropoiesis in this group. In this study, there were no differences in serious adverse events, including sepsis.[25]

In a recent multicenter trial, we observed,[26] until day 29, a more elevated reticulocyte count in 73 medicosurgical ICU patients receiving 40,000 units of EPO weekly plus 150 mg/d of iron compared to those receiving iron only. After day 29, the mean change in reticulocyte count remained identical, but the area under the curve for reticulocyte count in the initial and the last samples was greater in the EPO group, indicating an augmented erythropoietic response. In contrast to the study by Corwin et al,[25] iron metabolism was more altered at baseline in the EPO group than in the placebo group (serum iron concentration 24.4 ± 20.7 *v* 38.7 ± 42.5 μg/dL; ferritin 435 ± 299 *v* 642 ± 781 μg/L; transferrin saturation 16.5% ± 13.5% *v* 26.0% ± 26.2%).[26] Sepsis was the most frequently reported serious complication in both groups (12% in the placebo group and 6% in the EPO group).

Conclusion

In summary, iron metabolism is rapidly altered in ICU patients. Nevertheless, we need additional studies on selected patient populations (without RBC transfusions, without a long hospital stay before ICU admission, without hematologic disease) to better define the role of iron in the development of anemia in critically ill patients. Only then will we be able to study the effects of iron supplementation on anemia in non-infected critically ill patients.

References

1. Andrews T, Waterman H, Hillier V: Blood gas analysis: A study of blood loss in intensive care. J Adv Nurs 30:851-857, 1999
2. Vincent JL, Sakr Y, Creteur J: Anemia in the intensive care unit. Can J Anaesth 50:S53-S59, 2003
3. Weiss G, Goodnough LT: Anemia of chronic disease. N Engl J Med 352:1011-1023, 2005
4. Jurado RL: Iron, infections, and anemia of inflammation. Clin Infect Dis 25:888-895, 1997
5. Rogers JT: Ferritin translation by interleukin-1 and interleukin-6: The role of sequences upstream of the start codons of the heavy and light subunit genes. Blood 87:2525-2537, 1996
6. Andrews NC: Disorders of iron metabolism. N Engl J Med 341:1986-1995, 1999
7. Weiss G, Bogdan C, Hentze MW: Pathways for the regulation of macrophage iron metabolism by the anti-inflammatory cytokines IL-4 and IL-13. J Immunol 158:420-425, 1997
8. Lee TS, Chau LY: Heme oxygenase-1 mediates the anti-inflammatory effect of interleukin-10 in mice. Nat Med 8:240-246, 2002
9. Rafferty SP, Domachowske JB, Malech HL: Inhibition of hemoglobin expression by heterologous production of nitric oxide synthase in the K562 erythroleukemic cell line. Blood 88:1070-1078, 1996
10. Ganz T: Hepcidin, a key regulator of iron metabolism and mediator of anemia of inflammation. Blood 102:783-788, 2003
11. Delaby C, Pilard N, Goncalves AS, Beaumont C, Canonne-Hergaux F: Presence of the iron exporter ferroportin at the plasma membrane of macrophages is enhanced by iron loading and down-regulated by hepcidin. Blood 106:3979-3984, 2005
12. Kemna E, Pickkers P, Nemeth E, van der Hoeven H, Swinkels D: Time-course analysis of hepcidin, serum iron, and plasma cytokine levels in humans injected with LPS. Blood 106:1864-1866, 2005
13. Darveau M, Denault AY, Blais N, Notebaert E: Bench-to-bedside review: Iron metabolism in critically ill patients? Crit Care 8:356-362, 2004
14. Gutteridge JM, Quinlan GJ, Evans TW: Transient iron overload with bleomycin detectable iron in the plasma of patients with adult respiratory distress syndrome. Thorax 49:707-710, 1994
15. Gutteridge JM, Quinlan GJ, Mumby S, Heath A, Evans TW: Primary plasma antioxidants in adult respiratory distress syndrome patients: Changes in iron-oxidizing, iron-binding, and free radical-scavenging proteins. J Lab Clin Med 124:263-273, 1994
16. Connelly KG, Moss M, Parsons PE, Moore EE, Moore FA, Giclas PC, et al: Serum ferritin as a predictor of the acute respiratory distress syndrome. Am J Respir Crit Care Med 155:21-25, 1997
17. Sharkey RA, Donnelly SC, Connelly KG, Robertson CE, Haslett C, Repine JE: Initial serum ferritin levels in patients with multiple trauma and the subsequent development of acute respiratory distress syndrome. Am J Respir Crit Care Med 159:1506-1509, 1999
18. Hobisch-Hagen P, Wiedermann F, Mayr A, Fries D, Jelkmann W, Fuchs D, et al: Blunted erythropoietic response to anemia in multiply traumatized patients. Crit Care Med 29:743-747, 2001
19. Piagnerelli M, Boudjeltia KZ, Nuyens V, De Backer D, Su F, Wang Z, et al: Rapid alterations in transferrin sialylation during sepsis. Shock 24:48-52, 2005
20. Piagnerelli M, Herpain A, Cotton F, Gulbis B, Chatti R., Vincent JL: Le métabolisme du fer est rapidement altéré chez les patients septiques. Reanimation 15:SP30, 2006 (abstr)
21. van Iperen CE, Gaillard CA, Kraaijenhagen RJ, Braam BG, Marx JJ, van de Wiel A: Response of erythropoiesis and iron metabolism to recombinant human erythropoietin in intensive care unit patients. Crit Care Med 28:2773-2778, 2000
22. Muñoz M, Romero A, Morales M, Campos A, Garcia-Erce JA, Ramirez G: Iron metabolism, inflammation and anemia in critically ill patients. A cross-sectional study. Nutr Hosp 20:115-120, 2005
23. Piagnerelli M, Vincent JL: Role of iron in anemic critically ill patients: It's time to investigate! Crit Care 8:306-307, 2004
24. Corwin HL, Gettinger A, Rodriguez RM, Pearl RG, Gubler KD, Enny C, et al: Efficacy of recombinant human erythropoietin in the critically ill patient: A randomized, double-blind, placebo-controlled trial. Crit Care Med 27:2346-2350, 1999
25. Corwin HL, Gettinger A, Pearl RG, Fink MP, Levy MM, Shapiro MJ, et al: Efficacy of recombinant human erythropoietin in critically ill patients: A randomized controlled trial. JAMA 288:2827-2835, 2002
26. Vincent JL, Spapen HD, Creteur J, Piagnerelli M, Hubloue I, Diltoer M, et al: Pharmacokinetics and pharmacodynamics of once-weekly subcutaneous epoetin alfa in critically ill patients: Results of a randomized, double-blind, placebo-controlled trial. Crit Care Med 34:1661-1667, 2006
27. Patruta SI, Horl WH: Iron and infection. Kidney Int 69:S125-S130, 1999 (suppl)
28. Wizorek JJ, Turnbull IR, Buchman TG: Iron overload before cecal ligation and puncture increases mortality. Shock 20:52-55, 2003
29. Javadi P, Buchman TG, Stromberg PE, Husain KD, Dunne WM, Woolsey CA, et al: High-dose exogenous iron following cecal ligation and puncture increases mortality rate in mice and is associated with an increase in gut epithelial and splenic apoptosis. Crit Care Med 32: 1178-1185, 2004
30. Bobbio-Pallavicini F, Verde G, Spriano P, Losi R, Bosatra MG, Braschi A, et al: Body iron status in critically ill patients: significance of serum ferritin. Intensive Care Med 15:171-178, 1989
31. von Ahsen N, Muller C, Serke S, Frei U, Eckardt KU: Important role of nondiagnostic blood loss and blunted erythropoietic response in the anemia of medical intensive care patients. Crit Care Med 27:2630-2639, 1999

32. Rodriguez RM, Corwin HL, Gettinger A, Corwin MJ, Gubler D, Pearl RG: Nutritional deficiencies and blunted erythropoietin response as causes of the anemia of critical illness. J Crit Care 16:36-41, 2001
33. Patteril MV, Davey-Quinn AP, Gedney JA, Murdoch SD, Bellamy MC: Functional iron deficiency, infection and systemic inflammatory response syndrome in critical illness. Anaesth Intensive Care 29:473-478, 2001
34. Mumby S, Margarson M, Quinlan GJ, Evans TW, Gutteridge JM: Is bleomycin-detectable iron present in the plasma of patients with septic shock? Intensive Care Med 23:635-639, 1997

ELSEVIER
Seminars in
HEMATOLOGY

The Use of Iron Sucrose Complex for Anemia in Pregnancy and the Postpartum Period

Christian Breymann

Iron-deficiency anemia resulting in reduced blood reserves is one the most common problems in pregnancy. It is estimated that 20% to 50% of the world population is suffering from iron deficiency and iron-deficient states, pregnancy being one of the most important "risk factors" for iron deficiency and iron-deficiency anemia. The traditional treatments, ie, oral iron therapy and blood transfusion, involve significant drawbacks. High doses of oral iron frequently cause side effects, and noncompliance is common. Therefore, intravenous iron, alone or in association with recombinant human erythropoietin (rHuEPO) therapy, has been considered as an alternative in the management of iron deficiency in this setting. There is increasing evidence that iron sucrose is safe for the mother and the fetus using the recommended dosages and therapy regimens. Iron sucrose is effective in pregnant and postpartum patients who do not respond to oral iron, who are noncompliant to oral iron, or who are treated with rHuEPO. In both cases, according to the present data, the expected hemoglobin increase and time for therapy are predictable in responding patients. Whether it is reasonable to wait for a response to oral iron in moderate to severe anemia is therefore questionable. Indications for the use of iron sucrose complex are: preexisting (moderate–severe) anemia; no effect of oral iron; side effects of oral iron; refusal of blood transfusion (eg, Jehovah's Witness patients); limited time until delivery; coexisting risks (eg, bowel disease, renal disease); pre- and postoperative period and postpartum anemia. Future fields of research are the evaluation of patient satisfaction and quality of life, impact on costs and hospital stay, impact on blood transfusion frequency and mortality rate, and finally impact on other factors such as breast feeding behavior and neonatal outcome such as birth weight, prematurity and neonatal iron stores.
Semin Hematol 43(suppl 6):S28-S31

Iron-deficiency anemia is one the most common problems in pregnancy. It is estimated that 20% to 50% of the world population is suffering from iron deficiency and iron-deficient states, pregnancy being one of the most important "risk factors" for iron deficiency and iron-deficiency anemia.[1-3] According to World Health Organization (WHO) data presented at the Federation International d'Obstetrique e Gynecology (FIGO) meeting in 2003 in Chile, around 500,000 maternal death cases per year and 20,000,000 morbidity cases per year are related to iron deficiency and anemia. In view of the fetal and maternal risks associated with iron-deficiency anemia, it is obvious that treating anemia efficiently would lead to a considerable reduction in the risk factors affecting pregnancy and fetal outcome (Table 1).

Feto Maternal Medicine, Obstetric Research, Feto Maternal Hematology Research Group, University Hospital Zurich, Zurich, Switzerland.
Address correspondence to Christian Breymann, MD, University Hospital Zurich, Frauenklinikstr. 10, 8091 Zurich, Switzerland. E-mail: christian.breymann@usz.ch

The traditional treatments, ie, oral iron therapy and blood transfusion, involve significant drawbacks. High doses of oral iron frequently cause side effects, and noncompliance is common. In addition, such therapy has to be given for a long time in cases of severe iron deficiency, and absorption and red blood cell production are influenced by additional pathologies such as renal disease or chronic inflammatory bowel disease in pregnancy. As far as blood transfusions are concerned, because of the risk of infection (bacterial, viral, prions) and immunomodulation associated with allogeneic blood products, especially in this young and otherwise healthy population, transfusions are used only in the most severe cases and particularly in life-threatening situations.[4-6] Therefore, intravenous iron, alone or in association with recombinant human erythropoietin (rHuEPO), has been considered as an alternative in the management of iron deficiency in this setting.[7-15] Since the early 1990s, iron sucrose (Venofer®, Vifor, St. Gallen, Switzerland) has been the only parenteral iron preparation used during pregnancy and the puerperium at the Zurich University Hospital Obstetrics Clinic.

 0037-1963/06/$-see front matter
doi:10.1053/j.seminhematol.2006.08.002

Table 1 Fetal and Maternal Risks as a Consequence of Anemia

Fetus	Mother
Growth retardation	Quality of life
Prematurity	Anemia symptoms (dizziness, cardiovascular, etc)
Death in utero	Lactation habits (insufficient milk syndrome)
Amnion rupture	Physical performance
Infection	"Baby blues"
Fetal programming (feto-placental miss-ratio)	Infection rate
	Wound healing, fever
	Prolonged hospital stay

Data on the safety of the iron sucrose complex were first collected in a multicenter study in 1998. The side effect rate following the administration of 2000 ampoules, with a maximum single dose of 200 mg intravenously, was found to be less than 0.5%.[16] Our data are in accordance with previously published studies showing that iron sucrose complex produces no side effects during pregnancy.

In accordance with Obstetrics Clinic guidelines, an incremental treatment plan is used in anemia management.[4] Prerequisites for the use of parenteral iron include diagnostic investigations and fulfillment of the following inclusion criteria:

- Hemoglobin (Hb) <10 g/dL
- No effect of oral iron therapy (160–200 mg/d) over 2 weeks (ie, no Hb increase and/or reticulocyte response)
- Proven iron deficiency (serum ferritin <15 μg/L)
- Exclusion of hemoglobinopathy or other red cell disorders
- Exclusion of acute inflammatory state (C-reactive protein determination)
- Gestational age over 16 weeks

The first Hb determination is normally carried out during the first trimester, with oral iron prescribed in the first instance only if the Hb value is less than 10 g/dL. If the Hb level on oral iron treatment falls below 10 g/dL within 2 to 4 weeks, or if the Hb level on the first diagnostic test is already less than 10 g/dL, we use the iron sucrose complex as the treatment of first choice.

Practical Use of Iron Sucrose at the Zurich Clinic of Obstetrics

The substance is administered through a venous butterfly canula, once correct positioning in the vein has been tested with NaCl. Iron sucrose can be administered undiluted as a bolus or diluted, eg, to 100 to 200 mL of isotonic NaCl solution as a short infusion. Administration of a test dose (1 mL) is required in different countries. The bolus injection may be given over 5 to 10 minutes; however, a short infusion over approximately 20 minutes is considered safer. The maximum single dose is 200 mg. We generally give two doses a week to achieve a target Hb value of 11 g/dL. The treatment can be given on an outpatient basis without any problems; in our experience, a long period of monitoring is not usually necessary following administration.

Anemia of Pregnancy

Between 1992 and 2005, more than 500 pregnant women with anemia were treated at the Zurich Obstetrics Clinic. The mean treatment duration was 25 (8 to 29) days, with a mean total dose of 1,000 mg (400 to 1,600 mg) iron sucrose, corresponding to five doses of 200 mg. There are several studies on, and clinical experience with, the use of iron sucrose during pregnancy and in the postpartum period. Overall, a high level of efficacy and safety was demonstrated in all studies. Similarly, parenteral iron therapy with the iron sucrose complex was superior to oral iron in all studies so far. Concerning evidence of effectiveness of iron sucrose in pregnancy, it can be concluded that iron sucrose is effective:

- in patients not responding to oral iron
- in combination with rHuEPO, particularly in the case of a significant inflammatory state
- in severe anemia (Hb <9 g/dL)

Baseline hematologic values and results of intravenous iron sucrose therapy of pregnant anemic women are given in Table 2. The study of Bayoumeu et al showed no advantage of iron sucrose over oral iron with regard to Hb increase but an advantage concerning ferritin levels at the end of treatment.[7]

In the Cochrane Database Review (2001) of 54 studies on the use of intravenous iron during pregnancy, only one study showed a favorable Hb response at 36 weeks and pre-delivery, using intravenous iron compared to oral iron in anemic women.[17] It should be noted that this review includes only studies with other intravenous iron preparations such as iron dextran and ferric gluconate, while most positive experiences with iron sucrose complex in pregnancy were published from 2000 onwards. These studies should be included in a forthcoming new edition of this review.

Table 2 Baseline Hematologic Values and Values After Therapy of Pregnant Anemic Women With Iron Sucrose Complex (200 mg IV twice weekly)

	Baseline	End (day 25)
Hb (g/dL)	9.1	11.0*
Reticulocytes (%)	2.2	4.2*
MCV (fL)	79	87*
MCH (pg)	25	28*
Transferrin saturation (%)	6	20*
Ferritin (μg/L)	6	180*

Abbreviations: IV, intravenous; Hb, hemoglobin; MCV, mean corpuscular volume; MCH, mean corpuscular volume.
Data from Huch and Breymann.[4]
*$P < .01$ v baseline values.

Postpartum Anemia

The treatment of postpartum anemia depends on the severity of the anemia and/or additional maternal risk factors or co-morbidities. A young, healthy woman can compensate for heavy blood losses far better than a puerpera with a heart defect who may decompensate even after less severe losses. In addition, blood losses need to be viewed in relation to the body mass and the estimated total blood volume. Another consideration is that significant errors can be made particularly when estimating blood loss. Blood loss is often underestimated, which can readily be verified by comparing prepartum and postpartum Hb levels.

In addition to volume replacement, treatment options include the administration of oral iron, parenteral iron and allogeneic blood transfusion. Another option to be considered is the administration of rHuEPO.[4,11,18-23]

Oral iron should be prescribed at hemoglobin levels of over 9.5 g/dL; 80 to 100 mg/d is sufficient in such cases. The iron supplementation should be continued for a period of several months, so as to normalize not only the Hb but also the iron stores. In one study, we were able to show that puerperae with iron deficiency, but no anemia can replenish their iron stores through iron supplementation only.[24]

Thus, puerperae who have iron deficiency and anemia are particularly likely to have high iron requirements. We therefore continue to give iron for at least 6 months. In most cases, giving oral iron is not enough when treating severe anemia, since the endogenous iron stores are usually depleted and not enough iron is provided to ensure sufficient erythropoiesis. As mentioned earlier, the reasons for this include limited absorption, poor compliance at high doses due to adverse effects, and low plasma transferrin saturation levels, which lead to functional iron deficiency. In addition, an inflammatory reaction can occur, particularly following surgically assisted deliveries and cesarean section, leading to iron sequestration in the macrophages and decrease of intestinal absorption, so that the administered iron is not available for hemopoiesis.[10,18]

One alternative is the parenteral administration of iron sucrose. The high plasma iron concentrations that occur shortly after intravenous administration bypass the limited release of iron from the reticuloendothelial system and the inhibited absorption through the intestinal mucosa, thus delivering sufficient quantities of iron for erythropoiesis. As in pregnancy, we follow an incremental treatment plan using parenteral iron sucrose at Hb levels below 9.5 g/dL.[4]

Since 1996 we have published several studies on the use of iron sucrose (with or without rHuEPO) for postpartum anemia in various dosages between 100 and 800 mg (total dose). Depending on the selected total dose, Hb increases between 2.1 and 3.5 g/dL were observed after 14 days (Fig 1).[4,19,20,22,23] In our studies, a reduction of transfusion frequency was not detected since transfusion was not an outcome parameter, ie, we would consider transfusion only in emergency cases and not as a regular treatment option. Gravier et al showed a Hb increase of 3.8 g/dL after 14 days (400 to 600 mg total dose) and a time difference of 14 days versus 30 days (with oral iron) until target Hb was reached.[11]

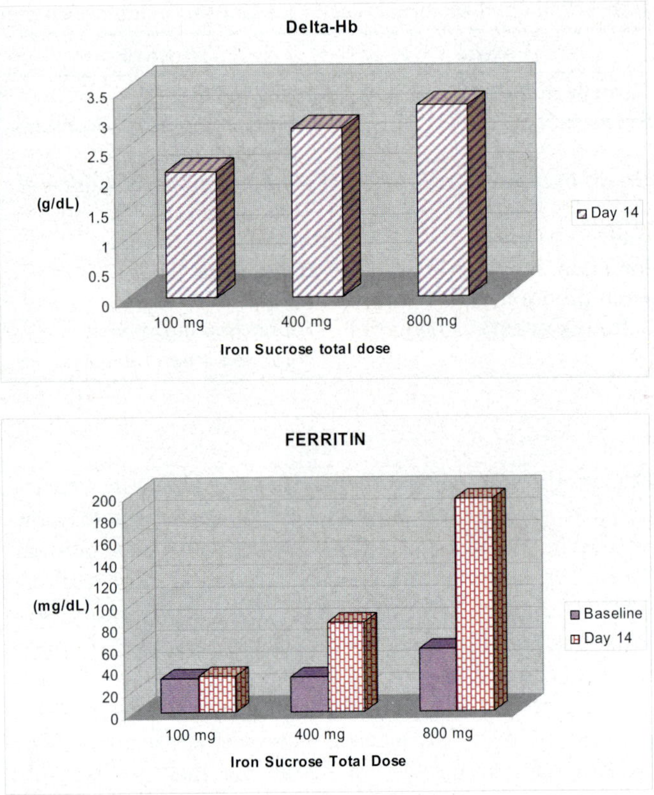

Figure 1 Hemoglobin increase (delta Hb from baseline) and ferritin (absolute increase) 14 days after therapy with iron sucrose complex in various total dosages in women with postpartum anemia.[18-20]

More recently, Broche et al retrospectively analyzed data from 4,292 patients who gave birth in their institution between April 2001 and March 2003. All patients who presented with postpartum anemia (Hb <8 g/dL) within 48 hours of delivery ($n = 217$, ie, 5% of all parturients), were included in the study. Two groups were distinguished based on the availability of intravenous iron sucrose in the institution at the time of delivery. The analysis comprised clinical and laboratory outcomes. Between April 2001 and March 2002, 103 patients received either blood transfusions ($n = 15$ [14.6%]) or oral iron ($n = 88$), whereas between April 2002 and March 2003, 114 patients received either blood transfusion ($n = 5$ [4.4%]), oral iron ($n = 66$), or intravenous iron sucrose ($n = 43$). The mean total dose of intravenous iron administered was 359 mg (range, 200 to 600 mg). The mean increase in Hb concentration over 7 days in patients who received iron sucrose was significantly higher compared to those who received oral iron exclusively (1.86 ± 0.91 [0 to 3.8] *v* 0.87 ± 0.65 [-0.4 to 1.8] g/dL; $P = 3.9 \times 10^{-8}$).

The authors concluded that since the availability of intravenous iron sucrose in their institution, the number of transfused patients had been divided by three; the increase in Hb concentrations was significantly higher with iron sucrose than with oral iron in patients with postpartum anemia. Iron sucrose was well tolerated.[25]

In summary, iron sucrose improves postpartum anemia in a dose-dependent manner with a maximum increase for an 800-mg total dose. Iron status is improved in all patients;

however, a lasting (depot) effect over several weeks has not been shown. Blood transfusion frequency was reduced in one study.[25] Two studies showed that iron sucrose is superior to oral iron already at day 7, again depending on the dosage.[11] In contrast, a recent study by Dede et al showed no difference between iron sucrose and oral iron until 28 days after delivery with regard to hematological parameters, although the effect on iron status was greater with iron sucrose.[26]

The Cochrane Collaboration reports on several trials comparing different iron compounds (with or without rHuEPO) for the treatment of postpartum anemia. The authors conclude that a favorable outcome was seen in patients who were additionally treated with rHuEPO, and that further trials, focusing on iron administration, the role of dietary iron and blood transfusion, are needed.[27]

Conclusion

With regard to the use of intravenous iron in obstetrics, there is increasing evidence that iron sucrose is safe for the mother and the fetus using the recommended dosages and therapy regimens. Iron sucrose is effective in pregnancy and in the postpartum period in patients who do not respond to oral iron, who are non-compliant to oral iron, or who are treated with rHuEPO (rHuEPO is not currently registered for use in pregnancy and postpartum). In both cases, according to the present data, the expected hemoglobin increase and time for therapy are predictable in responding patients. Whether it is reasonable to wait for a response to oral iron in moderate to severe anemia is therefore questionable.

Indications for the use of iron sucrose complex are: preexisting (moderate–severe) anemia; no effect of oral iron; side effects of oral iron; refusal of blood transfusion (eg, Jehovah's Witness patients); limited time until delivery; coexisting risks (eg, bowel disease, renal disease); and pre- and postoperative period and postpartum anemia. According to our experience, the effectiveness of iron sucrose is increased by the use of rHuEPO in patients with a profound postpartum inflammatory state such as anemic patients after cesarean section.[19]

Future fields of research are the evaluation of patient satisfaction and quality of life, impact on costs and hospital stay, impact on blood transfusion frequency and mortality rate, and finally impact on other factors such as breast feeding behavior and neonatal outcome such as birth weight, prematurity and neonatal iron stores.

References

1. Allen LH: Pregnancy and iron deficiency: unresolved issues. Nutr Rev 55:91-101, 1997
2. Hercberg S, Galan P, Preziosi P: Consequences of iron deficiency in pregnant women: Current issues. Clin Drug Invest 19:1-7, 2000 (suppl 1)
3. Hercberg S, Preziosi P, Galan P: Iron deficiency in Europe. Public Health Nutr 4:537-545, 2001
4. Huch R, Breymann C: Anaemia in Pregnancy and Postpartum (ed 1). Bremen, Germany, Uni-Med Verlag, 2005
5. Milman N, Agger AO, Nielson OJ: Iron supplementation during pregnancy. Effect on iron status markers, serum erythropoietin and human placental lactogen. A placebo controlled study in 207 Danish women. Dan Med Bull 38:471-476, 1991
6. Williamson L, Lowe S, Love E, Cohen H, Soldan K, McClelland DB, et al: Serious hazards of transfusion (SHOT) initiative: Analysis of the first two annual reports. BMJ 319:16-19, 1999
7. Bayoumeu F, Subiran-Buisset C, Baka NE, Legagneur H, Monnier-Barbarino P, Laxenaire MC: Iron therapy in iron deficiency anemia in pregnancy: Intravenous route versus oral route. Am J Obstet Gynecol 186:518-522, 2002
8. Breymann C, Major A, Richter C, Huch R, Huch A: Recombinant human erythropoietin and parenteral iron in the treatment of pregnancy anemia: A pilot study. J Perinat Med 23:89-98, 1995
9. Breymann C, Visca E, Huch R, Huch A: Efficacy and safety of intravenously administered iron sucrose with and without adjuvant recombinant human erythropoietin for the treatment of resistant iron-deficiency anemia during pregnancy. Am J Obstet Gynecol 184:662-667, 2000
10. Crichton R, Danielson B, Geisser P: Iron Therapy. Bremen, Germany, Uni-Med Verlag, 2005
11. Gravier A, Descargues G, Marpeau L: Comment éviter les transfusions dans le post-partum: intérêt d'une supplémentation martiale par voie intraveineuse. J Gynecol Obstet Biol Reprod (Paris) 28:77-78, 1999
12. Koenig HM, Levine EA, Resnick DJ, Meyer WJ: Use of recombinant human erythropoietin in a Jehovah's Witness. J Clin Anesth 5:244-247, 1993
13. Krafft A, Breymann C, Huch R, Huch A: Intravenous iron sucrose in two pregnant women with inflammatory bowel disease and severe iron deficiency anemia. Acta Obstet Gynecol Scand 79:720-722, 2000
14. al-Momen AK, al-Meshari A, al-Nuaim L, Saddique A, Abotalib Z, Khashogji T, et al: Intravenous iron sucrose complex in the treatment of iron deficiency anemia during pregnancy. Eur J Obstet Gynecol Reprod Biol 69:121-124, 1996
15. Polatti F, Mandelli B: Treatment with intravenous iron of hypochromic anemia in pregnancy. Boll Soc Medico Chir Pavia 97:13-16, 1983
16. Hoigné R, Breymann C, Künzi U, Brunner F: Parenteral iron therapy: problems and possible solutions. Schweiz Med Wochenschr 128:528-535, 1998
17. Cuervo L, Mahomed K: Treatments for iron deficiency anaemia in pregnancy. Cochrane Database Syst Rev (2):CD003094, 2001
18. Breymann C: Modern therapy concepts for severe anaemia in pregnancy and post partum. In: Huch A, Huch R, Breymann C (eds): Prevention and Management of Anaemia in Pregnancy and Postpartum Haemorrhage. Zurich, Switzerland, Schellenberg Druck AG, 1998, pp 107-122
19. Breymann C, Richter C, Hüttner C, Huch R, Huch A: Effectiveness of recombinant erythropoietin and iron sucrose vs. iron therapy only, in patients with postpartum anaemia and blunted erythropoiesis. Eur J Clin Invest 30:154-161, 2000
20. Breymann C, Zimmermann R, Huch R, Huch A: Use of recombinant human erythropoietin in combination with parenteral iron in the treatment of postpartum anaemia. Eur J Clin Invest 23:123-126, 1996
21. Treatment of iron deficiency anemia in pregnancy and the immediate puerperium and other ferropenic conditions with saccharated iron administered intravenously in fractionated doses. XIVth International Congress of Haematology, Sao Paolo, Brazil, 1972
22. Zimmermann R, Breymann C, Huch R, Huch A: rHuEPO in the treatment of postpartum anemia: Subcutaneous versus intravenous administration. Clin Investig 72:S25-S30, 1994 (suppl)
23. Zimmermann R, Breymann C, Richter C, Huch R, Huch A: rhEPO treatment of postpartum anemia. J Perinat Med 23:111-116, 1995
24. Krafft A, Perewusnyk G, Hänseler E, Quack K, Huch R, Breymann C: Effect of postpartum iron supplementation on red cell and iron parameters in non-anaemic iron-deficient women: A randomised placebo-controlled study. BJOG 112:445-450, 2005
25. Broche DE, Gay C, Armand-Branger S, Grangeasse L, Terzibachian JJ: Anémies sévères du post-partum immédiat. Pratique clinique et intérêt du fer par voie intraveineuse. Gynecol Obstet Fertil 32:613-619, 2004
26. Dede A, Uygur D, Yilmaz B, Mungan T, Ugur M: Intravenous iron sucrose complex vs. oral ferrous sulfate for postpartum iron deficiency anemia. Int J Gynecol Obstet 90:238-239, 2005
27. Dodd J, Dare MR, Middleton P: Treatment for women with postpartum iron deficiency anaemia. Cochrane Database Syst Rev (4):CD004222, 2004

ELSEVIER

Seminars in
HEMATOLOGY

Role of Intravenous Iron in Elective and Non-elective Orthopedic Surgery

José Antonio García-Erce,[a] Jorge Cuenca,[b] and Manuel Muñoz[c]

Perioperative anemia is a common condition among patients undergoing orthopedic surgery, and there was an inverse relationship between baseline hemoglobin and the probability of receiving allogeneic blood transfusion. Perioperative intravenous iron reduces the frequency and volume of allogenic blood transfusion in orthopedic surgery, facilitates autologous blood donation, and may hasten the recovery from postoperative anemia, while preserving iron stores. These effects seem to be augmented by the addition of a single dose of erythropoietin (EPO). In addition, iron sucrose administration seems to decrease infections and morbidity-mortality after hip fracture repair, although it should not be given to patients with ongoing bacteremia.
Semin Hematol 43(suppl 6):S32-S35

Perioperative anemia is a common condition among patients admitted to a Department of Orthopedic Surgery and Traumatology. Although it may already be present before surgery, perioperative blood loss is the main cause of anemia, which is aggravated by inflammation-induced blunted erythropoiesis.

When anemia is acutely developed due to perioperative blood loss, allogeneic red blood cell (RBC) transfusion is the method most commonly used to rapidly and effectively restore hemoglobin (Hb) levels and avoid the deleterious effects of anemia, especially in elderly patients whose compensatory mechanisms have a limited capacity of response. Thus, 30% to 70% of patients undergoing hip fracture repair or total hip or knee replacement receive allogeneic blood transfusions,[1,2] a low preoperative Hb level being one of the major predictive factors.[2,3] In a prospective survey of 3,996 patients, 30% of the patients scheduled for unilateral non-revision knee or hip arthroplasty, who did not receive erythropoietin (EPO), had a baseline Hb level less than 13 g/dL, and there was an inverse relationship between baseline Hb values and the probability of receiving an allogeneic RBC transfusion.[2]

However, allogeneic transfusion is an increasingly costly and scarce resource, and is not risk-free, as it may increase the risk of postoperative infection.[1,2] Overall, concerns about adverse effects of allogeneic transfusion have prompted the review of transfusion practice and the search for a safer and more biologically rational treatment of perioperative anemia, such as stimulation of erythropoiesis with intravenous iron, with or without EPO.

Intravenous Iron, With or Without Erythropoietin, in Non-elective Orthopedic Surgery

Recently, the safety and utility of iron sucrose, an intravenous iron formulation with fewer and milder side effects than iron dextran, for the treatment of acute anemia in pertrochanteric (PHF) and subcapital (SHF) hip fracture patients was assessed in four studies.

After evaluation of the safety of iron sucrose administration in a small number of patients with PHF,[4] the effectiveness of preoperative intravenous iron sucrose administration (200 to 300 mg) on the reduction of transfusion requirements and postoperative morbidity-mortality in patients with PHF and SHF was prospectively investigated.[5,6] No adverse reactions to iron administration were observed, and preoperative iron sucrose reduced postoperative infection rate when compared to a control group. In addition, there was a trend towards a lower percentage of transfused patients, a lower 30-day mortality and a shorter hospital stay in patients receiving iron sucrose (significant for SHF patients) (Table 1). On the other hand, data from patients with admission Hb ≤12 g/dL suggested that a benefit could be obtained if iron sucrose and EPO were administered jointly.

[a]Departments of Hematology, University Hospital "Miguel Servet," Zaragoza, Spain.
[b]Department of Orthopedic Surgery and Traumatology, University Hospital "Miguel Servet," Zaragoza, Spain.
[c]GIEMSA, School of Medicine, University of Málaga, Málaga, Spain.
Address correspondence to Manuel Muñoz, MD, PhD, GIEMSA, Facultad de Medicina, Universidad de Málaga, Campus de Teatinos, s/n, 29071 Málaga, Spain. E-mail: mmunoz@uma.es

 0037-1963/06/$-see front matter
doi:10.1053/j.seminhematol.2006.08.006

Table 1 Demographic and Clinical Characteristics of Patients (in three studies) Undergoing Surgery for Pertrochanteric and Subcapital Hip Fracture Repair Who Were Treated With IV Iron, With or Without EPO, or According to Standard of Care (Control)

	Cuenca, 2004, 2005		García-Erce, 2005	
	Control	IV Iron	Control	IV Iron ± EPO
Patients (n)	159	75	41	83
Age (yr)	83 ± 9	85 ± 7	84 ± 7	81 ± 8
Gender (M/F)	37/122	17/58	4/37	22/61*
Admission Hb (g/dL)	124 ± 16	124 ± 18	127 ± 21	125 ± 19
Patients transfused (n, %)	78 (49)	27 (36)	29 (71)	20 (24)*
Transfusion rate (U/patient)	1.09 ± 1.24	0.72 ± 0.83	1.27 ± 1.34	0.89 ± 1.22*
Infection (n, %)	53 (33)	12 (16)*	13 (31)	10 (13)*
30-day mortality (n, %)	28 (18)	5 (7)	6 (15)	6 (7)
Length of hospital stay (d)	14.2 ± 3.4	12.4 ± 3.4	15.0 ± 0.8	15.3 ± 0.6

Abbreviations: EPO, erythropoietin; IV, intravenous; M, male; F, female; Hb, hemoglobin.
*P <.05, treatment *v* control.

The effects of combined therapy with EPO and iron sucrose were explored in a fourth study in patients with PHF or SHF who received 600 mg iron sucrose (plus 40,000 IU EPO subcutaneously if Hb <13 g/dL) and were treated according to a restrictive transfusion protocol (transfusion trigger: Hb <8 g/dL and/or symptoms of acute anemia).[7] The treatment resulted in a reduction of the percentage of transfused patients, the number of transfused units and the postoperative infection rate compared to a control group (Table 1). In addition, there was a trend towards reduced 30-day mortality (Table 1), and no adverse reactions to iron administration were observed.

Intravenous Iron, With or Without Erythropoietin, in Elective Orthopedic Surgery

Preoperative Iron Administration

In addition to anemia, there seems to be a widespread underlying depletion of iron stores in patients scheduled for major joint replacement. Thus, patient review in pre-admission clinic before surgery and treatment of iron-deficiency anemia with oral or intravenous iron should be highly recommended. In this regard, the implementation of a blood-saving protocol for 156 consecutive total knee replacements (TKR), consisting of a restrictive transfusion trigger (Hb <8 g/dL) plus oral hematinics for 30 to 45 days prior to surgery, has proved to be useful since the transfusion rate (32 *v* 5.8%) and transfusion index (2.22 *v* 1.78 units per transfused patient) were reduced in comparison to a previous series of 156 matched patients treated in our institution.[8]

Although oral administration should be the preferred mode of iron supplementation, this is a time-consuming process. A person weighing 70 kg with a Hb of 8.5 g/dL would have a body iron deficit of about 1,700 mg. Even at the maximum daily iron absorption in the presence of iron deficiency (10 mg), nearly 6 months of oral iron replacement regimen would be required to correct the iron deficit in this patient. Such a time frame is unacceptable for most patients who require surgery.

If a patient's iron stores are depleted going into the procedure, the blood loss cannot be corrected by endogenous red cell production. Thus, preoperative intravenous iron administration might be considered when the time to surgery is too short for oral therapy. The administration of intravenous iron sucrose only (600 to 1,200 mg over 2 to 3 weeks) has been shown to increase Hb levels (1.8 g/dL) in patients with iron deficiency or inflammatory anemia scheduled for orthopedic surgery.[9]

Iron in Preoperative Autologous Blood Donation

Preoperative autologous blood donation (PABD) has been shown to decrease significantly the risk of exposure to allogeneic blood transfusion in patients undergoing elective orthopedic surgery, this effect being improved with the use of EPO to augment PABD yield, although the route of administration of concomitant iron supplement also seemed to play a role. In this regard, the administration of intravenous iron is recommended for female patients undergoing an aggressive PABD program (4 units) and for those with iron deficiency or inflammatory anemia receiving adjuvant EPO. In addition, intravenous iron might permit a reduction in the dose of EPO used to facilitate PABD.[10]

Perioperative Iron Administration

The effects on transfusion requirements of perioperative administration of intravenous iron sucrose (2 × 200 mg, days 0 and +2) plus folic acid and vitamin C until discharge, were evaluated in 311 patients undergoing surgery for TKR. In addition, patients with preoperative Hb less than 13 g/dL (n = 66) received one dose of EPO (40,000 IU subcutaneously, day 0), and allogeneic RBC transfusion was given if postoperative Hb value was lower than 8 g/dL (Hb <9 g/dL for patients with active cardiac disease) or if there were clinical symptoms of acute anemia. No adverse effects of iron sucrose or EPO administration were observed, and only 4%

of the patients received allogeneic blood.[11] No major differences in perioperative blood counts or iron metabolism parameters were observed between patient subgroups, but stimulation of erythropoiesis seemed to be more pronounced in those patients receiving EPO. Interestingly, the allogeneic transfusion rate in patients with preoperative Hb less than 13 g/dL (9%) was no different from that reported with the administration of 4 × 40,000 IU EPO (10.8%).[12]

Treatment of Postoperative Anemia

The administration of oral iron for anemia after orthopedic surgery does not appear to be worthwhile,[13] since postoperative erythropoiesis is limited by the inflammatory effects of surgery on iron metabolism. However, iron sucrose (3 mg/kg/d) was shown to be more effective than oral iron in restoring postoperative Hb levels after spinal surgery in children.[14]

Recently, the effect of postoperative administration of 300 mg of intravenous iron sucrose on allogeneic transfusion requirements in total hip replacement (THR) patients was evaluated.[15] The group given iron showed a lower transfusion index (0.96 *v* 1.68 units per patient; $P = .038$), and a trend towards a lower transfusion rate (46% *v* 73%; $P = .067$), in comparison to a previous series without iron therapy. This reduction cannot be related to changes in transfusion practice, since there were no differences in pretransfusion Hb levels between groups. The percentage of transfused patients in this study is higher than that reported in other studies, most probably due to the high prevalence of preoperative anemia (37%) in this series. However, it is worth noting that admission Hb levels for nontransfused patients were lower in the iron group than in the control group (127 ± 09 *v* 140 ± 12 g/L; $P = .017$), suggesting an erythropoietic effect of iron. Additionally, since 65% of transfusions were given on the third or fourth postoperative day or later, an extended postoperative iron administration schedule might be useful to further reduce late postoperative allogeneic transfusions.

More recently, we also evaluated the effectiveness of perioperative iron with or without EPO on the recovery from postoperative anemia in a series of 141 TKR patients. Despite a mean Hb loss of 3.6 g/dL at postoperative day 7, only seven patients (5%) were transfused. Preoperatively, 66 patients (45%) did not have enough stored iron (ferritin <100 μg/L) to compensate for this Hb loss. However, at postoperative day 30, only 15% were anemic, and 71% of Hb loss and 92% of preoperative Hb was recovered, although erythropoietin response was higher in patients receiving erythropoietin ($P < .05$).[16] Moreover, this Hb reconstitution was attained without a reduction of iron stores in any group, whereas Wallis et al,[17] using oral iron or no treatment, found a similar Hb reconstitution (80%), but at postoperative day 56. In addition, 40% of their patients received allogeneic blood and there was significant reduction of ferritin levels in those that were not transfused.[17] Hence, our protocol seems to reduce allogeneic blood exposure and may hasten the recovery from postoperative anemia in TKR patients, although further studies are needed to ascertain which patients may benefit from extended intravenous iron (eg, 3 × 200 mg) and/or EPO administration.

Conclusions

- Preoperative oral or intravenous iron corrects anemia and reduces the number of transfused units and the percentage of transfused patients.
- The administration of oral or intravenous iron, with or without EPO, facilitates autologous predonation, especially in patients with iron deficiency, reduced body weight, or inflammation. In addition, intravenous iron may reduce the dose of adjuvant EPO.
- Perioperative intravenous iron reduces the frequency and volume of allogenic blood transfusion in orthopedic and trauma surgery, and may hasten the recovery from postoperative anemia, while preserving iron stores. These effects seem to be augmented by the addition of a single dose of EPO.
- Iron sucrose is considered one of the safest intravenous iron formulations. Nevertheless, although iron sucrose administration seems to decrease infections and morbidity–mortality after hip fracture repair, it should not be given to patients with ongoing bacteremia.

References

1. Rosencher N, Kerkkamp HE, Macheras G, Munuera LM, Menichella G, Barton DM, et al: Orthopedic Surgery Transfusion Hemoglobin European Overview (OSTHEO) study: Blood management in elective knee and hip arthroplasty in Europe. Transfusion 43:459-469, 2003
2. Carson JL, Altman DG, Duff A, Noveck H, Weinstein MP, Sonnenberg FA, et al: Risk of bacterial infection associated with allogenic blood transfusion among patients undergoing hip fracture repair. Transfusion 39:694-700, 1999
3. García-Erce JA, Cuenca J, Solano VM: Factores predictivos de la necesidad de transfuseón en la fractura subcapital de cadera en pacientes mayores de 65 años. Med Clin (Barc) 120:161-166, 2003
4. Cuenca J, García-Erce JA, Martínez AA, Solano VM, Modrego JF: Seguridad y eficacia del hierro intravenoso en la anemia aguda por fractura trocantérea de cadera en el anciano. Med Clin (Barc) 123:281-285, 2004
5. Cuenca J, García-Erce JA, Muñoz M, Izuel M, Martínez AA, Herrera A: Patients with pertrochanteric hip fracture may benefit from preoperative intravenous iron therapy: A pilot study. Transfusion 44:1447-1452, 2004
6. Cuenca J, García-Erce JA, Martínez AA, Solano VM, Molina J, Muñoz M: Role of parenteral iron in the management of anaemia in the elderly patient undergoing displaced subcapital hip fracture repair. Preliminary data. Arch Orthop Trauma Surg 125:342-347, 2005
7. García-Erce JA, Cuenca J, Muñoz M, Izuel M, Martinez AA, Herrara A, et al: Perioperative stimulation of erythropoiesis with intravenous iron and erythropoietin reduces transfusion requirements in patients with hip fracture. A prospective observational study. Vox Sang 89:235-243, 2005
8. Cuenca J, García-Erce JA, Martínez F, Cardona R, Pérez-Serrano L, Muñoz M: Preoperative haematinics and transfusion protocol reduce the need for transfusion after total knee replacement. Int J Surg (in press)
9. Bisbe E, Rodríguez C, Ruiz A, Sáez M, Castillo J, Santiveri X: Uso preoperatorio de hierro endovenoso. Una nueva terapéutica en medicina transfusional. Rev Esp Anestesiol Reanim 52:536-540, 2005
10. Messmer K: Consensus statement: Using epoetin alfa to decrease the risk of allogeneic blood transfusion in the surgical setting. Roundtable of Experts in Surgery Blood Management. Semin Hematol 33:78-80, 1996 (suppl 2)

11. Cuenca J, García-Erce JA, Martínez F, Pérez-Serrano L, Herrera A, Muñoz M: Perioperative intravenous iron, with or without erythropoietin, plus restrictive transfusion protocol reduce the need for allogeneic blood after knee replacement surgery. Transfusion 46:1112-1119, 2006
12. Weber EW, Slappendel R, Hémon Y, Mähler S, Dalen T, Rowet E, et al: Effects of epoetin alfa on blood transfusions and postoperative recovery in orthopaedic surgery: The European Epoetin Alfa Surgery Trial (EEST). Eur J Anaesthesiol 22:249-257, 2005
13. Mundy GM, Birtwistle SJ, Power RA: The effect of iron supplementation on the level of haemoglobin after lower limb arthroplasty. J Bone Joint Surg Br 87:213-217, 2005
14. Bernière J, Dehullu JP, Gall O, Murat I: Intravenous iron in the treatment of postoperative anemia in surgery of the spine in infants and adolescents. Rev Chir Orthop 84:319-322, 1998
15. Muñoz M, Naveira E, Seara J, Palmer JH, Cuenca J, García-Erce JA: Role of parenteral iron on transfusion requirements after total hip replacement. A pilot study. Transfus Med 16:137-142, 2006
16. García-Erce JA, Cuenca J, Martínez F, Cardona R, Pérez-Serrano L, Muñoz M: Perioperative intravenous iron preserves iron stores and may hasten the recovery from postoperative anaemia after knee replacement surgery. Transfus Med (in press)
17. Wallis JP, Wells AW, Whitehead S, Brewster N: Recovery from postoperative anaemia. Transfus Med 15:413-418, 2005

Seminars in
HEMATOLOGY

Intravenous Iron in Colorectal Cancer Surgery

Manuel Muñoz,[a] Arturo Campos,[b] and José Antonio García-Erce[c]

Patients requiring elective colorectal cancer surgery have a high prevalence of anemia and iron deficiency. Intravenous iron therapy, with or without recombinant erythropoietin (EPO), may play an important role in the correction of perioperative anemia and facilitate preoperative autologous donation, thus reducing the risk of patient exposure to allogeneic red blood cell (RBC) transfusion and improving patient outcomes. In addition, the use of intravenous iron allows for a significant reduction in EPO dose requirements. However, large and well-conducted randomized controlled trials are needed to define more cost-effective intravenous iron and EPO regimens.
Semin Hematol 43(suppl 6):S36-S38 © 2006 Elsevier Inc. All rights reserved.

Anemia is one of the main signs of colorectal cancer. The incidence of anemia in these patients may vary from 25% to 70%, depending on the hemoglobin (Hb) cut-off, and is related to patient's age, tumor site and size, and Dukes stage.[1-3] However, more than half of these patients present with iron deficiency, with or without anemia, due to chronic blood loss, which in turn is related to tumor site and size.[1-3] Thus, anemia of chronic disease plus iron deficiency is a common finding in colorectal cancer.

On the other hand, it is well established that preoperative anemia is associated with increased requirements for allogeneic red blood cell (RBC) transfusion, which has been controversially linked to increased postoperative infection, recurrence rates, and mortality in patients with colorectal cancer, even after the introduction of universal leukoreduction.[4,5] Longer hospital stays and higher health care costs have also been linked to allogeneic RBC transfusion.[6] Thus, attempts have been made to reduce the use of transfusion in colorectal cancer patients using perioperative iron therapy with or without erythropoietin (EPO) administration and with or without preoperative autologous blood donation (PABD).

Perioperative Treatment With Iron and Erythropoietin

Okuyama et al[7] studied 116 anemic patients (Hb ≤10 g/dL) who underwent colorectal cancer surgery: 32 who received oral iron supplementation (200 mg/d) for at least 2 weeks before surgery, and 84 who did not. Patients receiving iron had a significantly higher Hb level immediately before surgery and received fewer intraoperative RBC transfusions (9.4% *v* 27.4%; $P < .05$). In another study,[8] 43 colorectal cancer patients received preoperative treatment with oral iron if they had a Hb greater than 14 g/dL and iron deficiency; iron sucrose (200 mg/wk) if Hb was 10 to 14 g/dL; or iron sucrose (200 mg twice per week) if Hb was less than 10 g/dL, during 2 to 3 weeks. Seventeen of these patients also received postoperative iron sucrose (200 mg on days 0, 2, and 4) in addition to the preoperative treatment. A retrospective series of patients not receiving iron was used as a control group (n = 66). Despite a lower baseline Hb (12.3 *v* 11.5 g/dL; $P < .05$), iron therapy reduced the transfusion index (4.0 *v* 1.3 units per patient; $P < .05$) and the percentage of patients who received preoperative transfusions (33% *v* 9%; $P < .05$), but not the percentage of patients administered perioperative transfusions (48% *v* 35%; $P = .161$). However, the treatment was ineffective in patients with a high transfusion index (>5 units per patient).[8]

Most probably, the effectiveness of perioperative iron treatment could be enhanced by concomitant EPO administration. Thus, in patients with moderate anemia (Hb >8.5 g/dL and ≤13 g/dL) scheduled for colorectal cancer surgery, perioperative treatment with EPO reduced the risk of exposure to allogeneic transfusion (100/263, 38% *v* 97/207, 47%) (relative risk [RR], 0.81; 95% confidence interval [CI], 0.61 to 1.00; $P = .054$), although there was great variability in total EPO dose and iron supplementation, as well as in outcomes (Table 1).Thus, EPO plus oral iron resulted in either no effect[9] or a reduction in the number of transfused units only.[10,11] In contrast, the administration of EPO plus intravenous iron resulted in a reduction of both the percentage of transfused patients and the number of transfused units.[12,13]

[a]GIEMSA, School of Medicine, University of Málaga, Málaga, Spain.
[b]Department of Hematology, University Hospital "Virgen de la Victoria," Málaga, Spain.
[c]Department of Hematology, University Hospital "Miguel Servet," Zaragoza, Spain.
Address correspondence to Manuel Muñoz, MD, PhD, GIEMSA, Facultad de Medicina, Universidad de Málaga, Campus de Teatinos, s/n, 29071 Málaga, Spain. E-mail: mmunoz@uma.es

 0037-1963/06/$-see front matter © 2006 Elsevier Inc. All rights reserved.
doi:10.1053/j.seminhematol.2006.08.005

Table 1 Effects of Perioperative Administration of Erythropoietin and Iron on Transfusion Requirements in Patients Undergoing Elective Colorectal Cancer Resection

Study	+ EPO n	+ EPO % Transfused	Placebo n	Placebo % Transfused	Iron (type, dose, days)	EPO‡ (IU/kg, route)
Braga (1997)[12]	10	10	10	50*	IV, 125 mg/d, 4 d	500, SC
Kettelhack (1998)[10]	48	33	54	28	Oral, NS, 5–10 d pre IV, 40 mg, 1 d post	3,000–4,500, SC
Qvist (1999)[11]	38	34	43	54†	Oral, 200 mg/d, 4 d	1,350, SC
Kosmadakis (2003)[13]	31	29	32	59*	IV, 100 mg/d, 14 d	4,200, SC
Christodoulakis (2005)[9]	69	49	68	52	Oral, 200 mg/d, 10 d	1,800, SC
Christodoulakis (2005)[9]	67	40	68	52†	Oral, 200 mg/d, 10 d	3,600, SC

Abbreviations: EPO, erythropoietin; IV, intravenous; SC, subcutaneous.
*Reduction in both percentage of transfused patients and number of transfused units.
†Reduction in the number of transfused units only.
‡EPO: total dose of recombinant human erythropoietin.

Additionally, the use of intravenous iron allowed for a significant reduction in the total dose of EPO (Table 1). Similar results were reported by two small trials in 30 patients undergoing surgery for gastric cancer.[14,15]

Preoperative Autologous Blood Donation

PABD is considered as one of the most safe and effective alternatives to allogeneic RBC transfusion in patients scheduled for surgical tumor resection. The results of four randomized controlled trials involving 1,067 patients undergoing colorectal cancer surgery showed that PABD significantly reduces allogeneic RBC transfusion requirements (RR, 0.44; 95% CI, 0.38 to 0.53; $P < .001$) (Table 2).[16-19] However, the presence of anemia in many of these patients precludes their inclusion in a PABD program. Since perioperative treatment with EPO significantly increases Hb levels preoperatively, a combination of EPO and PABD seems a reasonable approach to reducing transfusion exposure in these patients. In fact, the result of two small trials (76 patients) showed a lower allogeneic transfusion rate in patients treated with PABD and EPO, compared to those treated with PABD alone (RR, 0.34; 95% CI, 0.14 to 0.85; $P < .012$).[20,21] Again, the use of intravenous iron, as compared with oral iron, resulted in a reduction in the total dose of EPO oral iron (600 IU/kg *v* 2,200 IU/kg) (Table 2).

Conclusions

Patients requiring elective colorectal cancer surgery have a high prevalence of anemia and iron deficiency, which increases with patient age and tumor size, site, and stage.

Intravenous iron therapy, with or without EPO, may play an important role in the correction of perioperative anemia and facilitate PABD, thus reducing the risk of patient exposure to allogeneic RBC transfusion and improving patient outcomes. In addition, the use of intravenous iron allows for a significant reduction in EPO dose requirements.

Intravenous iron sucrose may be safely used in cancer surgical patients. As a short-term therapy, it does not put the patient at risk for long-term iatrogenic effects. However, large and well-conducted randomized controlled trials are needed to define more cost-effective intravenous iron and EPO regimens.

Table 2 Effects of Preoperative Autologous Blood Donation, With or Without Erythropoietin, on Transfusion Requirements in Patients Undergoing Elective Colorectal Cancer Resection

Study	PABD n	PABD % Transfused	Control n	Control % Transfused	Iron (route)	EPO† (IU/kg, route)
Hoynck van Papendrecht (1992)[16]	150	23	160	61*	Oral	—
Heiss (1993)[17]	58	35	63	60*	Oral	—
Busch (1993)[18]	239	28	236	56*	Oral	—
Vignali (1995)[19]	53	4	108	44*	IV	—
Study	**PABD n**	**PABD % Transfused**	**PABD + EPO n**	**PABD + EPO % Transfused**	**Iron (route)**	**EPO† (IU/kg, route)**
Braga (1995)[20]	11	36	11	0*	IV	600, SC
Rau (1998)[21]	26	39	28	18*	Oral	2,200, SC

Abbreviations: EPO, erythropoietin; IV, intravenous; PABD, preoperative autologous blood donation; SC, subcutaneous.
*Reduction in both percentage of transfused patients and number of transfused units.
†EPO: total dose of recombinant human erythropoietin.

References

1. Sadahiro S, Suzuki T, Tokunaga N, Mukai M, Tajima T, Makuuchi H, et al: Anemia in patients with colorectal cancer. J Gastroenterol 33:488-494, 1998
2. Beale AL, Penney MD, Allison MC: The prevalence of iron deficiency among patients presenting with colorectal cancer. Colorectal Dis 7:398-402, 2005
3. Prutki M, Poljak-Blazi M, Jakopovic M, Tomas D, Stipancic I, Zarkovic N: Altered iron metabolism, transferrin receptor 1 and ferritin in patients with colon cancer. Cancer Lett 238:188-196, 2006
4. Li F, Kishida T, Kobayashi M: Serum iron and ferritin levels in patients with colorectal cancer in relation to the size, site, and disease stage of cancer. J Gastroenterol 34:195-199, 1999
5. Jensen LS, Puho E, Pedersen L, Mortensen FV, Sorensen HT: Long-term survival after colorectal surgery associated with buffy-coat-poor and leucocyte-depleted blood transfusion: A follow-up study. Lancet 365: 681-682, 2005
6. Vamvakas EC, Carven JH: Allogeneic blood transfusion, hospital charges, and length of hospitalization: A study of 487 consecutive patients undergoing colorectal cancer resection. Arch Pathol Lab Med 122:145-151, 1998
7. Okuyama M, Ikeda K, Shibata T, Tsukahara Y, Kitada M, Shimano T: Preoperative iron supplementation and intraoperative transfusion during colorectal cancer surgery. Surg Today 35:36-40, 2005
8. Campos A, Sevilla I, Baca JJ, Romero A, Ramírez G, Muñoz M: Perioperative iron therapy and transfusion requirements in patients undergoing surgery for colon cancer. Preliminary results. Transfusion Alternatives Transfusion Med 7:96, 2005 (suppl, abstr)
9. Christodoulakis M, Tsiftsis DD, Hellenic Surgical Oncology Perioperative EPO Study Group: Preoperative epoetin alfa in colorectal surgery: A randomized, controlled study. Ann Surg Oncol 12:718-725, 2005
10. Kettelhack C, Hones C, Messinger D, Schlag PM: Randomized multicentre trial of the influence of recombinant human erythropoietin on intraoperative and postoperative transfusion need in anaemic patients undergoing right hemicolectomy for carcinoma. Br J Surg 85:63-67, 1998
11. Qvist N, Boesby S, Wolff B, Hansen CP: Recombinant human erythropoietin and hemoglobin concentration at operation and during the postoperative period: Reduced need for blood transfusions in patients undergoing colorectal surgery—Prospective double-blind placebo-controlled study. World J Surg 23:30-35, 1999
12. Braga M, Gianotti L, Gentilini O, Vignali A, Di Carlo V: Erythropietic response induced by recombinant human erythropoietin in anemic cancer patients candidate to major abdominal surgery. Hepatogastroenterology 44:685-690, 1997
13. Kosmadakis N, Messaris E, Maris A, Katsaragakis S, Leandros E, Konstadoulakis MM, et al: Perioperative erythropoietin administration in patients with gastrointestinal tract cancer: prospective randomized double-blind study. Ann Surg 237:417-421, 2003
14. Tsuji Y, Kambayashi J, Shiba E, Sakon M, Kawasaki T, Mori T: Effect of recombinant human erythropoietin on anaemia after gastrectomy: A pilot study. Eur J Surg 161:29-33, 1995
15. Heiss MM, Tarabichi A, Delanoff C, Allgayer H, Jauch KW, Hernandez-Richter T, et al: Perisurgical erythropoietin application in anemic patients with colorectal cancer: A double-blind randomized study. Surgery 119:523-527, 1996
16. Hoynck van Papendrecht MA, Hop W, Langenhorst BL, Kothe FC, Marquet RL, Jeekel J: Feasibility of a predeposit autologous blood donation program in colorectal cancer patients: Results from a randomized clinical study. Vox Sang 62:102-107, 1992
17. Heiss MM, Mempel W, Jauch KW, Delanoff C, Mayer G, Mempel M, et al: Beneficial effect of autologous blood transfusion on infectious complications after colorectal cancer surgery. Lancet 342:1328-1333, 1993
18. Busch OR, Hop WC, Hoynck van Papendrecht MA, Marquet RL, Jeekel J: Blood transfusions and prognosis in colorectal cancer. N Engl J Med 328:1372-1376, 1993
19. Vignali A, Braga M, Dionigi P, Radaelli G, Gentilini O, Bellini A, et al: Impact of a programme of autologous blood donation on the incidence of infection in patients with colorectal cancer. Eur J Surg 161:487-492, 1995
20. Braga M, Gianotti L, Vignali A, Gentilini O, Servida P, Bordignon C, et al: Evaluation of recombinant human erythropoietin to facilitate autologous blood donation before surgery in anaemic patients with cancer of the gastrointestinal tract. Br J Surg 82:1637-1640, 1995
21. Rau B, Schlag PM, Willeke F, Herfarth C, Stephan P, Franke W: Increased autologous blood donation in rectal cancer by recombinant human erythropoietin (rhEPO). Eur J Cancer 34:992-998, 1998

ELSEVIER

Seminars in
HEMATOLOGY

Intravenous Iron in Cardiac Surgery

Manuel Muñoz,[a] Ramón Leal-Noval,[b] and José Antonio García-Erce[c]

In patients presenting for elective cardiac surgery, preoperative anemia is associated with increased risk of postoperative transfusion, morbidity, and mortality. Intravenous iron therapy, with or without erythropoietin (EPO), may play an important role in the correction of preoperative anemia, as well as in facilitating autologous blood donation, thus reducing the risk of patient exposure to allogeneic blood transfusions. In addition, postoperative intravenous iron may act by treating decreased iron availability, thus increasing the action of both endogenous and exogenous EPO and improving the quality of postoperative recovery. As a short-term therapy, intravenous iron does not put the patient at risk for long-term iatrogenic effects.
Semin Hematol 43(suppl 6):S39-S42

Cardiac surgery, with or without cardiopulmonary bypass (CPB), results in a significant blood loss that predisposes the patient to perioperative allogeneic blood transfusions, which may result in increased postoperative morbidity.[1] If patients at high risk for requiring perioperative transfusions (eg, anemic patients) can be identified in the preoperative period, prophylactic and therapeutic modalities can be targeted to those patients who might benefit from such treatments.

Moreover, preoperative anemia has been associated not only with an increased risk of allogeneic transfusion,[2] but also with a greater risk for lower survival after coronary artery bypass grafting.[3] Disease severity and comorbidity have the greatest effect on mortality in anemic patients, which may be aggravated by transfusion of stored blood, anemia being just a consequence of some other disorders such as acute or chronic blood loss, nutritional iron deficiency, renal failure, malignancy, or chronic inflammatory disease. Consequently, the first step to be taken in the setting of elective cardiac surgery will be the preoperative identification and evaluation of anemia early enough to implement the appropriate treatment. Whenever possible, preoperative pharmacologic treatment of anemia should be used, rather than transfusion.[4]

Postoperative anemia may occur in up to 90% of patients, most probably due to perioperative blood loss and blunted erythropoietic response. It is well known that major surgery is followed by a systemic inflammatory response whose humoral mediators (eg, interleukin [IL]-1, interferon-γ, and tumor necrosis factor-α) inhibit erythropoiesis both directly by suppressing erythroid colony growth and indirectly by suppressing erythropoietin (EPO) production. These inflammatory cytokines also induce a status of decreased iron availability, ie, a clinical situation where the iron stores in the bone marrow macrophages is normal but this iron is not available for erythropoiesis, due to an alteration of its release from the macrophages. Also, intestinal iron absorption is inhibited, due to a reduction of its release through the enterocytic basolateral membrane. Hepcidin, a hepatic acute-phase protein, seems to play a major role in both alterations.[5]

Intravenous iron emerges as a timely therapeutic option for the treatment of decreased iron availability in these patients, since once injected in vivo the iron–carbohydrate complexes are metabolized, the iron is released and binds to transferrin in the plasma, and the redundant carbohydrate moiety is then cleared via the liver. Hence, intravenous iron therapy, with or without EPO, may play an important role in perioperative anemia management in order to decrease the need for allogeneic blood transfusions and improve patient outcomes.

Perioperative Treatment With Iron and Erythropoietin

Recently, we performed a study of the prevalence of anemia and alteration of iron metabolism in a series of 60 consecutive patients undergoing cardiac surgery. There were 30 myocardial revascularizations without CPB, and 16 valve prostheses and 14 mixed surgeries with CPB. Preoperatively, 27 (45%)

[a]GIEMSA, School of Medicine, University of Málaga, Málaga, Spain.
[b]Department of Intensive Care, University Hospital "Virgen del Rocio," Seville, Spain.
[c]Department of Hematology, University Hospital "Miguel Servet," Zaragoza, Spain.
Address correspondence to Manuel Muñoz, MD, PhD, GIEMSA, Facultad de Medicina, Universidad de Málaga, Campus de Teatinos, s/n, 29071 Málaga, Spain. E-mail: mmunoz@uma.es

0037-1963/06/$-see front matter
doi:10.1053/j.seminhematol.2006.08.009

patients were anemic, 13 (22%) had serum iron less than 50 μg/dL, 25 (42%) ferritin less than 100 μg/L, 17 (28%) transferrin saturation less than 20%, 13 (22%) C-reactive protein greater than 1 mg/dL, and 10 (17%) IL-6 greater than 10 pg/mL.[6] In addition, patients treated with angiotensin-converting enzyme (ACE) inhibitors had lower hemoglobin (Hb) levels, erythropoietin concentrations, and reticulocyte indices, and a higher incidence of anemia.[7] Thus, chronic administration of ACE inhibitors to patients with coronary artery disease or cardiac valve pathology seems to be associated with a higher incidence of preoperative anemia, most probably due to a reduced EPO synthesis. These data suggest that anemic patients scheduled for cardiac surgery might benefit from treatment with iron and EPO.

In adult patients scheduled for cardiac surgery, perioperative treatment with EPO reduced the risk of exposure to allogeneic blood transfusion (60/195, 31% *v* 56/104, 54%) (relative risk [RR], 0.57; 95% confidence interval [CI], 0.43 to 0.75; *P* <.001), but there was a great variability in total EPO dose and iron supplementation, as well as in outcomes (Table 1). EPO plus oral iron resulted in either a reduction of the percentage of transfused patients and the number of transfused units,[8,9] or had no significant effect[10] (Table 1). In pediatric cardiac surgery, perioperative administration of EPO plus intravenous iron resulted in a reduction of both the percentage of transfused patients and the number of transfused units.[11] Overall, the use of intravenous iron seems to allow for a reduction in the total dose of EPO (Table 1).

Preoperative Autologous Blood Donation

Preoperative autologous blood donation (PABD) before elective cardiac surgery has proved to be an effective measure to reduce the exposure of patients to allogeneic blood transfusion. However, in patients who are unable to compensate the Hb drop due to repeated phlebotomy, the subsequent reduction in oxygen delivery to the myocardium may aggravate myocardial ischemia.

In a small trial (n = 32), anemic adult patients (Hb <11 g/dL) who received EPO (3 × 500 IU/kg subcutaneously) and oral iron (plus intravenous iron, in hospitalized patients, if ferritin <100 μg/L) donated 2 to 3 blood units, and only 25% received allogeneic transfusions. In contrast, patients in the control group who received oral iron only were not able to donate blood and 100% received allogeneic transfusions (*P* <.05).[12] Similar data have been reported for the use of EPO to facilitate PABD in a series of children (n = 78) undergoing open-heart surgery (Table 2).[13] Overall, the administration of iron, with or without EPO, to anemic patients scheduled for cardiac surgery allowed them to enter the PABD program and reduced the exposure to allogeneic blood transfusions (RR, 0.17; 95% CI, 0.09 to 0.16; *P* <.001).

The combined results of seven clinical trials (318 patients) showed that, for patients included in a PABD program, EPO administration facilitates collection of the required units and prevents a preoperative Hb drop. In addition, exposure to allogeneic transfusion was less likely among patients who received EPO than among those who did not (RR, 0.40; 95% CI, 0.26 to 0.60; *P* <.001) (Table 2).[8,14-19] There were no differences in either the allogeneic transfusion rate or the total EPO dose administered between patients receiving oral iron and those receiving intravenous iron (Table 2).

Postoperative Anemia

In the postoperative period, several studies have evaluated the effectiveness of oral[20] or intravenous iron replacement therapy[21-23] for treatment of acute anemia after cardiac surgery. The administration of oral iron after uncomplicated coronary artery bypass surgery did not help to restore red blood cell mass nor to maintain total body iron stores.[20] In contrast, postoperative intravenous iron alone preserved iron stores during recovery from anemia,[21,22] whereas postoperative iron plus EPO also resulted in increased reticulocyte counts during the first 2 postoperative weeks.[21] In addition, the increase in Hb level from postoperative day 4 (nadir) to postoperative day 30 was 1 g/dL higher in patients who received intravenous iron supplements compared to those who received placebo.[21]

More recently, Karkouti et al[23] conducted a double-blind, placebo-controlled randomized study in patients undergoing cardiac (42%) or orthopedic surgery to determine if early recovery from severe postoperative anemia is accelerated by

Table 1 Effects of Perioperative Administration of Erythropoietin and Iron on Transfusion Requirements in Patients Undergoing Elective Cardiac Surgery

Study	+ EPO		Placebo		Iron (type, dose, days)	EPO† (IU/kg, route)
	n	% Transfused	n	% Transfused		
Kyo (1992)[8]	40	50	16	75*	IV, 80–120 mg/wk, 4 wk	500–1,500, IV
Sowade (1997)[9]	36	11	36	53*	Oral, 300 mg/d, 14 d	2,500, IV
D'Ambra (1997)[10]	60	28	52	48	Oral, 975 mg/d, >8 d	1,200, SC
D'Ambra (1997)[10]	59	32	52	48	Oral, 975 mg/d, >8 d	2,400, SC
Shimpo (1997)[11]	11[a]	9	16[b]	31	[a]IV, NS, 4 d	600, IV
Shimpo (1997)[11]	21[a]	0	16[b]	31*	[b]Oral, NS, 28 d	1,200, IV

Abbreviations: EPO, erythropoietin; IV, intravenous; NS, not stated; SC, subcutaneous.
*Reduction in both percentage of transfused patients and number of transfused units.
†EPO: total dose of recombinant human erythropoietin.
[a]Patients receiving IV iron; [b]patients receiving oral iron.

Table 2 Effects of Preoperative Autologous Blood Donation, With or Without Erythropoietin, on Transfusion Requirements in Patients Undergoing Elective Cardiac Surgery

	Control		PABD + rHuEPO			
Study	n	% Transfused (allogeneic)	n	% Transfused (allogeneic)	Iron (route)	EPO† (IU/kg, route)
Kiyama (1999)[12]	16	100	16	25*	Oral ± IV	1,500, SC
Sonzogni (2001)[13]	39	61	39	8*	Oral	1,000, SC + IV
	PABD		PABD + EPO			
Study	n	% Transfused (allogeneic)	n	% Transfused (allogeneic)	Iron (route)	EPO† (IU/kg, route)
Watanable (1992)[14]	14	29	12	0*	IV	1,400, IV
Watanable (1992)[14]	14	29	14	0*	Oral	1,200, SC
Kyo (1992)[8]	5	40	62	21*	IV	600–1,900, IV
Schmoeckel (1993)[15]	6	17	37	19	Oral	800–6,400, IV
Kulier (1993)[16]	12	67	12	8*	Oral	1,600, SC
Hayashi (1994)[17]	28	36	58	10*	Oral	600–1,200, SC
Walpoth (1996)[18]	10	20	21	19	Oral	600–1,200, SC
Kobayashi (2001)[19]	11	27	16	12	Oral	600, SC

Abbreviations: EPO, erythropoietin; IV, intravenous; PABD, preoperative autologous blood donation; SC, subcutaneous.
*Reduction in both percentage of transfused patients and number of transfused units.
†EPO: total dose of recombinant human erythropoietin.

intravenous iron therapy alone (n = 11) or in combination with EPO (n = 10), compared to oral iron (n = 10). They concluded that treatment with intravenous iron alone or in combination with EPO does not appear to accelerate early recovery from postoperative anemia, although reticulocyte counts and ferritin levels at postoperative day 7 were higher in the combination group and there was a trend towards lower transfusion requirements and better Hb recovery at postoperative day 42. However, the authors admitted several weaknesses in their study and did not exclude the possibility that higher doses or different timing of postoperative intravenous iron and EPO may be effective in accelerating correction of postoperative anemia.

Conclusions

In patients presenting for elective cardiac surgery, there is a high prevalence of anemia, which is linked to increase postoperative morbidity and mortality. Hence, preoperative anemia needs to be identified and evaluated early enough to implement the appropriate treatment.

Intravenous iron therapy, with or without EPO, may play an important role in the correction of perioperative anemia, as well as in facilitating PABD, thus reducing the risk of patient exposure to allogeneic blood transfusions.

Postoperative anemia is even more frequent than preoperative anemia, and systemic inflammation is probably the factor which impairs the effectiveness of oral iron therapy. Parenteral iron may act by treating decreased iron availability, thus increasing the action of both endogenous and exogenous erythropoietin. Although results are controversial, a faster reversion of anemia following intravenous iron injection might improve the quality of postoperative recovery.

As a short-term therapy, iron sucrose does not put the patient at risk for long-term iatrogenic effects. However, large and well-conducted randomized controlled trials are needed to define more cost-effective intravenous iron and EPO regimens.

References

1. Leal-Noval SR, Jara-López I, García-Garmendia JL, Marín-Niebla A, Herruzo-Avilés A, Camacho-Laraña P, et al: Influence of erythrocyte concentrate storage time on postsurgical morbidity in cardiac surgery patients. Anesthesiology 98:815-822, 2003
2. Khanna MP, Hebert PC, Fergusson DA: Review of the clinical practice literature on patient characteristics associated with perioperative allogeneic red blood cell transfusion. Transfus Med Rev 17:110-119, 2003
3. Koch CG, Weng Y, Zhou SX, Savino JS, Mathew JP, Hsu PH, et al: Prevalence of risk factors, and not gender per se, determines short- and long-term survival alter coronary artery bypass surgery. J Cardiothorac Vasc Anesth 17:585-593, 2003
4. Muñoz M, Garcia-Erce JA, Leal-Noval SR: Perioperative transfusion in anaemic patients undergoing coronary artery bypass. Lancet 360:1427-1428, 2002
5. Muñoz M, Campos A, García-Erce JA, Ramírez G: Fisiopatología del metabolismo del hierro: Implicaciones diagnósticas y terapéuticas. Nefrología 25:9-19, 2005
6. Fernández MA, Cobos A, Ariza D, Muñoz E, Ramírez G, Muñoz M: Postoperative erythropoiesis is blunted in patients undergoing cardiac surgery. Transfusion Alternatives Transfusion Med 8:61, 2006 (suppl, abstr)
7. Fernández MA, García-Pinilla JM, Jiménez M, Muñoz E, Campos A, Muñoz M: Preoperative anemia in cardiac surgery. Role of angiotensin-converting enzyme inhibitors. TATM 8:60, 2006 (suppl, abstr)
8. Kyo S, Omoto R, Hirashima K, Eguchi S, Fujita T: Effect of human recombinant erythropoietin on reduction of homologous blood transfusion in open-heart surgery. A Japanese multicenter study. Circulation 86:II413-II418, 1992 (suppl)
9. Sowade O, Messinger D, Franke W, Sowade B, Scigalla P, Warnke H: The estimation of efficacy of oral iron supplementation during treatment with epoetin beta (recombinant human erythropoietin) in patients undergoing cardiac surgery. Eur J Haematol 60:252-259, 1998
10. D'Ambra MN, Gray RJ, Hillman R, Jones JW, Kim HC, Rawitscher R,

et al: Effect of recombinant human erythropoietin on transfusion risk in coronary bypass patients. Ann Thorac Surg 64:1686-1693, 1997
11. Shimpo H, Mizumoto T, Onoda K, Yuasa H, Yada I: Erythropoietin in pediatric cardiac surgery: Clinical efficacy and effective dose. Chest 111:1565-1570, 1997
12. Kiyama H, Ohshima N, Imazeki T, Yamada T: Autologous blood donation with recombinant human erythropoietin in anemic patients. Ann Thorac Surg 68:1652-1656, 1999
13. Sonzogni V, Crupi G, Poma R, Annechino F, Ferri F, Filisetti P, et al: Erythropoietin therapy and preoperative autologous blood donation in children undergoing open heart surgery. Br J Anaesth 87:429-434, 2001
14. Watanabe Y, Fuse K, Naruse Y, Kobayashi T, Yamamoto S, Konishi H, et al: Subcutaneous use of erythropoietin in heart surgery. Ann Thorac Surg 54:479-483, 1992
15. Schmoeckel M, Nollert G, Mempel M, Mempel W, Reichart B: Effects of recombinant human erythropoietin on autologous blood donation before open heart surgery. Thorac Cardiovasc Surg 41:364-368, 1993
16. Kulier AH, Gombotz H, Fuchs G, Vuckovic U, Metzler H: Subcutaneous recombinant human erythropoietin and autologous blood donation before coronary artery bypass surgery. Anesth Analg 76:102-106, 1993
17. Hayashi J, Kumon K, Takanashi S, Kawashima Y, Eguchi S, Takaku F, et al: Subcutaneous administration of recombinant human erythropoietin before cardiac surgery: A double-blind, multicenter trial in Japan. Transfusion 34:142-146, 1994
18. Walpoth B, Galliker B, Spirig P, Haeberli A, Rosenmund A, Althaus U, et al: Use of epoetin alfa in autologous blood donation programs for patients scheduled for elective cardiac surgery. Semin Hematol 33:75-76, 1996 (suppl 2)
19. Kobayashi T, Makuuchi H, Takahashi K, Furuse A, Shibata Y, Tsuno H, et al. Effects of recombinant human erythropoietin therapy on blood coagulation and fibrinolysis system. Ann Thorac Cardiovasc Surg 7:273-277, 2001
20. Crosby L, Palarski VA, Cottington E, Cmolik B: Iron supplementation for acute blood loss anemia after coronary artery bypass surgery: A randomized, placebo-controlled study. Heart Lung 23:493-499, 1994
21. Madi-Jebara S, Sleilaty GS, Achouh PE, Yazigi AG, Haddad FA, Hayek GM, et al: Postoperative intravenous iron used alone or in combination with low-dose erythropoietin in not effective for correction of anemia after cardiac surgery. J Cardiothorac Vasc Anesth 18:59-63, 2004
22. Hulin S, Durandy Y: Intérět du fer intraveineux dans les anémies induites par l'hémodilution en chirurgie cardiaque pédiatrique. Ann Fran Anesth Reanim 24:1262-1265, 2005
23. Karkouti K, McCluskey SA, Ghannam M, Salpeter MJ, Quirt I, Yau TM: Intravenous iron and recombinant erythropoietin for the treatment of postoperative anemia. Can J Anesth 53:11-19, 2006

ELSEVIER
SAUNDERS
email: reprints@elsevier.com